CLINICAL MAGNETIC RESONANCE IMAGING

CLINICAL MAGNETIC RESONANCE IMAGING

Edited by

VAL M. RUNGE, M.D.

Professor of Diagnostic Radiology
Director of the Magnetic Resonance Imaging and Spectroscopy Center
University of Kentucky
Lexington, Kentucky

WITH 16 CONTRIBUTORS

1792

J.B. LIPPINCOTT COMPANY
Philadelphia

Grand Rapids New York St. Louis San Francisco
London Sydney Tokyo

Acquisitions Editor: Charles McCormick, Jr.
Project Editor: Mary Rose Muccie
Copy Editor: Ann Morris
Indexer: Alexandra Nickerson
Art Director: Susan Hess Blaker
Designer: Doug Smock
Production Manager: Helen Ewan
Production Coordinator: Pamela Milcos
Compositor: Progressive Typographers
Printer/Binder: Halliday Lithograph Corporation

6 5 4 3 2 1

Library of Congress Cataloging-in-Publication Data
Clinical magnetic resonance imaging / edited by Val M. Runge: with 16 contributors.
p. cm.
Includes bibliographies and index.
ISBN 0-397-50989-8
1. Magnetic resonance imaging. I. Runge, Val M.
[DNLM: 1. Magnetic Resonance Imaging. WN 445 C6407]
RC78.7.N83C55 1990
616.07′548—dc20
DNLM/DLC
for Library of Congress 89-12810
CIP

The authors and publisher have exerted every effort to ensure that drug selection and dosage set forth in this text are in accord with current recommendations and practice at the time of publication. However, in view of ongoing research, changes in government regulations, and the constant flow of information relating to drug therapy and drug reactions, the reader is urged to check the package insert for each drug for any change in indications and dosage and for added warnings and precautions. This is particularly important when the recommended agent is a new or infrequently employed drug.

To B.J. and Sadie, with all my love today and every tomorrow
and to the MRI Staff at Tufts University, in recognition of their work and dedication.

CONTRIBUTORS

Gregory V. Babigian, M.D.

Fellow, Neuroradiology, Albany Medical Center, Albany, New York

Mark R. Bankoff, M.D.

Associate Professor of Radiology, Tufts University—New England Medical Center Hospitals, Boston, Massachusetts

Bert R. Carollo, M.D.

Radiologist, Department of Radiology, Salem Hospital, Salem, Oregon

Barbara L. Carter, M.D.

Professor of Radiology and Otolaryngology, Tufts University—New England Medical Center Hospitals, Boston, Massachusetts

Madeleine R. Fisher, M.D.

Professor of Radiology, Director of Magnetic Resonance Imaging Services, Hospital of the Good Samaritan, Los Angeles, California

Daphna Y. Gelblum, M.S.

Research Associate, Tufts University—New England Medical Center Hospitals, Boston, Massachusetts

Kevin L. Nelson, PHARM.D., M.D.

Director, Magnetic Resonance Imaging, Clarkson Memorial Hospital, Omaha, Nebraska

Martha L. Pacetti, R.N.

Magnetic Resonance Imaging Nurse, Tufts University—New England Medical Center Hospitals, Boston, Massachusetts

Ann C. Price, M.D.

Associate Professor of Radiology, Albany Medical Center, Albany, New York

Stephen J. Robertson, M.D.

Neuroradiologist, Delray Community Hospital, Delray Beach, Florida

Val M. Runge, M.D.

Professor of Diagnostic Radiology, Director of the Magnetic Resonance Imaging and Spectroscopy Center, University of Kentucky, Lexington, Kentucky

David D. Stark, M.D.

Associate Professor of Radiology, Massachusetts General Hospital, Boston, Massachusetts

Clifford R. Wolf, M.D.

Clinical Assistant Professor, University of Illinois, Chicago, and Radiologist, Department of Radiology, Northwest Community Hospital, Arlington Heights, Illinois

Samuel M. Wolpert, M.D.

Professor of Radiology and Neurology, New England Medical Center Hospitals, Boston, Massachusetts

Michael L. Wood, M.D.

Assistant Professor of Radiation Oncology and Radiology, New England Medical Center Hospitals, Boston, Massachusetts

E. Kent Yucel, M.D.

Instructor, Vascular Radiology, Massachusetts General Hospital, Boston, Massachusetts

PREFACE

This text is intended to serve as a practical guide for clinical magnetic resonance imaging (MRI). The first 12 chapters are organized along anatomic lines and discuss disease entities commonly encountered in clinical practice. In the review of magnetic resonance physics (Chapter 13), attention has been focused on practical concerns with respect to imaging technique. Chapter 14 provides information on image quality, patient safety, and sedation. The use of contrast media is discussed in detail in Chapter 15, in addition to the integration of this material in each of the first 12 chapters. Chapter 16 summarizes the clinical indications for MRI using a teaching case approach.

Emphasis is placed on disease entities that routinely present for MRI. The text focuses on common examinations, covering both the technical approach and clinical interpretation. Clinical cases serve as a backbone for this discussion.

Advances in instrumentation and new developments in contrast media continue to impact on the use of magnetic resonance. Techniques such as presaturation, gradient moment nulling, and gradient echo imaging represent relatively new advances that can improve significantly routine clinical image quality. These and other techniques are discussed in an integrated fashion according to organ system. Scan times continue to decrease with subsequent advances in instrumentation and software, analogous to the evolution of computed tomography (CT). The development of pulse sequences acquired during breath holding will lead to increased applications for MRI, particularly in the abdomen and pelvis.

Newer instrumentation has lifted many of the technical restrictions imposed on pulse techniques in the past. For example, the number of phase encoding steps can now be varied between 128 and 512 by increments of 1. Echo times of less than 5 ms for gradient echo techniques are possible. Half-Fourier imaging and asymmetrical matrices can be employed routinely. With the use of improved computer technology, set-up and reconstruction times have been minimized. Significant advances also have been made in coil design, including the implementation of quadrature detection and the development of dual coils for evaluation of the temporomandibular joint.

Gadolinium DTPA (Gd DTPA) has had a major impact on both the choice of imaging technique and the use of MRI. For example, before the advent of intravenous contrast media, drop metastases were visualized poorly. Recent clinical studies, however, recommend the replacement of both myelography and x-ray CT by Gd DTPA-enhanced MRI in the study of this disease. It is likely that, in the future, a large percentage of central nervous system examinations will be performed with a contrast agent such as Gd DTPA. Currently under clinical evaluation are new contrast agents such as SQ 32,692 (Gd HP-DO3A, a nonionic gadolinium chelate of the tetraazacyclododecane-triacetate family, developed by Squibb Diagnostics). In less than 10 years, MRI has witnessed the development of *nonionic* contrast media (within an entirely new class of pharmaceuticals), a process that took conventional radiology nearly 100 years. New agents are more stable, can be used at higher doses, and can be derivatized. In the future, such agents may find significant application in the study of liver and cardiac disease. These developments also may make qualitative measurements of organ perfusion possible.

The clinical applications of magnetic resonance continue to expand with both new technical developments and greater availability. Progress in magnetic resonance *imaging* has dominated the field of radiology for the past 10 years. Unfortunately, spectroscopy remains primarily a research technique. Today magnetic resonance stands as a major new diagnostic subspecialty. The complexity of this technique and the continued advances dictate that magnetic resonance will continue to play a dominant role in clinical medicine.

Val M. Runge

CONTENTS

CLINICAL MAGNETIC RESONANCE IMAGING

1

Brain: White Matter Disease/Infection

Val M. Runge

Since the early 1980s, magnetic resonance imaging (MRI) has been the technique of choice for visualizing white matter lesions in the brain, especially for those brain lesions found in multiple sclerosis (MS). Many conditions can be confused clinically and radiologically with MS, including cerebral vascular disease, sarcoidosis, and cerebellar degeneration, but careful inspection of images and the use of pattern recognition markedly improves diagnostic specificity (Table 1-1).

Although sensitive to disease, MRI cannot always provide a specific diagnosis, and clinical presentation is then critical for differentiation. In MS, periventricular changes are typically punctate and asymmetric. Postmortem studies have confirmed that the white matter abnormalities demonstrated by MRI correspond to MS plaques. Edema associated with acute lesions and gliosis with chronic lesions permit visualization on MRI. Demyelination does not contribute significantly to alterations in proton density or relaxation. In other conditions that mimic MS, such as cerebrovascular disease, periventricular changes are often milder and smoother in contour. However, the white matter changes found in dementia can resemble those of advanced MS.

In very ill patients with intracranial infection, the duration of the MRI scan and the relative inaccessibility of the patient often compel the use of computed tomography (CT). However, MRI offers the advantage of direct, high-resolution, multiplanar imaging with superior sensitivity to inflammatory change. In a mature abscess, the capsule can be differentiated from inner debris and surrounding edema on unenhanced MRI. CT offers advantages in detecting calcifications, such as those associated with chronic infections (cysticercosis) and end-stage congenital infection. However, MRI is more sensitive to parenchymal hemorrhage, regardless of stage. MRI can detect hemorrhage long after CT scans become normal, allowing more complete characterization of certain infectious diseases. In disease of the medial temporal lobe, such as herpes simplex type 1, MRI is markedly more sensitive than CT.

The initial superiority of CT for the diagnosis of meningeal disease, as in tuberculosis, has been negated due to clinical introduction of an FDA-approved intravenous contrast agent for MRI, gadolinium DTPA (Gd DTPA). Studies have demonstrated that enhanced MRI is superior to enhanced CT for detecting meningeal disease.

There are guidelines for the clinician deciding between MRI and CT for patients with intracranial infection. If detection of calcifications is important for diagnosis, CT is advocated. However, MRI is superior for demonstrating soft tissue lesions due to increased free water and associated vasogenic edema. Differential diagnosis can be made on the basis of the pattern of disease involvement (Table 1-2).

Table 1-1 **White Matter Disease—Differential Diagnosis**

DISEASE	DISTRIBUTION	COMMENTS
Multiple sclerosis	Primarily periventricular, asymmetric	Inactive lesions—small, "punctate" Acute lesions—large, "fluffy"
Optic neuritis	Can be identical to MS	Monophasic illness, demonstration of optic nerve lesions requires specialized technique (STIR)
Dilated perivascular spaces	Adjacent to anterior commissure, supraventricular white matter	CSF signal intensity
Deep white matter ischemia (DWMI)	Immediate periventricular and peripheral white matter, symmetric	Smooth, confluent lesions
Periventricular leukomalacia	Resembles DWMI	Pediatric population
Leukodystrophies	White matter tracts, focal contiguous involvement	Enzymatic defect, familial
Hypoxemia	Basal ganglia, deep white matter	
Systemic lupus erythematosus	Gray and white matter involvement	Wedge-shaped lesions
Radiation injury	Focal (port) or diffuse	If diffuse, abuts cortical gray matter

Table 1-2 **Infection**

DISEASE	COMMENTS
Parenchymal	Improved detection and assessment of activity with Gd DTPA. Acute disseminated encephalomyelitis can resemble acute MS.
Meningeal	Gd DTPA required in most instances for detection. Other causes can be neoplastic, traumatic, and postoperative.
Herpes Encephalitis (type 1)	Temporal lobe, may also involve frontal or parietal lobes. Meningeal enhancement can occur.
Sarcoidosis	Parenchymal and meningeal disease. White matter lesions can resemble MS.
AIDS	Small discrete lesions, as depicted by MRI, most commonly due to toxoplasmosis.

WHITE MATTER DISEASE

Multiple Sclerosis

MS is characterized clinically by multiple neurologic episodes separated in time. Two-thirds of patients are female. The disease progresses in a relentless stepwise fashion, marked by exacerbations and remissions. MS is highly variable in its course. A study from the Mayo Clinic documented that 75% of patients were alive 25 years after onset, 55% without significant disability.

The diagnosis of MS by MRI hinges on pattern recognition. Most lesions are small, usually 1 to 5 mm in diameter. The most common location of MS plaques is in the periventricular region, particularly adjacent to the superolateral angles of the lateral ventricles (Fig. 1-1). There is often a marked asymmetry in lesion distribution, a distinguishing factor from ischemic disease that is often encountered in the elderly patient. Other common locations for lesions include the centrum semiovale, the atrial trigone, occipital horns, forceps major and minor, colliculi, and temporal lobes (Figs. 1-2 and 1-3). Approximately 30% of patients demonstrate brain stem and cerebellar lesions, with the middle cerebellar peduncles a preferred location.

Corpus callosum involvement by MS is common, with 30% of patients demonstrating focal lesions both on MRI and pathologic examination.[1] Long, inner callosal-subcallosal lesions also have been imaged. Focal or diffuse atrophy of the corpus callosum is seen in 40% of patients.[1] Thinning of the corpus callosum results from general cerebral atrophy and accompanying Wallerian degeneration. Changes in the corpus callosum are most prominent in patients with longstanding and extensive disease.

Although MS is commonly thought of as a white matter disease, 5 to 10% of plaques occur in gray matter. These can be seen in the cortex and in the basal ganglia (Fig. 1-2).

Among MRI techniques, spin echo sequences with moderate T2 weighting are preferred for visualizing MS plaques within the brain (Fig. 1-4). The scans are typically performed in the axial plane with relatively thin sections ($\leq$5 mm) for improved lesion detection,

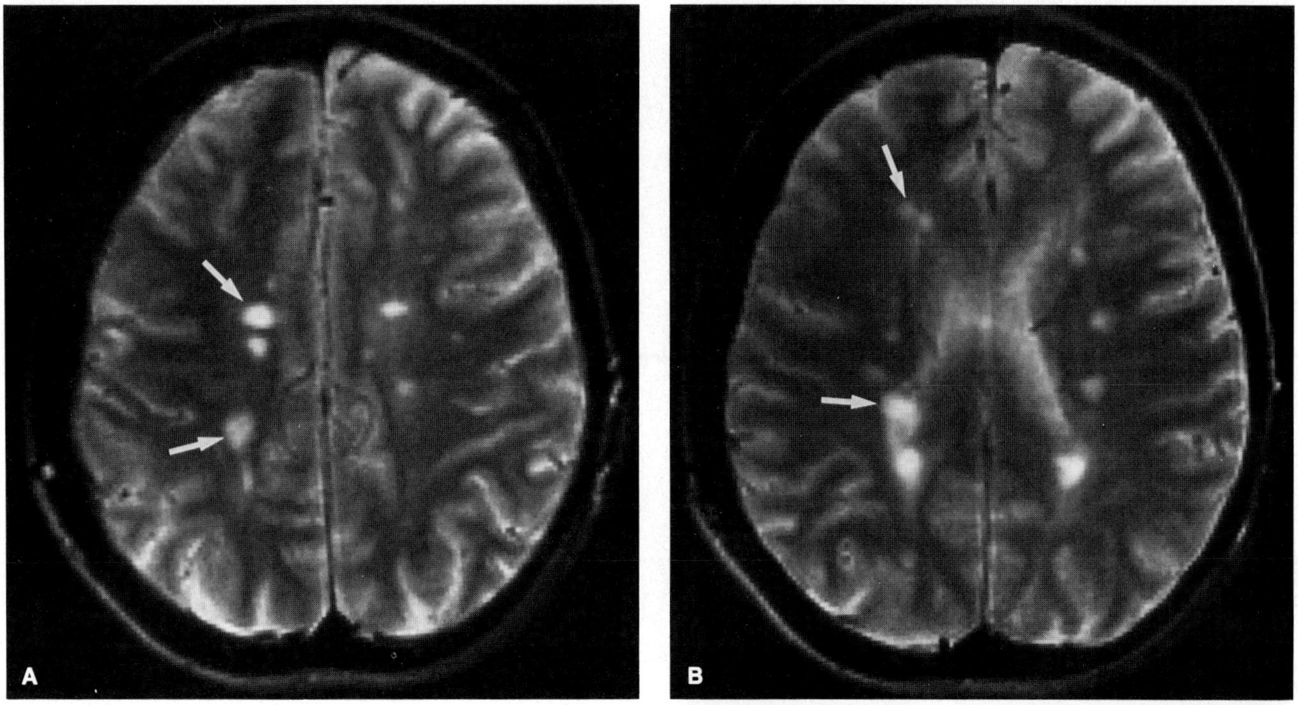

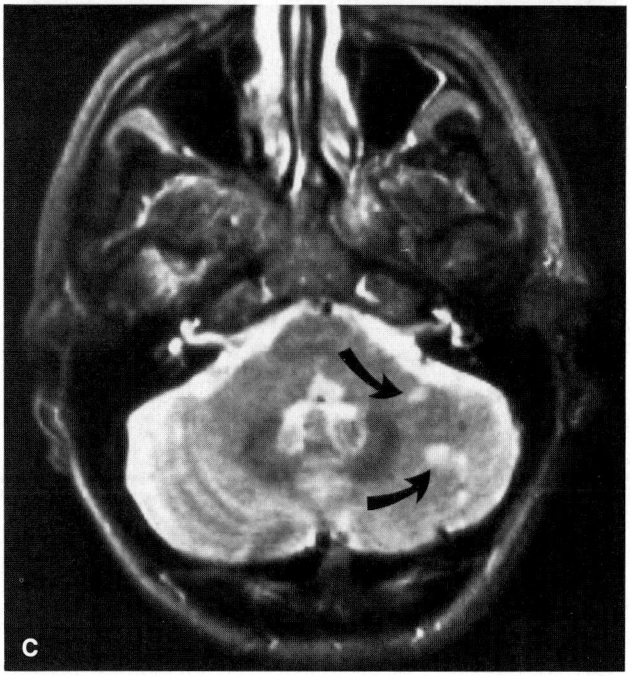

FIGURE 1 – 1. MS. T2-weighted images from two patients demonstrate the appearance of periventricular lesions **(A,B)**. Multiple punctate periventricular plaques (arrows) in an asymmetric distribution, combined with the appropriate clinical presentation, permit a definitive diagnosis. Each section should be carefully inspected, because additional plaques in other characteristic locations improve diagnostic confidence. Lesions **(C)** can be identified in the cerebellar hemisphere and middle cerebellar peduncle (curved arrows).

minimizing partial volume effects. The appearance of MS plaques on both spin echo and inversion recovery images was described early in the development of MRI.[2–4] MS plaques are characterized by prolonged T1 and T2 relaxation times and by increased proton density. Low-intensity lesions can be demonstrated by heavily T1-weighted inversion recovery (IR) techniques, which provide excellent contrast between the lesions and normal surrounding white matter (Fig. 1–5). However, inversion recovery techniques are insensitive to lesions adjacent to the ventricles or gray matter, due to the lack of signal contrast between the structures.[5] T2-weighted techniques, which depict

(text continues on page 7)

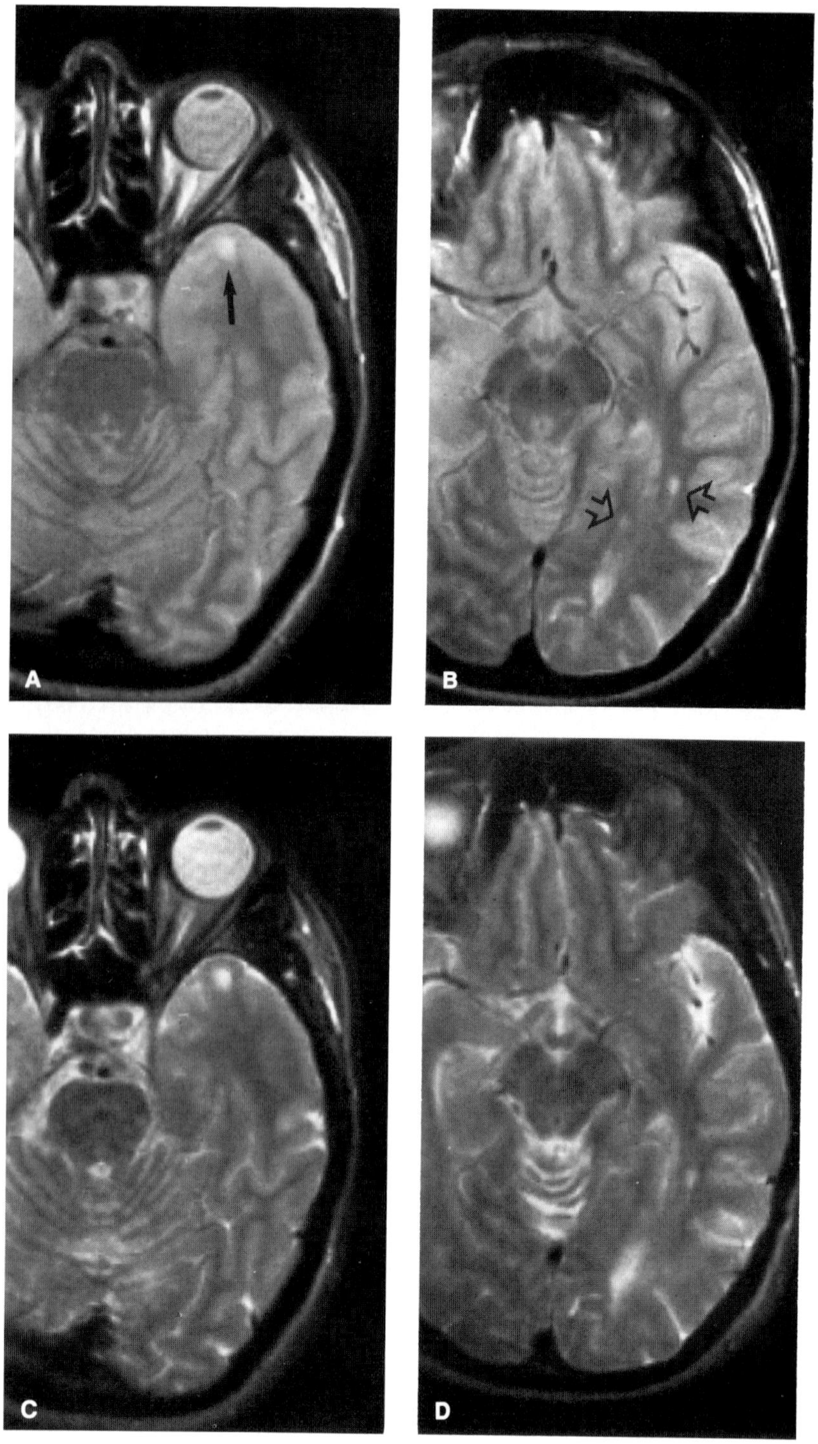

FIGURE 1 – 2. Temporal and occipital lobe lesions occur in MS. **(A,B)** Mildly T2-weighted images (TR/TE = 3000/45) and **(C,D)** heavily T2-weighted images (TR/TE = 3000/90) are from a 44-year-old woman with a 10-year history of intermittent left optic neuritis. There is a lesion (closed arrow) at the gray-white matter junction in the left temporal lobe, with multiple lesions (open arrows) lining the left occipital horn. These lesions are easier to detect and confirm on the first echo of the T2-weighted scan because of the isointense signal characteristics of CSF at this ratio of TR and TE values.

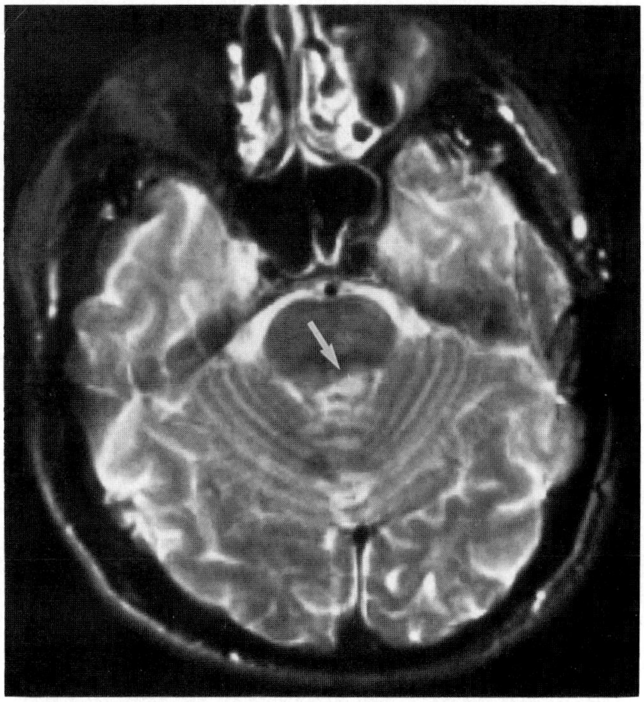

FIGURE 1 – 3. Collicular lesion (arrow) in MS demonstrated in a T2-weighted image (TR/TE = 3000/90). This represents another common location for MS plaques.

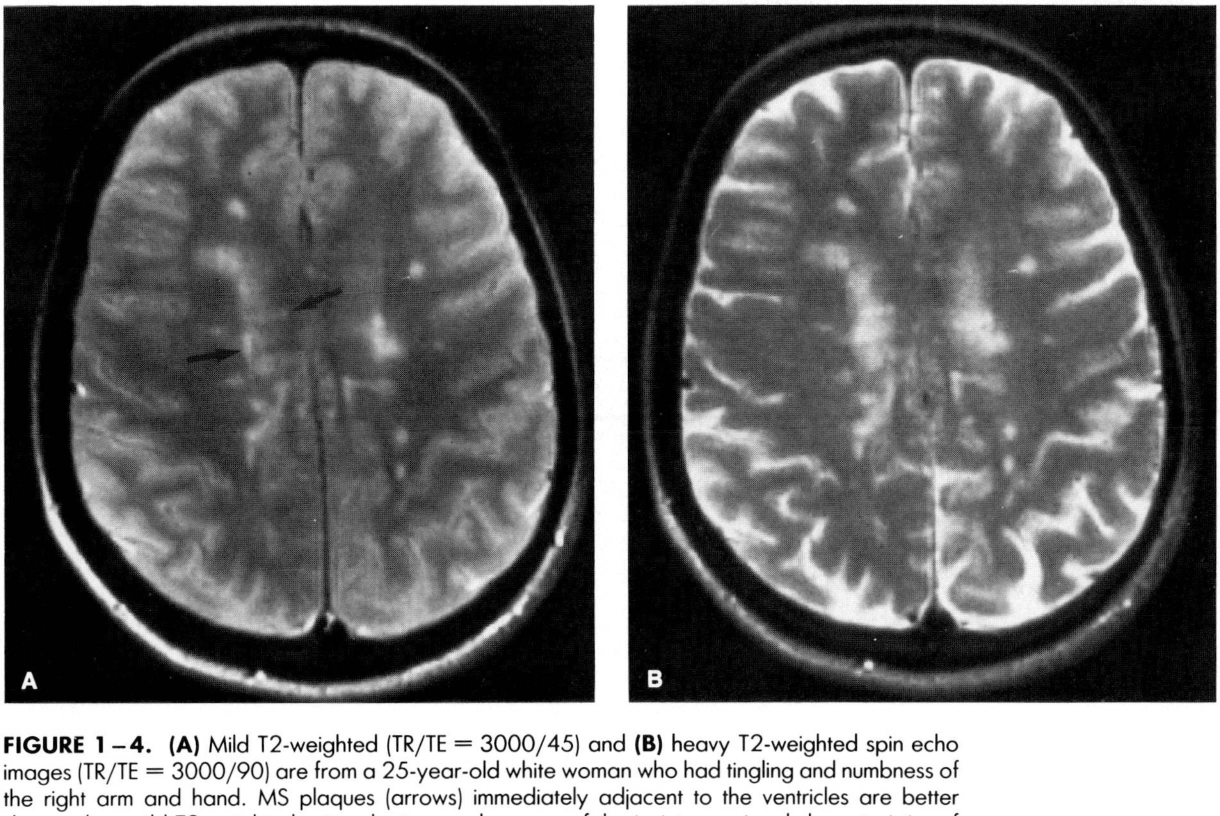

FIGURE 1 – 4. **(A)** Mild T2-weighted (TR/TE = 3000/45) and **(B)** heavy T2-weighted spin echo images (TR/TE = 3000/90) are from a 25-year-old white woman who had tingling and numbness of the right arm and hand. MS plaques (arrows) immediately adjacent to the ventricles are better detected on mild T2-weighted spin echo images because of the isointense signal characteristics of CSF.

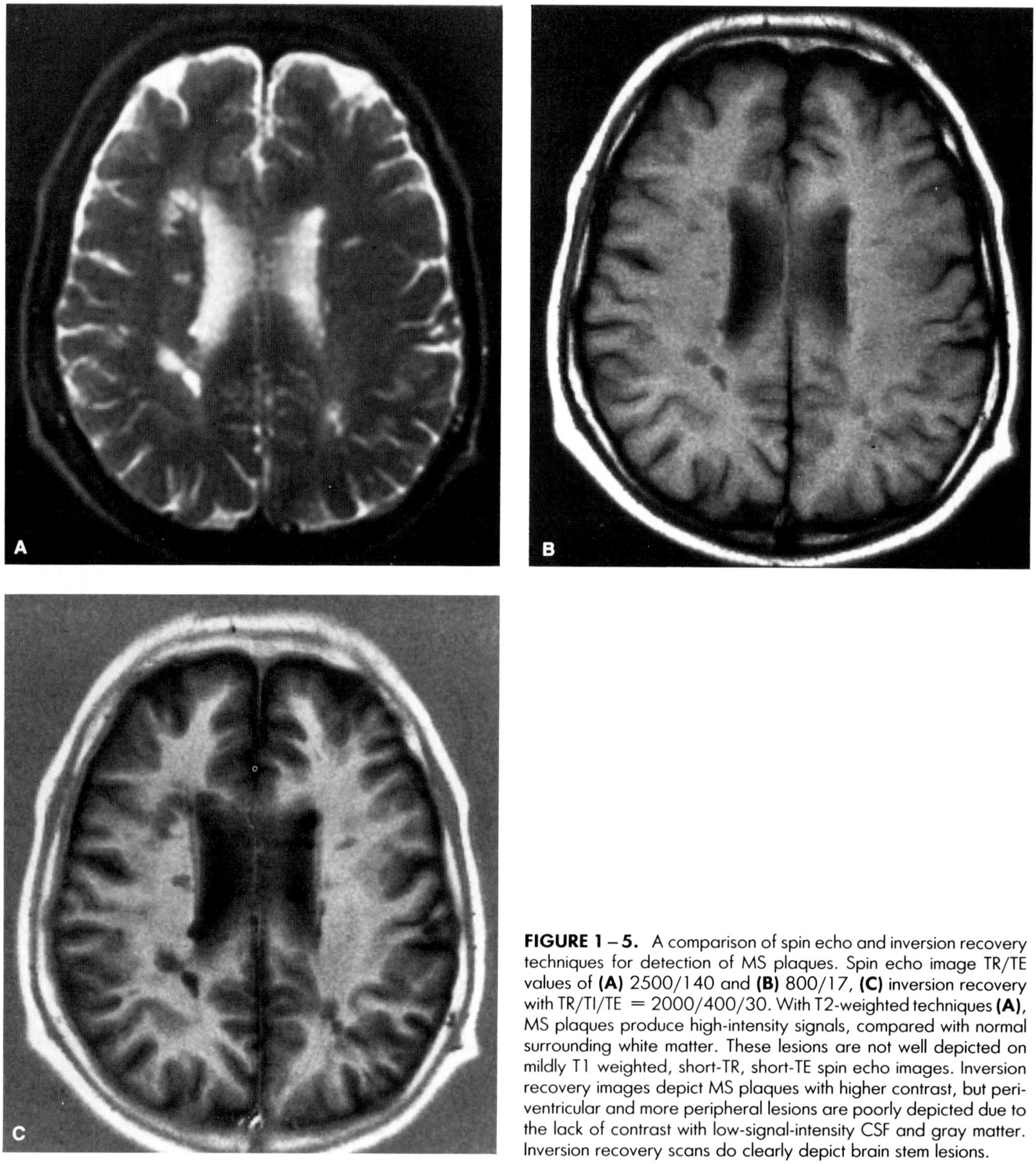

FIGURE 1–5. A comparison of spin echo and inversion recovery techniques for detection of MS plaques. Spin echo image TR/TE values of **(A)** 2500/140 and **(B)** 800/17, **(C)** inversion recovery with TR/TI/TE = 2000/400/30. With T2-weighted techniques **(A)**, MS plaques produce high-intensity signals, compared with normal surrounding white matter. These lesions are not well depicted on mildly T1 weighted, short-TR, short-TE spin echo images. Inversion recovery images depict MS plaques with higher contrast, but periventricular and more peripheral lesions are poorly depicted due to the lack of contrast with low-signal-intensity CSF and gray matter. Inversion recovery scans do clearly depict brain stem lesions.

plaques as high-signal-intensity foci compared with surrounding normal brain, are preferred for lesion detection in the brain.[3-6]

It has been reported that brain stem lesions are more readily assessed using inversion recovery sequences.[5,6] These results were obtained before the advent of gradient moment nulling for reduction of CSF pulsation artifacts. Thus T2-weighted scans on current-generation equipment, employing at least two-axis first-order gradient moment nulling, are probably more sensitive to brain stem lesions than published reports indicate.

Two studies in the literature describe the inherent sensitivity of magnetic resonance for detecting MS plaques and its superiority to x-ray CT.[2,4] At Hammersmith Hospital, examinations of five patients with MS revealed 8 lesions on postcontrast x-ray CT, 33 on IR scans, and 44 on T2-weighted spin echo scans. Less severe disease is generally undetected by CT.[5] Heavily T2-weighted scans (TE $\geq$ 80 msec) can fail to detect some MS lesions due to their proximity to high-signal-intensity cerebrospinal fluid (CSF). This problem is not encountered with mildly T2-weighted spin echo technique, because the CSF signal is isointense relative to white matter.

MS plaques tend to appear slightly smaller on IR scans compared with T2-weighted spin echo scans.[6] Multi-echo scans can confirm the presence of lesions. Short TI Inversion Recovery (STIR) is a relatively new technique that can suppress the signal from fat. Although this method can detect parenchymal lesions (Fig. 1-6), it has been specifically advocated for detecting optic nerve lesions.[7] Surrounding orbital fat impedes recognition of optic nerve lesions because of chemical-shift artifacts and loss of lesion contrast.

Periventricular abnormalities in MS typically have irregular outlines. This "lumpy-bumpy" appearance can distinguish MS from cerebrovascular disease. Ischemic disease in the elderly patient typically produces milder abnormalities with smooth outlines in the immediate periventricular area.[8] Confluent periventricular high signal intensity can be seen in patients with severe disability and long-standing MS. However, chronic MS tends to differ in pattern from deep white matter ischemia, presenting as an irregular, "lumpy-bumpy," confluent mass of plaques with marked asymmetry between right and left sides.

Acute or clinically active plaques in MS tend to be large (>1 cm) with indistinct margins (Fig. 1-7). This contrasts sharply with the well-demarcated small punctate plaques seen by MRI in patients with quiescent disease.

In MS, lesions larger than 1 cm can represent confluent plaques of different ages or clinically active foci (Figs. 1-8 and 1-9). MS plaques demonstrate a wide

(text continues on page 10)

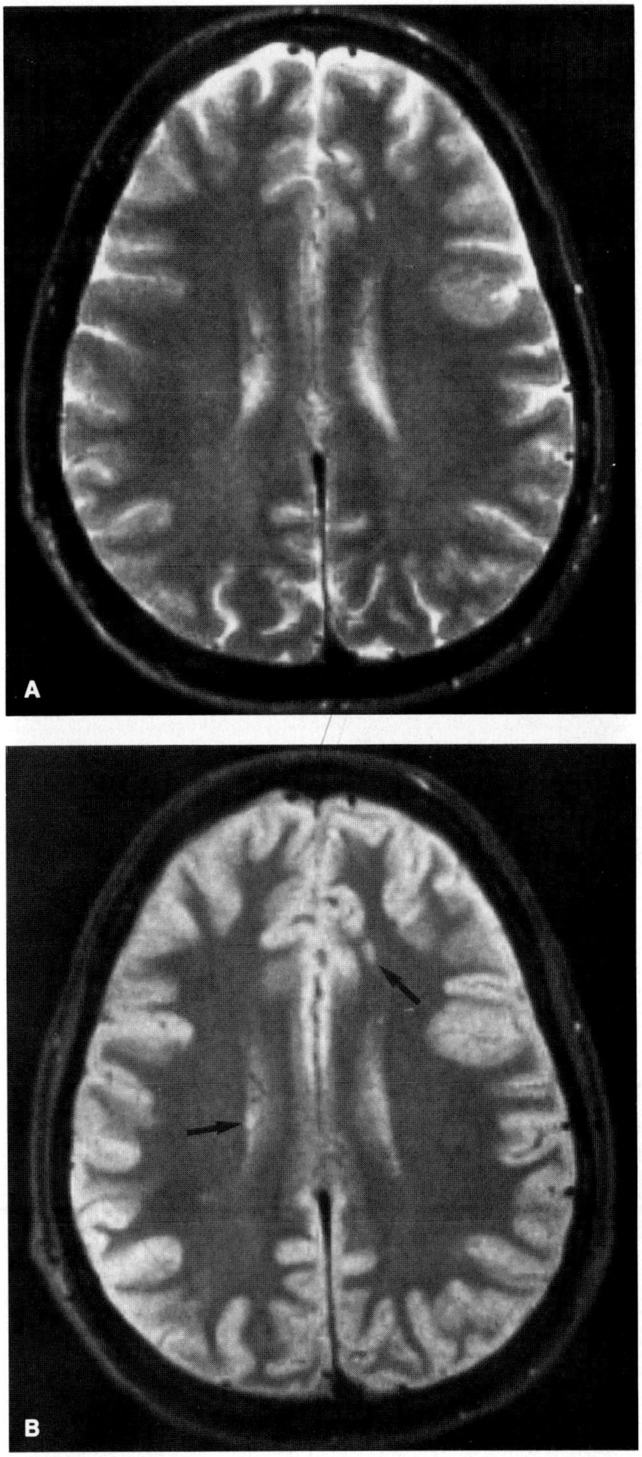

FIGURE 1-6. **(A)** T2-weighted technique (TR/TE = 3000/90) is compared with **(B)** short-TI inversion recovery (STIR) technique (TR/TI/TE = 2000/125/28) for detecting MS plaques. Several punctate white matter lesions (arrows) can be identified. With STIR, the TI can be chosen so that orbital fat has no signal intensity, improving depiction of the optic nerve. Unlike spin echo technique, the effect of prolongation of T1 and T2 on signal intensity is additive, further improving lesion detection.

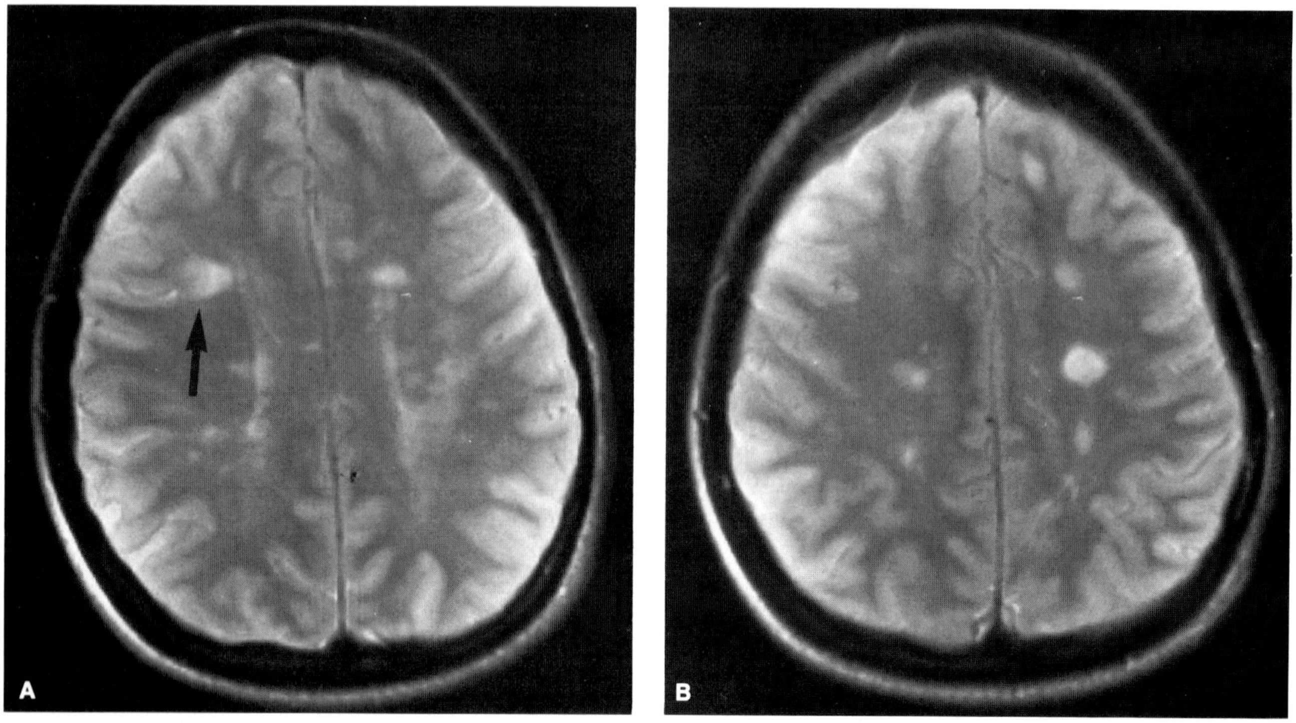

FIGURE 1–7. In patients with clinically active MS, large lesions and lesions with indistinct borders can be seen. **(A,B)** T2-weighted sections (TR/TE = 3000/45) at two anatomic levels in a 23-year-old woman who had left optic neuritis. Many small punctate lesions in a periventricular distribution occur with several large lesions in the left centrum semiovale. A large lesion with indistinct peripheral borders (arrow) is adjacent to the right frontal horn.

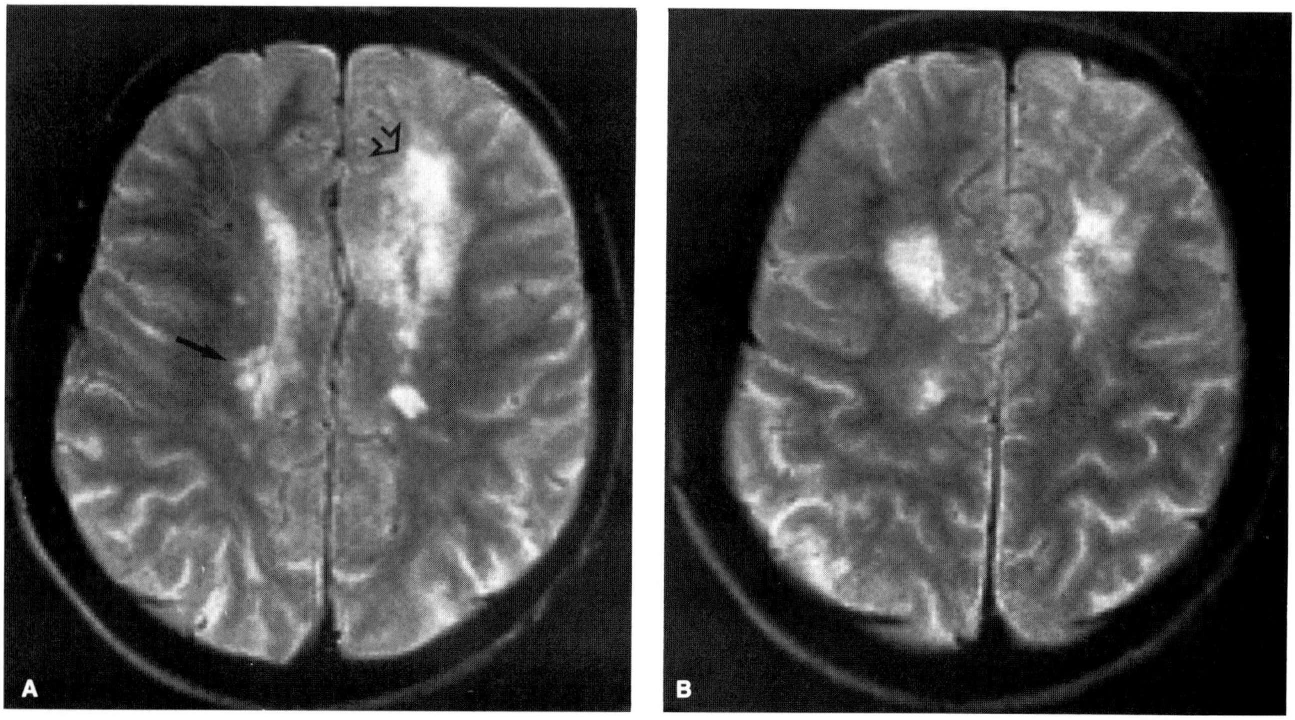

FIGURE 1–8. In MS, extensive white matter abnormalities are demonstrated **(A,B)** in two anatomic sections (TR/TE = 3000/60). In advanced disease and in clinically symptomatic patients, large confluent white matter lesions (open arrow) can occur. Detection of periventricular, discrete, punctate lesions (closed arrow) assists in the diagnosis of these patients.

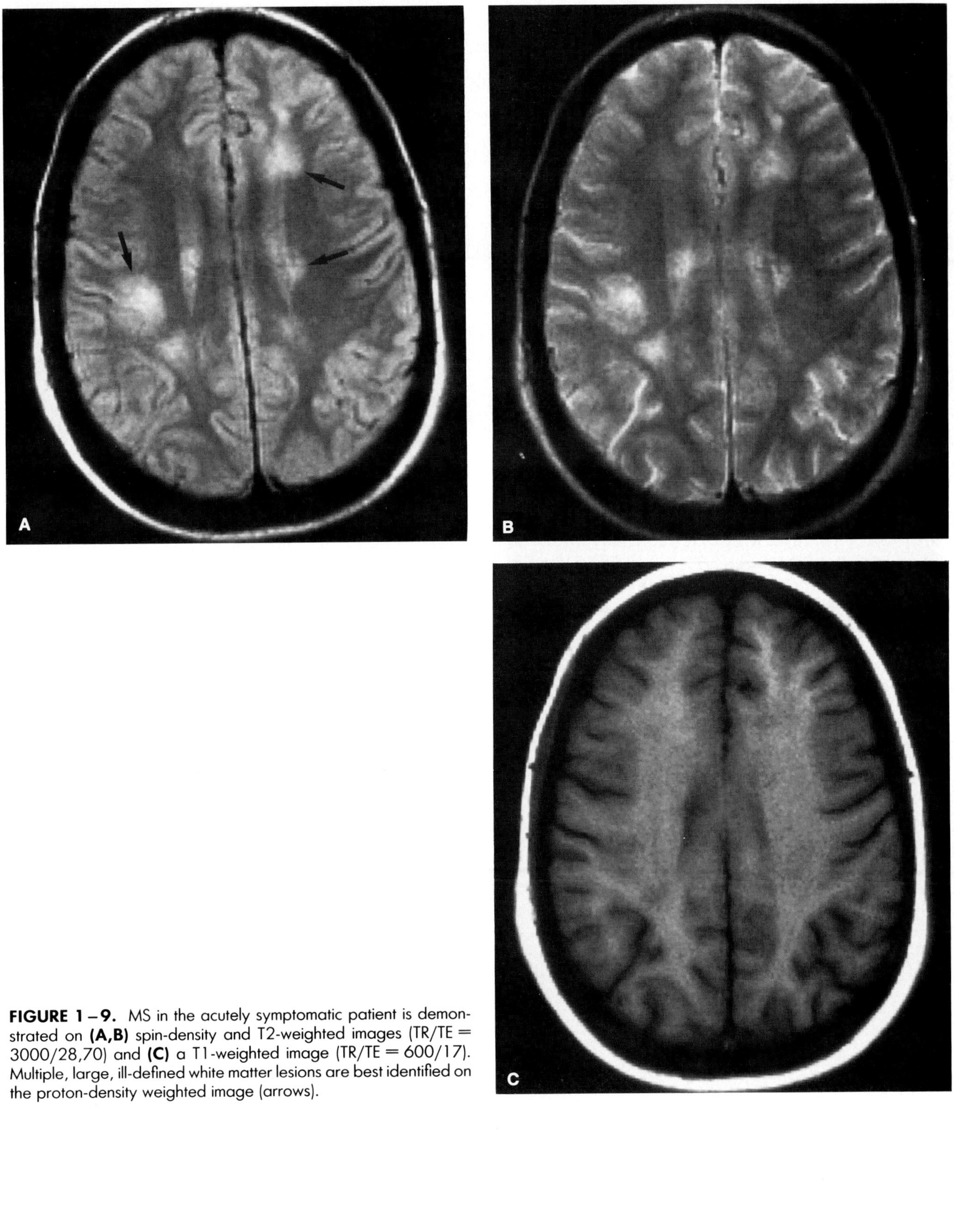

FIGURE 1–9. MS in the acutely symptomatic patient is demonstrated on **(A,B)** spin-density and T2-weighted images (TR/TE = 3000/28,70) and **(C)** a T1-weighted image (TR/TE = 600/17). Multiple, large, ill-defined white matter lesions are best identified on the proton-density weighted image (arrows).

range of T1 and T2 relaxation times.[9] The prolongation of T1 and T2 observed in imaging acute plaques is probably caused by edema. Chronic plaques demonstrate gliosis, consisting of a cellular fibroglial tissue. Demyelination (lipid loss) does not contribute significantly to the changes in relaxation times with MRI. The T2 of apparently normal white matter is also significantly prolonged in MS patients.[8,9]

MS plaques are not necessarily homogeneous in appearance. Both T1- and T2-weighted scans can demonstrate inhomogeneity, commonly permitting differentiation between the border of a lesion and its center (Fig. 1-10). T1 shortening also has been described at the edge of MS lesions.[10] On T1-weighted images, including both spin echo and IR techniques, a thin line of high signal intensity can be seen encircling low signal intensity plaques in certain instances. In a study using Gd DTPA, this thin line of high signal intensity on precontrast images corresponded to the edge of the enhancing region.[10] Pathologically, this appearance may be due to the accumulation of myelin breakdown products at the edge of active lesions.

MRI can detect characteristic MS lesions in 80 to 100% of patients, compared with 23 to 33% detected with x-ray CT.[11-13] CT usually detects only the larger lesions demonstrated on MRI. X-ray CT is relatively insensitive and nonspecific for detecting and diagnosing MS.

The severity of disease, as assessed by size and number of lesions on MRI, does correlate with the likelihood of a positive CT scan, but not with the degree of disability, duration of disease, or positive CSF oligoclonal banding.[14] MRI is sensitive for detecting MS lesions, but clinical assessment continues to be crucial for diagnosis. MRI is more sensitive than somatosensory evoked potentials, although brainstem auditory evoked potentials may be slightly better for detecting brainstem lesions.[15] MRI is superior to CSF testing and visual evoked potentials in establishing the diagnosis of MS, but it can be negative in a small percentage of patients with clinically proven MS.[16] Clinical diagnosis of MS, although only 95% accurate, remains the gold standard.[17] This is particularly true given the relative nonspecificity of lesions found by MRI.

Confluent abnormalities in the periventricular region correlate with long-standing disease. Most lesions (72-79%) remain unchanged on follow-up examinations.[16] However, new lesions are often observed with the apparent resolution of older lesions.[18]

Using the sensitivity of MRI for detecting MS lesions, clinical studies have assessed the correlation between clinical function and the pattern of disease depicted on MRI scans.[19-21] MRI also has been used to assess responses to administration of cyclosporin A and azathioprine.[22] The consensus from these studies is that there is no correlation between functional disability and the number of brain lesions depicted on MRI scans. Patients with more severe disease tend to have a larger number of plaques and more confluent white matter disease, and in long-standing disease, MRI and CT demonstrate thinning of the corpus callosum and generalized parenchymal atrophy.[23] However, many lesions depicted by MRI are clinically silent. Occasionally, lesions correlating with specific clinical symptoms can be identified (Fig. 1-11). MRI is more sensitive for detecting disease and demonstrating disease activity than physical examination.

Experimental allergic encephalomyelitis (EAE) has been studied in canines and guinea pigs, animals that provide a model of demyelinating disease with marked similarity to MS. This relapsing-remitting disease resembles MS clinically and pathologically.[24] This model suggests that the high signal intensity observed on T2-weighted images is caused by inflammatory change rather than demyelination.[25] On T2-weighted images, acute lesions were indistinguishable from older, chronic lesions, which was similar to the clinical experience with MS. However, after IV injection of Gd DTPA, enhancement was seen only in acute lesions.[26] This work has formed the basis for subsequent clinical trials with Gd DTPA in an attempt to differentiate acute demyelinating lesions from chronic inactive disease.

The role of Gd DTPA in the study of MS has been investigated primarily at two centers.[27-31] These trials examined principally patients with clinically active disease. It is the minority of patients with MS who demonstrate enhanced lesions on MRI after Gd DTPA administration (Figs. 1-12 and 1-13). Results from these clinical trials reveal that enhancement is more sensitive than clinical examination in detecting active disease. Enhancement with Gd DTPA is a consistent finding in new lesions. Serial comparisons revealed some lesions reverting to normal signal intensity on T2-weighted scans, suggesting resolution of transient inflammatory changes.

MS is a dynamic disease, with lesions demonstrating dramatic changes during longitudinal study. Gd DTPA can be used as a marker of biologically active lesions, suggesting its use for monitoring therapy. Both the pattern and time course of enhancement may provide information. A recent study suggests that older lesions enhance less rapidly than new lesions and may demonstrate ring enhancement, differing from acute lesions, which enhance uniformly.[31]

MS plaques in the cervical (Fig. 1-14) and thoracic cord can be demonstrated by MRI.[32] These lesions often do not respect gray-white boundaries, nor do they follow specific fiber tracks. Lesions may be elon-

(text continues on page 13)

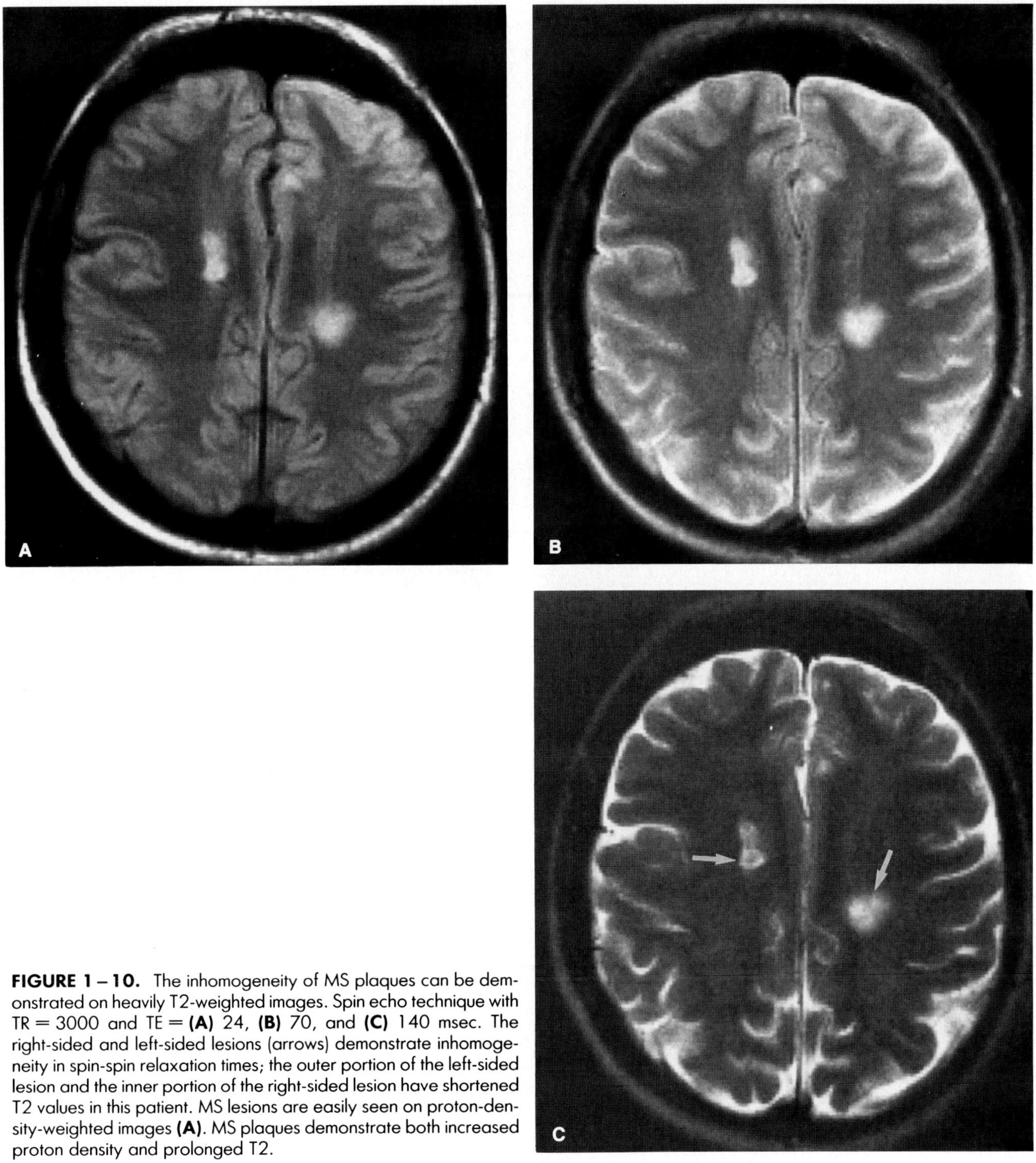

FIGURE 1 – 10. The inhomogeneity of MS plaques can be demonstrated on heavily T2-weighted images. Spin echo technique with TR = 3000 and TE = **(A)** 24, **(B)** 70, and **(C)** 140 msec. The right-sided and left-sided lesions (arrows) demonstrate inhomogeneity in spin-spin relaxation times; the outer portion of the left-sided lesion and the inner portion of the right-sided lesion have shortened T2 values in this patient. MS lesions are easily seen on proton-density-weighted images **(A)**. MS plaques demonstrate both increased proton density and prolonged T2.

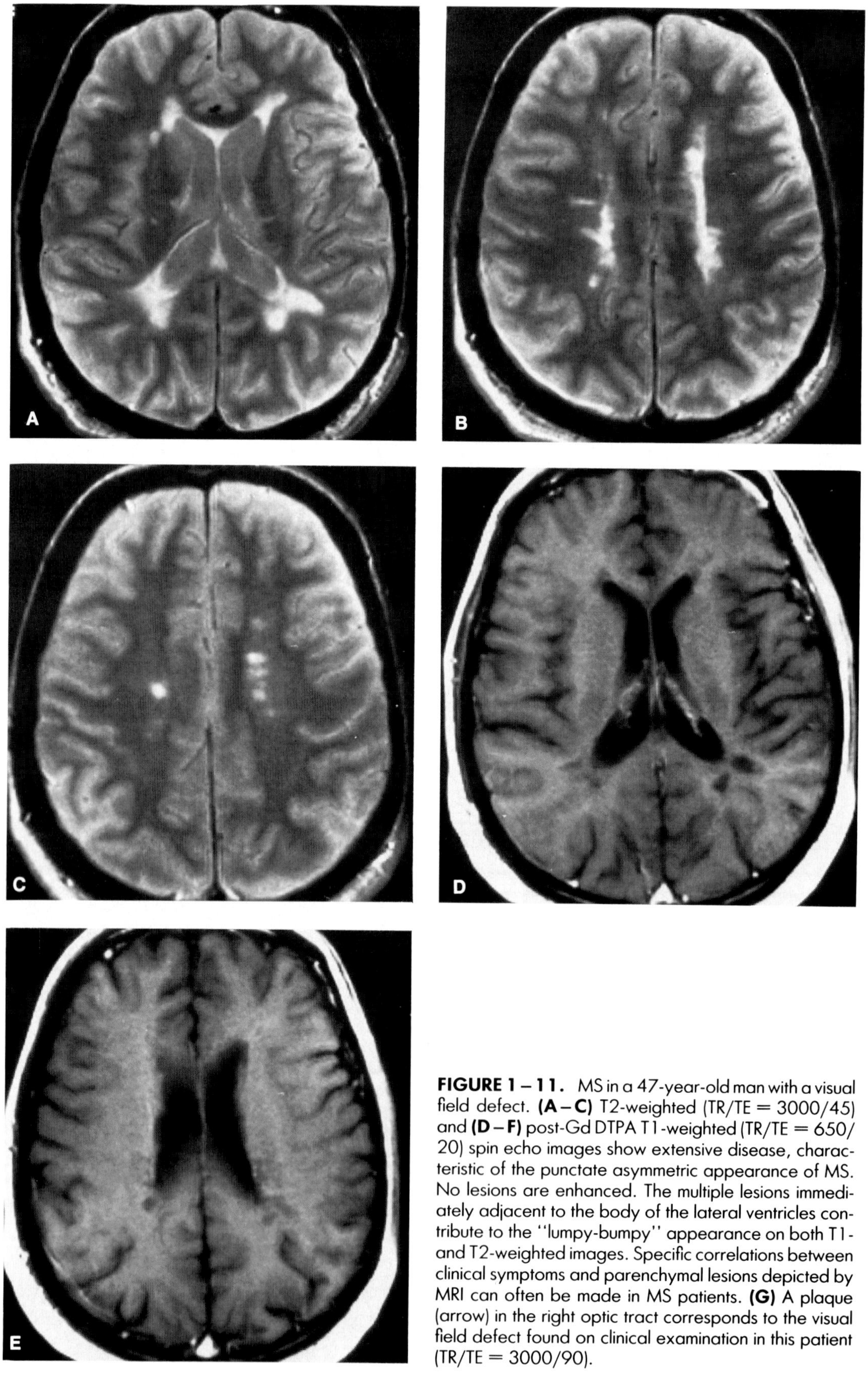

FIGURE 1–11. MS in a 47-year-old man with a visual field defect. **(A–C)** T2-weighted (TR/TE = 3000/45) and **(D–F)** post-Gd DTPA T1-weighted (TR/TE = 650/20) spin echo images show extensive disease, characteristic of the punctate asymmetric appearance of MS. No lesions are enhanced. The multiple lesions immediately adjacent to the body of the lateral ventricles contribute to the "lumpy-bumpy" appearance on both T1- and T2-weighted images. Specific correlations between clinical symptoms and parenchymal lesions depicted by MRI can often be made in MS patients. **(G)** A plaque (arrow) in the right optic tract corresponds to the visual field defect found on clinical examination in this patient (TR/TE = 3000/90).

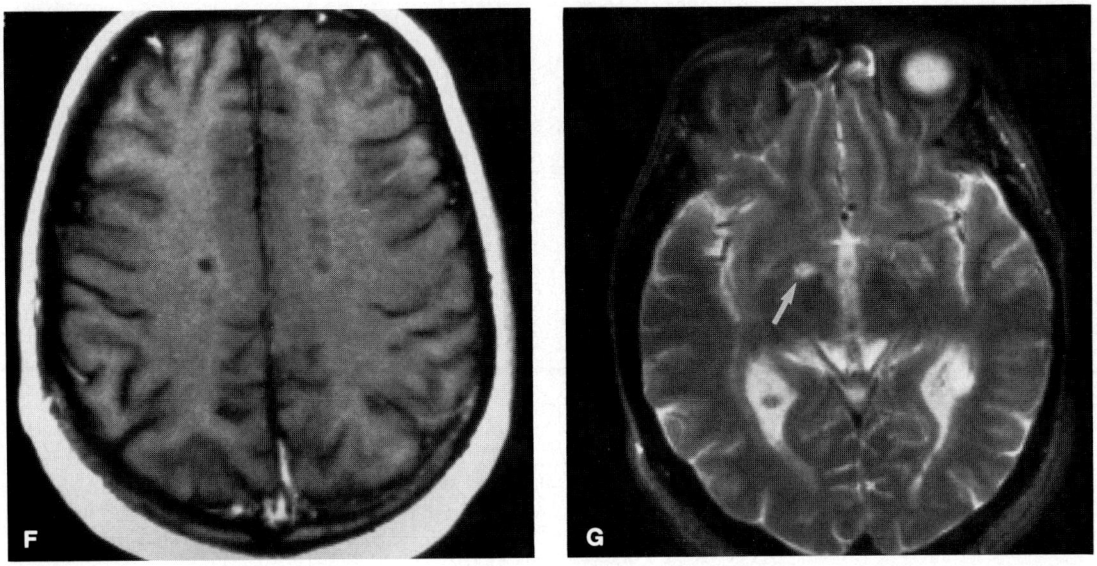

FIGURE 1–11. (Continued)

gated, paralleling the axis of the cord, and they are more common dorsally and laterally within the cord (Fig. 1–15). Before the advent of MRI, these lesions were rarely detected by radiologic means. Cervical lesions are detected more commonly than thoracic lesions, a finding that may be related to technique. Imaging of the thoracic cord is still inferior to that of the cervical cord, due to differences in coil design and problems caused by cardiac pulsation. T2-weighted imaging may be necessary in the sagittal and axial planes to confirm the presence of lesions. Gradient echo imaging is not satisfactory for detection of MS plaques within the cord, due to the relatively poor T2 contrast inherent in most techniques. Transverse myelitis may be indistinguishable from MS on spinal MRI scans (Fig. 1–16). Differentiation may be possible in certain cases only on clinical grounds.

Although lesions can be demonstrated in the cervical and thoracic cord, cranial MRI is suggested for the first examination in patients with isolated spinal cord symptoms.[33] MRI technique is more sensitive to intracranial lesions. The demonstration of characteristic periventricular plaques can confirm the diagnosis of MS, while spinal imaging may reveal only one or two nonspecific lesions.

Optic Neuritis

MRI is valuable for the study and follow-up of patients with optic neuritis.[34] Disseminated demyelinated areas can be observed in a pattern similar to that seen with MS.[35,36] The frequency with which patients with isolated optic neuritis subsequently develop MS is controversial.[37] Pediatric studies have demonstrated diffuse disease in optic neuritis, but MS can begin in childhood, making differentiation difficult.[38] The actual demonstration of optic nerve lesions can be difficult on MRI scans. Results have been most promising using STIR, with abnormalities demonstrated in 84% of symptomatic nerves.[39] Despite refined imaging techniques, visual evoked potentials remain more sensitive than MRI for detecting optic nerve lesions in optic neuritis.

(text continues on page 17)

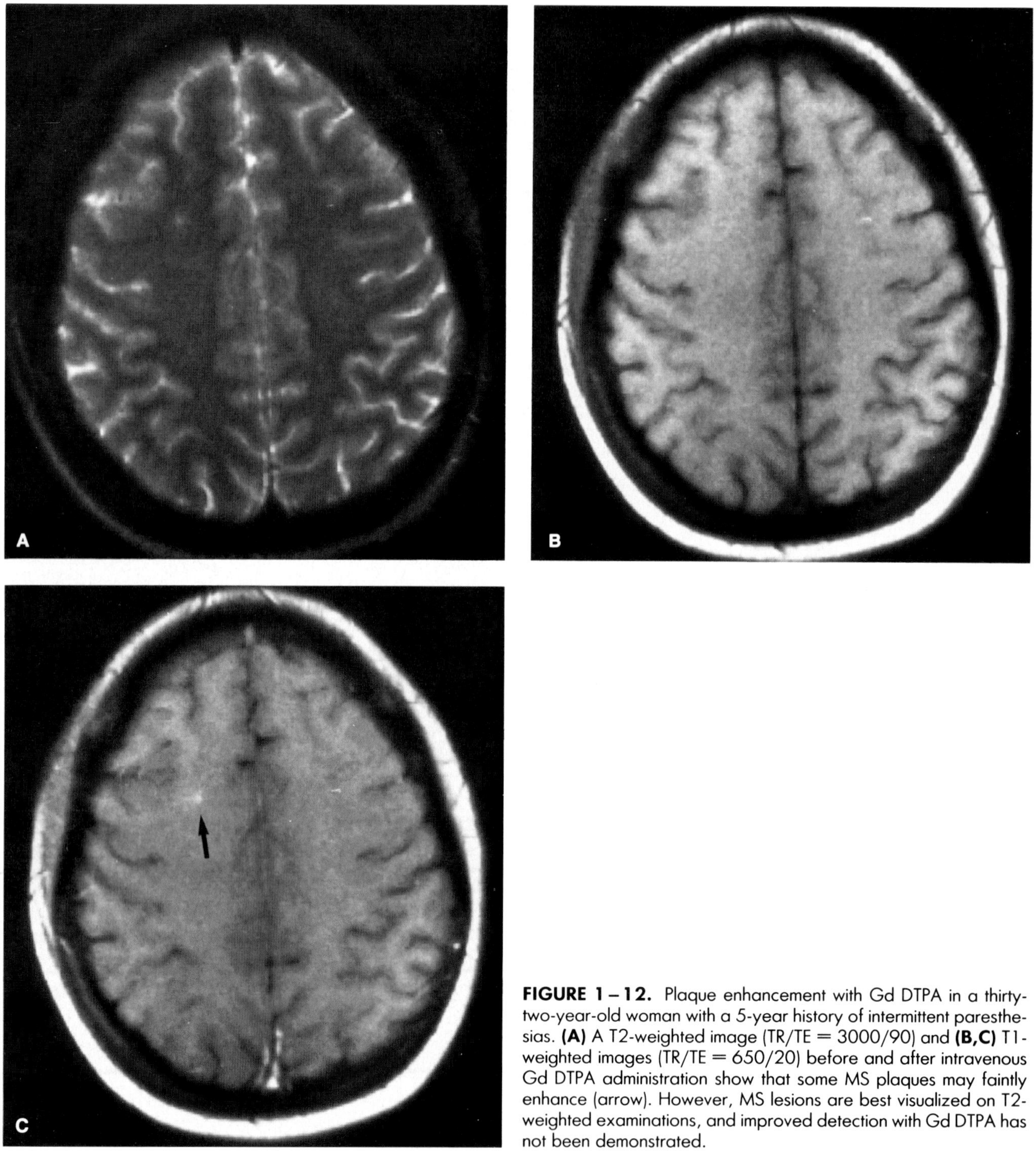

FIGURE 1–12. Plaque enhancement with Gd DTPA in a thirty-two-year-old woman with a 5-year history of intermittent paresthesias. **(A)** A T2-weighted image (TR/TE = 3000/90) and **(B,C)** T1-weighted images (TR/TE = 650/20) before and after intravenous Gd DTPA administration show that some MS plaques may faintly enhance (arrow). However, MS lesions are best visualized on T2-weighted examinations, and improved detection with Gd DTPA has not been demonstrated.

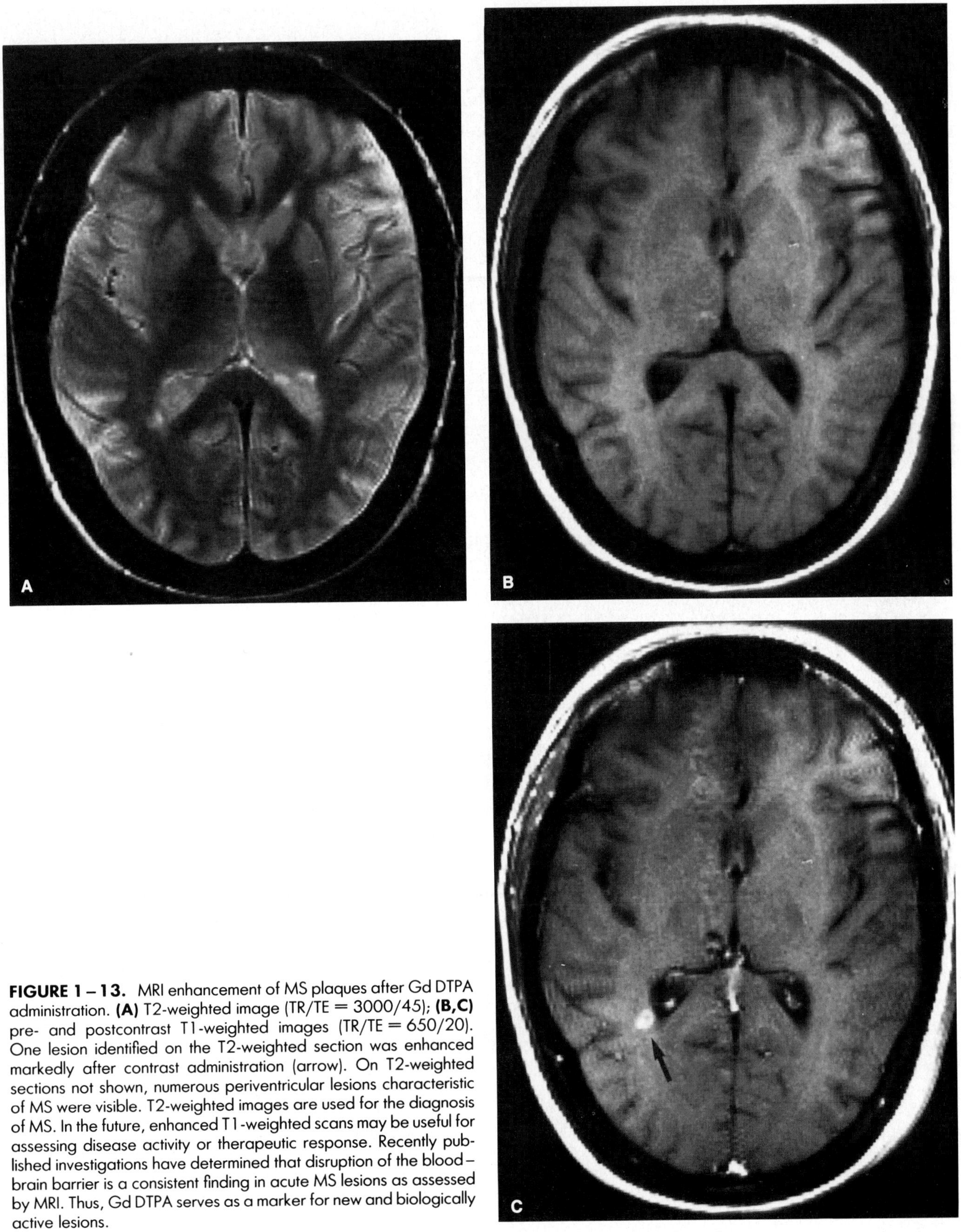

FIGURE 1 – 13. MRI enhancement of MS plaques after Gd DTPA administration. **(A)** T2-weighted image (TR/TE = 3000/45); **(B,C)** pre- and postcontrast T1-weighted images (TR/TE = 650/20). One lesion identified on the T2-weighted section was enhanced markedly after contrast administration (arrow). On T2-weighted sections not shown, numerous periventricular lesions characteristic of MS were visible. T2-weighted images are used for the diagnosis of MS. In the future, enhanced T1-weighted scans may be useful for assessing disease activity or therapeutic response. Recently published investigations have determined that disruption of the blood–brain barrier is a consistent finding in acute MS lesions as assessed by MRI. Thus, Gd DTPA serves as a marker for new and biologically active lesions.

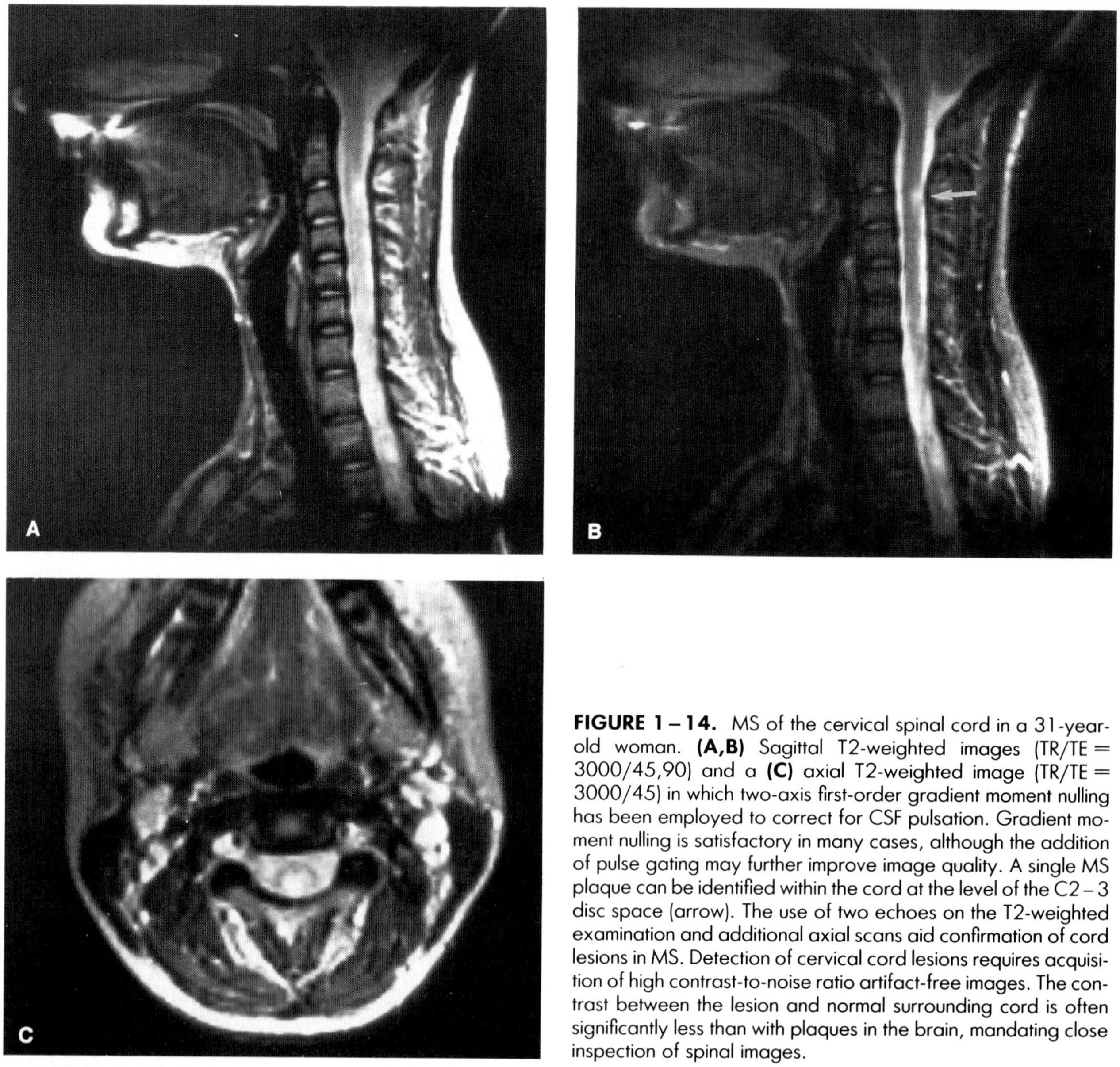

FIGURE 1–14. MS of the cervical spinal cord in a 31-year-old woman. **(A,B)** Sagittal T2-weighted images (TR/TE = 3000/45,90) and a **(C)** axial T2-weighted image (TR/TE = 3000/45) in which two-axis first-order gradient moment nulling has been employed to correct for CSF pulsation. Gradient moment nulling is satisfactory in many cases, although the addition of pulse gating may further improve image quality. A single MS plaque can be identified within the cord at the level of the C2–3 disc space (arrow). The use of two echoes on the T2-weighted examination and additional axial scans aid confirmation of cord lesions in MS. Detection of cervical cord lesions requires acquisition of high contrast-to-noise ratio artifact-free images. The contrast between the lesion and normal surrounding cord is often significantly less than with plaques in the brain, mandating close inspection of spinal images.

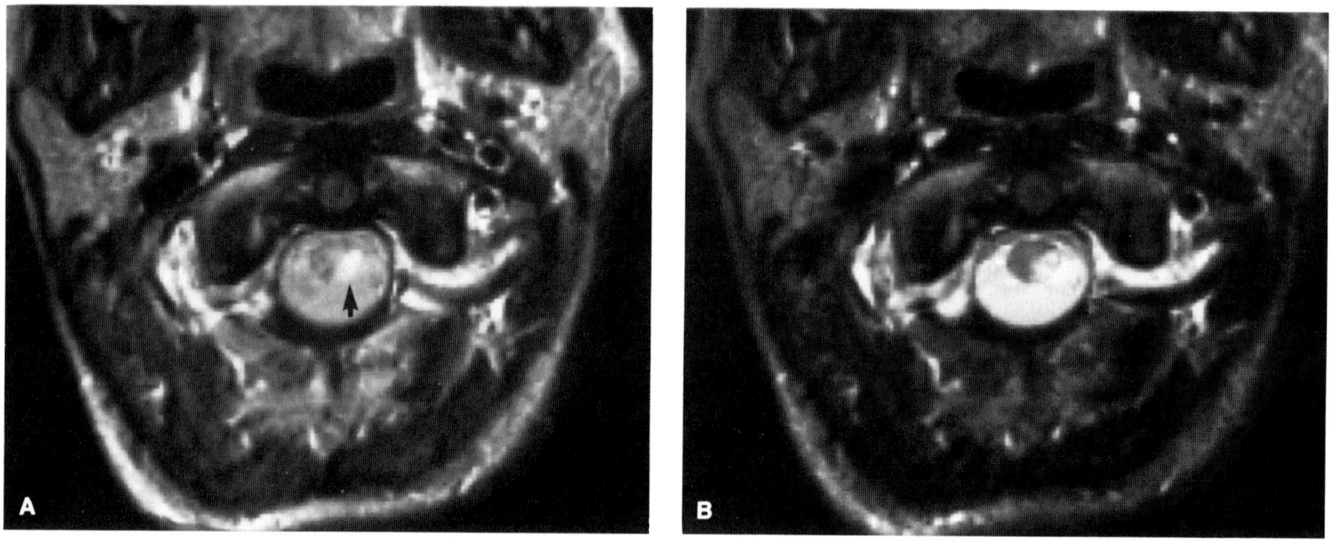

FIGURE 1–15. **(A,B)** T2-weighted images (TR/TE = 3000/45,90) are used to identify an MS plaque in the left side of the spinal cord at the level of C1 (arrow).

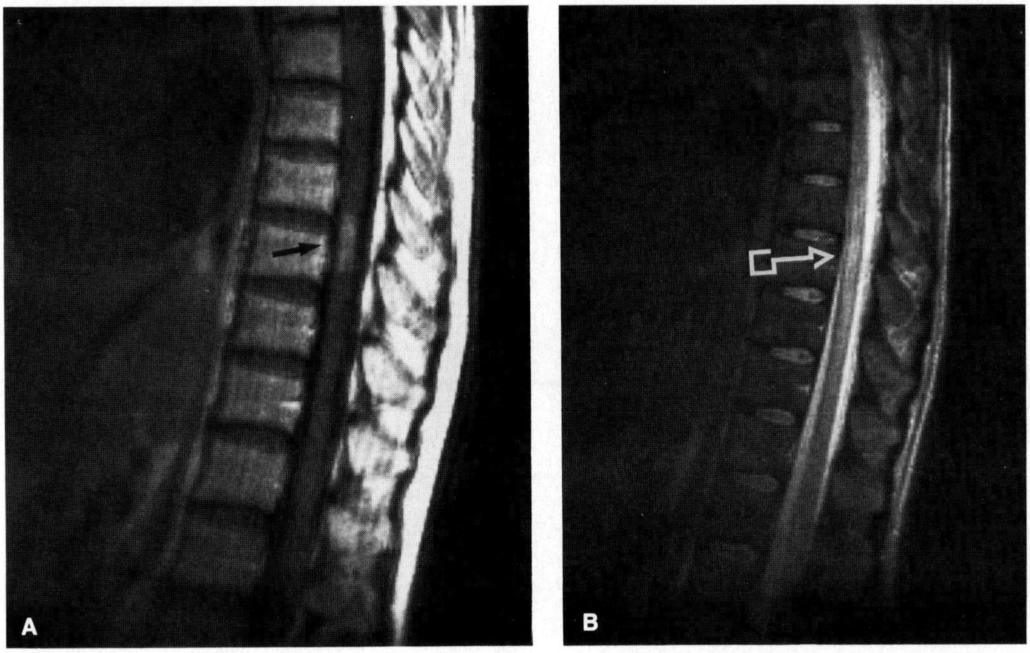

FIGURE 1 – 16. Transverse myelitis (presumptive diagnosis) in a 39-year-old white woman, who had mid-back pain, right leg weakness, and left leg numbness. Postmyelographic CT of the thoracic spine and cranial MRI findings were within normal limits. **(A)** Gd DTPA-enhanced T1-weighted image (TR/TE = 450/20) and **(B)** motion-compensated T2-weighted image (TR/TE = 3000/90) show an enhanced lesion in the cord at T9 (closed arrow) and high signal intensity (open arrow), presumably representing edema. There is no cord deformity. With the advent of surface coils, cord lesions in multiple sclerosis and transverse myelitis can be readily identified.

DIFFERENTIAL DIAGNOSIS

There are many pitfalls in the MRI diagnosis of MS.[40] Differentiation from other clinically diverse entities that mimic MS on MRI scans depends on pattern recognition and clinical history.

Dilated Perivascular Spaces

Dilated perivascular spaces can be a normal finding on MRI (Fig. 1–17). It is important to distinguish this common variant from other pathologic entities, such as lacunar infarction, that carry more serious clinical implications. Dilated perivascular spaces (Virchow-Robin spaces) are isointense compared with CSF on all pulse sequences.[41] In general, these are smaller than lacunar infarcts. They are commonly located in the basal ganglia adjacent to the anterior commissure and in the supraventricular white matter.

Deep White Matter Ischemia

Patchy white matter lesions, common in the elderly patient, must be differentiated from MS (Figs. 1–18 and 1–19).[42–45] These periventricular abnormalities, commonly noted in patients with cerebrovascular disease, are often symmetric with smooth margins, allowing differentiation from MS.[8] Three studies have been performed with postmortem specimens to establish the cause of these lesions.[46–48] Patchy white matter lesions occurred in 20 to 30% of elderly patients in good general medical health. In these patients, areas

(text continues on page 20)

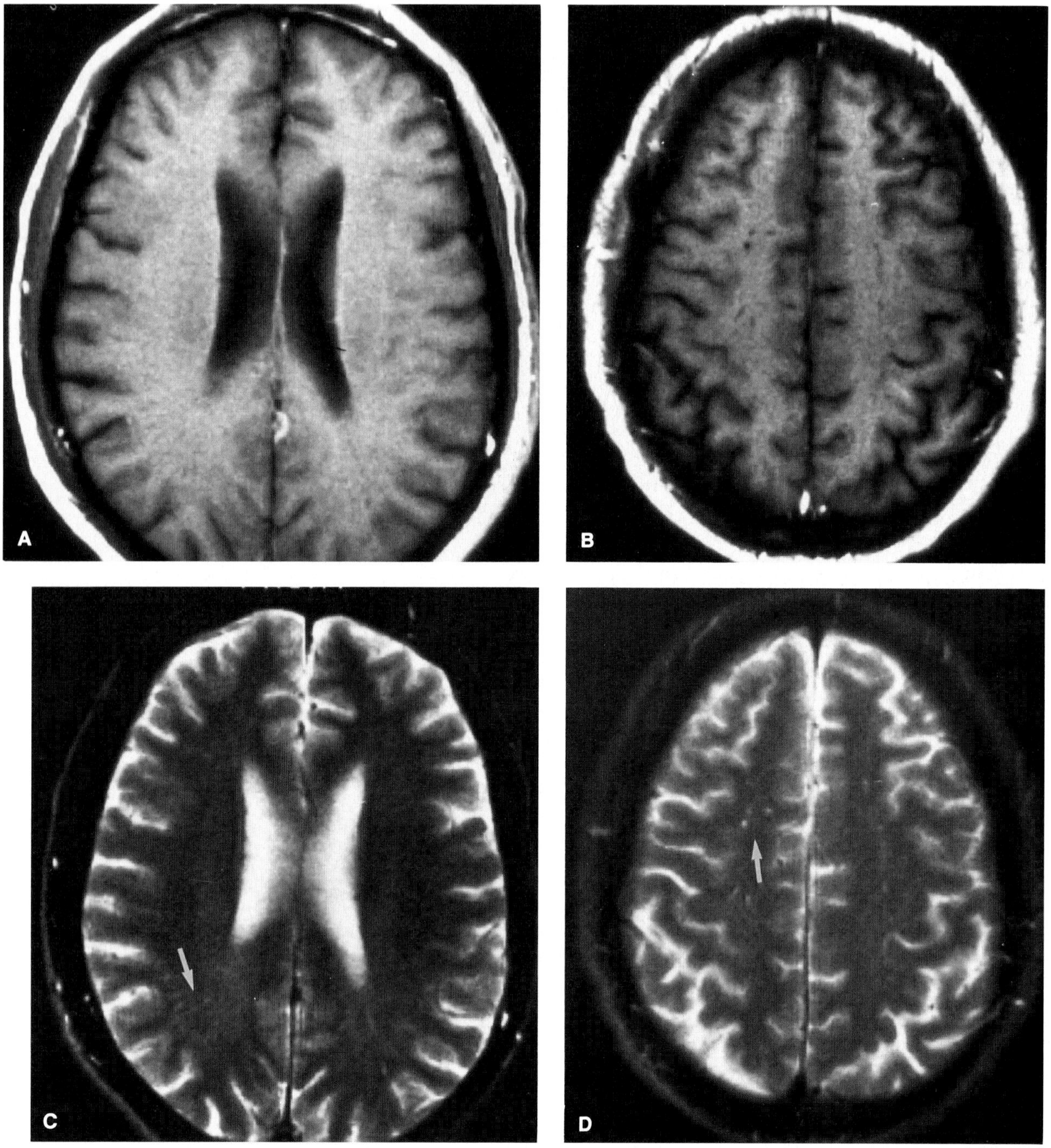

FIGURE 1–17. Dilated perivascular spaces (arrows) in a 57-year-old man. Sections are presented at two anatomic levels: **(A,B)** T1 weighted (TR/TE = 650/20) and **(C,D)** T2 weighted (TR/TE = 3000/90). Differentiation can be made from ischemic disease on the basis of anatomic appearance and location. Dilated perivascular spaces are considered to be a normal variant.

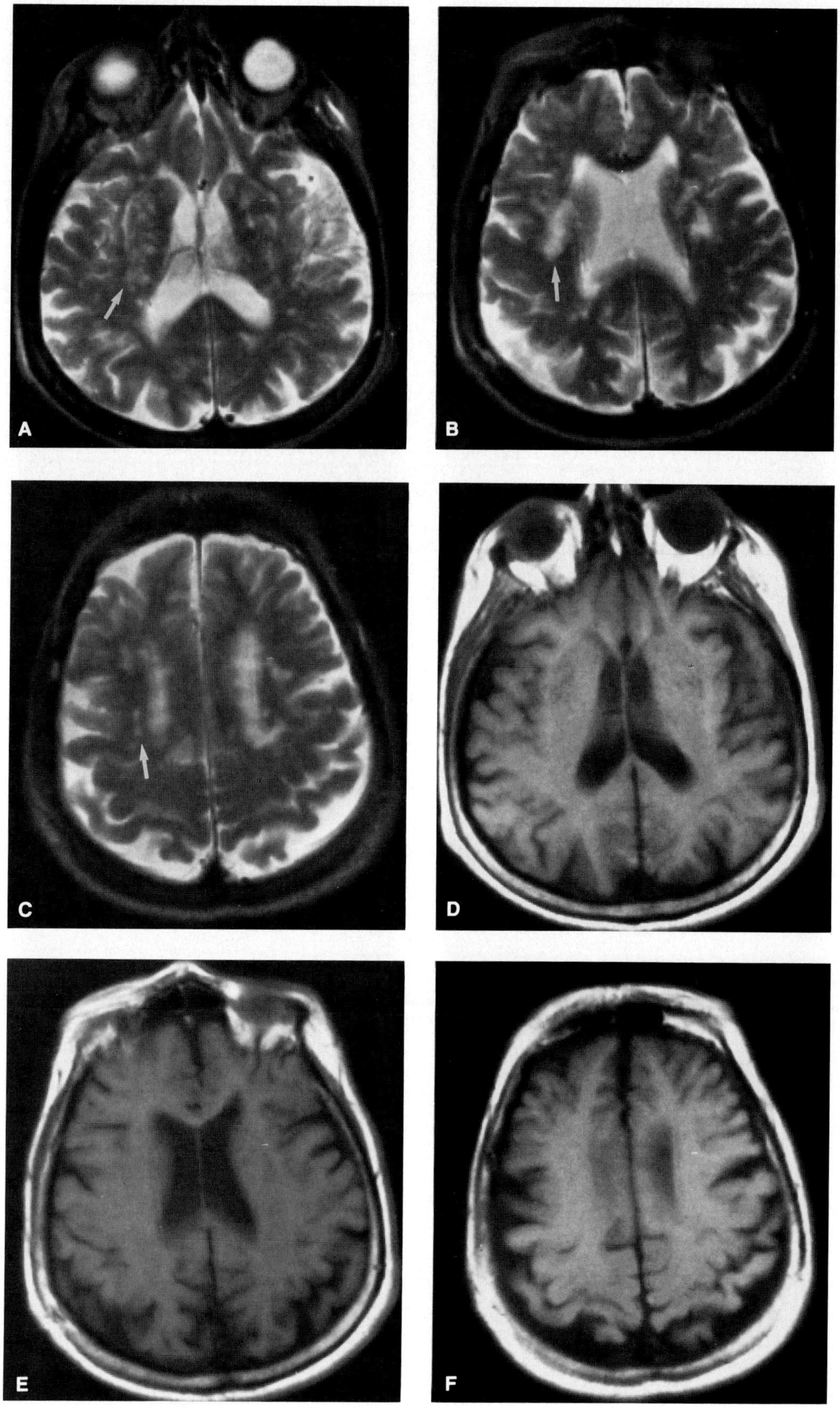

FIGURE 1–18. Deep white matter ischemia in an 80-year-old woman at three anatomic levels is depicted with **(A–C)** heavy T2 weighting and **(D–F)** T1 weighting. Pathologic studies conclude that gliosis, demyelination, or frank infarction, presumably on the basis of chronic vascular insufficiency, account for the majority of white matter lesions seen on MRI scans in elderly patients. These (arrows) are best depicted on T2-weighted scans. Periventricular lesions are best depicted with intermediate T2 weighting. In such scans, lesions appear as high-intensity signals, contrasting well with the isointense signal of adjacent CSF. Symmetry of disease and involvement of more peripheral white matter are characteristic for vascular disease and must be differentiated from multiple sclerosis, which typically is asymmetric and displays lesions more closely confined to the immediate periventricular area.

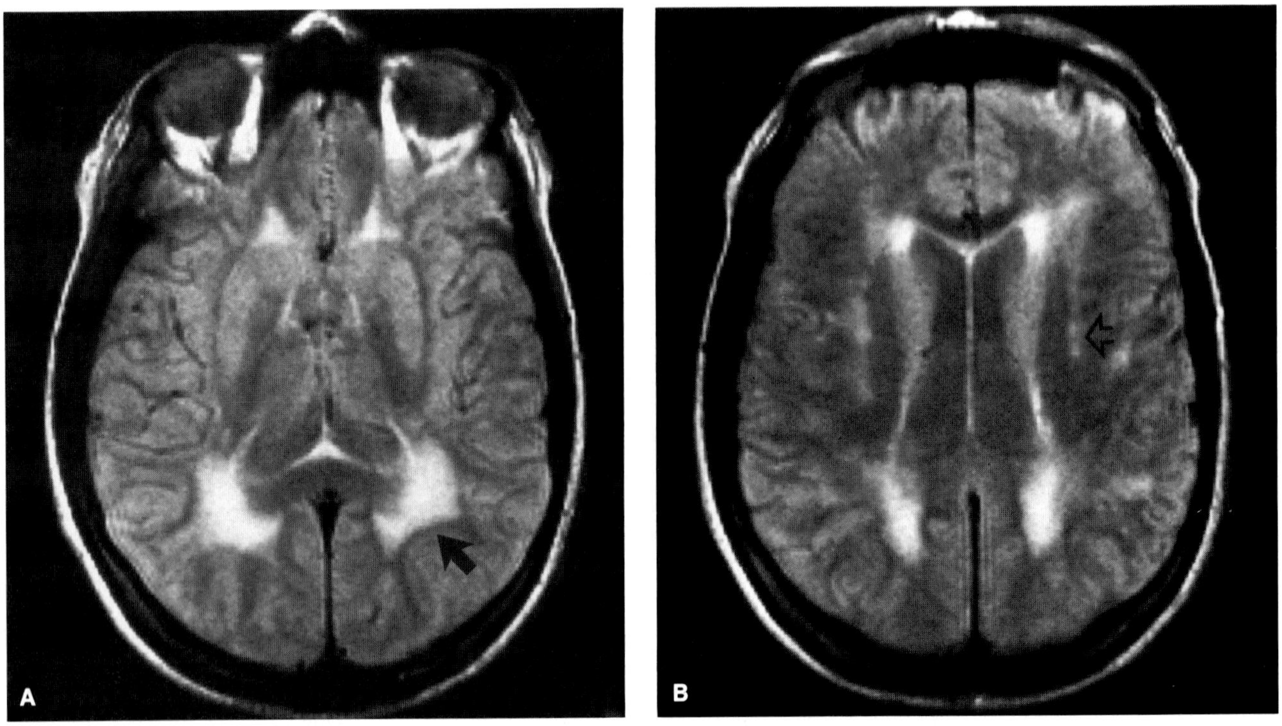

FIGURE 1–19. Deep white matter ischemia is shown by **(A,B)** proton density weighting (TR/TE = 3000/28) at two anatomic levels. The pattern and distribution of the white matter abnormality is different from that encountered in MS. Confluent symmetric abnormalities, commonly seen in the peri-atrial area (open arrow), and more peripheral white matter involvement (closed arrow) are characteristic.

of gliosis and demyelination were presumably caused by chronic vascular insufficiency. Larger lesions may demonstrate necrosis, axonal loss, and demyelination, therefore representing true infarcts. These lesions and those of frank infarction account for the majority of white matter lesions seen on MRI scans in the elderly population.[49] CT examination may fail to reveal these lesions. Focal gliosis and encephalomalacia commonly surround ventricular shunts (Fig. 1–20) and are unrelated to the patchy white matter lesions of the elderly.

Periventricular Leukomalacia

Periventricular leukomalacia (PVL) in the infant can resemble the pattern of deep white matter ischemia in the elderly (Fig. 1–21). Age and clinical history clearly differentiate these two populations. Although neurosonography is used for evaluation of the neonate, the sensitivity of this modality is low in mild or moderate disease. Follow-up MRI in symptomatic infants can confirm the diagnosis of PVL in spite of a negative neonatal ultrasound examination.

Leukodystrophies

Dysmyelinating diseases can be identified and differentiated on MRI scans from MS and ischemic disease in the elderly (Table 1–3). Dysmyelinating diseases, which include the leukodystrophies, are presumed to be genetically determined (causing defective myelin) and appear early in life. MRI is extremely sensitive to white matter disease, anticipating its use in detecting and evaluating the extent of disease in the leukodystrophies. Enhancement with Gd DTPA provides definition of areas of active demyelination on the basis of focal blood-brain barrier disruption.

Adrenoleukodystrophy (Fig. 1–22) can be easily differentiated from MS by the confluent involvement of specific white matter tracts. Auditory and visual pathway involvement is characteristic. Lesions are more clearly identified and delineated by MRI (i.e., better demarcation between abnormal and normal white matter) than by CT. MRI can also identify subcortical white matter abnormalities.

In more clinically severe disease (Fig. 1–23), white matter can be diffusely involved. The precise reason

(text continues on page 24)

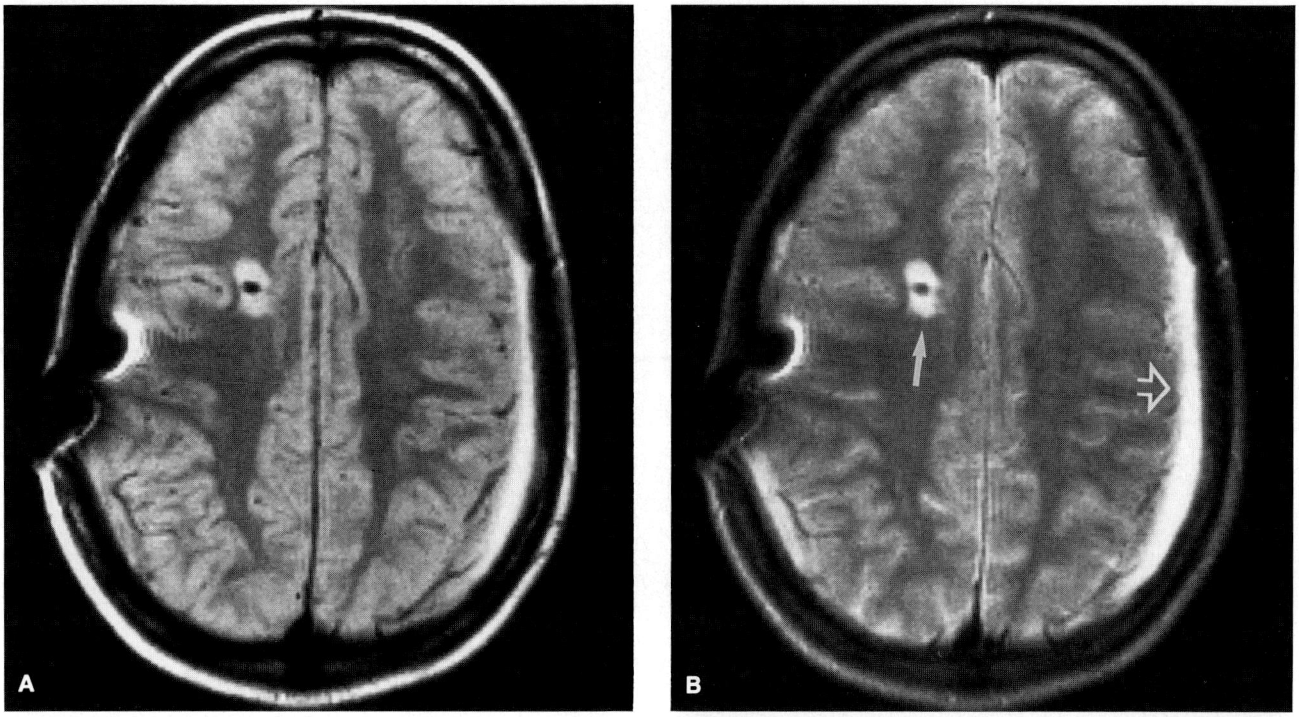

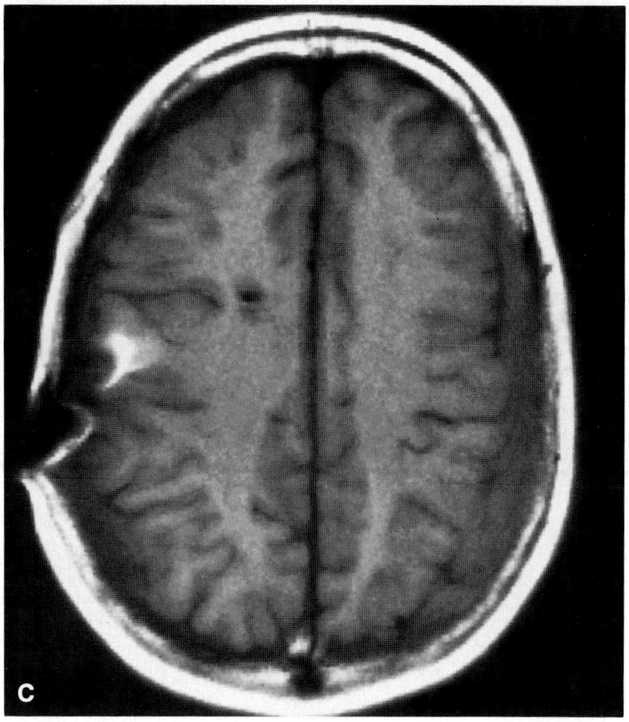

FIGURE 1–20. Leukomalacia (closed arrow) surrounding a ventricular shunt placed for obstructive hydrocephalus is shown in **(A,B)** T2-weighted scans (TR/TE = 3000/28,70) and a **(C)** T1-weighted scan (TR/TE = 600/17). There is also a left-sided subdural fluid collection (open arrow).

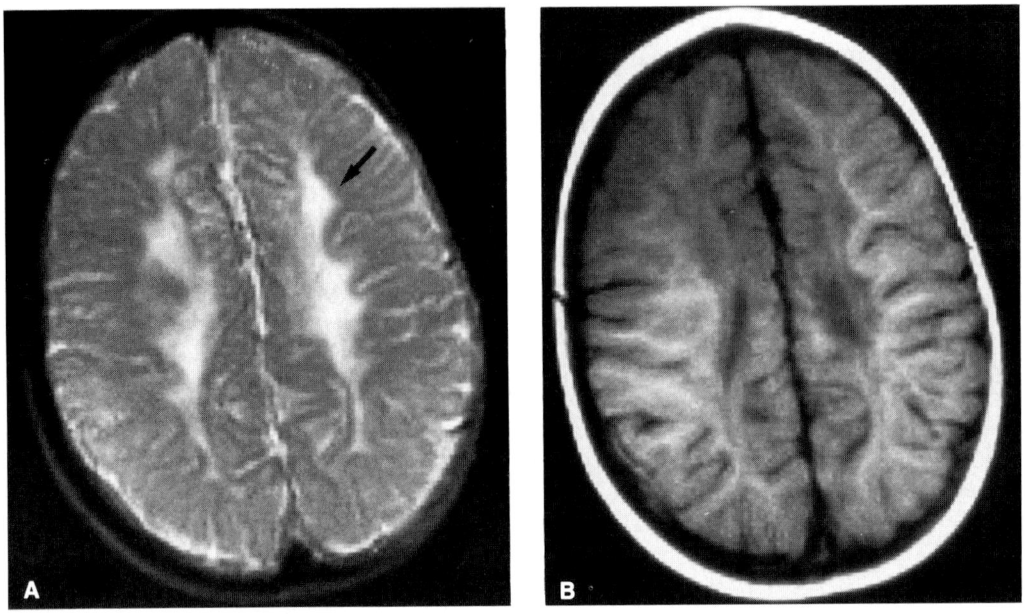

FIGURE 1 – 21. Periventricular leukomalacia in a 15-month-old infant is shown in a **(A)** T2-weighted image (TR/TE = 3000/90) and **(B)** T1-weighted image (TR/TE = 650/20). There is periventricular high signal intensity on the T2-weighted scan, corresponding to low signal intensity on the T1-weighted scan, which is most prominent anteriorly (arrow). In end-stage periventricular leukomalacia, the most common finding is abnormal signal intensity in the peri-atrial regions. Poor clinical outcome is correlated with lesions involving all four cerebral lobes, delay in myelination, and cortical atrophy.

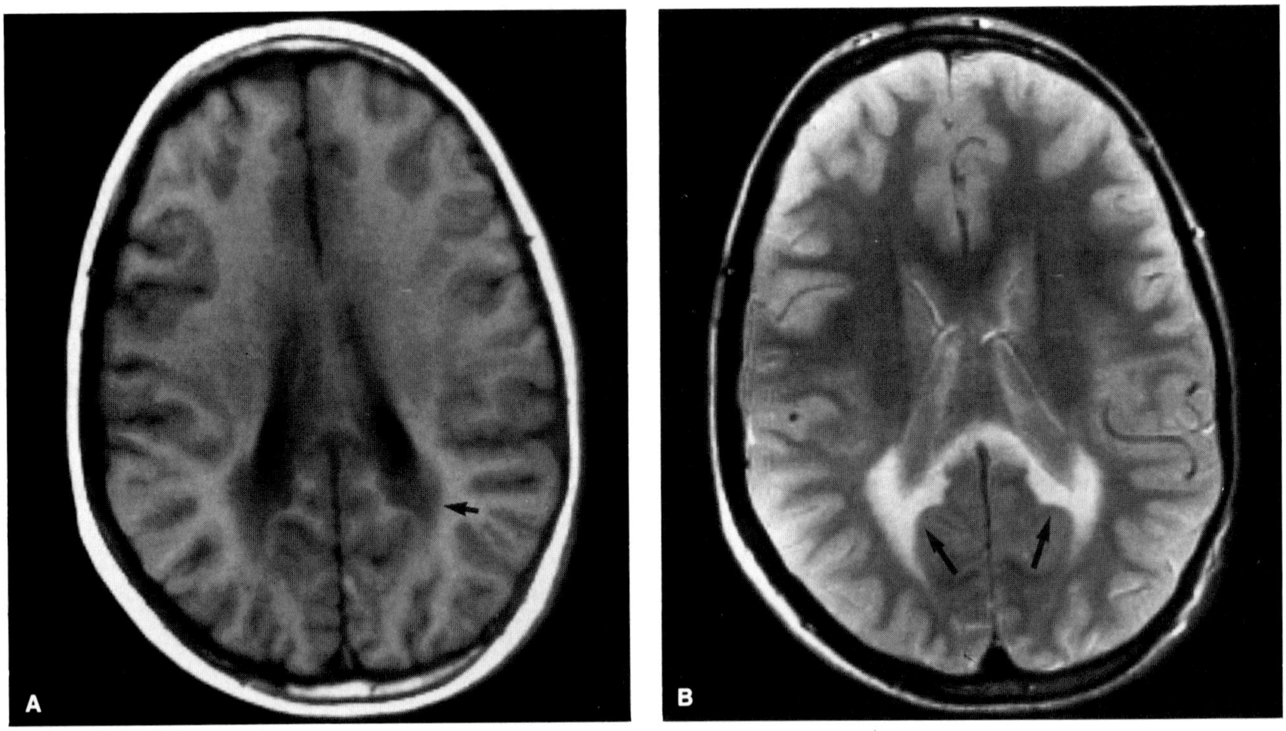

FIGURE 1 – 22. Adrenoleukodystrophy (X-linked) in a 12-year-old boy with Addison's disease is demonstrated by **(A)** T1-weighted (TR/TE = 650/20) and **(B)** T2-weighted (TR/TE = 3000/90) spin echo techniques. Involvement of the splenium of the corpus callosum and the parieto-occipital white matter is visualized as abnormal high signal intensity on a T2-weighted scan and as low signal intensity on a T1-weighted scan (arrows). MRI is exquisitely sensitive to white matter disease in adrenoleukodystrophy. No enhancement occurred with IV Gd DTPA administration. Contrast enhancement is necessary to depict disease activity.

Table 1 – 3 **Dysmyelinating Diseases**

DISEASE*	ETIOLOGY	INVOLVED REGIONS	AGE	SEX
Adrenoleukodystrophy				
X-linked	Peroxisomal disorder, impaired capacity to degrade VLCFA† due to deficient beta-oxidation of VLCFA	Centrum semiovale, parieto-occipital white matter, posterior corpus callosum, fornix, posterior limbs of internal capsule	Child	M (X-linked)
Neonatal	Reduced number and size of peroxisomes, impaired synthesis of ether phospholipids, reduced activity of dihydroxyacetone phosphate acyltransferase, elevated levels of pipecolic acid, accumulation of bile intermediates, decreased activity of phytanic acid oxidase	Peri-Sylvian and adjacent fronto-parietal convexity, olivary nuclei and cerebellum; also abnormalities in neuronal migration	Infant	M/F (recessive)
Metachromatic leukodystrophy	Aryl-sulfatase A deficiency causing sulfatide storage	Diffuse cerebral and cerebellar white matter (nonadult type)	Type I 6 – 24 months Type II 4 – 8 years Type III ≥ 15 years Type IV 6 – 18 months	M/F (recessive)
Krabbe	Defective galactosylceramidase	Caudate, thalami, corona radiata, brainstem, and cerebellum	Type I infant Type II 1 – 3 years Type III adult	M/F (recessive)
Pelizaeus-Merzbacher	Defective synthesis of proteolipid proteins	Bilateral diffuse white matter loss	Type I infancy & early childhood Type II neonatal & early infancy	M (X-linked) M/F (recessive)
Canavan	Deficiency of aspartoacylase causing N-acetylaspartic aciduria	Bilateral cerebral white matter	Infantile — 1st few months of life; juvenile — after 5 years	M/F (recessive)
Alexander	No enzymatic or biochemical defect found to date	Periventricular frontal regions, caudate, thalami	Infantile — 6 months; juvenile — 7 – 14 years	(sporadic)
Leigh	Pyruvate dehydrogenase complex, NADH-CoQ reductase, and cytochrome-c oxidase deficiencies	Putamen, thalamus, cerebellum	Infant	(recessive)

* Diseases listed in decreasing order of incidence.
† VLCFA: very long chain fatty acid.

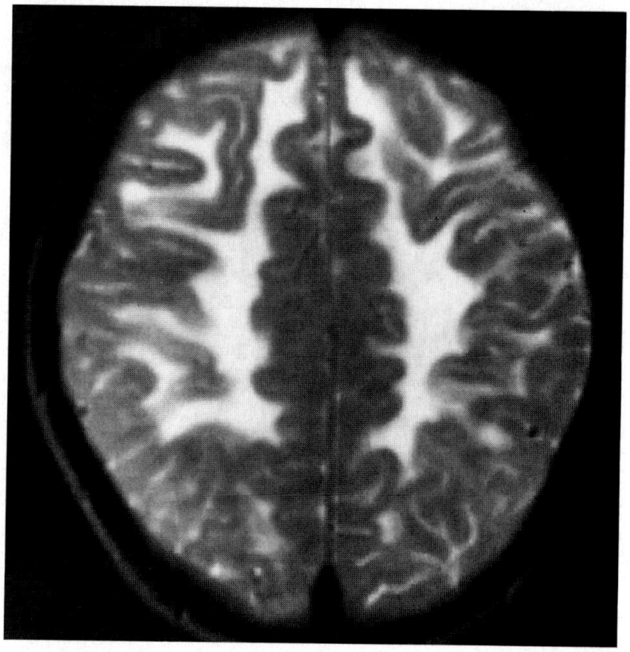

FIGURE 1 – 23. Unexplained, progressive leukodystrophy in an 8-year-old girl. Enzyme studies were negative for metachromatic leukodystrophy and Canavan's disease. The T2-weighted image (TR/TE = 3000/90) shows diffusely abnormal supraventricular white matter.

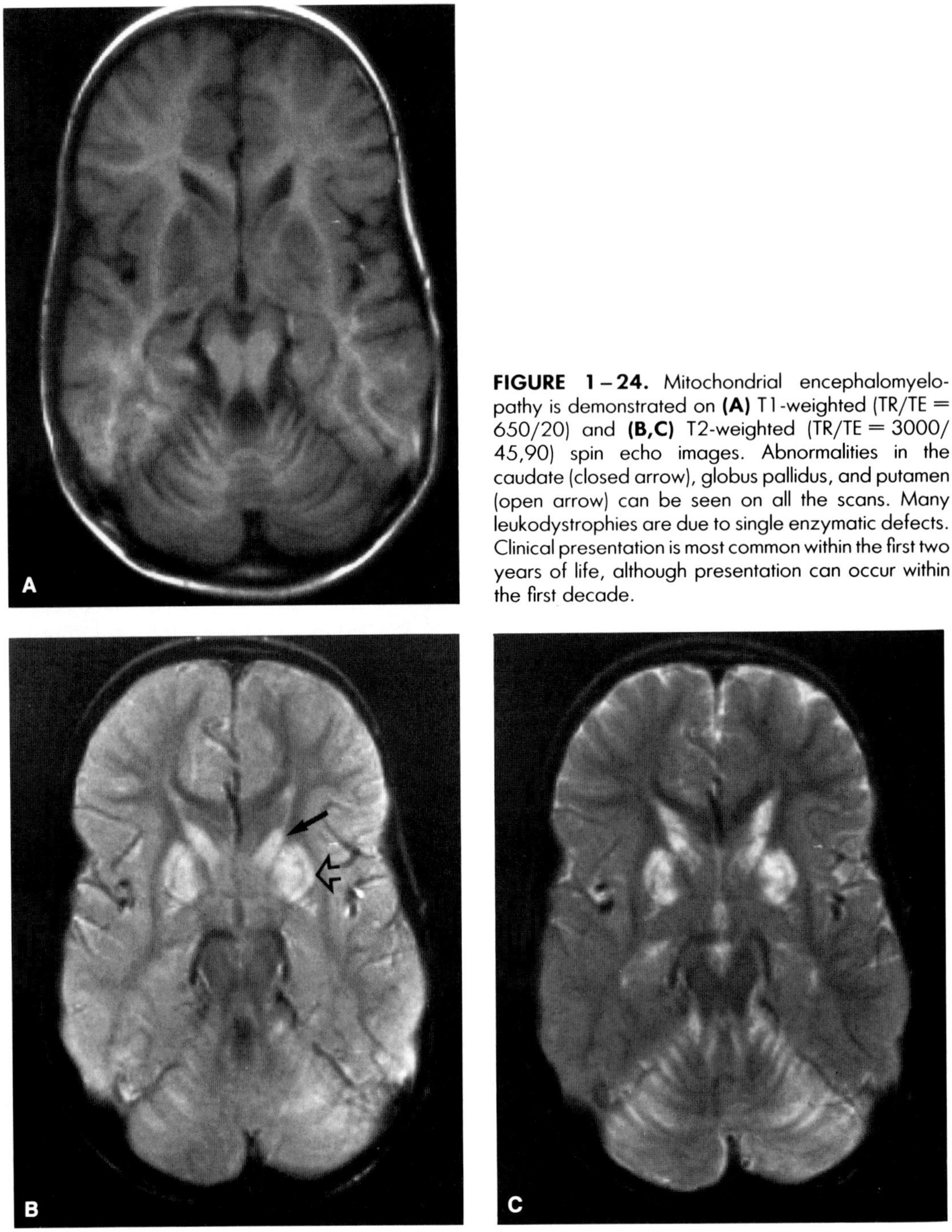

FIGURE 1–24. Mitochondrial encephalomyelopathy is demonstrated on **(A)** T1-weighted (TR/TE = 650/20) and **(B,C)** T2-weighted (TR/TE = 3000/45,90) spin echo images. Abnormalities in the caudate (closed arrow), globus pallidus, and putamen (open arrow) can be seen on all the scans. Many leukodystrophies are due to single enzymatic defects. Clinical presentation is most common within the first two years of life, although presentation can occur within the first decade.

for prolongation of T1 and T2 on a cellular level is not known, although white matter edema contributes to the appearance. Leigh's disease and related entities are characterized by involvement of the basal ganglia (Fig. 1–24).

Hypoxemia

The white matter diseases discussed previously should not be confused with ischemia due to hypoperfusion or anoxia (Fig. 1–25). Hypoxemia from near-drowning, cardiorespiratory arrest, and other causes can produce irreversible brain damage. Deep white matter, cortical gray matter, and the basal ganglia are commonly involved.

Systemic Lupus Erythematosus

The sensitivity of MRI for detecting cerebral lesions in systemic lupus erythematosus (SLE) and its superiority to x-ray CT was first demonstrated in 1983.[50] Subsequent studies have confirmed this ability in larger patient populations.[51–53] Patients with SLE demonstrate many patterns of disease involvement, from perivascular microinfarctions to discrete cerebral infarction. Partial or complete resolution of gray matter lesions can be seen on follow-up examinations. The wedge-shaped pattern of lesions in many patients and the significant involvement of gray and white matter enable differentiation from MS (Fig. 1–26). MRI is an important technique for detecting the extent of cere-

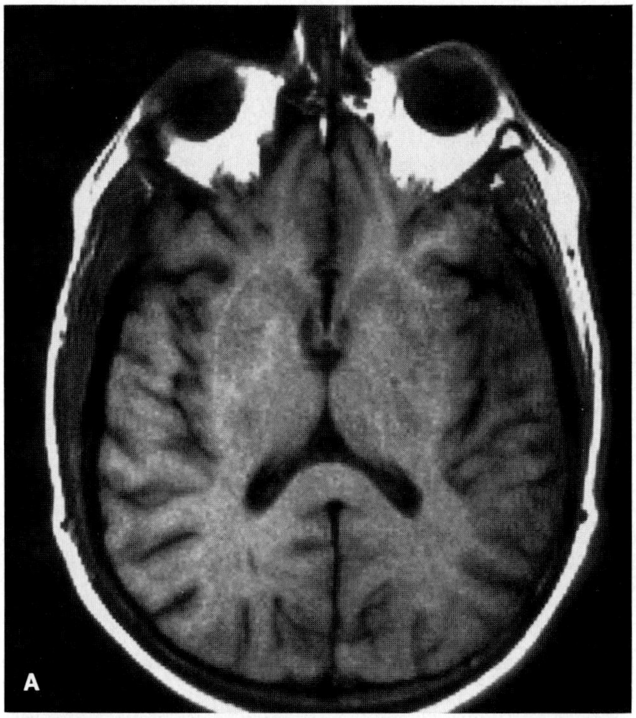

FIGURE 1 – 25. Bilateral caudate and lentiform nucleus infarction secondary to severe anoxia occurred in a patient who was resuscitated after an episode of hypoxia due to aspiration. **(A)** T1-weighted (TR/TE = 650/20) and **(B,C)** T2-weighted (TR/TE = 3000/45,90) spin echo images. Without a contrast agent, ischemia is best appreciated on T2-weighted studies. Both anoxia and hypoperfusion can produce irreversible brain damage, with the basal ganglia, cortex, and deep white matter predominantly involved.

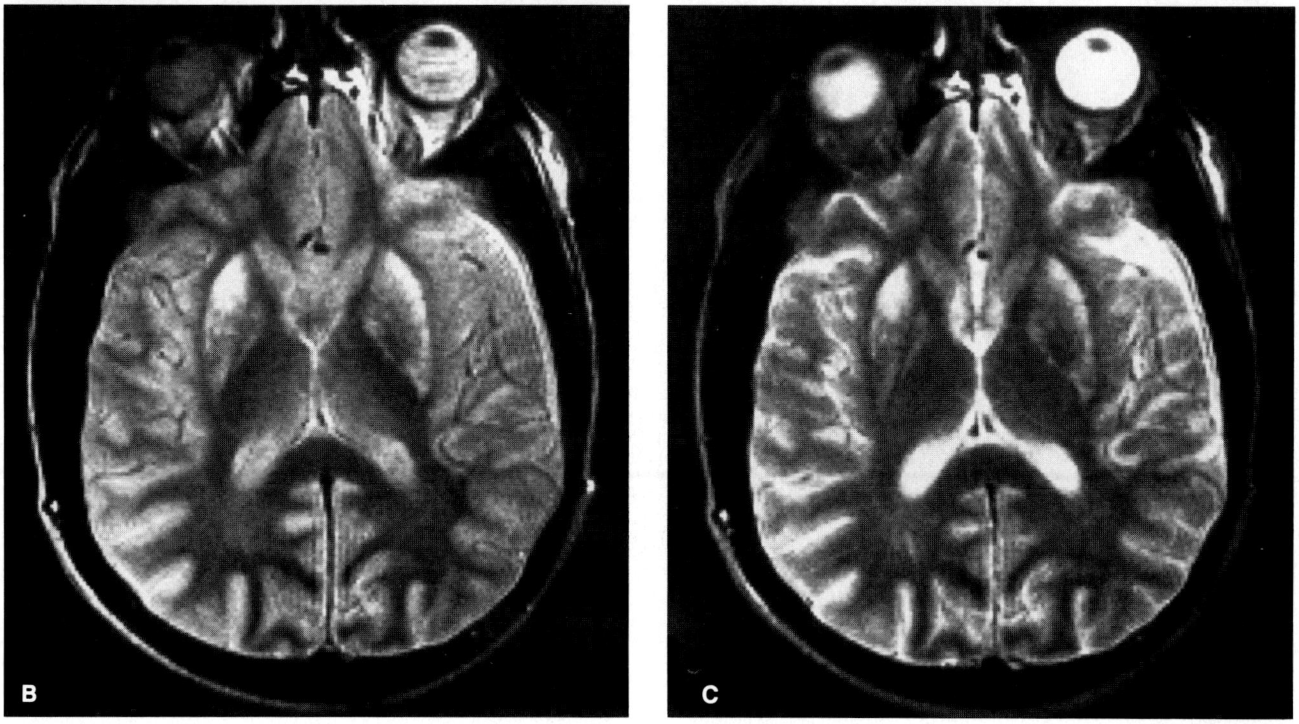

bral injury in SLE. These lesions are often occult on x-ray CT scans.

Normal Variants

In most patients, some degree of periventricular hyperintensity can be recognized on MRI scans.[54] A very fine line of high signal intensity adjacent to the ventricular system, often most prominent near the frontal horns, should be considered a normal finding and not indicative of demyelinating disease or hydrocephalus, but this pattern must be distinguished from that seen with transependymal flow in obstructive hydrocephalus.

Radiation Injury

Symmetric periventricular white matter lesions are a typical finding in radiation injury to the brain (Fig. 1 – 27). MRI evidence of injury is more likely to be seen

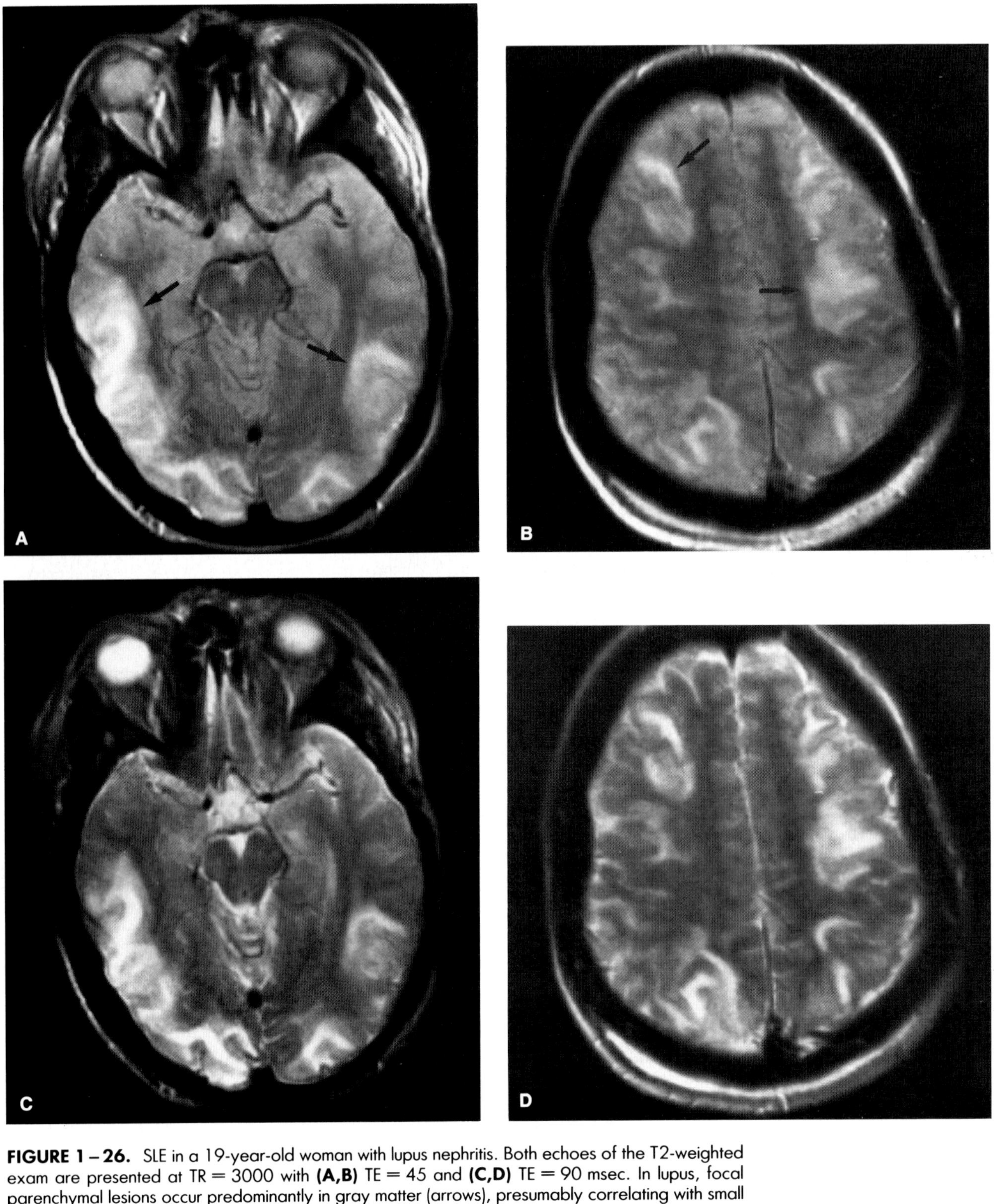

FIGURE 1–26. SLE in a 19-year-old woman with lupus nephritis. Both echoes of the T2-weighted exam are presented at TR = 3000 with **(A,B)** TE = 45 and **(C,D)** TE = 90 msec. In lupus, focal parenchymal lesions occur predominantly in gray matter (arrows), presumably correlating with small vessel disease. Two other patterns can be observed, discrete cerebral infarction and multiple small areas of high signal intensity (on T2-weighted scans). The latter pattern is presumed to be caused by microinfarctions.

in older patients or in those receiving combined radiation and chemotherapy. The injury of white matter by radiation consists of demyelination, edema, and fibrillary gliosis. The pattern may be focal, if radiation is restricted to a port, or diffuse. In the diffuse pattern of disease, involvement of the white matter may abut cortical gray matter. The corpus callosum is usually spared. Diffuse white matter disease is also caused by inhalation of organic solvents (Fig. 1–28). Although experience is limited, uniform involvement of both central and peripheral white matter is more characteristic of radiation injury. MRI demonstrates high

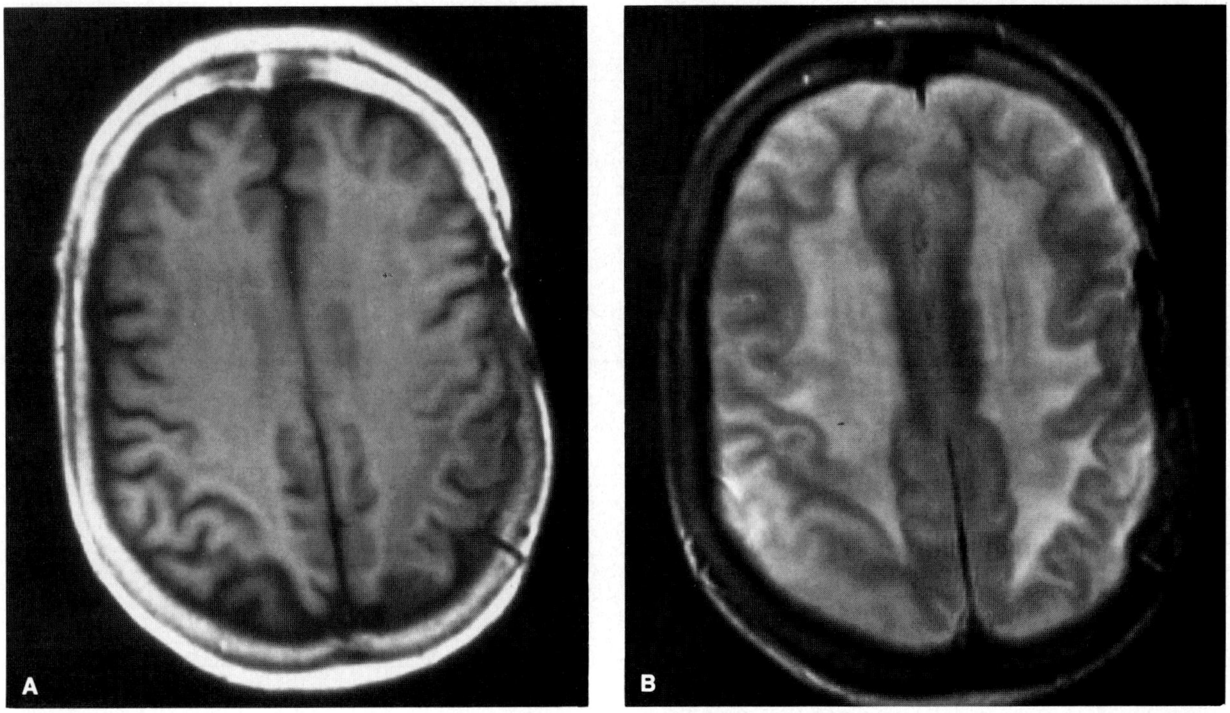

FIGURE 1 – 27. Radiation injury to the brain of a 68-year-old woman. Resection of a left temporal glioma, followed by radiation therapy, occurred 3 years before MRI, and aphasia developed 1 year before the examination. In **(A)** T1-weighted and **(B)** T2-weighted spin echo images, the supraventricular white matter is diffusely abnormal. A uniform high signal intensity is seen on the T2-weighted scan, but this abnormality is easily missed on the T1-weighted spin echo image. High-dose whole brain irradiation can lead to demyelination without necrosis, as in this case. Enhancement with Gd DTPA can occur in areas of radiation-induced necrosis.

sensitivity to radiation-induced changes, but low specificity. Examination of a model of brain radiation injury in cats demonstrated that the high signal intensity seen on T2-weighted images represented areas of edema and demyelination without necrosis.[55,56] Enhancement with Gd DTPA on T1-weighted images was found in areas of radiation-induced necrosis and Wallerian degeneration.

Patient studies confirm that radiation-related lesions are characterized by symmetric, diffuse high signal intensity in the periventricular white matter.[57,58] The neuropathologic consequences of therapeutic radiation include demyelination, microvascular occlusion, and disruption of the blood-brain barrier. CT is relatively insensitive for detecting radiation damage, and visualization of abnormalities is confined primarily to patients with severe disease.[59] Of 41 patients with radiation-induced changes demonstrated on MRI, CT detected abnormal regions in only 14 (35%).[60] Both MRI and CT can demonstrate sulci enlargement and ventriculomegaly.

White matter abnormalities on MRI are more common with higher dosages and radiation to larger volumes. Older patients also have more severe abnormalities after brain irradiation. However, some patients receiving high radiation dosages do not demonstrate white matter changes on MRI scans. In other patients, severe white matter changes may be found that are not expressed clinically. Radiation-induced changes can mask recurrent tumors and other pathologic findings.[61] MRI lacks specificity in discriminating a recurrent brain tumor from radiation-induced necrosis.

The scalloped appearance of radiation injury at the junction of the gray-white matter represents extensive white matter damage involving the more peripheral arcuate fibers. This pattern can be differentiated from transependymal absorption, which does not extend to the gray-white matter junction and demonstrates a sharp, rounded margin (Fig. 1–29).

INFECTION

Infection may reach the intracranial contents by hematogenous spread, direct extension (e.g., from sinusitis), and spread along peripheral nerves (e.g., herpes encephalitis). In parenchymal disease (Fig. 1–30), MRI is valuable for early detection.[62,63] Dystrophic calcification represents the primary finding on x-ray CT in chronic and congenital infections; MRI is relatively insensitive to calcification.

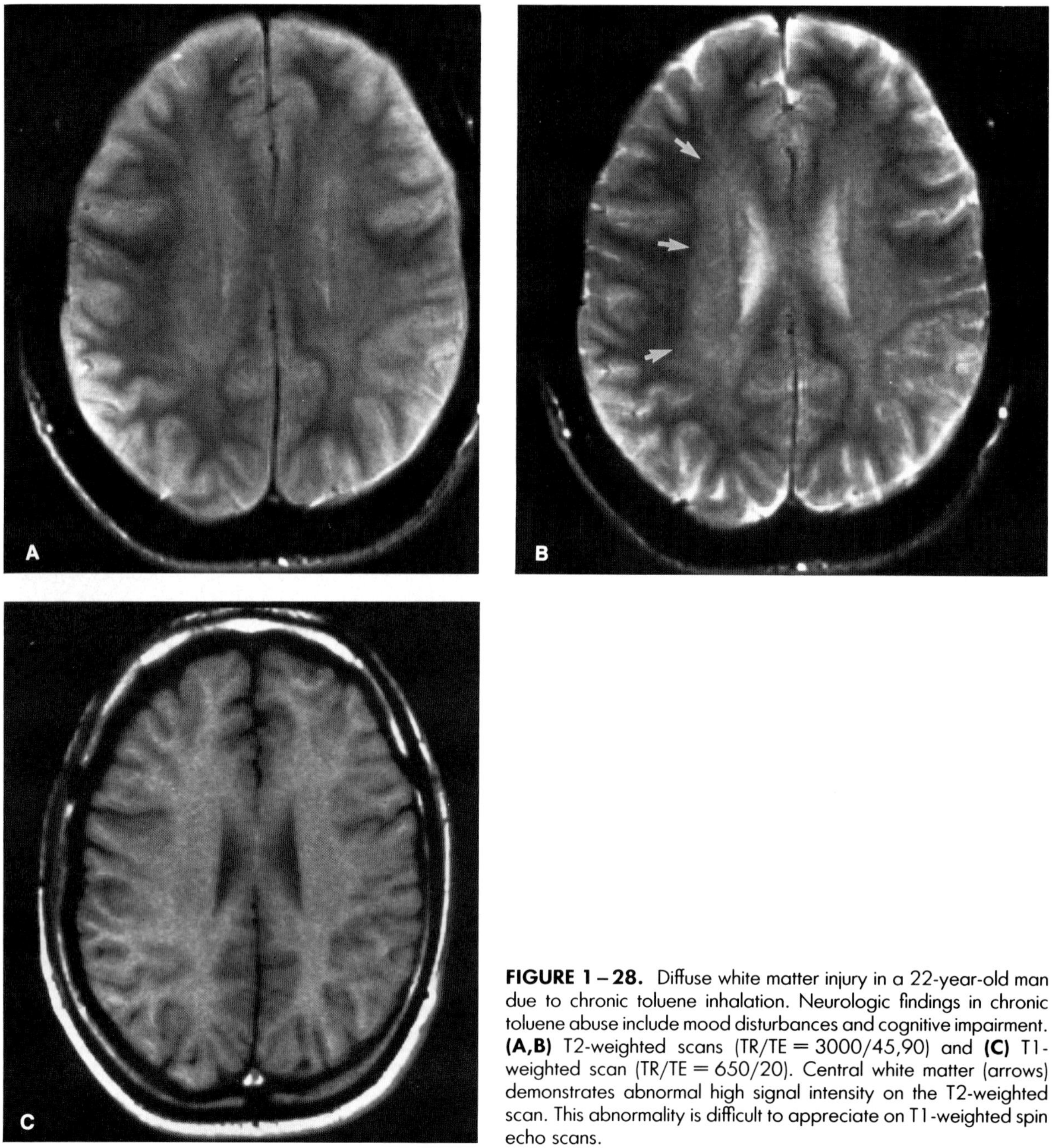

FIGURE 1–28. Diffuse white matter injury in a 22-year-old man due to chronic toluene inhalation. Neurologic findings in chronic toluene abuse include mood disturbances and cognitive impairment. **(A,B)** T2-weighted scans (TR/TE = 3000/45,90) and **(C)** T1-weighted scan (TR/TE = 650/20). Central white matter (arrows) demonstrates abnormal high signal intensity on the T2-weighted scan. This abnormality is difficult to appreciate on T1-weighted spin echo scans.

Parenchymal Disease

Staphylococcus, streptococcus, and more recently toxoplasmosis (in AIDS) are the common organisms responsible for focal parenchymal brain infections. The evolution of brain infection has been carefully studied in both animal and human investigations by CT and MRI.[64] An abscess evolves from a focus of cerebritis to formation of a discrete capsule. Extracellular agents, such as Gd DTPA, enhance contrast due to identification of blood-brain-barrier disruption and permit differentiation of cerebritis and capsule stages. Animal investigations established that contrast-enhanced MRI is superior to unenhanced MRI and enhanced CT for detecting intracranial infection.[64] Subsequent clinical experience confirmed that MRI is superior for early detection of cerebral infection and for more precise delineation of extension.[65] The evolution of intracranial infection, whether treated by antibiotic therapy or neurosurgical drainage, also is well evaluated by MRI.

The most common cause for diffuse parenchymal infection is viral infection (Fig. 1–31). The brain responds to insult with an inflammatory infiltration of

(text continues on page 33)

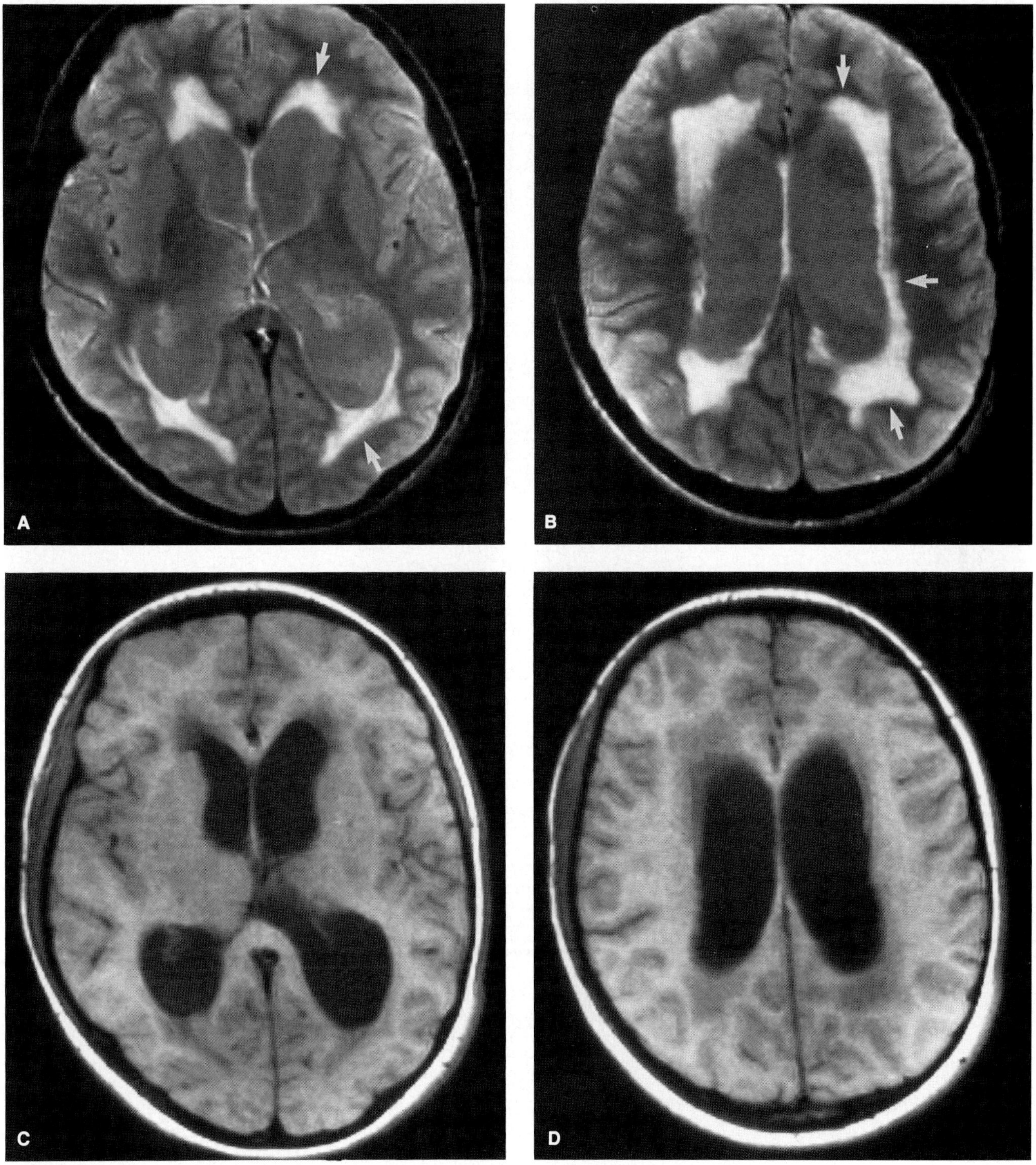

FIGURE 1 – 29. Transependymal resorption of CSF in a 14-year-old patient with a pineal region tumor. **(A,B)** T2-weighted sections (TR/TE = 3000/45) and **(C,D)** T1-weighted sections (TR/TE = 650/20) are presented for two anatomic levels. Transependymal flow (arrows), best seen on T2-weighted images, can be differentiated from other white matter disease by contiguity with the ventricular system, homogeneous signal intensity, and sharp margination from adjacent, more peripheral white matter.

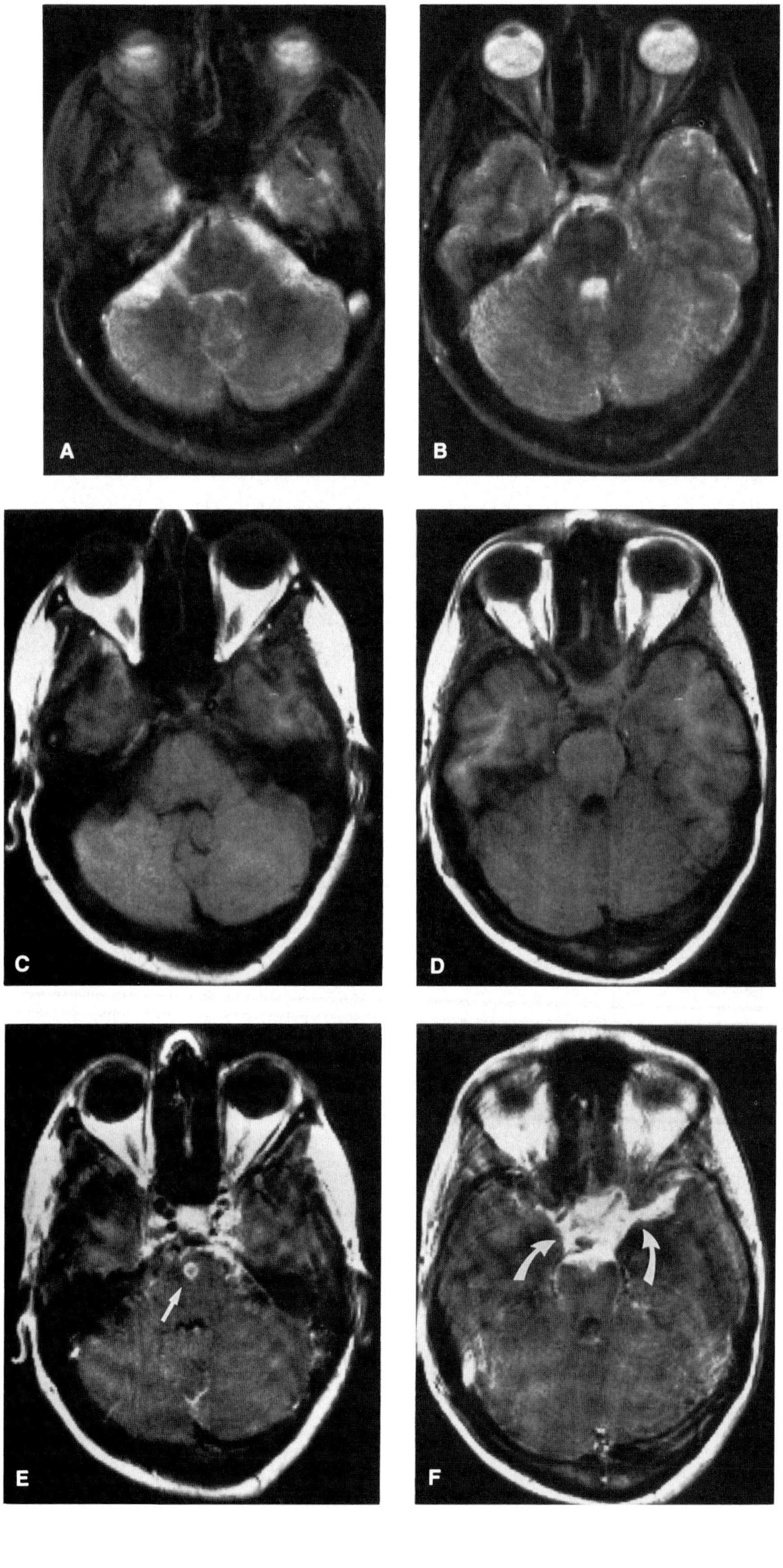

FIGURE 1–30. Tuberculous meningitis (curved arrows) and pontine tuberculoma (arrow) can be detected in **(A,B)** T2-weighted sections (TR/TE = 3000/90) and **(C,D)** precontrast and **(E,F)** postcontrast T1-weighted sections (TR/TE = 650/20). Contrast-enhanced MRI is superior to unenhanced MRI and enhanced CT for detecting parenchymal and meningeal inflammatory disease.

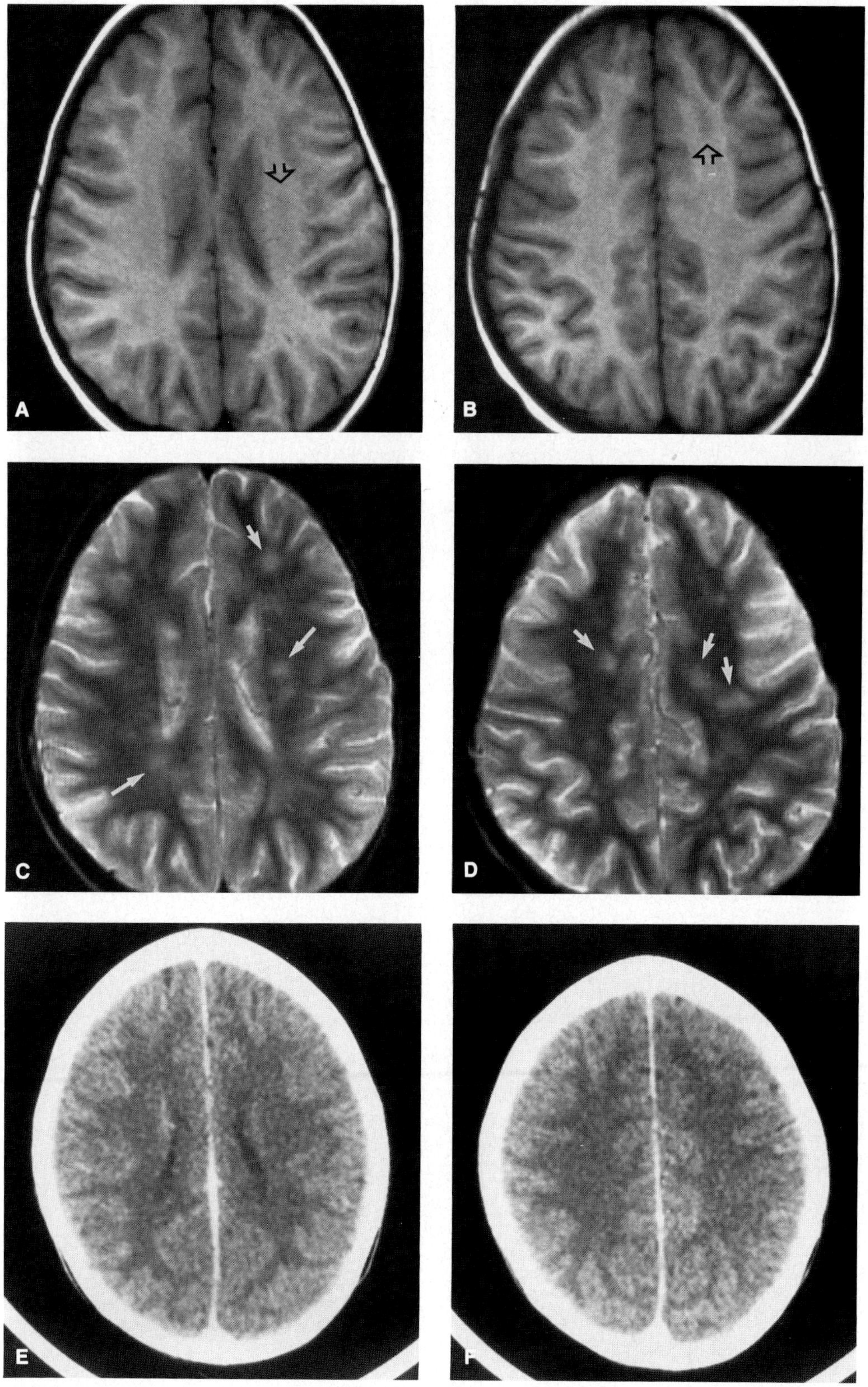

FIGURE 1–31. Viral encephalitis in a 5-year-old girl with a history of rash, lethargy, and upper extremity weakness. Two levels are illustrated in **(A,B)** T1-weighted images (TR/TE = 650/20), **(C,D)** T2-weighted images (TR/TE = 3000/90), and **(E,F)** enhanced CT scans. Many poorly marginated white matter lesions (closed arrows) are seen on the T2-weighted image. These are difficult to detect with T1 weighting, although some lesions appear as areas of low signal intensity (open arrows). The CT examinations with and without contrast were normal. MRI is more sensitive than CT for detecting white matter lesions in viral encephalitis.

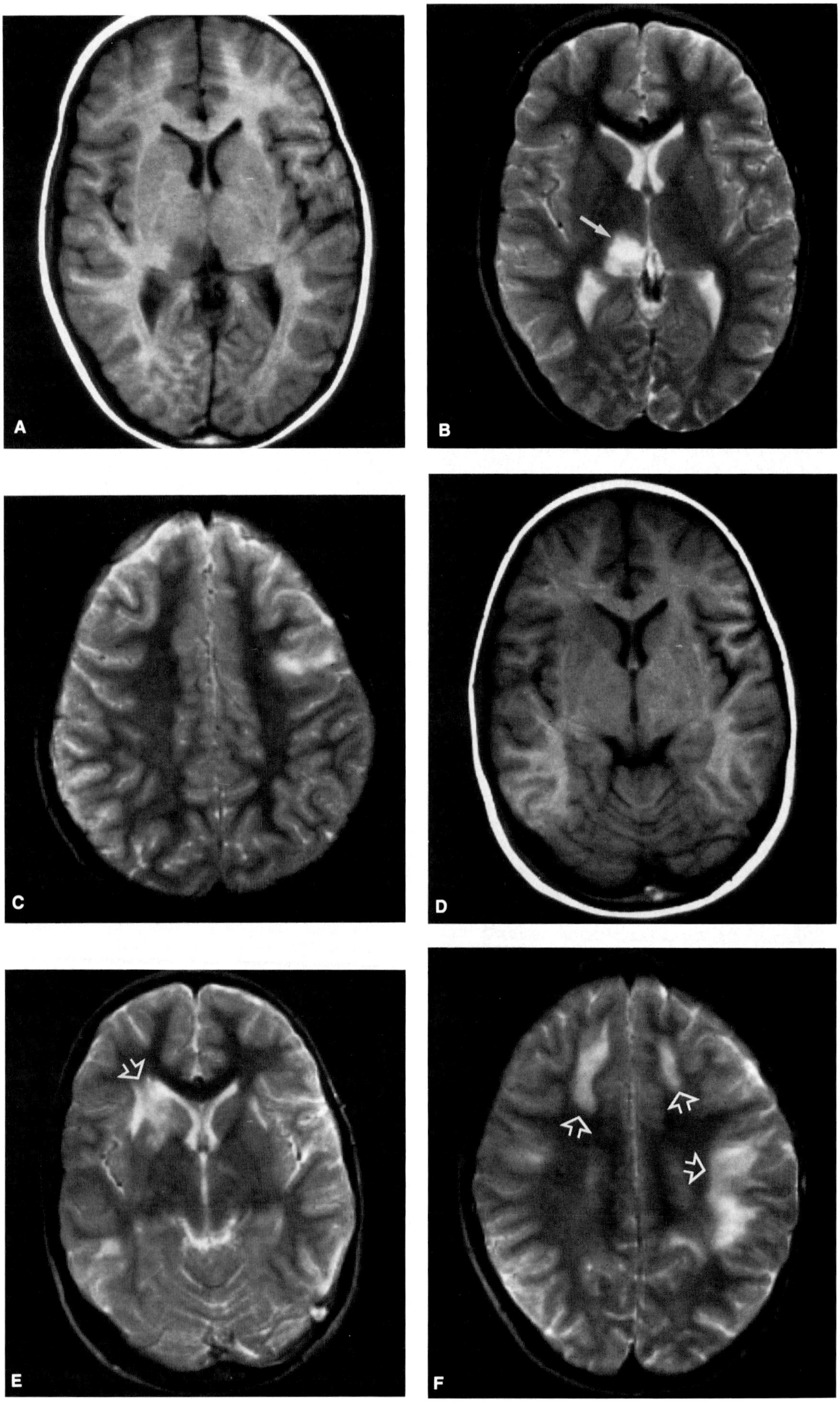

FIGURE 1–32.

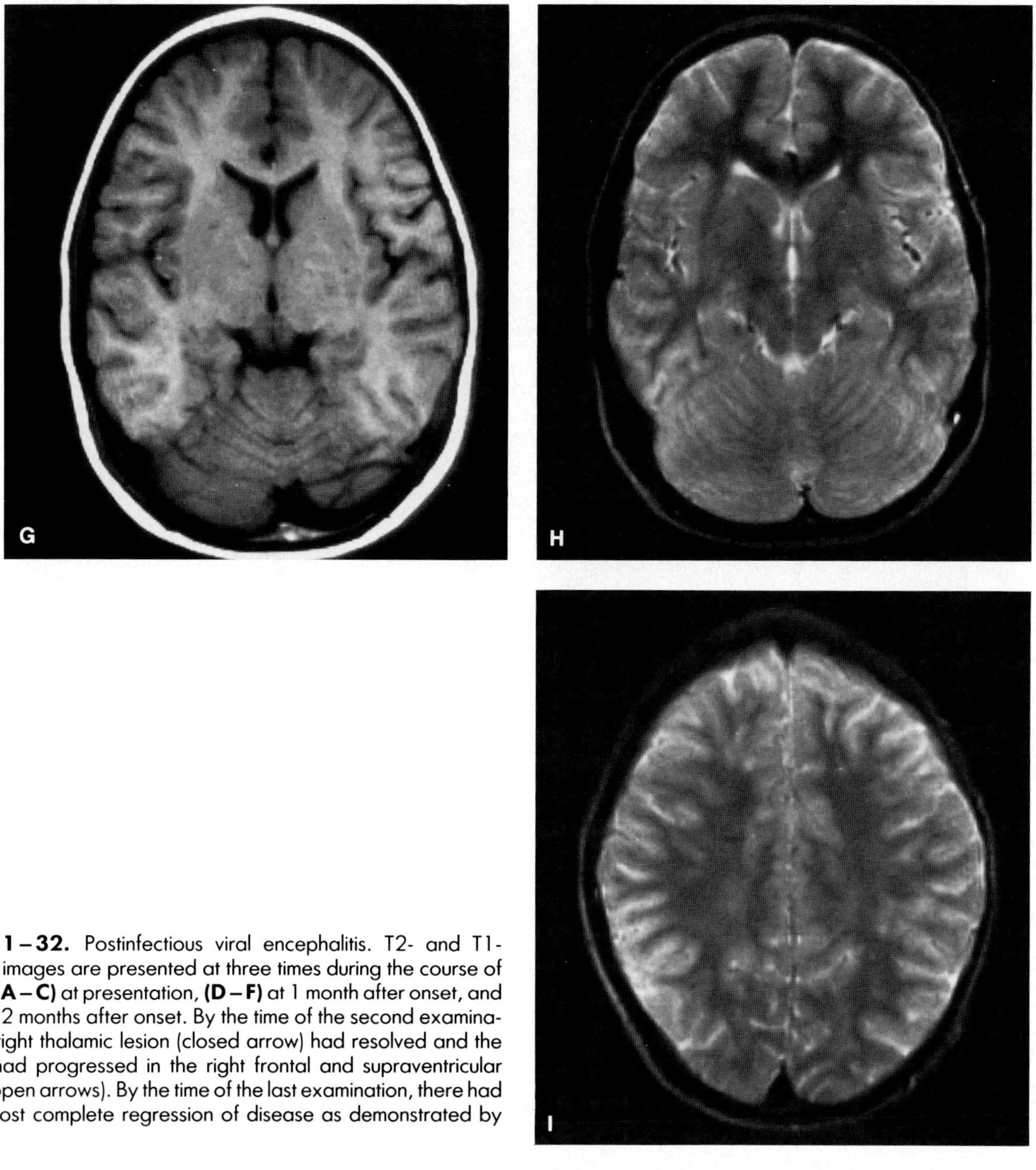

FIGURE 1–32. Postinfectious viral encephalitis. T2- and T1-weighted images are presented at three times during the course of disease: **(A–C)** at presentation, **(D–F)** at 1 month after onset, and **(G–I)** at 2 months after onset. By the time of the second examination, the right thalamic lesion (closed arrow) had resolved and the disease had progressed in the right frontal and supraventricular regions (open arrows). By the time of the last examination, there had been almost complete regression of disease as demonstrated by MRI.

lymphocytes and mononuclear cells. Petechial hemorrhage can result from vascular necrosis.

Acute, disseminated encephalomyelitis is an inflammatory and demyelinating disorder of white matter, which can occur after a childhood viral infection. CT is usually nondiagnostic. MRI can demonstrate multiple foci of demyelination in the brain stem, cerebellum, and cerebrum. Lesions are relatively few, nonhemorrhagic, and asymmetric, and they correlate with clinical symptoms. Follow-up MRI examinations can demonstrate resolution of these lesions (Fig. 1–32) in conjunction with clinical improvement.[66,67] MRI is an important modality for diagnosing acute, disseminated encephalomyelitis due to its ability to identify the sites and extent of involvement and response to therapy.

Herpes Encephalitis

Herpes simplex type 1 encephalitis typically involves the temporal lobe, although involvement may extend to the frontal or parietal lobes (Fig. 1–33). The basal ganglia are typically spared. MRI allows early diagnosis and can document effective response to therapy.[68] Coronal imaging may benefit visualization of

(text continues on page 36)

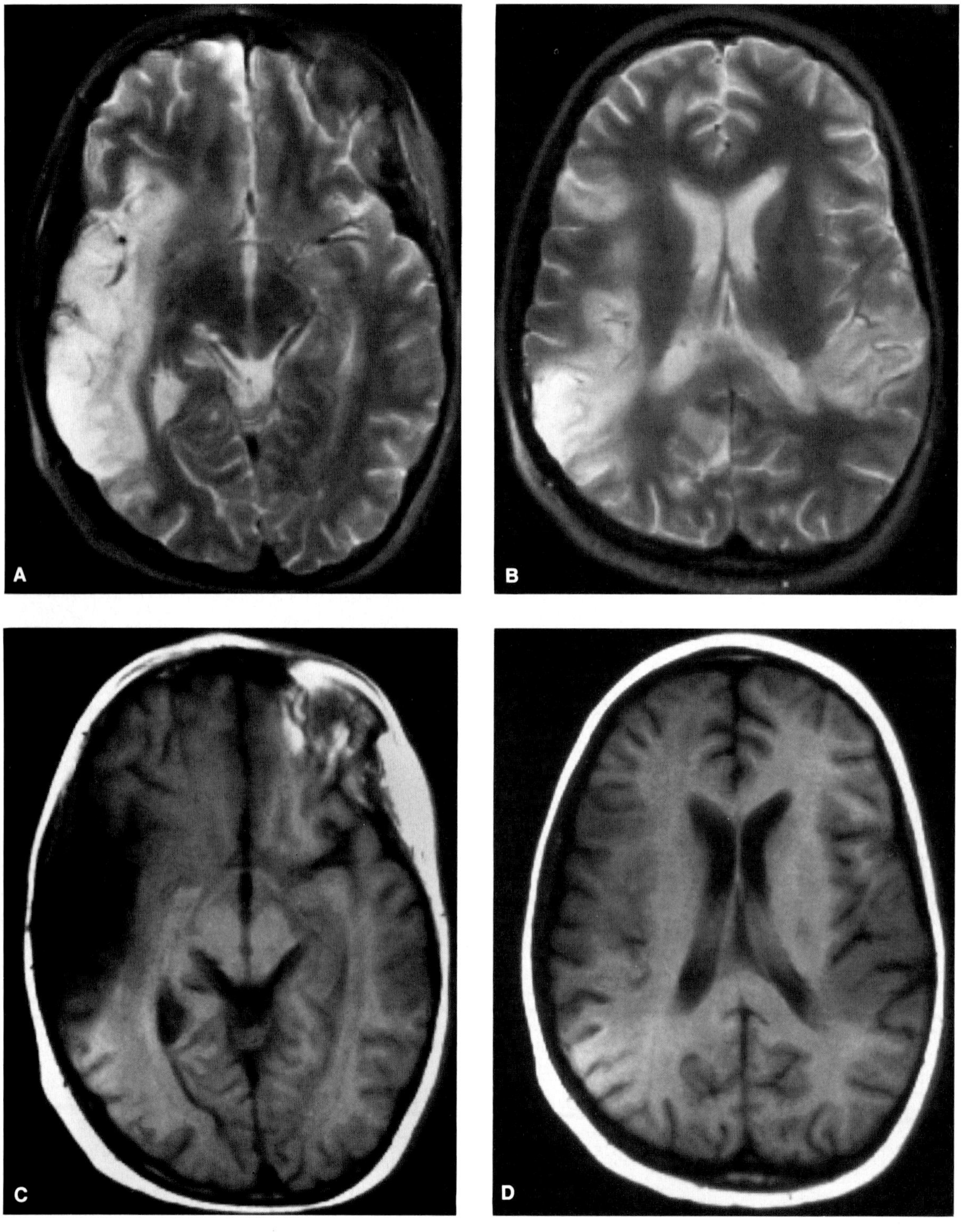

FIGURE 1 – 33. Biopsy-proven herpes encephalitis in a 12-year-old girl. Two anatomic levels are presented in **(A,B)** T2-weighted images (TR/TE = 3000/90), **(C,D)** precontrast and **(E,F)** postcontrast T1-weighted images (TR/TE = 650/20), and **(G,H)** enhanced CT scans. Although bilateral lesions were detected on CT, recognition of disease and definition of its extent are improved with MRI. Only faint enhancement occurs on CT, compared with the prominent enhancement with Gd DTPA on MRI. Enhancement also identifies disease in the frontal and occipital lobes (arrows), not seen on CT or unenhanced MRI. The classic pathologic changes associated with herpes simplex type 1 infection include hemorrhagic necrotizing involvement of the frontal or temporal lobes. Contrast enhancement is not seen on CT scans during the first week after the onset of symptoms.

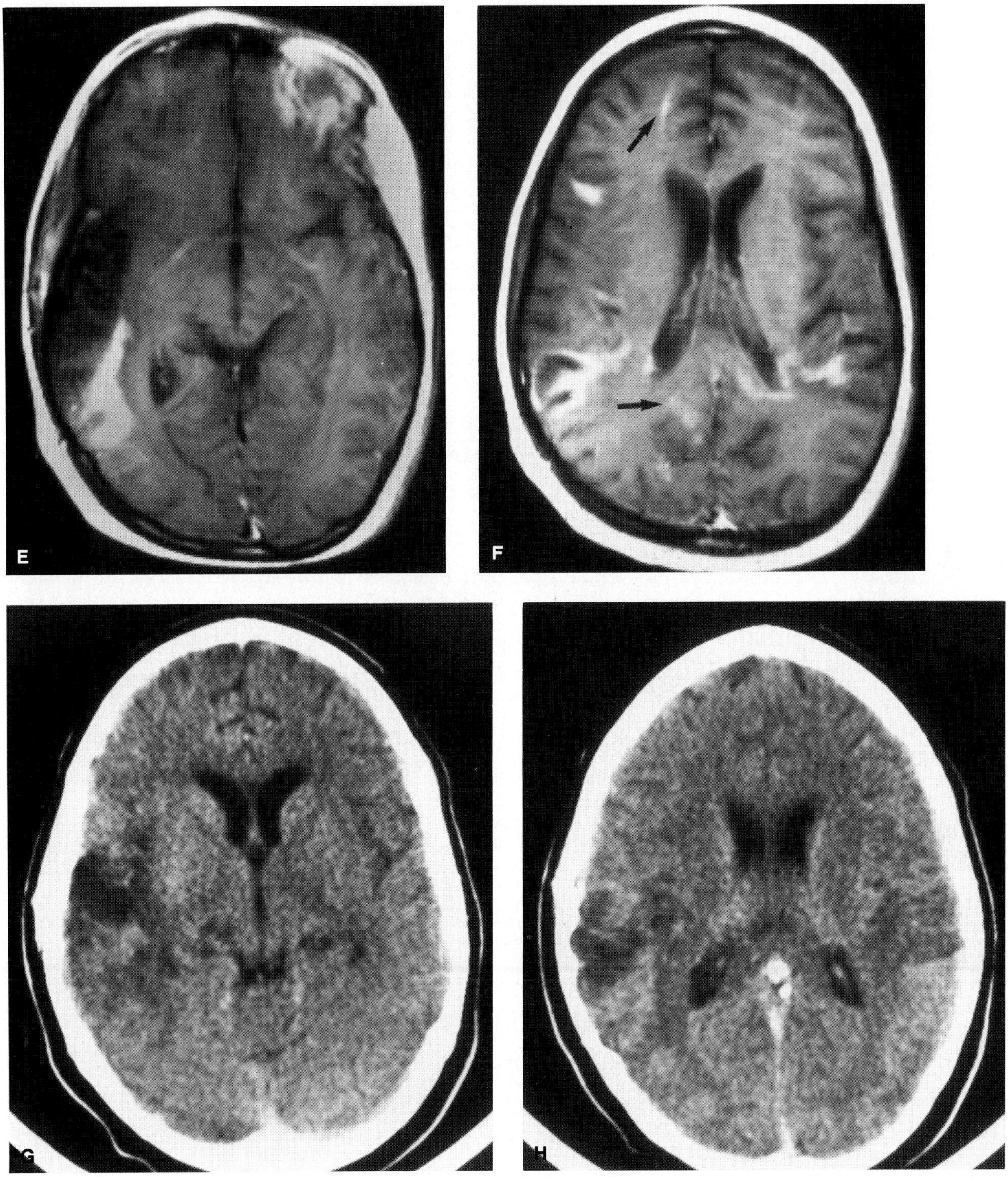

FIGURE 1 – 33. (Continued)

temporal lobe pathology in this and other diseases (Fig. 1-34). Following neonatal infection (type 2), atrophic changes can appear rapidly (Fig. 1-35).

Meningeal Disease

Enhanced MRI is highly sensitive to meningeal disease (Fig. 1-36). Unfortunately, neoplastic, inflammatory, and traumatic changes cannot be differentiated (Fig. 1-37).[69] MRI is superior to x-ray CT in demonstrating meningeal disease. Although T2-weighted imaging can be used in certain cases, detection of meningeal disease is possible in some patients only after Gd DTPA injection. In a canine model of experimental bacterial meningitis, abnormal leptomeningeal enhancement was consistently demonstrated on MRI scans after Gd DTPA administration, but contrast enhancement on CT scans occurred in only one of four dogs. Enhanced MRI also can be used to identify the complications of meningitis, including ventriculitis and cerebritis, more effectively than x-ray CT. Abnormal areas of contrast enhancement

(text continues on page 38)

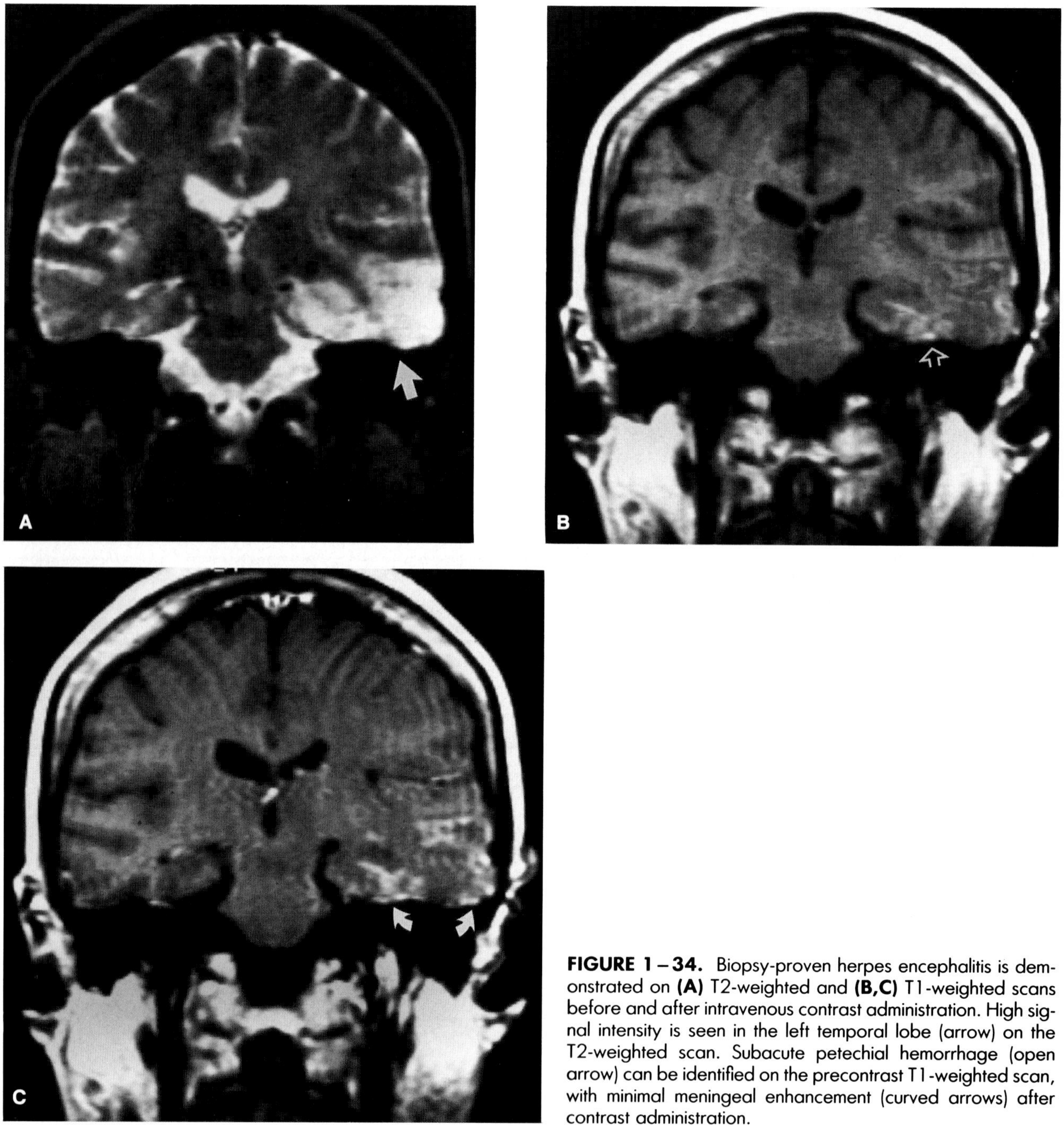

FIGURE 1-34. Biopsy-proven herpes encephalitis is demonstrated on **(A)** T2-weighted and **(B,C)** T1-weighted scans before and after intravenous contrast administration. High signal intensity is seen in the left temporal lobe (arrow) on the T2-weighted scan. Subacute petechial hemorrhage (open arrow) can be identified on the precontrast T1-weighted scan, with minimal meningeal enhancement (curved arrows) after contrast administration.

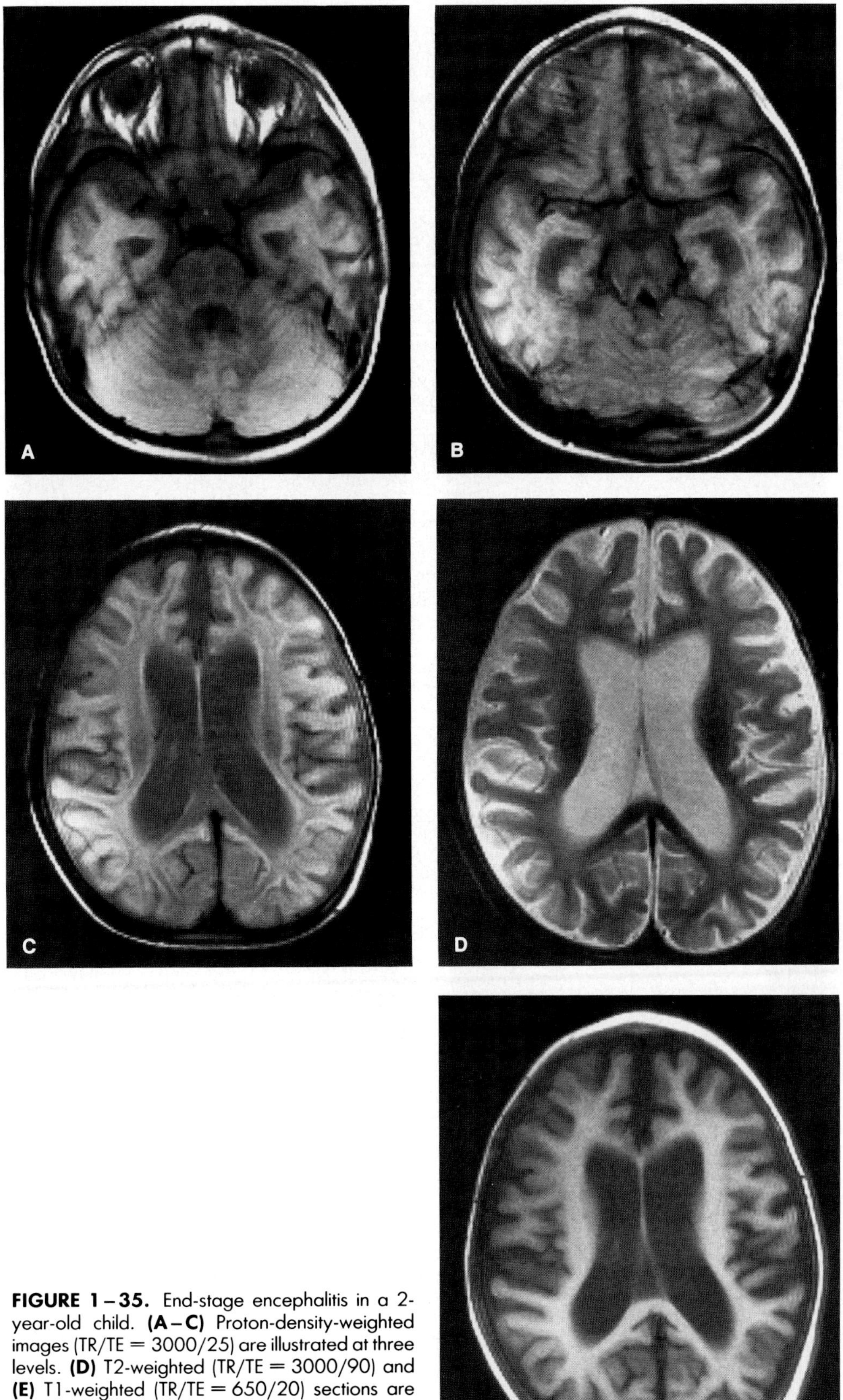

FIGURE 1–35. End-stage encephalitis in a 2-year-old child. **(A–C)** Proton-density-weighted images (TR/TE = 3000/25) are illustrated at three levels. **(D)** T2-weighted (TR/TE = 3000/90) and **(E)** T1-weighted (TR/TE = 650/20) sections are presented for comparison at the level of the lateral ventricles. There is extensive brain atrophy and an increase in CSF space surrounding the brain.

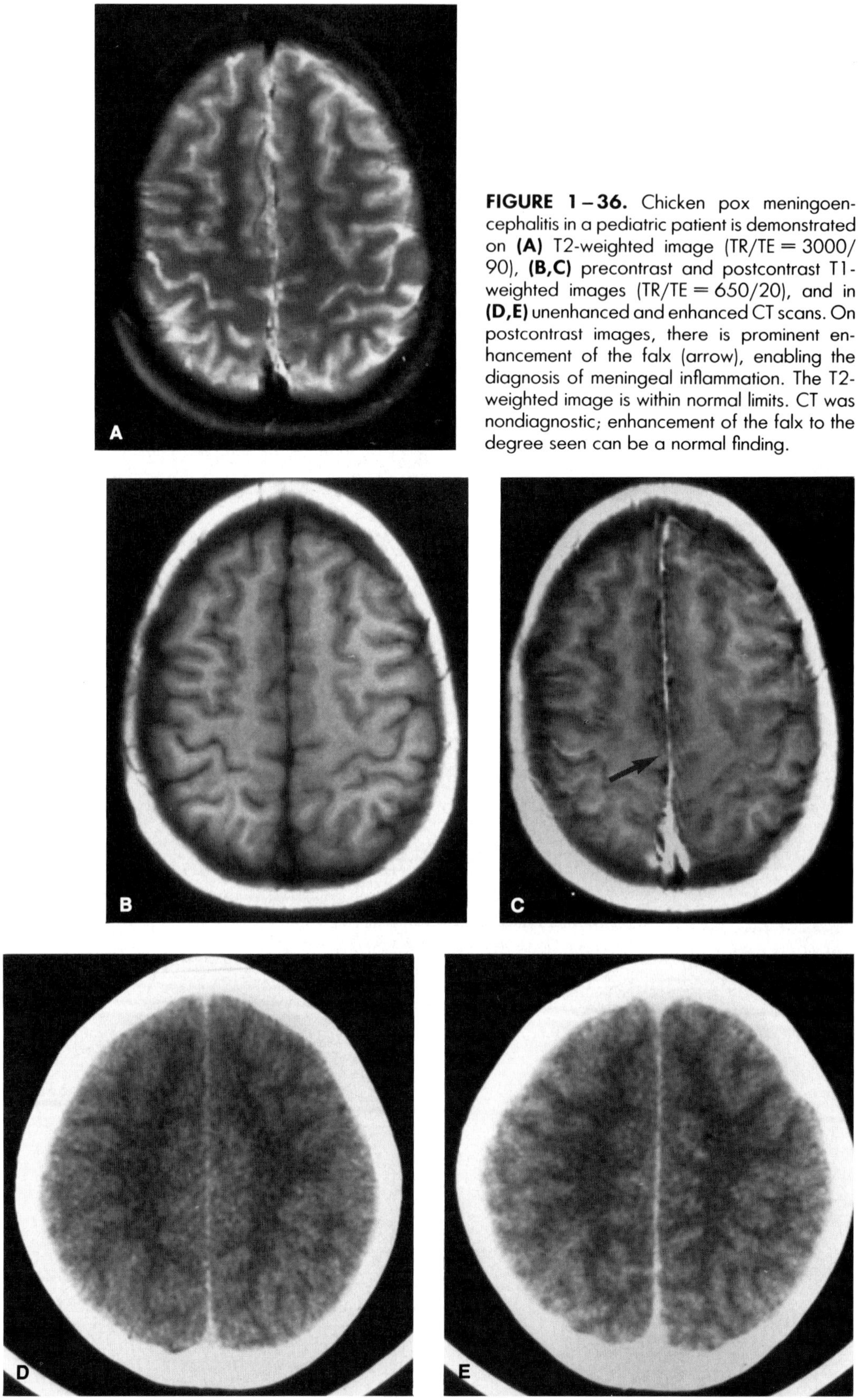

FIGURE 1–36. Chicken pox meningoencephalitis in a pediatric patient is demonstrated on **(A)** T2-weighted image (TR/TE = 3000/90), **(B,C)** precontrast and postcontrast T1-weighted images (TR/TE = 650/20), and in **(D,E)** unenhanced and enhanced CT scans. On postcontrast images, there is prominent enhancement of the falx (arrow), enabling the diagnosis of meningeal inflammation. The T2-weighted image is within normal limits. CT was nondiagnostic; enhancement of the falx to the degree seen can be a normal finding.

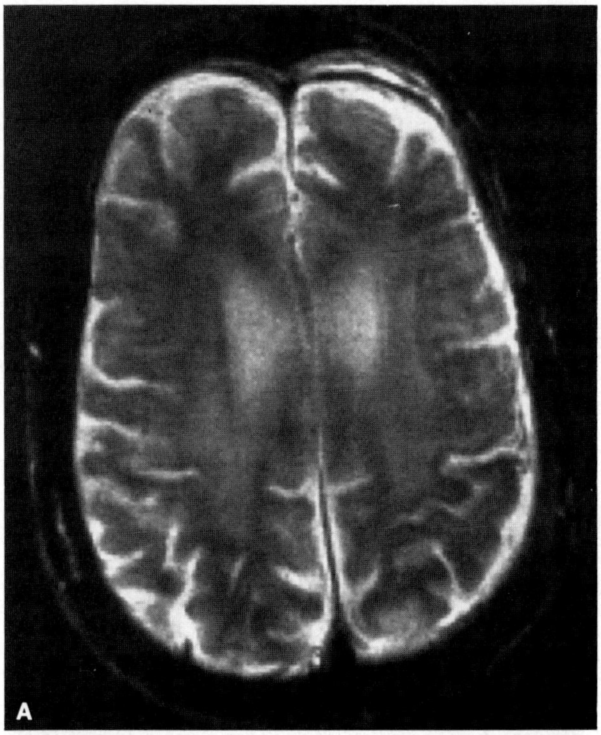

FIGURE 1–37. Communicating hydrocephalus in an 18-year-old woman with a remote history of significant head trauma. **(A)** T2-weighted image (TR/TE = 3000/90); **(B,C)** T1-weighted images (TR/TE = 650/20) before and after Gd DTPA administration. There is diffuse cerebral atrophy with marked dural (arrows) enhancement.

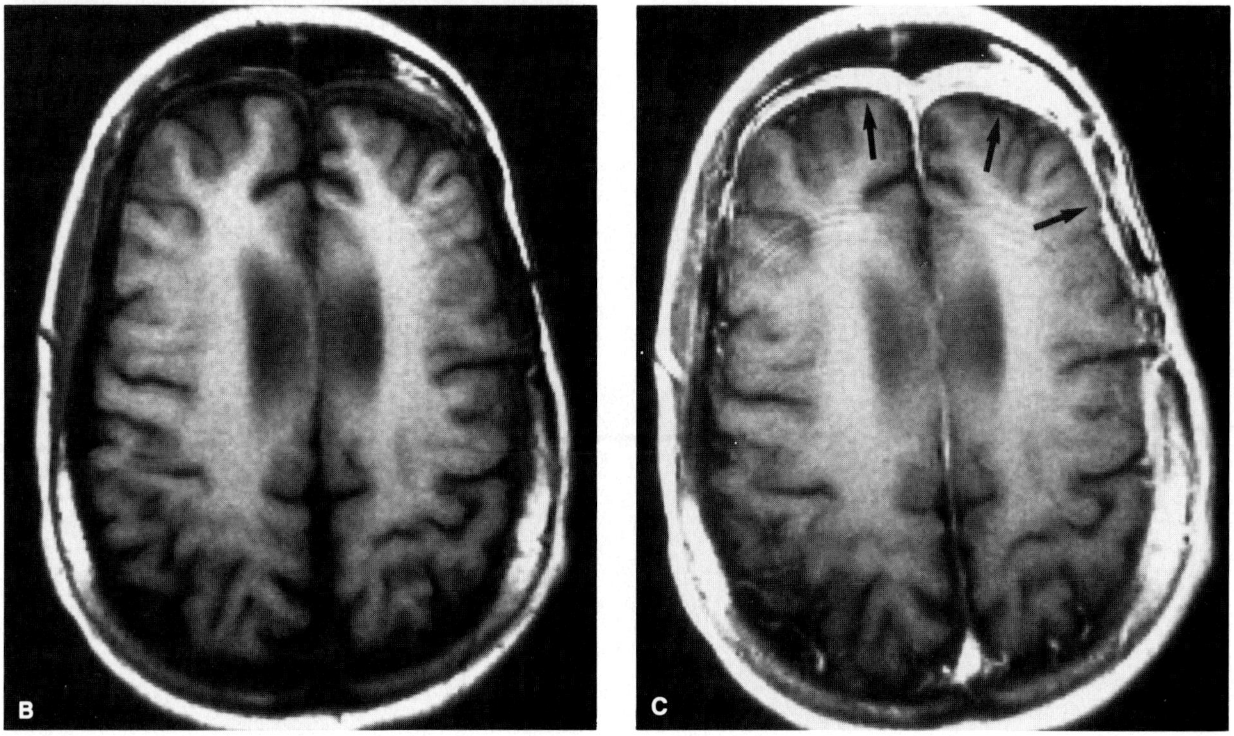

correlate pathologically with inflammatory cell infiltration. Unfortunately, enhancement does not identify the full extent of leptomeningitis.[70]

Meningeal enhancement is common after intracranial surgery (Fig. 1–38). This has occurred as late as 12 years after an operation.[71] Enhancement may be the result of local inflammation or chemical arachnoiditis caused by blood. Enhancement after surgery or trauma must be differentiated from inflammatory and neoplastic meningeal disease.[72]

Sarcoidosis

Both parenchymal and meningeal disease (Fig. 1–39) can be identified by MRI in patients with central ner-

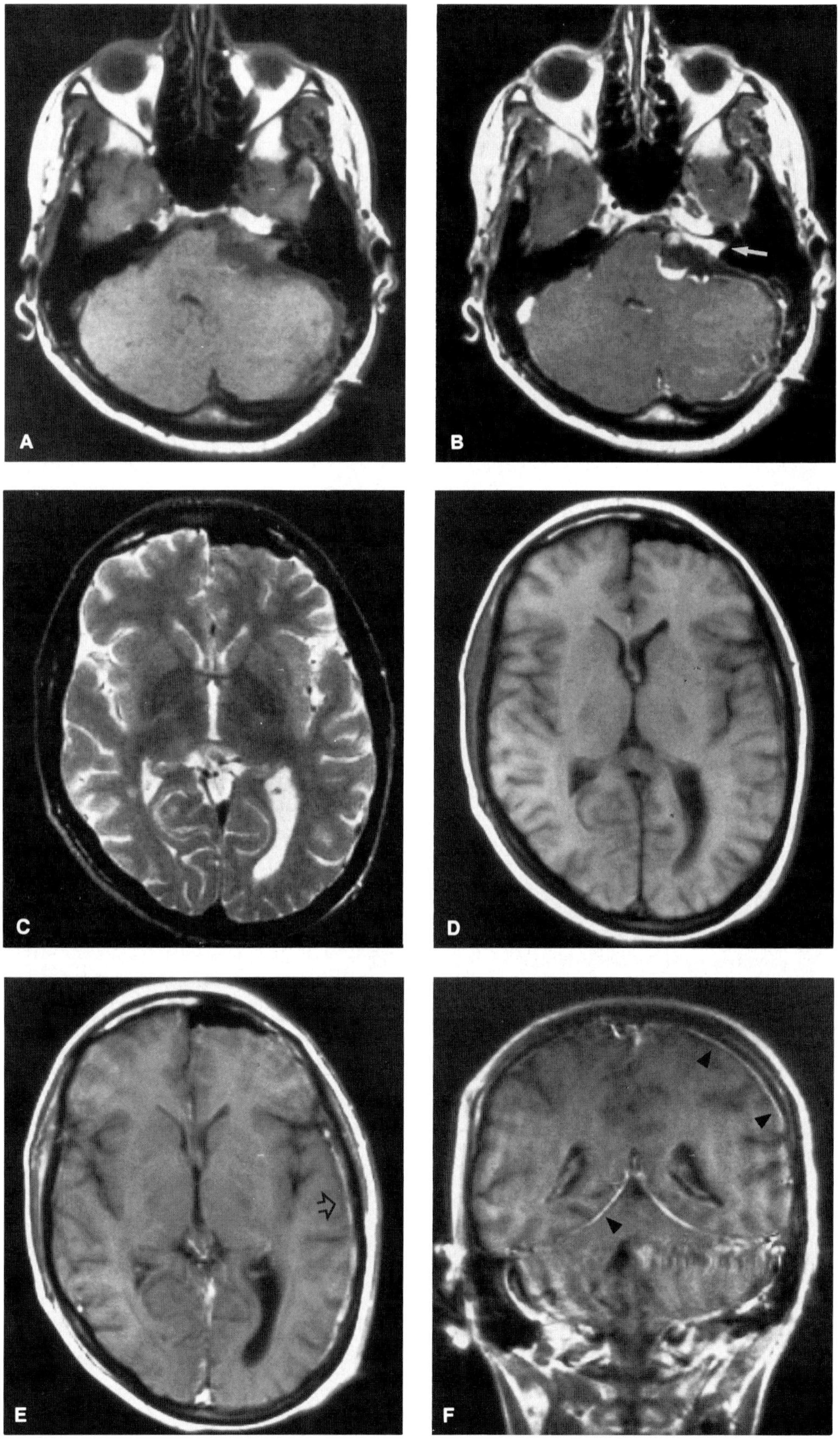

FIGURE 1–38. Meningeal inflammation with enhancement after contrast administration can be seen in postsurgical patients. Scans are presented from a 42-year-old woman, 4 days after partial resection of a large, left-sided acoustic neuroma. **(A,B)** Precontrast and postcontrast axial T1-weighted scans at the level of the internal auditory canal. Axial sections at the level of the basal ganglia used a **(C)** T2-weighted technique and **(D,E)** precontrast and postcontrast T1-weighted techniques. Residual neoplastic disease (closed arrow) can be identified on the contrast-enhanced scan at the level of the internal auditory canal. Dural inflammation (open arrow) can be detected on the postcontrast scan due to enhancement. No abnormality is identified on the precontrast T2-weighted scan. As in many cases, the coronal scan **(F)** is superior to the axial scan for depicting enhancement of the dura and tentorium (arrowheads).

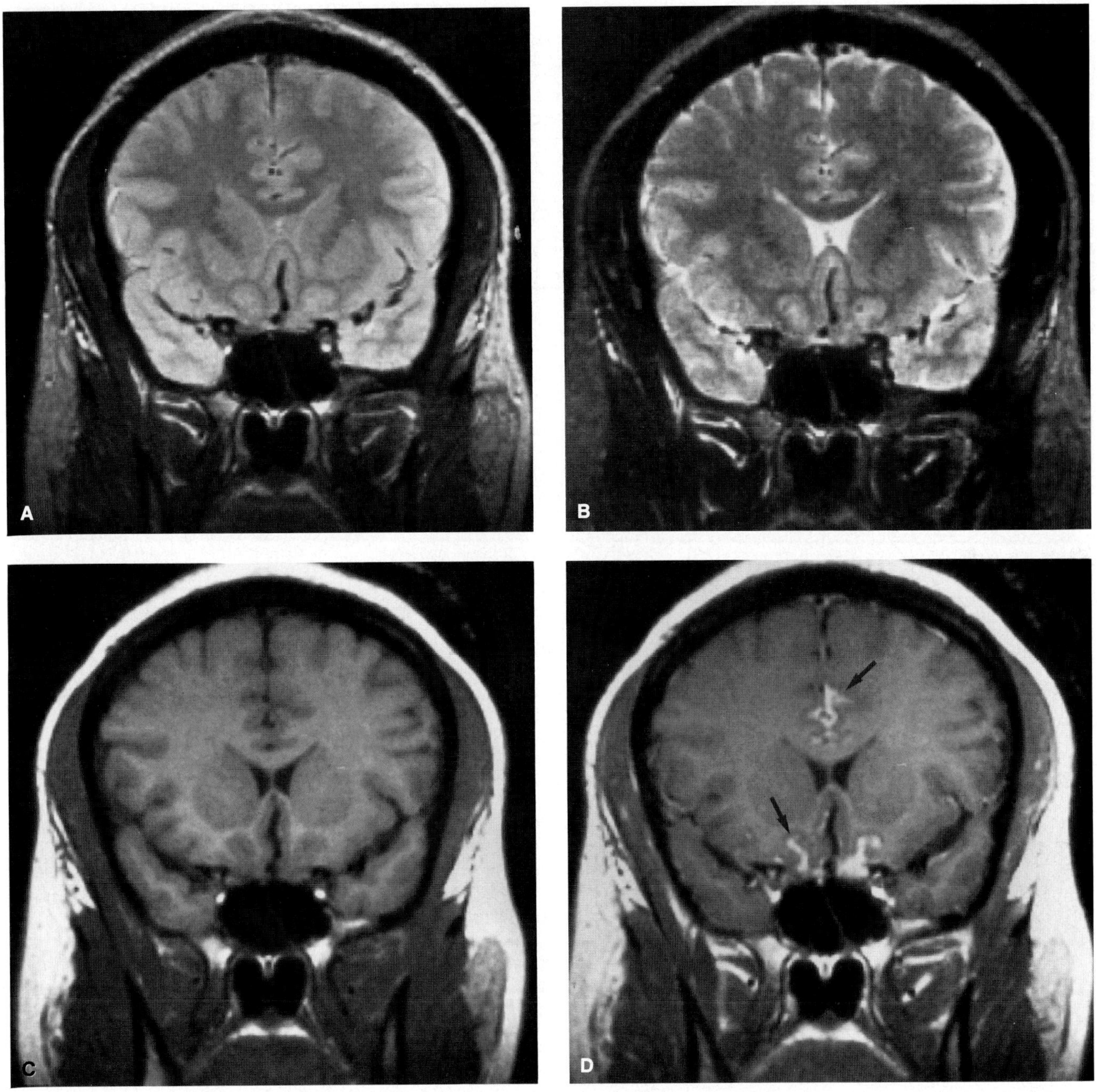

FIGURE 1–39. Intracranial sarcoidosis in a 31-year-old woman presenting with hypersomnolence is demonstrated on **(A,B)** T2-weighted (TR/TE = 3000/45,90) and **(C,D)** precontrast and postcontrast T1-weighted (TR/TE = 650/20) spin echo images. Meningeal infiltration by granulomas in sarcoidosis is a common pathologic finding, which can manifest clinically as aseptic meningitis. The post-Gd DTPA T1-weighted image demonstrates marked meningeal enhancement (arrows). Meningeal involvement can be focal or diffuse. This appearance in sarcoid is indistinguishable from meningeal carcinomatosis, bacterial meningitis, and fungal meningitis. Parenchymal disease causing hypothalamic dysfunction also was present in this case (scans not shown).

vous system (CNS) sarcoidosis.[73] As with other CNS infections, MRI is more sensitive than CT and better demonstrates the extent of disease. Periventricular and multifocal white matter lesions can be seen in CNS sarcoidosis. This pattern in certain instances may be indistinguishable from that of MS.

Extracerebral Fluid Collections

MRI is superior to CT for detecting extracerebral fluid collections, and MRI should be useful for the early diagnosis and follow-up of subdural empyemas. Early diagnosis is critical in this disease, due to the possible

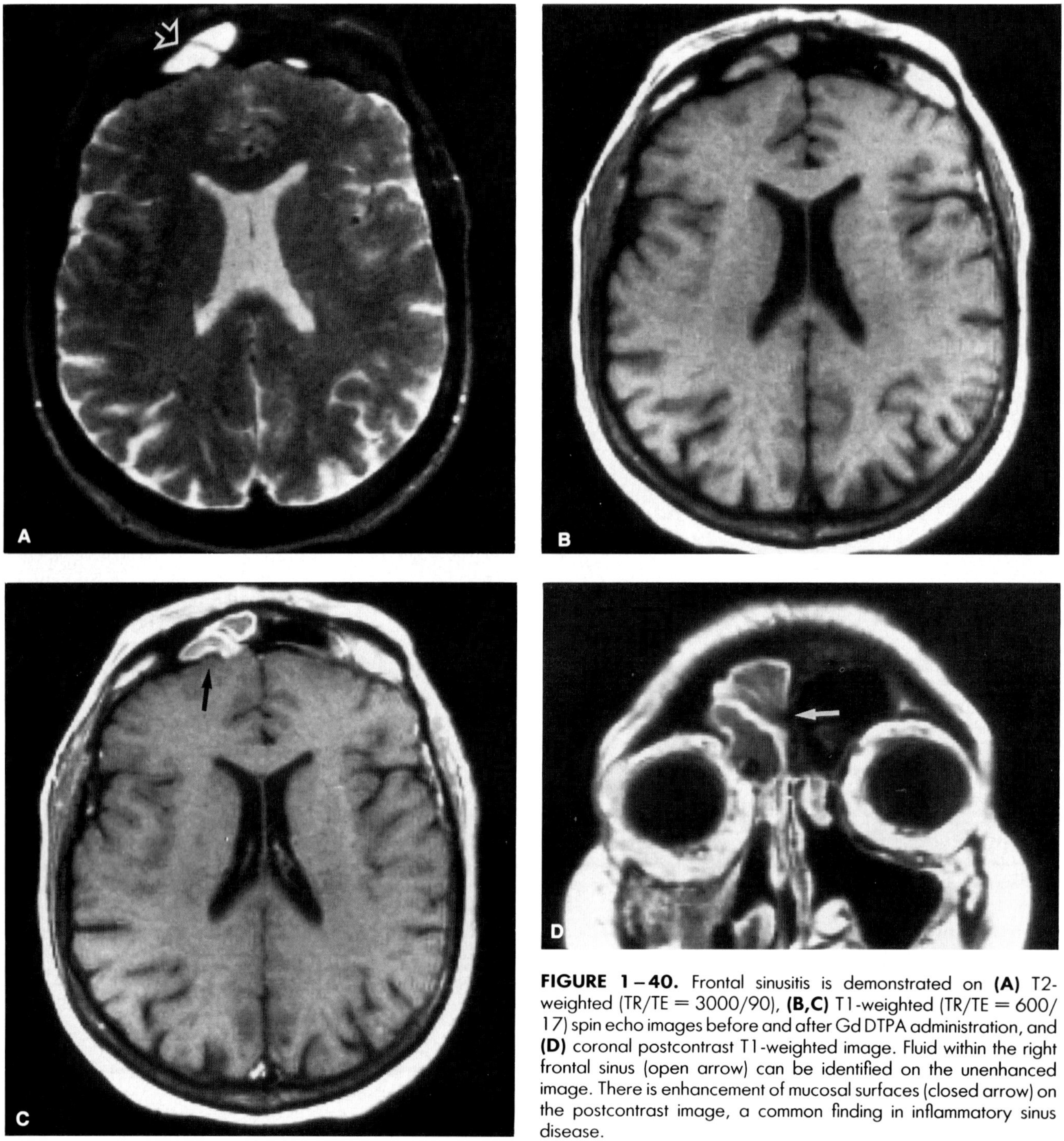

FIGURE 1–40. Frontal sinusitis is demonstrated on **(A)** T2-weighted (TR/TE = 3000/90), **(B,C)** T1-weighted (TR/TE = 600/17) spin echo images before and after Gd DTPA administration, and **(D)** coronal postcontrast T1-weighted image. Fluid within the right frontal sinus (open arrow) can be identified on the unenhanced image. There is enhancement of mucosal surfaces (closed arrow) on the postcontrast image, a common finding in inflammatory sinus disease.

sequelae of cortical venous thrombosis and infarction. If all pulse sequences are compared, purulent fluid can be distinguished from CSF due to the shortening of T1 and T2. Epidural empyemas may be caused by the extension of sinus or ear disease or may occur as a complication after neurosurgical intervention.

Sinus Disease

MRI is very sensitive to inflammatory sinus disease. Inflamed mucosa is of high signal intensity on T2-weighted images. In the paranasal sinuses, mucoperiosteal thickening and inflammation of the mucosal lining enhance markedly after Gd DTPA administration (Fig. 1–40).

Retained secretions within an obstructed sinus typically do not enhance. Mastoid sinus disease, like paranasal sinus inflammation, is also commonly encountered (Fig. 1–41). The nasal turbinates normally demonstrate prominent enhancement and, combined with the enhancement of inflammatory sinus disease, this can mask more significant pathology.

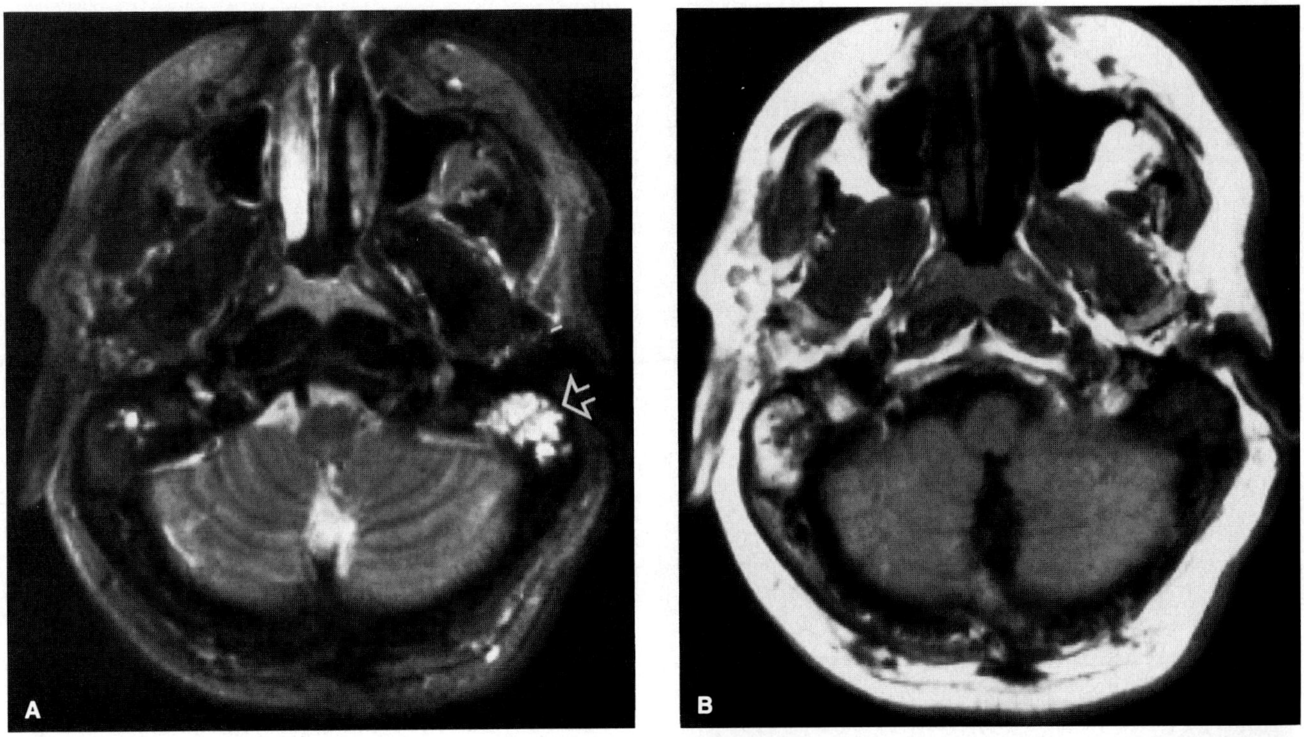

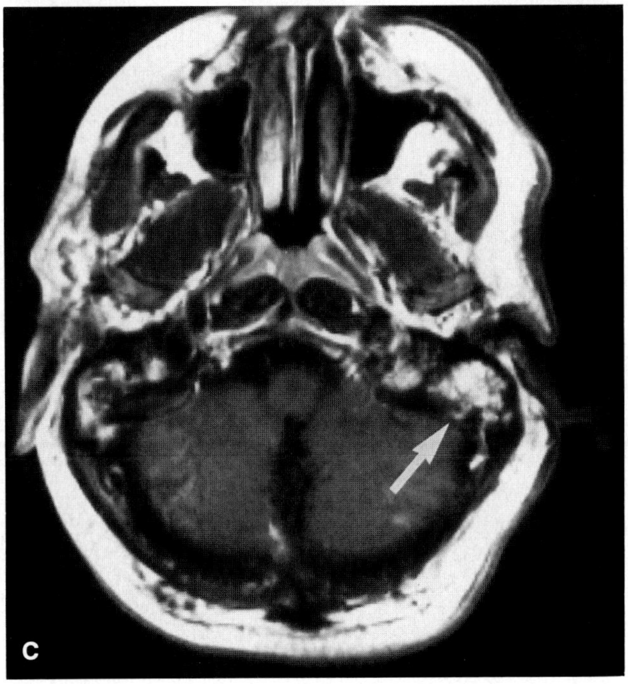

FIGURE 1–41. Inflammatory disease of the mastoid air cells on a **(A)** T2-weighted image (TR/TE = 3000/90) and **(B,C)** precontrast and postcontrast T1-weighted images (TR/TE = 650/20). High signal intensity due to fluid and inflammatory reaction is seen on the precontrast T2-weighted image (open arrow), with enhancement after (closed arrow) Gd DTPA administration (on the T1-weighted image).

AIDS

The superior contrast resolution of MRI, compared with x-ray CT, combined with the use of Gd DTPA, will probably make it the imaging mode of choice for the examination of acquired immune deficiency syndrome (AIDS) and its CNS complications.[74] MRI is superior to CT in detecting white matter lesions in AIDS.[75] Before the advent of contrast enhancement, CT was superior for biopsy localization, judging lesion activity, and detecting small cortical lesions with minimal surrounding edema. Cortical atrophy is found in virtually all patients with HIV encephalitis. HIV-induced foci of demyelination can also be observed better with MRI.[76]

In toxoplasmosis, multiple small lesions (<2 cm) appear as discrete high-signal-intensity foci on T2-weighted images (Fig. 1–42). There may be variable enhancement. In acute parenchymal lesions, enhancement slowly progresses with time after Gd

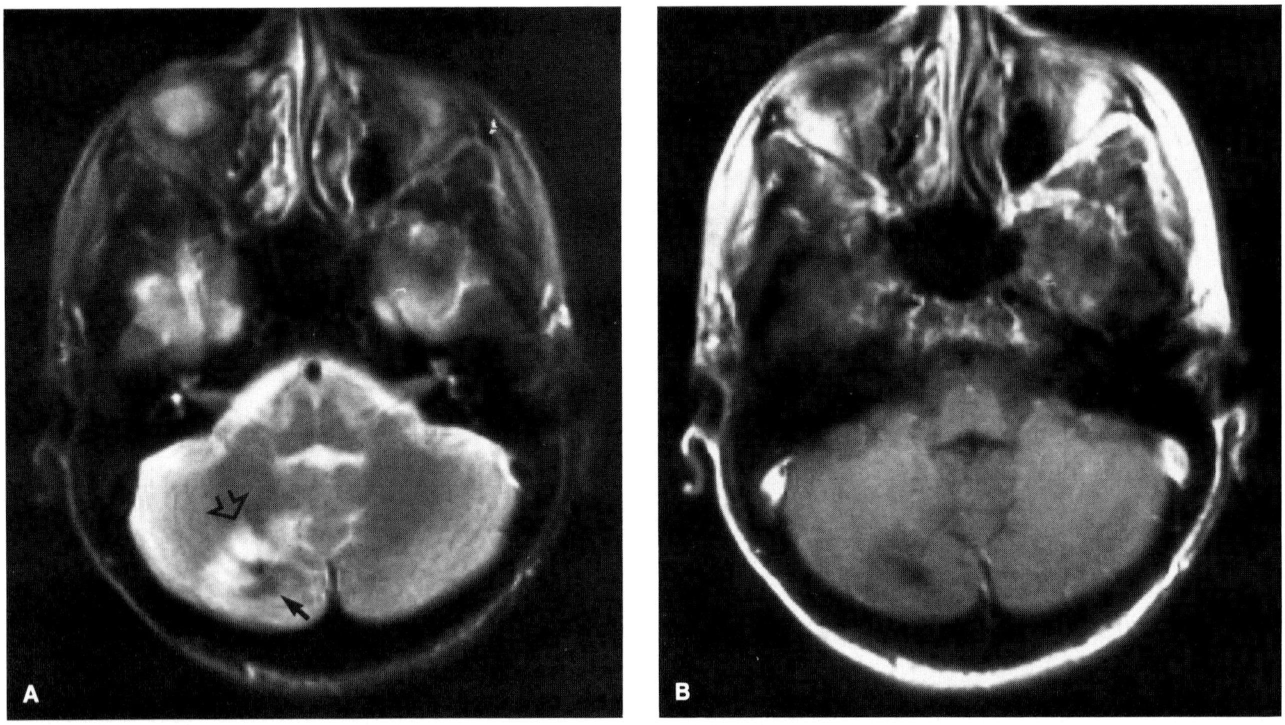

FIGURE 1-42. Toxoplasmosis in AIDS. This 41-year-old woman developed AIDS as a complication of renal transplant. **(A)** T2-weighted image and **(B)** post-Gd DTPA T1-weighted image. On T2-weighted images, a lesion with high signal intensity (open arrow) is seen in the right cerebellum. An area of low signal intensity (closed arrow) is due to hemosiderin deposition from a previous biopsy-associated hemorrhage. The lack of enhancement with Gd DTPA confirms the inactivity of this lesion, with the patient presenting for routine follow-up examination.

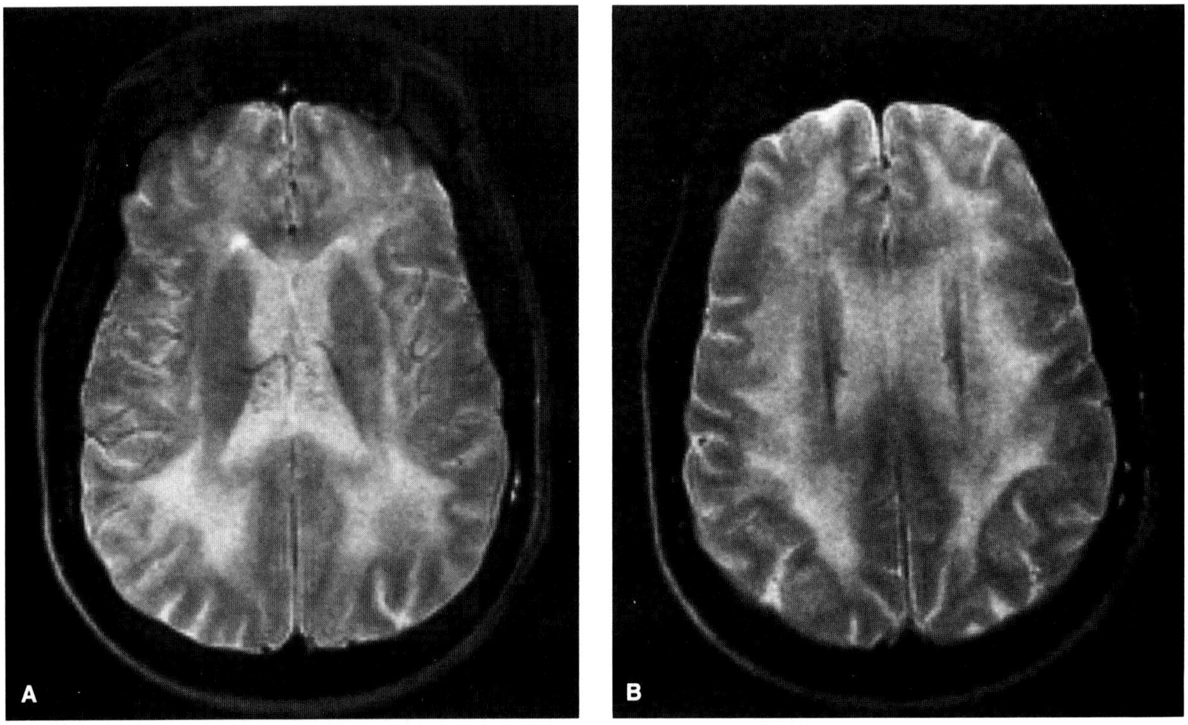

FIGURE 1-43. PML in AIDS is demonstrated in **(A,B)** T2-weighted images (TR/TE = 3000/70) at two anatomic levels. Involvement is confined primarily to white matter. PML is a diffuse, parenchymal infection, which typically involves the parietal and occipital lobes and may have multifocal distribution.

DTPA administration.[77] Lymphoma, commonly a single lesion (>3 cm), also may demonstrate enhancement.[78,79] Both multiplicity and size are useful in differentiating these two pathologic processes. Generalized enlargement of sulci and the ventricular system reflect atrophic changes from chronic HIV infection and prolonged debilitation. Focal white matter lesions are typical of progressive multifocal leukoencephalopathy (PML). These lesions may first be round or oval, subsequently enlarging and becoming confluent with absence of mass effect (Fig. 1–43). Involvement is often asymmetric and distant from the ventricular system.[80,81]

CONCLUSION

Initial clinical results in 1981 demonstrating MRI's sensitivity in MS led to immediate recognition of this technique as a significant new imaging modality. Subsequent experience confirmed the sensitivity to white matter diseases and intracranial infection.[64] Many diseases, especially deep white matter ischemia, can mimic MS radiologically. Pattern recognition and clinical presentation can aid differentiation. Intravenous contrast media such as Gd DTPA play a vital role in improving the sensitivity of MRI to intracranial infection, in particular meningitis. As scan times continue to decrease due to improvements in hardware and software, MRI will find greater application in seriously ill patients, in particular those with intracranial infectious diseases. The role of MRI is also likely to expand further as CNS involvement in AIDS becomes more common.

REFERENCES

1. Simon JH, Holtas SL, Schiffer RB, et al. Corpus callosum and subcallosal-periventricular lesions in multiple sclerosis: detection with MR. Radiology 1986;160:363.
2. Young IR, Hall AS, Pallis CA, et al. Nuclear magnetic resonance imaging of the brain in multiple sclerosis. Lancet 1981;2:1063.
3. Young IR, Randell CP, Kaplan PW, et al. Nuclear magnetic resonance (NMR) imaging in white matter disease of the brain using spin-echo sequences. J Comput Assist Tomogr 1983;7:290.
4. Lukes SA, Crooks LE, Aminoff MJ, et al. Nuclear magnetic resonance imaging in multiple sclerosis. Ann Neurol 1983;12:592.
5. Runge VM, Price AC, Kirschner HS, et al. Magnetic resonance imaging of multiple sclerosis: a study of pulse-technique efficacy. AJR 1984;143:1015.
6. Robertson WD, Li DK, Mayo JR, et al. Assessment of multiple sclerosis lesions by magnetic resonance imaging. J Can Assoc Radiol 1987;38:177.
7. Johnson G, Miller DH, MacManus D, et al. STIR sequences in NMR imaging of the optic nerve. Neuroradiology 1987;29:238.
8. Ormerod IE, Miller DH, McDonald WI. The role of NMR imaging in the assessment of multiple sclerosis and isolated neurologic lesions. A quantitative study. Brain 1987;110:1579.
9. Larsson HB, Frederiksen J, Kjaer L. In vivo determination of T1 and T2 in the brain of patients with severe but stable multiple sclerosis. Magn Reson Med 1988;7:43.
10. Kermode AG, Tofts PS, MacManus DG, et al. Shortened T1 at the edge of multiple sclerosis lesions. SMRI 1989: 7th Annual Meeting Program and Abstracts, 168.
11. Bone G, Ladurner G, Artmann W, et al. Correlations between clinical and magnetic resonance imaging findings in multiple sclerosis. Eur Neurol 1988;28:212.
12. Stewart JM, Houser OW, Baker HL, et al. Magnetic resonance imaging and clinical relationships in multiple sclerosis. Mayo Clin Proc 1987;62:174.
13. Scotti G, Scialfa G, Biondi A, et al. Magnetic resonance in multiple sclerosis. Neuroradiology 1986;28:319.
14. Kirshner HS, Tsai SI, Runge VM, et al. Magnetic resonance imaging and other techniques in the diagnosis of multiple sclerosis. Arch Neurol 1985;42:859.
15. Cutler JR, Aminoff MJ, Brant-Zawadzki M. Evaluation of patients with multiple sclerosis by evoked potentials and magnetic resonance imaging: a comparative study. Ann Neurol 1986;20:645.
16. Uhlenbrock D, Seidel D, Gehlen W, et al. MR imaging in multiple sclerosis: comparison with clinical, CSF, and visual evoked potential findings. AJNR 1988;9:59.
17. Paty DW, Oger JJ, Kastrukoff LF, et al. MRI in the diagnosis of MS: a prospective study with comparison of clinical evaluation, evoked potentials, oliogoclonal banding, and CT. Neurology 1988;38:180.
18. Johnson MA, Li DBK, Bryant DJ, et al. Magnetic resonance imaging: serial observations in multiple sclerosis. AJNR 1984;5:495.
19. Reese L, Carr TJ, Nicholson RL, et al. Magnetic resonance imaging for detecting lesions of multiple sclerosis: comparison with computed tomography and clinical assessment. Can Med Assoc J 1986;135:639.
20. Isaac C, Li DK, Genton M, et al. Multiple sclerosis: a serial study using MRI in relapsing patients. Neurology 1988;38:1511.
21. Huber SJ, Paulson GW, Chakeres D, et al. Magnetic resonance imaging and clinical correlations in multiple sclerosis. J Neurol Sci 1988;86:1.
22. Jacobs L, Kinkel PR, Kinkel WR. Impact of nuclear magnetic resonance imaging on the assessment of multiple sclerosis patients. Semin Neurol 1986;6:24.
23. Simon JH, Schiffer RB, Rudick RA, et al. Quantitative determination of MS-induced corpus callosum atrophy in vivo using MR imaging. AJNR 1987;8:599.
24. Karlik SJ, Wong C, Gilbert JJ, et al. NMR studies in the relapsing-remitting model of EAE. SMRI 1989: 7th Annual Meeting Program and Abstracts, 168.
25. Grossman RI, Lisak RP, Macchi PJ, et al. MR of acute experimental allergic encephalomyelitis. AJNR 1987;8:1045.
26. Kuharik MA, Edwards MK, Farlow MR, et al. Gd-enhanced MR imaging of acute and chronic experimental demyelinating lesions. AJNR 1988;9:643.
27. Grossman RI, Gonzalez-Scarano F, Atlas SW, et al. Multiple sclerosis: gadolinium enhancement in MR imaging. Radiology 1986;161:721.
28. Gonzalez-Scarano F, Grossman RI, Galetta S, et al. Multiple sclerosis disease activity correlates with gadolinium-enhanced magnetic resonance imaging. Ann Neurol 1987;21:300.
29. Grossman RI, Braffman BH, Brorson JR, et al. Multiple sclerosis: serial study of gadolinium-enhanced MR imaging. Radiology 1988;169:117.
30. Miller DH, Rudge P, Johnson G, et al. Serial gadolinium-enhanced magnetic resonance imaging in multiple sclerosis. Brain 1988;111:927.
31. Kermode AG, Tofts PS, MacManus DG, et al. Quantitative dynamic Gd-DTPA-enhanced MRI (QDEM) in multiple sclerosis. SMRI 1989: 7th Annual Meeting Program and Abstracts, 518.
32. Maravilla KR, Weinreb JC, Suss R, et al. Magnetic resonance demonstration of multiple sclerosis plaques in the cervical cord. AJR 1985;144:381.

33. Edwards MK, Farlow MR, Stevens JC. Cranial MR in spinal cord MS: diagnosing patients with isolated spinal cord symptoms. AJNR 1986;7:1003.
34. Riikonen R, Ketonen L, Sipponen J. Magnetic resonance imaging, evoked responses and cerebrospinal fluid findings in a follow-up study of children with optic neuritis. Acta Neurol Scand 1988;77:44.
35. Leys D, Petit H, Block AM, et al. Devic's optic neuromyelitis. 4 cases. Rev Neurol (Paris) 1987;143:722.
36. Guthoff R, Terwey B, Bragelmann L, et al. Role of nuclear magnetic resonance imaging in the diagnosis of monosymptomatic optic neuritis. Klin Monatsbl Augenheilkd 1988;192:311.
37. Rudick RA, Jacobs L, Kinkel PR, et al. Isolated idiopathic optic neuritis. Analysis of free kappa-light chains in cerebrospinal fluid and correlation with nuclear magnetic resonance findings. Arch Neurol 1986;43:456.
38. Riikonen R, Donner M, Erkkila H. Optic neuritis in children and its relationship to multiple sclerosis: a clinical study of 21 children. Dev Med Child Neurol 1988;30:349.
39. Miller DH, Newton MR, van der Poel JC, et al. Magnetic resonance imaging of the optic nerve in optic neuritis. Neurology 1988;38:175.
40. Miller DH, et al. MR brain scanning in patients with vasculitis: differentiation from multiple sclerosis. Neuroradiology 1987;29:226.
41. Braffman BH, Zimmerman RA, Trojanowski JQ, et al. Brain MR: pathologic correlation with gross and histopathology. 2. Hyperintense white-matter foci in the elderly. AJR 1988;151:559.
42. Awad IA, Spetzler RF, et al. Incidental subcortical lesions identified on magnetic resonance imaging in the elderly. I. Correlation with age and cerebrovascular risk factors. Stroke 1986;17:1084.
43. Awad IA, Johnson PC, et al. Incidental subcortical lesions identified on magnetic resonance imaging in the elderly. II. Postmortem pathological correlations. Stroke 1986;17:1090.
44. Bradley WG, et al. Patchy, periventricular white matter lesions in the elderly: a common observation during NMR imaging. Noninv Med Imaging 1984;1:35.
45. Brant-Zawadzki M, et al. MR imaging of the aging brain: patchy white-matter lesions and dementia. AJR 1985;6:675.
46. Braffman BH, Zimmerman RA, Trojanowski JQ, et al. Brain MR: pathologic correlation with gross and histopathology. 1. Lacunar infarction and Virchow-Robin spaces. AJR 1988;151:551.
47. Marshall VG, Bradley WB, Marshall CE, et al. Deep white matter infarction: correlation of MR imaging and histopathologic findings. Radiology 1988;167:517.
48. Kirkpatrick JB, Hayman LA. White matter lesions in MR imaging clinically healthy brains of elderly subjects: possible pathologic basis. Radiology 1987;162:509.
49. Drayer BF: Imaging of the aging brain. Part I. Normal findings and Part II. Pathologic conditions. Radiology 1988;166:785.
50. Vermess M, et al. Nuclear magnetic resonance (NMR) imaging of the brain in systemic lupus erythematosus. JCAT 1983;73:461.
51. Jacobs L, Kinkel PR, Costello PB, et al. Central nervous system lupus erythematosus: the value of magnetic resonance imaging. J Rheumatol 1988;15:601.
52. Aisen AM, Gabrielsen TO, McCune WJ. MR imaging of systemic lupus erythematosus involving the brain. AJR 1985;144:1027.
53. McCune WJ, MacGuire A, Aisen A, et al. Identification of brain lesions in neuropsychiatric systemic lupus erythematosus by magnetic resonance scanning. Arthritis Rheum 1988;31:159.
54. Zimmerman RD, Fleming CA, Lee BC, et al. Periventricular hyperintensity as seen by magnetic resonance: prevalence and significance. AJR 1986;146:443.
55. Grossman RI, Hecht-Leavitt CM, Evans SM, et al. Experimental radiation injury: combined MR imaging and spectroscopy. Radiology 1988;169:305.
56. Hecht-Leavitt C, Grossman RI, Curran WJ, et al. MR of brain radiation injury: experimental studies in cats. AJNR 1987;8:427.
57. Curnes JT, Laster DW, Ball MR, et al. Magnetic resonance imaging of radiation injury to the brain. AJR 1986;147:119.
58. Tsuruda JS, Kortman KE, Bradley WG, et al. Radiation effects on cerebral white matter: MR evaluation. AJR 1987;149:165.
59. Curran WJ, Hecht-Leavitt C, Schut L, et al. Magnetic resonance imaging of cranial radiation lesions. Int J Radiat Oncol Biol Phys 1987;13:1093.
60. Constine LS, Konski A, Ekholm S, et al. Adverse effects of brain irradiation correlated with MR and CT imaging. Int J Radiat Oncol Biol Phys 1988;15:319.
61. Dooms GC, Hecht S, Brandt-Zawadzki, et al. Brain radiation lesions: MR imaging. Radiology 1986;158:149.
62. Zimmerman RA, et al. Intracranial infection. In: Brant-Zawadski M, Norman D, eds. MRI of the central nervous system. New York: Raven Press, 1987.
63. Davidson HD, et al. Magnetic resonance imaging in infections of the central nervous system. AJNR 1985;6:499.
64. Runge VM, Clanton JA, Price AC, et al. Evaluation of contrast-enhanced MR imaging in a brain-abscess model. AJNR 1985;6:139.
65. Schroth G, Kretzschmar K, Gawehn J, et al. Advantage of magnetic resonance imaging in the diagnosis of cerebral infections. Neuroradiology 1987;29:120.
66. Dun V, Bale JF, Zimmerman RA, et al. MRI in children with postinfectious disseminated encephalomyelitis. Magn Reson Imag 1986;4:25.
67. Atlas SW, Grossman RI, Goldberg HI, et al. MR diagnosis of acute disseminated encephalomyelitis. J Comput Assist Tomogr 1986;10:798.
68. Lester JW, Carter MP, Reynolds TL. Herpes encephalitis: MR monitoring of response to acyclovir therapy. J Comput Assist Tomogr 1988;12:941.
69. Henkes H, Schoerner W, Sander B, et al. MR imaging of the meninges. SMRI 1989: 7th Annual Meeting Program and Abstracts, 108.
70. Mathews VP, Kuharik MA, Edwards MK, et al. Dyke Award. Gd-DTPA-enhanced MR imaging of experimental bacterial meningitis: evaluation and comparison with CT. AJNR 1988;9:1045.
71. Burke JW, Podrasky AE, Bradley WG. Meningeal enhancement by Gd DTPA in postoperative brain MR imaging. SMRI 1989: 7th Annual Meeting Program and Abstracts, 107.
72. Frank JA, Girton M, Dwyer AJ, et al. Meningeal carcinomatosis in the VX2 rabbit tumor model: detection with Gd DTPA-enhanced MR imaging. Radiology 1988;167:825.
73. Miller DH, Kendall BE, Barter S, et al. Magnetic resonance imaging in central nervous system sarcoidosis. Neurology 1988;38:378.
74. Ramsey RG, Geremia GK. CNS complications of AIDS: CT and MR findings. AJR 1988;151:449.
75. Post MJ, Sheldon JJ, Hensley GT, et al. Central nervous system disease in acquired immunodeficiency syndrome: prospective correlation using CT, MR imaging, and pathologic studies. Radiology 1986;158:141.
76. Post MJ, Tate LG, Quencer RM, et al. CT, MR, and pathology in HIV encephalitis and meningitis. AJR 1988;151:373.
77. Henkes H, Schoerner W, Bittner R, et al. Gd-DTPA-enhanced MRI in inflammatory brain disease. SMRI 1989: 7th Annual Meeting Program and Abstracts, 105.
78. Jarvik J, Hesselink JR, Kennedy C, et al. Acquired immunodeficiency syndrome. Magnetic resonance patterns of brain involvement with pathologic correlation. Arch Neurol 1988;45:731.
79. Gill PS, Graham RA, Boswell W, et al. A comparison of imaging, clinical, and pathologic aspects of space-occupying lesions within the brain in patients with acquired immune deficiency syndrome. Am J Physiol Imag 1986;1:134.
80. Olsen WL, Longo FM, Mills CM, et al. White matter disease in AIDS: findings at MR imaging. Radiology 1988;169:445.
81. Guilleux MH, Steiner RE, Young IR. MR imaging in progressive multifocal leukoencephalopathy. AJNR 1986;7:1033.

2

Brain: Vascular Disease

Bert R. Carollo
Val M. Runge

Diseases of the cerebrovascular system are the most common cause of pathology affecting the brain. Structural vascular anomalies, which include aneurysms and vascular malformations, and vascular disease causing cerebral ischemia or infarction comprise the major pathologic subgroups of cerebrovascular disease. Cerebrovascular disease is often heralded by intracranial hemorrhage.

Magnetic resonance imaging (MRI) has emerged as a sensitive modality for evaluating hemorrhage, vascular anomalies, and cerebral infarction. The noninvasive MR examination often obviates the need for other imaging modalities, including invasive angiography. This chapter will initially focus on the MR principles of intracranial hemorrhage and the appearance of intra-axial and extra-axial hemorrhage. Then the two major subgroups of cerebrovascular disease, vascular anomalies and cerebral ischemia, will be considered.

HEMORRHAGE

MRI provides exquisite identification of intracranial hemorrhage in its various stages. Compared with computerized tomography (CT), in which identifying hemorrhage depends upon x-ray attenuation, clinical MR images protons and the effects of other substances on the behavior of these protons. Understanding the MR appearance of hemorrhage requires a knowledge of how different forms of blood affect the local proton environment. Relaxation time (TR), echo time (TE), field strength, imaging sequence, oxygen tension, rate of clot formation, and the integrity of the blood-brain barrier and the red blood cell membrane also affect the MRI appearance of hemorrhage.[1-4] The evolving hemorrhage follows an orderly progression of changes, although the exact timing of these changes is variable. For these reasons, intracranial hemorrhage often has a confusing appearance.

PROTON RELAXATION ENHANCEMENT

To understand the effects of different forms of hemoglobin on the proton environment after hemorrhage, proton relaxation enhancement (PRE) must be considered.

A single proton composes the nucleus of each hydrogen atom in a water molecule. This unpaired proton possesses angular momentum or spin, producing a magnetic moment, which is a vector quantity with direction and magnitude that defines a magnetic dipole. The resulting magnetic field surrounds the nucleus (proton) and is analogous to a microscopic bar magnet. The interactions between the magnetic dipoles of protons in water molecules are called proton-proton dipole-dipole interactions.[1,2]

The hydrogen nuclei that form the basis for MRI are in constant motion, which is characterized by rotational, translational, and vibrational components.[5,6] In pure water, T1 and T2 relaxation occurs by proton-proton dipole-dipole interactions among water molecules. These interactions are proportional to the frequency of motion of water molecules. Because water is a small molecule with a high frequency of motion compared with the Larmour frequency used for MRI, in pure water there is inefficient T1 and T2 relaxation, resulting in long T1 and T2 relaxation times. A long T1 relaxation time (the characteristic time constant for

* The author gratefully acknowledges Dr. Robert I. Grossman, University of Pennsylvania, for his review of the chapter.

spins to align with the external magnetic field) yields low signal intensity on images with relative T1 weighting (i.e., short relaxation time [TR], short echo time [TE]). A long T2 relaxation time (the characteristic time constant for loss of transverse magnetization or equivalently loss of phase coherence among spins) yields high signal intensity on images with relative T2 weighting (i.e., long TR, long TE).

Many of the breakdown products of hemoglobin are paramagnetic substances, which have unpaired electrons. An unpaired electron is the dominant factor in a magnetic moment created by a proton (positive charge) and an electron (negative charge). An electron has a mass equal to 1/1000th of the mass of a proton, and it therefore has a magnetic moment 1000 times that of a proton.[2] The addition of a paramagnetic substance to water or to a proton environment can change the predominant proton relaxation mechanism from a proton-proton dipole-dipole interaction to a proton-electron dipole-dipole interaction. For a proton-electron dipole-dipole interaction to occur, the proton of the water molecule must approach within 3 angstroms of the paramagnetic center (unpaired electrons). If this occurs, the frequency of motion of water decreases (e.g., a bulkier complex is formed), which yields a more efficient energy transfer (relaxation) and shortens both T1 and T2 relaxation times.[1,6,7] This process is called proton-electron dipole-dipole proton relaxation enhancement (PEDD PRE).

A paramagnetic substance, such as a component of hemorrhage, can be confined within a red blood cell by the red blood cell membrane and have a heterogeneous distribution. If there is a heterogeneous distribution of the paramagnetic substance and the protons of water molecules cannot approach within 3 angstroms of the paramagnetic center, a proton-electron dipole-dipole interaction cannot occur. A higher intracellular concentration of the paramagnetic substance causes local magnetic inhomogeneity. The precession rate of water molecules (Larmour frequency) is proportional to the local field strength, and the local field strength varies with local magnetic inhomogeneity.[2,7,8] Water protons diffusing through this local magnetic inhomogeneity precess at different rates and lose coherence.[3,7] These dephased protons cannot be refocused by the 180° spin echo pulse, and transverse phase coherence is lost. This causes a shorter transverse relaxation time (T2), without affecting T1. This process is called preferential T2 proton relaxation enhancement (T2 PRE).[7] T2 PRE is proportional to the square of the magnetic field and therefore is more pronounced at higher field strengths.[2,3,7,8] T2 PRE is also proportional to the square of the concentration of the paramagnetic substance and is increased by lengthening the interecho interval (i.e., the time between the 180° refocusing pulses in a spin echo sequence).[2,3,7,8] Lengthening the interecho interval allows the diffusing water molecules to encounter greater local magnetic inhomogeneity, which increases dephasing and further shortens T2 (Fig. 2–1).

THE MR APPEARANCE OF HEMORRHAGE

Using knowledge about PRE, it is possible to predict the appearance of hemorrhage on standard spin echo sequences. Hemorrhage is composed of different forms of the hemoglobin molecule, some of which are paramagnetic. As a hemorrhage ages, the hemoglobin molecule undergoes the following degradation pattern: oxyhemoglobin to deoxyhemoglobin to methemoglobin to hemosiderin (Table 2–1).

Before describing each of these forms of hemoglobin, a brief discussion of standard MR terminology is appropriate. Sequences with relative T1 weighting (i.e., short TR, short TE) are called T1-weighted images. Sequences with relative T2 weighting (i.e., long TR, long TE) are called T2-weighted images. Long TR, short TE sequences are called proton density images. Even though a sequence is "T1-weighted" or "T2-weighted," it is composed of both T1 and T2 effects, and either effect may predominate and yield a particular signal intensity on a given image.[9] Cranial

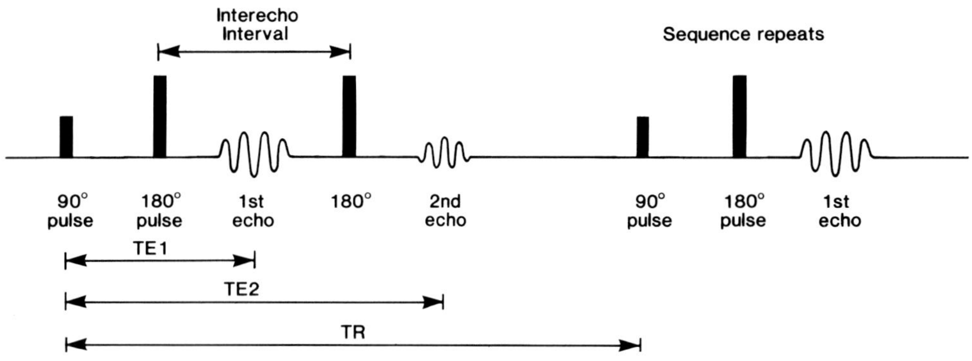

FIGURE 2–1. Double echo spin-echo MR sequence consisting of a 90° pulse followed by two 180° refocusing pulses. The interecho interval is the time between the 180° pulses. The interecho interval can be increased by decreasing TE1 or by increasing TE2.

Table 2–1

HEMOGLOBIN DEGRADATION PATTERNS					
CHARACTERISTICS	***Oxyhemoglobin***	***Deoxyhemoglobin***	***Methemoglobin***		***Hemosiderin***
Compartment	Intracellular	Intracellular	Intracellular	Extracellular	Intralysosomal
Water solubility	+	+	+	+	–
Iron state	Ferrous (Fe^{+2})	Ferrous (Fe^{+2})	Ferric (Fe^{+3})	Ferric (Fe^{+3})	Ferric (Fe^{+3})
Number of unpaired electrons	0	4	5	5	~10,000
Magnetism	Diamagnetic	Paramagnetic	Paramagnetic	Paramagnetic	Paramagnetic
PEDD PRE	–	–	+	+	–
T2 PRE	–	+	+	–	+
Effect on relaxation times					
T1	Increased T1		Decreased T1	Decreased T1	
T2	Increased T2	Decreased T2	Decreased T2	Decreased T2*	Decreased T2
Signal Characteristics					
T1-weighted image (short TR, short TE)	Low or isointense	Low or isointense	High	High	Low or isointense
Proton density weighted image (long TR, short TE)	Isointense or high	Low	High or isointense	High	Low
T2 weighted image (long TR, long TE)	High	Very low	Very low	High	Very low

PEDD PRE, Proton-electron dipole-dipole proton relaxation enhancement;
T2 PRE, preferential T2 proton relaxation enhancement.
* Proton density and T1 effects predominate, causing high signal intensity on long TR images.

lesions are described as hypointense (i.e., low signal intensity), isointense (i.e., similar signal intensity), or hyperintense (i.e., high signal intensity). On T1-weighted images, cranial lesions are compared with gray matter as a reference. On T2-weighted images, cranial lesions are compared with white matter as a reference.

Oxyhemoglobin

A simple intraparenchymal hemorrhage initially is composed of intact red blood cells containing oxygenated hemoglobin. Oxyhemoglobin contains iron in the ferrous state (Fe^{+2}) and has no unpaired electrons.[8] Oxyhemoglobin is not paramagnetic and is classified as a diamagnetic substance, which produces essentially no magnetic moment.[3,6,8] Therefore, there is no PRE. The hyperacute hematoma containing oxyhemoglobin exhibits prolongation of T1 and T2 relaxation times and is hypointense or isointense on T1-weighted images and high signal intensity on T2-weighted images. This is the expected MR appearance of a protein-containing fluid (Fig. 2–2). Oxyhemoglobin is often isointense with other intracranial mass lesions.[6] Fortunately, the intra-axial oxyhemoglobin lasts only a few hours, and it is uncommon to visualize only oxyhemoglobin within an intraparenchymal hemorrhage. However, the poor discrimination of oxyhemoglobin accounts for the limited detection of acute subarachnoid hemorrhage by MR.

Deoxyhemoglobin

Within the next few hours, the red blood cells forming the hemorrhage become desaturated, and oxyhemoglobin is converted to deoxyhemoglobin. Iron remains in the ferrous state (Fe^{+2}) in the deoxyhemoglobin molecule, but there are four unpaired electrons, making deoxyhemoglobin paramagnetic.[2,6–8] Intracellular deoxyhemoglobin is confined by the red blood cell membrane and is heterogeneously distributed. Water protons cannot approach within 3 angstroms of the paramagnetic center of deoxyhemoglobin, probably because of a slight change in the configuration of the hemoglobin molecule.[10] Preferential T2 PRE shortens T2 but not T1. As a result, intracellular deoxyhemoglobin is slightly hypointense or isointense on T1-weighted images and has low signal intensity on T2-weighted images (Fig. 2–3). The low signal intensity on T2-weighted images becomes more pronounced with increasing field strength, increasing the interecho interval (i.e., diffusion effects), and increasing the amount of the paramagnetic substance.

Methemoglobin

The intracellular deoxyhemoglobin within the hemorrhage is oxidized to methemoglobin. This process depends on the partial pressure of oxygen.[6,11] The rate of oxidation is maximal at a Po_2 of about 20 and de-

(text continues on page 52)

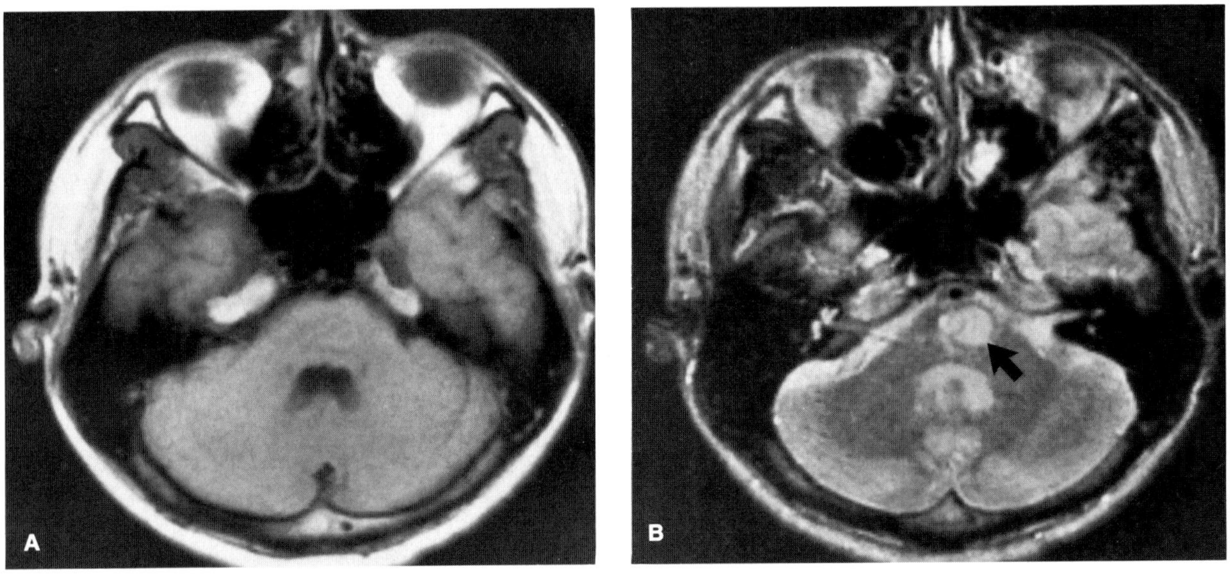

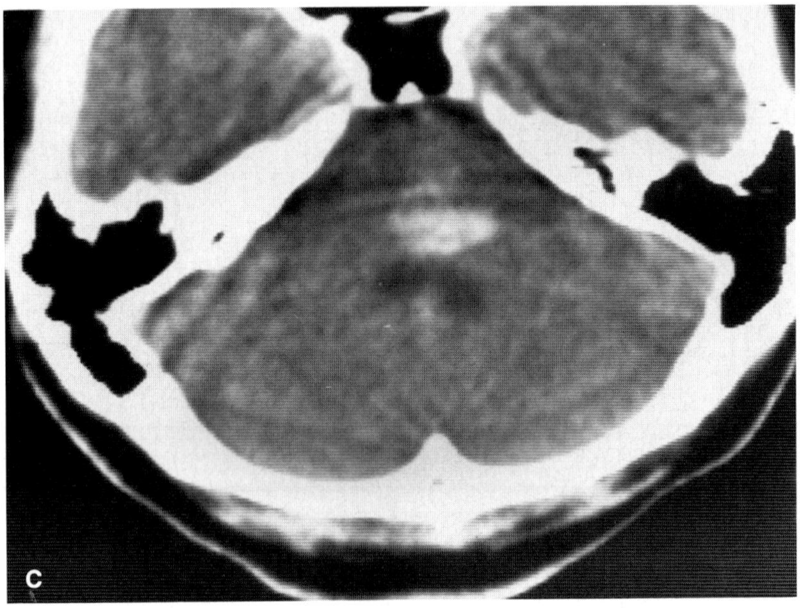

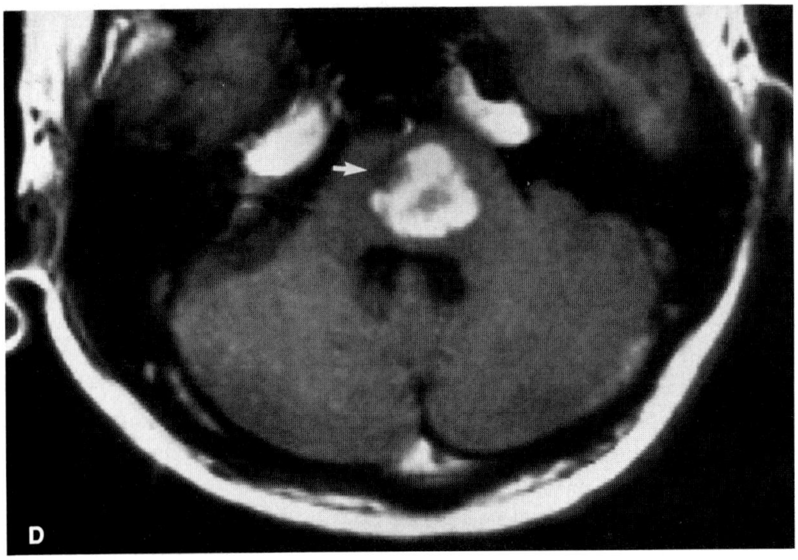

FIGURE 2–2. A 26-year-old Oriental man with an acute pontine hemorrhage. **(A)** Axial T1-weighted image (TR/TE = 600/30) and **(B)** axial T2-weighted image (TR/TE = 3000/80); 0.35 Tesla system. **(D,F)** Axial T1-weighted images (TR/TE = 650/20) and **(E,G)** axial T2-weighted images (TR/TE = 3000/90); 1.0 Tesla system. The initial MR images **(A,B)** demonstrate a focal area of increased signal intensity involving the pons at the level of the middle cerebellar peduncles (arrow). Differential diagnosis included neoplasm, demyelination, or hyperacute hemorrhage. A noninfused axial CT **(C)** through this level 5 days later demonstrates increased density compatible with acute hemorrhage. Nine days after the initial MR scans, the patient's clinical condition deteriorated. A repeat scan through the level of the middle cerebellar peduncles **(D,E)** demonstrates a subacute hematoma, which displaced the fourth ventricle posteriorly. Intracellular methemoglobin constitutes the posterior portion and extracellular methemoglobin forms the anterior portion of this hematoma. A hemosiderin rim (open arrow) has started to form, and edema (closed arrows) surrounds the hematoma. Images through the medulla **(F,G)** demonstrates a new component of acute hemorrhage. Hyperintense intracellular methemoglobin forms the peripheral margin of the hematoma on the T1-weighted image **(F)**. There is deoxyhemoglobin centrally, and edema (arrows) surrounds the hematoma.

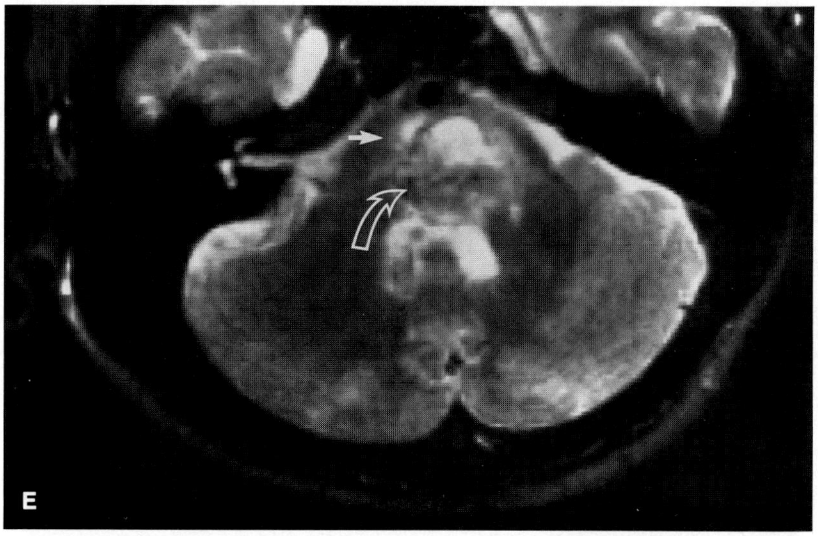

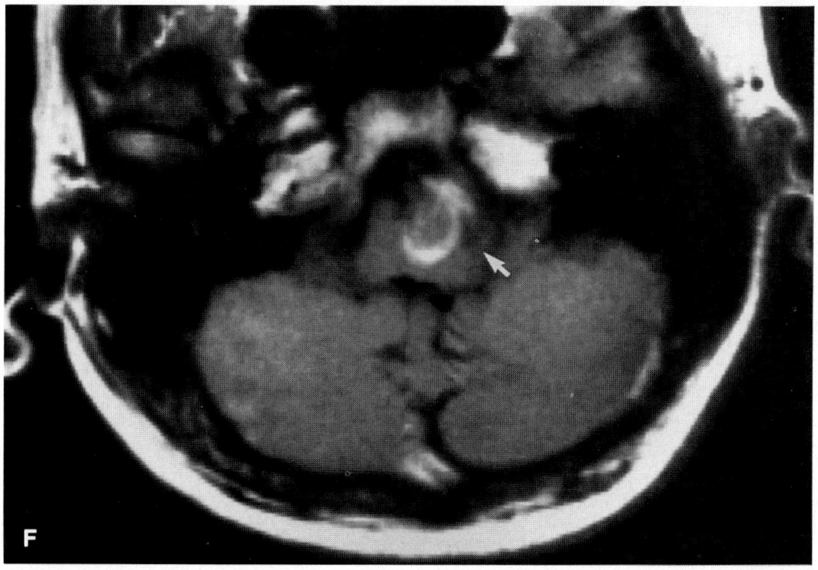

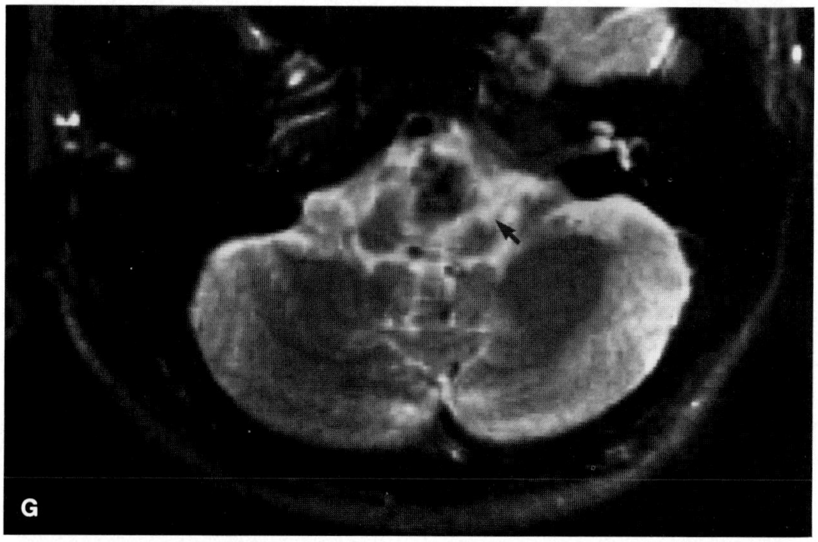

FIGURE 2–2. (Continued)

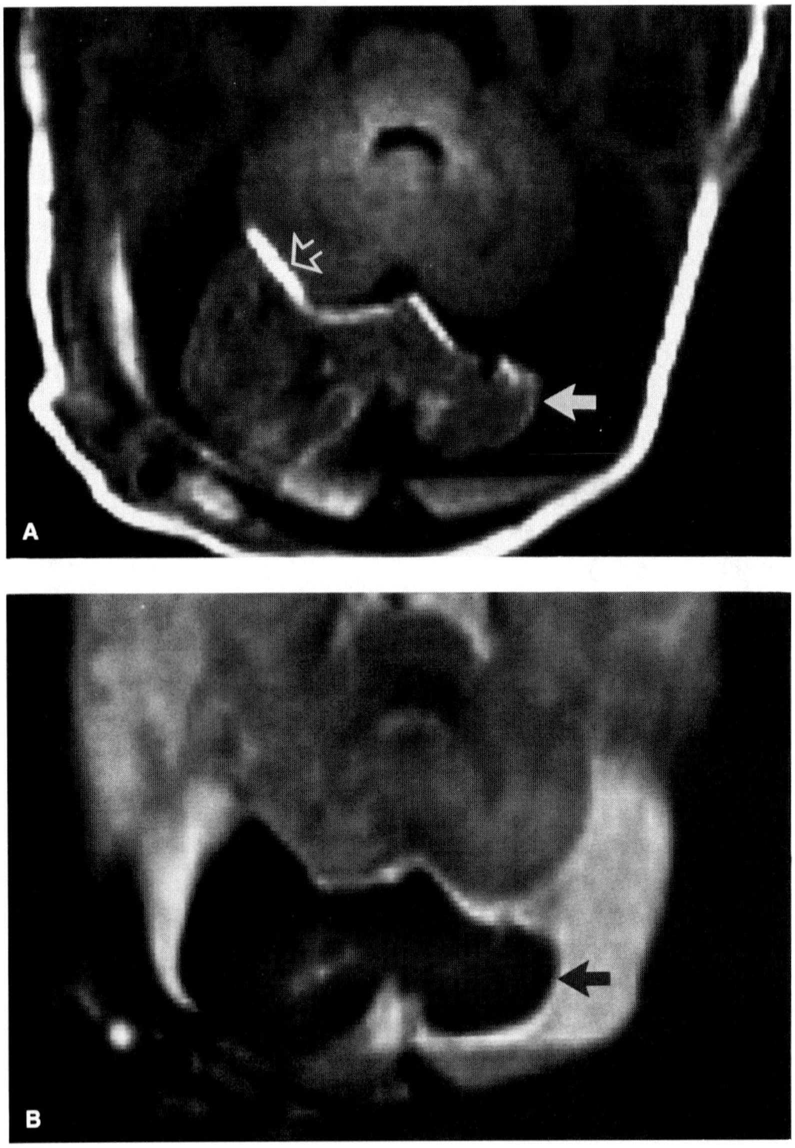

FIGURE 2–3. A 14-day-old boy with surgical drainage of a retrocerebellar cyst shown on an **(A)** axial T1-weighted image (TR/TE = 650/20) and **(B)** axial T2-weighted image (TR/TE = 3000/90). Deoxyhemoglobin fills the extra-axial retrocerebellar cyst (closed arrows). The bright thin rim (open arrow) on the T1-weighted image represents intracellular methemoglobin.

creases significantly at very low or very high oxygen tensions.[6,8,11] These factors result in a variable temporal formation of methemoglobin, which typically is identified at about 2 to 14 days.

In the formation of methemoglobin, the heme iron is oxidized to the ferric state (Fe^{+3}). Methemoglobin has five unpaired electrons and is highly paramagnetic.[2,5–7,12] The molecular configuration of methemoglobin allows the water protons to approach within 3 angstroms of the protein's paramagnetic center. A proton-electron dipole-dipole interaction shortens both T1 and T2. The heterogeneous distribution of methemoglobin in the intracellular state accentuates T2 relaxation (T2 PRE), causing intracellular methemoglobin to appear as high signal intensity on T1-weighted images and low signal intensity on T2-weighted images (Fig. 2–4).

Soon after methemoglobin forms within the red blood cell, glucose reserves become depleted, which causes a loss of red blood cell membrane integrity, increased permeability, and lysis. Extracellular (free) methemoglobin accumulates in the hematoma cavity, and the distribution of methemoglobin is no longer heterogeneous (i.e., partitioned by a red blood cell membrane), causing a loss of T2 PRE.[2,3,12] With red blood cell lysis, extracellular methemoglobin produces PEDD PRE, which decreases T1 relaxation times.[3,12] Therefore, extracellular methemoglobin is typically high in signal intensity on T1-weighted images.

The signal intensity of extracellular methemoglobin on T1-weighted images is also affected by concentration (i.e., dilutional effects). The signal intensities of various dilutions of free methemoglobin can vary from hyperintense to hypointense on a given T1-weighted image.[12] As free methemoglobin is progres-

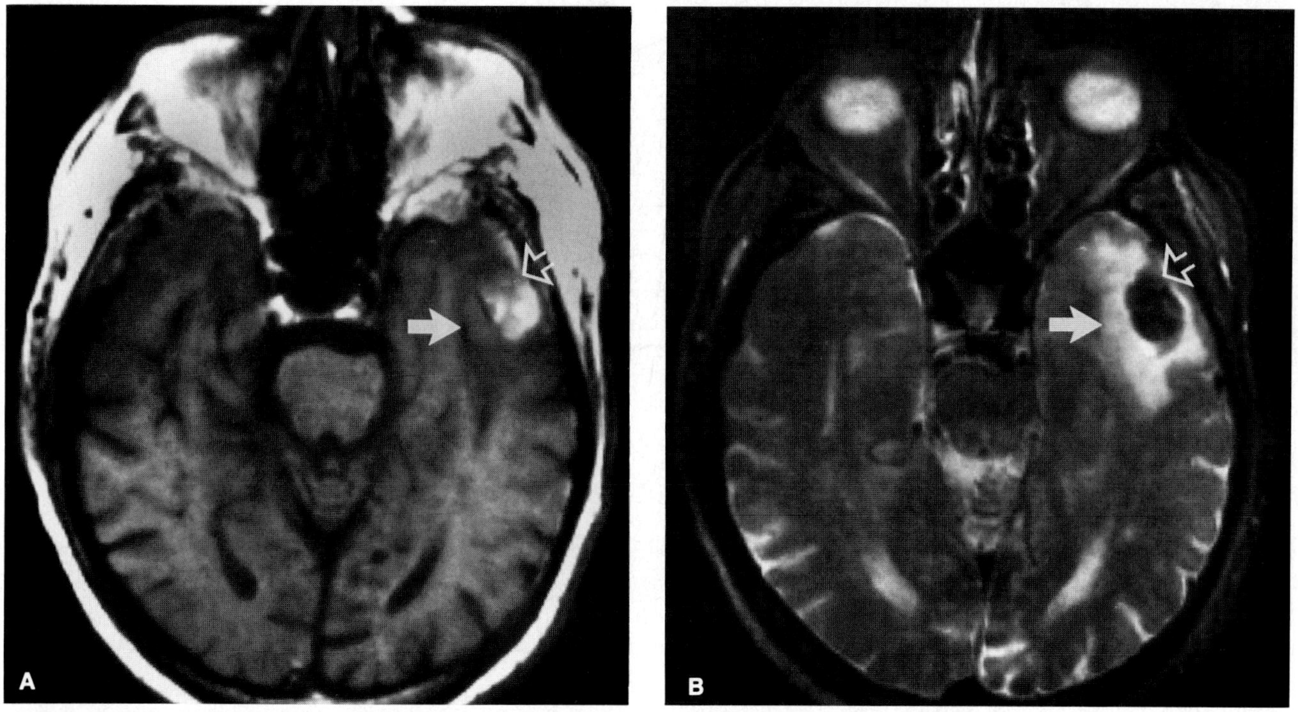

FIGURE 2–4. A 71-year-old man with an acute-subacute left temporal hematoma shown on an **(A)** axial T1-weighted image (TR/TE = 650/20) and an **(B)** axial T2-weighted image (TR/TE = 3000/90). Edema (solid arrows) surrounds a left temporal hematoma. The hematoma is anteriorly composed of deoxyhemoglobin (open arrows). The remainder of the hematoma is composed of intracellular methemoglobin.

sively diluted, it loses its PEDD PRE, and its proton density and signal characteristics approach those of cerebrospinal fluid (CSF).[12] This dilute solution of free methemoglobin has high proton density.[8,9,12] The T1 shortening and effects of the high proton density of free methemoglobin overwhelm the T2 shortening produced by the PEDD interaction. Therefore, on proton density and T2-weighted images, extracellular methemoglobin appears as high signal intensity. As methemoglobin is resorbed, a protein-containing fluid is formed, and actual prolongation of T2 occurs, which also accounts for increased signal intensity on T2-weighted images.[13] In review, red blood cell lysis yields extracellular methemoglobin, which is typically high in signal intensity on both T1-weighted and T2-weighted images (Fig. 2–5).

Hemosiderin

Extracellular methemoglobin is oxidized to a series of compounds called hemichromes, which are degraded into hemosiderin. Hemosiderin is phagocytized and accumulates in the lysosomes of macrophages. Hemosiderin contains iron in the ferric state (Fe^{+3}) and is strongly paramagnetic.[2,6–8] Hemosiderin is insoluble in water and, therefore, no dipole-dipole interaction occurs. However, because hemosiderin has an inhomogeneous distribution, T2 PRE causes a low signal intensity on T2-weighted images.[7] This strong T2 effect may be appreciated as slightly low signal intensity on T1-weighted images.

Hemosiderin (iron) and other paramagnetic substances can often be distinguished from calcium because their T2 PRE effects are proportional to the interecho interval and the TE of the second echo. Hemosiderin is slightly low in signal intensity on T1-weighted images, moderately low in signal intensity on the first echo of T2 (i.e., long TR, short TE), and very low in signal intensity on the second echo of T2 (i.e., long TR, long TE). Thus, there is an orderly progression in the loss of signal intensity if the T1-weighted image, the first echo of T2, and the second echo of T2 are compared (Fig. 2–5). Calcium has no mobile protons and does not change in signal intensity on T1-weighted, proton density, or T2-weighted images. However, calcium is sometimes mixed with hemosiderin, and the iron in the mixture produces a T2 PRE effect. Because T2 PRE is proportional to the square of field strength, these effects are most pronounced at higher field strengths ($\geq$1.0T).

Hemosiderin can persist indefinitely in a lesion with an intact blood-brain barrier and is a landmark for identifying chronic hemorrhage. However, in lesions without an intact blood-brain barrier, the hemo-

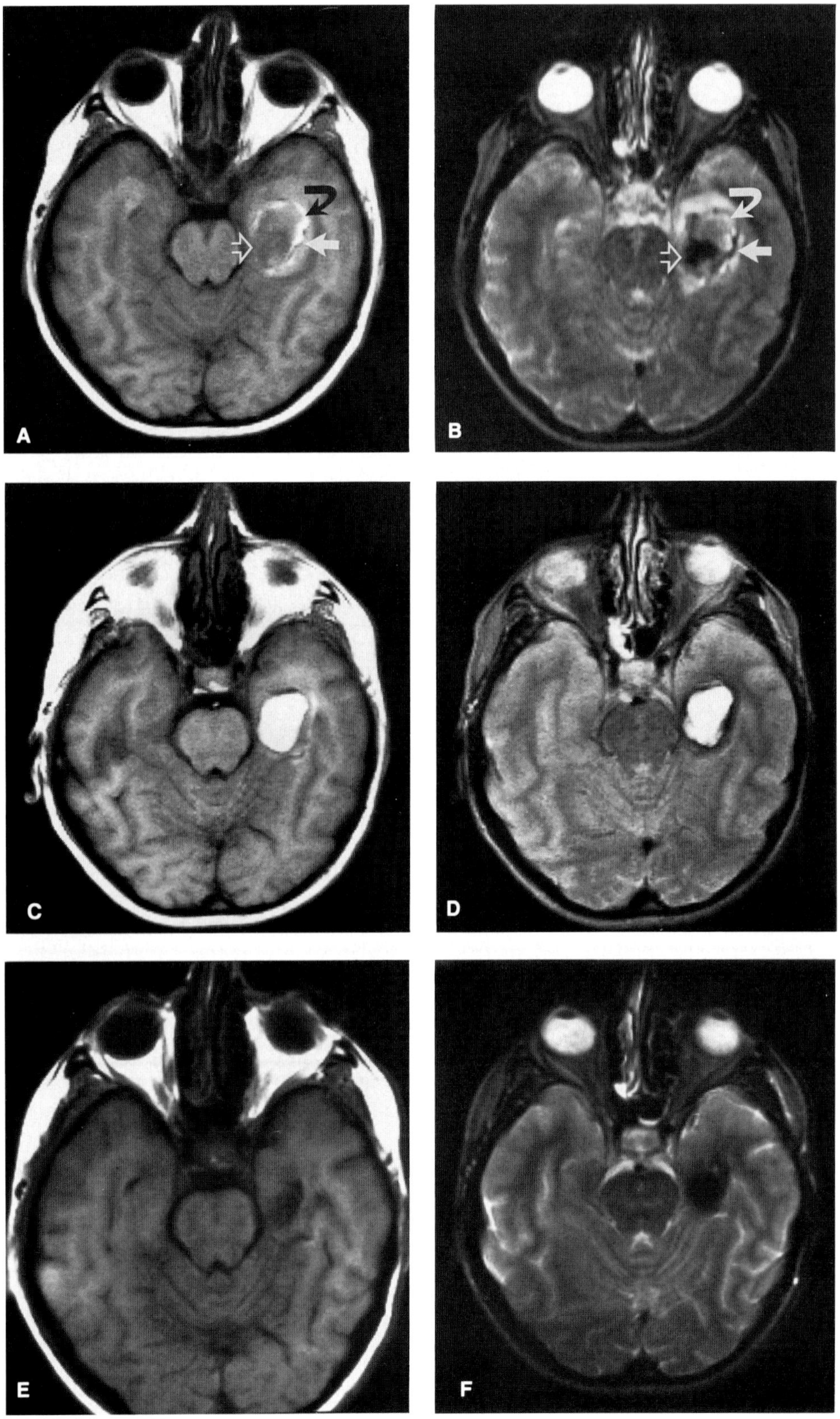

FIGURE 2–5. Resolution of a left medial temporal hematoma in a 32-year-old woman is demonstrated in **(A,C,E)** axial T1-weighted images and **(B,D,F)** axial T2-weighted images. The initial MR images **(A,B)** demonstrate an acute left medial temporal hematoma. Deoxyhemoglobin forms the posterior component of this hematoma (open arrows), and a hyperintense rim of extracellular methemoglobin (curved arrows) marginates the anterior component. Dilute free methemoglobin forms the central portion of this anterior component. A hemosiderin rim (closed arrows) has started to form, and edema surrounds the hematoma. Two months later, a repeat MRI examination was performed **(C,D)**. The hematoma was hyperintense on both T1- and T2-weighted images, compatible with extracellular methemoglobin. A hemosiderin rim surrounds the hematoma and was more pronounced on the T2-weighted image **(D)**. The surrounding edema has resolved. Twenty months after the initial scans, a follow-up examination was performed **(E,F)**. A residual hemosiderin cleft was identified in the left medial temporal region. The residual hemosiderin was more evident on the T2-weighted image **(F)**, an effect caused by the preferential T2 PRE.

siderin-laden macrophages have access to the bloodstream, and the hemosiderin is reabsorbed.[8] The configuration of the hemosiderin rim can be an important feature in differentiating a simple intraparenchymal hematoma from intratumoral hemorrhage. In hemorrhage associated with neoplasm, hemosiderin deposition is discontinuous or inconspicuous because the blood-brain barrier is not intact. In a simple intraparenchymal hematoma, the hemosiderin rim is characteristically well-defined and continuous.

INTRACEREBRAL HEMATOMA

The evolution of an intraparenchymal hematoma is depicted by a characteristic sequence of MRI changes. These changes depend on many factors, including size, compartmentalization, oxygen tension, and blood-brain barrier integrity. Therefore, the staging of intracerebral hematomas is not rigid. For example, several components of hemoglobin can be seen concurrently within a large hematoma. Although the timing and appearance of these changes is variable, a temporal sequence of changes can be described that provides a conceptual framework for identifying the stages of an intracerebral hematoma.[5,6,8,14] Four stages in the evolving hematoma can be described: hyperacute (first few hours), acute (first few hours to 2 days), subacute (2 days to 4 weeks), and chronic (>4 weeks).

In the hyperacute stage, a simple intraparenchymal hematoma is composed of a mixture of oxyhemoglobin and deoxyhemoglobin. The formation of deoxyhemoglobin depends on the local oxygen tension.[3,6] For example, hemorrhagic cortical infarcts are in a high local oxygen environment (i.e., arterial perfusion), and the formation of deoxyhemoglobin may be retarded, but in hemorrhagic venous infarction or in a large intraparenchymal hematoma, the oxygen tension is lower and deoxyhemoglobin predominates. In a hyperacute intraparenchymal hematoma in which oxyhemoglobin predominates, the hematoma is characterized by a hypointense or isointense lesion relative to gray matter on T1-weighted images and a hyperintense lesion relative to white matter on T2-weighted images (Fig. 2-2). This hyperacute intraparenchymal hematoma containing oxyhemoglobin is indistinguishable from other intracranial mass lesions, and its signal may be nearly isointense with CSF. Fortunately, this hyperacute stage is not commonly imaged, but because oxyhemoglobin can have signal intensities similar to other lesions, an inaccurate characterization of the lesion could result. CT is more accurate in detecting this hyperacute hematoma stage.[5,6]

Generally, within the first few hours of the formation of a hematoma, oxyhemoglobin is converted into deoxyhemoglobin, which corresponds to the acute stage. The acute intraparenchymal hematoma containing deoxyhemoglobin within intact red blood cells is characterized by a slightly hypointense or isointense lesion on T1-weighted images and a hypointense lesion on T2-weighted images. The degree of hypointensity on images with relative T2 weighting increases with the increasing field strength (i.e., proportional to the square of the applied field strength). Consequently, on low-field-strength systems, an acute hematoma can be nearly isointense with the brain on T2-weighted images.

Acute hemorrhage is surrounded by extracellular water, which initially is serum extruded by the retracting clot and later is edema fluid.[2] This increased water content causes a low-intensity margin on T1-weighted images and a high-intensity margin on T2-weighted images (Fig. 2-5).

During the subacute stage, intracellular deoxyhemoglobin is oxidized to intracellular methemoglobin, a process that particularly depends on the local oxygen tension.[6,11] The formation of intracellular methemoglobin begins at the periphery of the hematoma, where the conditions for its formation are optimal, and progresses inwards toward the center of the hematoma.[7] Intracellular methemoglobin results in a hyperintense periphery of a hematoma on T1-weighted images and a hypointense periphery of the hematoma on T2-weighted images, which progress centrally as deoxyhemoglobin is oxidized. On T1-weighted images, the subacute hematoma could have a low-intensity surrounding margin (i.e., reactive edema), a hyperintense periphery (i.e., intracellular methemoglobin), and a hypointense or isointense center (i.e., intracellular deoxyhemoglobin). The corresponding appearance on T2-weighted images is a high-intensity surrounding margin, a low-intensity periphery, and a hypointense center of the hematoma. With time, the entire hematoma fills in (i.e., intracellular methemoglobin) and demonstrates a high signal intensity on T1-weighted images.

After 1 week to 1 month, red blood cell lysis occurs, and intracellular methemoglobin becomes extracellular. This typically causes high signal intensity within the hematoma, corresponding to free methemoglobin on both T1-weighted and T2-weighted images. Because of dilutional effects, the signal of dilute free methemoglobin in the central portion of a hematoma can be low or isointense on T1-weighted images.[12] The typical change in the appearance of the hematoma after red blood cell lysis with the formation of free methemoglobin, compared with the hematoma containing intracellular methemoglobin, is that T2-weighted images demonstrate high signal intensity.

At about the same time that methemoglobin becomes extracellular, the hematoma develops a periph-

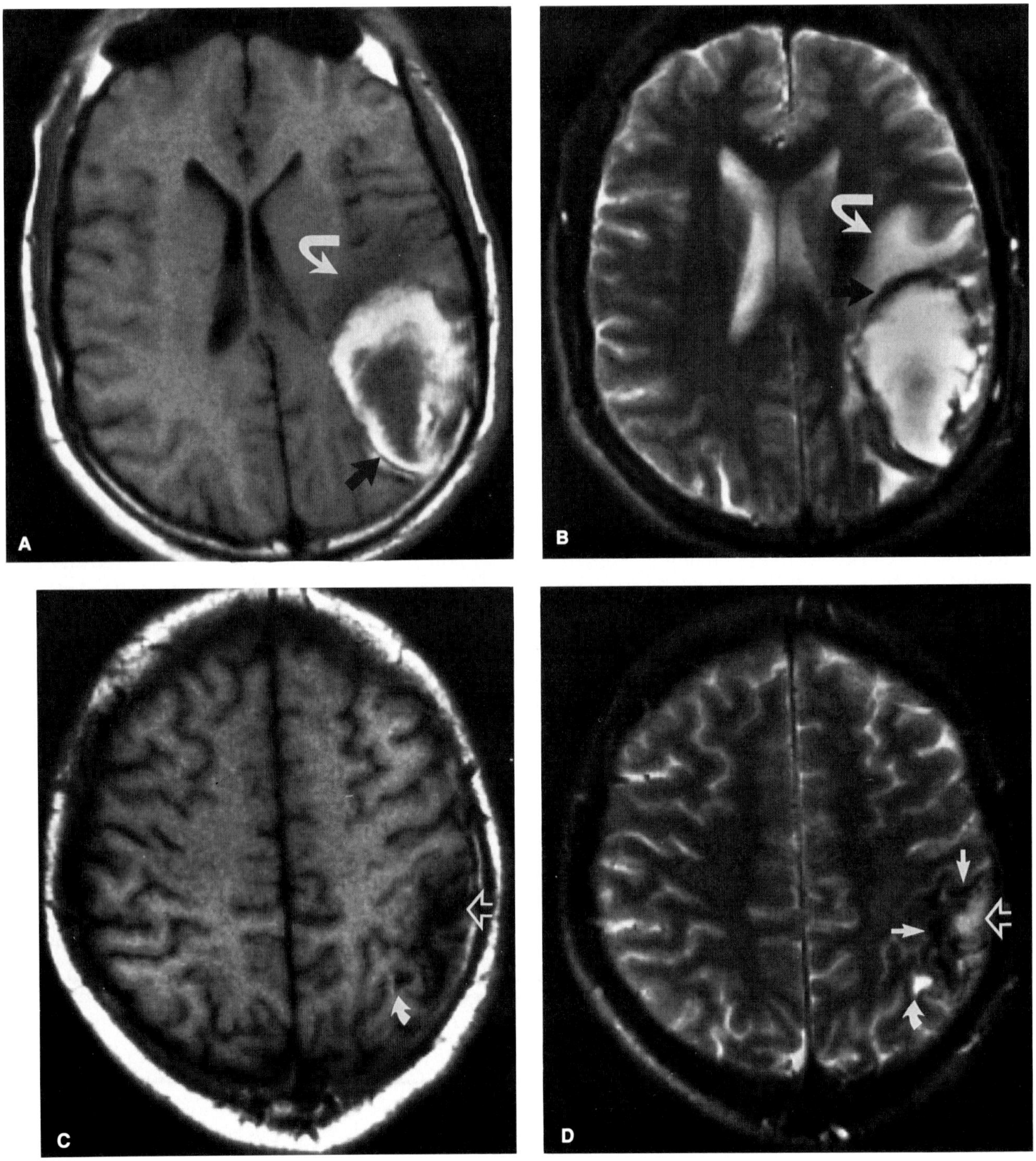

FIGURE 2–6. A 36-year-old man with idiopathic thrombocytopenic purpura (ITP), shown on **(A,C)** T1-weighted images (TR/TE = 650/20) and **(B,D)** T2-weighted images (TR/TE = 3000/90). On the initial exam, **(A,B)** there is a large, subacute, left posterior parietal hematoma. A hemosiderin rim outlines the hematoma (straight arrows). Extracellular methemoglobin forms the hyperintense peripheral components of the hematoma. The central component of the hematoma has signal characteristics compatible with dilute free methemoglobin. Edema (curved arrows) surrounds the hematoma. In a follow-up examination performed 6 months later **(C,D)**, the edema had resolved, and there were linear hemosiderin clefts (straight solid arrows) in the left posterior parietal region. There were also small areas of cystic encephalomalacia (curved arrows) and gliosis (open arrows) in this region.

eral rim of low intensity, which is more easily seen on T2-weighted images and corresponds to hemosiderin in macrophages (Fig. 2–6). The formation of the hemosiderin rim requires an intact blood-brain barrier. As the hematoma resorbs, the hemosiderin rim increases in thickness. The low-intensity hemosiderin rim becomes more pronounced with increasing field strength.[2,7,8] The reactive edema that surrounds the hematoma and marginates the forming hemosiderin rim begins to resolve.

After the surrounding edema has resolved, the late-stage subacute hematoma is characterized by a low-intensity rim of hemosiderin and central high-intensity area of extracellular methemoglobin (Fig. 2–7). This appearance is similar on T1-weighted and T2-weighted images, except the hemosiderin rim is more pronounced on images with T2 weighting.

In the chronic stage (>4 weeks), the methemoglobin within the center of the hematoma is broken down and resorbed.[15] As this occurs, the T1 shortening produced by methemoglobin is lost as a central protein-containing fluid that is isointense with CSF is formed. This central fluid may be resorbed, leaving only hemosiderin. Thus, the appearance of a chronic hematoma is variable and can have the following features: a high-intensity center (i.e., methemoglobin) and a peripheral low-intensity rim (i.e., hemosiderin); a central area isointense with CSF (i.e., resorbed methemoglobin) and a peripheral low-intensity rim (i.e., hemosiderin); and a residual, low-intensity hemosiderin cleft (i.e., the central methemoglobin and fluid have been completely resorbed).[6]

SUBDURAL AND EPIDURAL HEMATOMAS

Subdural Hematoma

Subdural hematomas result from a venous injury in which blood marginates the brain parenchyma between the dura and arachnoid. Like intraparenchymal hematomas, four stages in the evolution of subdural hematomas can be described: hyperacute, acute, subacute, and chronic.[1,6,16]

Hyperacute subdural hematomas are composed of a mixture of oxyhemoglobin and deoxyhemoglobin and are hypointense or isointense relative to brain tissue on T1-weighted images and hyperintense on T2-weighted images. The acute subdural hematoma is composed of deoxyhemoglobin in intact red blood cells, causing preferential T2 PRE. The acute subdural

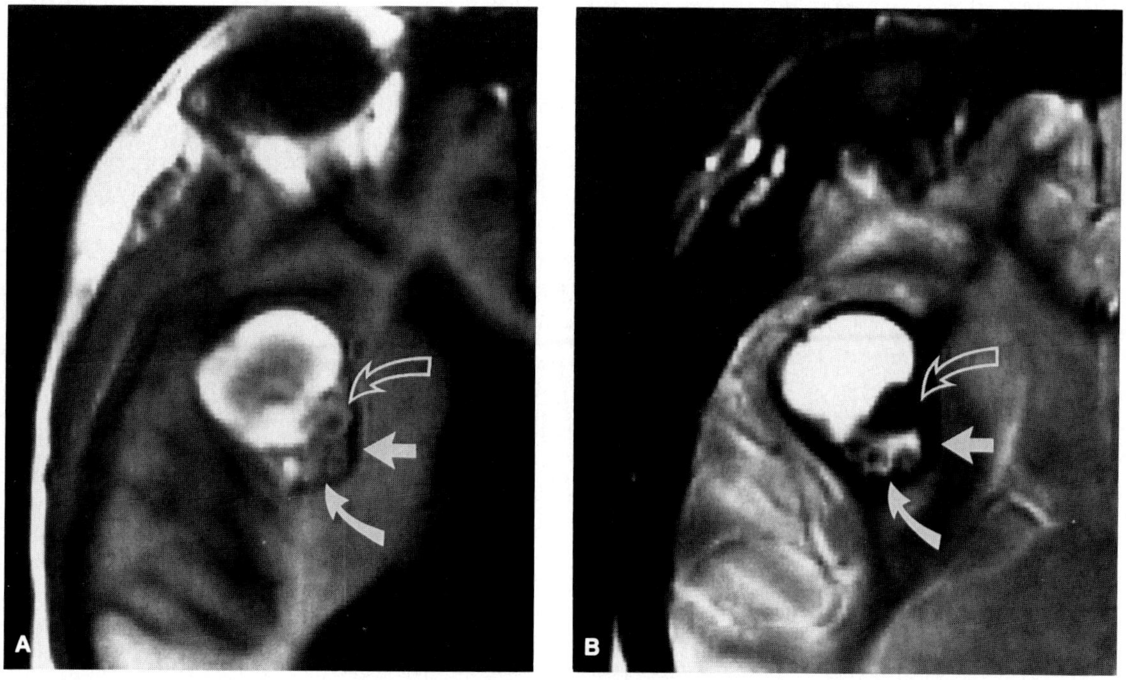

FIGURE 2–7. A 52-year-old woman with a ring-enhancing lesion in the right temporal region, which was identified by previous CT. **(A)** Axial T1-weighted image (TR/TE = 650/20); **(B)** axial T2-weighted image (TR/TE = 3000/90). There is a right temporal hematoma with a thick hemosiderin rim (solid straight arrows). Deoxyhemoglobin (open arrows) forms the medial component of this hematoma. Extracellular methemoglobin forms the hyperintense circular rim anteriorly. The central portion of this anterior component has signal characteristics compatible with dilute free methemoglobin. The smaller posterior component (curved arrows) has signal characteristics compatible with both intracellular and extracellular methemoglobin.

hematoma is hypointense or isointense relative to brain tissue on T1-weighted images and is hypointense on T2-weighted images.

In the subacute subdural hematoma, intracellular deoxyhemoglobin is oxidized to methemoglobin, which appears hyperintense on T1-weighted images and hypointense on T2-weighted images. By 14 days, red blood cell lysis results in free methemoglobin, causing hyperintensity on T1-weighted and T2-weighted images. As methemoglobin is slowly broken down in the chronic phase and hemichromes are formed, the subdural hematoma becomes intermediate in signal intensity compared with methemoglobin and CSF on T1-weighted images and high signal intensity, but lower than CSF on T2-weighted images. These are the expected characteristics of a protein-containing extra-axial fluid collection. These important characteristics distinguish a chronic subdural hematoma from the prominent CSF spaces seen with atrophy (Fig. 2-8).

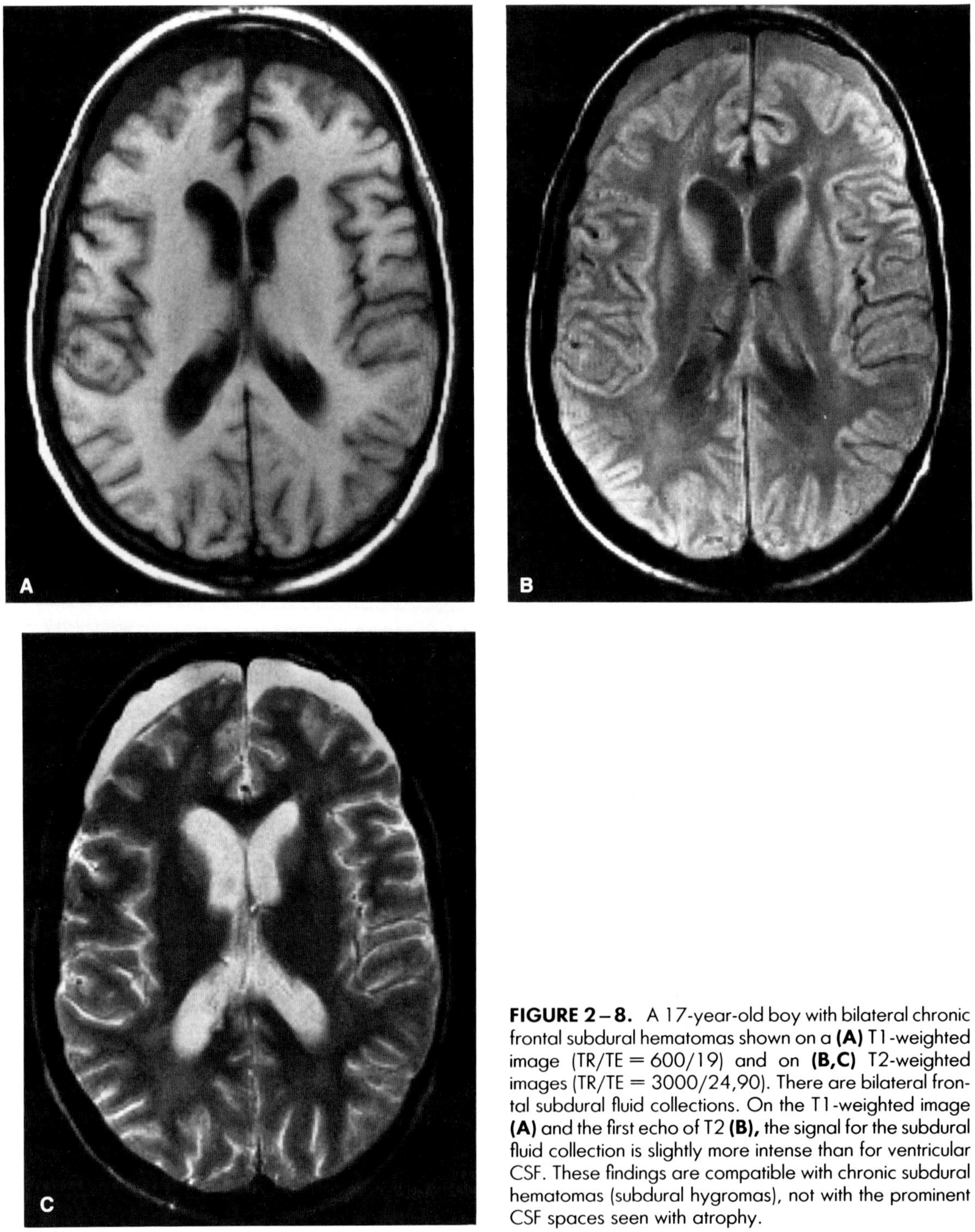

FIGURE 2-8. A 17-year-old boy with bilateral chronic frontal subdural hematomas shown on a **(A)** T1-weighted image (TR/TE = 600/19) and on **(B,C)** T2-weighted images (TR/TE = 3000/24,90). There are bilateral frontal subdural fluid collections. On the T1-weighted image **(A)** and the first echo of T2 **(B)**, the signal for the subdural fluid collection is slightly more intense than for ventricular CSF. These findings are compatible with chronic subdural hematomas (subdural hygromas), not with the prominent CSF spaces seen with atrophy.

In the chronic phase, the membrane delimiting the subdural hematoma may enhance with intravascular paramagnetic contrast agents like gadolinium DTPA (Gd DTPA).[17] Subdural hematomas may have acute and subacute-chronic components, which appear as fluid–fluid layers of the different forms of hemoglobin comprising the hematoma (Fig. 2–9). Hemosiderin accumulation is typically absent in extra-axial fluid collections, presumably because of the absence of a blood-brain barrier in the dura and access of hemosiderin-laden macrophages to the bloodstream. On rare occasions, hemosiderin can be identified in patients with recurrent bleeds into chronic subdural hematomas.

Epidural Hematoma

Epidural hematomas usually occur after an arterial injury, and blood dissects between the calvarium and dura, resulting in a biconvex lentiform configuration. Epidural hematomas follow the same pattern of evolution as a subdural hematoma.[1,5,6] An epidural hematoma can be distinguished from a subdural hematoma by its configuration and by the low-intensity fibrous dura that demarcates the margin of the hematoma from the brain parenchyma. However, in the acute phase, the low-intensity dura may not be visualized as a separate structure from the low-intensity hematoma (i.e., deoxyhemoglobin), and the diagnosis of an epidural hematoma or subdural hematoma may be difficult if the configuration of the extra-axial fluid collection is atypical.

During the subacute to chronic phase of an extra-axial hematoma, MR is especially sensitive and is superior to CT.[12,18] In the chronic phase, these fluid collections are low-density on CT and may be indistinguishable from large CSF spaces seen with atrophy. Moreover, CT bone artifact can obscure small extra-axial fluid collections, even in the acute phase. In comparing a CT and an MR image of a patient with a stable extra-axial fluid collection, it may appear larger on MR because of bone artifact and soft tissue windowing, which tend to reduce the apparent size of the fluid collection on CT. The hyperintensity of methemoglobin in the subacute or chronic phases makes these extra-axial hematomas readily identifiable on MR. Only occasionally can flow-related enhancement in a cortical vein or a chemical shift artifact at the margin of the brain mimic the appearance of a small subdural fluid collection on a single imaging se-

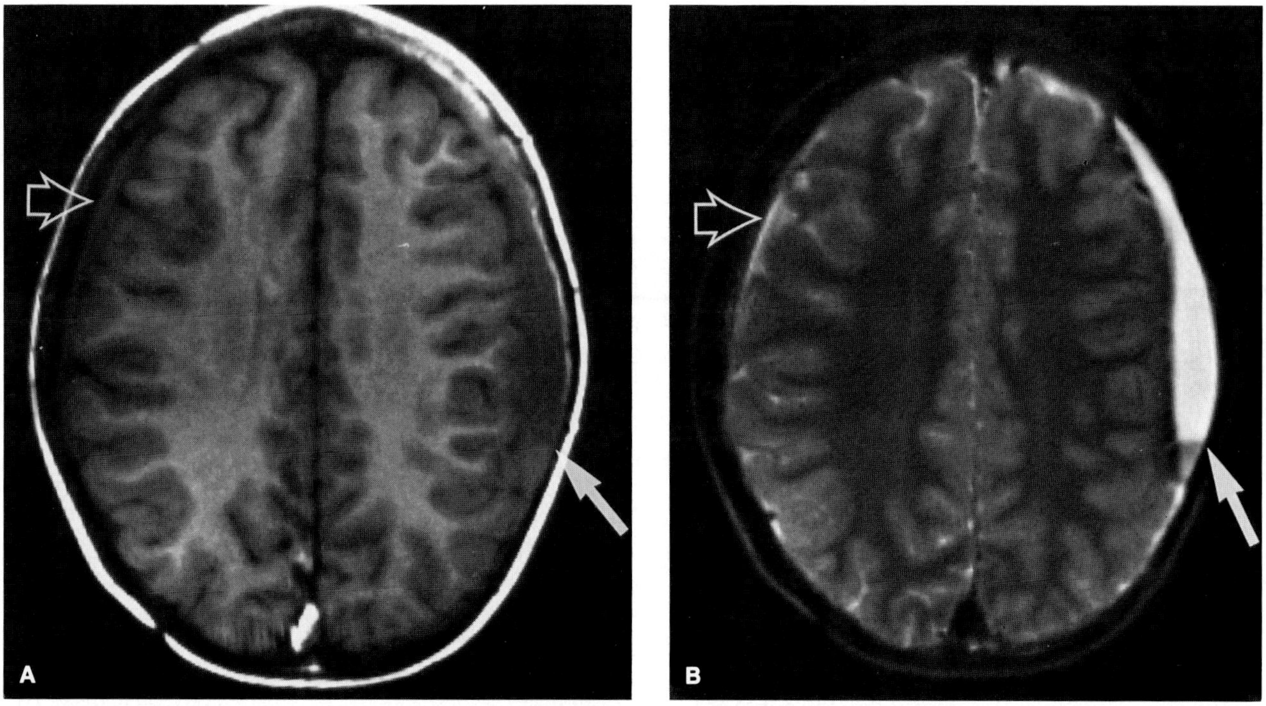

FIGURE 2–9. An 8-year-old girl with bilateral postsurgical subdural hematomas shown on an **(A)** axial T1-weighted image (TR/TE = 650/20) and an **(B)** axial T2-weighted image (TR/TE = 3000/90). There is a moderate-sized left frontal-parietal subdural hematoma and a very small, right posterior frontal subdural hematoma (open arrows). Dependent components layer in the left-sided subdural hematoma (closed arrows). The larger, superior component of the left subdural hematoma has signal characteristics compatible with proteinaceous fluid. The smaller, inferior component is probably composed of dilute free methemoglobin.

quence. These entities are easily distinguished from a subdural hematoma, because they change in appearance on different sequences.

SUBARACHNOID HEMORRHAGE

Subarachnoid hemorrhage, commonly secondary to rupture of an intracranial aneurysm or an arteriovenous malformation, is a potentially life-threatening event that requires prompt diagnosis and therapy. Unfortunately, hyperacute and acute subarachnoid hemorrhages are not successfully imaged by current spin echo techniques.[2,5,6,8] The conditions in the subarachnoid space are different from other intracranial locations, and the expected pattern of evolution of hemorrhage does not occur.

The acute subarachnoid hemorrhage is bathed by CSF, and this compartment has an average Po_2 of 43 mm Hg, and 72% of the hemoglobin is in the saturated oxyhemoglobin state.[8] Oxyhemoglobin has signal characteristics that are almost isointense to CSF and therefore would not be imaged. The contribution of deoxyhemoglobin, which causes preferential T2 PRE, to T2 shortening during this phase is negligible. Because T2 shortening is proportional to the square of the concentration of the paramagnetic compound, deoxyhemoglobin in a concentration of 28% (100–72%) contributes only 8% (0.28^2) to T2 shortening.[8] The T2 shortening of deoxyhemoglobin, which decreases signal intensity on T1-weighted and T2-weighted images, is also masked by the significant dilutional and pulsational effects of CSF. Therefore, it is not surprising that oxyhemoglobin and deoxyhemoglobin in the acute subarachnoid hemorrhage are not routinely imaged. Clearly, CT remains the modality of choice in the identification and diagnosis of acute subarachnoid hemorrhage.[8,19]

In the subacute phase of subarachnoid hemorrhage, an isointense or hyperintense signal can occasionally be identified on T1-weighted and T2-weighted images, presumably corresponding to methemoglobin within thrombus.[20] In rare instances, deoxyhemoglobin within thrombus in the acute phase can be visualized. However, this appearance of subarachnoid hemorrhage is not reliably present. In chronic or recurrent subarachnoid hemorrhage, hemosiderin deposition can occur in a subpial location, which is called "superficial hemosiderosis" or "superficial siderosis."[21,22] Superficial siderosis is characterized by thin rims of marked hypointensity that marginate the parenchymal surface, which is best visualized on T2-weighted images (Fig. 2–10). This condition can be caused by hemorrhage from vascular abnormalities, intracranial tumors, ependymoma of the conus medullaris, or neonatal hemorrhage. Occasionally, patients develop hearing loss with eighth cranial nerve involvement, other cranial nerve abnormalities, and cerebellar ataxia.[21,22]

GRADIENT ECHO IMAGING OF HEMORRHAGE

Gradient refocused echo (GRE) acquisition is a relatively new type of MR pulse sequence that is characterized by reduced flip angle radio-frequency (RF) pulses and applied gradients that refocus the echo, rather than the 90° radio-frequency pulse and 180° refocusing pulse that is used in routine spin echo (SE) imaging. GRE, also known as fast scan imaging, is particularly sensitive to the magnetic susceptibility effects of paramagnetic substances.[1,2,6]

Magnetic susceptibility is defined as the ratio of the induced magnetic field to the main magnetic field.[2] Magnetic susceptibility occurs when, under the influence of an externally applied field, substances are induced to form their own weak magnetic fields. Three classes of substances exhibit this type of magnetic behavior: paramagnetic, superparamagnetic, and ferromagnetic substances, all characterized by unpaired electrons in their outer orbitals. Superparamagnetic and ferromagnetic substances can acquire large magnetic moments, even if exposed to very weak external magnetic fields. Ferromagnetic substances, unlike paramagnetic and superparamagnetic substances, retain their magnetism after the external magnetic field is removed.

Paramagnetic substances have a high degree of magnetic susceptibility. Since many of the degradation products of hemoglobin (i.e., deoxyhemoglobin, methemoglobin, and hemosiderin) are paramagnetic, they are visualized with increased sensitivity on GRE compared with SE imaging. Small amounts of these paramagnetic hemoglobin compounds can be detected with GRE that may not be visualized with standard SE imaging or CT. For example, small cortical petechial hemorrhages or small amounts of residual hemosiderin from old hemorrhagic angiomas can be identified as areas of focal signal loss on GRE. However, these susceptibility effects can also overwhelm other signal characteristics of a lesion and obscure important diagnostic features. The central high-intensity area in a cavernous angioma could be obscured by the susceptibility effects of the hemosiderin rim. The boundary between deoxyhemoglobin or intracellular methemoglobin and the surrounding brain can appear as a hypointense rim on GRE, possibly obscuring the identification of a hemosiderin rim. This effect is important in evaluating hemorrhagic intracranial

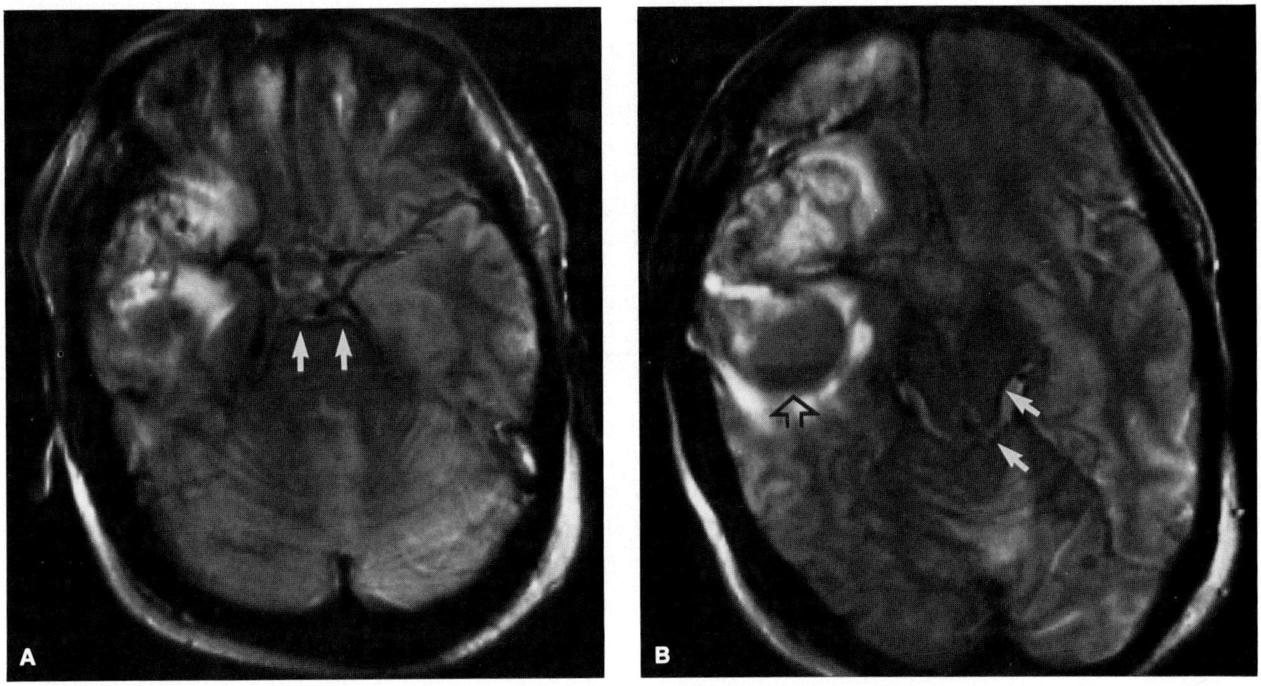

FIGURE 2–10. A 36-year-old man with a recurrent right frontal-temporal oligodendroglioma shown in axial T2-weighted images (TR/TE = 3000/45). Images through the pons **(A)** and cerebral peduncles **(B)** demonstrate thin rims of hypointensity outlining the pons, brain stem, and folea of the cerebellum (arrows), compatible with hemosiderin deposition from recurrent subarachnoid hemorrhage (superficial siderosis). The large, right frontal intra-axial neoplasm is easily visualized. The spheric, posterior component of the neoplasm **(B)** represents a hemorrhagic component (open arrow).

tumors, which typically have an incomplete surrounding hemosiderin rim because of their lack of an intact blood-brain barrier.[8]

CEREBROVASCULAR ANOMALIES

Intracranial aneurysms and vascular malformations comprise the major subgroups of cerebrovascular anomalies. The clinical presentation of patients with cerebrovascular anomalies varies. However, these patients can present with acute intracranial hemorrhage, either secondary to subarachnoid hemorrhage or an intraparenchymal hematoma (see the display on this page). In acute cases, CT remains the modality of choice for evaluation because MR cannot detect acute-stage subarachnoid blood and poorly characterizes hyperacute intraparenchymal hematoma. Despite this limitation, MR has emerged as an accurate noninvasive technique for characterizing intracranial vascular pathology. MR has replaced CT as a screening modality for detecting vascular malformations and intracranial aneurysms and associated mural thrombi.

Intracranial Aneurysms

An aneurysm is a focal dilatation of a vessel. Aneurysms can be characterized by their configuration as fusiform, a progressive, spindle-shaped dilatation of a vessel, or saccular, a sharply circumscribed, spheric

Causes of Nonneoplastic Intraparenchymal Hemorrhage

- Trauma
- After surgery
- Vascular anomalies
  - Aneurysms
  - Vascular malformations
- Vascular occlusive disease
  - Hypertensive hemorrhage (arteriosclerosis)
  - Hemorrhagic infarction
    - Arterial
    - Venous
- Vasculitis
- Anticoagulation and hematologic disorders
- Amyloid angiopathy
- Neonatal intracranial hemorrhage

sac. Fusiform aneurysms are commonly secondary to arteriosclerosis and often involve the basilar artery and intracranial carotid arteries. The vast majority of aneurysms are saccular (berry aneurysms) and are thought to be congenital.[23] They commonly arise at arterial branch points and are secondary to an inherent defect in the tunica media.[23-25] Fewer than 5% of aneurysms are caused by mycotic infection, trauma, or neoplasm. These aneurysms typically occur at peripheral locations rather than branch points.

In the general population, the incidence of intracranial aneurysms is approximately 3%.[26,27] The common congenital saccular aneurysm involves the anterior carotid circulation in 85 to 90% of cases and the posterior basilar circulation in 10 to 15% of cases.[23,24,26] In the anterior circulation, the most common locations of saccular aneurysms are the anterior communicating artery (30%), the posterior communicating artery (25%), and the middle cerebral artery bifurcation/trifurcation (20%).[24,26,28] In the posterior circulation, the basilar artery trunk and bifurcation (10%) and the vertebral-posterior inferior cerebellar artery (3%) are the most common sites.[29] In 20% of patients, multiple aneurysms are identified at angiography.[23,24,26,28]

A ruptured intracranial aneurysm is the most common cause (75%) of subarachnoid hemorrhage; vascular malformations cause 5% of the cases.[30] These patients commonly present with the acute onset of a severe headache that may progress to coma. In the patient with a suspected acute subarachnoid hemorrhage caused by a ruptured aneurysm, CT remains the screening modality of choice. CT readily visualizes acute hemorrhage as high-density, and CT is more easily performed in the uncooperative patient.

MR is often initially performed for patients without intracranial hemorrhage or in patients with intracranial hemorrhages and with atypical symptoms. In these patients, MR can often demonstrate and characterize the aneurysm itself. In approximately 20% of aneurysms that bleed, there is an associated intraparenchymal hematoma.[31] Beyond the hyperacute stage, MR exquisitely demonstrates intraparenchymal hematomas, and their location can suggest the diagnosis of a ruptured aneurysm. For example, an intraparenchymal hematoma adjacent to the anterior interhemispheric fissure suggests a ruptured anterior communicating artery aneurysm, and an intraparenchymal hematoma adjacent to the sylvian cistern suggests a ruptured middle cerebral artery aneurysm. In patients with known aneurysms, MR can identify the bleeding site by demonstrating a subacute hemorrhage adjacent to the aneurysm.[32] In some cases, MR can identify subacute and chronic subarachnoid hemorrhages caused by ruptured aneurysms.

A unique feature of MR is its ability to detect vascular flow, particularly in the arterial system. High-velocity flow in arteries or veins typically appears as a flow void on MR images, which is called high-velocity signal loss (HVSL). HVSL occurs when protons in flowing blood do not remain within the selected slice long enough to acquire both the 90° and 180° pulses to produce a spin echo.[33] Saccular aneurysms appear as regions of flow void in a typical configuration and location (Fig. 2-11).

Another supporting finding seen with pulsatile flow in patent aneurysms is a pulsation artifact that propagates in the plane of the aneurysm along the phase-encoding axis (Fig. 2-12). These pulsation artifacts are typically more pronounced on Gd-DTPA-enhanced images because of the increased signal of the contrast in the vascular space. Depending on imaging parameters (e.g., TR, TE, slice thickness, location) and the effects of turbulence and rephasing, slow flowing blood within a tubular vessel or an aneurysm can have high or mixed signal intensity, rather than a flow void. High velocity, turbulence, flow-related enhancement, and even echo rephasing are processes that cause increased signal intensity within vascular structures. These phenomena have been described in detail and should be recognized as possible pitfalls in the recognition of intracranial aneurysms (Fig. 2-13).[33,34] Another less common pitfall in the diagnosis of basilar artery aneurysms is CSF pulsation artifacts in the prepontine cistern that can simulate a basilar artery aneurysm.[35] This artifact is more pronounced with increased slice thickness.

MR routinely visualizes large intracranial aneurysms (1.0-2.5 cm in diameter) and giant aneurysms, which are defined as aneurysms greater than 2.5 cm in diameter. These aneurysms commonly present with symptoms related to mass effect rather than subarachnoid hemorrhage.[36-38] Large and giant aneurysms are often partially thrombosed and can be confused with an intraparenchymal hematoma. MR provides an elegant, noninvasive method for diagnosing partially thrombosed giant intracranial aneurysms.[39] MR is superior to CT and angiography in characterizing this type of aneurysm.[39]

The MR findings in partially thrombosed large or giant intracranial aneurysms include a flow void in the residual patent lumen of the aneurysm. A high-intensity rim is immediately adjacent to this signal void on both T1-weighted and T2-weighted images, which corresponds to free methemoglobin. This finding contrasts with the formation of methemoglobin in an intraparenchymal hematoma, in which methemoglobin first forms at the periphery rather than centrally. Mixed, laminated signal intensity surrounds the high-intensity methemoglobin rim, which represents different stages of organized clot (i.e., methemoglobin and hemosiderin) in the thrombosed portion of the aneurysm. Perianeurysmal hemorrhage and adjacent

(text continues on page 66)

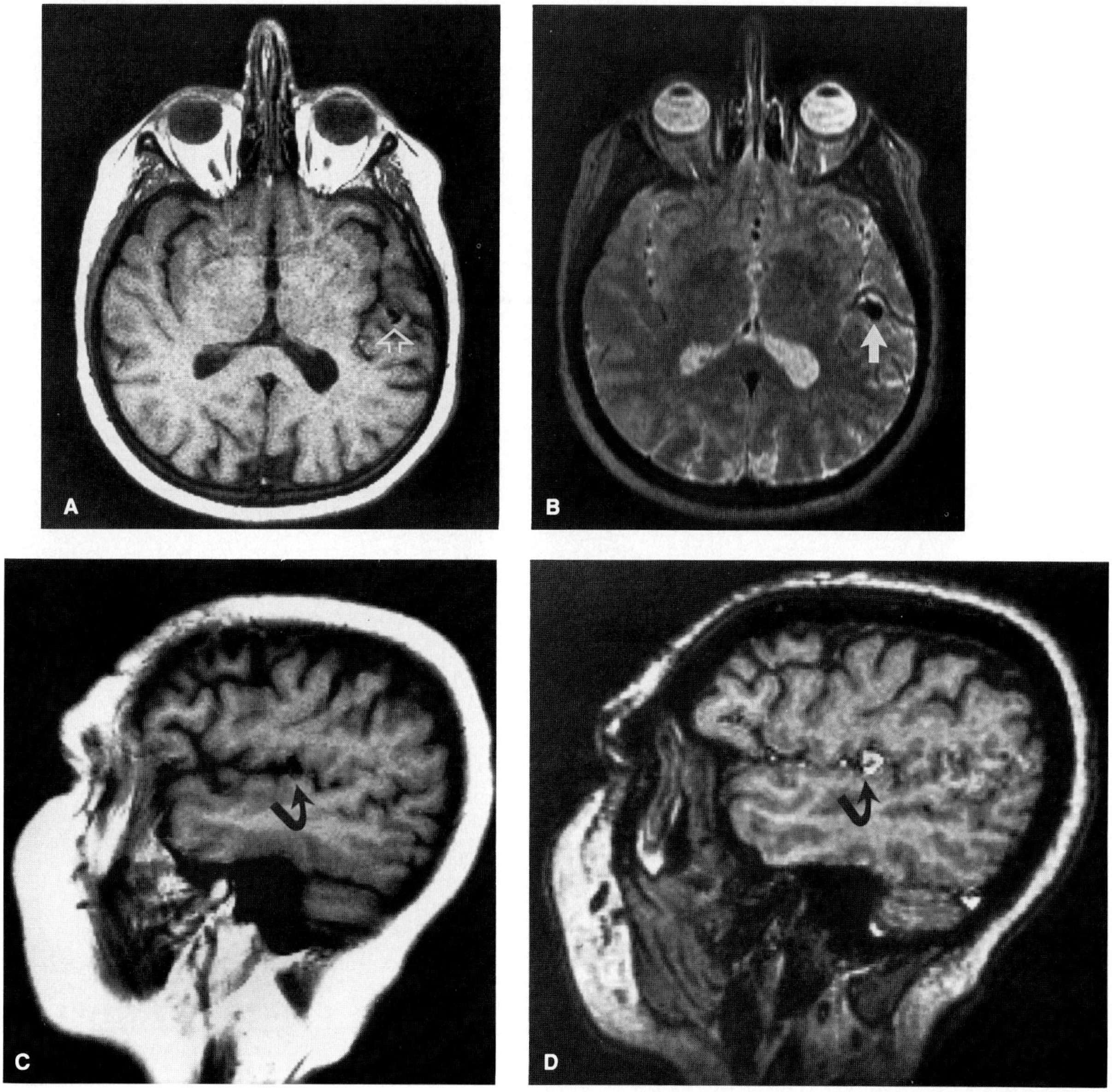

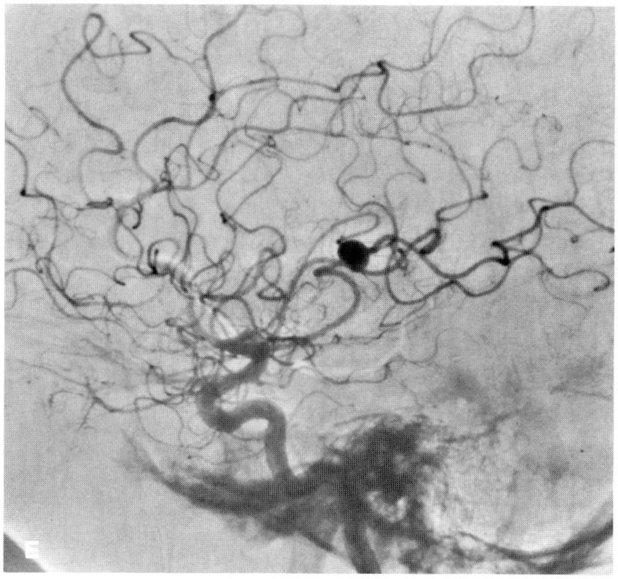

FIGURE 2–11. A 53-year-old woman with an asymptomatic left-middle cerebral artery aneurysm shown in **(A,C)** axial and sagittal T1-weighted images (TR/TE = 600/17), **(B)** axial T2-weighted image (TR/TE = 3000/70); and **(D)** sagittal GRE (FLASH) image (TR/TE/Flip angle = 60/18/40). Axial images **(A,C)** demonstrate a focal signal void (arrow) involving a left-middle cerebral artery branch and are compatible with an aneurysm. The aneurysm is best visualized on the T2-weighted image **(B).** On the T1-weighted image **(A)** through the same level, the aneurysm (open arrow) is only partially imaged because of volume averaging. To confirm the presence of flow, sagittal T1-weighted and GRE images were compared. The sagittal GRE image demonstrates an increased signal in the aneurysm (curved arrow), confirming flow. A left carotid arteriogram **(E),** lateral view, demonstrates a saccular aneurysm involving a left-middle cerebral artery branch.

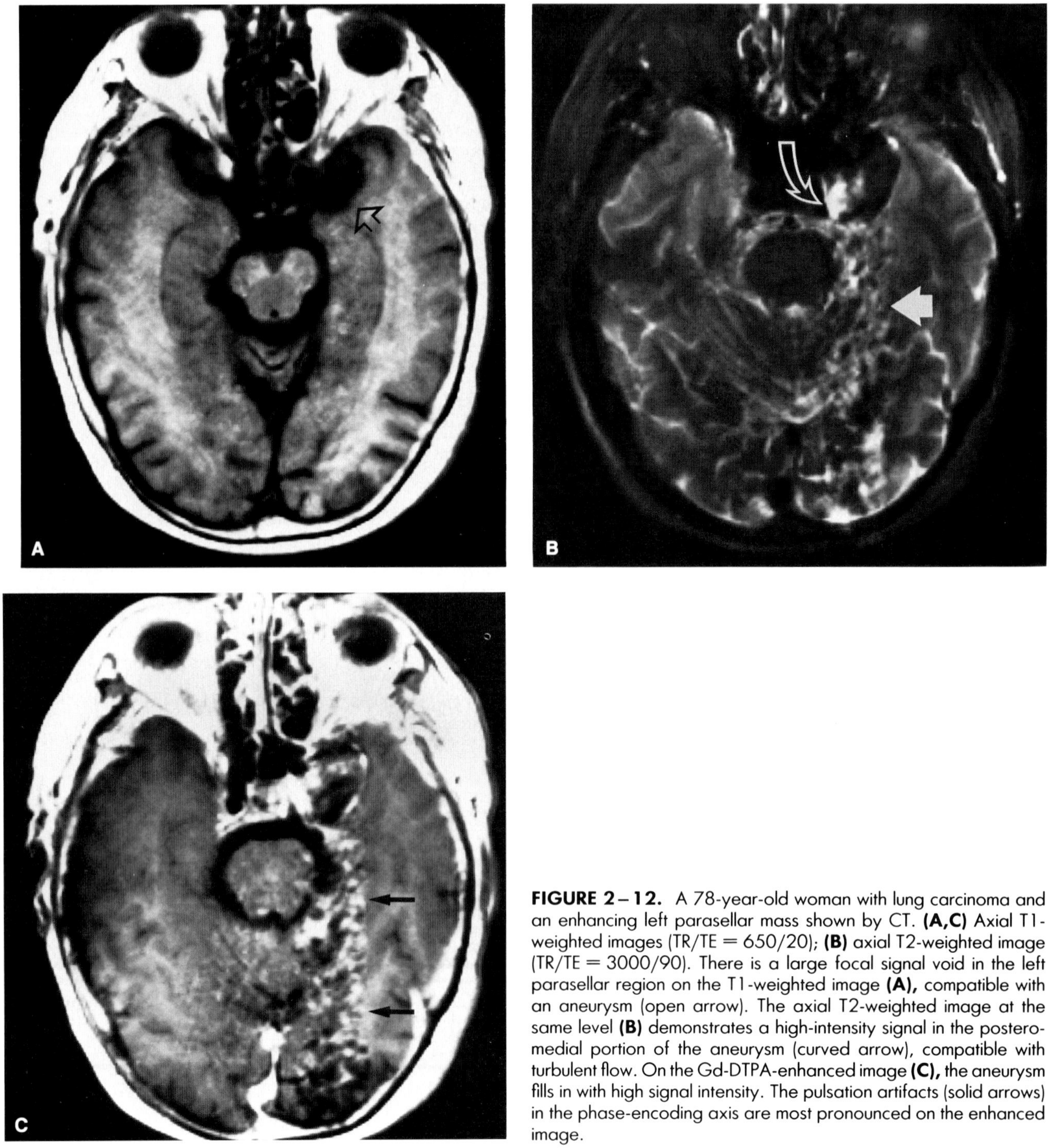

FIGURE 2–12. A 78-year-old woman with lung carcinoma and an enhancing left parasellar mass shown by CT. **(A,C)** Axial T1-weighted images (TR/TE = 650/20); **(B)** axial T2-weighted image (TR/TE = 3000/90). There is a large focal signal void in the left parasellar region on the T1-weighted image **(A),** compatible with an aneurysm (open arrow). The axial T2-weighted image at the same level **(B)** demonstrates a high-intensity signal in the posteromedial portion of the aneurysm (curved arrow), compatible with turbulent flow. On the Gd-DTPA-enhanced image **(C),** the aneurysm fills in with high signal intensity. The pulsation artifacts (solid arrows) in the phase-encoding axis are most pronounced on the enhanced image.

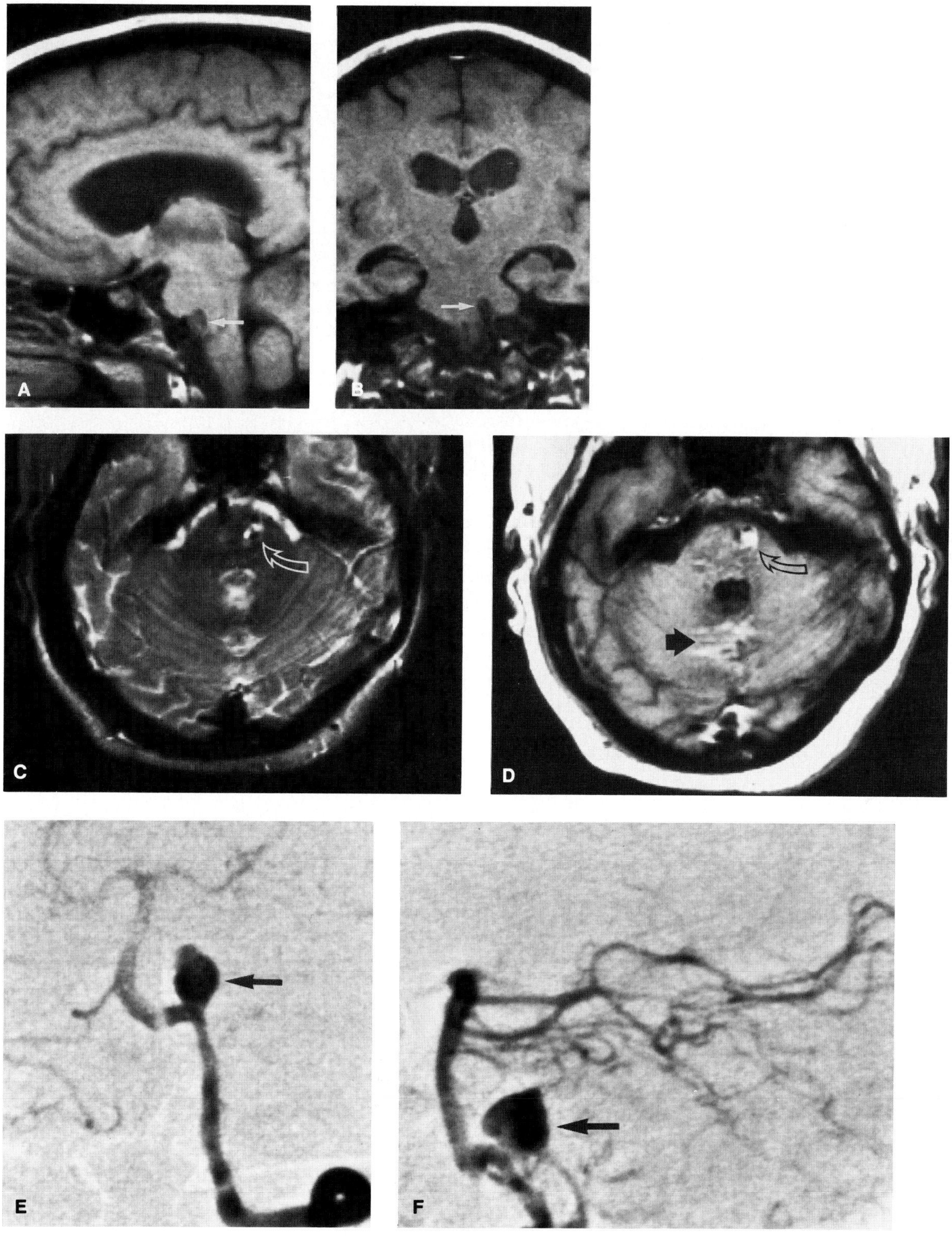

FIGURE 2–13. A 46-year-old woman with a left PICA aneurysm shown in **(A,B,D)** sagittal, coronal, and axial T1-weighted images (TR/TE = 650/20) and in an **(C)** axial T2-weighted image (TR/TE = 3000/90). Unenhanced T1-weighted images **(A,B)** demonstrate an intermediate-signal-intensity lesion (arrows) anterior and inferior to the left pons. An axial T2-weighted image through this region **(C)** demonstrates high and low signal intensity, suggesting the presence of flow (open arrow), and a Gd-DTPA-enhanced axial image **(D)** through the same level demonstrates enhancement of the inferior portion of this lesion (open arrow). The high signal intensity posterior to the fourth ventricle (arrow) is caused by pulsation artifacts in the phase-encoding axis from the contrast-enhanced torcula. A digital subtraction angiogram, in anteroposterior **(E)** and lateral **(F)** views, confirms a left PICA aneurysm (arrows).

edema within the brain may occur and can be distinguished from the aneurysm (Fig. 2-14). Perianeurysmal hemorrhage in the brain parenchyma appears as areas of hyperintensity on T1-weighted images and either hypointensity or hyperintensity on T2-weighted images because of the presence of intracellular and extracellular forms of methemoglobin. Edema within the brain parenchyma is hypointense on T1-weighted images and hyperintense on T2-weighted images (Fig. 2-15).

MR is sensitive in demonstrating complete thrombosis of large aneurysms. An old, organized thrombus commonly has a signal that is isointense with soft tissue or a protein-containing fluid (e.g., isointense on T1-weighted images and hyperintense on T2-weighted images) (Fig. 2-16). Other soft tissue masses, including neoplasms, can have similar appearances and should be considered in the differential diagnosis. Patency or thrombosis of the adjacent major intracranial vessels can also be determined by the presence or absence of arterial flow voids. MR is also useful in evaluating thrombosis of an aneurysm after balloon embolization (Fig. 2-17).

Although current cross-sectional MRI can identify and characterize intracranial aneurysms, it cannot definitively exclude an aneurysm. Aneurysms are often multiple, and the majority of them are small (< 1.0 cm in diameter).[28] Furthermore, patients with these small aneurysms commonly present with acute subarachnoid hemorrhage. MR may fail to visualize these small structures because of the inherent resolution of this cross-sectional imaging technique, volume averaging, and variation and tortuosity of normal vascular anatomy. Angiography remains the gold standard for evaluating intracranial aneurysms. However, a new volumetric MR imaging technique, 3D MR angiography, holds promise as a noninvasive way to evaluate the vascular tree.

MR is contraindicated in the evaluation of the post-surgical patient with ferromagnetic aneurysm clips. However, nonferromagnetic aneurysm clips are commercially available, and patients with these clips have been successfully scanned.[40,41] Shellock and Crues have studied a group of surgical clips, including aneurysm clips, and have determined which have ferromagnetic properties and which can safely be scanned (Fig. 2-18).[42] An easy way to determine if a surgical clip is ferromagnetic is to suspend it from a string or place it in a plastic bag and see if the clip is deflected when placed in the bore of the machine's magnet.

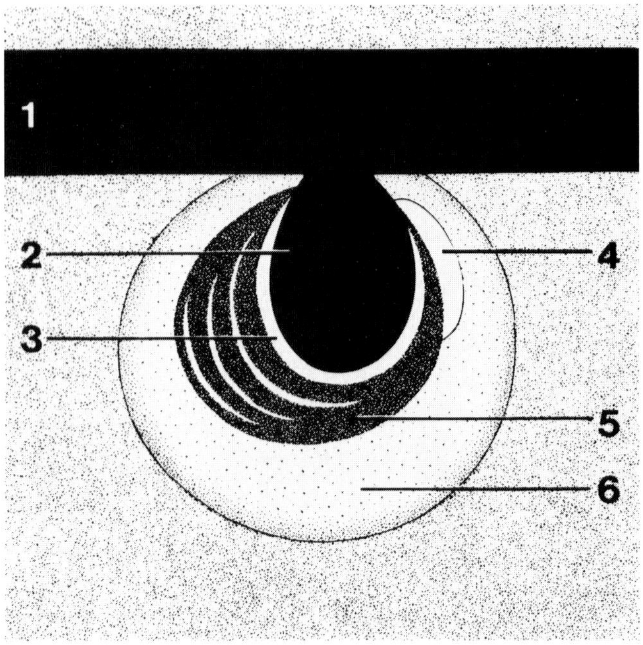

FIGURE 2-14. Schematic diagram of the MR signal intensities in a partially thrombosed giant aneurysm: *1*, signal void in the parent vessel; *2*, signal void in the patent portion of the aneurysm lumen; *3*, rim of hyperintense methemoglobin surrounding the patent lumen; *4*, perianeurysmal hemorrhage; *5*, mixed signal intensity in the thrombosed portion of the aneurysm lumen; *6*, perianeurysmal edema in the brain parenchyma. (Atlas SW. Partially thrombosed giant intracranial aneurysms: Correlation of MR and pathologic findings. Radiology 1987;162:111)

Vascular Malformations

Vascular malformations are congenital developmental abnormalities of the vascular system. Cerebrovascular malformations are divided into four major pathologic categories: arteriovenous malformations (AVM); venous angioma; capillary telangiectasia; and cavernous angioma.[43] AVMs and venous angiomas can be routinely visualized with angiography, CT, and MR. Capillary telangiectasias and cavernous angiomas are not directly visualized with current imaging modalities, but are detected because of hemorrhage associated with the lesion.[44] Thrombosed AVMs and venous angiomas may also be detected only by the presence of hemorrhage if their abnormal vessels become obliterated. These vascular malformations, detected by the presence of recurrent or chronic hemorrhage, in which the vascular anomaly is not visualized angiographically, are called occult cerebrovascular malformations (OCVM). Based on current imaging studies, the majority of vascular malformations are divided into three major radiologic groups: AVM, venous angioma, and OCVM.[24]

Arteriovenous Malformation

AVMs are the most common type of vascular malformation, with an incidence of approximately 0.14% in the general population.[45] The clinical presentation is variable and includes headaches, seizures, neurologic deficits, and symptoms related to hemorrhage. Occasionally AVMs are discovered as incidental findings during the evaluation of an unrelated problem. All age

(text continues on page 70)

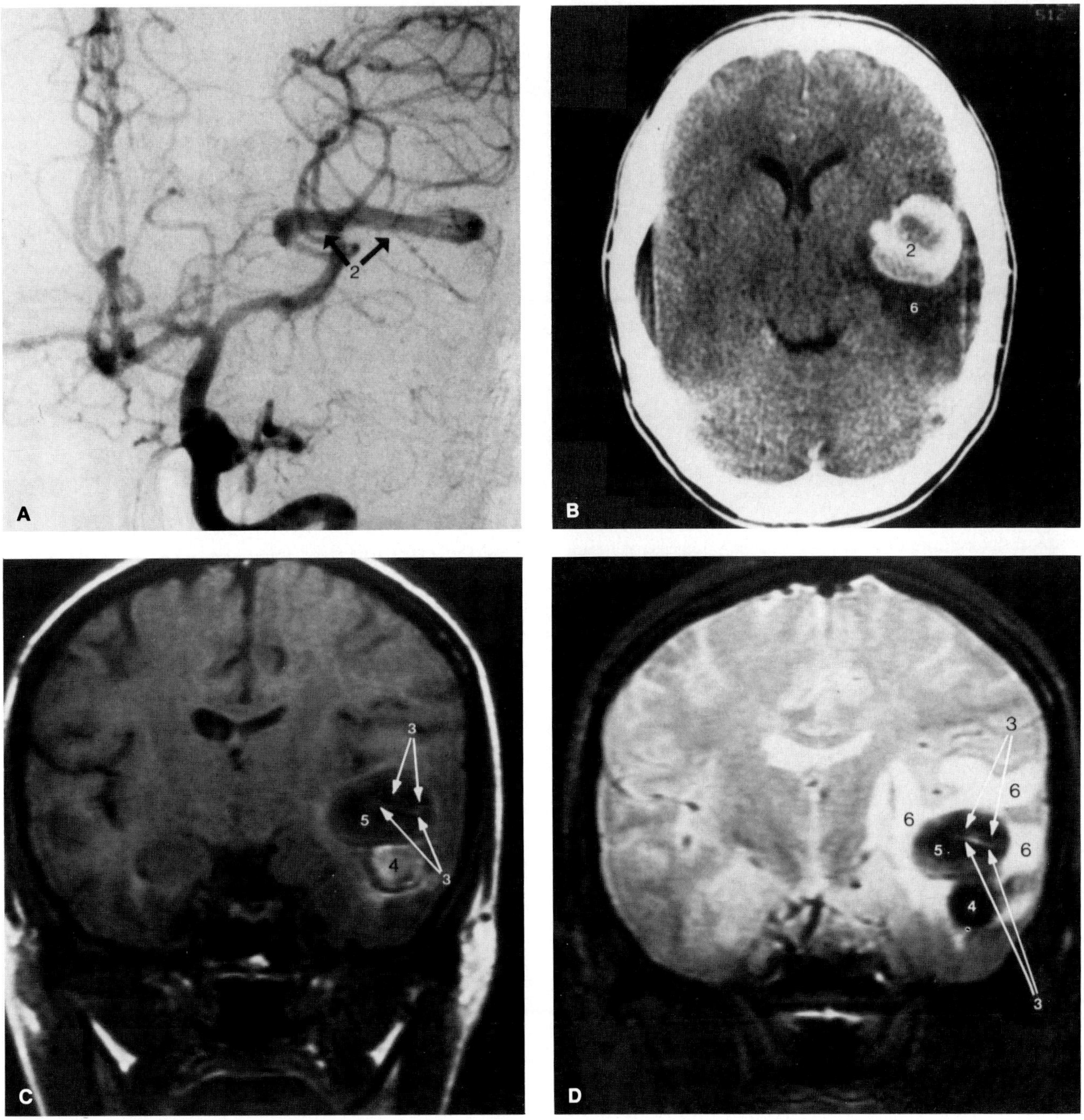

FIGURE 2–15. A 32-year-old woman with a giant aneurysm involving the left-middle cerebral artery. A left internal carotid arteriogram **(A)**, anteroposterior view, demonstrates the serpiginous patent portion of the aneurysm lumen *(2)*. On a contrast-enhanced axial CT image **(B)**, there is high attenuation of a left temporal lobe mass with partial enhancement *(2)* and a surrounding region of low attenuation *(6)*. Coronal T1-weighted **(C)** and T2-weighted **(D)** MR images demonstrate a bilobed left temporal mass with complex internal signal characteristics. A thin, horizontally oriented region of signal void (the patent portion of the aneurysm lumen) is surrounded by an adjacent rim of hyperintense methemoglobin *(3)*. The large area of layered signal intensity *(5)* represents the thrombosed portion of the aneurysm lumen. Extra-aneurysmal hemorrhage *(4)* is centrally hyperintense with a rim of hypointensity **(C)** or markedly hypointense **(D)**. On the T2-weighted image **(D)**, there is hyperintense perianeurysmal edema *(6)*. (Atlas SW. Partially thrombosed giant intracranial aneurysms: Correlation of MR and pathologic findings. Radiology 1987;162:111)

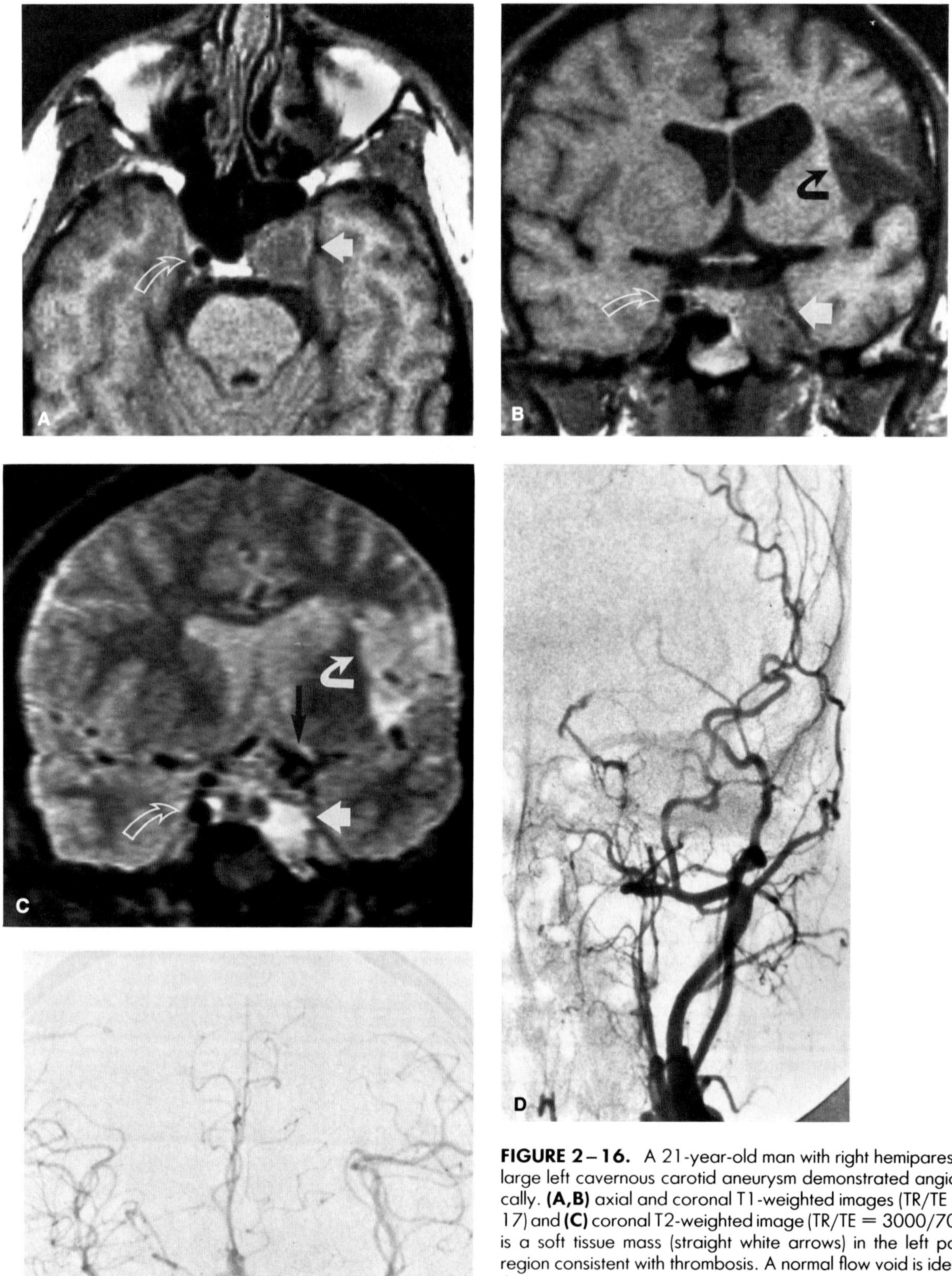

FIGURE 2–16. A 21-year-old man with right hemiparesis and a large left cavernous carotid aneurysm demonstrated angiographically. **(A,B)** axial and coronal T1-weighted images (TR/TE = 600/17) and **(C)** coronal T2-weighted image (TR/TE = 3000/70). There is a soft tissue mass (straight white arrows) in the left parasellar region consistent with thrombosis. A normal flow void is identified in the cavernous segment of the right internal carotid artery (open curved arrows). Flow voids compatible with vascular patency **(C)** involve the distal supraclinoid segment of the left internal carotid artery and the proximal portions of the left anterior and middle cerebral arteries (straight black arrow). There is an old left middle cerebral artery infarct (curved arrows), with focal dilatation of the left lateral ventricle. A left common carotid artery arteriogram **(D),** anteroposterior view, confirms occlusion of the left internal carotid artery and filling of left external carotid artery branches. A right common carotid artery arteriogram **(E),** anteroposterior view, demonstrates cross-filling of the left anterior and middle cerebral arteries.

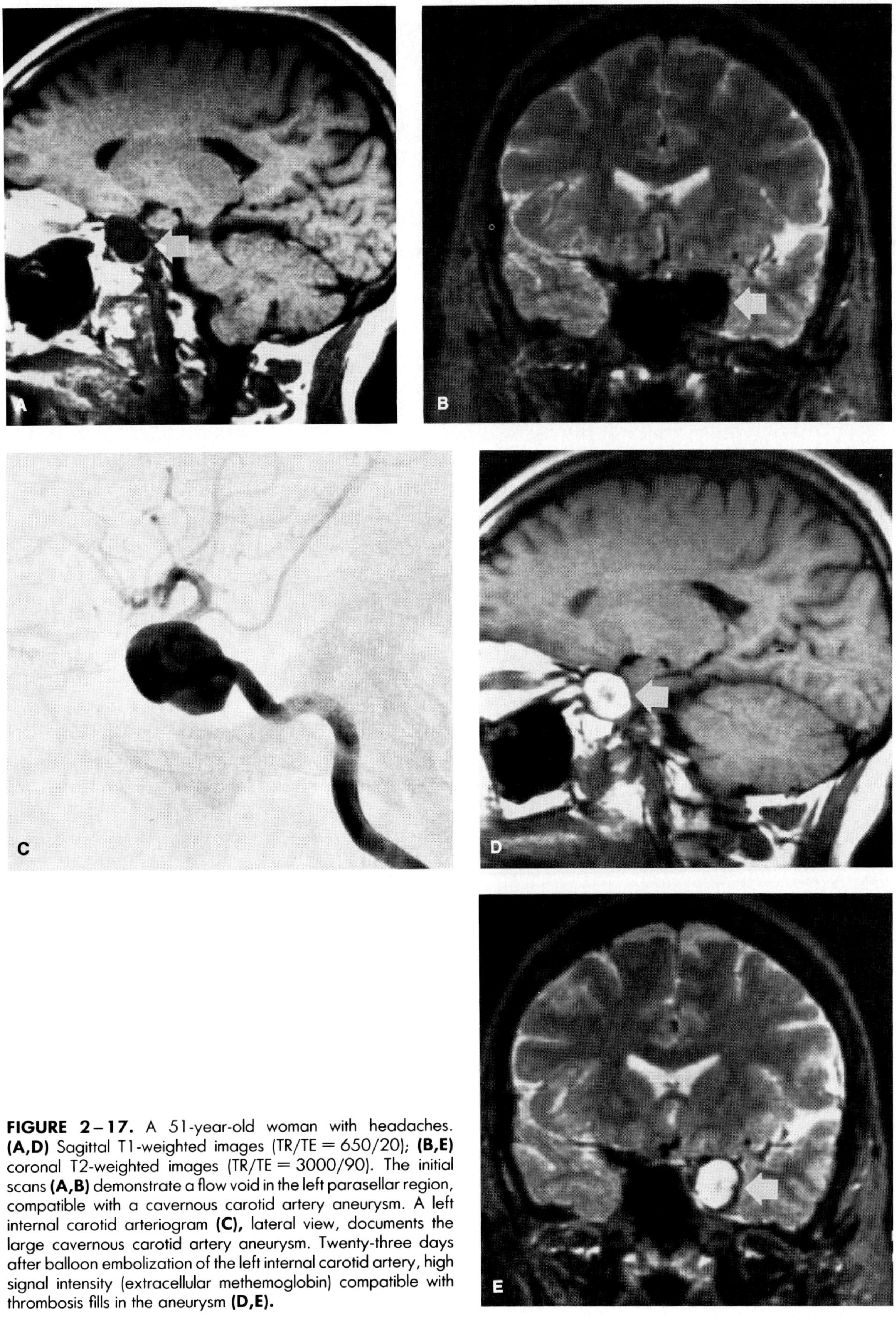

FIGURE 2–17. A 51-year-old woman with headaches. **(A,D)** Sagittal T1-weighted images (TR/TE = 650/20); **(B,E)** coronal T2-weighted images (TR/TE = 3000/90). The initial scans **(A,B)** demonstrate a flow void in the left parasellar region, compatible with a cavernous carotid artery aneurysm. A left internal carotid arteriogram **(C),** lateral view, documents the large cavernous carotid artery aneurysm. Twenty-three days after balloon embolization of the left internal carotid artery, high signal intensity (extracellular methemoglobin) compatible with thrombosis fills in the aneurysm **(D,E).**

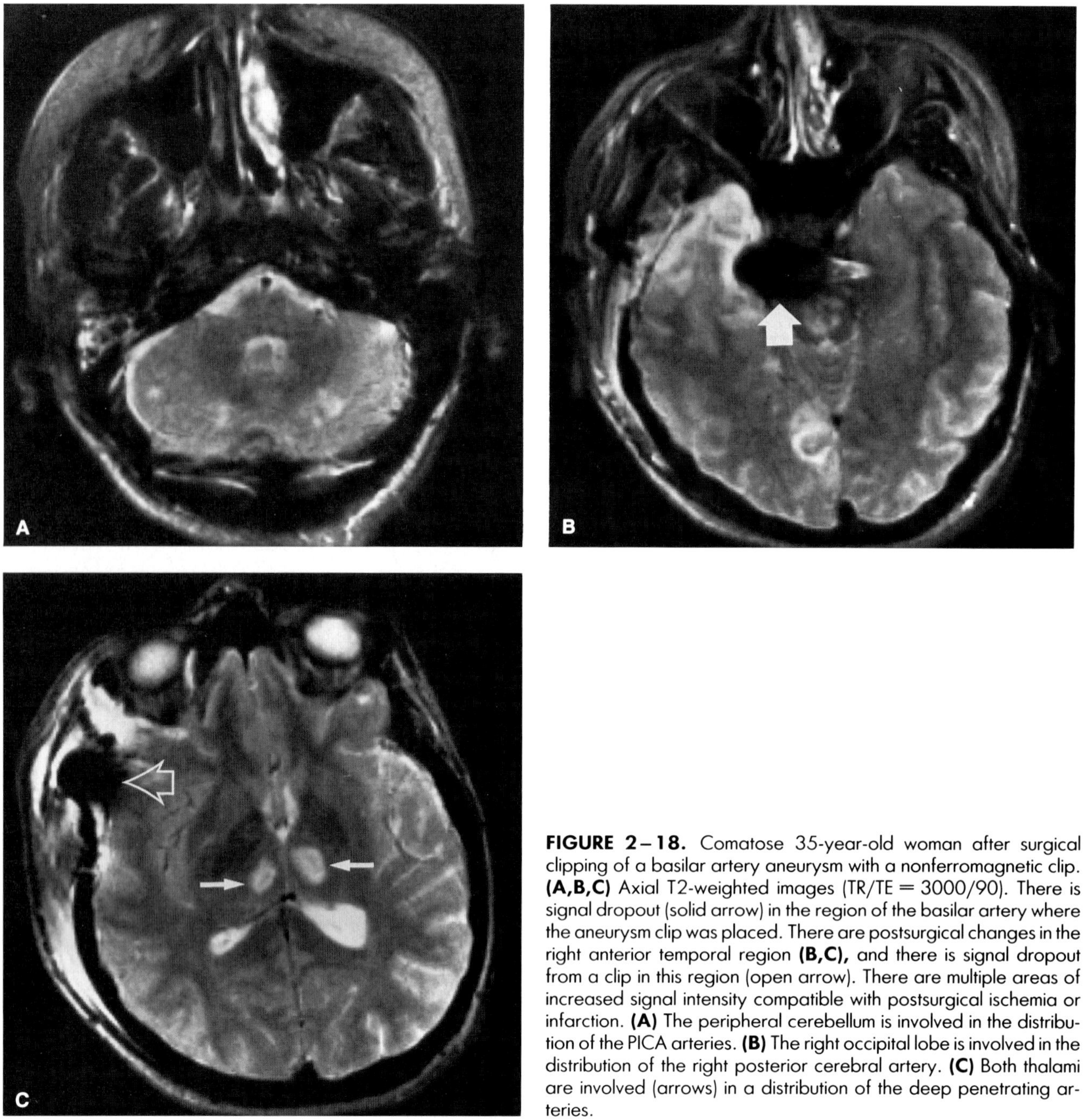

FIGURE 2–18. Comatose 35-year-old woman after surgical clipping of a basilar artery aneurysm with a nonferromagnetic clip. **(A,B,C)** Axial T2-weighted images (TR/TE = 3000/90). There is signal dropout (solid arrow) in the region of the basilar artery where the aneurysm clip was placed. There are postsurgical changes in the right anterior temporal region **(B,C)**, and there is signal dropout from a clip in this region (open arrow). There are multiple areas of increased signal intensity compatible with postsurgical ischemia or infarction. **(A)** The peripheral cerebellum is involved in the distribution of the PICA arteries. **(B)** The right occipital lobe is involved in the distribution of the right posterior cerebral artery. **(C)** Both thalami are involved (arrows) in a distribution of the deep penetrating arteries.

groups are affected, with most patients presenting with symptoms between the third and fourth decades (44% of patients).[46]

AVMs occur throughout the central nervous system and are characterized pathologically by a direct communication between the arterial and venous circulations, without an intervening capillary bed. Intracranial AVMs are most commonly supratentorial (80%) and involve the peripheral branches of the middle cerebral artery.[47] Angiographically, AVMs consist of a racemose tangled group of dilated vessels supplied by enlarged tortuous feeding arteries and draining veins. Most commonly, the arterial supply of AVMs is pial, arising from the cerebral or cerebellar arteries. In some AVMs, there is a mixed pial-dural or dural blood supply. Half of the infratentorial lesions and approximately 20% of the supratentorial lesions have a dural component to their blood supply.[47] Aneurysms are associated with the feeding arteries of AVMs in approximately 10% of patients.[48]

Spin echo MR imaging accurately defines the vascular channels forming AVMs as flow voids. Typically, the arterial-venous shunting is so rapid in these lesions that an increased intravascular signal related to slow flow is not visualized (Fig. 2–19). As with intracranial aneurysms, pulsation artifacts can be

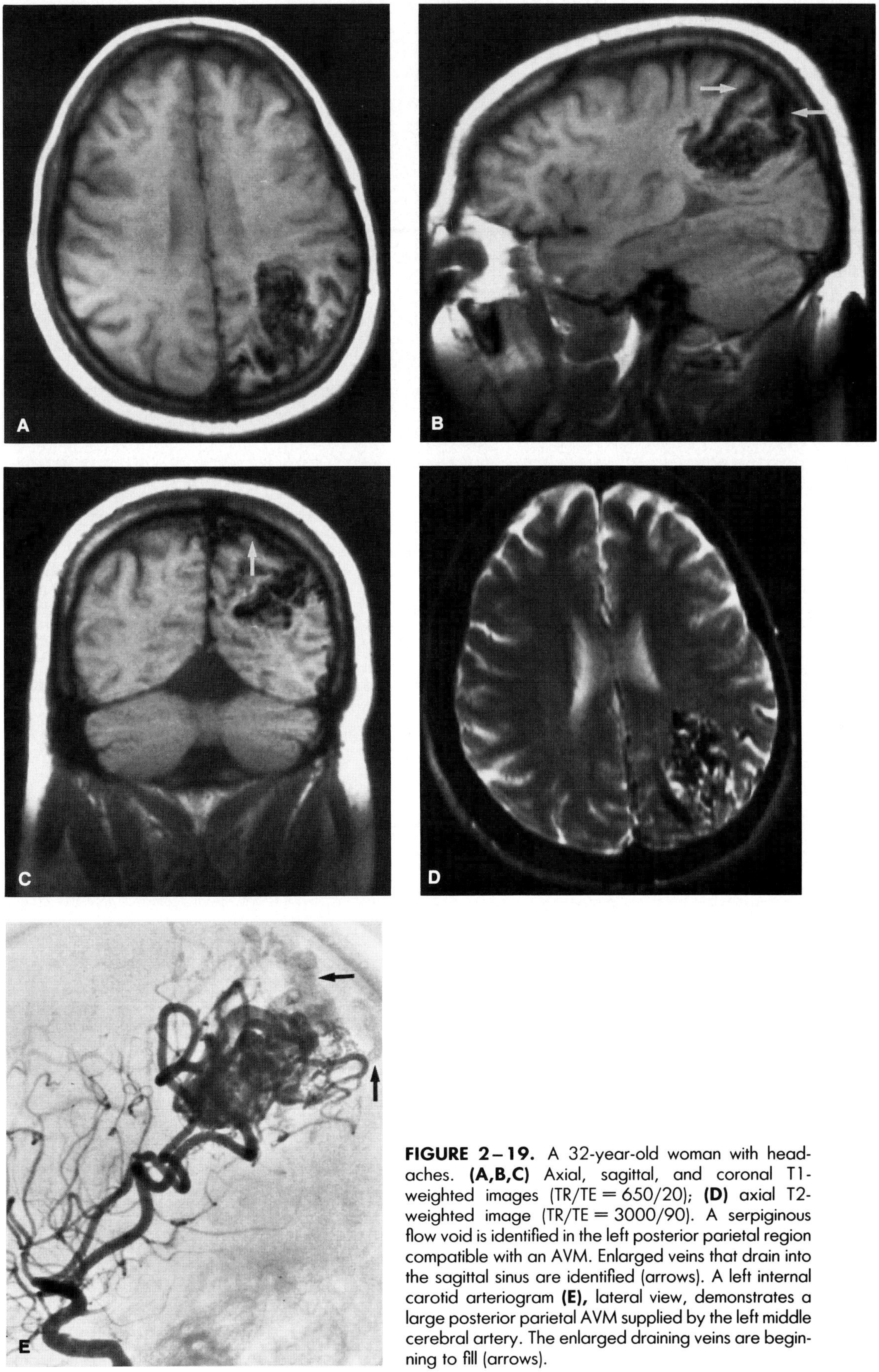

FIGURE 2–19. A 32-year-old woman with headaches. **(A,B,C)** Axial, sagittal, and coronal T1-weighted images (TR/TE = 650/20); **(D)** axial T2-weighted image (TR/TE = 3000/90). A serpiginous flow void is identified in the left posterior parietal region compatible with an AVM. Enlarged veins that drain into the sagittal sinus are identified (arrows). A left internal carotid arteriogram **(E),** lateral view, demonstrates a large posterior parietal AVM supplied by the left middle cerebral artery. The enlarged draining veins are beginning to fill (arrows).

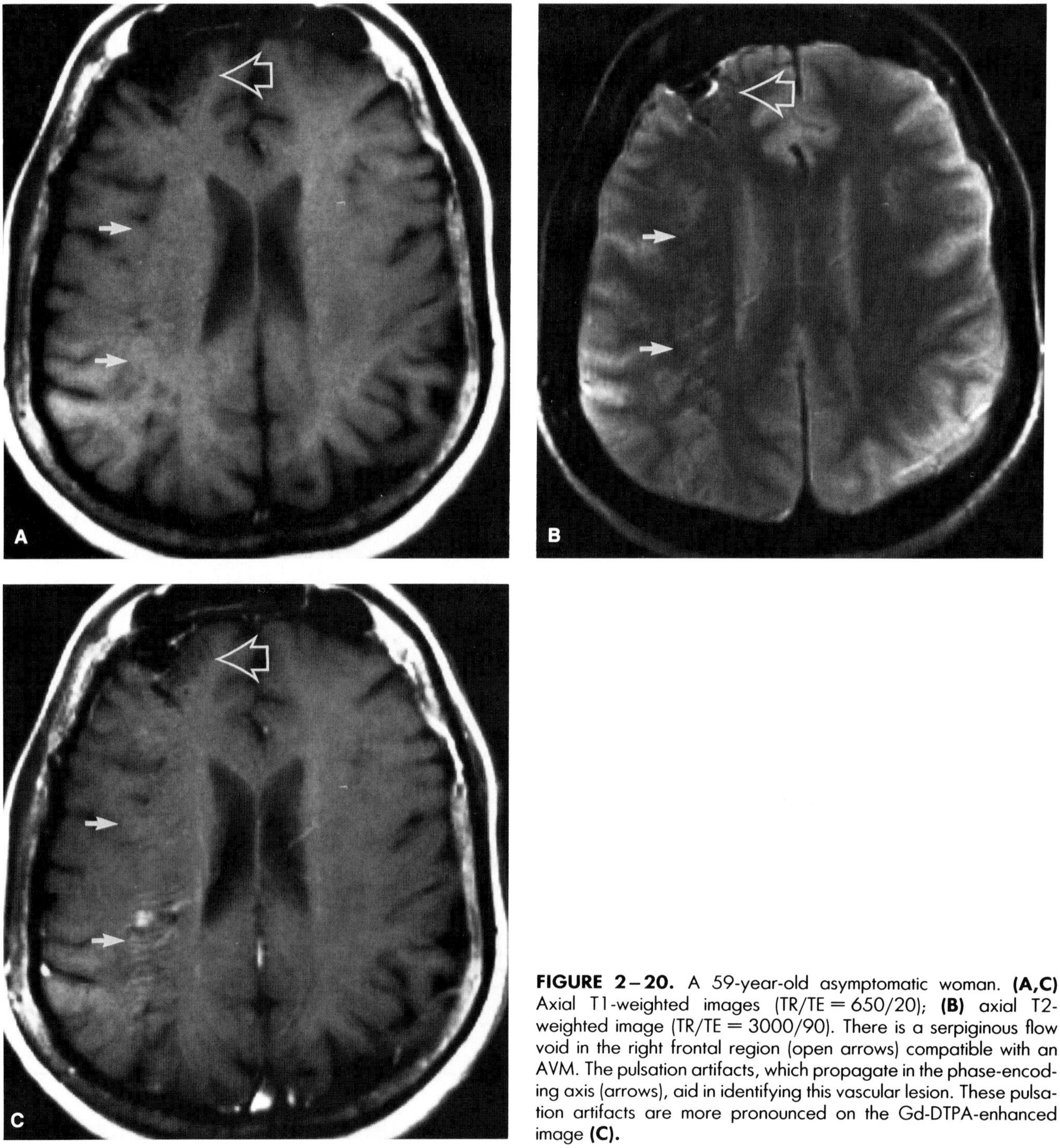

FIGURE 2–20. A 59-year-old asymptomatic woman. **(A,C)** Axial T1-weighted images (TR/TE = 650/20); **(B)** axial T2-weighted image (TR/TE = 3000/90). There is a serpiginous flow void in the right frontal region (open arrows) compatible with an AVM. The pulsation artifacts, which propagate in the phase-encoding axis (arrows), aid in identifying this vascular lesion. These pulsation artifacts are more pronounced on the Gd-DTPA-enhanced image **(C)**.

seen with AVMs, and these artifacts become more pronounced on Gd-DTPA-enhanced images (Fig. 2–20). The origins of feeding arteries are often delineated. Draining veins are identified by their caliber (i.e., larger than the arteries) and their drainage pattern into deep or cortical veins (Fig. 2–21).[44] Motion-compensated T2-weighted images (gradient moment nulling) can potentially obscure an AVM or any vascular anomaly because the motion-compensation gradients attempt to restore signal within the flow void created by moving blood. Therefore, the use of a nonmotion-compensated sequence should be considered in patients being evaluated for vascular anomalies. MRI accurately depicts and ages intraparenchymal hematomas associated with AVMs (Fig. 2–22).[7,44,49] MRI also detects superficial siderosis related to chronic

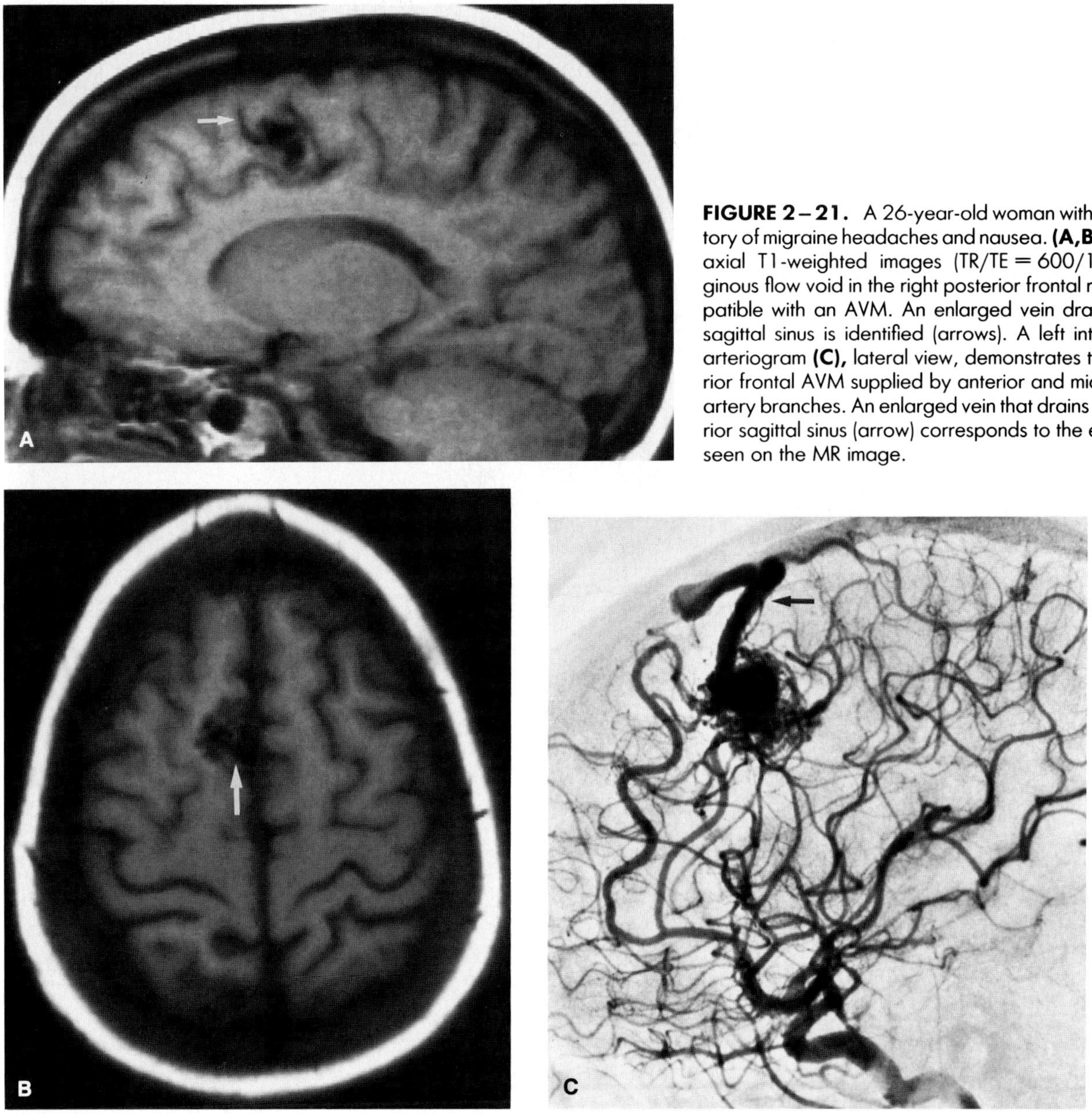

FIGURE 2–21. A 26-year-old woman with a 6-year history of migraine headaches and nausea. **(A,B)** Sagittal and axial T1-weighted images (TR/TE = 600/17). A serpiginous flow void in the right posterior frontal region is compatible with an AVM. An enlarged vein draining into the sagittal sinus is identified (arrows). A left internal carotid arteriogram **(C),** lateral view, demonstrates the left posterior frontal AVM supplied by anterior and middle cerebral artery branches. An enlarged vein that drains into the superior sagittal sinus (arrow) corresponds to the enlarged vein seen on the MR image.

subarachnoid hemorrhage, which is frequently associated with vascular malformations. This entity is not generally visualized by CT.

In contrast to congenital AVMs, pure dural-based AVMs are often acquired during trauma or inflammatory disease.[26] These lesions drain into the venous sinuses or cortical veins and commonly have associated intracranial or subarachnoid hemorrhage. MRI may have difficulty in detecting these lesions adjacent to the inner table of the skull because vascular flow and cortical bone both appear as signal voids. CT also has difficulty in detecting these lesions.[26] GRE imaging does not provide additional information because the magnetic susceptibility artifact from cortical bone and the sinuses associated with this technique obscures this region.[50] MRI, however, does identify hemorrhage complicating these lesions.

AVMs can have calcified components, and CT is more sensitive than MRI in detecting calcium.[7,51] Calcium has no mobile protons and appears as a signal void on MR sequences, which can be confused with flowing blood. In difficult cases in which accurate

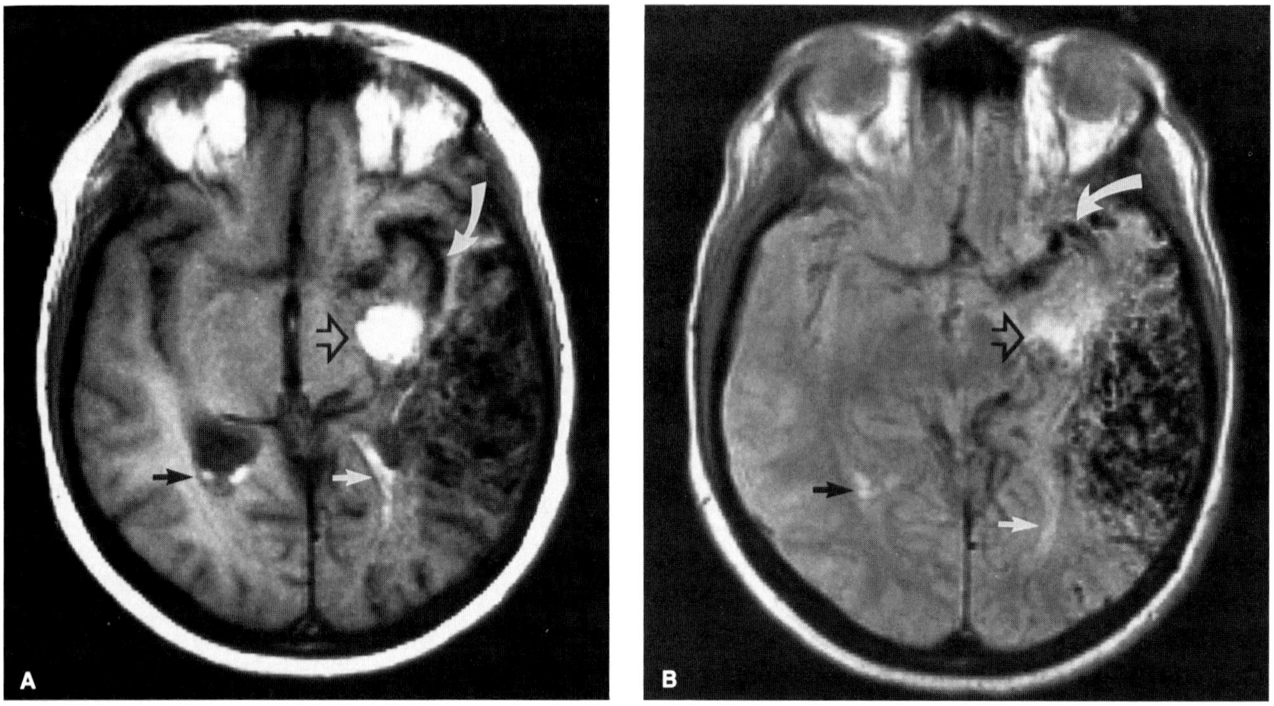

FIGURE 2–22. A 46-year-old woman with a complicated AVM. **(A)** Axial T1-weighted image (TR/TE = 600/17); **(B)** axial T2-weighted image (TR/TE = 3000/28). Flow voids identified in the left temporal parietal region are compatible with an extensive AVM. The left middle cerebral artery is enlarged (curved arrow). There is a circular hemorrhage (extracellular methemoglobin) involving the left basal ganglia (open arrow). There are increased signals in the dependent portions of the occipital horns (straight arrows), compatible with intraventricular blood (extracellular methemoglobin).

characterization of calcium, blood flow, and hemorrhagic components is desired, GRE techniques may be employed as a helpful adjunct to spin echo imaging.[49,50] On these sequences, flowing blood generally has increased signal intensity and can be distinguished from calcium or hemosiderin. Occasionally, however, flowing blood can also have low signal intensity on GRE images because of turbulent, in-plane, or very slow flow, and this potential pitfall should be recognized.[50]

The brain parenchyma adjacent to vessels forming the AVM can be affected by gliosis, edema, or ischemia. These parenchymal changes can be best detected as high signal intensity marginating a lesion on T2-weighted images.[44] This increased signal cannot definitely be differentiated from other causes, including neoplasm, of high signal intensity on T2-weighted images. However, the absence of a soft tissue mass favors a benign process, such as gliosis, edema, or ischemia.

VEIN OF GALEN ANEURYSM

Included in the spectrum of AVMs is the rare congenital anomaly, the vein of Galen aneurysm. Dilatation of the vein of Galen occurs if there is a downstream venous obstruction and there is increased flow through the vein of Galen secondary to an arteriovenous shunt.[26] Hydrocephalus often develops. Infants usually present with cardiac failure, and older children present with hydrocephalus and increased intracranial pressure.[52] MRI is useful in defining the anatomic extent of the abnormality and also evaluating blood flow patterns or thrombus within the aneurysm.[53] Preoperative angiography remains essential because the precise identification of the feeding arteries is necessary.

WYBURN MASON SYNDROME

This rare syndrome consists of a midbrain AVM, a facial cutaneous nevus in the distribution of the trigeminal nerve, and a retinal angioma ipsilateral to the facial nevus. MRI can noninvasively evaluate the retinal and midbrain components of this syndrome.[24,49]

Venous Angioma

Venous angiomas are vascular malformations involving only the venous side of the circulation. They occur throughout the central nervous system. Patients with venous angiomas are most commonly asymptomatic, although some patients may present with seizures or intracranial hemorrhage, including subarachnoid hemorrhage.[54] Cerebellar venous angiomas are more likely to hemorrhage.[55] Venous angiomas consist of a group of dilated medullary venous tributaries, often arranged in a radial "spoke-wheel" pattern, which typically drain into a large transcerebral vein. This large transcerebral vein drains into a venous sinus, a cortical vein, or a subependymal ventricular vein.

On spin echo MRI, venous angiomas typically appear as tubular flow voids with a radial configuration in the white matter (Fig. 2–23). An enlarged draining vein and its site of drainage are often visualized as well. Both T1-weighted and T2-weighted images are necessary to detect venous angiomas, and T2-weighted sequences are often the most sensitive.[56] Because of slow venous flow, which can cause an increased intravascular signal, these lesions may be inapparent (i.e., isointense to adjacent brain) on some imaging sequences. In particular, periventricular lesions can be difficult to identify.[57] MRI also best demonstrates parenchymal changes of ischemia or gliosis adjacent to the venous angioma. Intravascular contrast agents will further improve the ability of MRI to detect venous angiomas. We have identified venous angiomas on T1-weighted images after Gd DTPA administration that were difficult to visualize on the noncontrast images (Fig. 2–24).

Sturge-Weber Syndrome

Included in the spectrum of venous malformations is a neurocutaneous syndrome called Sturge-Weber syndrome or encephalotrigeminal angiomatosis. This syndrome consists of a cutaneous facial nevus (i.e., port wine stain), usually in the ophthalmic distribution of the trigeminal nerve, ipsilateral leptomeningeal angiomatosis, and ipsilateral cortical atrophy with linear cortical gyral calcifications in a tram-track configuration.[24,49,58] An ipsilateral choroid plexus an-

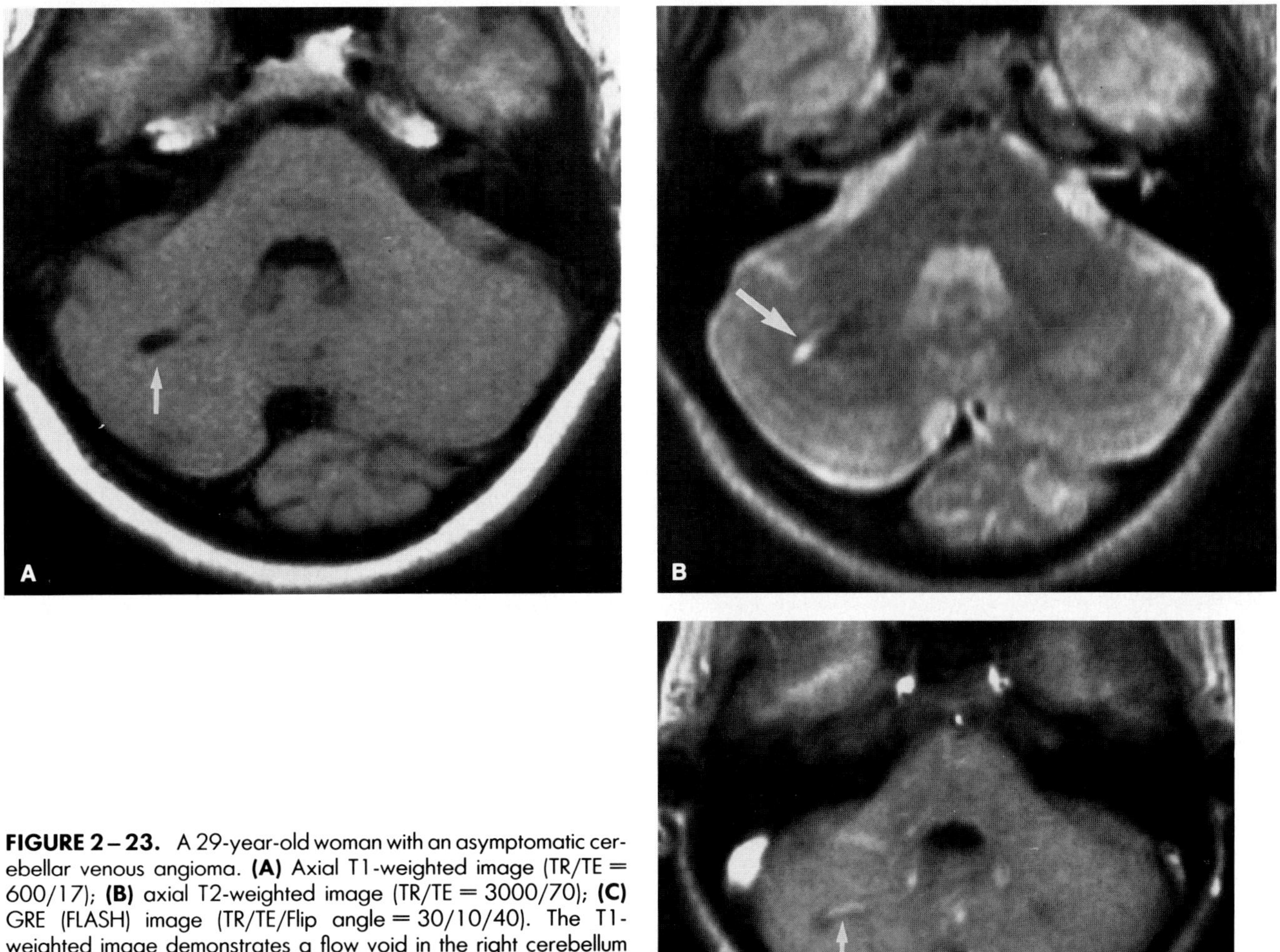

FIGURE 2–23. A 29-year-old woman with an asymptomatic cerebellar venous angioma. **(A)** Axial T1-weighted image (TR/TE = 600/17); **(B)** axial T2-weighted image (TR/TE = 3000/70); **(C)** GRE (FLASH) image (TR/TE/Flip angle = 30/10/40). The T1-weighted image demonstrates a flow void in the right cerebellum with a branching, spoke-wheel pattern in the white matter that is compatible with a venous angioma. The T2-weighted image demonstrates an intense signal in the peripheral portion of the angioma, compatible with slow flow (arrow). The GRE image demonstrates high signal intensity within the lesion, compatible with flow (arrow). Notice the high-signal-intensity flow within the transverse sinus, basilar artery, and internal carotid arteries **(C)**.

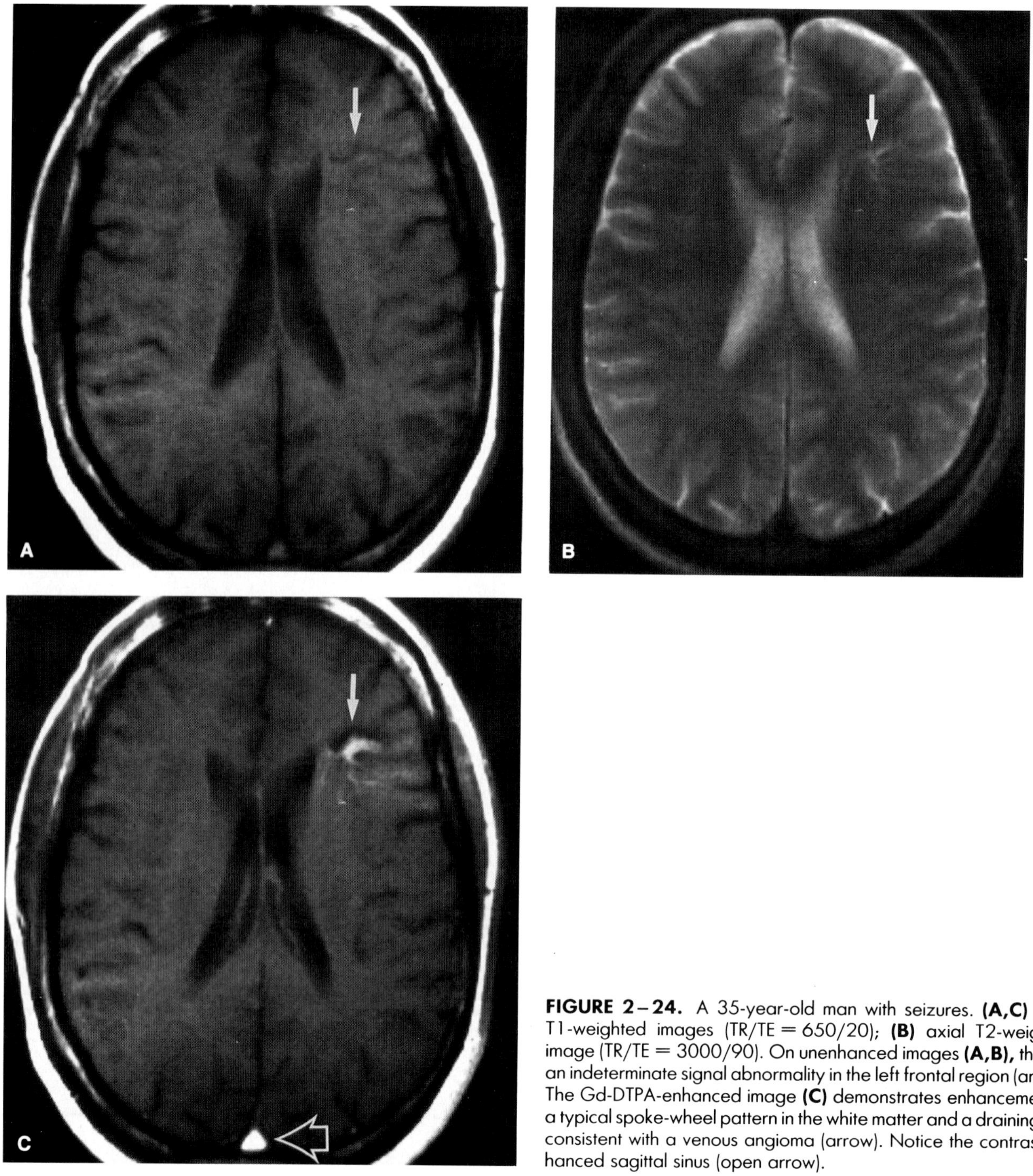

FIGURE 2–24. A 35-year-old man with seizures. **(A,C)** Axial T1-weighted images (TR/TE = 650/20); **(B)** axial T2-weighted image (TR/TE = 3000/90). On unenhanced images **(A,B),** there is an indeterminate signal abnormality in the left frontal region (arrow). The Gd-DTPA-enhanced image **(C)** demonstrates enhancement of a typical spoke-wheel pattern in the white matter and a draining vein consistent with a venous angioma (arrow). Notice the contrast-enhanced sagittal sinus (open arrow).

gioma is a common finding. Spin echo MR can successfully detect the vascular components of this syndrome.[58] The cortical and choroid plexus lesions characteristically enhance with contrast-enhanced CT, and similar findings are expected with contrast-enhanced MRI. GRE MRI can be useful in detecting the cortical gyral calcifications.[59]

Cavernous Angioma

A cavernous angioma (cavernous malformation or cavernous hemangioma) is a collection of endothelial-lined vascular spaces, which has no intervening brain parenchyma between these vessels.[43] They occur throughout the central nervous system but are more common in supratentorial and subcortical locations. Cavernous angiomas occur as multiple lesions in as many as 33% of cases.[43] These lesions are usually asymptomatic, but some patients present with seizures. There are two forms of cavernous angioma; the sporadic and familial forms. The familial form has a high incidence of multiple lesions, is autosomal dominant in transmission, and appears to have an increased frequency in Mexican-American families.[60]

Capillary Telangiectasia

Capillary telangiectasias (capillary angioma) are small, solitary lesions frequently found in the pons. In contrast to cavernous angiomas, capillary telangiectasia consists of dilated capillaries with intervening brain parenchyma between the vessels.[61] Most of these lesions are asymptomatic clinically, but can occasionally be associated with hemorrhage.[62]

Occult Cerebrovascular Malformations

Any of the four previously described pathologic entities comprising cerebrovascular malformations can be categorized as an OCVM if the lesion is angiographically occult. These lesions comprising the vascular malformations probably represent a continuum of abnormality. Venous angiomas, for example, can coexist with other occult cerebrovascular malformations.[49] MRI has become the primary screening modality in detecting these lesions because of its exquisite ability to detect the components of hemorrhage.[60,63]

OCVMs are characterized by multiple, recurrent, small hemorrhages and a central, nonresorbable nidus. A characteristic MR appearance of OCVMs has been described.[49,63] These characteristic features are rounded focal areas of increased signal intensity on T1-weighted and T2-weighted images corresponding to extracellular methemoglobin in subacute-chronic hemorrhage; a smooth, continuous rim of hypointensity, which is more pronounced on T2-weighted images than on T1-weighted images, that surrounds the high-intensity component and corresponds to hemosiderin; and no evidence of mass effect, edema, or associated enlarged arteries or veins (Fig. 2-25). Lesions with these characteristics are commonly cavernous angiomas on pathologic examination. After an acute hemorrhage, OCVMs may be difficult to distinguish from an intraparenchymal hematoma, particularly those caused by neoplasm. Beyond this acute stage, OCVMs can be distinguished from hematomas of other causes by their continuous hemosiderin rim, the absence of parenchymal mass effect or edema, the location of the lesion, and the expected temporal evolution of hemorrhage in a simple hematoma.[57,62]

The detection of very small OCVMs by MR depends on identifying the characteristic circumferential low-intensity hemosiderin rim. The preferential T2 PRE of hemosiderin is proportional to the square of magnetic field strength. High-field MR is more sensitive in detecting hemosiderin and, therefore, OCVM.[60,63] Ancillary GRE imaging can be used to improve the detection of small OCVMs because of the increased sensitivity of this technique to magnetic suspectibility effects.[50]

MRI is less sensitive than CT in detecting calcium.[7,51] Routine spin echo MRI may miss the small OCVMs with only small focal calcifications that are detected by CT.[64] In some OCVMs, contrast-enhanced CT also demonstrates various degrees of peripheral enhancement, which often has a ring configuration. Similar findings are expected with MRI after the administration of intravascular contrast agents (e.g., Gd DTPA), assuming that there is associated breakdown of the blood-brain barrier.

Flow Imaging Techniques

The use of MRI to depict flowing blood in the vascular system holds promise as a noninvasive method to evaluate the arterial and venous circulations throughout the body. Two processes primarily affect the appearance of flowing blood in the MR image: phase shifts of protons in moving blood with respect to stationary protons, and time-of-flight effects, which can cause decreased signal (i.e., high-velocity signal loss) or increased signal (i.e., flow-related enhancement).[65]

One technique called "flow imaging by phase display" or "phase imaging" is based on the phase shift of moving blood as it courses through the plane of section. In an MR exam, protons oscillate like spinning tops, and phase is the dimension used to describe each subdivision of this oscillation.[66] A change in phase within a voxel is called a phase shift, and it is specific for motion.[66] Each spin echo MR signal has both phase and magnitude. Therefore, a phase image, in addition to the standard magnitude image, can be reconstructed for any preselected spin echo sequence. T1-weighted sequences are often selected because of the short TE and the signal generated for moving blood. The application of gradient moment nulling with phase imaging may potentially obscure signal from slow flow. However, for detection of higher velocity flow, the use of partially rephased techniques is recommended.

In a phase image, areas with constant phase are represented by a homogeneous grey intensity or a "zebra-stripe" pattern of alternating bright and dark bands. A phase shift or flow will appear as a bright or dark intensity in relation to the grey background or as a distortion of the zebra-stripe pattern. Areas that contain no signal (e.g., air and bone) are also represented as a dark intensity, even though there is no

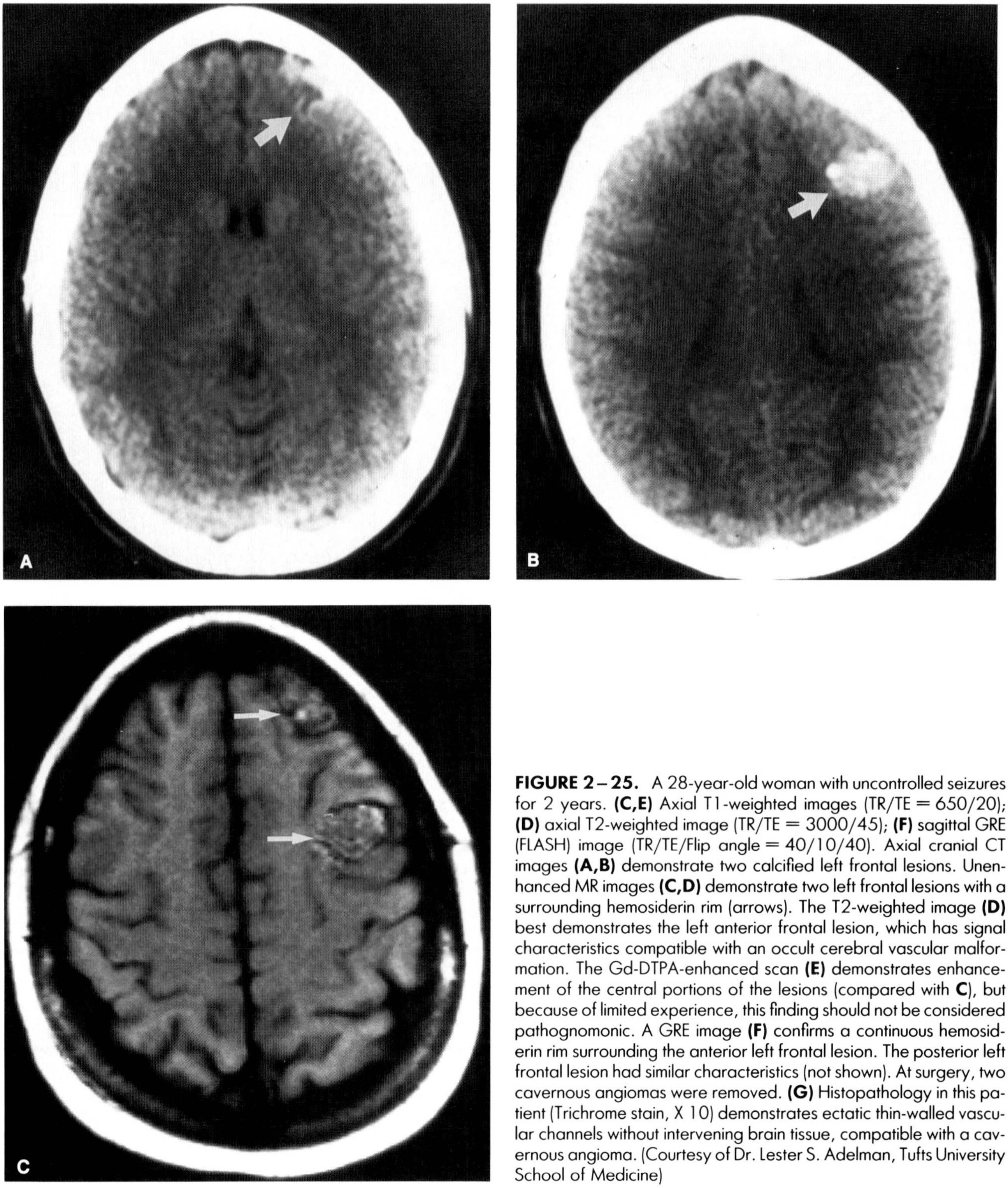

FIGURE 2–25. A 28-year-old woman with uncontrolled seizures for 2 years. **(C,E)** Axial T1-weighted images (TR/TE = 650/20); **(D)** axial T2-weighted image (TR/TE = 3000/45); **(F)** sagittal GRE (FLASH) image (TR/TE/Flip angle = 40/10/40). Axial cranial CT images **(A,B)** demonstrate two calcified left frontal lesions. Unenhanced MR images **(C,D)** demonstrate two left frontal lesions with a surrounding hemosiderin rim (arrows). The T2-weighted image **(D)** best demonstrates the left anterior frontal lesion, which has signal characteristics compatible with an occult cerebral vascular malformation. The Gd-DTPA-enhanced scan **(E)** demonstrates enhancement of the central portions of the lesions (compared with **C**), but because of limited experience, this finding should not be considered pathognomonic. A GRE image **(F)** confirms a continuous hemosiderin rim surrounding the anterior left frontal lesion. The posterior left frontal lesion had similar characteristics (not shown). At surgery, two cavernous angiomas were removed. **(G)** Histopathology in this patient (Trichrome stain, X 10) demonstrates ectatic thin-walled vascular channels without intervening brain tissue, compatible with a cavernous angioma. (Courtesy of Dr. Lester S. Adelman, Tufts University School of Medicine)

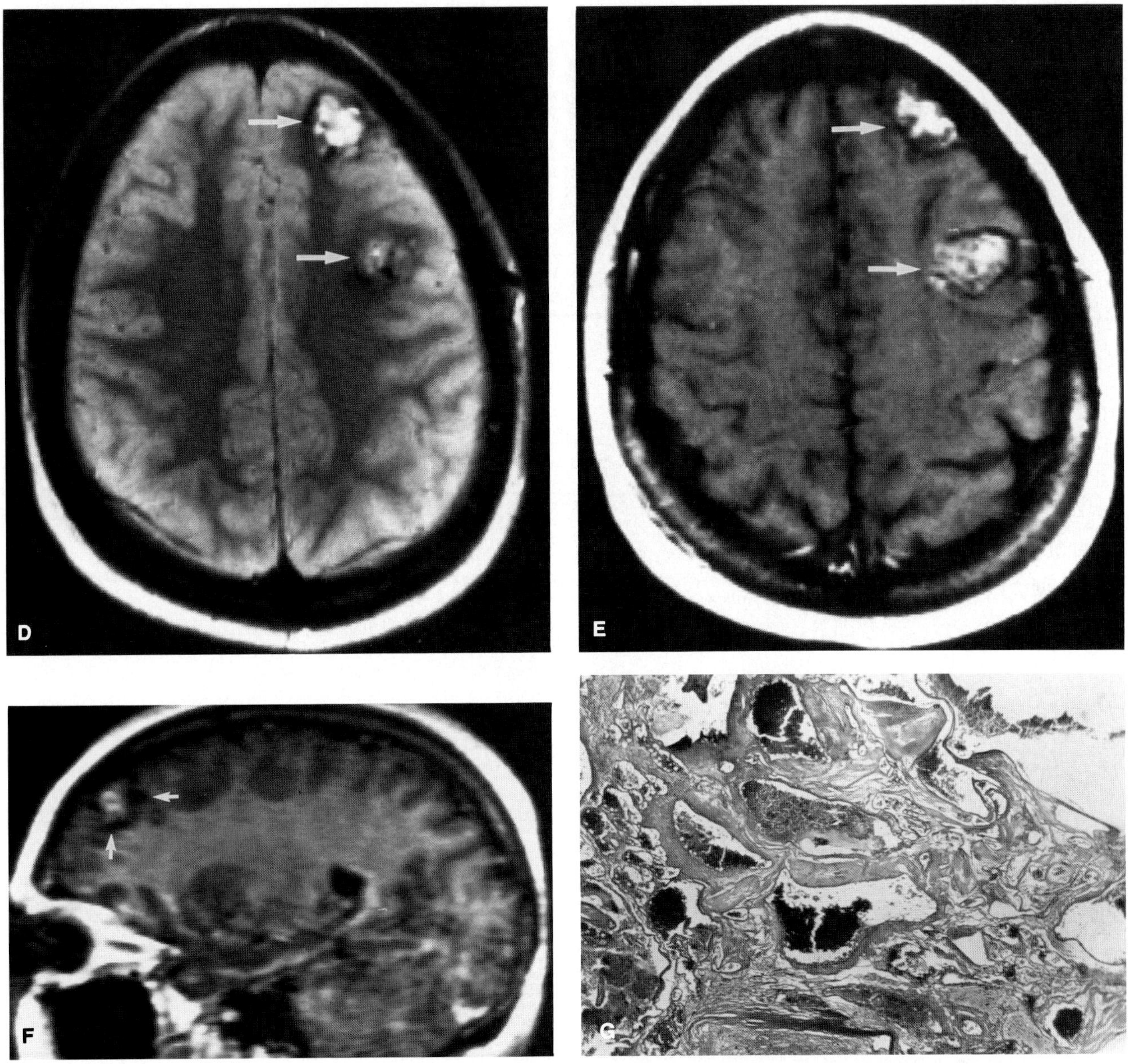

FIGURE 2–25. (Continued)

phase shift. For this reason, the phase image must be correlated with the anatomic magnitude image to avoid confusing air or bone with flowing blood (Fig. 2–26).

Another MR flow imaging technique, MR angiography, exploits the time-of-flight effects and phase shifts of moving blood to form an angiographic image. Time-of-flight effects include high-velocity signal loss (HVSL) and flow-related enhancement (FRE). HVSL causes decreased signal intensity from moving blood because protons do not remain within the selected slice long enough to acquire the 90° and 180° pulses of a spin echo MR sequence.[33,34,65] FRE occurs when unsaturated blood, which has zero net longitudinal magnetization and is fully magnetized, enters the selected slice and generates a stronger signal than the partially saturated protons in the adjacent tissue.[33,34,65] To counteract the FRE effect, a saturation RF pulse can be applied to a volume upstream of the selected slice. In this case, the moving blood entering the slice is saturated and does not generate a signal. Additional gradients can also be applied to further dephase the protons of flowing blood. This is an example of a dephased image.

Another phenomena that increases intravascular signal intensity is even-echo rephasing.[33,34,65] In a double-echo MR sequence, the first echo has motion-induced loss of phase coherence (i.e., dephasing), which

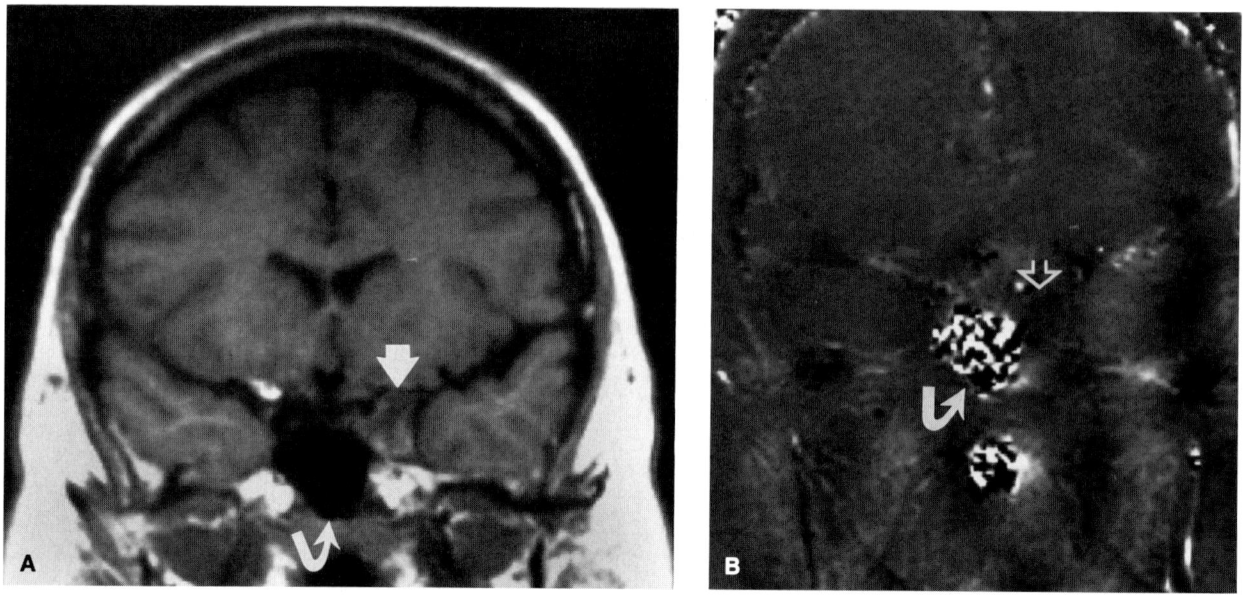

FIGURE 2–26. A 51-year-old woman with headaches and a bruit after embolization of a left cavernous carotid artery aneurysm (same patient as Fig. 2–17). **(A)** Coronal T1-weighted image (TR/TE = 650/20); **(B)** coronal phase image. The T1-weighted image demonstrates intermediate signal intensity in the region of the previously thrombosed left cavernous aneurysm (arrow). The phase image through the same level demonstrates no high or low signal intensity in this region (open arrows), confirming the absence of flow. The central low signal intensity (curved arrows) represents air in the sphenoid sinuses.

causes a loss of signal.[66,67] The addition of a second symmetric and selective 180°RF gradient (e.g., TE2 = 2 TE1) can compensate for the motion-induced phase changes of moving blood. The selective gradient refocuses the signal at the time of the second echo, which causes an increased intravascular signal.[68–70] This is the simplest example of the application of rephasing gradients to recapture or refocus the signal loss of moving blood. A more precise rephased image can be obtained by adding additional gradients to more perfectly refocus and restore intravascular signal. These gradients can correct for the velocity and acceleration of moving blood and are commonly oriented in the frequency-encoding (read) and/or the slice-select direction. These rephased sequences are identical to the motion-compensated sequences (i.e., gradient moment nulling) used in routine imaging.

The rephased image (i.e., high signal in the vascular space) and dephased image (i.e., low signal in the vascular space) can be subtracted to form a subtraction MR angiogram. Because stationary protons have no change in location or phase, their signals will cancel. Typically these sequences are gated to the cardiac cycle (i.e., R wave of the EKG) to control the phase changes and selectively image the arteries.[70] Dephased images are usually obtained at systole, which produces maximal motion-induced signal loss. The rephased images are obtained at diastole to obtain maximal intravascular signal (i.e., minimum of motion-induced signal loss). Presaturation pulses can be applied to selectively saturate portions of the vascular tree. Accurate manipulation of the TE, gradients, saturation pulses, and the volume imaged (voxel) are critical for quality images.[65,66] This type of MR angiography can either be performed in two dimensions (i.e., individual slices) or in three dimensions (i.e., a volumetric study); 2D MR angiography is commonly used to image the carotid bifurcation, and 3D MR angiography is commonly used to image the brain.

Flowing blood can also have increased signal intensity on certain GRE sequences. Another 3D MR angiographic technique, gradient-echo volume imaging, uses a single GRE acquisition instead of separate rephased and dephased sequences.[65] Computer tracing algorithms and thresholding techniques are used to display the high signal intensity in the vessels (Figs. 2–27 and 2–28).

In the cranial circulation, MR angiography may soon provide a noninvasive evaluation of the carotid arteries and intracranial vascular pathology, including aneurysms and vascular malformations, but some problems remain. Signal loss from turbulent flow at branch points or from slow flowing blood causes inaccurate delineation of vascular anatomy, and the resolution of MR angiography is inferior to conventional

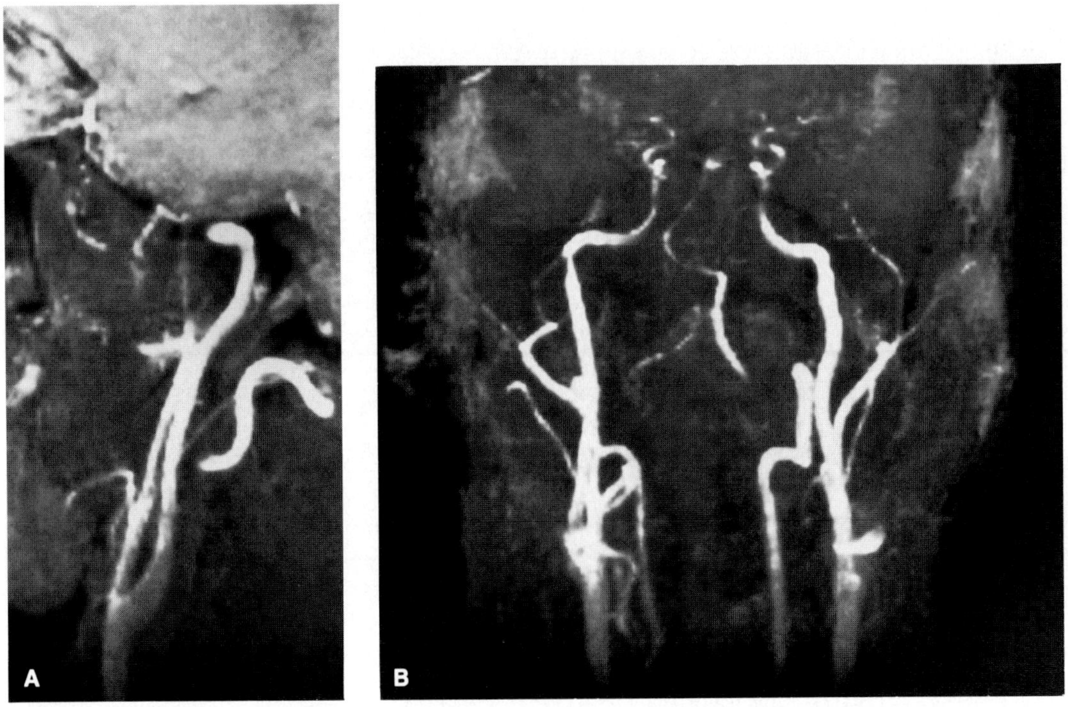

FIGURE 2–27. MR angiography of the neck. Gradient-echo volume imaging. **(A)** Normal carotid bifurcation (TR/TE/Flip angle = 80/11/20); **(B)** normal four vessels in the neck (TR/TE/Flip angle = 40/11/15). (Courtesy of University Radiology Clinics, Muenster, West Germany)

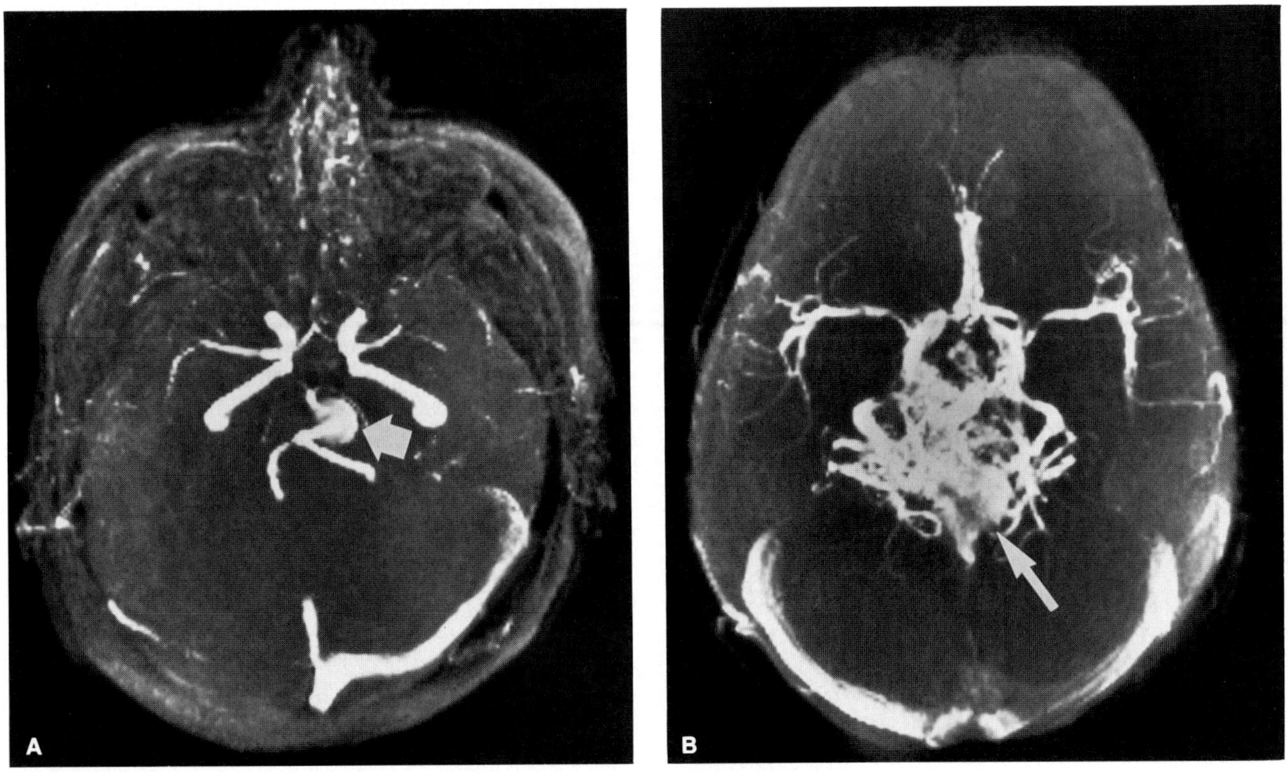

FIGURE 2–28. 3D MR angiography of the brain in two patients by gradient-echo volume imaging. Submental vertex projections (TR/TE/Flip angle = 40/7/15) demonstrate **(A)** a large aneurysm (arrow) involving the tip of the basilar artery and **(B)** an extensive midbrain AVM, which drains into an enlarged vein of Galen (arrow). (Courtesy of University Radiology Clinics, Muenster, West Germany)

angiography. Despite these problems, the future of MR angiography is promising. Other sources provide a more detailed discussion of this topic.[65-70]

CEREBRAL ISCHEMIA AND INFARCTION

Cerebrovascular occlusive disease causing cerebral ischemia or infarction is the most common disease affecting the brain. It is the most common neurologic disease seen by the radiologist in daily practice. Cerebrovascular disease is an important health care problem, particularly in a population over 55 years of age. It affects approximately 400,000 Americans annually and is the third leading cause of death, following cancer and myocardial infarction.[71,72] Almost half of the affected patients will have permanent neurologic deficits, and there are over 2 million survivors of cerebral infarction.[29,72]

MR is the imaging modality that most completely characterizes cerebrovascular occlusive disease by providing information concerning pathophysiology, anatomic localization, and vascular patency.

Clinical Considerations

Stroke is a general term describing an acute neurologic insult with a permanent deficit caused by a disease of the blood vessels. Cerebrovascular accident (CVA) is synonymous with stroke. The clinical presentation of patients with stroke is variable and nonspecific. Patients with a ruptured aneurysm, subdural hematoma, or hemorrhage into a tumor can present with stroke-like symptoms similar to patients with cerebral ischemia or infarction. The role of the radiologist is to employ the imaging modality that most effectively determines the cause of the symptoms in the individual patient.

In patients with ischemia or infarction, there is often a disparity between the pathophysiology and the clinical manifestations of the disease.[73] Therefore, the accurate use of terminology describing ischemic disease is important. Cerebral ischemia and infarction describe pathophysiologic processes.[73,74] Cerebral ischemia describes global or regional reduction of blood flow to the brain. Cerebral infarction occurs when the reduction of blood flow causes irreversible cellular damage (i.e., cell death).

The clinical terminology describing ischemic neurologic events is based on clinical presentation and evolution.[71] A transient ischemic attack (TIA) is a transient loss of neurologic function that resolves in 24 hours. Reversible ischemic neurologic deficit (RIND) indicates loss of neurologic function that resolves within 21 days. A progressing stroke or stroke in evolution describes a changing neurologic state. A completed stroke indicates a permanent and fixed neurologic deficit. A patient with a cerebral infarction may present with any of these clinical states, even though permanent tissue damage has occurred. Subclinical cerebral ischemia and infarction are often only detected by the current sensitive imaging modalities, particularly MRI.

Pathophysiology

In the normal state, the brain receives 15 to 20% of the cardiac output, and the brain extracts 50% of the available oxygen and 10% of the available glucose for cerebral metabolism.[73,75] After an ischemic event, the tissue oxygen concentration decreases more than the glucose concentration. Prolonged lack of oxygen reduces energy production, decreasing ATP levels and building lactic acid levels. The sodium-potassium pump fueled by ATP fails, and as sodium moves into cells, potassium leaks out. Tissue osmolality increases because of the continued presence of glucose. Water accumulates in cells because of the osmotic gradient and increased intracellular sodium. This process in which fluid accumulates in the intracellular spaces is called cytotoxic edema.[73] Within 30 minutes after the insult, mitochondria are destroyed. Disruption of cytoplasmic and endothelial membranes follow, and by 6 hours, there is disruption of the blood-brain barrier.[72,73] These pathophysiologic changes suggest that reversible ischemia occurs within the first hour, before the disruption of the blood-brain barrier.[72,73]

Disruption of the blood-brain barrier causes leakage of water and protein into the extracellular compartment. Reperfusion of the infarcted region can occur within the first 30 minutes, by reestablishing the native circulation or by development of collaterals.[76] The degree of reperfusion of the infarcted region determines the amount of fluid that enters the extracellular compartment. This increase in extracellular fluid is called vasogenic edema.[73] The vasogenic edema can progress with continued reperfusion and create an expanding mass that compresses the adjacent microcirculation. There may be extension of the infarct by this process, and irreversible cellular damage (infarction) may result at the margins of the original ischemic region.[73,74]

In general, the mass effect caused by vasogenic edema progresses the first 3 to 7 days, stabilizes in the second week, and begins to resolve by the third week.[73,74] Blood-brain-barrier disruption can be seen up to 6 weeks after the ischemic insult.[77] The development of secondary hemorrhagic foci (i.e., petechial hemorrhage) occurs in as many as 40% of cases, typically during the second week.[73,74] These hemorrhages are usually clinically occult. Intraparenchymal hemorrhage can occasionally present clinically in the first few days, and in this situation the hemorrhage is commonly secondary to embolic infarction.[74]

In the completed infarct, there is gliosis, loss of tissue, and associated focal atrophy. There may be residual cystic areas (i.e., macrocystic encephalomalacia) in the infarcted territory. If there has been associated hemorrhage, hemosiderin may be detected. Dystrophic calcification of the infarcted brain rarely occurs.[73,74] In large supratentorial territory infarcts, anterograde degeneration of descending pathways in the cerebral peduncles, pons, or brain stem can be visualized and is called Wallerian degeneration.[78]

Basic MR Principles of Cerebral Infarction

The pathophysiology provides a conceptual framework for understanding the appearance of cerebral ischemia and infarction on spin echo MR images. Cerebral ischemia and infarction produce fluid changes in the intracellular and extracellular spaces (i.e., cytotoxic and vasogenic edema). MRI provides exquisite sensitivity in detecting cerebral ischemia and infarction because of its ability to detect small changes in tissue water content. Increased water content causes prolongation of both T1 and T2 relaxation times. Thus, the edema of cerebral ischemia or infarction appears as a low or isointense signal intensity on T1-weighted images and high signal intensity on T2-weighted images. T2-weighted images have proven to be the most sensitive in the detection of cerebral infarction.[73,79] The signal-intensity changes of infarction are more easily recognized on T2-weighted spin echo images because they are high in signal intensity. Commonly used "T1-weighted" spin echo sequences (i.e., short TR, short TE) do not have optimal T1 contrast, and the low-intensity T1 changes are less obvious. Inversion recovery sequences or GRE sequences providing T1 contrast (i.e., 3D FLASH) will have more T1 weighting, or more T1 contrast, and the low-intensity changes of ischemia or infarction will be better visualized than with spin echo imaging (Fig. 2–29).

Clinical studies have demonstrated the increased sensitivity of MRI compared with CT in detecting cerebral infarction, particularly in the acute phase (0–3 days).[73,80] In animals, MRI detected cerebral ischemia as early as 30 minutes after vascular occlusion.[81] MRI routinely demonstrates ischemic changes by 4 to 6 hours.[77,81–83] The reported CT detection of cerebral

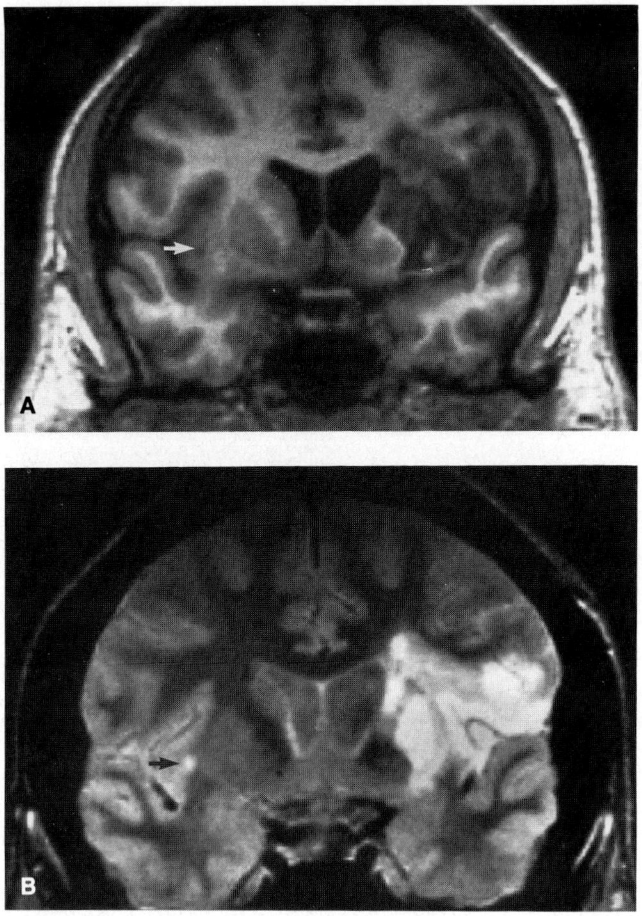

FIGURE 2–29. A 38-year-old woman with right hemiparesis and aphasia. **(A)** Coronal 3D GRE (FLASH) image (TR/TE/Flip angle = 40/15/40); **(B)** coronal T2-weighted image (TR/TE = 3000/45). There is a wedge-shaped left parietal lesion that extends to the cortical surface and is consistent with a thrombotic infarct in the distribution of the left middle cerebral artery. There is involvement of deep structures, including the head of the caudate nucleus, the anterior limb of the internal capsule, and the putamen. The GRE sequence demonstrates excellent T1 contrast, and the low-intensity T1 changes of infarction are easily visualized. The focal dilatation of the frontal horn of the left lateral ventricle is compatible with chronic infarction. A small focal area of ischemia and gliosis occurs in the right temporal region (arrows).

infarction is only 20% in the first 6 hours and 79% in the first 24 hours.[84] In the immediate period after infarction, MRI may be the most sensitive. During this phase, the prolongation of T1 and T2 is the greatest, because there is only the accumulation of bulk water (i.e., cytotoxic edema). After the blood-brain barrier is disrupted, the influx of protein into the tissues (i.e., vasogenic edema) decreases the degree of T1 and T2 prolongation because a protein-containing fluid is

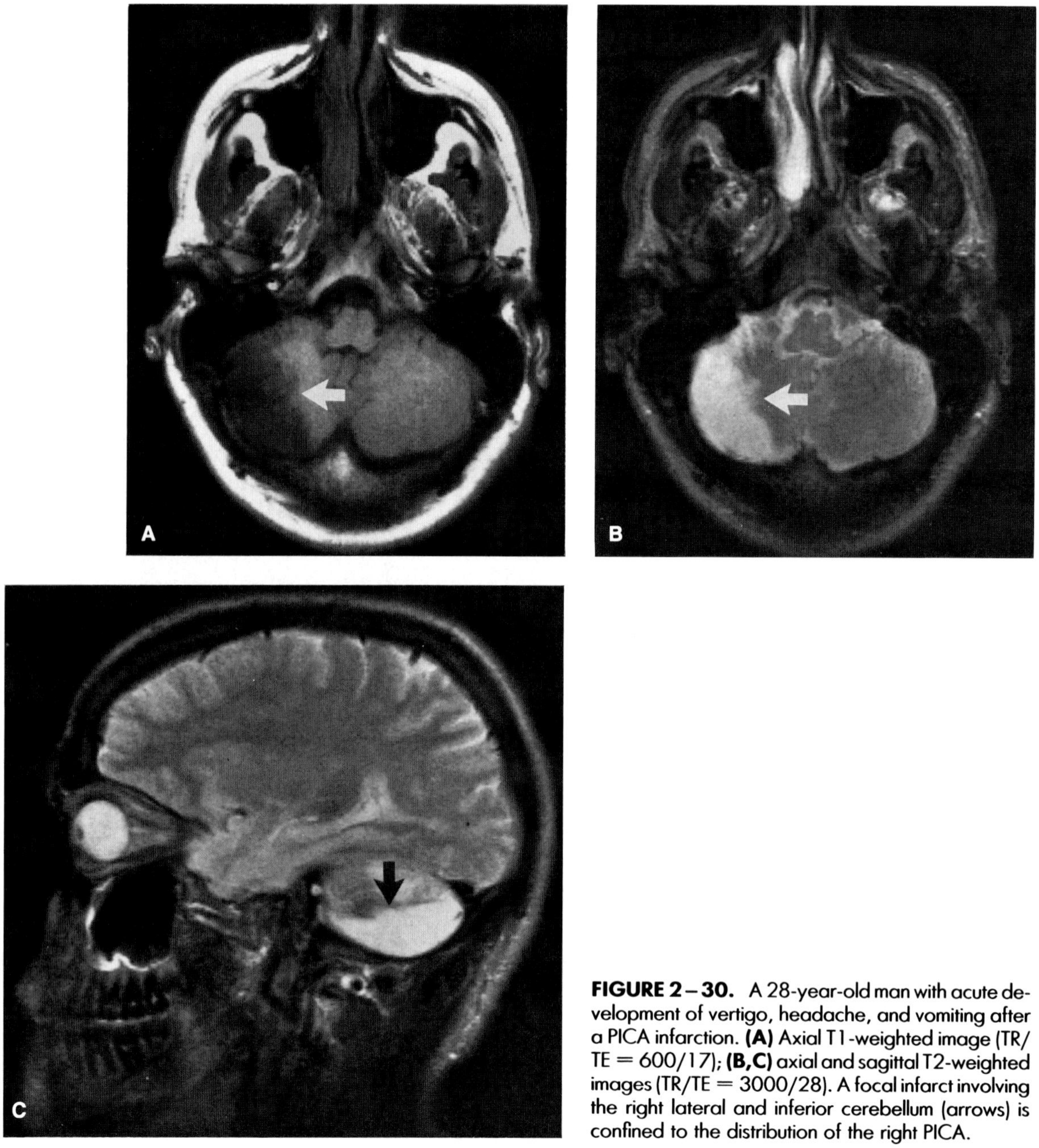

FIGURE 2–30. A 28-year-old man with acute development of vertigo, headache, and vomiting after a PICA infarction. **(A)** Axial T1-weighted image (TR/TE = 600/17); **(B,C)** axial and sagittal T2-weighted images (TR/TE = 3000/28). A focal infarct involving the right lateral and inferior cerebellum (arrows) is confined to the distribution of the right PICA.

formed that may decrease the contrast of the lesion compared with the surrounding normal tissue.[77,82] MRI is also superior to CT in detecting posterior fossa and brain stem infarcts because, unlike CT, these regions are not obscured by beam-hardening artifacts (Fig. 2–30).

Intravenous paramagnetic contrast agents (e.g., Gd DTPA) provide a sensitive marker of blood-brain-barrier disruption.[77] Paramagnetic contrast agents decrease T1 relaxation times, increasing signal intensity on T1-weighted images. Enhancement after cerebral infarction can be detected as early as the first day.[77,82] Peak enhancement usually occurs at 30 minutes after injection.[76] MRI is at least as sensitive as CT in detecting blood-brain-barrier disruption caused by cerebral infarction.[76] Accurate, early detection has clinical im-

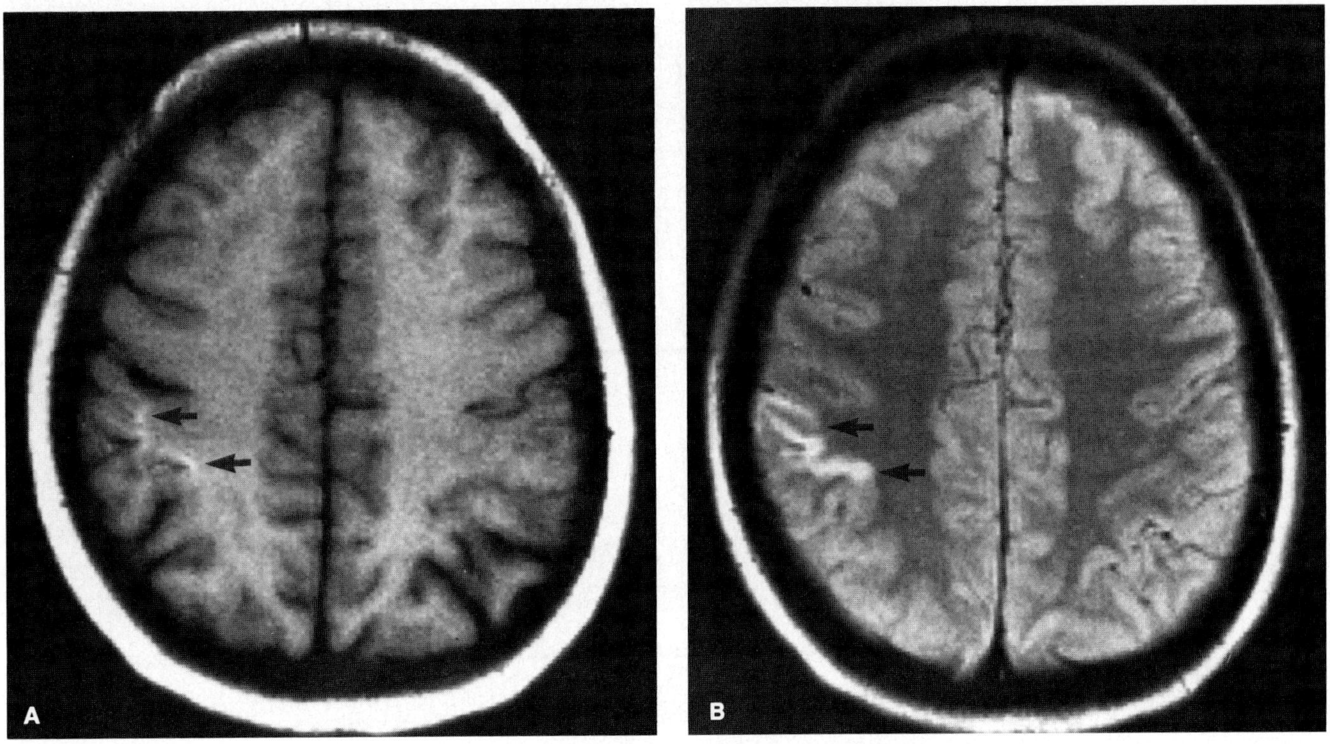

FIGURE 2–31. A 39-year-old woman with a left hemisensory deficit and a hemorrhagic cortical infarction. **(A)** Axial T1-weighted image (TR/TE = 600/17); **(B)** axial T2-weighted image (TR/TE = 3000,28). Serpiginous linear areas of increased signal intensity (arrows) marginate cortical gyri in the right parietal region. These findings are compatible with extracellular methemoglobin in a hemorrhagic infarct.

plications, because the loss of blood-brain-barrier integrity indicates an irreversible lesion (i.e., infarction), and therapy attempting to reestablish perfusion may have an adverse outcome in these cases.[72]

In the subacute phase (3 days to 3 weeks), cerebral infarction continues to be characterized by increased signal intensity on T2-weighted images and isointense or decreased signal intensity on T1-weighted images. MRI accurately defines the mass effect associated with infarction, which is often most pronounced in the early, subacute phase. These findings include compression and effacement of the sulci or ventricular system and displacement of midline structures.

MRI is particularly sensitive in detecting petechial hemorrhage, which commonly complicates infarction, particularly in the subacute phase. Petechial hemorrhage or cortical hemorrhagic infarction is most commonly identified as high signal intensity on T1-weighted images because of methemoglobin (Fig. 2–31). Acute and chronic stages of cortical hemorrhagic infarction also have been described.[85] In the acute phase, cortical low signal intensity produced by deoxyhemoglobin is identified on T2-weighted images, which is outlined by the subcortical high-intensity edema of the infarct. The cortical signal changes produced by deoxyhemoglobin are isointense with brain on T1-weighted images (Fig. 2–32). In the chronic phase, there is marked cortical low signal intensity on T2-weighted images produced by hemosiderin deposition that outlines the deep cortical gyri. Corresponding low signal intensity can be identified on T1-weighted images in the chronic phase as well, which is characteristic of this chronic phase and is produced by a dominant T2 PRE effect. Because the T2 PRE effects of deoxyhemoglobin and hemosiderin are proportional to field strength, these findings are most pronounced at high field strengths and may not be detected at low field strengths.

In the chronic stage of infarction (>3 weeks), the edema subsides, and there is subsequent glial proliferation with brain shrinkage. Gliosis causes increased brain water content and appears as high signal inten-

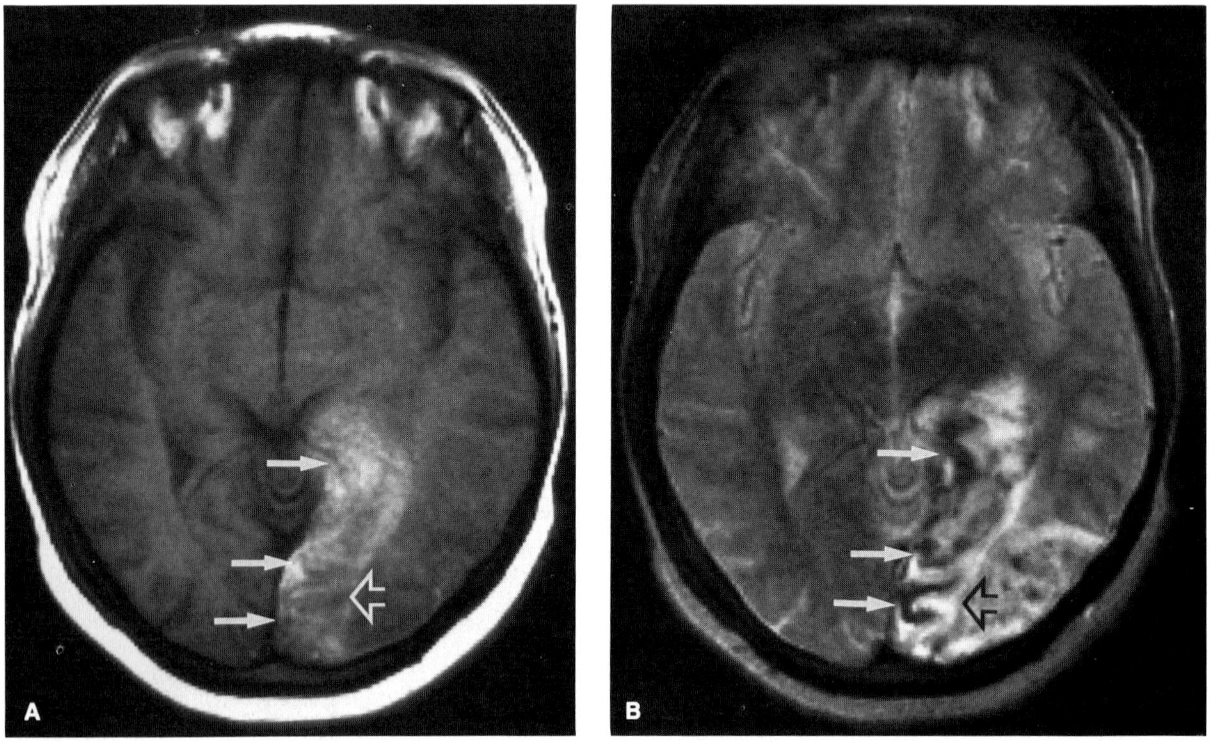

FIGURE 2–32. A 19-year-old woman with right homonymous hemianopsia for 1 week. **(A)** Axial T1-weighted image (TR/TE = 600/17); **(B)** axial T2-weighted image (TR/TE = 3000/70). The T1-weighted image demonstrates increased signal intensity in the right occipital region compatible with methemoglobin in a hemorrhagic infarction. The T2-weighted image demonstrates linear areas of low signal intensity (arrows) that outline the cortex and represent deoxyhemoglobin. These regions are isointense with brain tissue (arrows) on the T1-weighted image. Just deep to the cortical deoxyhemoglobin is subcortical edema (open arrows). These findings represent a subacute hemorrhagic infarction in the distribution of the left posterior cerebral artery and the left posterior-middle cerebral artery watershed region.

sity on T2-weighted images and as low signal intensity on T1-weighted images. Focal atrophy is identified as enlargement of adjacent sulci or portions of the ventricular system. Cystic changes (e.g., macrocystic encephalomalacia), if present, are characterized by a fluid intensity that follows CSF (Fig. 2–33). Typically, disruption of the blood-brain barrier, as detected by Gd DTPA, is not visualized beyond 6 weeks.[72]

Causes of Cerebral Ischemia and Infarction

The cause of cerebral ischemia is often multifactorial. The efficiency of the heart, the integrity of vessels supplying the brain, and the state of the blood itself in supplying oxygen at the cellular level (e.g., oxygen carrying capacity, viscosity, coagulability) can contribute to cerebral ischemia or infarction.[73] Lesions of the vascular tree are commonly the dominant factor in the development of cerebrovascular insufficiency that leads to infarction.[71] The display on page 88 lists the major causes of cerebral infarction and provides a framework for the following discussion.

Thrombotic Infarction

Arterial thrombotic infarction occurs when the arterial lumen is narrowed significantly and blood clots form that occlude the artery. Degenerative atherosclerotic disease, inflammatory disease, or arterial dissection can cause arterial narrowing, although atherosclerotic disease is by far the most common cause.[29,71] Atherosclerosis is a degeneration of the intima and media of the arterial wall, with associated

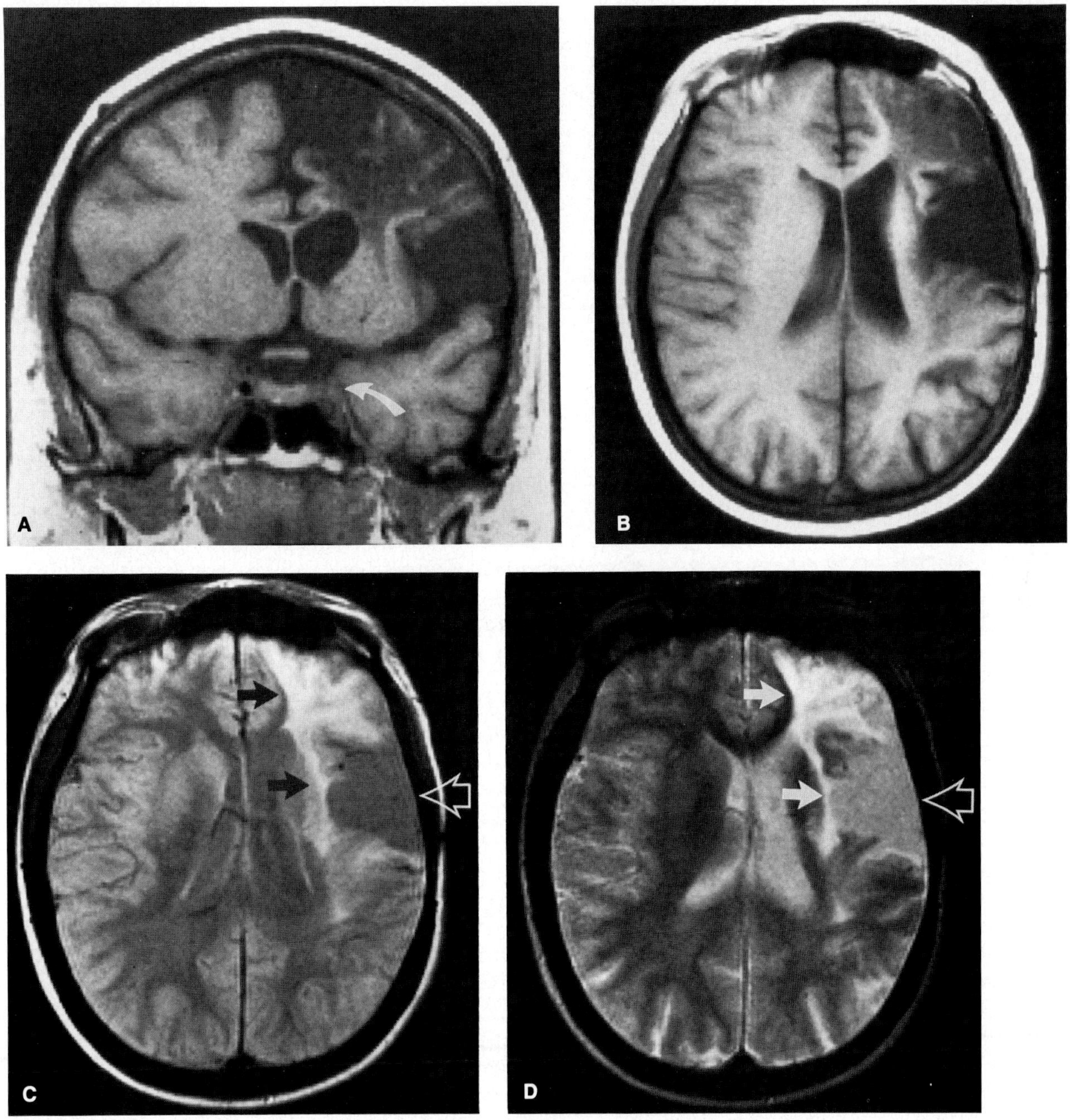

FIGURE 2–33. A 37-year-old woman with a left hemispheric CVA 8 years ago and residual right lower extremity weakness. **(A,B)** Coronal and axial T1-weighted images (TR/TE = 600/17); **(C,D)** axial T2-weighted images (TR/TE = 3000/28,70). There is absence of the normal flow void in the cavernous and supraclinoid segments of the left internal carotid artery (curved arrow). A chronic left frontal-parietal infarct involves the distribution of the left middle cerebral artery and the watershed zone of the left anterior-middle cerebral artery. Gliosis (closed arrows) and associated dilatation of the left lateral ventricle are shown. Posteriorly and inferiorly, fluid intensity (open arrows) parallels CSF signal intensity and represents cystic encephalomalacia.

Causes of Cerebral Infarction

Arterial Disease

Thrombotic (atherosclerotic) infarction
Embolic infarction
Hemodynamic infarction
Microangiopathy
  Lacunar infarction
  White matter ischemia—gliosis
Arteritis
Vasospasm
Anoxia and carbon monoxide poisoning
Arterial dissection
Other
  Moyamoya
  Amyloid angiopathy

Veno-occlusive Disease

Venous thrombosis

proliferation of these elements and lipid deposition.[29,71,86] Atherosclerotic lesions or plaques occur at arterial branch points, which are the sites of greatest mechanical stress and turbulence.[86] As an atherosclerotic plaque slowly enlarges, a critical size is reached at which the surface of the plaque may fissure and ulcerate. Platelets adhere to the irregular plaque surface and release prostaglandins, which promote deposition of additional platelet-fibrin plugs and clot on the plaque surface.[29,71] Thrombosis then occurs, which results in arterial occlusion.

Atherosclerotic thrombotic infarction typically involves large arteries and causes major arterial branch distribution ischemic infarction. Atherosclerotic thrombosis most commonly involves the middle cerebral artery (50%), the internal carotid artery (25%), and the vertebrobasilar system (25%).[75] The extent of the infarction is determined by the location of the obstruction (i.e., the more proximal the lesion, the less likely the development of infarction), the availability of collateral circulation, the extent of the occlusion, and the state of the systemic circulation.[75,87]

Atherosclerotic disease occurs more commonly in patients with hypertension, hypercholesterolemia, or hyperlipidemia and in those who smoke.[29] The common locations of atherosclerotic lesions are related to sex and race. In white men, atherosclerotic lesions predominate at the carotid bifurcation, the carotid siphon, and the vertebrobasilar system.[88] White men also have a high incidence of vascular occlusive disease, hypertension, and hyperlipidemia. In women, blacks, and persons of Chinese or Japanese ancestry, atherosclerotic lesions predominate in the intracranial arteries. The common locations are the supraclinoid internal carotid arteries; the anterior, middle, and posterior cerebral arteries; and the vertebrobasilar branches supplying the cerebellum.[88] These patients also have a high incidence of diabetes and hypertension.

MR FINDINGS IN THROMBOTIC INFARCTION

The MR findings in thrombotic cerebral infarction are an area of increased water content, causing high signal intensity on T2-weighted images and low or isointense signal intensity on T1-weighted images that is strictly confined to a major cerebral arterial vascular distribution. The distribution of this abnormality corresponds to the occluded artery. Characteristically, thrombotic infarcts are sharply demarcated, wedge-shaped lesions that extend to the cortical surface (Fig. 2–29). However, depending on the extent and location of the occlusion and the status of the collateral circulation, thrombotic infarcts can have a variety of configurations, but the signal changes remain confined to a vascular distribution (Fig. 2–34). For this reason, a knowledge of the arterial territories of the brain is necessary (see the Arterial Vascular Territories display on pages 90–93).

Because the signal characteristics of other parenchymal lesions, including hyperacute hemorrhage, neoplasm, and inflammatory disease, can be similar to that of thrombotic infarction, other MR findings can aid in the discrimination of these entities. A hyperacute intraparenchymal hematoma is typically a spheric focal mass that may not be localized to an arteriovascular distribution. An intraparenchymal hematoma has a characteristic temporal progression, which can distinguish this lesion from a bland infarct. Most thrombotic cerebral infarctions involve both gray and white matter. In contrast, primary or secondary neoplasms or inflammatory disease (abscesses) are usually centered in the white matter, although they can extend to the cortex. The edema associated with neoplasm or inflammatory disease spreads diffusely in the white matter in finger-like projections, has ill-defined margins, and may not be restricted to an arterial distribution.

Contrast enhancement can add specificity to the MR examination.[75–77] Neoplasm and inflammatory disease are often characterized by a central enhancing mass. The configuration of enhancement in cerebral infarction is often variable but conforms to the wedge-shaped distribution of the lesion. Peripheral linear gyral enhancement can also be seen. We have seen early cortical infarction that is identified only by

(text continues on page 94)

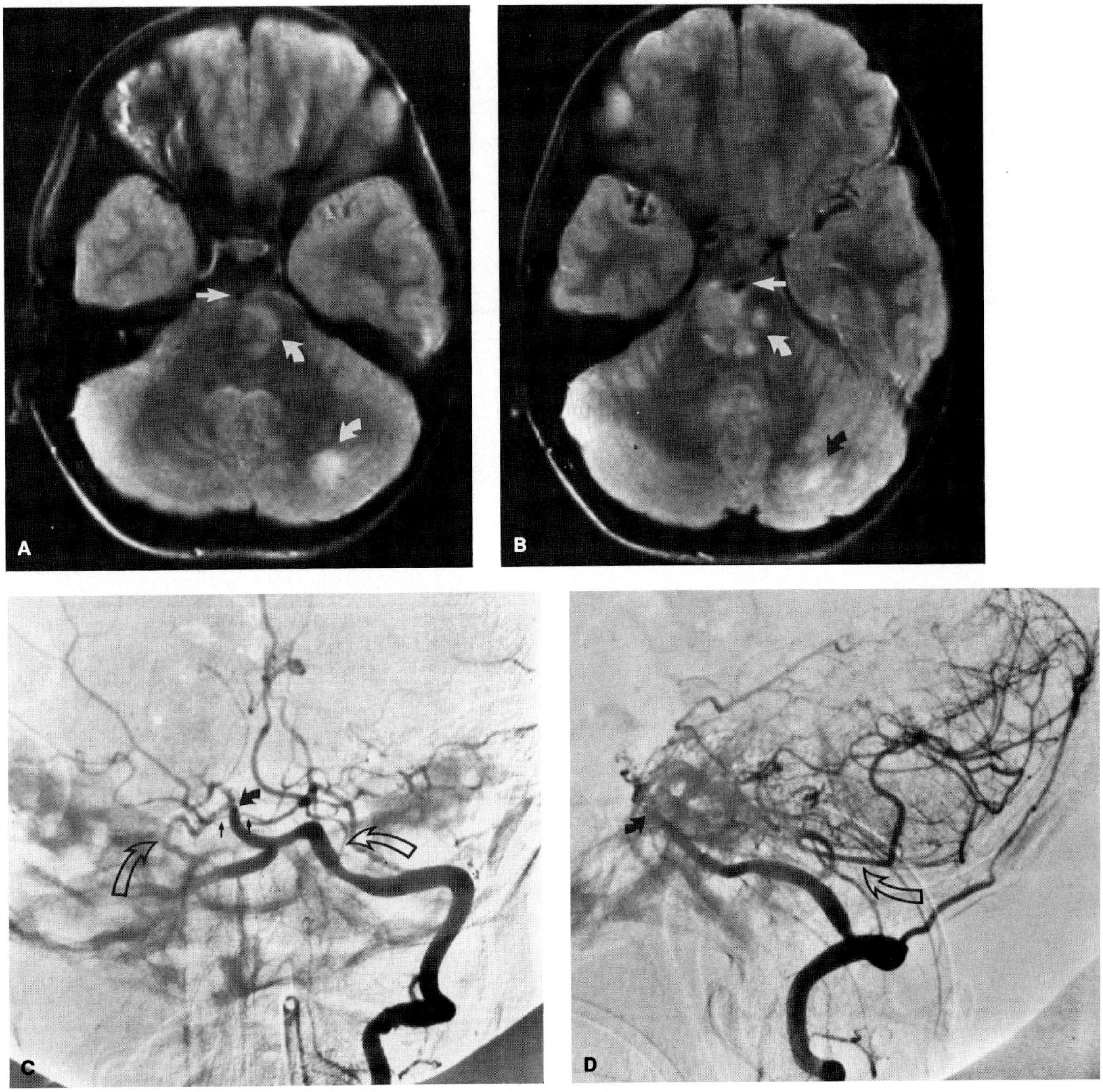

FIGURE 2–34. A 6-year-old boy with acute development of headache, left hemiparesis, incontinence, and lethargy. **(A,B)** Axial T2-weighted images (TR/TE = 3000/45) through the level of the pons and middle cerebellar peduncles demonstrate focal areas of signal intensity involving the pons and the gray-white matter junction of the left cerebellum (curved arrows). A small flow void is identified in the basilar artery (straight arrows). Differential diagnosis included neoplasm, demyelination, and infarction. A left vertebral arteriogram, anteroposterior **(C)** and lateral **(D)** views, 8 days later demonstrates a sharply marginated occlusion involving the proximal basilar artery (curved solid arrow) just beyond the origins of the anterior inferior cerebellar arteries (small straight arrows). PICA are filled bilaterally (curved open arrows). Bilateral internal carotid arteriograms (not shown) demonstrated filling of both posterior cerebral arteries through the patent posterior communicating arteries. The pontine infarction is in the distribution of the penetrating branches of the basilar artery and the left cerebellar infarction is at the border zone of the left superior cerebellar and posterior inferior cerebellar arteries.

ARTERIAL VASCULAR TERRITORIES—AXIAL PLANE

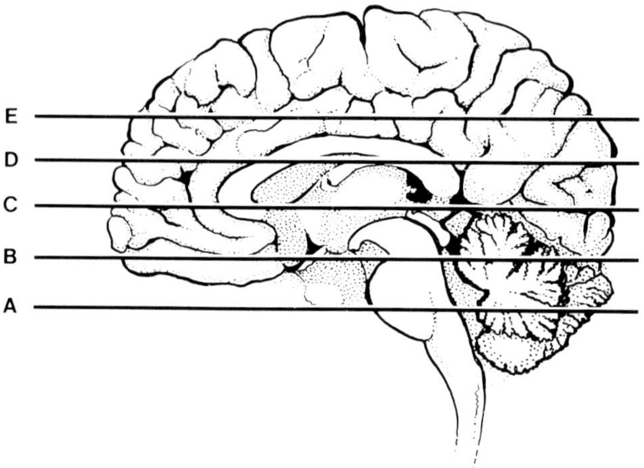

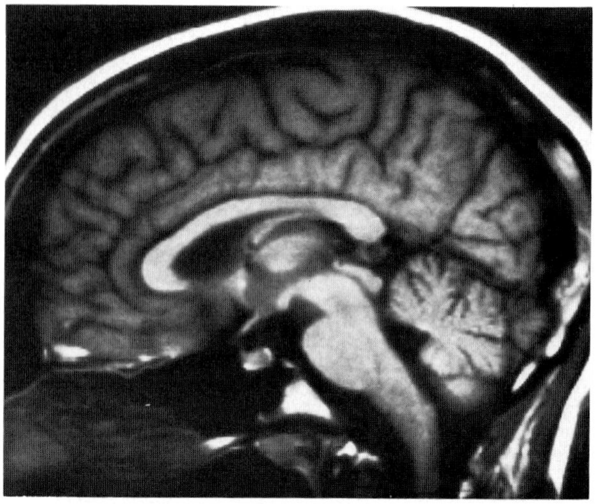

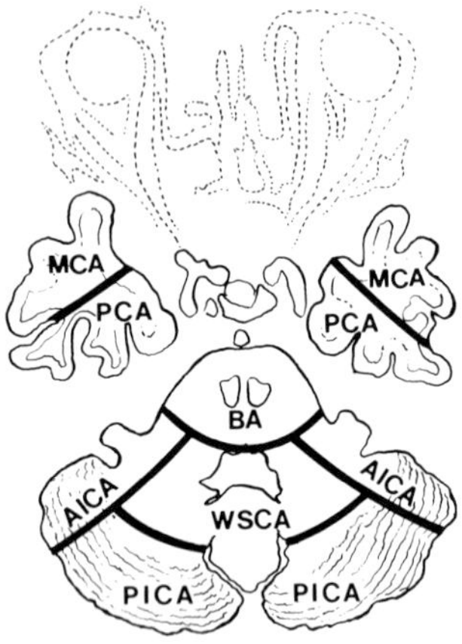

A

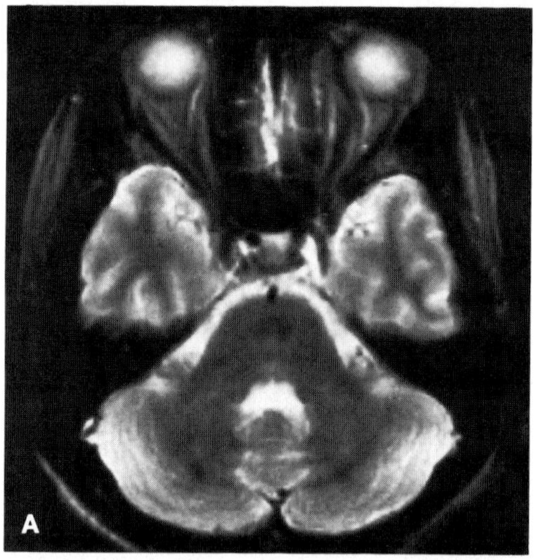

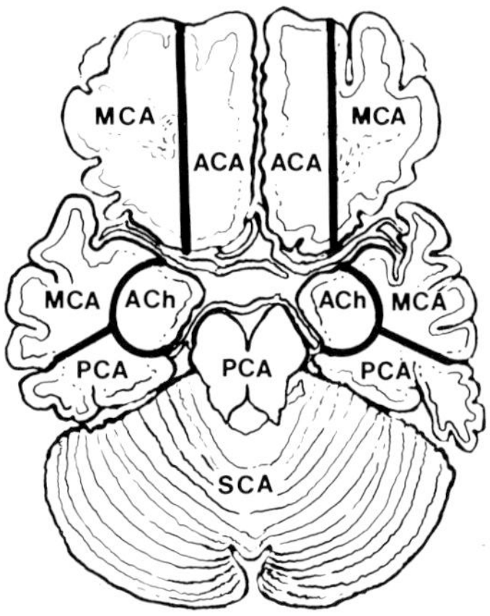

B

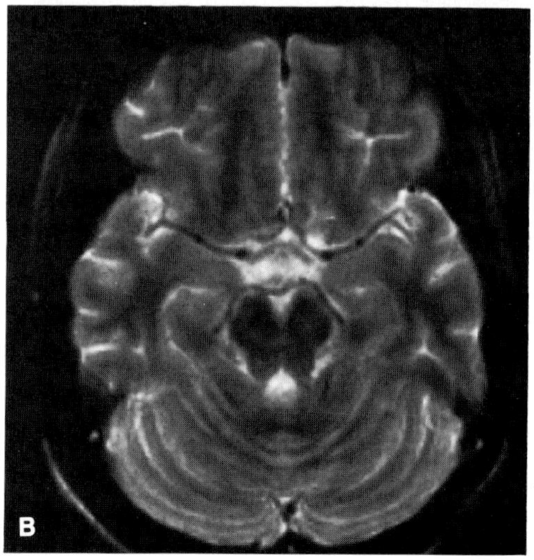

ARTERIAL VASCULAR TERRITORIES

- ACA = Anterior cerebral artery
- H = Recurrent artery of Heubner
- MCA = Middle cerebral artery
- ACh = Anterior choroidal artery
- LSA = Lenticulostriate arteries
- BA = Perforating branches of the basilar artery
- PCA = Posterior cerebral artery
- SCA = Superior cerebellar artery
- WSCA = Watershed region supplied predominantly by the SCA
- AICA = Anterior inferior cerebellar artery
- PICA = Posterior inferior cerebellar artery

ARTERIAL VASCULAR TERRITORIES—AXIAL PLANE

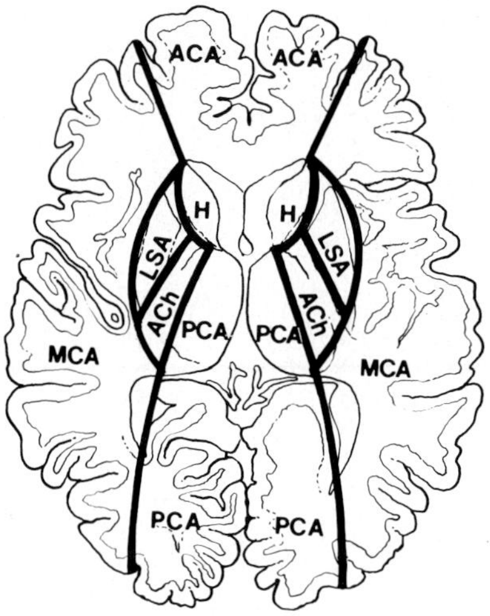

C

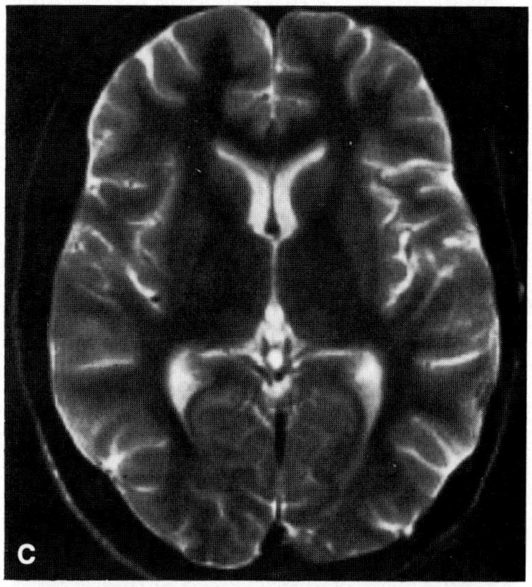

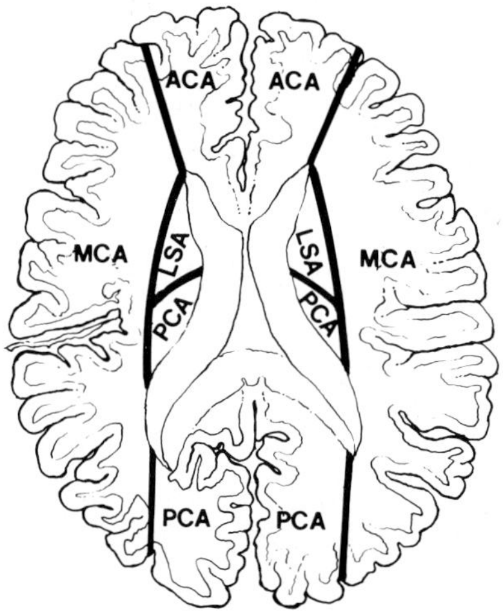

D

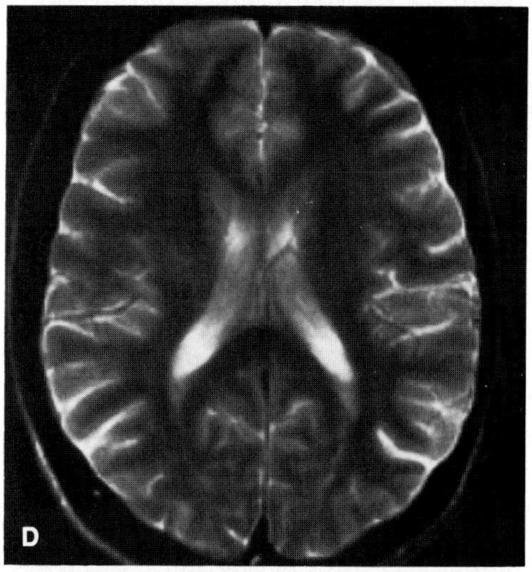

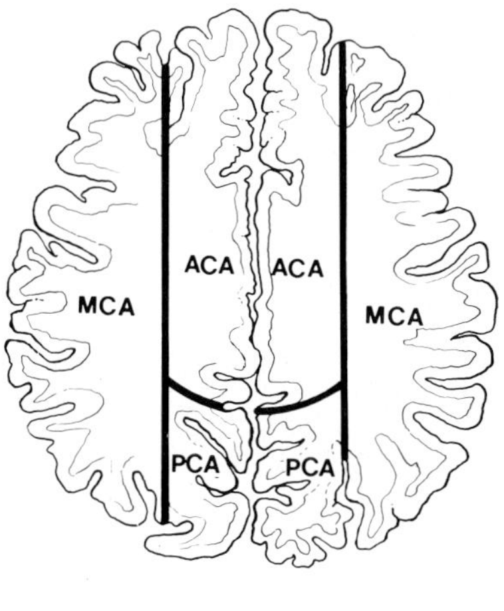

E

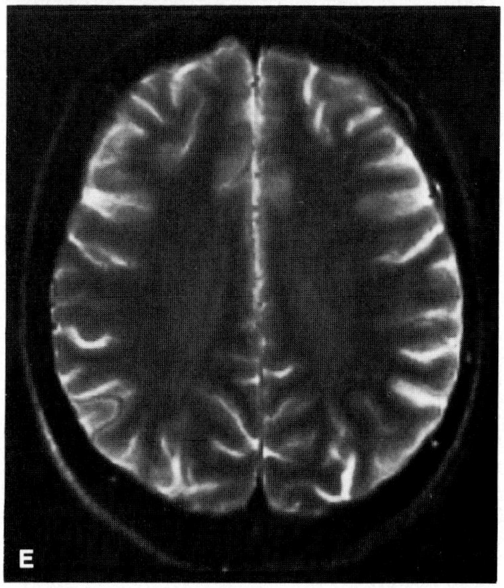

ARTERIAL VASCULAR TERRITORIES—CORONAL PLANE

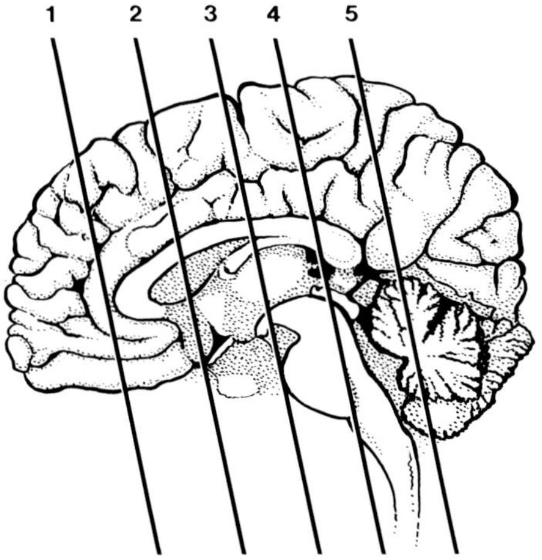

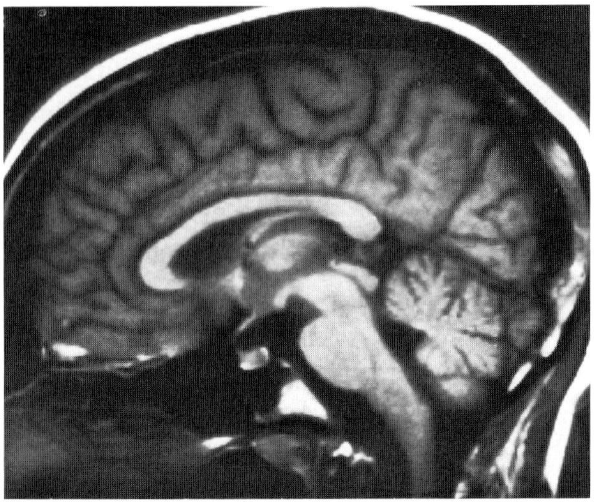

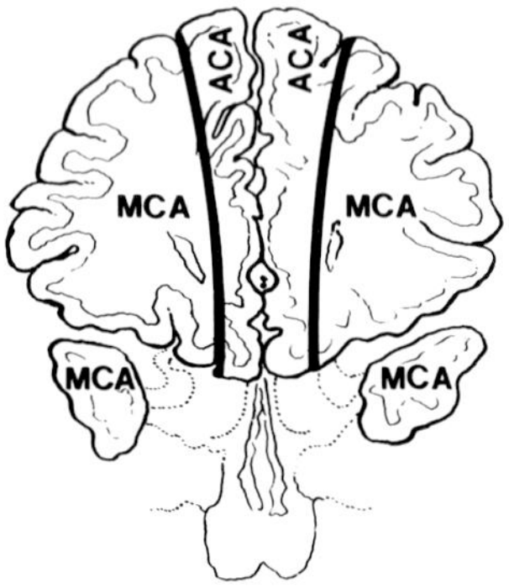

1

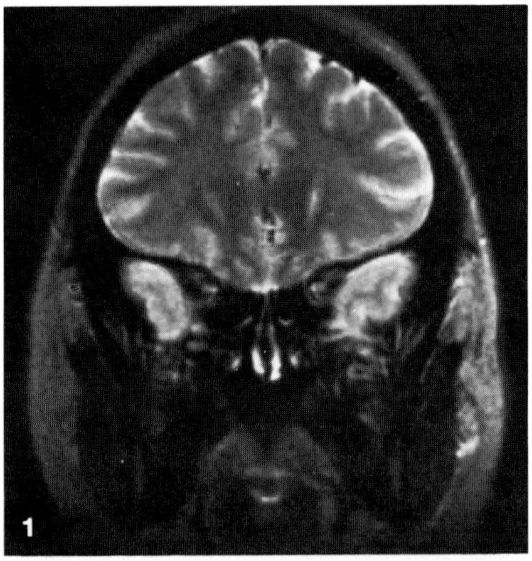

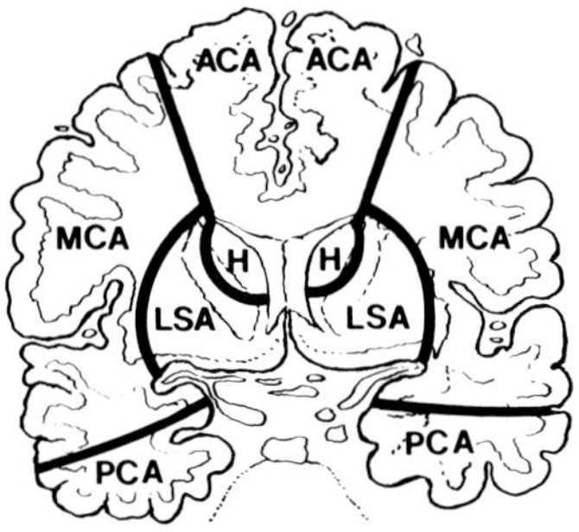

2

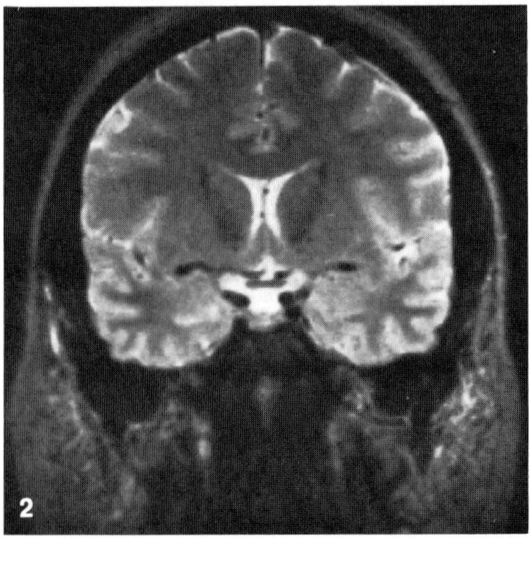

ARTERIAL VASCULAR TERRITORIES
ACA = Anterior cerebral artery
H = Recurrent artery of Heubner
MCA = Middle cerebral artery
ACh = Anterior choroidal artery

LSA = Lenticulostriate arteries
BA = Perforating branches of the basilar artery
PCA = Posterior cerebral artery
SCA = Superior cerebellar artery

WSCA = Watershed region supplied predominantly by the SCA
AICA = Anterior inferior cerebellar artery
PICA = Posterior inferior cerebellar artery

ARTERIAL VASCULAR TERRITORIES—CORONAL PLANE

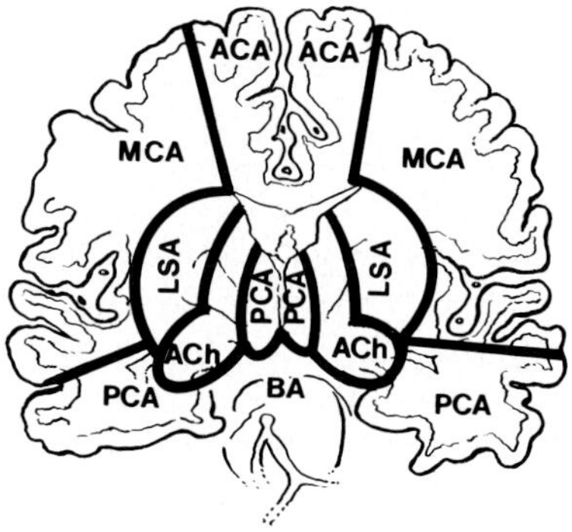

3

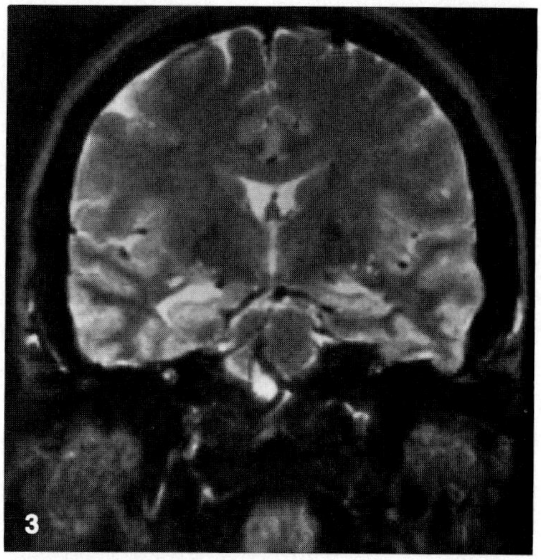

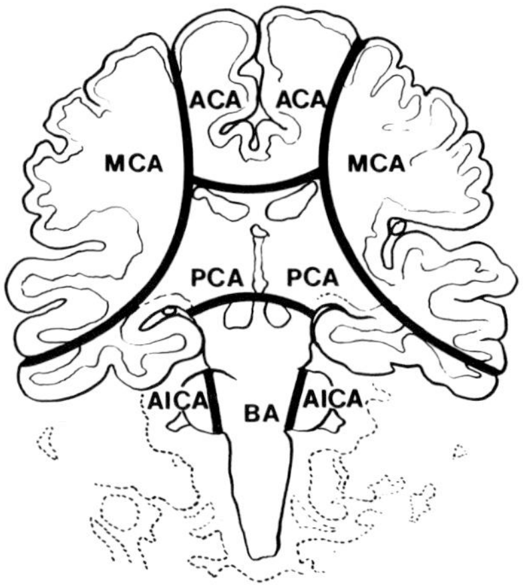

4

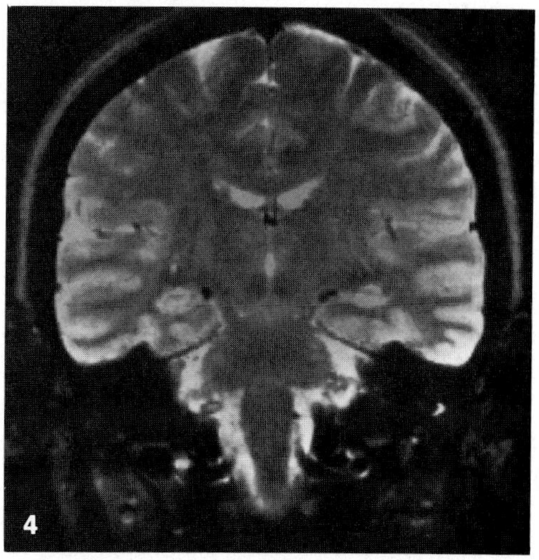

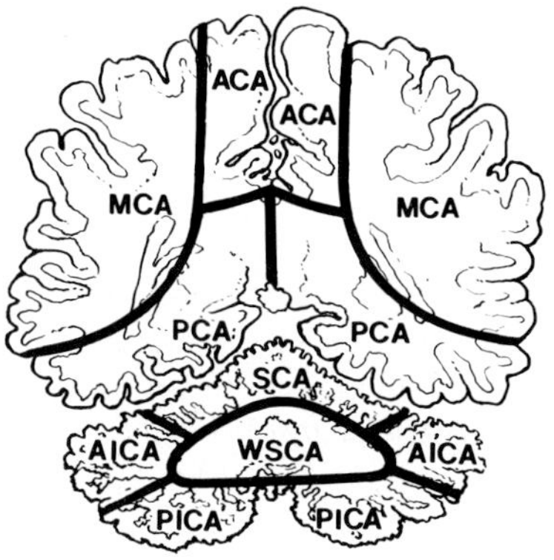

5

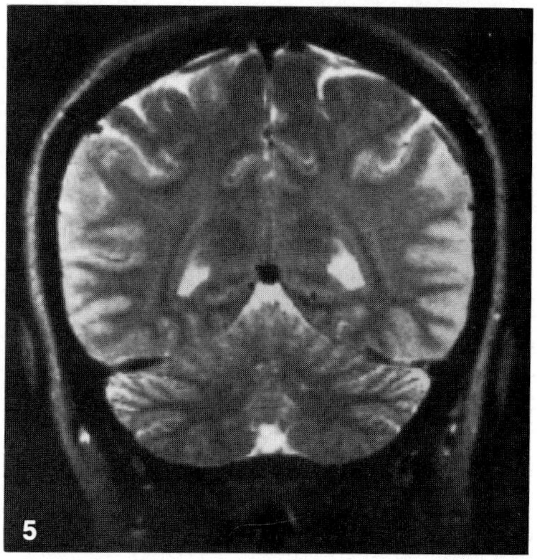

the presence of gyriform enhancement (Fig. 2-35). Despite these features, some lesions, particularly demyelinating disease, may be difficult to distinguish from bland thrombotic infarction.

MRI can also provide information about vascular patency. The major cerebral arteries are consistently visualized as signal voids because of rapid blood flow on the standard spin echo MR exam. The absence of a normal flow void in a major cerebral vessel is presumptive evidence of occlusion (Fig. 2-33). In the future, MR angiography may more elegantly characterize the patency of the cerebral arterial tree.

Embolic Infarction

In embolic cerebral infarction, the occlusive material arises proximal to the occluded artery. These emboli most frequently arise from the heart or from atherosclerotic plaques involving the carotid bifurcation or vertebral arteries.[29,71] The common causes of cardiac emboli include thrombi associated with myocardial infarction or cardiac arrhythmias, valvular disease (including prosthetic valves), bacterial or nonbacterial (marantic) endocarditis, and atrial myxomas.[29,75] The ulceration of atherosclerotic plaques produces cholesterol or calcific emboli.[89] Rare embolic causes of infarction are nitrogen emboli from rapid decompensation, fat emboli from long bone fractures, and iatrogenic air emboli.

The location and temporal evolution of embolic infarction differs from thrombotic infarction. Embolic particles shower the intracranial cerebral circulation, which often causes multiple peripheral infarcts in different major arterial distributions. Embolic occlusions frequently fragment and lyse between the first and fifth day, which reestablishes normal circulation.[90] These findings differ from the relatively permanent occlusion of a single major vascular distribution with atherosclerotic thrombotic infarction. Fragmentation and lysis of embolic occlusion produces a higher perfusion pressure than the occluded state that relied on collaterals for circulation.[90] There is also a loss of normal autoregulation of the cerebral vasculature, which can persist for several weeks. These factors produce hyperemia or luxury perfusion because the blood flow to the infarcted region is greater than its metabolic requirements. This higher perfusion pressure can also cause hemorrhage into the infarction and conversion of a bland anemic infarct into a hemorrhagic one.[91] This hemorrhage usually occurs between 6 hours and 2 weeks after the embolic event.[75] Anticoagulant treatment of bland anemic infarcts can also result in hemorrhage.

MR FINDINGS IN EMBOLIC INFARCTION

Before the lysis of the embolus, the MR changes in embolic infarction are similar to the findings in thrombotic infarction. However, in contrast to the relatively permanent ischemic lesion in thrombotic infarction, embolic infarctions are often multiple, may be located in more than one vascular distribution, and are approximately of the same age (Fig. 2-35). After fragmentation of the embolus occurs with resultant increase in perfusion pressure, a hemorrhagic infarction often develops (Fig. 2-31).[73,85] Most commonly, the hemorrhage in a hemorrhagic embolic infarction is a petechial cortical hemorrhage, although occasionally an intraparenchymal hematoma develops in the infarcted region. Development of a secondary hemorrhage is characteristic of embolic infarction, but occasionally it can be seen with thrombotic infarction or hemodynamic infarction (Fig. 2-36).

Hemodynamic Infarction

Hemodynamic infarction occurs because of the failure of the heart to pump sufficient blood to oxygenate the brain. This hypoperfusion is most commonly caused by cardiac failure, cardiac arrhythmias, or hypovolemia after blood loss. Patients may have concomitant systemic hypertension, a subcritical arterial stenosis, or even arterial occlusion that had been adequately perfused by collaterals. With the development of systemic hypoperfusion and decreased perfusion pressure to the brain, areas of the brain that were adequately perfused are now underperfused, which causes cerebral ischemia or infarction. In many patients, this ischemic event occurs at night while they are asleep, probably because of a nocturnal reduction in blood pressure.[90]

The areas of the brain that are most severely involved in hemodynamic infarction are the watershed areas of the brain occurring at the margins of the major arterial distributions.[92] These regions are the terminal areas supplied by each major artery, and they have the lowest perfusion pressure in that vascular distribution.[90] These watershed regions are more prone to ischemic insults caused by systemic hypoperfusion. A knowledge of the anatomic distributions of the major arterial blood supplies to the brain is necessary to recognize these hemodynamic watershed infarcts (see the Arterial Vascular Territories display on pages 90-93). In the cerebral cortex, these watershed areas are located at the junctions of the regions supplied by the anterior, middle, and posterior cerebral arteries.[29,90] Watershed regions occur at the junctions of the superior cerebellar and inferior cerebellar arteries in the cerebellum.[29,77,90,92] The parietal-occipital watershed region is particularly susceptible to hemodynamic ischemic injury, because this region is at the peripheral junction of the anterior, middle, and posterior cerebral arterial distributions (Fig. 2-35).[90,92]

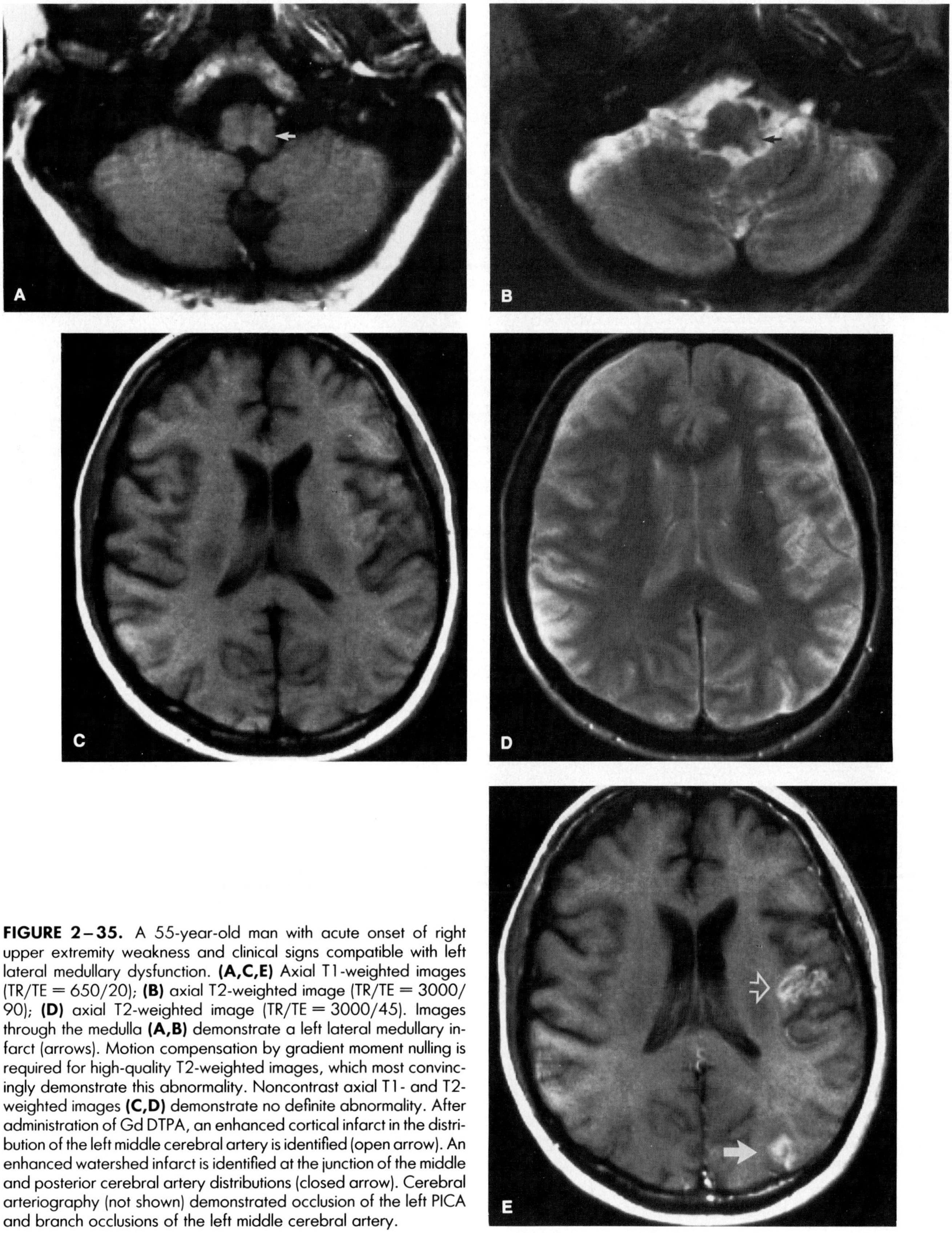

FIGURE 2–35. A 55-year-old man with acute onset of right upper extremity weakness and clinical signs compatible with left lateral medullary dysfunction. **(A,C,E)** Axial T1-weighted images (TR/TE = 650/20); **(B)** axial T2-weighted image (TR/TE = 3000/90); **(D)** axial T2-weighted image (TR/TE = 3000/45). Images through the medulla **(A,B)** demonstrate a left lateral medullary infarct (arrows). Motion compensation by gradient moment nulling is required for high-quality T2-weighted images, which most convincingly demonstrate this abnormality. Noncontrast axial T1- and T2-weighted images **(C,D)** demonstrate no definite abnormality. After administration of Gd DTPA, an enhanced cortical infarct in the distribution of the left middle cerebral artery is identified (open arrow). An enhanced watershed infarct is identified at the junction of the middle and posterior cerebral artery distributions (closed arrow). Cerebral arteriography (not shown) demonstrated occlusion of the left PICA and branch occlusions of the left middle cerebral artery.

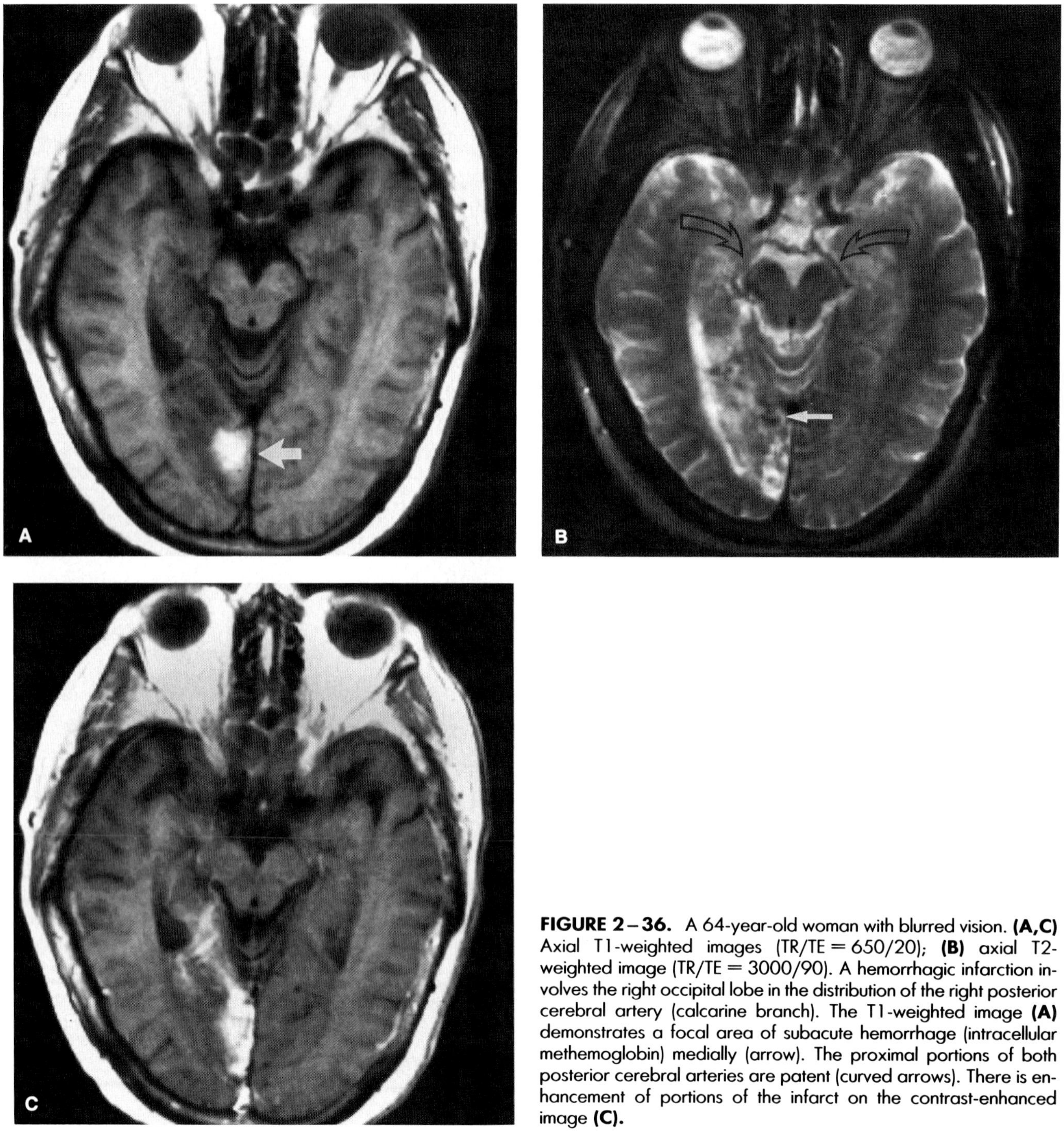

FIGURE 2–36. A 64-year-old woman with blurred vision. **(A,C)** Axial T1-weighted images (TR/TE = 650/20); **(B)** axial T2-weighted image (TR/TE = 3000/90). A hemorrhagic infarction involves the right occipital lobe in the distribution of the right posterior cerebral artery (calcarine branch). The T1-weighted image **(A)** demonstrates a focal area of subacute hemorrhage (intracellular methemoglobin) medially (arrow). The proximal portions of both posterior cerebral arteries are patent (curved arrows). There is enhancement of portions of the infarct on the contrast-enhanced image **(C)**.

MR FINDINGS IN HEMODYNAMIC INFARCTION

The MR findings in hemodynamic infarction are increased tissue water content in the distribution of the watershed or border zones of the major arterial vascular distributions. Often the deep periventricular white matter is preferentially involved.[90] The white matter receives approximately 25% of the blood flow, compared with the gray matter and is probably more susceptible to ischemia with a decrease in perfusion.[75] Common locations of white matter hemodynamic infarctions are superior and lateral to the body and trigone of the lateral ventricles.[90,93] The deep basal ganglia supplied by the lenticulostriate arteries can be similarly affected.[90]

Lacunar Infarction

Lacunar infarcts or lacunes are small, deep cerebral infarcts involving the penetrating arteries that supply the basal ganglia, internal capsule, thalamus, and brain stem. These small arteries arise from the major cerebral arteries and include the lenticulostriate branches of the anterior and middle cerebral arteries, the thalamo-perforating branches of the posterior cerebral arteries, and the paramedian branches of the basilar artery.[94] These penetrating arteries are small-end arteries (100–500 μm in diameter) that are difficult to evaluate angiographically. Most of these arteries are unbranching single vessels with essentially no collateral circulation. For these anatomic reasons, deep lacunar infarcts typically are spherical in shape and range from 0.3 to 2.5 cm in diameter.[90,95] The larger lacunes typically result from more proximal obstructions.[75]

Lacunar infarcts are commonly seen in patients older than 60 years of age with hypertension.[95] Chronic hypertension causes degeneration of the tunica media (i.e., arteriosclerosis), with hyalin deposition in the artery wall that narrows the lumen.[29,90,95] Plaque or thrombosis, called microatheroma, may subsequently occlude these vessels, particularly the larger vessels.[96] The weakened tunica media also predisposes to the formation of microaneurysms that can rupture, causing an intraparenchymal hematoma. A hypertensive hemorrhage or hypertensive hemorrhagic infarction has a characteristic location in the deep cerebral structures supplied by these deep, penetrating arteries. Other uncommon causes of lacunar infarction include a secondary arteritis caused by meningitis, microemboli, and arterial dissection.[96]

Lacunar infarction is often recognized by a distinctive clinical presentation. A pure motor stroke is the most common clinical syndrome, accounting for 30 to 60% of lacunar infarcts. A pure sensory stroke, combined sensorimotor stroke, ataxic hemiparesis, dysarthria or clumsy hand syndrome, and brain stem syndromes are the other characteristic clinical presentations of lacunar infarction.[96] Patients with lacunar infarction often have a gradual progression of symptoms.[96] An antecedent TIA occurs in approximately 25% of patients with lacunar infarction.[97]

MR FINDINGS IN LACUNAR INFARCTION

MRI accurately demonstrates lacunar infarction involving deep structures as focal slit-like or ovoid areas of increased water content in tissue (i.e., high signal intensity on proton density and T2-weighted images and isointense or low signal intensity on T1-weighted images) (Fig. 2–37).[98] The T2-weighted sequence is the most sensitive in detecting lacunar infarction.[94] The use of an intermediate T2-weighted echo (TE $\approx$ 45) is particularly helpful in distinguishing these small lacunes from the adjacent brain parenchyma and CSF. On this sequence, small high-intensity focal lesions can be discriminated from the intermediate signal intensity of normal surrounding brain and CSF. MRI is more sensitive than CT in detecting lacunar infarction.[94] Enhancement of small lacunar infarcts with Gd DTPA can indicate a recent lesion with blood-brain-barrier disruption.[99] Chronic lacunar infarcts are characterized by focal cavitation and a more pronounced decreased signal intensity on T1-weighted images than in the earlier stages of lacunar infarction. These chronic lacunar infarcts are isointense with CSF signal intensity on all imaging sequences (Fig. 2–38).[74,100,101]

Dilated Perivascular Spaces

Dilated perivascular spaces (DPVS) or Virchow-Robin spaces are invaginations of the subarachnoid

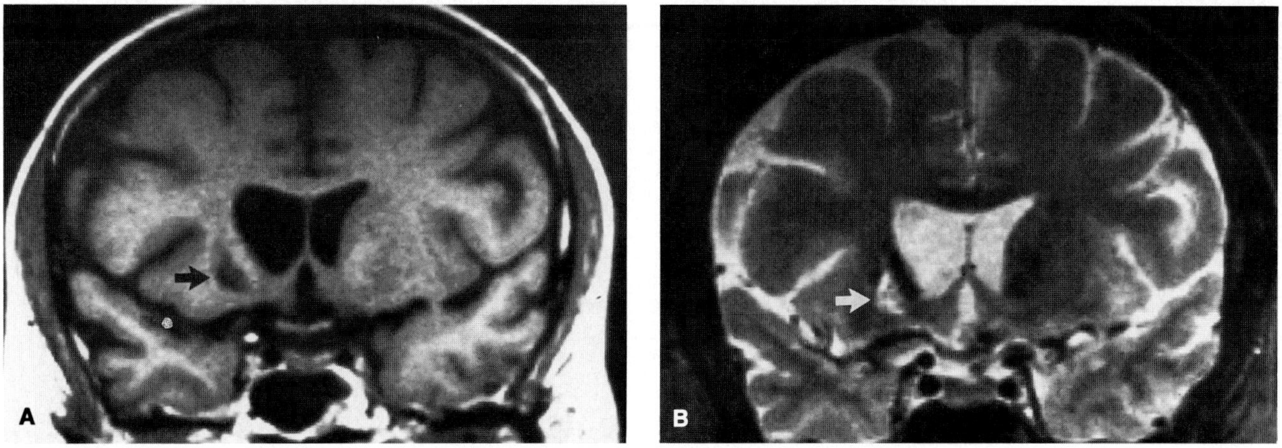

FIGURE 2–37. A 39-year-old woman after transphenoidal hypophysectomy for craniopharyngioma. **(A)** Coronal T1-weighted image (TR/TE = 650/20); **(B)** coronal T2-weighted image (TR/TE = 3000/90). A lacunar infarct involves the right putamen (arrows). The low intensity of the lesion on the T1-weighted image and the focal dilatation of the right lateral ventricle indicate a chronic lacunar infarct.

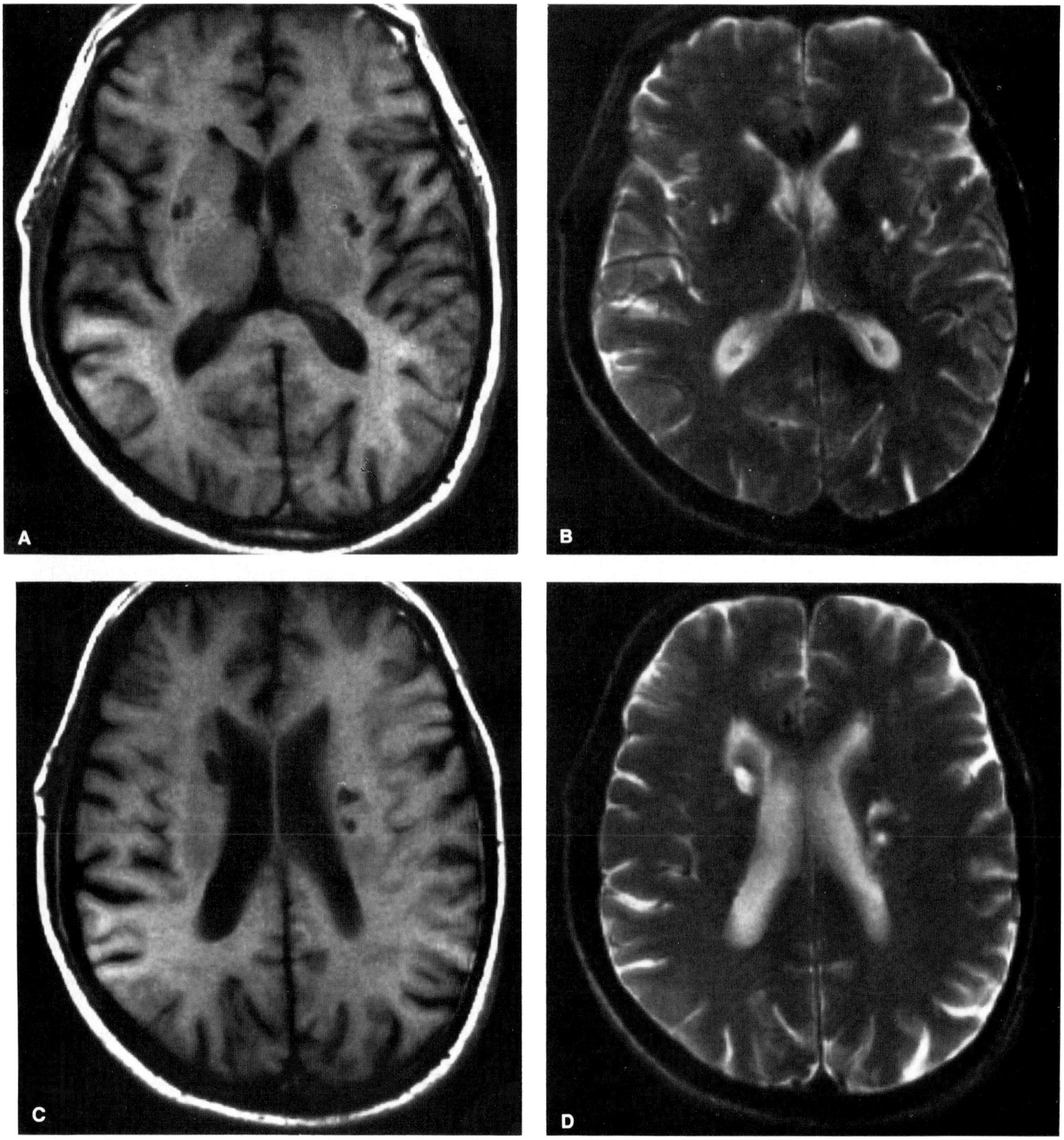

FIGURE 2–38. A 69-year-old man with memory loss, confusion, and ataxia. **(A,C)** Axial T1-weighted images (TR/TE = 650/20); **(B,D)** axial T2-weighted images (TR/TE = 3000/90). Chronic lacunar infarcts involve the putamen and periventricular white matter (centrum semiovale) bilaterally. The low-intensity-signal characteristics of the lesions on the T1-weighted images indicate a chronic lacunar infarct.

space that surrounds vessels as they course from the subarachnoid space through the brain. DPVS are commonly found in the basal ganglia, white matter, and medial temporal lobes.[100,102] DPVS are small, rounded or linear fluid collections that course along the penetrating vessels and have signal intensities that strictly follow the intensity of CSF (Fig. 2–39). Because of their location and appearance, they can mimic lacunar infarction. Therefore, correlation of the anatomic MR abnormality consistent with lacunar infarction and the clinical history is mandatory before definitive diagnosis can be made.

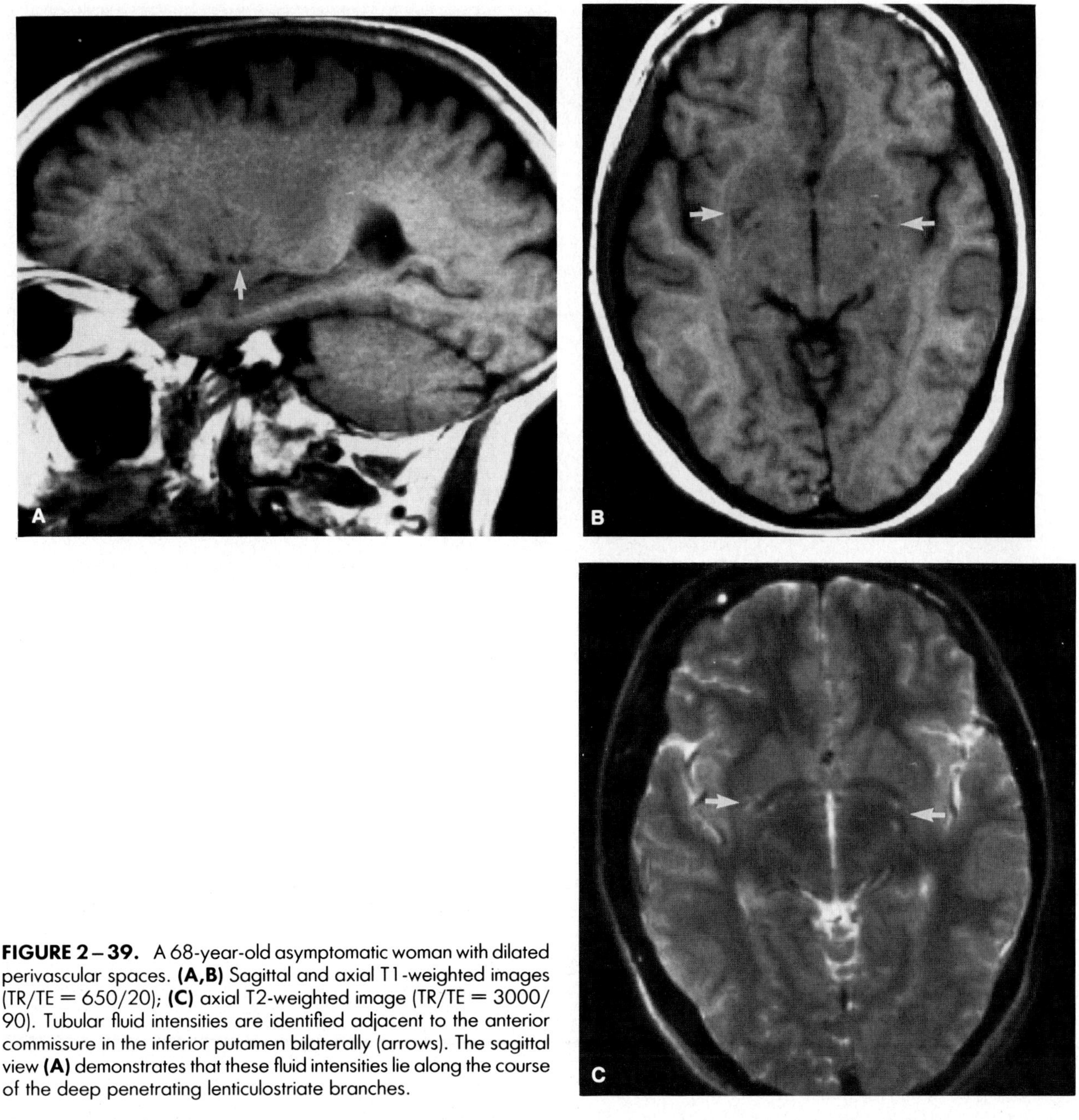

FIGURE 2–39. A 68-year-old asymptomatic woman with dilated perivascular spaces. **(A,B)** Sagittal and axial T1-weighted images (TR/TE = 650/20); **(C)** axial T2-weighted image (TR/TE = 3000/90). Tubular fluid intensities are identified adjacent to the anterior commissure in the inferior putamen bilaterally (arrows). The sagittal view **(A)** demonstrates that these fluid intensities lie along the course of the deep penetrating lenticulostriate branches.

DPVS that involve the lenticulostriate arteries supplying the basal ganglia are commonly located adjacent to the lateral aspect of the anterior commissure (Fig. 2–40).[102] Pathologically, focal fluid intensities in the region of the inferior one-third of the putamen invariably proved to be DPVS, but lesions in the upper two-thirds are commonly lacunar infarctions.[102] DPVS that surround middle cerebral artery branches located in the white matter of the centrum semiovale are seen with equal frequency in patients younger and older than 40 years of age.[102] DPVS in this location should be considered in the differential diagnosis of lacunar infarction, ischemic-gliotic white matter disease, and multiple sclerosis (Fig. 2–41).

DPVS often have MR characteristics that allow their differentiation from lacunar infarction and other small focal lesions. DPVS are commonly spheric or tubular, but lacunar infarcts are slit-like or ovoid. On sagittal or coronal images, the tubular configuration of DPVS along the course of the penetrating arteries can often be appreciated (Fig. 2–39). DPVS strictly follow CSF characteristics on T1-weighted and T2-weighted images, although volume averaging of small lesions with the adjacent brain can alter signal characteristics. Lacunar infarcts are frequently higher in signal intensity than CSF on T1-weighted images and on balanced or proton density images.

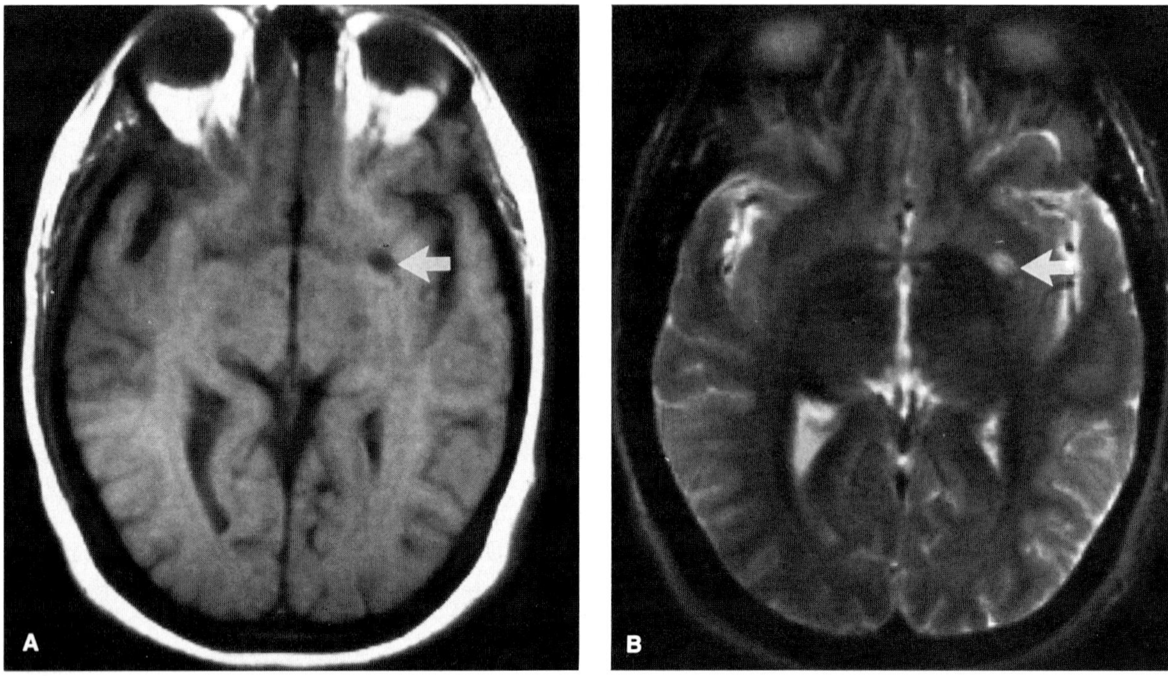

FIGURE 2–40. A 34-year-old woman with syncope. **(A)** Axial T1-weighted image (TR/TE = 650/20); **(B)** axial T2-weighted image (TR/TE = 3000/90). The circular fluid intensity in the left putamen just anterior to the anterior commissure is compatible with a large dilated perivascular space (arrows). Dilated perivascular spaces are frequently found in this region and can be large. A dilated perivascular space should be considered in the differential diagnosis of this lesion, particularly in the absence of classic clinical symptoms of lacunar syndrome.

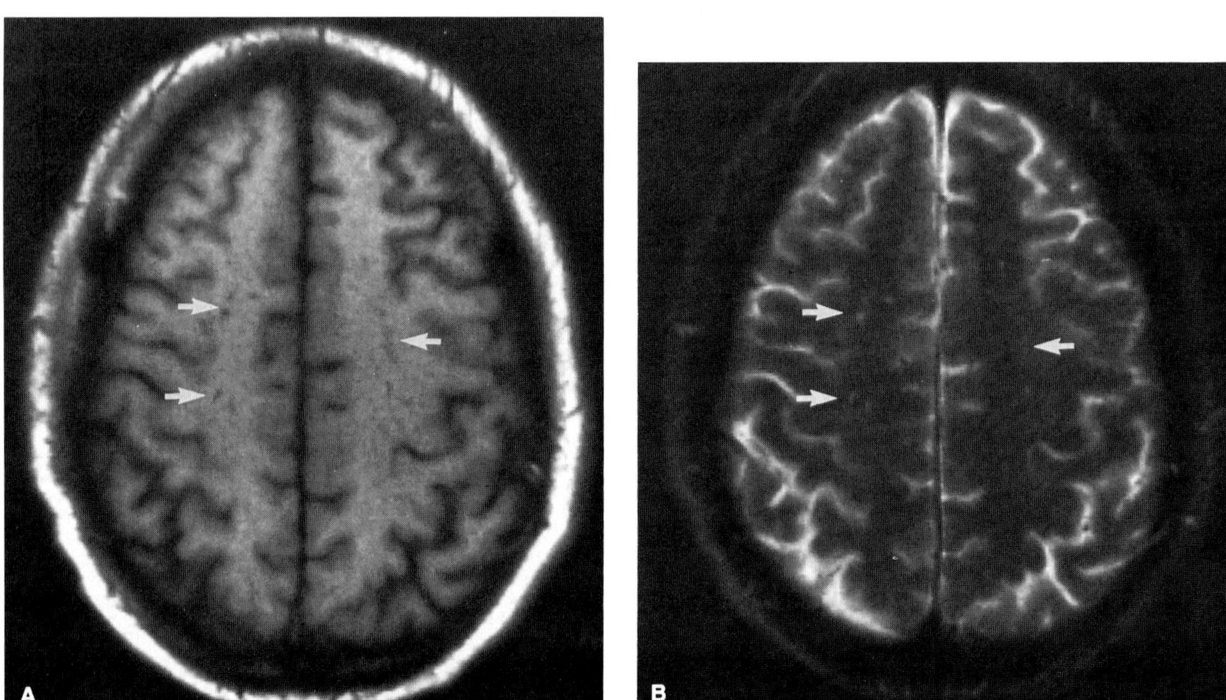

FIGURE 2–41. Dilated perivascular spaces in a 58-year-old man with Lyme disease and multiple neurologic complaints. **(A)** Axial T1-weighted image (TR/TE = 650/20); **(B)** axial T2-weighted image (TR/TE = 3000/90). There are multiple tubular structures (arrows) in the white matter of the centrum semiovale bilaterally (middle cerebral artery distribution) compatible with dilated perivascular spaces.

White Matter Ischemia — Gliosis

Punctate or confluent areas of increased signal intensity are commonly seen in the white matter of older patients on long TR images. These hyperintense white matter foci can be seen in as many as 30% of asymptomatic patients over the age of 65.[98,103] Approximately 79% of geriatric patients with cardiovascular risk factors and a history of completed stroke or ischemia (e.g., RIND or TIA) have hyperintense white matter foci.[98] These lesions often create problems in diagnostic interpretation because of their prevalence, particularly in the asymptomatic patient, and their similarity to other lesions.

Recent pathologic evidence correlated with MR abnormalities suggest that the majority of these lesions are produced by ischemia or infarction.[101,102,104,105] Although the terminology describing these lesions is different, the pathophysiologic basis for the majority of them is similar. Kirkpatrick and Hayman found white matter atrophy with shrinking of axons and myelin and gliosis surrounding thickened vessels in the region of the hyperintense MR white matter foci.[104] They called this process atrophic perivascular demyelination (APD) and postulated that increased extracellular water is responsible for the increased signal on long TR images. These authors state that the cause of APD is probably chronic, mild vascular insufficiency rather than thrombotic or embolic occlusive infarction, which would produce acute necrosis. Braffman and colleagues found that true white matter infarction was commonly the cause of hyperintense MR white matter foci.[100] Marshall and coworkers also described central necrosis, axonal loss, and demyelination compatible with true infarction.[101] They described reactive astrocytes that orient along the degenerated axons, which they called isomorphic gliosis. The protein and water content associated with this gliosis increases the apparent size of the lesion on long TR images.[101]

Because ischemia and infarction appear to be the predominant causes of hyperintense white matter foci in older patients, and because infarction often has a significant component of gliosis, we refer to these lesions as ischemic-gliotic changes and describe the degree of disease as mild, moderate, or severe. In mild cases, there are a few scattered, small white matter hyperintensities on long TR images (Fig. 2–42). In severe cases, there can be confluent increased signal intensity in the white matter. In moderate cases, the changes are intermediate (Fig. 2–43). In patients with diffuse white matter disease, the Gd-DTPA-enhanced exam can be useful in distinguishing areas of acute infarction from chronic disease (Fig. 2–44).

There are other, less common causes of hyperintense white matter lesions that should be recognized. Plaques of multiple sclerosis can occur with minimal or no clinical symptoms.[106] In these subclinical cases, the lesions tend to be small and involve only the supratentorial white matter and spare the brain stem and cerebellum. Brain cysts and congenital ventricu-

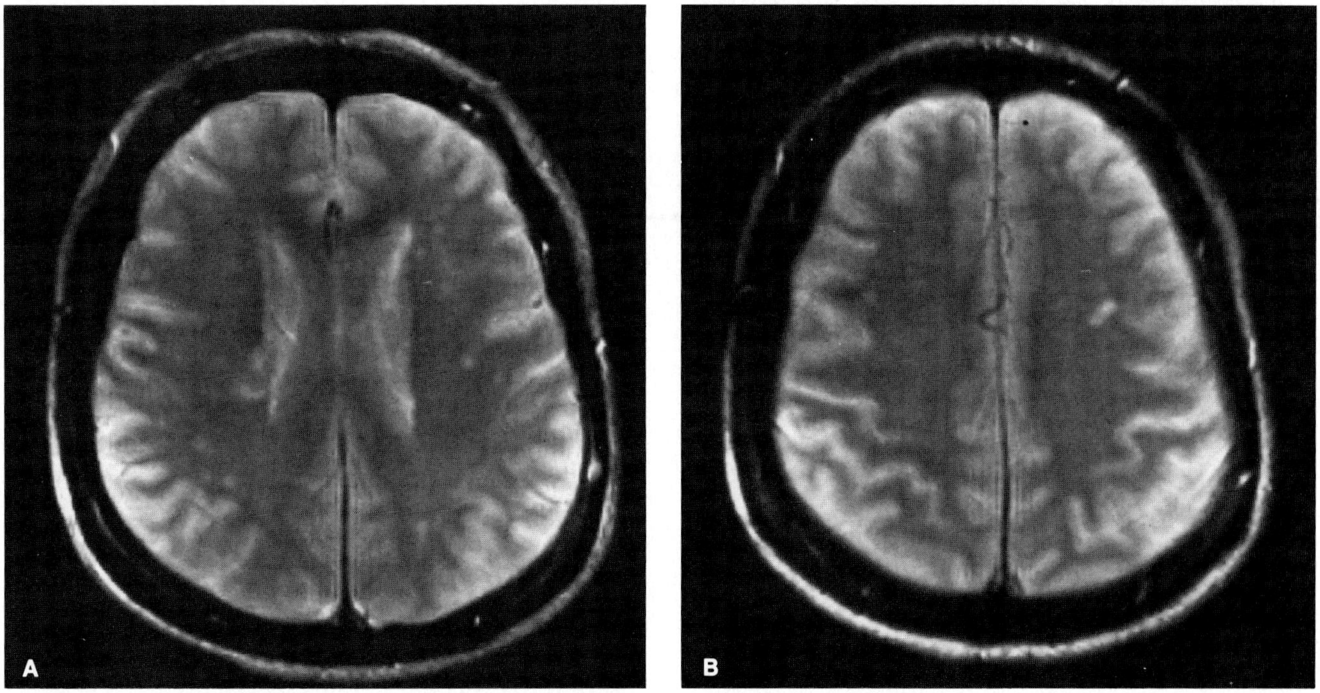

FIGURE 2–42. A 60-year-old man with headaches. **(A,B)** Axial T2-weighted images (TR/TE = 3000/45) show small focal areas of increased signal intensity involving periventricular white matter (centrum semiovale), compatible with mild ischemic-gliotic changes.

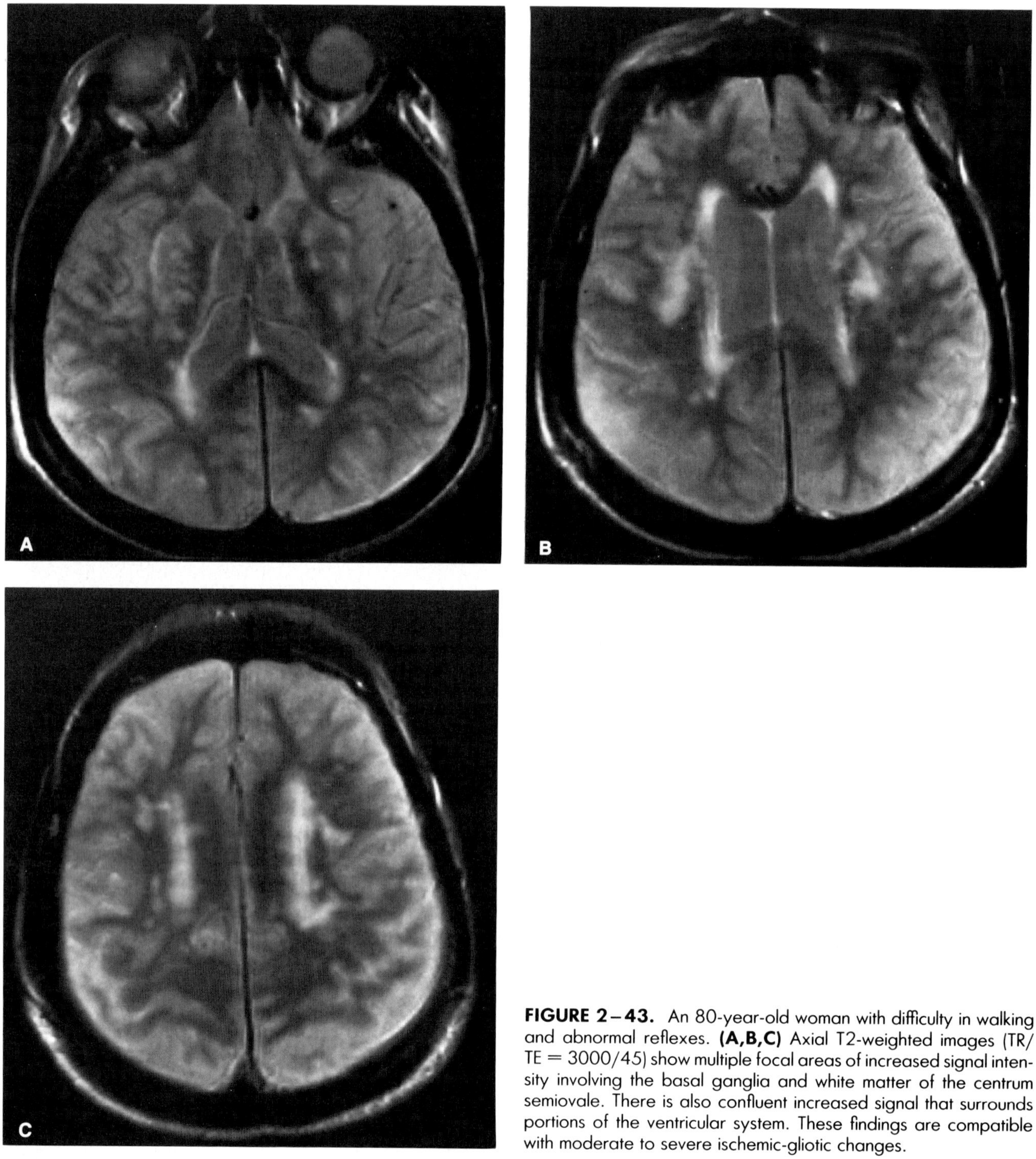

FIGURE 2–43. An 80-year-old woman with difficulty in walking and abnormal reflexes. **(A,B,C)** Axial T2-weighted images (TR/TE = 3000/45) show multiple focal areas of increased signal intensity involving the basal ganglia and white matter of the centrum semiovale. There is also confluent increased signal that surrounds portions of the ventricular system. These findings are compatible with moderate to severe ischemic-gliotic changes.

lar diverticula are increased in intensity on long TR images, but are uncommon.[98] They characteristically border the ventricular system or subarachnoid space, have a smooth rounded configuration, and are like CSF in signal intensity. Occasionally a cavitated infarct becomes cystic and displays CSF characteristics similar to these lesions.[74,100,101] DPVS can simulate focal white matter lesions and lacunar infarcts.

Binswanger's disease (i.e., subcortical arteriosclerotic encephalopathy) represents a distinct clinical entity with characteristic clinical findings in patients with hypertension, hydrocephalus, and dementia.[107] These patients have a rapid deterioration of their cognitive ability, a gradual development of neurologic symptoms, and a lengthy clinical course with long plateau periods. Occasionally patients develop seizures. Cranial MR demonstrates focal or confluent white matter lesions on T2-weighted images.[103] Cra-

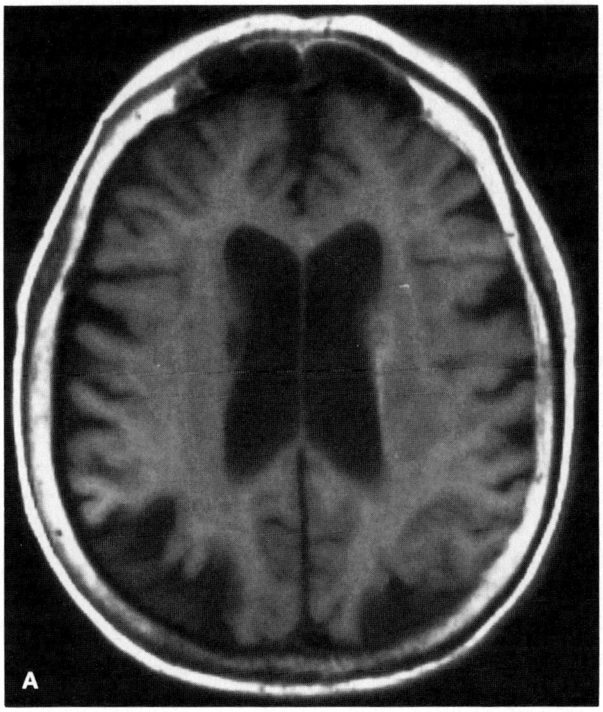

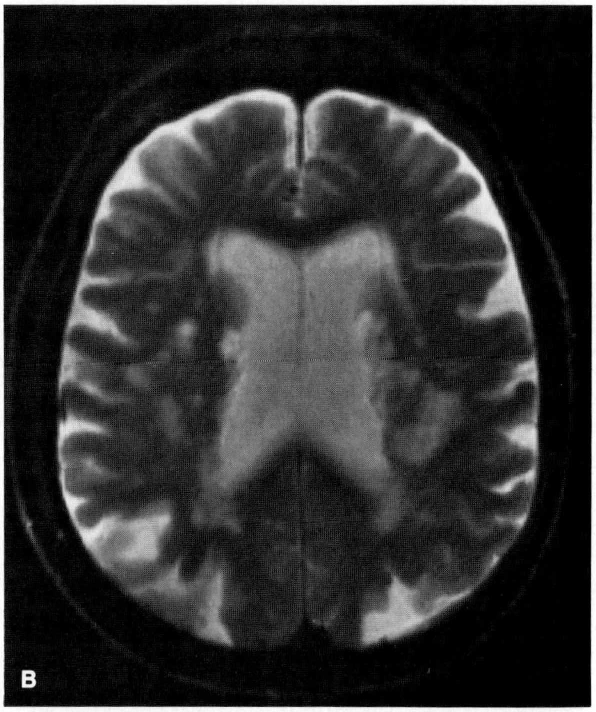

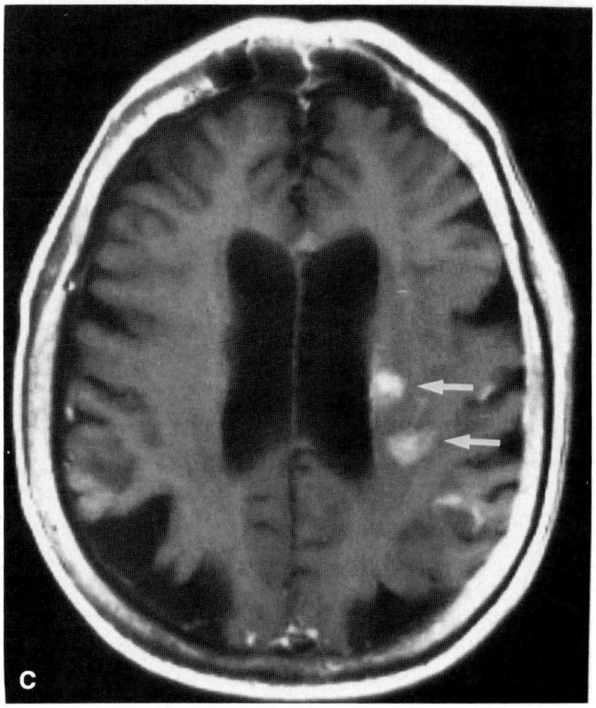

FIGURE 2–44. A 79-year-old woman with a 20-year history of hypertension and with recent development of right hemiparesis and aphasia. **(A,C)** Axial T1-weighted images (TR/TE = 650/20); **(B)** axial T2-weighted image (TR/TE = 3000/90). Unenhanced images **(A,B)** demonstrate moderate or severe ischemic-gliotic changes in the deep white matter. Focal areas of enhancement after Gd DTPA administration **(C)** identify areas of acute infarction (arrows).

nial MRI is a confirmatory examination of this disease in patients with the appropriate clinical presentation. Hypertensive encephalopathy (HTE) is an acute neurologic syndrome with a characteristic clinical presentation. In patients with HTE, T2-weighted images demonstrate hyperintense lesions in the white matter and cerebral cortex, particularly involving the occipital lobes.[108] A recent report describes reversibility of these lesions after treatment.[108]

Arteritis

Cerebral arteritis may be classified as primary or secondary. In the primary form, the inflammatory process originates in the arteries. In the secondary form, the inflammatory process starts in the brain parenchyma or meninges, and the arteries are involved secondarily.

Primary cerebral arteritis often presents with many relapsing neurologic symptoms that may simulate multiple sclerosis.[109,110] This disease tends to affect a younger age group than arteriosclerotic vascular disease. Primary cerebral arteritis is usually caused by a systemic disorder. Systemic lupus erythematosis (SLE), other collagen-vascular diseases, polyarteritis nodosa, giant cell arteritis, Behcet's disease, and sarcoidosis can cause this form of arteritis.

The MR findings in SLE have been described and include both white and gray matter involvement.[109,110] Two types of white matter involvement can be seen. One pattern consists of large, confluent areas of high signal intensity on T2-weighted images consistent with infarction. The other pattern consists of small focal punctate white matter lesions that probably represent small microinfarcts. High-signal-intensity lesions on T2-weighted images can also involve the gray matter. In some patients with gray matter involvement, the clinical findings resolve with resolution of these lesions (Fig. 2-45).[109]

Findings similar to SLE are seen in other vasculities, including polyarteritis nodosa.[110] Focal brain stem infarction has been described in Behcet's disease (Fig. 2-46).[110,111] Some MR findings may differentiate the lesions of arteritis from multiple sclerosis.[110] Periventricular white matter involvement is less extensive and may be absent in primary cerebral arteritis. Multiple sclerosis is typically characterized by irregular, punctate, asymmetric, and extensive periventricular white matter involvement. A lesion in a major cerebral artery vascular territory or cortical involvement also favor a vascular disease process.

The cause of secondary cerebral arteritis is commonly meningitis. Bacterial or fungal organisms, including tuberculosis, are common causes (Fig. 2-47). A contrast-enhanced MR examination should be performed to identify the location and extent of the meningeal disease. The T2-weighted sequence demonstrates high-signal-intensity lesions compatible with ischemia or infarction in the vascular distribution involved by the meningeal process.

Vasospasm and Migraine Headaches

Spasm of the intracranial arteries can be associated with subarachnoid hemorrhage or migraine headaches. Subarachnoid hemorrhage is commonly caused by a ruptured intracranial aneurysm (75% of cases).[26] The arteries in the affected subarachnoid space can experience varying degrees of spasm, which may progress to complete occlusion. MRI demonstrates findings compatible with ischemia or infarction involving major arterial distributions or their watershed regions, corresponding to the distribution of the artery in spasm.

Migraine headaches are thought to be produced by an initial vasoconstriction of extracranial and intracranial arteries, which cause ischemia, presenting clinically as neurologic deficits or an aura. This vasoconstriction is followed by vasodilatation, which produces the headache.[112,113] CT and MR findings consistent with ischemia or infarction have been described in these patients.[114-116] MR exams demonstrate focal lesions of increased signal intensity on T2-weighted images, predominantly involving periventricular white matter, but also involving the cortex. In a few of these lesions, corresponding hypointensity is identified on T1-weighted spin echo images.[114]

Patients with the classic or common form of migraine—a visual aura that responds to ergotamine, followed by a unilateral throbbing headache—had focal periventricular lesions. Patients with neurologic deficits or complicated migraine had larger periventricular lesions and often had cortical lesions. All the cortical lesions were associated with neurologic deficits.[114]

Anoxia and Carbon Monoxide Poisoning

Cerebral anoxia can have many causes, including primary or secondary respiratory failure, drowning, and carbon monoxide poisoning. The cerebral ischemia or infarction that develops initially involves the regions of the brain in which the blood supply is most tenuous. The watershed regions of the cortex, periventricular white matter, and the basal ganglia are particularly prone to ischemic injury.[73,90] In severe cases, the cortex, white matter, and basal ganglia can be diffusely involved.[90] Patients with irreversible injury demonstrate focal areas of necrosis or demyelination.

In children, the distribution of hypoxic-ischemic brain injury is related to the degree of development.[117] In premature infants, the periventricular corona radiata is most predisposed to ischemic injury.[118] These patients may later develop delayed myelination, periventricular leukomalacia, cerebral atrophy, and hydrocephalus.[117] In full-term infants and in young children, the cortical and subcortical regions are most prone to infarction. The full-term infant and older child no longer have the collaterals between the meninges and cerebral arteries that protect the cortex in the premature infant.[117,118]

MRI demonstrates increased signal intensity on T2-weighted images and isointense or low signal intensity on T1-weighted images in the ischemic or infarcted regions. In premature infants, MRI cannot separate the edema of an infarct from the normal water content of the white matter at this age. In the premature infant, ultrasound is a more useful modality for evaluating ischemic disease.[117] Increased iron deposition in infarcted regions in children who survived a severe ischemic-anoxic insult has been described.[119] This iron deposition may be produced by disruption of normal axonal transport of brain iron by injury. It is more evident at higher field strengths and with GRE imaging.

Carbon monoxide poisoning is characterized by

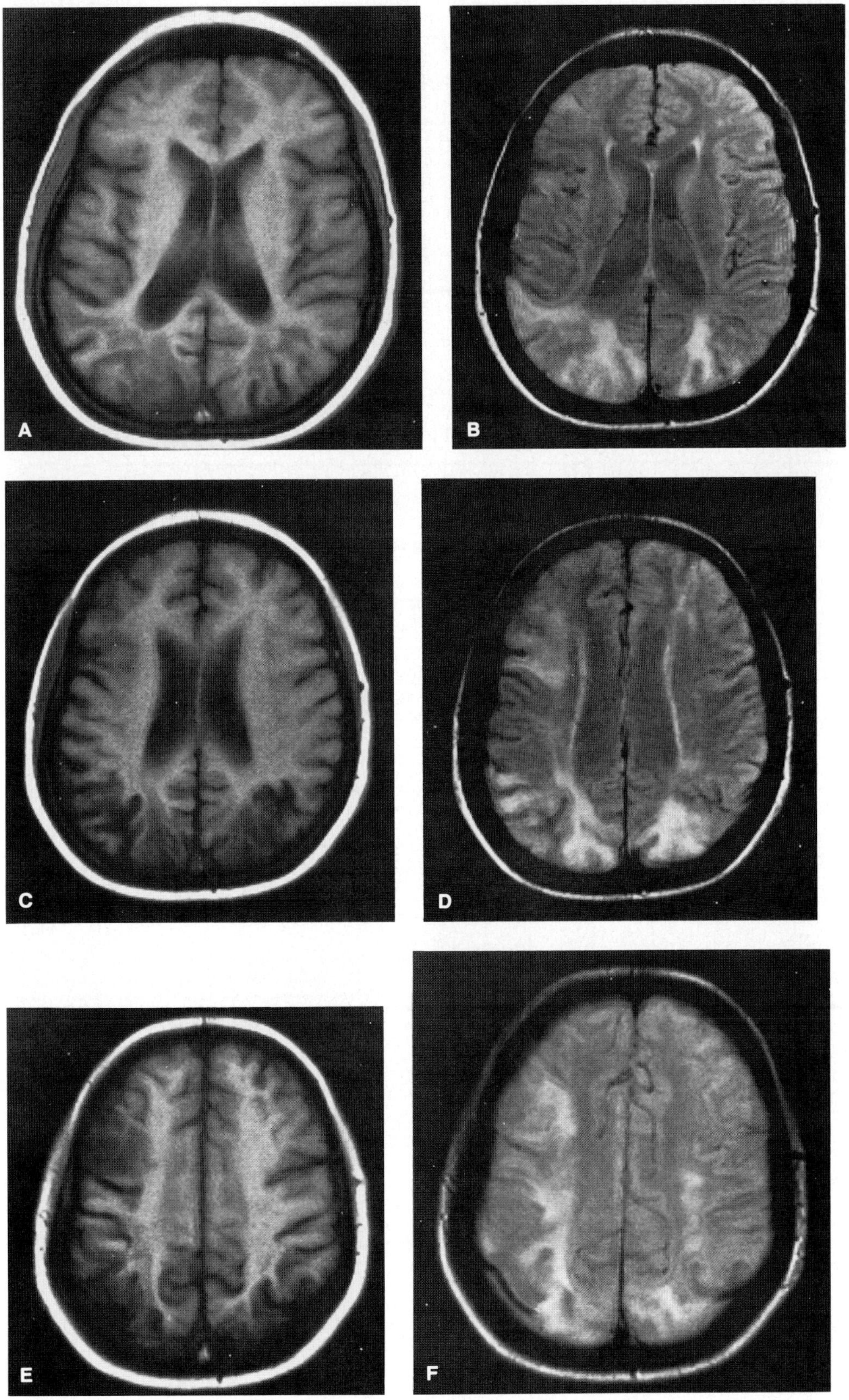

FIGURE 2–45. A 43-year-old woman with SLE and difficulty with spatial perception. **(A,C,E)** Axial, T1-weighted images (TR/TE = 600/17); **(B,D,F)** axial T2-weighted images (TR/TE = 3000/28). There are areas of increased water content in both gray and white matter, particularly in the occipital lobes and right posterior frontal lobe. The serpiginous peripheral contour of these lesions is characteristic of ischemia and infarction caused by a CNS vasculitis, particularly in SLE.

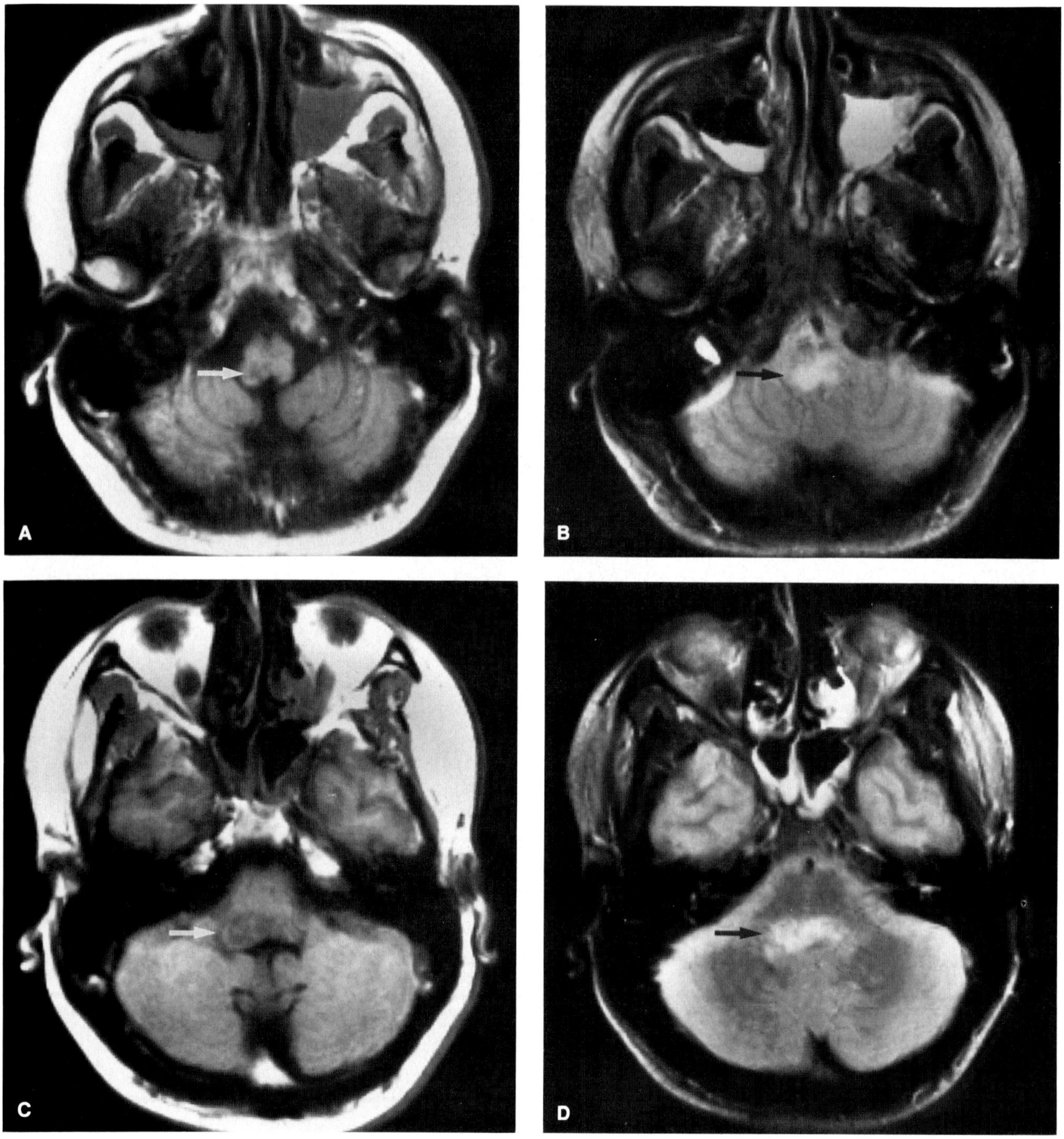

FIGURE 2–46. A 26-year-old man with Bechet's disease and dysarthria, dysphagia, ataxia, and increased deep tendon refluxes. **(A,C)** Axial T1-weighted images (TR/TE = 650/20) and **(B,D)** axial T2-weighted images (TR/TE = 3000/45) show focal areas of increased water content (arrows) in the medulla and posterior pons (tegmentum). These findings are compatible with brain stem ischemia and infarction in patients with Bechet's disease. There is also disease of the maxillary and sphenoid sinuses.

focal areas of ischemic necrosis. The intracranial lesions of carbon monoxide poisoning have been classified as four pathologic types: necrotic lesions of the globus pallidus, focal necrotic white matter lesions or confluent demyelination, spongy lesions in the cerebral cortex, and necrotic lesions of the hippocampus.[120] Frequently, MRI demonstrates only high-signal-intensity lesions on T2-weighted images confined bilaterally to the globus pallidus.[121] Cerebral white matter and globus pallidus involvement have been reported as low-density lesions on CT.[122] The increased sensitivity of MRI to subtle changes in tissue

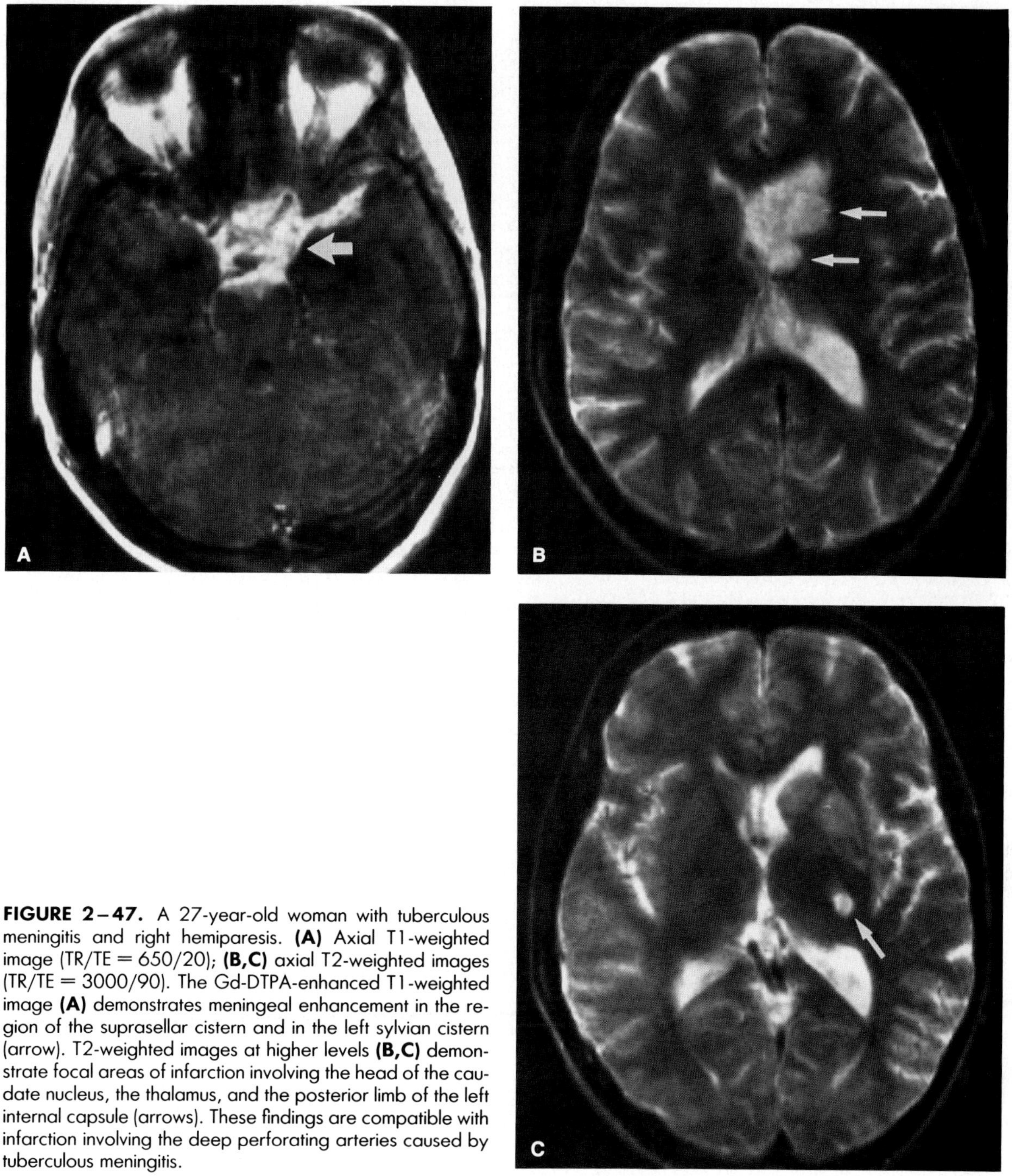

FIGURE 2–47. A 27-year-old woman with tuberculous meningitis and right hemiparesis. **(A)** Axial T1-weighted image (TR/TE = 650/20); **(B,C)** axial T2-weighted images (TR/TE = 3000/90). The Gd-DTPA-enhanced T1-weighted image **(A)** demonstrates meningeal enhancement in the region of the suprasellar cistern and in the left sylvian cistern (arrow). T2-weighted images at higher levels **(B,C)** demonstrate focal areas of infarction involving the head of the caudate nucleus, the thalamus, and the posterior limb of the left internal capsule (arrows). These findings are compatible with infarction involving the deep perforating arteries caused by tuberculous meningitis.

water content allows identification of the four types of lesions that characterize carbon monoxide poisoning.[120]

Arterial Dissection

Arterial dissection is often overlooked as a cause of cerebral ischemia or infarction. Arterial dissection may be caused by trauma, diseases intrinsic to the arterial wall, or local inflammatory disease, or it may have a spontaneous onset. Arteriography has been the best modality for diagnosing arterial dissection, but the findings may be nonspecific.[123,124] MR is a sensitive and noninvasive method for identifying the hemorrhagic component of a dissection, because MRI can effectively detect the components of hemorrhage. MRI can provide a definitive diagnosis in patients with nonspecific arteriographic findings and is useful in monitoring the resolution of these lesions.

The sequence of MR changes of intramural hemorrhage in an arterial dissection is similar to that of an intraparenchymal hematoma.[124,125] Hemosiderin does not deposit because a blood-brain barrier is lacking. Subacute intramural hemorrhage (i.e., extracellular methemoglobin) has been demonstrated in the internal carotid artery 12 days after a spontaneous dissection.[124] A subacute hemorrhagic dissection appears as a hyperintense lesion on T1-weighted, proton density, and T2-weighted images that expands the wall of the vessel and narrows its lumen. Axial images best demonstrate an intramural hemorrhage because the artery is visualized in cross-section. Sagittal images are difficult to interpret because of vascular tortuosity, volume averaging of the vessel, and the similarity of the linear, hyperintense intramural hematoma to an interstitial fat plane.[124]

An acute intramural hemorrhage may be difficult to diagnose because deoxyhemoglobin has low signal intensity on long TR images and may simulate a flow void. On T1-weighted images, an absence of the normal flow void indicates thrombosis. Phase images or GRE images emphasizing flow are useful in detecting the presence or absence of flow in these cases.

Moyamoya

Moyamoya, an ischemic vascular disease of unknown cause, is characterized by progressive stenosis or occlusion of the supraclinoid segments of the internal carotid arteries, with the development of lenticulostriate and thalamoperforate collaterals.[126] The proximal portions of the anterior, middle, and posterior cerebral arteries may be involved as well.[90] There is endothelial hyperplasia and fibrosis, but no evidence of inflammatory disease.[126] The disease usually develops during childhood, and children typically present with ischemic symptoms. Adults with the disease commonly present with subarachnoid or intracranial hemorrhage.[90] There is an increased prevalence in the Japanese population.[90]

Angiography has been the procedure of choice in confirming the diagnosis. Arterial stenoses and occlusions and the vascular blush of the collaterals are characteristic of the disease. This vascular blush is called moyamoya, or puff of smoke, in Japanese.

Characteristic MR findings have been described for moyamoya.[126–128] These include multiple bilateral infarctions involving the watershed regions of the carotid circulations, absence of the signal flow void in the supraclinoid internal carotid artery or middle cerebral artery, and visualization of the dilated collateral moyamoya vessels as multiple signal flow voids.

Amyloid Angiopathy

Amyloid angiopathy is an uncommon cause of nonhypertensive hemorrhage in older patients. Amyloid deposits are identified in the medium and small sized arteries and arterioles only in the cerebral cortex.[90,129] The temporal, parietal, and occipital lobes are the areas of the brain most frequently involved.[129,130] In particular, the calcarine region of the occipital lobe is commonly involved. These pathologic findings probably reflect changes of aging. The amyloid deposition in the vessel wall presumably increases vessel fragility, which predisposes to rupture of the vessel and hemorrhage. The autopsy incidence of this disease is 40% in patients over 70 years of age and 60% or greater in patients over 80 years of age.[90,129] Noncortical arteries of the brain are not involved. Cortical hemorrhages, which may extend into subcortical locations, suggest this disease in older patients. Subarachnoid hemorrhage is commonly an associated finding because of the peripheral location of the cortical hemorrhages.

Cerebral Venous Thrombosis

Cerebral venous thrombosis may involve any of the cerebral veins, including the major venous sinuses, cortical veins, or deep veins. The clinical diagnosis of this disease is difficult because the clinical manifestations are nonspecific. Because there is a high instance of morbidity and mortality with this disease, prompt recognition can improve patient survival.

Cerebral venous thrombosis can be divided into two major etiologic categories: inflammatory and noninflammatory. Before the advent of antibiotics, inflammatory causes, particularly mastoid sinus disease, were common causes of cerebral veno-occlusive disease. Inflammatory causes are relatively uncommon today, but there are many noninflammatory causes. Venous thrombosis associated with pregnancy and the puerperium, trauma, dehydration, neoplasm, the use of oral contraceptives, or L-asparginase therapy are currently the most common causes.[131]

MRI provides a sensitive, noninvasive means for evaluating cerebral venous thrombosis. An orderly temporal evolution of MR findings in this disease has been described.[131,132] Initially, the absence of a normal flow void is identified on T1-weighted images. In this stage, the thrombosis appears as an intermediate signal on T1-weighted images along the normal course of the vein. On T2-weighted images, there is low signal intensity in the corresponding region. These findings are produced by the paramagnetic effects of deoxyhemoglobin. The low-intensity area on T2-weighted images is more pronounced with increased field strength. A supportive finding is the identification of venous collaterals bypassing the obstruction. In the intermediate stages, the thrombus becomes high signal intensity, initially on T1-weighted images and later on T2-weighted images (Fig. 2–48). These findings are secondary to the formation of methemoglobin. In the late stage, the vessel can recanalize, and flow voids are again visualized.

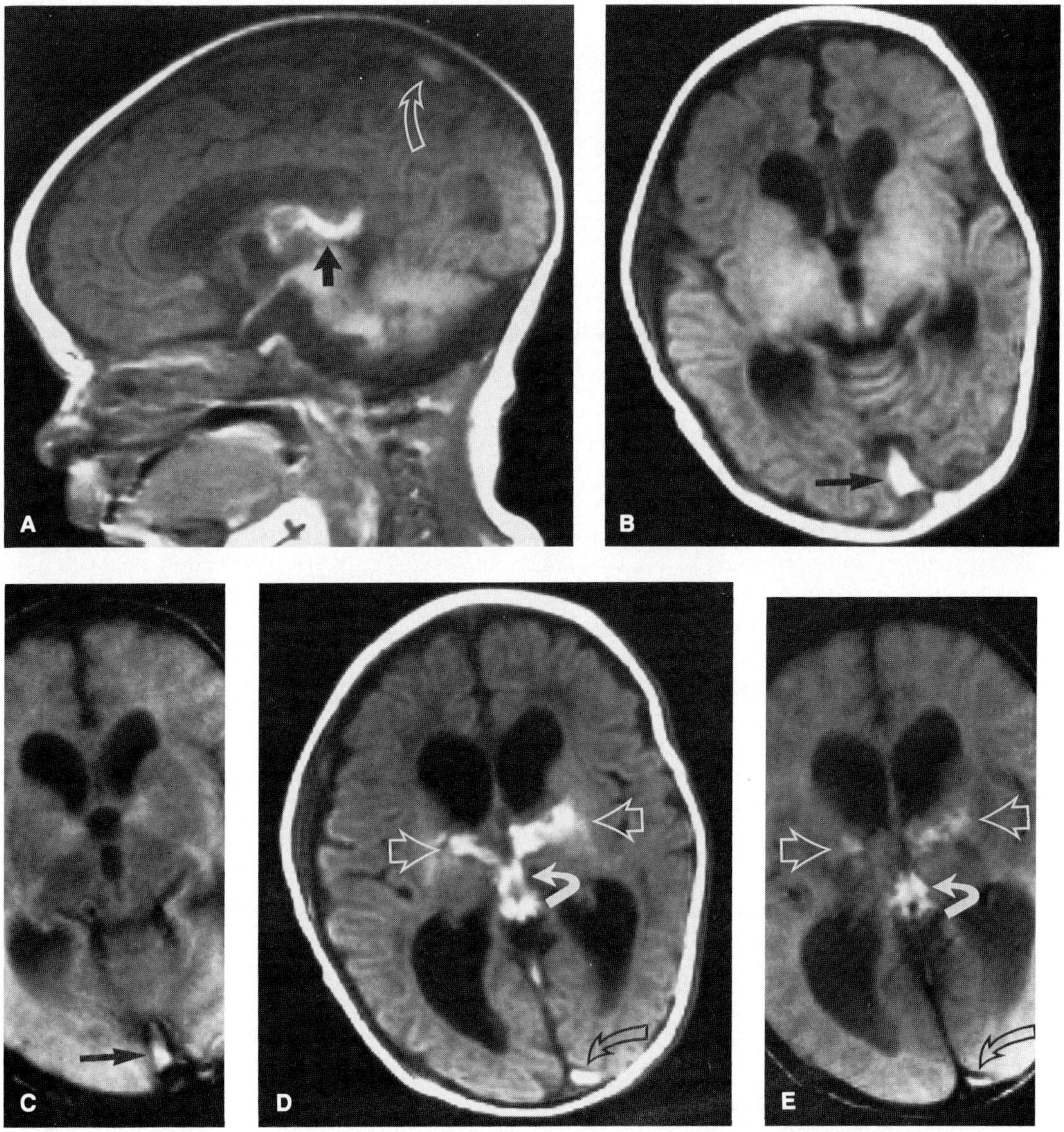

FIGURE 2–48. Venous thrombosis in a 3-week-old girl with bacterial meningitis and seizures. **(A)** Sagittal T1-weighted image (TR/TE = 650/20); **(B,D)** axial T1-weighted images (TR/TE = 650/20); **(C,E)** axial T2-weighted images (TR/TE = 3000/45). On T1- and T2-weighted images, there is increased signal intensity within the venous sinuses and the deep cerebral veins compatible with extracellular methemoglobin in thrombi. A sagittal T1-weighted image **(A)** demonstrates a thrombus involving the deep cerebral veins (the internal cerebral vein, the basal vein of Rosenthal, and the vein of Galen) (straight arrow) and the superior sagittal sinus (open curved arrow). Axial images **(B,C,D,E)** demonstrate high signal intensity thrombus in the straight sinus (straight arrows), the internal cerebral veins (curved closed arrows), and the sagittal sinus (curved open arrows). There are bilateral hemorrhagic (extracellular methemoglobin) thalamic infarcts (open arrows).

Slow flow in a normally patent vein can produce high or intermediate signal intensity and can have the appearance of a thrombus on a single sequence. Flow-related enhancement and even echo rephasing must be recognized as such and identified as representing normal venous flow.[33,34] However, a thrombus will maintain the same signal characteristics in any plane and on sequences done at different times. These features generally distinguish a thrombus from slow flow with high signal intensity.

Venous thrombosis is often associated with infarction. Venous infarction can involve the cortex and white matter (Fig. 2-48). A common pattern seen with superior sagittal sinus thrombosis is multiple bilateral, parasagittal, high-convexity infarcts. CT often identifies cortical gyral enhancement in venous infarcts associated with blood-brain-barrier disruption.[133] Similar findings should be expected with contrast-enhanced MRI. Hemorrhage is frequently associated with venous infarction. Hemorrhagic venous infarction commonly involves the cortex and often has a gyriform configuration.[90,133] Hemorrhage can occur in the white matter, with or without associated cortical hemorrhage.

REFERENCES

1. Bradley WG. Pathophysiological correlates of signal alterations. In: Brandt-Zawadski M, Norman D, eds. Magnetic resonance of the central nervous system. New York: Raven Press, 1987.
2. Gomori JM, Grossman RI. Mechanisms responsible for the MR appearance and evolution of intracranial hemorrhage. Radiographics 1988;8:427.
3. Gomori JM, Grossman RI, Ya-Ip C, et al. NMR relaxation times of blood: dependence of field strength, oxidation state and cell integrity. J Comput Assist Tomogr 1987;11:684.
4. Cohen MD, McGuire W, Cory DA, et al. MR appearance of blood and blood products: an in vitro study. AJR 1986;146:1293.
5. Bradley WG. MRI of hemorrhage and iron and in the brain. In: Stark DD, Bradley WG, eds. Magnetic resonance imaging. St. Louis: CV Mosby, 1988.
6. Barkovich JA, Atlas SW. Magnetic resonance imaging of intracranial hemorrhage: imaging in neuroradiology, part I. Radiol Clin North Am 1988;26:801.
7. Gomori JM, Grossman RI, Goldberg HI, et al. Intracranial hematomas: imaging by high-field MR. Radiology 1985; 157:87.
8. Grossman RI. MR highlights hemorrhage but can be misleading. Diagnostic Imaging 1988;10:126.
9. Hackney DB, Atlas SW, Grossman RI, et al. Subacute intracranial hemorrhage: contribution of spin density to appearance on spin-echo MR images. Radiology 1987;165:199.
10. William WJ, Beutler E, Erslev AJ, et al. Hematology. 3rd ed. New York: McGraw-Hill, 1983:35.
11. Neill JM, Hasting AB. The influence of the tension of molecular oxygen upon certain oxidations of hemoglobin. J Biol Chem 1925;63:479.
12. Gomori JM, Grossman RI, Hackney DB, et al. Variable appearances of subacute intracranial hematomas on high-field spin-echo MR. AJR 1988;150:171.
13. Di Chiro G, Brooks RA, Girton ME, et al. Sequential MR studies of intracerebral hematomas in monkeys. AJNR 1986;7:193.
14. Dooms GD, Uske A, Brant-Zawadzki M, et al. Spin echo MR imaging of intracranial hemorrhage. Neuroradiology 1988;28:132.
15. Bradley WG, Schmidt PG. Effect of methemoglobin formation on the MR appearance of subarachnoid hemorrhage. Radiology 1985;156:99.
16. Young IR, Bydder GM, Hall AS, et al. Extracerebral collections: recognition by NMR imaging. AJNR 1983;4:833.
17. Bydder GM. Clinical application of gadolinium DTPA. In: Stark DD, Bradley WG, eds. Magnetic resonance imaging. St. Louis: CV Mosby, 1988.
18. McArdle CB, Richardson CJ, Hayden CK, et al. Abnormalities of the neonatal brain: MR imaging. Part 1. Intracranial hemorrhage. Radiology 1987;163:387.
19. Chakeres DW, Bryan RN. Acute subarachnoid hemorrhage: in vitro comparison of magnetic resonance and computed tomography. AJNR 1986;7:223.
20. Yoon HC, Lufkin RB, Vinuela F, et al. MR of acute subarachnoid hemorrhage. AJNR 1988;9:404.
21. Gomori JM, Bilaniuk LT, Zimmerman RA, et al. High-field MR imaging of superficial siderosis of the central nervous system. J Comput Assist Tomogr 1985;9:972.
22. Gomori JM, Grossman RI, Goldberg HI, et al. High-field spin echo MR imaging of superficial and subependymal siderosis secondary to neonatal intraventricular hemorrhage. Neuroradiology 1987;29:339.
23. Huber P. Arterial aneurysms. In: Cerebral angiography. 2nd ed. New York: Thieme-Stratton, 1982.
24. Rao KC, Lee SH. Cerebrovascular anomalies. In: Stark DD, Bradley WG, eds. Magnetic resonance imaging. St. Louis: CV Mosby, 1988.
25. Crompton MR. Mechanism of growth and rupture in cerebral berry aneurysm. Br Med J 1966;1:1138.
26. TerBrugge K, Rao KC, Lee SH. Cerebral vascular anomalies. In: Lee SH, Rao KC, eds. Cranial computed tomography and MRI. 2nd ed. New York: McGraw Hill, 1987.
27. Chason JC, Hindman WM. Berry aneurysms of the circle of Willis: results of a planned autopsy study. Neurology 1958;8:41.
28. Locksley HB. Report on the cooperative study of intracranial aneurysms and subarachnoid hemorrhage. J Neurosurg 1966;25:219.
29. Caplan LR. Stroke. Clin Symp 1988;40:4.
30. Bradley WG. MRI of the central nervous system. Neurol Res 1984;6:91.
31. Heros RL, Zervas NT. Subarachnoid hemorrhage. Ann Rev Med 1983;34:367.
32. Hackney DB, Lesnick JE, Zimmerman RA, et al. MR identification of bleeding site in subarachnoid hemorrhage with multiple intracranial aneurysms. J Comput Assist Tomogr 1986;10:878.
33. Bradley WG, Waluch V, Lai KS, et al. The appearance of rapidly flowing blood on magnetic resonance images. AJR 1984;143:1167.
34. Avel L. Blood flow effects in magnetic resonance imaging. AJR 1984;143:1157.
35. Burt TB. MR of CSF flow phenomenon mimicking basilar artery aneurym. AJNR 1987;8:55.
36. Bull J. Massive aneurysms at the base of the brain. Brain 1969;92:535.
37. Nadjmi M, Ratzka M, Wodarz M. Giant aneurysms in CT and angiography. Neuroradiology 1978;16:284.
38. Scotti G, Ethier R, Melancon D, et al. Computed tomography in the evaluation of intracranial aneurysms and subarachnoid hemorrhage. Radiology 1977;123:85.
39. Atlas SW, Grossman RI, Goldberg HI, et al. Partially thrombosed giant intracranial aneurysms: correlation of MR and pathologic findings. Radiology 1987;162:11.
40. Becker RL, Norfray JF, Teitelbaum GP, et al. MR imaging in patients with intracranial aneurysm clips. AJNR 1988;9:885.
41. Holtas S, Olsson M, Romner B, et al. Comparison of MR imaging and CT in patients with intracranial aneurysm clips. AJNR 1988;9:891.

42. Shellock FG, Crues JV. High field strength MR imaging and metallic biomedical implants: an ex vivo evaluation of deflection forces. AJR 1988;151:389.
43. Stehbens WE. Pathology of the cerebral blood vessels. St. Louis: CV Mosby, 1972.
44. Lee BC, Herzberg L, Zimmerman RD, et al. MR imaging of cerebral vascular malformations. AJNR 1985;6:863.
45. Mickelsen WJ. Natural history and pathophysiology of arteriovenous malformations. Clin Neurosurg 1979;26:307.
46. Perret G, Nishioka H. Arteriovenous malformations: report on the cooperative study of intracranial aneurysms and subarachnoid hemorrhage. J Neurosurg 1966;25:467.
47. Huber P. Arteriovenous malformations. In: Cerebral angiography. 2nd ed. New York: Thieme-Stratton, 1982.
48. Miyasaka K, Wolpert SM, Prager RJ. The association of cerebral aneurysms, infundibula and intracranial arteriovenous malformations. Stroke 1982;13:196.
49. Atlas SW. Intracranial vascular malformations and aneurysms; current imaging applications; imaging in neuroradiology, part I. Radiol Clin North Am 1988;26:821.
50. Atlas SW, Mark AS, Fram EK, et al. Vascular intracranial lesions: applications of gradient echo MR imaging. Radiology 1988;169:455.
51. Kucharczyk W, Lemme-Pleghos L, Uske A, et al. Intracranial vascular malformations: MR and CT imaging. Radiology 1985;156:383.
52. Males LI. Arteriovenous malformations of the brain. In: Youmans JR, ed. Neurological surgery. 2nd ed. Philadelphia: WB Saunders, 1982.
53. Roosen N, Schirmer M, Lins E, et al. MRI of an aneurysm of the vein of Galen. AJNR 1986;7:733.
54. Wendling LR, Moore JS, Kieffer SA, et al. Intracerebral venous angioma. Radiology 1976;119:141.
55. Rothfus WE, Albright AL, Casey KF, et al. Cerebellar venous angioma: "benign" entity? AJNR 1984;5:61.
56. Augustyn GT, Scott JA, Olson E, et al. Cerebral venous angiomas: MR imaging. Radiology 1985;156:391.
57. Cammarata C, Han JS, Haaga JR, et al. Cerebral venous angiomas imaged by MR. Radiology 1985;155:639.
58. Stimac GK, Soloman MA, Newton TH. CT and MR of angiomatous malformations of the choroid plexus in patients with Sturge-Weber disease. AJNR 1986;7:623.
59. Atlas SW, Grossman RI, Hackney DB, et al. Calcified intracranial lesions: detection with gradient echo acquisition rapid MR imaging. AJNR 1988;9:253.
60. Rigamonti D, Hadley MN, Drayer BP, et al. Cerebral cavernous malformations, incidence and familial occurrence. N Engl J Med 1988;319:343.
61. Okazaki H: Fundamentals of neuropathology. New York: Igaku-Shain, 1983.
62. Atlas SW, Grossman RI, Gomori JM, et al. Spin echo MR imaging of hemorrhagic intracranial malignant neoplasms. Radiology 1987;164:71.
63. Gomori JM, Grossman RI, Goldberg HI, et al. Occult cerebral vascular malformations: high-field MR imaging. Radiology 1986;158:707.
64. Lemure-Plaghos L, Kucharczgk W, Brant-Zawadzki M, et al. MRI of angiographically occult vascular malformations. AJR 1986;145:1223.
65. Ross JS. MR angiography furnishes detailed vascular images. Diagnostic Imaging 1988;10:96.
66. Weeden VJ. Flow MRI holds promise in vascular diagnosis. Diagnostic Imaging 1986;8:84.
67. Dumaulin CL, Souza SP, Hart HR. Rapid scan magnetic resonance angiography. Magn Reson Med 1987;5:238.
68. Dumaulin CL, Hart HR. Magnetic resonance angiography. Radiology 1986;161:717.
69. Masaryk TJ, Ross JS, Modic MT, et al. Carotid bifurcation: MR imaging. Radiology 1988;166:461.
70. Alfidi RJ, Masaryk TJ, Haacke EM, et al. MR angiography of peripheral, carotid and coronary arteries. AJR 1987;149:1097.
71. Kricheff II. Arteriosclerotic ischemic cerebrovascular disease. Radiology 1987;162:101.
72. Price AC, Runge VM, Nelson KL. Nonneoplastic disease. In: Runge VM, ed. Enhanced magnetic resonance imaging. St. Louis: CV Mosby, 1989.
73. Brant-Zawadzki M, Weinstein P, Bartkowski H, et al. MR imaging and spectroscopy in clinical and experimental cerebral ischemia: a review. AJR 1987;148:579.
74. Brant-Zawadzki M. Ischemia. In: Stark DD, Bradley WG, eds. Magnetic resonance imaging. St. Louis: CV Mosby, 1988.
75. Drayer BP. Brain infarction. In: Stark DD, Bradley WG Jr, eds. MR imaging, a categorical course in diagnostic radiology. Radiological Society of North America, 1988:39.
76. Virapongse C, Mancuso A, Quisling R. Human brain infarcts: Gd DTPA-enhanced MR imaging. Radiology 1986;161:785.
77. Drayer BP, Muraki A, Osborne D, et al. Gd DTPA enhanced magnetic resonance imaging for study of blood-brain-barrier permeability in naturally occurring and experimentally induced brain infarction. In: Runge VM, Claussen C, Felix R, James AE, eds. Contrast agents in magnetic resonance imaging. Princeton: Excerpta Medica, 1986.
78. Kuhn MJ, Johnson KA, Davis KR. Wallerian degeneration: evaluation with MR imaging. Radiology 1988;168:199.
79. Brant-Zawadzki M, Norman D, Newton TH, et al. Magnetic resonance of the brain: the optimal screening technique. Radiology 1984;152:71.
80. Unger E, Littlefield J, Gado M. Water content and water structure in CT and MR signal changes; possible influence in detection of early stroke. AJNR 1988;9:687.
81. Brant-Zawadzki M, Pereira B, Weinstein P, et al. MR imaging of acute experimental ischemia in cats. AJNR 1986;7:7.
82. McNamara MT, Brant-Zawadski M, Berry I, et al. Acute experimental ischemia: MRI enhancement using Gd DTPA. Radiology 1986;158:701.
83. Spetzler RF, Zabramski JM, Kaufman B, et al. Acute NMR changes during MCA occlusion: a preliminary study in primates. Stroke 1983;14:185.
84. Wall SD, Brant-Zawadazki M, Jeffrey RB, et al. High-frequency CT findings within 24 hours after cerebral infarction. AJR 1982;138:307.
85. Hecht-Leavitt C, Gomori JM, Grossman RI. High-field MRI of hemorrhagic cortical infarction. AJNR 1986;7:581.
86. Grady PA. Pathophysiology of extracranial cerebral arterial stenosis: a critical review. Stroke 1984;15:224.
87. Drayer BP. Diseases of the cerebral vascular system. In: Rosenberg RN, Heinz ER, eds. The clinical neurosciences. New York: Churchill Livingstone, 1984.
88. Caplan LR, Gorelick PB, Hier DB. Race, sex, and occlusive vascular disease, a review. Stroke 1986;17:648.
89. Imparato AM, Riles RS, Gorstein F. The carotid bifurcation plaque: pathologic findings associated with cerebral ischemia. Stroke 1979;53:665.
90. Goldberg HI, Lee SH. Stroke. In: Lee SH, Rao KC, eds. Cranial computed tomography and MRI. New York: McGraw-Hill, 1987.
91. Bralet AM, Belay A, Belay P, et al. Brain edema and blood-brain-barrier permeability following quantitative cerebral microembolism. Stroke 1979;10:34.
92. Romanul FC, Abramowicz A. Changes in brain and pial vessels in arterial border zones. Arch Neurol 1964;11:40.
93. DeReuck J. The human periventricular arterial blood supply and the anatomy of cerebral infarctions. Eur Neurol 1971;5:321.
94. Brown JJ, Hesselink JR, Rothrock JF. MR and CT of lacunar infarcts. AJNR 1988;9:477.
95. Fisher CM. Lacunar strokes and infarcts: a review. Neurology 1982;32:871.
96. Mohr JP. Lacunes. Neurol Clin 1983;1:201.
97. Mohr JP, Caplan LR, Melski JW, et al. The Harvard cooperative stroke registry: a prospective study. Neurology 1978;28:754.
98. Braffman BH, Zimmerman RA, Trojanowski JQ. Brain MR: pathologic correlation with gross and histopathology. Hyperintense white-matter foci in the elderly. AJR 1988;151:559.
99. Miyashita K, Naritomi H, Sawada T, et al. Identification of recent lacunar lesions in cases of multiple small infarctions by magnetic resonance imaging. Stroke 1988;19:834.
100. Braffman BH, Zimmerman RA, Trojanowski TQ, et al. Brain

MR: pathologic correlation with gross and histopathology. Lacunar infarction and Virchow-Robin spaces. AJR 1988;151:551.

101. Marshall VG, Bradley WB, Marshall CE, et al. Deep white matter infarction: correlation of MR imaging and histopathologic findings. Radiology 1988;167:517.

102. Jangreis CA, Kanal E, Hirsch WL, et al. Normal perivascular spaces mimicking lacunar infarction: MR imaging. Radiology 1988;169:101.

103. Brant-Zawadzki M, Fein G, Van Dyke C, et al. MR imaging of the aging brain: patchy white matter lesions and dementia. AJNR 1985;6:675.

104. Kirkpatrick JB, Hayman LA. White matter lesions in MR imaging of clinically healthy brains of elderly subjects: possible pathologic basis. Radiology 1987;162:509.

105. Issam AA, Johnson PC, Spetzler RF, et al. Incidental subcortical lesions identified on magnetic resonance imaging in the elderly. Postmortem pathological correlations. Stroke 1986;17:1090.

106. Gilbert JJ, Sadler M. Unsuspected multiple sclerosis. Arch Neurol 1983;40:533.

107. Caplan LR, Schoene WC. Clinical features of subcortical arteriosclerotic encephalopathy (Binswanger disease). Neurology 1978;28:1206.

108. Hauser RA, Lacey M, Knight MR. Hypertensive encephalopathy. Magnetic resonance imaging demonstration of reversible cortical and white matter lesions. Arch Neurol 1988;45:1078.

109. Aisen AM, Gabrielsen TO, McCune WJ. MR imaging of systemic lupus erythematosus involving the brain. AJNR 1985;6:197.

110. Miller DH, Ormerod IE, Gibson A, et al. MR brain scanning in patients with vasculitis: differentiation from multiple sclerosis. Neuroradiology 1987;29:226.

111. Willeit J, Schmutzhard E, Aichner F, et al. CT and MR imaging in neuro-Behcet disease. J Comput Assist Tomogr 1986;10:313.

112. Simard D, Paulson OB. Cerebral vasomotor paralysis during migraine attack. Arch Neurol 1973;29:207.

113. Blan JN. Migraine: a vasomotor instability of the meningeal circulation. Lancet 1978;2:1136.

114. Soges LJ, Cacayorin ED, Petro GR, et al. Migraine: evaluation by MR. AJNR 1988;9:425.

115. Blousser MG, Baron JC, Chiras J. Ischemic strokes and migraine. Neuroradiology 1985;27:583.

116. Mathews NT, Meyer JS, Welch KM. Abnormal CT scans in migraine. Headache 1977;16:272.

117. McArdle CB, Richardson CJ, Hayden CK, et al. Abnormalities of the neonatal brain: MR imaging. Part II. Hypoxic-ischemic brain injury. Radiology 1987;163:395.

118. Volpe JJ. Neonatal hypoxic-ischemic brain injury. Pediatr Clin North Am 1976;23:383.

119. Dietrich RB, Bradley WG. Iron accumulation in the basal ganglia following severe ischemic-anoxic insults in children. Radiology 1988;168:203.

120. Horowitz AL, Kaplan R, Sarpel G. Carbon monoxide toxicity: MR imaging in the brain. Radiology 1987;162:787.

121. Davis PL: The magnetic resonance imaging appearances of basal ganglia lesions in carbon monoxide poisoning. Magn Reson Imaging 1986;4:489.

122. Miura T, Mitomo M, Kawai R, et al. CT of the brain in acute carbon monoxide intoxication: characteristic features and prognosis. AJNR 1985;6:739.

123. O'Dwyer JA, Moscow N, Trevor R, et al. Spontaneous dissection of the carotid artery. Radiology 1980;137:379.

124. Goldberg HI, Grossman RI, Gomori JM, et al. Cervical internal carotid artery dissecting hemorrhage: diagnosis using MR. Radiology 1986;158:157.

125. Grossman RI. Hemorrhage. In: Stark DD, Bradley WG Jr, eds. MR imaging, a categorical course in diagnostic radiology. Radiological Society of North America, 1988:189.

126. Bruno A, Yuh WT, Biller J, et al. Magnetic resonance imaging in young adults with cerebral infarction due to moyamoya. Arch Neurol 1988;45:303.

127. Brooks BS, Gammal TE, Adams RJ, et al. MR imaging of moyamoya in neurofibromatosis. AJNR 1987;8:178.

128. Fujisawa I, Asato R, Nishimura K, et al. Moyamoya disease: MR imaging. Radiology 1987;164:103.

129. Wagle WA, Smith TW, Weiner M. Intracerebral hemorrhage caused by cerebral amyloid angiopathy: radiographic-pathologic correlation. AJNR 1984;5:171.

130. Vinters HV, Gilbert JJ. Amyloid angiopathy: its incidence and complications in the aging brain. Stroke 1981;12:118.

131. McMurdo KS, Brant-Zawadzki M, Bradley WG, et al. Dural sinus thrombosis: study using intermediate field strength MR imaging. Radiology 1986;161:83.

132. Macchi DJ, Grossman RI, Gomori JM, et al. High field MR imaging of cerebral venous thrombosis. J Comput Assist Tomogr 1986;10:10.

133. Rao KC, Knipp HC, Wagner EJ. Computed tomographic findings in cerebral sinus and venous thrombosis. Radiology 1981;140:391.

3

Brain: Neoplastic Disease

Ann C. Price
Val M. Runge
Gregory V. Babigian

In the few short years since its introduction and widespread clinical usage, magnetic resonance imaging (MRI) has proven its utility in evaluating a diversity of intracranial abnormalities, including intracranial neoplastic disease.[1-3] Superior resolution of soft tissue planes, absence of bone artifact, direct multiplanar imaging capability, and multiple sequence imaging parameters have led to a highly sensitive and versatile imaging technique. As a result, MRI has become the principal or primary imaging modality in intracranial tumor detection and evaluation.

The sensitivity of MRI in demonstrating most brain neoplasms is due to the ease of detecting extracellular fluid that results from blood-brain-barrier (BBB) disruption.[1] Although both T1 and T2 parameters are prolonged, it is the increase in signal intensity occurring on T2-weighted images that allows early tumor detection. MR diagnosis is possible even if tumors are small or cause few or no changes detected by computed tomography (CT) (Fig. 3-1). Some brain tumors without a BBB, such as neurofibromas, have an increased water content and produce similar but less pronounced prolongation of T1 and T2 parameters.

Despite the sensitivity and versatility of MRI, the visualization and characterization of many tumors was not possible before the development of MR contrast agents (e.g., Gd DTPA). Principal clinical examples include the separation of tumor nidus from the edema it produces, the consistent visualization of tumors without a BBB (e.g., meningiomas), and the detection of metastatic lesions that are not associated with significant edema.[4-13] MR contrast agents have largely overcome these drawbacks by providing information about BBB integrity and tissue vascularity.

CONTRAST AGENTS

Iodinated contrast agents that are essential in other phases of radiologic imaging are not effective at clinical doses in MRI. This would be expected because of the difference in physical principles of the two imaging modalities. Iodinated contrast agents attenuate the x-ray beam, whereas MR contrast agents must sufficiently alter the microchemical environment to shorten T1 or T2 parameters. It is the greater shortening of T1 that is most important in producing contrast enhancement in clinical MRI. A more detailed discussion of contrast media is offered in Chapter 15, but a few clinically important aspects are considered here.

Several agents have been used experimentally.[6,7] Gd DTPA has emerged as the principal agent to date. It is safe and clinically well tolerated.[8-12] Extensive clinical and laboratory studies have failed to show toxicity for any organ, including the kidney, liver, heart, and brain.[4,5,8-12] These would be the target organs if decomplexation of this highly stable agent occurred. There is a transient but significant elevation of serum iron (up to 15 mg/dL above normal) in a few patients.[9] The reason for this has not been explained, nor does it appear to have any clinical relevance.

Renal excretion is rapid, with approximately 80% of the contrast agent appearing in the urine of laboratory animals within the first 3 hours after intravenous injection.[7] Because Gd DTPA is renally excreted, patients with poor renal function or advanced renal disease may not be candidates for contrast enhancement.

No allergic reactions have been reported with Gd DTPA.[4,5,8-13] We have observed hives after injection, but they occur in less than 1% of cases. This represents a significant advantage over iodinated contrast

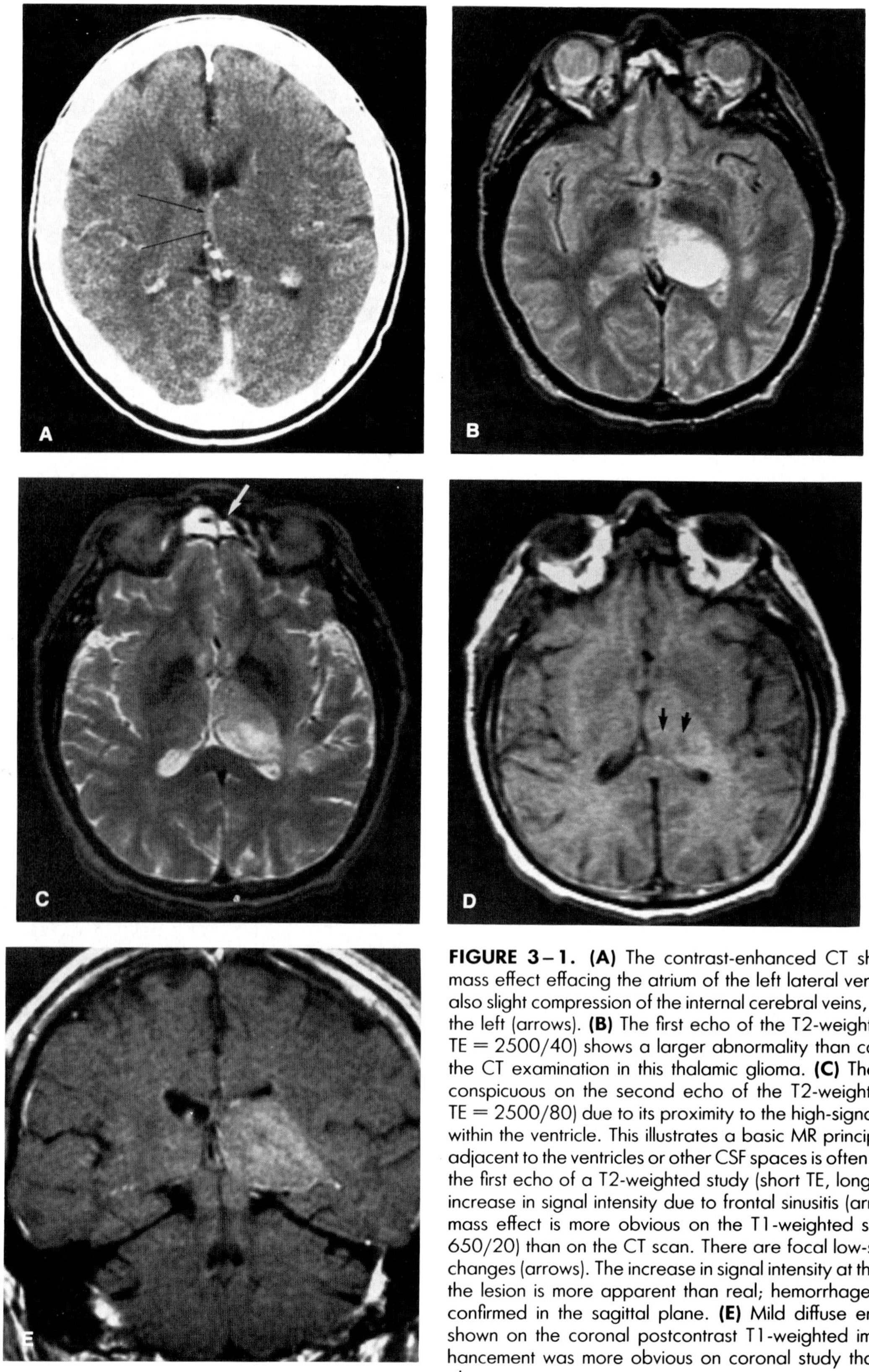

FIGURE 3–1. **(A)** The contrast-enhanced CT shows a vague mass effect effacing the atrium of the left lateral ventricle. There is also slight compression of the internal cerebral veins, particularly on the left (arrows). **(B)** The first echo of the T2-weighted series (TR/TE = 2500/40) shows a larger abnormality than can be seen on the CT examination in this thalamic glioma. **(C)** The tumor is less conspicuous on the second echo of the T2-weighted study (TR/TE = 2500/80) due to its proximity to the high-signal-intensity CSF within the ventricle. This illustrates a basic MR principle. Pathology adjacent to the ventricles or other CSF spaces is often better seen on the first echo of a T2-weighted study (short TE, long TR). Note the increase in signal intensity due to frontal sinusitis (arrows). **(D)** The mass effect is more obvious on the T1-weighted study (TR/TE = 650/20) than on the CT scan. There are focal low-signal-intensity changes (arrows). The increase in signal intensity at the periphery of the lesion is more apparent than real; hemorrhage could not be confirmed in the sagittal plane. **(E)** Mild diffuse enhancement is shown on the coronal postcontrast T1-weighted image. The enhancement was more obvious on coronal study than in the axial plane.

agents, which commonly produce allergic reactions. The steroids administered for reaction prophylaxis to iodinated contrast agents alter and transiently close the BBB, so that the degree of enhancing of the abnormality may not be precisely shown.[14] Contrast-enhanced MRI, therefore, provides a safer and more accurate alternative to contrast-enhanced CT.

Due to the expense of Gd DTPA and the concern for cost containment, a recent clinical study has addressed the issue of reducing the current standard dose by one-half.[15] Unfortunately, the study was too small to adequately assess the effectiveness of this reduced dosage in detecting a spectrum of abnormalities. The currently accepted dosage of 0.1 mmol/kg conforms to FDA guidelines, which are based on clinical studies of safety and efficacy. Further documentation will be necessary before widespread clinical adaptation of a reduced dosage.

With larger doses (0.2 mmol/kg), additional metastatic lesions have been demonstrated.[16] Dosage increases above this level may have a negative effect because of the decreased signal intensity produced by greater T2 shortening.

Mechanisms of Enhancement

The mechanism of tumor enhancement with MR contrast agents is similar to iodinated contrast agents used in CT. Enhancement with both agents occurs due to an alteration in local vascularity and the BBB. Due to its sensitivity and greater resolution of soft tissue planes, contrast-enhanced MRI usually shows smaller abnormalities earlier than CT.[17]

The enhancement of most neoplasms depends on the degree of BBB disruption. Histologic studies have shown a structural alteration in the capillary walls of the tumor that allows extravascular or interstitial accumulation of contrast.[18] Generally, the more aggressive the tumor, the greater the BBB breakdown and the greater the contrast enhancement.[19,20]

Runge and colleagues confirmed a similar basis of enhancement with paramagnetic agents using a model of reversible BBB disruption by hyperosmolar mannitol and an animal brain abscess model.[17,21] In each case, Gd DTPA enhancement marked the BBB disruption. The animal brain abscess model fulfilled an additional purpose in showing a localized area of BBB disruption as a focal area of enhancement. This occurred in the early cerebritis stage of abscess evolution, which was much earlier than could be shown by CT.[17]

The degree of vascularity plays an important role in tumors that do not have a BBB. These are usually tumors that do not arise within the brain parenchyma and include meningiomas, schwannomas, neurinomas, neuromas, pituitary-origin tumors, and some parasellar tumors like chordomas.[10,12]

Imaging Considerations

Contrast enhancement is better visualized on T1-weighted sequences. This has been documented by clinical usage and contrast-enhancement curves, calculation of contrast-to-noise ratios, and calculation of T1 and T2 parameters. Although both T1 and T2 relaxation times are shortened, T1 is shortened to a greater extent.[22,23]

Contrast enhancement can occasionally be visualized on T2-weighted images, with greater detection at higher field strengths, presumably due to the prolongation of T1. Many meningiomas and some pituitary-origin tumors do not show an increase in signal on unenhanced T2-weighted images. Because of this, enhancement can frequently be visualized in these tumors on T2-weighted sequences.[9,23,24]

Therefore, if enhancement and signal-intensity change are to be clearly distinguished, T2-weighted sequences should be obtained before contrast enhancement. One exception to this may be in the evaluation of metastatic disease where greater lesion conspicuity has been seen on the first echo of the post-contrast T2-weighted study.[37] Precontrast T1-weighted images are necessary to differentiate enhancement from hemorrhage or a lipid component of the suspected tumor. Examination in similar planes (e.g., axial) is necessary for accurate comparisons. Supplementary coronal or sagittal planes may be used for further evaluation of the abnormality.

T1-Weighted Sequences

The relaxation time (TR) selected should remain within the manufacturer's suggested guidelines for the field strength. Most of the images used in this chapter were obtained at 1.0 T. A TR of ≤0.7 seconds will provide sufficient slices to cover the head from base to vertex at 5- to 7-mm intervals, with an appropriate gap (30%). A gap between slices prevents image degradation from "cross-talk." With a 256^2 matrix and 1 average (NEX), excellent clinical images are generated in less than 3 minutes.

Other TRs may be used but must take into consideration the available slices, slice widths, averages, matrix size, and image resolution (see Chapter 5). Although routine imaging of the head is not as complex as that for the cervical spine, the same imaging principles apply.

T2-Weighted Sequences

The TR for these sequences are usually selected for time efficiency. It is particularly important to leave adequate time for contrast-enhanced T1-weighted sequences and not exceed the patient's customarily allowed time period (≤1 hour). A TR of 2.5 seconds may require 2 averages on some instrumentation for sufficient SNR with a 256 × 256 matrix. This yields an imaging time of 21.3 minutes. A TR of 3.0 has a sufficient signal-to-noise ratio (SNR) to require only one average and reduce the imaging time to 12.8 minutes. This substantial time savings allows a postcontrast study in multiple planes if an abnormality needs further delineation.

On T2-weighted sequences, cerebrospinal fluid (CSF) motion artifact is an important imaging consideration, particularly at field strengths of 1.0 T and above. Techniques that suppress motion must be used to prevent image degradation by dephasing artifacts. Cardiac gating or gradient motion suppression can be used. CSF motion predominately affects the temporal lobe and suprasellar regions, but image degradation also occurs at the convexities.

Gradient Echo

New gradient echo sequences with very short TEs and TRs and flip angles of 90° or less are increasingly used with and without Gd DTPA enhancement.[24,26] Preliminary results indicate that images generated with this technique are of high diagnostic quality and can add additional clinical information in tumor imaging (Fig. 3-2). The considerable reduction in examination time has the potential for increasing throughput.

Time Course of Enhancement

The time course of Gd DTPA enhancement differs from iodinated contrast. An early peak and relatively rapid decline over 1 hour occurs with iodinated CT contrast agents. With Gd DTPA, there is a rapid rise to maximum in the first 4 to 8 minutes, followed by a nearly flat enhancement curve to 60 minutes, which shows only a slight decline from the maximum.[9,23,27] This allows a greater latitude in scan time than for CT, and a visible decline in enhancement should not occur, even if the abnormality is evaluated in multiple planes.

INTRA-AXIAL TUMORS

Gliomas

Astrocytomas and glioblastoma multiforme (GBM) are the most common brain tumors, accounting for 50% of all intracranial neoplasms.[1,2] As the name implies, astrocytomas arise from the astrocyte or its primitive precursor. These tumors arise in the white matter, where astrocytes are abundant. In adults, these are more frequent above the tentorium in the cerebral hemispheres, while in youth and childhood these arise more commonly in the cerebellar hemispheres and brain stem (Fig. 3-3).[28]

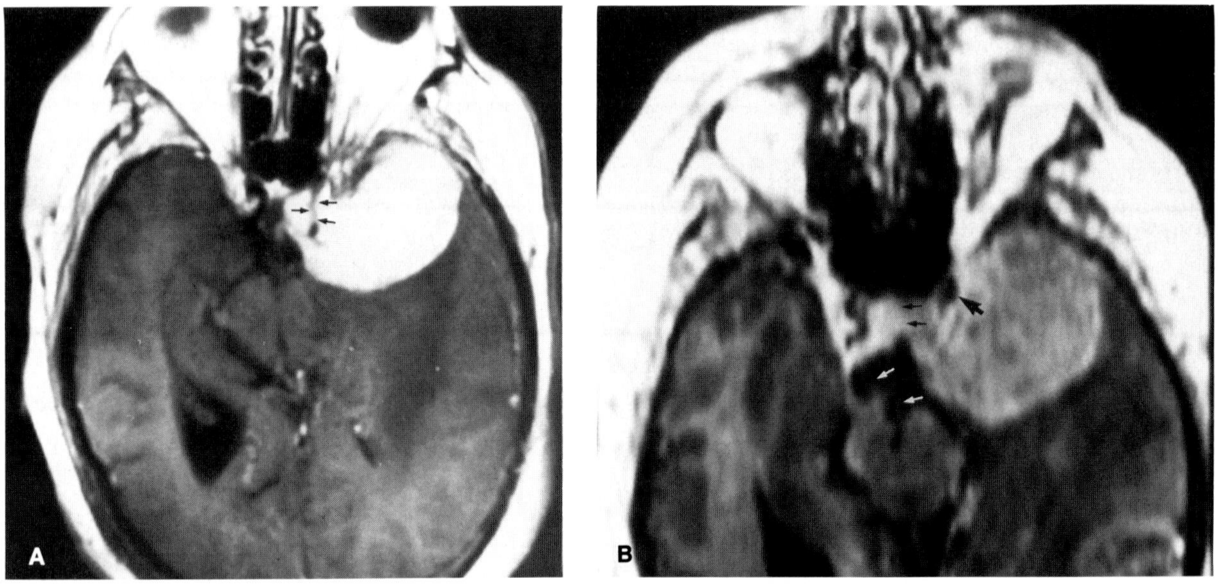

FIGURE 3-2. (A) An enhancing left sphenoid wing meningioma is shown on this T1-weighted spin-echo (TR/TE = 700/17) axial section. Cavernous sinus invasion is suspected due to the irregularity of the internal carotid artery (arrows). **(B)** An axial view reformatted from a 3D volume examination obtained with the FLASH technique (50°, TR = 40, TE = 8) more clearly shows the cavernous sinus invasion with displacement of the internal carotid artery (arrowhead) and compression of the pituitary (small arrows). The resolution is sufficient to show the CN III (white arrows). The mass effaces the brain stem. The enhancing rim is more intense than the remainder of the tumor.

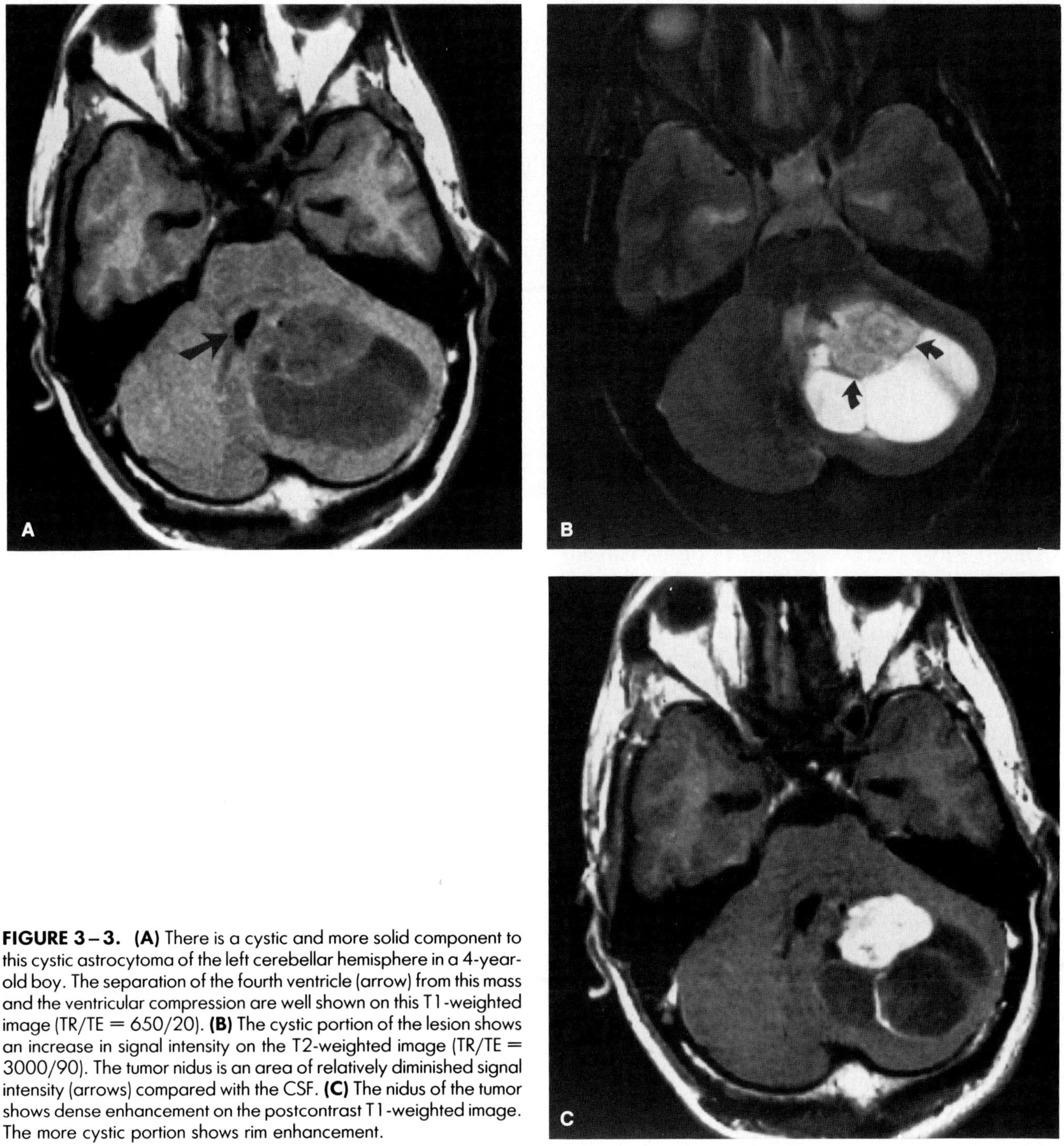

FIGURE 3–3. **(A)** There is a cystic and more solid component to this cystic astrocytoma of the left cerebellar hemisphere in a 4-year-old boy. The separation of the fourth ventricle (arrow) from this mass and the ventricular compression are well shown on this T1-weighted image (TR/TE = 650/20). **(B)** The cystic portion of the lesion shows an increase in signal intensity on the T2-weighted image (TR/TE = 3000/90). The tumor nidus is an area of relatively diminished signal intensity (arrows) compared with the CSF. **(C)** The nidus of the tumor shows dense enhancement on the postcontrast T1-weighted image. The more cystic portion shows rim enhancement.

The gliomas have been classified by Kernohan as Grades I through IV, based on their increasingly aggressive behavior, with Grades III and IV being the most malignant. Rubenstein has divided these tumors into three categories: the astrocytoma (Kernohan Grade I), the malignant astrocytoma (Kernohan Grade II), and the GBM (Kernohan Grade III and IV).[28] The Rubenstein classification is a little easier to correlate with imaging findings.

Although the lower-grade classification implies a lesser degree of malignancy, the outcome of these tumors is generally poor due to the infiltrative pattern of growth. Complete tumor resection is often impossible, resulting in a greater risk of tumor recurrence. The cystic cerebellar astrocytoma of childhood is the one major exception. Surgical removal of these tumors usually produces a clinical cure (Fig. 3–3).

MRI is the most sensitive imaging modality for detecting gliomas.[1,2] The alteration of the BBB causes an accumulation of extracellular fluid or vasogenic edema, which can be easily identified on T2-weighted sequences as an area of increase in signal intensity. This change may be the only or most convincing indication of a tumor. The alteration in T1 relaxation parameters may be difficult to visualize in some tumors, and the CT scan may be nearly normal or show only a subtle mass effect (Fig. 3–1).

The GBM has the most profound and nearly typical imaging change. Thus, it is the most readily diagnosed and least frequently confused with other neoplasms, such as large necrotic solitary metastases (Fig. 3–4). The GBM usually has a considerable amount of mass effect, margin irregularity, and signal intensity heterogeneity on T1-weighted and T2-weighted sequences.[2,29,30] The low-signal-intensity abnormality on T1 weighted images is due to cystic change and necrosis. The latter alteration occurs as the tumor outgrows its blood supply. The increase in signal intensity on T2 weighted images occurs in conjunction with marked amounts of associated vasogenic edema. Hemorrhage may occur in higher-grade gliomas; these are more frequently microhemorrhages (Fig. 3–5). Rarely, large areas of hemorrhage may obscure the underlying disease. Precontrast T1-weighted sequences are best for evaluating hemorrhage. These tumors spread through white matter tracts and frequently cross the corpus callosum to the opposite hemisphere (Fig. 3–6).[2,29] Bifrontal corpus callosum tumors are frequently referred to as "butterfly" gliomas.

Areas of ring enhancement occur after contrast administration in the higher-grade tumors and reflect the greater degree of BBB disruption (Fig. 3–4). Other patterns of enhancement include homogenous, garland-shaped, mixed or patchy, linear, and central (Figs. 3–1, 3–3, 3–5 through 3–9).[4,13] These enhancement patterns may occur in any tumor, and are not grade specific. Occasionally, high-grade tumors will show little or no tumor enhancement. Thus, a completely accurate prediction of tumor grade by the imaging appearance is not possible.

Contrast administration should be routinely used in the assessment of all tumors. Because it improves visualization, localization, and delineation of tumor margins, a higher level of diagnostic confidence results.[4,8,13,31] This is partially due to the separation of the tumor nidus from the surrounding edema (Figs. 3–4 and 3–6), because edema does not measurably enhance.[6,27] Comparative CT and histologic studies show that enhancement does not represent the entirety of the tumor (Figs. 3–4, 3–6, and 3–9), but the maximal site of BBB disruption.[4,6,7,32] The area of maximal enhancement provides the most accurate site for diagnostic stereotactic biopsy. The irregular, finger-like pattern of tumor extension or infiltrative growth pattern produces areas that are relatively uninvolved with tumor. If these areas are selected for biopsy, the histologic diagnosis may be normal although the imaging changes are consistent with tumor. This produces a management quandary for the surgeon or radiation oncologist.

Patterns of enhancement can be used to separate more viable tumor from frankly necrotic components. The necrotic portion of the tumor shows less enhancement than the remainder of the tumor. When serial images are obtained over a 1-hour period, there is gradual enhancement from the periphery inward in the more viable portions of the tumor. Areas of necrosis maintain low signal intensity without evidence of enhancement.[27,31]

Necrotic central portions of tumors may be difficult to distinguish from cystic change. With cyst formation, a fairly well-circumscribed area of prolonged relaxation time occurs on T1-weighted and T2-weighted sequences (Figs. 3–3 and 3–8). The inner margin is smooth, and enhancement occurs at the periphery. This may be associated with a fluid-debris level or a contrast-fluid level, the latter indicating a degree of BBB disruption sufficient to allow the formation of this type of fluid level.[16] The distinction of cysts from necrosis may prove useful when selecting optimal sites for decompressive surgery or diagnostic biopsy.

Because all portions of the tumor may not enhance (Figs. 3–9 and 3–10), precontrast T2-weighted sequences are necessary to determine the full extent of the abnormality. Thus, a suitable imaging protocol includes T1-weighted and T2-weighted sequences before contrast, followed by postcontrast T1-weighted sequences. To avoid confusion of preexisting signal intensity changes and enhancement, the precontrast and postcontrast study should be obtained in similar planes (i.e., axial with additional supplementary views in another orthogonal plane). Coronal views are helpful with temporal lobe abnormalities (Figs. 3–4 and 3–11), and sagittal views assist in evaluation of brain stem and craniovertebral junction abnormalities.

Intermediate-grade tumors or malignant astrocytomas usually present with less severe imaging changes, compared with the GBM. The margins are not as irregular, there is less mass effect, and the signal intensity changes on T1-weighted and T2-weighted images are not as profound or heterogeneous (Fig. 3–11). Hemorrhage is less frequently found. Tissue necrosis and cyst formation may occur, but to a lesser degree than for GBM.[2,29]

The enhancement patterns are variable (Fig. 3–9). Contrast enhancement may provide a higher level of diagnostic confidence and assist in differentiation

(text continues on page 124)

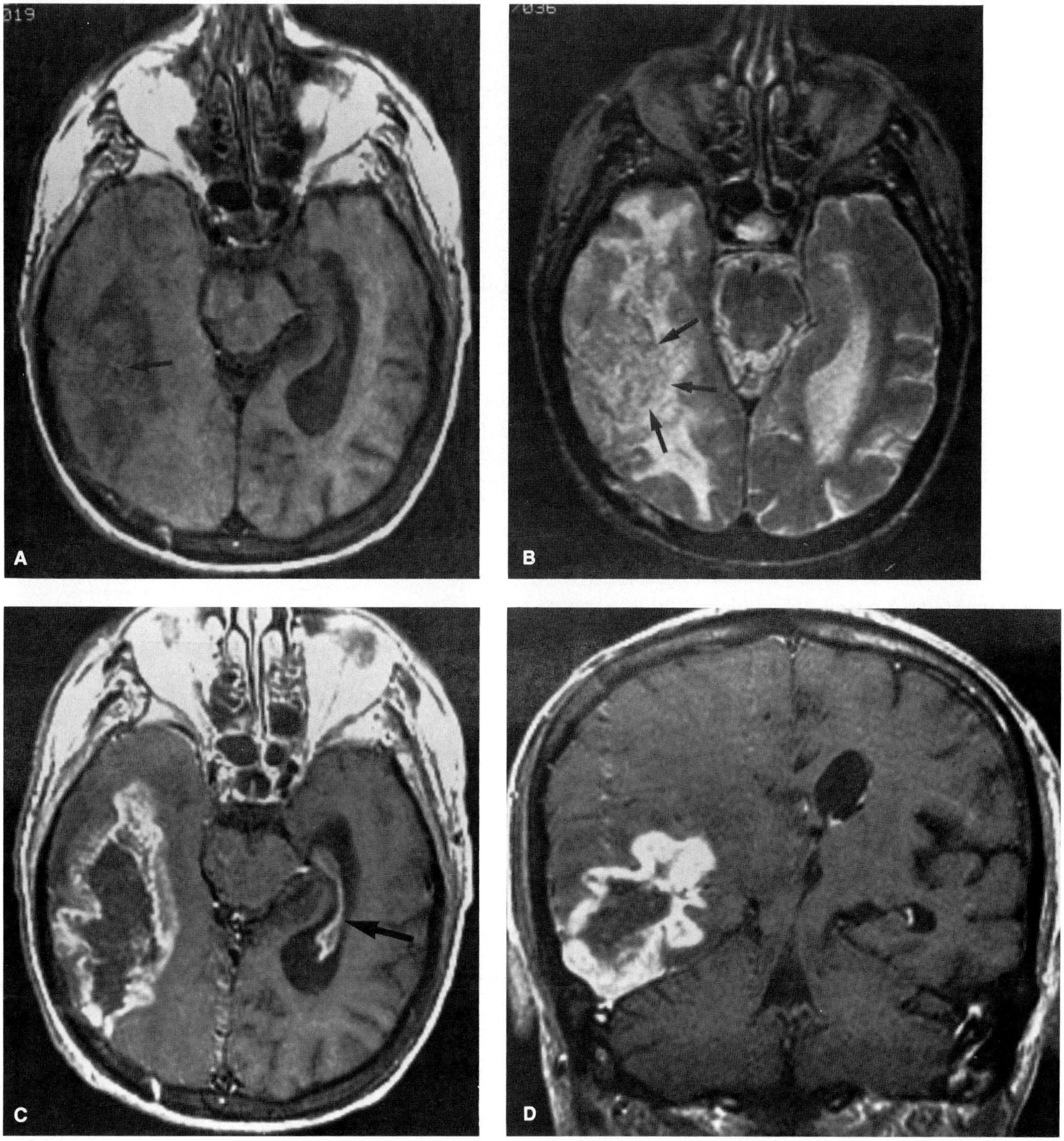

FIGURE 3–4. **(A)** There is a diffuse right temporal lobe low-signal-intensity change on this T1-weighted image (TR/TE = 500/20). Heterogeneous signal intensity (arrow) effaces and partially obliterates the temporal horn. **(B)** The T2-weighted image (TR/TE = 2000/80) more clearly shows the heterogeneous central portion of the tumor (arrows). The surrounding increase in signal intensity is attributed to vasogenic edema. **(C)** Irregular ring enhancement on this postcontrast T1-weighted image is consistent with the surgical diagnosis of glioblastoma multiforme. The choroid plexus of the left temporal horn is also enhanced (arrow). **(D)** The coronal view shows the ring enhancement and a greater degree of mass effect, ventricular effacement, and midline shift. This illustrates the benefit of coronal imaging in temporal lobe tumors.

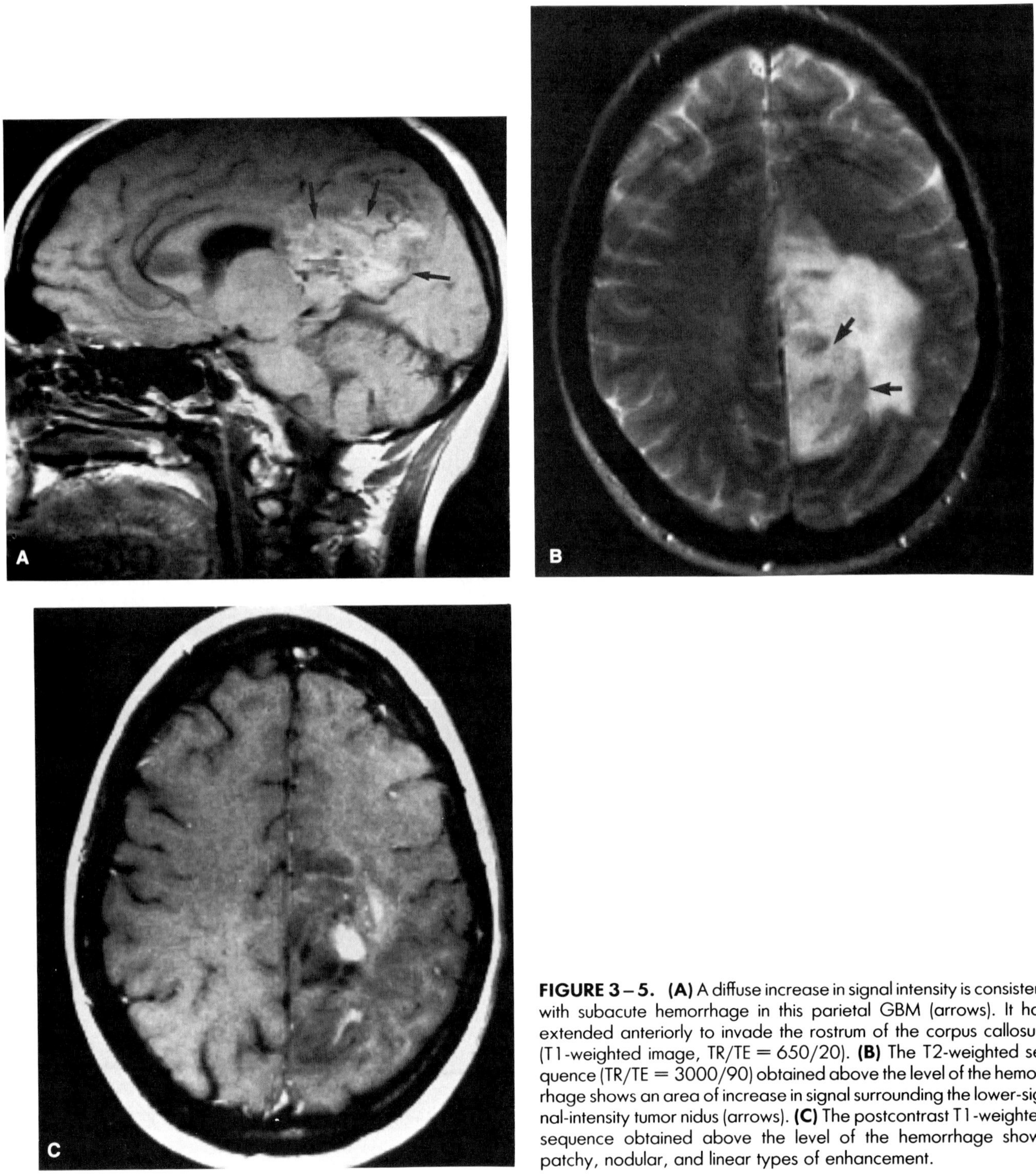

FIGURE 3–5. **(A)** A diffuse increase in signal intensity is consistent with subacute hemorrhage in this parietal GBM (arrows). It has extended anteriorly to invade the rostrum of the corpus callosum (T1-weighted image, TR/TE = 650/20). **(B)** The T2-weighted sequence (TR/TE = 3000/90) obtained above the level of the hemorrhage shows an area of increase in signal surrounding the lower-signal-intensity tumor nidus (arrows). **(C)** The postcontrast T1-weighted sequence obtained above the level of the hemorrhage shows patchy, nodular, and linear types of enhancement.

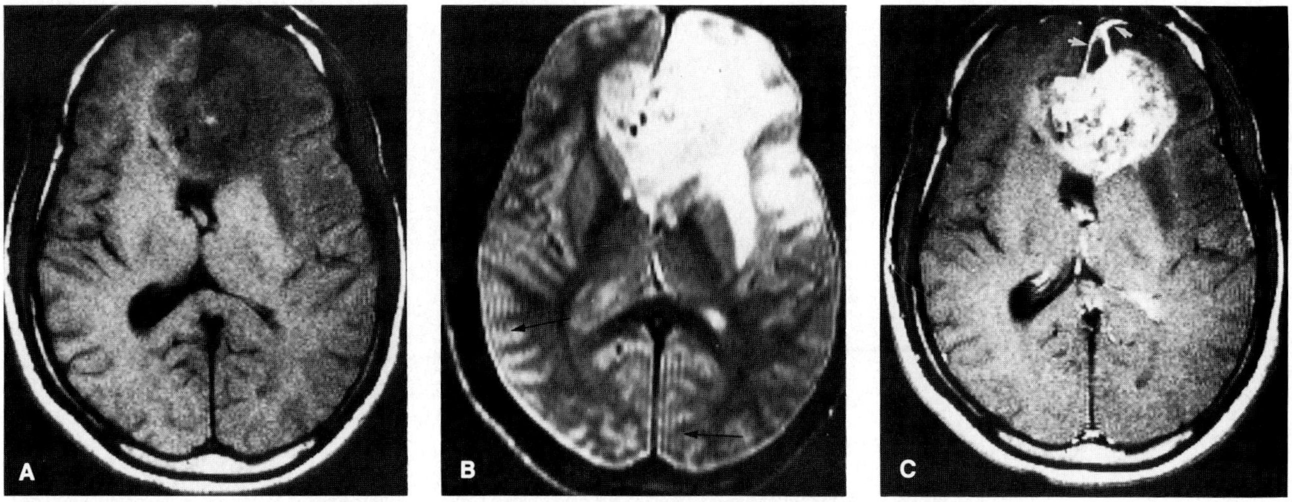

FIGURE 3–6. **(A)** A large, low-signal-intensity abnormality in the left frontal lobe extends across the midline on this T1-weighted image (TR/TE = 700/17). **(B)** There is a greater extent of the abnormality on the T2-weighted image (TR/TE = 3000/40). Although tumor extension across the corpus callosum may be suspected, it is difficult to distinguish from edema. A 128 × 256 matrix was used to obtain this image. Compare the resolution of this image to that in Fig. 3–3B. Notice the linear and curvilinear lines due to the smaller matrix (arrows). **(C)** The enhancement confirms the spread of the tumor across the corpus callosum. The dural enhancement (arrows) is due to previous surgery for this recurrent malignant astrocytoma.

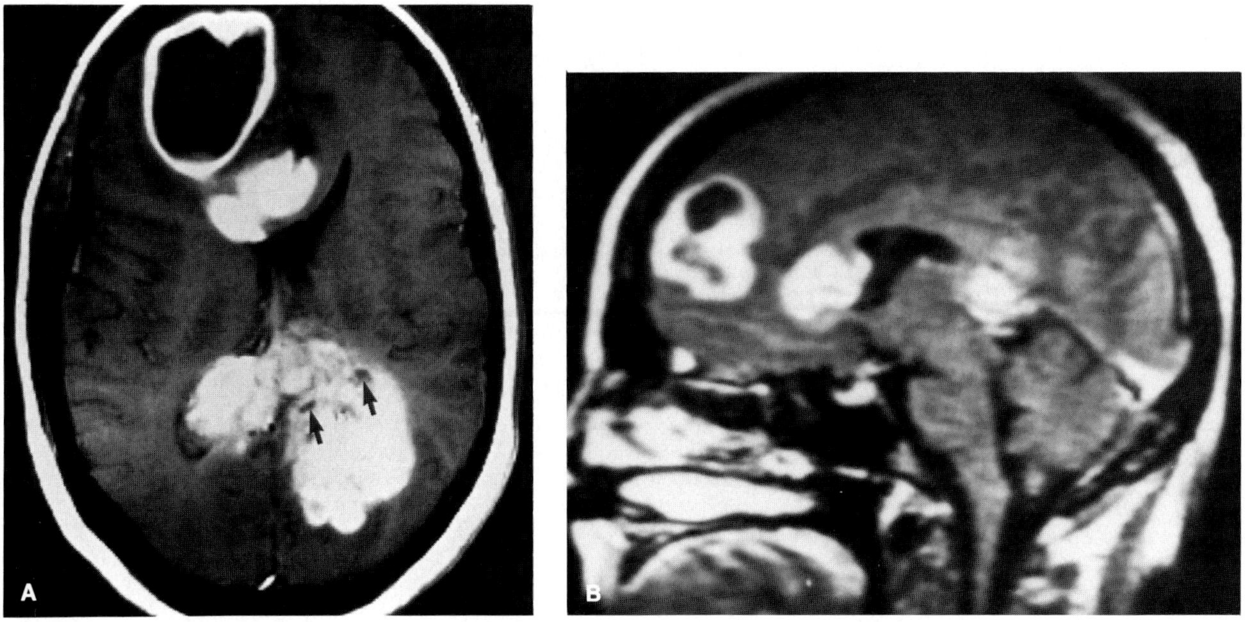

FIGURE 3–7. **(A)** This postcontrast T1-weighted image shows multiple patterns of enhancement. There is ring enhancement in the right frontal lobe, diffuse enhancement in the genu of the corpus callosum, and patchy enhancement in the rostrum. This was thought to represent either a multicentric glioma or extensive spread from a corpus callosum glioma. The mottled appearance (arrows) is due to calcifications that are common in corpus callosum gliomas. **(B)** This midline sagittal view from a T1-weighted postcontrast 3D volume study confirms the location of these abnormalities. This is a 1-mm section from which high resolution reformatted views can be obtained in any plane, as in Figure 3–2B.

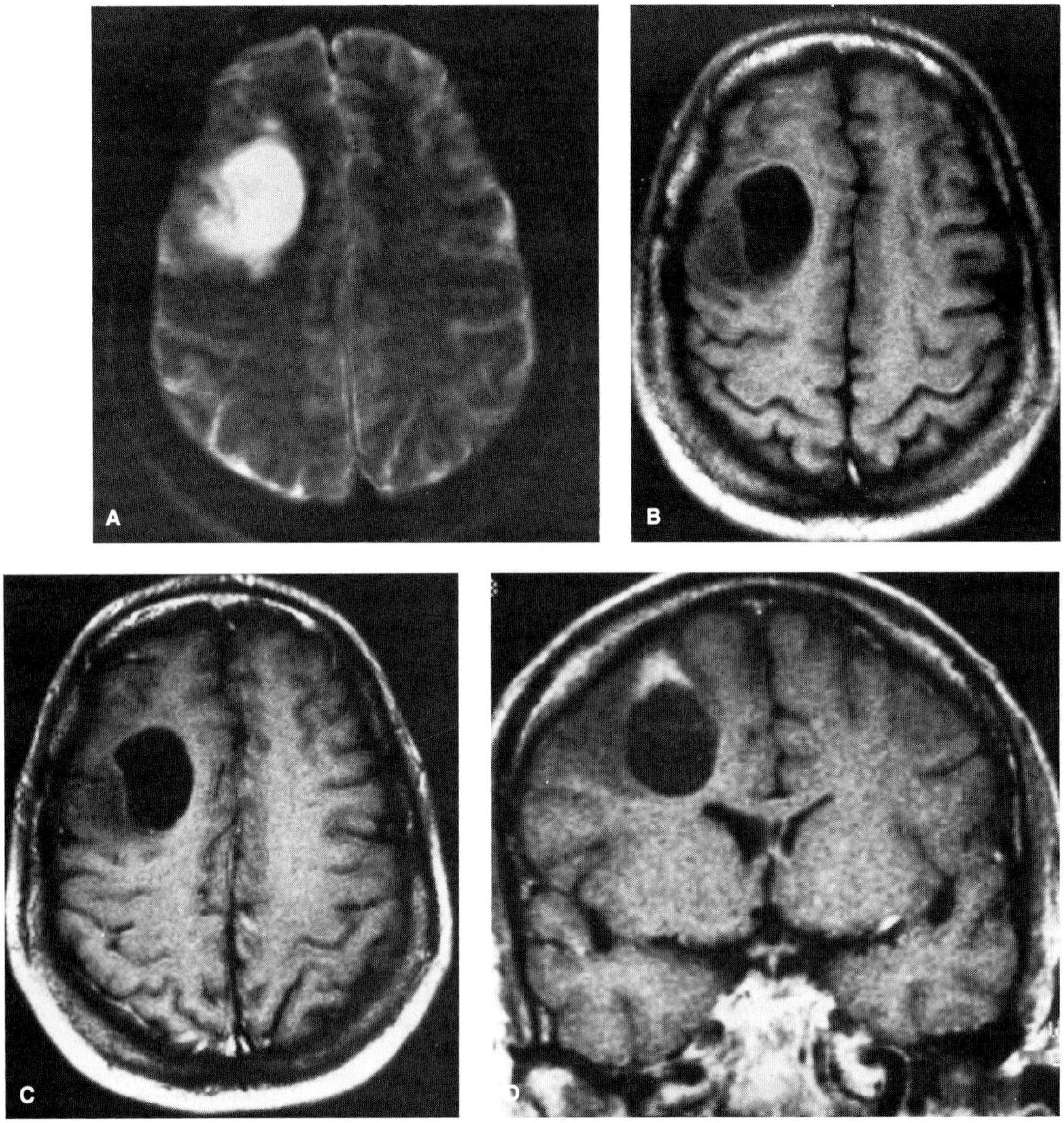

FIGURE 3–8. **(A)** The T2-weighted image (TR/TE = 3000/90) shows a well-defined area of increase in signal intensity near the right parietal convexity in this cystic astrocytoma. **(B)** A well-defined cystic lesion is shown on the T1-weighted image (TR/TE = 700/17) without contrast. The margins are smooth, and there is decrease in signal intensity in the central portion of the lesion. **(C)** No definite enhancement was seen in the margins of the cyst on the axial T1-weighted postcontrast image. Enhancement near the convexity was questionable. **(D)** The coronal postcontrast image shows this enhancement more clearly. A more confident diagnosis of tumor was thus possible. The cystic change was less obvious by CT (not shown), and the abnormality was thought to represent posttraumatic encephalomalacia.

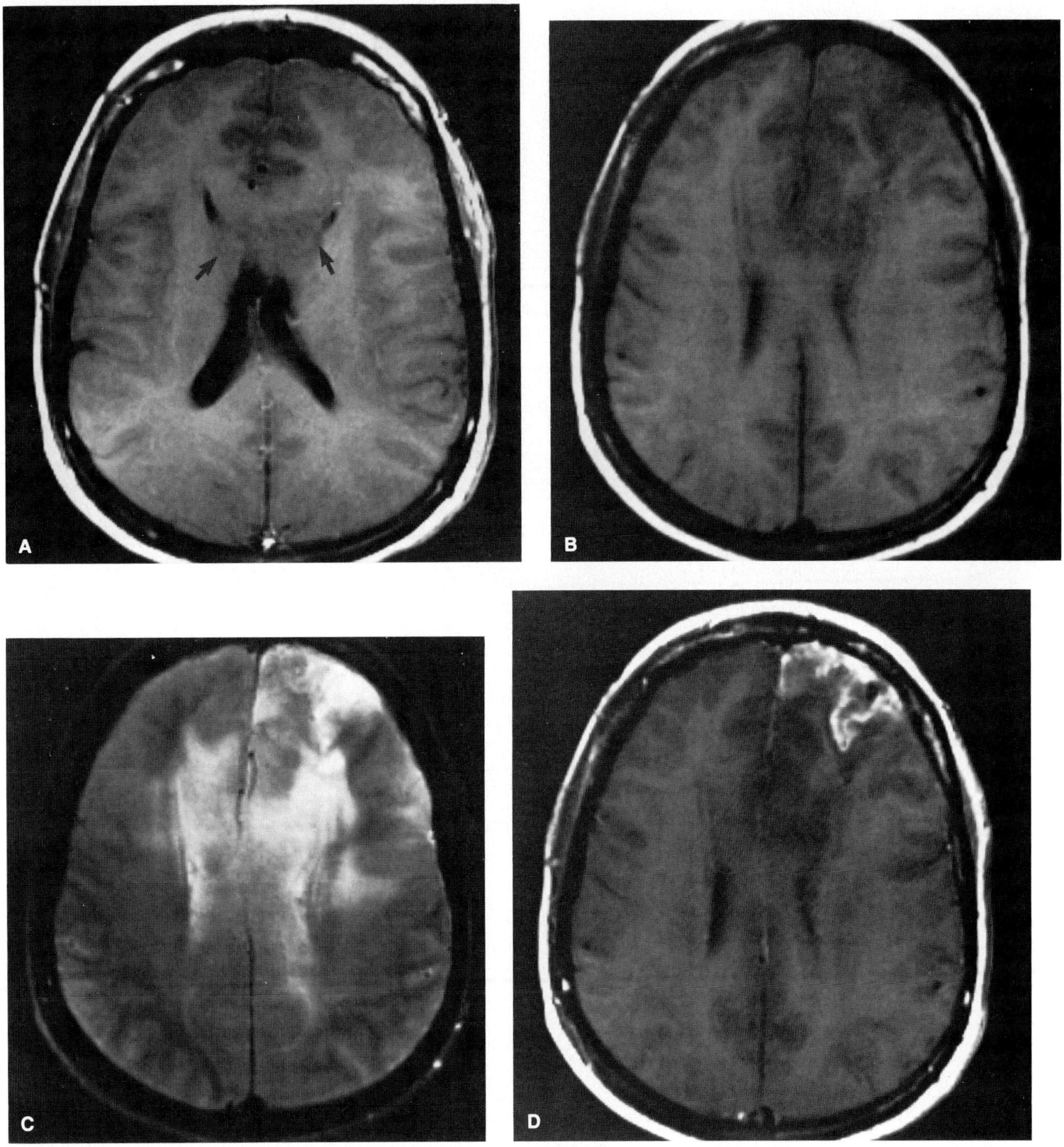

FIGURE 3–9. **(A)** An irregular mass effaces both frontal horns of the lateral ventricles (arrows) in this pre-contrast T1-weighted study. **(B)** At a slightly higher level of the T1-weighted study (TR/TE = 700/17), the mass effect is more diffuse, with irregular-signal-intensity changes extending into the left frontal lobe. **(C)** Increase in signal intensity occurs on the T2-weighted study (TR/TE = 3000/90) in these areas in this corpus callosum or "butterfly" glioma. There is minimal motion on this study. Motion frequently occurs in patients who are uncooperative due to their frontal lobe involvement. **(D)** Only the left frontal extension of this tumor is affected by contrast enhancement. The lower-grade portion of this mixed tumor involves the corpus callosum and did not enhance.

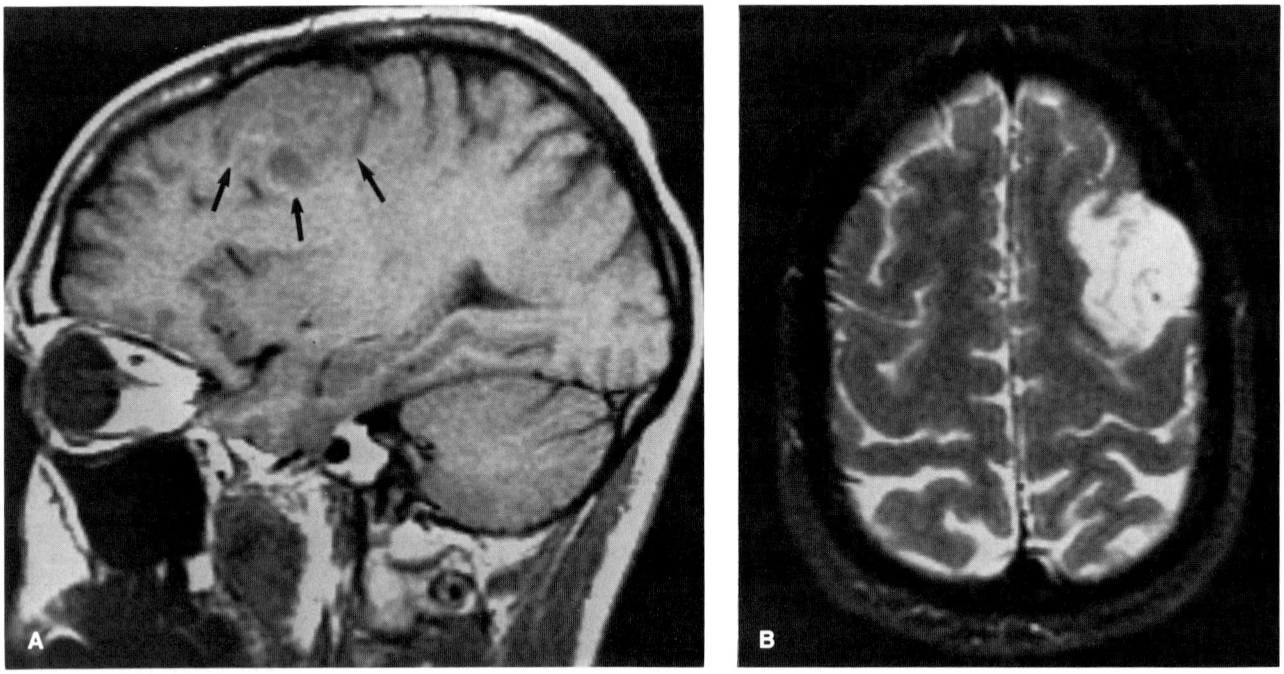

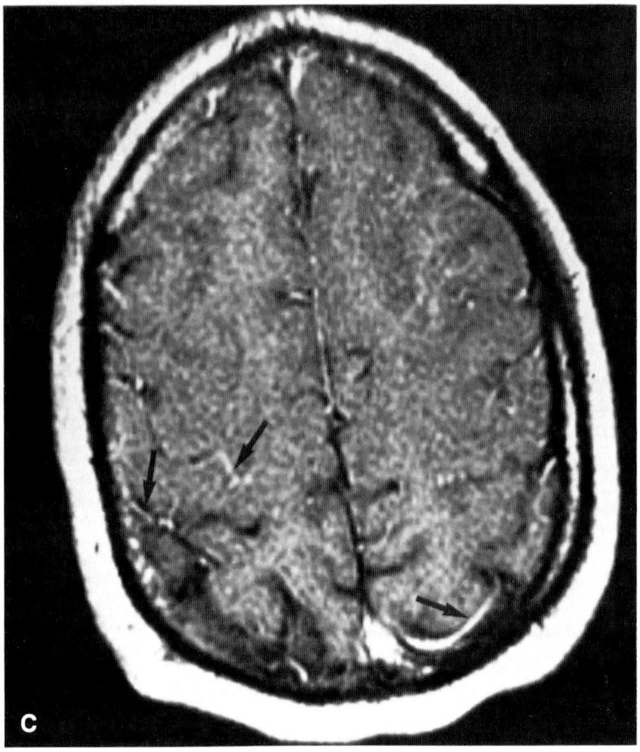

FIGURE 3–10. (A) The sagittal T1-weighted image (TR/TE = 500/20) demonstrates a low-signal-intensity lesion with mass effect on the posterior frontal convexity (arrows). **(B)** Increase in signal intensity occurs on the T2-weighted image (TR/TE = 2600/80) in this low-grade glioma. Compare the smooth margins of this astrocytoma with the GBM in Fig. 3-4. **(C)** There is little enhancement on the T1-weighted axial image. This image also shows the result of adding unnecessary imaging options, such as gradient moment nulling. Contrast agent is seen in vascular structures due to the use of this motion compensation technique (arrows). The field of view was decreased without compensatory increase in averages. A noisy image yields an abnormality that is poorly defined.

from other abnormalities. The differential diagnosis of the malignant astrocytoma includes infarction, abscess, and resolving hematoma.[28] If the tumor lies near a convexity, the enhancement may be difficult to assess without imaging in a second plane (Fig. 3–8).

The astrocytoma has the least severe degree of imaging changes. The margin may be slightly irregular and mass effect minimal (Figs. 3–1, 3–8, and 3–10). Cystic changes and necrosis are infrequent, and contrast enhancement may not occur. Calcifications are more frequent but are not usually visualized with spin echo imaging. These tumors may not be visualized by CT, particularly if they are located in the temporal lobe. Thus, a patient with temporal lobe seizures and a normal CT should have an MR study for complete evaluation (Fig. 3–11).[2,29]

It may be impossible to distinguish these low-grade tumors from infarcts on a single study. Serial studies

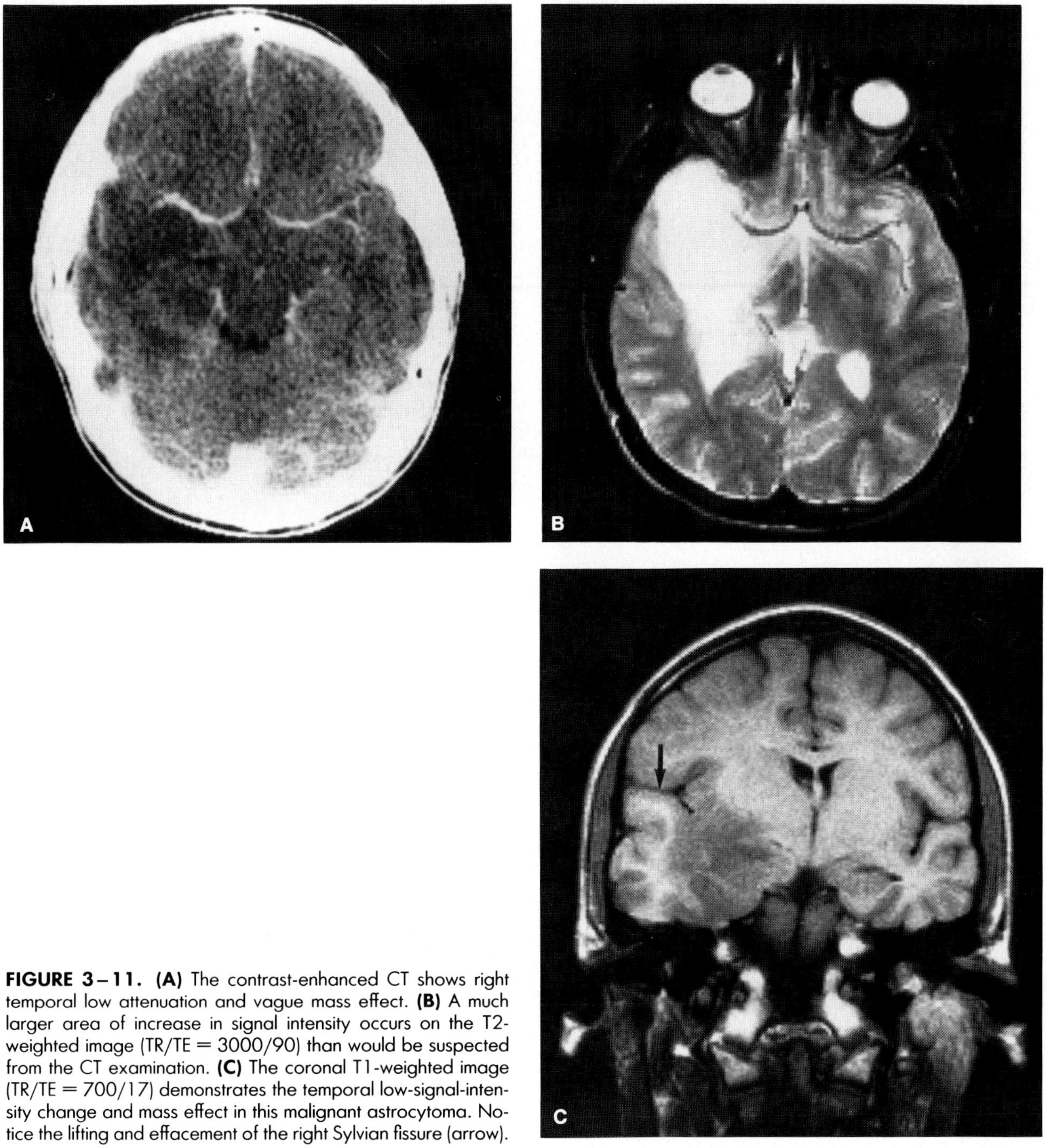

FIGURE 3–11. **(A)** The contrast-enhanced CT shows right temporal low attenuation and vague mass effect. **(B)** A much larger area of increase in signal intensity occurs on the T2-weighted image (TR/TE = 3000/90) than would be suspected from the CT examination. **(C)** The coronal T1-weighted image (TR/TE = 700/17) demonstrates the temporal low-signal-intensity change and mass effect in this malignant astrocytoma. Notice the lifting and effacement of the right Sylvian fissure (arrow).

may be necessary to establish the diagnosis. Infarctions show a decline in mass effect over time and an increase in encephalomalacic changes. Tumors show a progressive increase in mass effect and may show enhancement over time.

Oligodendrogliomas

Oligodendrogliomas are relatively rare, accounting for 4 to 7% of all intracranial neoplasms. These slow-growing tumors are characteristically large and calcified, and tend to involve the anterior cerebrum (Fig. 3–12). They are round or oval but rarely multilobulated, and they generally have fairly well-defined margins.

Calcifications are more common in oligodendrogliomas than in other glial-origin tumors, occurring in 50 to 90% of cases.[28,33,34] Because of this, CT has the diagnostic advantage. Gradient-echo imaging, which advantageously uses magnetic susceptibility changes, may prove to be as useful in the demonstration of calcifications by MRI.[35] If the tumor is not calcified, it may be difficult to differentiate from other large gliomas. Although the margins tend to be fairly well-

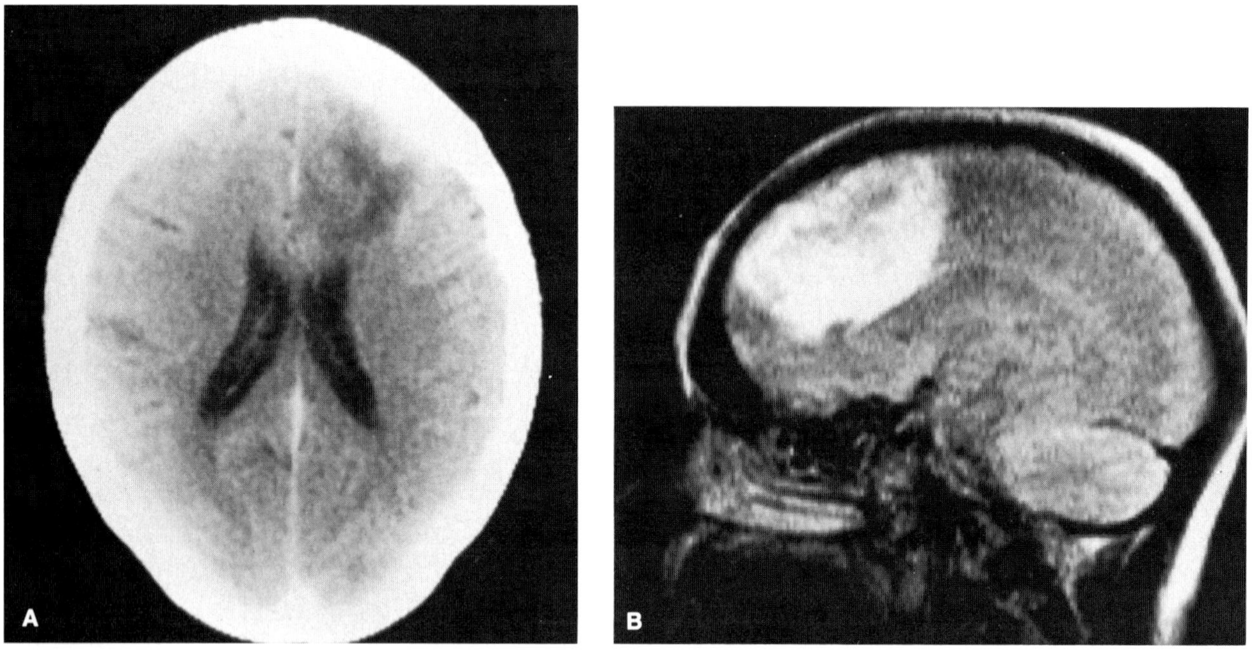

FIGURE 3–12. (A) There is a nonenhancing left frontal lobe low attenuation mass on this contrast-enhanced CT. This was a surgically proven oligodendroglioma. **(B)** A larger area of increase in signal intensity is shown on this T2-weighted image (TR/TE = 1000/120; 0.5 T). Notice the sharp definition of the tumor margins.

defined by MR, the signal intensity changes and enhancement patterns are not characteristic.[28,33]

The MR evaluation of these tumors before radiation therapy has been advocated. The sharper definition of the tumor margin allows more accurate treatment planning. This minimizes radiation necrosis, which occurs in proportion to the amount of normal tissue treated by megavoltage therapy.[34]

Metastases

Metastases comprise almost 40% of intracranial tumors. The most common tumors that metastasize intracranially are lung, breast, melanoma, colon, rectum, and kidney. Multiplicity is the hallmark that distinguishes metastases from gliomas or other primary tumors. Other imaging findings that suggest metastases are a gray-white-matter junction location, a small tumor nidus with a large amount of associated vasogenic edema, and a lesser degree of margin irregularity.[28]

MRI is superior to CT in detecting metastatic disease, particularly if MR contrast agents are used. Recent investigations have shown that many more metastatic lesions can be shown with contrast-enhanced MRI than with CT or MRI without contrast.[36,37]

Although T2-weighted sequences are quite sensitive in demonstrating the vasogenic edema as areas of increased signal intensity, not all metastatic lesions have sufficient edema to be identified (Fig. 3–13). The failure of MRI to demonstrate the edema around these cortical and subcortical metastases has been attributed to the ultrastructure of the edema and the anatomic arrangement of the myelinated fibers.[36] The lesions not visualized by MRI without contrast are typically small (< 5 mm), may lie adjacent to a larger metastatic lesion, and are located in the temporal lobes or in the cortical or subcortical regions. Thus, a complete initial evaluation of metastatic disease requires precontrast and postcontrast T1-weighted studies. Because some authors have noticed increased metastatic lesion conspicuity on post-contrast T2-weighted sequences, the evaluation of metastatic disease may be one exception to the generally accepted protocol of obtaining the T2-weighted study before enhancement.[25,37]

Sufficiently large metastatic lesions appear as areas of diminished signal intensity on T1-weighted sequences, while small lesions may be difficult to visualize.[37] The primary purpose of the precontrast T1-weighted image is to distinguish areas of enhancement from subacute hemorrhage (Fig. 3–14). The MR appearance of the various stages of hemorrhage is covered in detail in Chapter 2.

MRI also surpasses CT in its demonstration of subacute hemorrhage in typically hemorrhagic metastases, including melanoma, choriocarcinoma, lung tumors (oat cell), kidney, colon, and thyroid.[28] Pa-

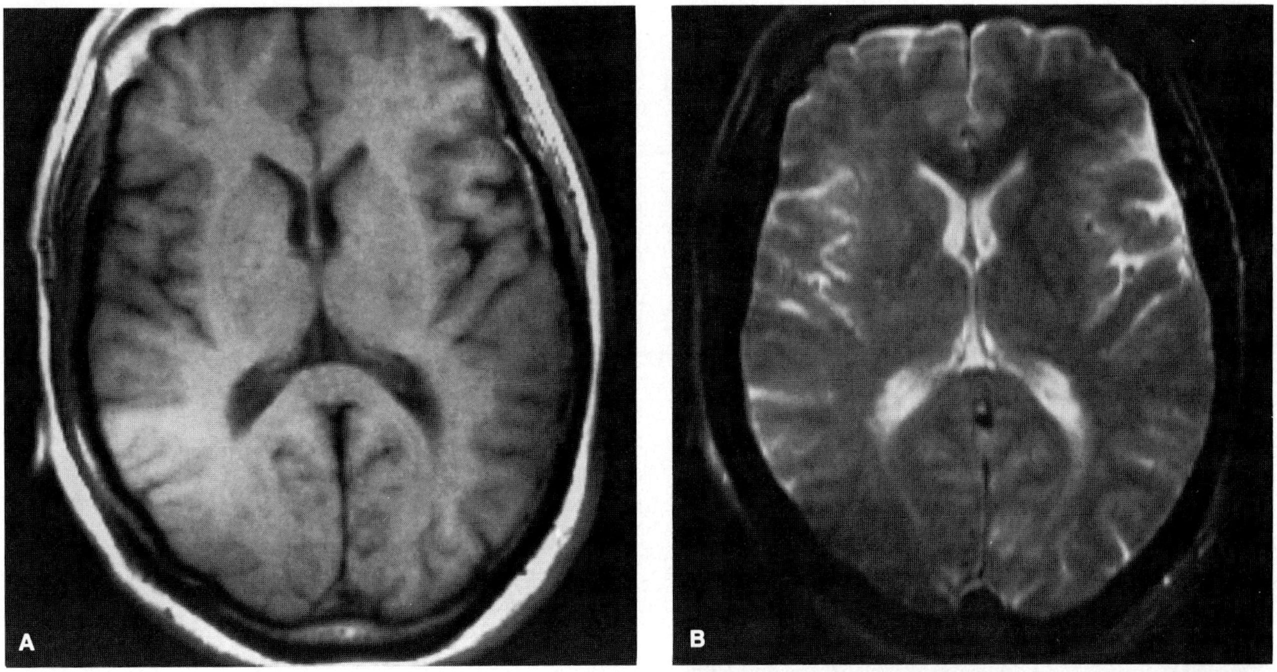

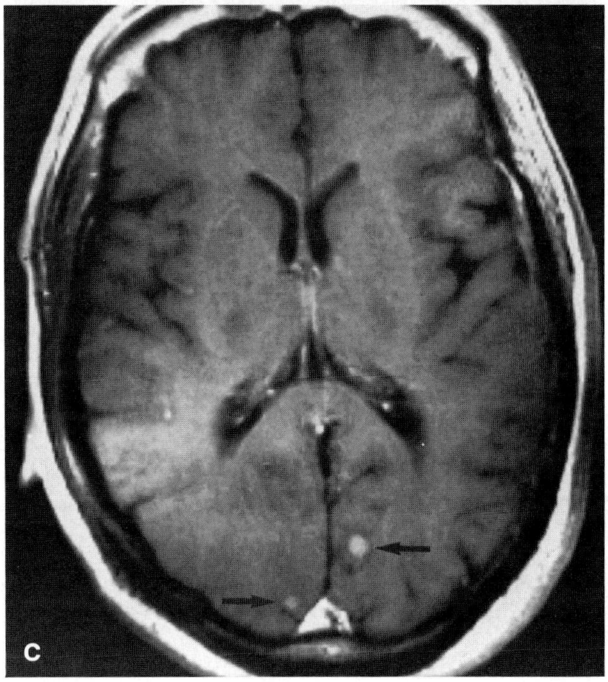

FIGURE 3–13. **(A)** No abnormality is seen on the T1-weighted axial section (TR/TE = 650/20). **(B)** Any signal intensity change on this T2-weighted image (TR/TE = 3000/90) could be due to focal sulcal enlargement. There was an obvious lesion at a slightly higher level that could also be seen by CT. **(C)** There are two abnormal areas of enhancement (arrows) on this postcontrast T1-weighted image. The multiplicity confirmed the diagnosis of metastases in a patient with known melanoma.

tients receiving chemotherapy may occasionally develop coagulopathies. Ensuing intracranial hemorrhage may produce a sudden decline in mental status similar to the effect of a significant hemorrhage into an intracranial metastasis. These hemorrhages may remain undiagnosed by CT, as do many subacute hemorrhages.

The mechanism of enhancement for intraaxial metastases is similar to gliomas in that the site of BBB disruption is marked, separating tumor nidus from surrounding edema. For most metastases reported, the contrast-enhanced MR image is superior to the contrast-enhanced CT scan.[36,37]

Various types of enhancement have been reported, including focal dot-like, larger rounded, and variable-sized areas of ring enhancement. Perhaps the greatest importance of contrast in evaluating metastases is the greater number of lesions depicted.[36] The diagnostic and therapeutic impact is immense. The demonstration of multiple lesions may indicate radiation or

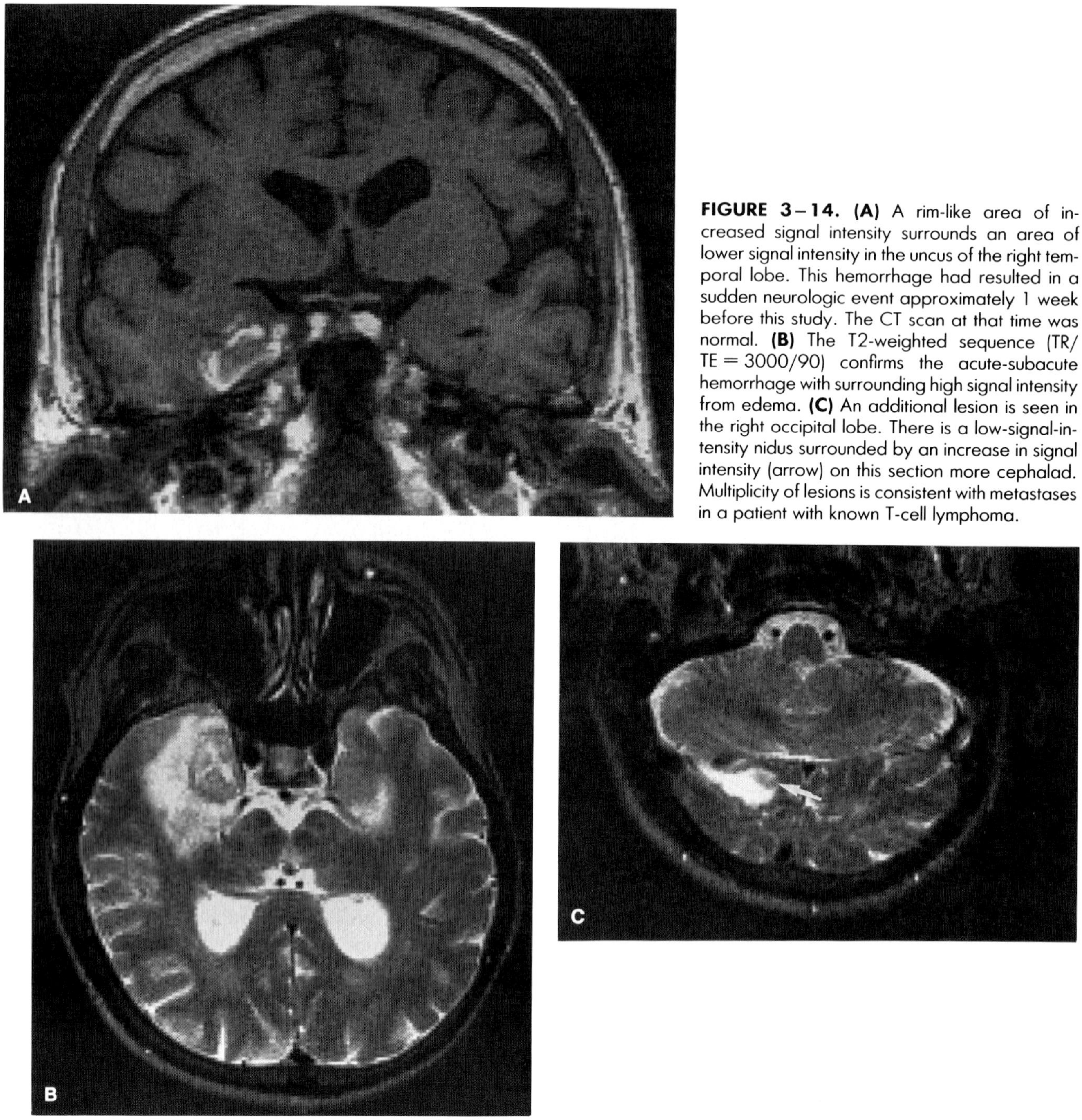

FIGURE 3–14. **(A)** A rim-like area of increased signal intensity surrounds an area of lower signal intensity in the uncus of the right temporal lobe. This hemorrhage had resulted in a sudden neurologic event approximately 1 week before this study. The CT scan at that time was normal. **(B)** The T2-weighted sequence (TR/TE = 3000/90) confirms the acute-subacute hemorrhage with surrounding high signal intensity from edema. **(C)** An additional lesion is seen in the right occipital lobe. There is a low-signal-intensity nidus surrounded by an increase in signal intensity (arrow) on this section more cephalad. Multiplicity of lesions is consistent with metastases in a patient with known T-cell lymphoma.

chemotherapy, while a solitary lesion may be more effectively treated with surgical extirpation.

Contrast-enhanced MR images may be mandatory for many elderly individuals with age-related white matter changes. These areas of increase in signal intensity on T2-weighted images associated with demyelination may be impossible to distinguish from the signal intensity change of a metastatic lesion.

Higher-dose, delayed-imaging techniques have been used with CT to maximize the visualization of metastatic lesions.[38] Whether these techniques are financially feasible or will contribute significantly to additional lesion detection by MRI awaits further investigation.

Leptomeningeal Metastases

Tumors that have access to cortical or ventricular surfaces may spread or seed through the CSF or along the meninges. Examples of tumors that typically spread

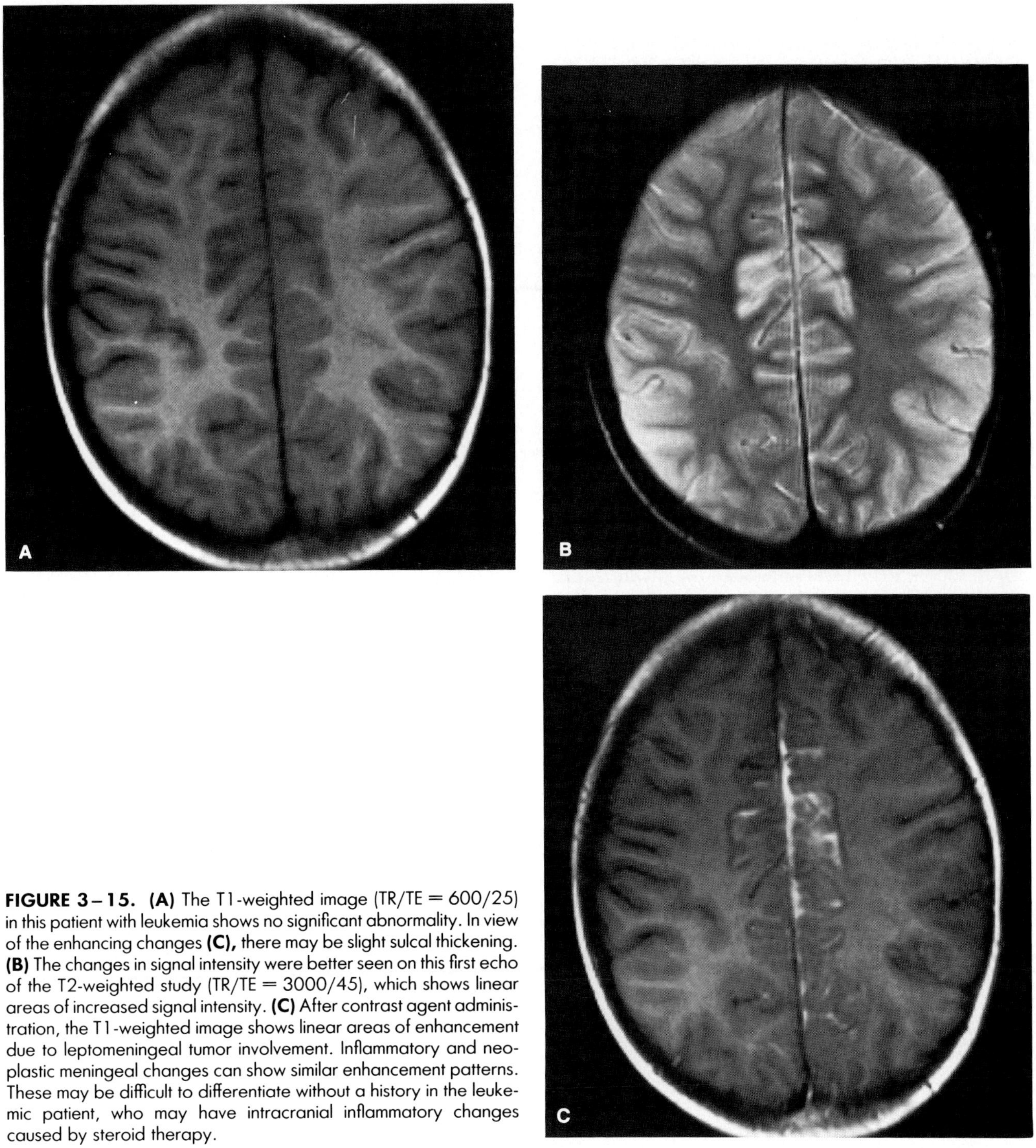

FIGURE 3–15. **(A)** The T1-weighted image (TR/TE = 600/25) in this patient with leukemia shows no significant abnormality. In view of the enhancing changes **(C)**, there may be slight sulcal thickening. **(B)** The changes in signal intensity were better seen on this first echo of the T2-weighted study (TR/TE = 3000/45), which shows linear areas of increased signal intensity. **(C)** After contrast agent administration, the T1-weighted image shows linear areas of enhancement due to leptomeningeal tumor involvement. Inflammatory and neoplastic meningeal changes can show similar enhancement patterns. These may be difficult to differentiate without a history in the leukemic patient, who may have intracranial inflammatory changes caused by steroid therapy.

through CSF pathways due to their origin in or near the ventricular system are ependymomas, medulloblastomas, pineal region tumors, and occasionally glioblastomas.[28] These metastases, often called "drop metastases," seed more commonly to the spine (Fig. 5–6).

Tumors that spread through cortical or meningeal involvement are metastatic breast carcinoma, melanoma, lymphoma, leukemia, and calvarial metastases with secondary meningeal involvement (Fig. 3–15). Diffuse meningeal changes may be followed by parenchymal deposits which occur after the malignant meningeal lesions dip into the perivascular spaces of Virchow-Robin and spread to the parenchyma, forming nodular metastases.[28]

Before Gd DTPA, these metastases were difficult or impossible to visualize.[39] With contrast, enhancement of linear and nodular metastases parallels the meningeal surfaces and extends into sulci and cisterns (Fig. 3-15). Because this form of metastatic disease is difficult to assess by CT, enhanced MRI is the modality of choice.

Lymphoma

Primary lymphomas of the brain are rare. Also known as reticulum cell sarcomas or microgliomas, these tumors are derived from microglial cells that histologically resemble lymphocytes. The basal ganglia, thalamus, and corpus callosum are the most frequently affected sites.[28]

Lymphomas are commonly associated with immunosuppression and, therefore, can be found after organ transplantation (Fig. 3-16). They are being increasingly encountered in AIDS-related diseases. In association with this disease complex, the appearance can be indistinguishable from the ring-enhancing lesions of toxoplasmosis.[5,40] Lesions not associated with AIDS may show a more homogenous, periventricular or parenchymal enhancement.[40] Lymphomas may be difficult to distinguish from abscesses, metastases, or glial tumors. The periventricular location and the absence of significant edema are additional differential features.[28]

Pineal Region Tumors

Pinealoma is a general term that has been applied to all tumors that arise in the posterior third ventricle. Tumor location and most secondary changes are adequately assessed by CT, but their differentiation is more difficult.[28] Whether MRI will be more accurate in the characterization of these rare tumors awaits further investigation. Tumors in this region are more easily understood if categorized by the cell of origin, the pineal cell, or the germ cell.

Pineal Cell Tumors

The pineocytoma and pineoblastoma are less common than other tumors in this region, particularly the germinoma. There is no sex predilection, and these tumors may calcify. The pineoblastoma is the more malignant of the two types and arises from a more primitive cell type (Fig. 3-17).[28]

MRI is particularly helpful in assessing the extent of these rather large, bulky tumors and the degree of involvement of adjacent structures. The signal intensity is diminished on the T1-weighted image and increased on early echoes of the T2-weighted image. Both the MR signal intensity changes and enhancement patterns await further clarification in a large patient population.

Germ Cell Tumors

Germ cell tumors include the germinoma, teratoma, and teratocarcinoma. All of these occur more commonly in male patients. The germinoma is the most common of these abnormalities and occurs almost exclusively in males (Fig. 3-18).[28] These tumors may be large and engulf the pineal region. The margins are better defined by MRI than by CT. There is a slightly

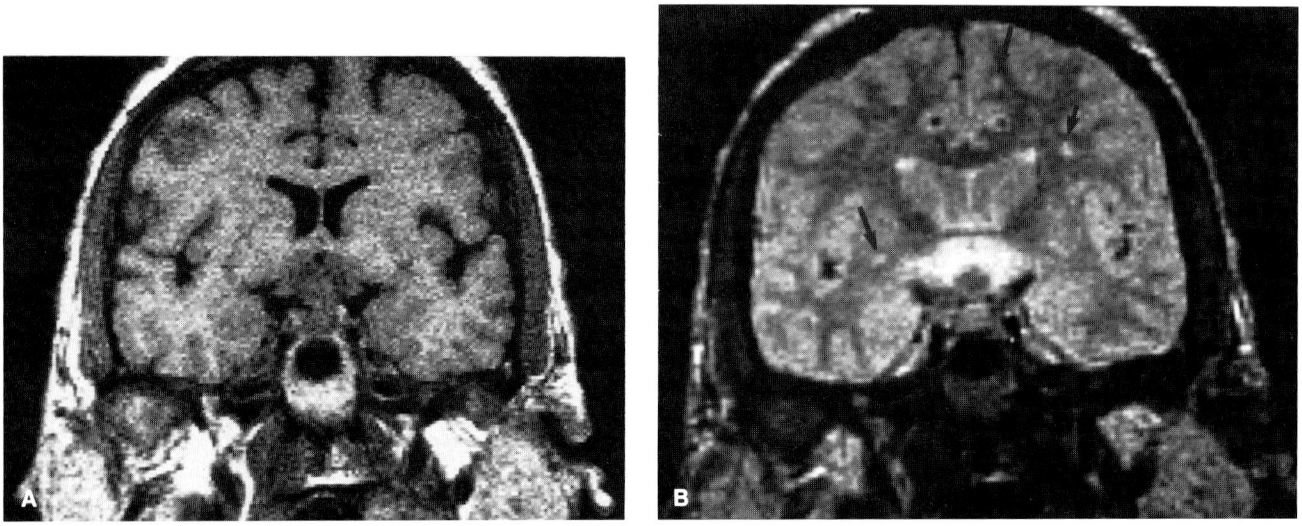

FIGURE 3-16. **(A)** There is a low-signal-intensity hypothalamic mass on the T1-weighted image (TR/TE = 700/17) of this patient after renal transplantation. **(B)** The first echo of the T2-weighted sequence (TR/TE = 3000/40) shows a slightly larger area of increased signal intensity. This was a hypothalamic lymphoma. Contrast agents were not given because of the patient's poor renal status. There are several additional areas of nonspecific, white matter disease (arrows).

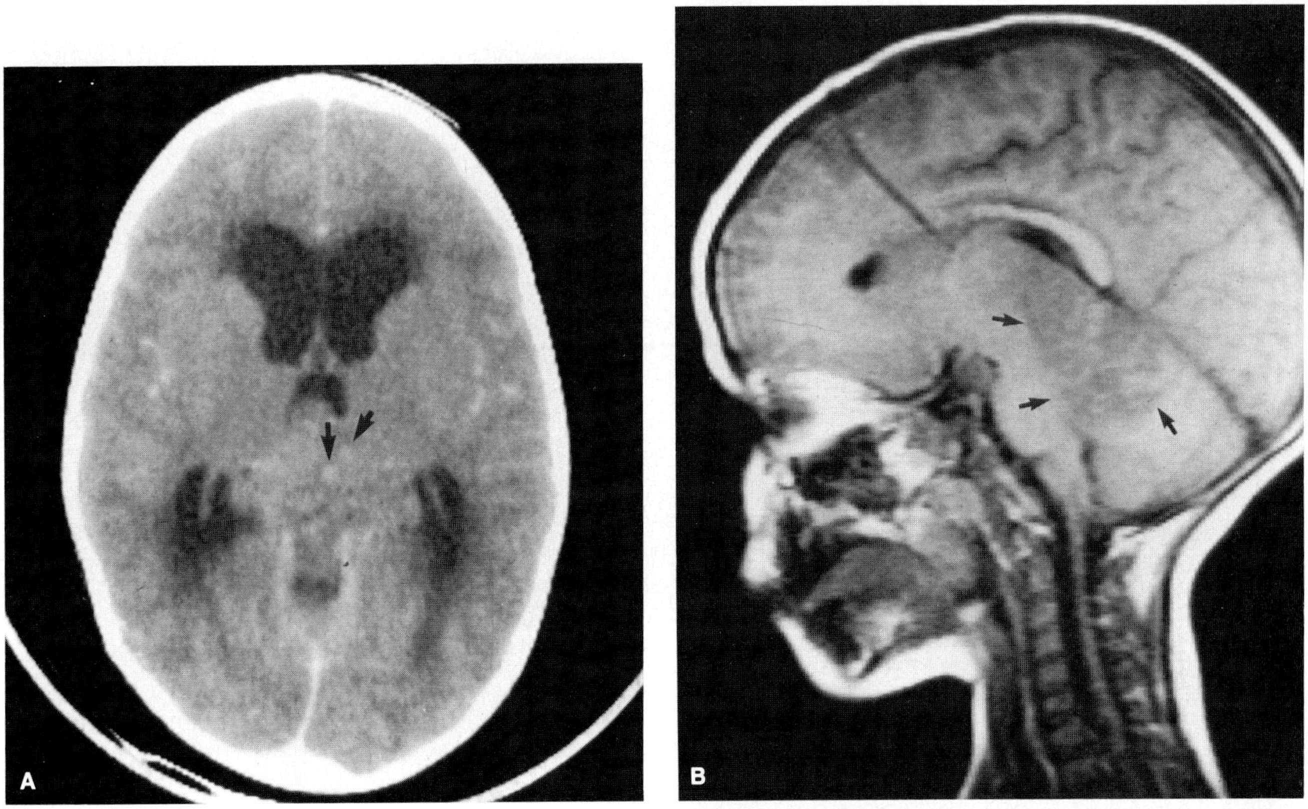

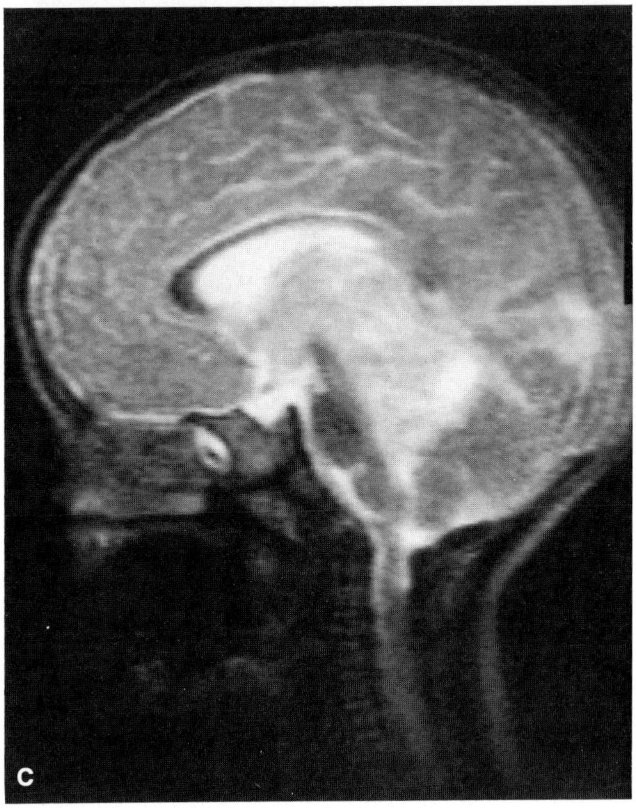

FIGURE 3–17. **(A)** The contrast-enhanced CT scan shows a large, bulky tumor with poorly defined margins and small areas of punctate calcification (arrows). Despite the minimal enhancement in this usually densely enhancing tumor, it was confirmed to be a pineoblastoma at surgery. Notice the ventricular enlargement from obstructive hydrocephalus. **(B)** The T1-weighted image (TR/TE = 500/30, 0.5 T) shows an extensive low-signal-intensity lesion invading the thalamus and posterior brain stem. It extends below the tentorium and impresses the cerebellum. **(C)** The heavily T2-weighted image (TR/TE = 2000/240) shows the tumor as a relatively lower-signal-intensity lesion outlined by the bright CSF, similar in extent to the previous image **(B)**.

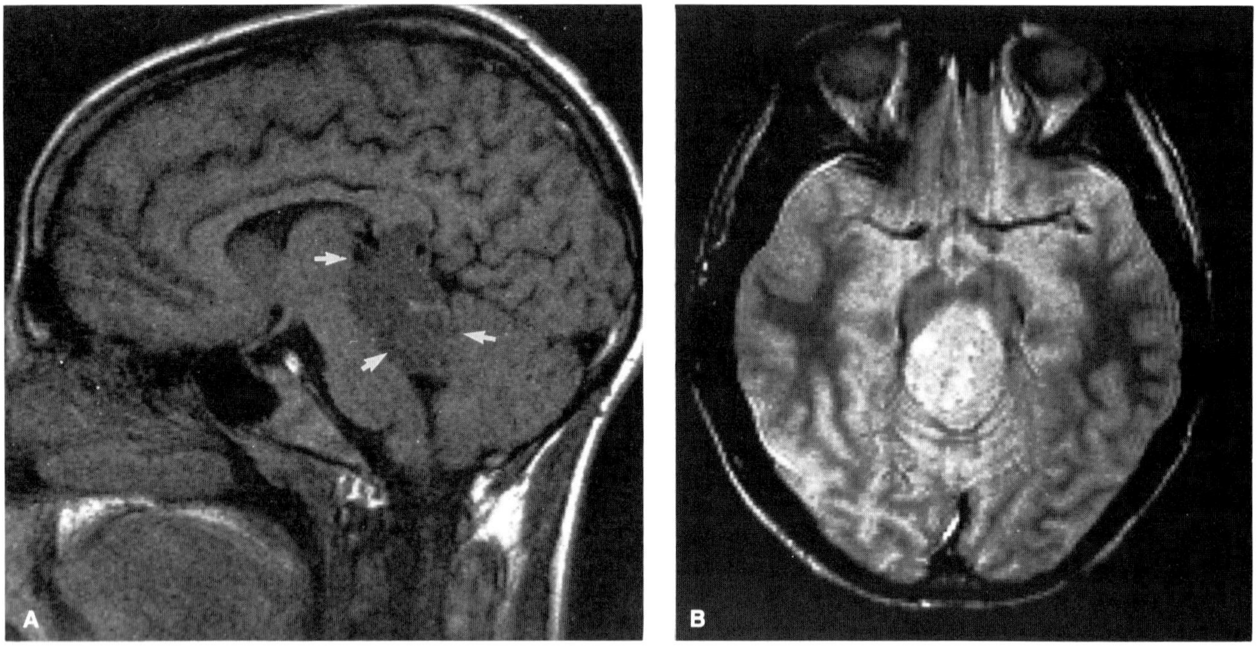

FIGURE 3–18. **(A)** The sagittal T1-weighted image (TR/TE = 700/17) shows a low-signal-intensity abnormality in the pineal region (arrows). This surgically proven germinoma occurred in an adolescent male. **(B)** The abnormality was more clearly shown as an area of increased signal intensity on the first echo of the T2-weighted study (TR/TE = 3000/40). The bright signal intensity of the CSF in the adjacent ventricles and cisterns obscured some of the tumor margin on the second echo.

diminished signal intensity on T1-weighted images. The lack of calcifications may explain the lesser degree of heterogeneity in signal intensity in germ cell tumors than in the pineal cell tumors. On T2-weighted images, there is an increase in signal intensity. Dense, homogenous enhancement occurs with contrast-enhanced CT. Characterization of MR enhancement awaits further experience.

Metastases and gliomas may also occur in the pineal region. Obstructive hydrocephalus may accompany large tumors. All but the teratoma are notorious for seeding by CSF pathways. More benign pineal cysts may occasionally cause difficulty in differential diagnosis (Fig. 3–19).

INTRAVENTRICULAR TUMORS

Colloid Cyst

The colloid cyst is a rare benign cyst that originates in the primitive neuroepithelium that forms the roof plate of the tela choroidea.[41] These lesions are well defined and vary from a few millimeters to several centimeters in diameter (Fig. 3–20). Colloid cysts that produce hydrocephalus are usually larger than 1 cm and obstruct the foramen of Monro.[28] These congenital cysts grow slowly and may not become symptomatic until adult life.

Colloid cysts are easily identified on MR images by their location and by increased signal intensity on T1-weighted images. The signal intensity will depend on the concentration of lipids, cholesterol, or mucin and the state of hydration. If it is predominantly lipid, the signal intensity will be bright on T1-weighted images and will fade to low signal intensity on T2-weighted images (Fig. 3–20). The diminished signal intensity of T2-weighted images may also be due to the high ionic concentrations of sodium, calcium, magnesium, copper, and iron within the mucinous cyst fluid.[41] If there is less lipid content and more complex cholesterol or mucin, the signal intensity will be increased on both T1-weighted and T2-weighted images; however, the signal intensity on T1-weighted images will not be as bright as that shown in Figure 3–20.

Because of their characteristic location and appearance, colloid cysts are seldom confused with other intraventricular tumors. MR contrast administration will likely offer little additional information, since these lesions are often bright on T1-weighted images without contrast. Furthermore, by CT, these lesions do not enhance.

Choroid Plexus Papilloma

Choroid plexus papillomas originate from the ependymal layer. These are more common during the first decade of life, showing a slight male preponderance. These tumors most frequently arise in the lateral ven-

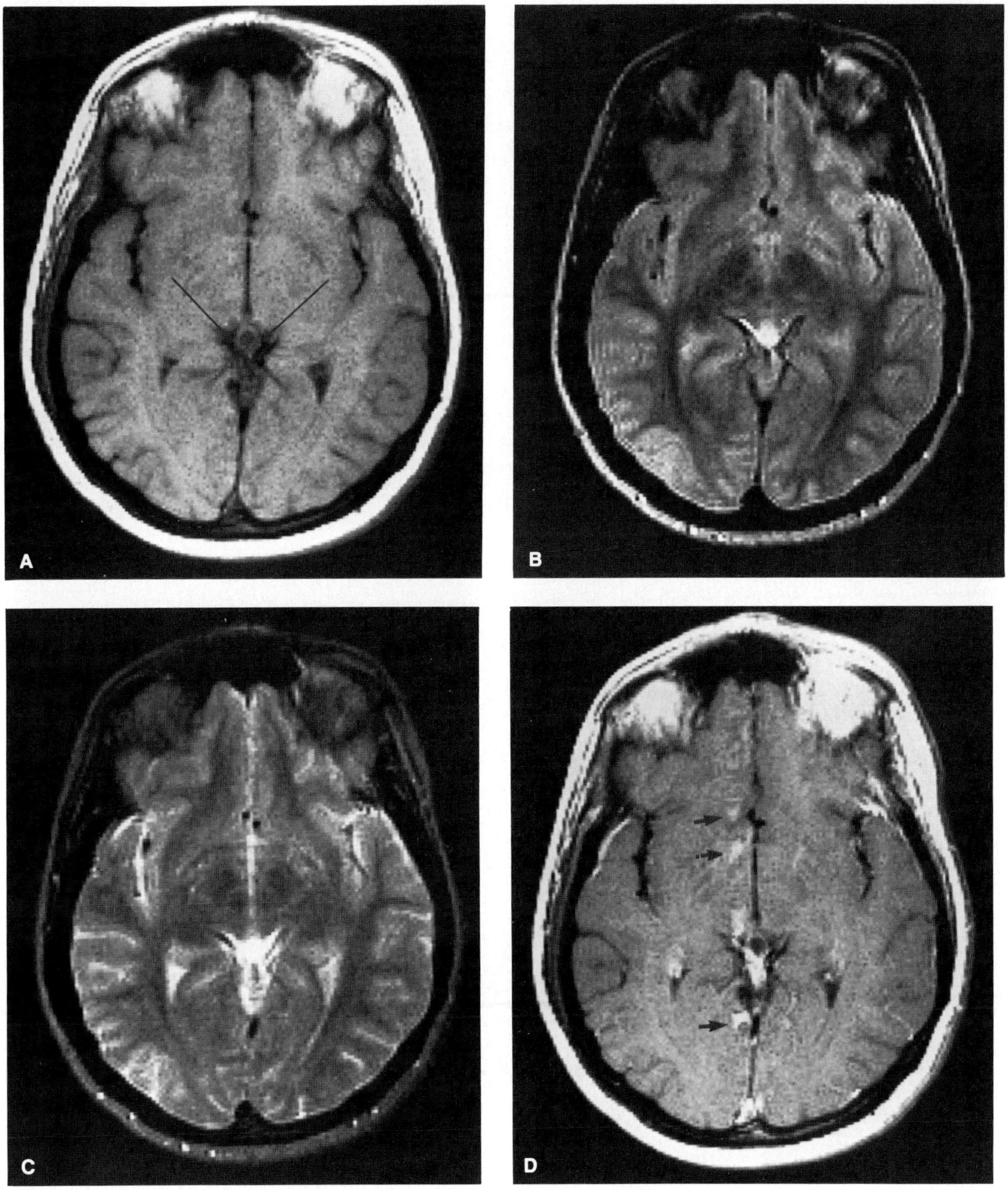

FIGURE 3–19. (A) There is a small cystic lesion of the pineal on the T1-weighted image (TR/TE = 700/20), which has a thin soft tissue intensity rim (arrows). **(B)** The first echo of the T2-weighted scan (TR/TE = 3000/40) shows a small focal area of increased signal intensity in this pineal cyst. **(C)** On the second echo (TR/TE = 3000/90), the cyst is obscured by the increase in signal intensity in the adjacent cistern. **(D)** The rim of the cyst is enhanced on the postcontrast T1-weighted image. Notice the artifact in the phase-encoding direction. This vascular pulsation artifact is more prominent on postcontrast examinations (arrows) and can occasionally be mistaken for an abnormality. (Courtesy of Dr. Fred Laine, Medical College of Virginia, Richmond, VA)

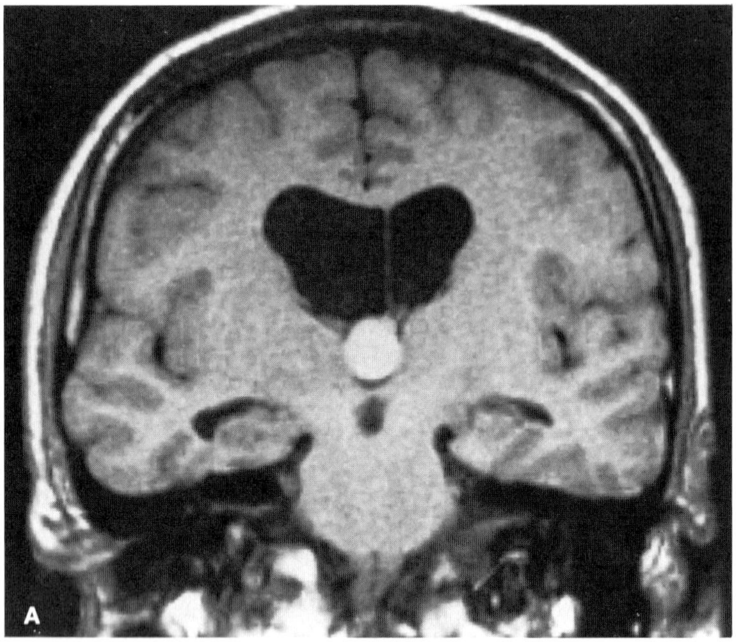

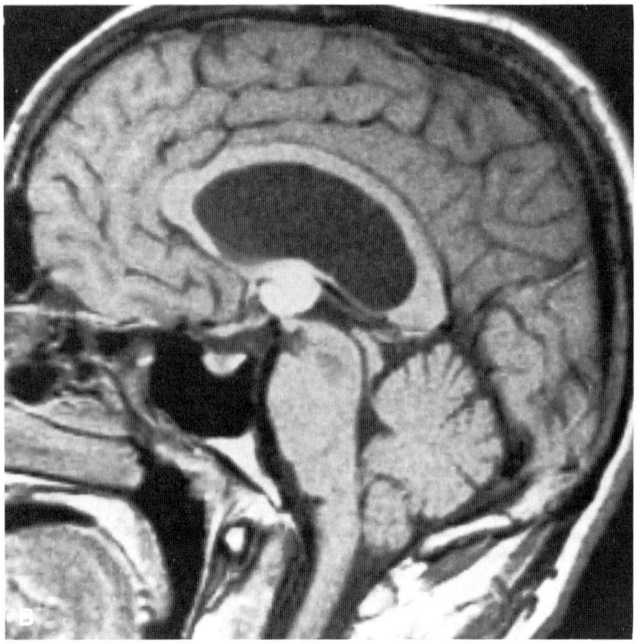

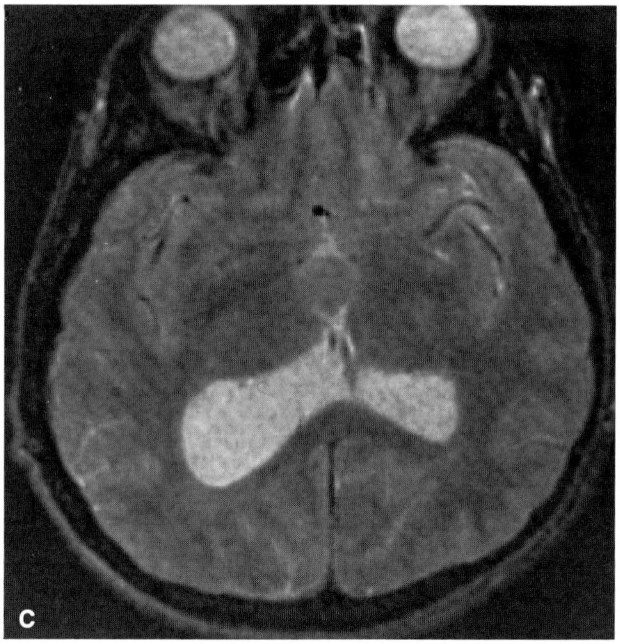

FIGURE 3–20. **(A)** A rounded area of increased signal intensity is seen in the anterior third ventricle near the foramen of Monro on this T1-weighted coronal image (TR/TE = 650/20). This mass results in moderately severe hydrocephalus. **(B)** The sagittal image confirms the location of this colloid cyst. **(C)** A decrease in signal intensity on the second echo of the axial T2-weighted image (TR/TE = 3000/90) indicates a greater fatty component in this abnormality.

tricle, particularly the left lateral ventricle. Hydrocephalus is asymmetric but bilateral and results from outlet obstruction of the ventricle, overproduction of CSF, or a combination of these two factors (Fig. 3–21). Intermittent hemorrhage into these tumors is not uncommon and may contribute to the obstructive hydrocephalus.[28] In the adolescent or young adult, a choroid plexus papilloma often occurs in the fourth ventricle (Fig. 3–22). Hydrocephalus in this case is symmetrical. Focal calcifications are frequently found within the lobulated tumor. Enhancement on CT and MR scans is intense.

There is little difference in appearance between the choroid plexus papilloma and the choroid plexus carcinoma, except the latter produces changes in the adjacent brain parenchyma. The differential diagnosis includes ependymoma, meningioma, and metastases, all of which are more common in the adult population.

Meningiomas

Intraventricular meningiomas are rare, occurring in the atrium of the lateral ventricle more commonly than in the third or fourth ventricles. They can occur

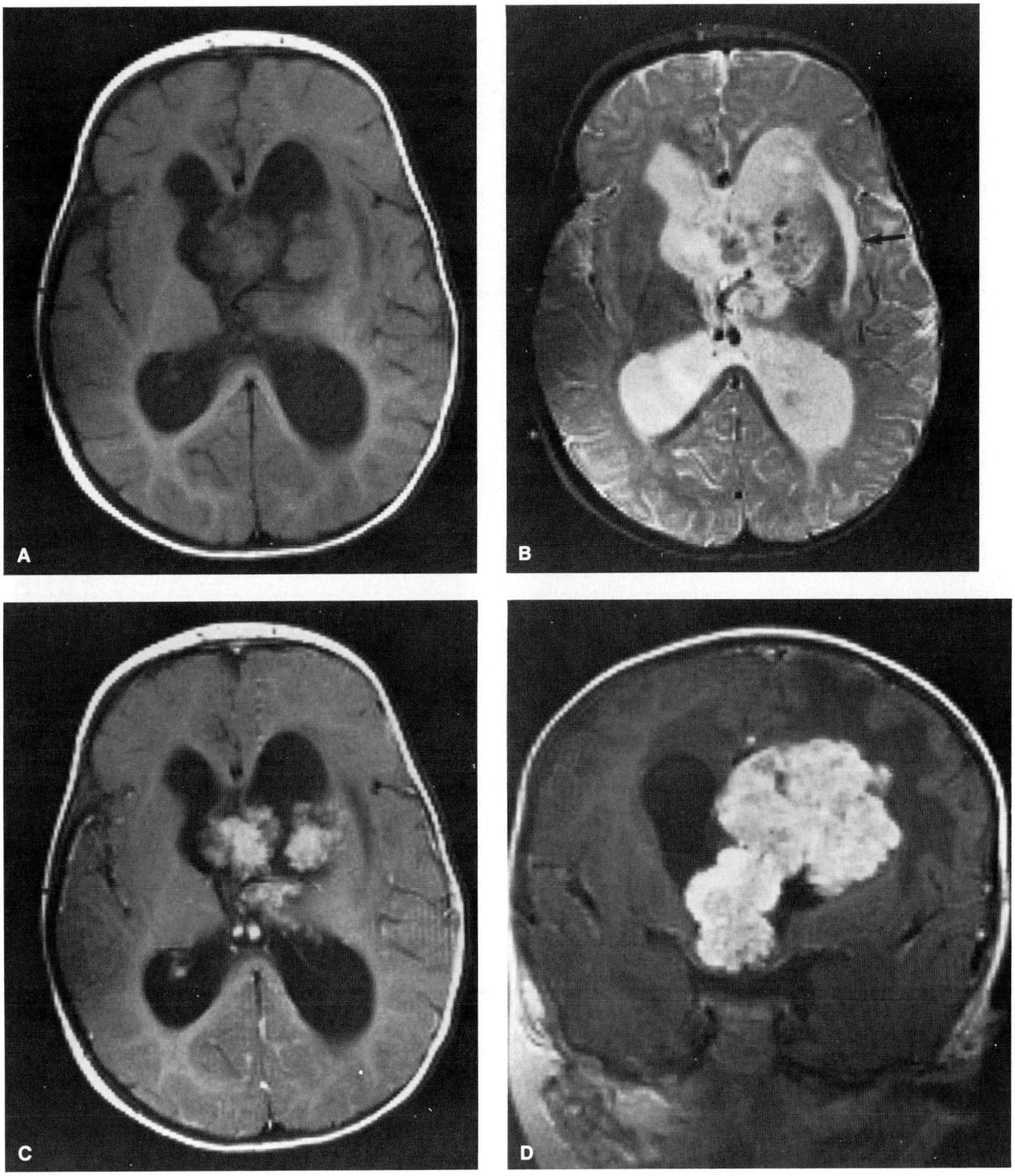

FIGURE 3–21. **(A)** There is a lobulated mass in the left lateral ventricle on the T1-weighted image (TR/TE = 700/20). Ventricular enlargement is asymmetric in this surgically proven choroid plexus papilloma. **(B)** On the T2-weighted image (TR/TE = 3000/90), the mass contains areas of low signal intensity caused by calcifications or hemosiderin from an old hemorrhage. A high-signal-intensity area in the external capsule (arrow) is due to edema or ischemia. **(C)** The mass is intensely enhanced on the postcontrast T1-weighted image. **(D)** A more extensive abnormality is shown in this young male patient on the coronal postcontrast view. (Courtesy of Dr. Fred Laine, Medical College of Virginia, Richmond, VA)

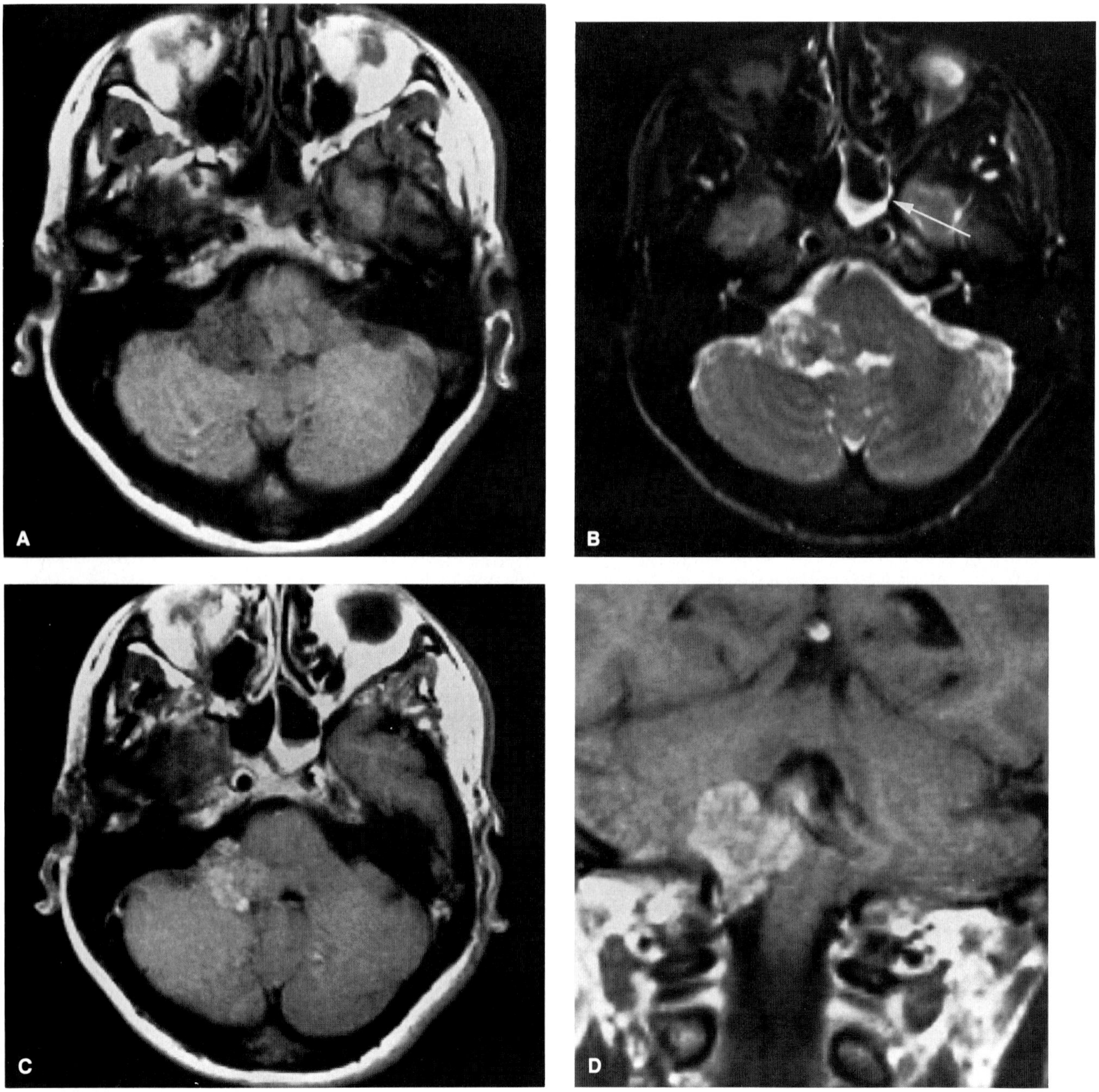

FIGURE 3–22. (A) There is an irregular, low-signal-intensity abnormality extending from the fourth ventricle toward the right CP angle on this T1-weighted image. This patient was a female adolescent. **(B)** A mixed, low-signal-intensity mass is surrounded by an area of high signal intensity on the T2-weighted image (TR/TE = 3000/90). The increase in signal intensity rimming the left sphenoid sinus is consistent with sinusitis (arrow). **(C)** There is faint enhancement on the axial T1-weighted image (TR/TE = 650/20). **(D)** The coronal postcontrast image better shows the lobulated contour and intraventricular component of the choroid plexus papilloma. The position simulates a meningioma, but the enhancement is not as intense. Notice the brain stem displacement to the left.

at all ages, but show a predilection for older adults.[28] As with other meningiomas, there is an increased incidence in neurofibromatosis.

These are usually large, lobulated masses, which may show areas of calcifications on CT. Slight ventricular dilatation may be unilateral or bilateral. Similar to meningiomas in other locations, these tumors have a mottled appearance that may be due to a combination of hypervascularity and calcifications. Dense enhancement occurs after contrast administration. With multiplanar imaging, MRI more accurately assesses the intraventricular location (Fig. 3–23). The differ-

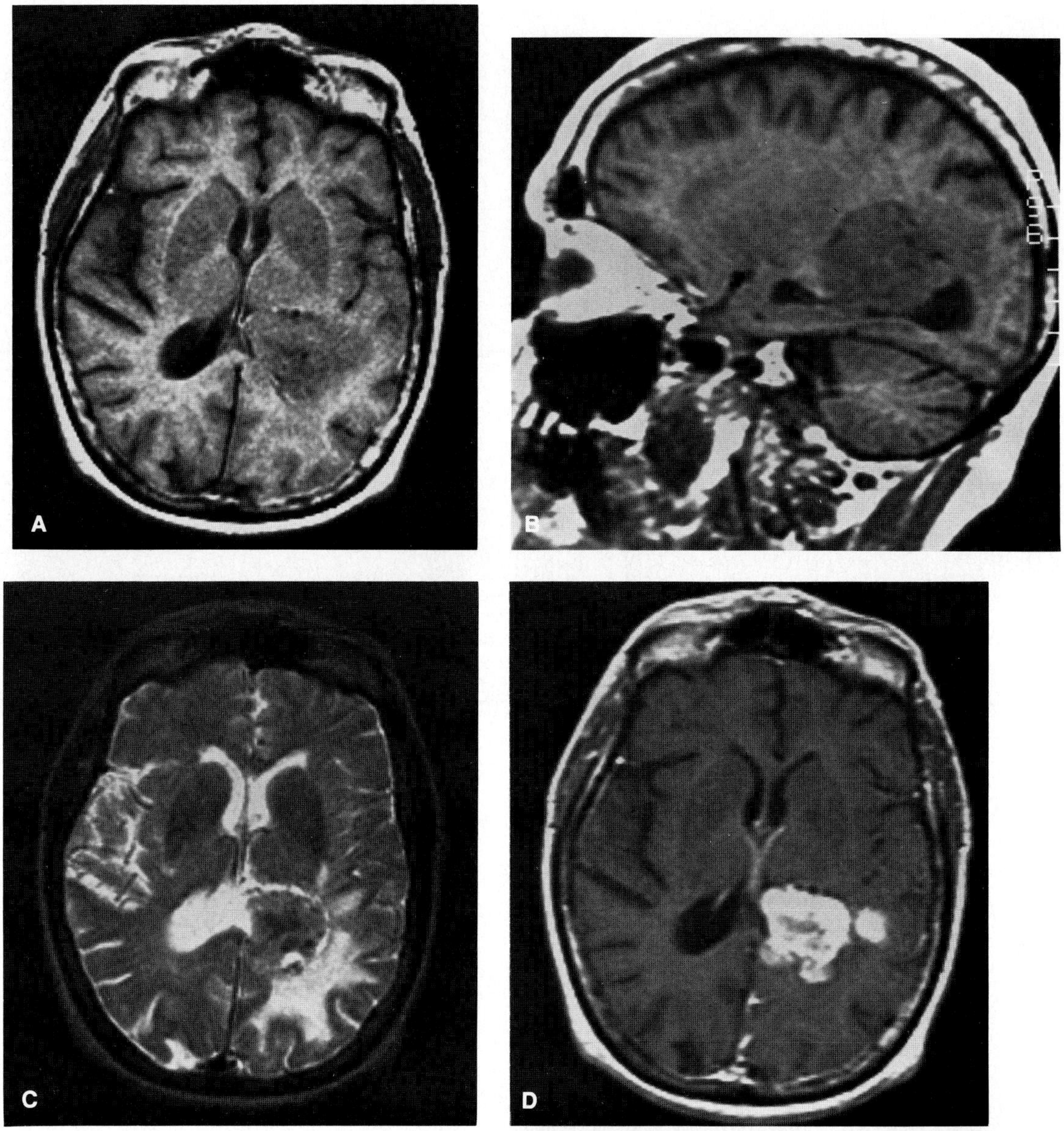

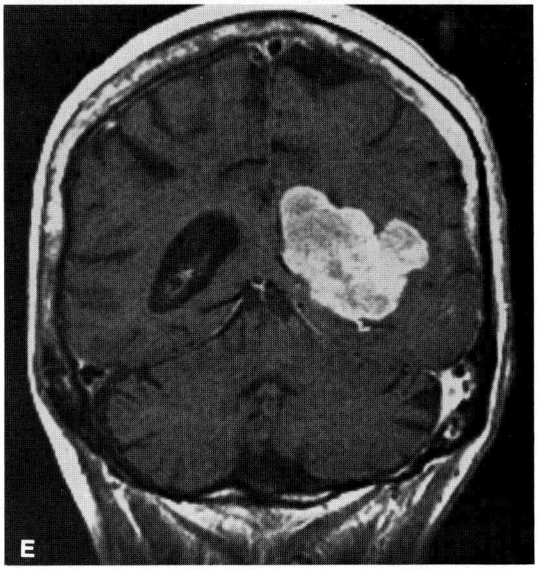

FIGURE 3 – 23. **(A)** A mottled, low-signal-intensity abnormality is noted in the atrium of the left lateral ventricle on the T1-weighted axial image (TR/TE = 750/20). **(B)** The intraventricular location of this meningioma is better shown on the sagittal T1-weighted image. This lesion was heavily calcified on CT scans. **(C)** The mass remains low-intensity on the T2-weighted image (TR/TE = 2500/80). There is an extraventricular signal intensity change that is presumably due to edema. **(D)** Intense enhancement occurs on the postcontrast T1-weighted image. **(E)** The coronal postcontrast view more clearly shows the intraventricular position of all portions of the enhancing abnormality.

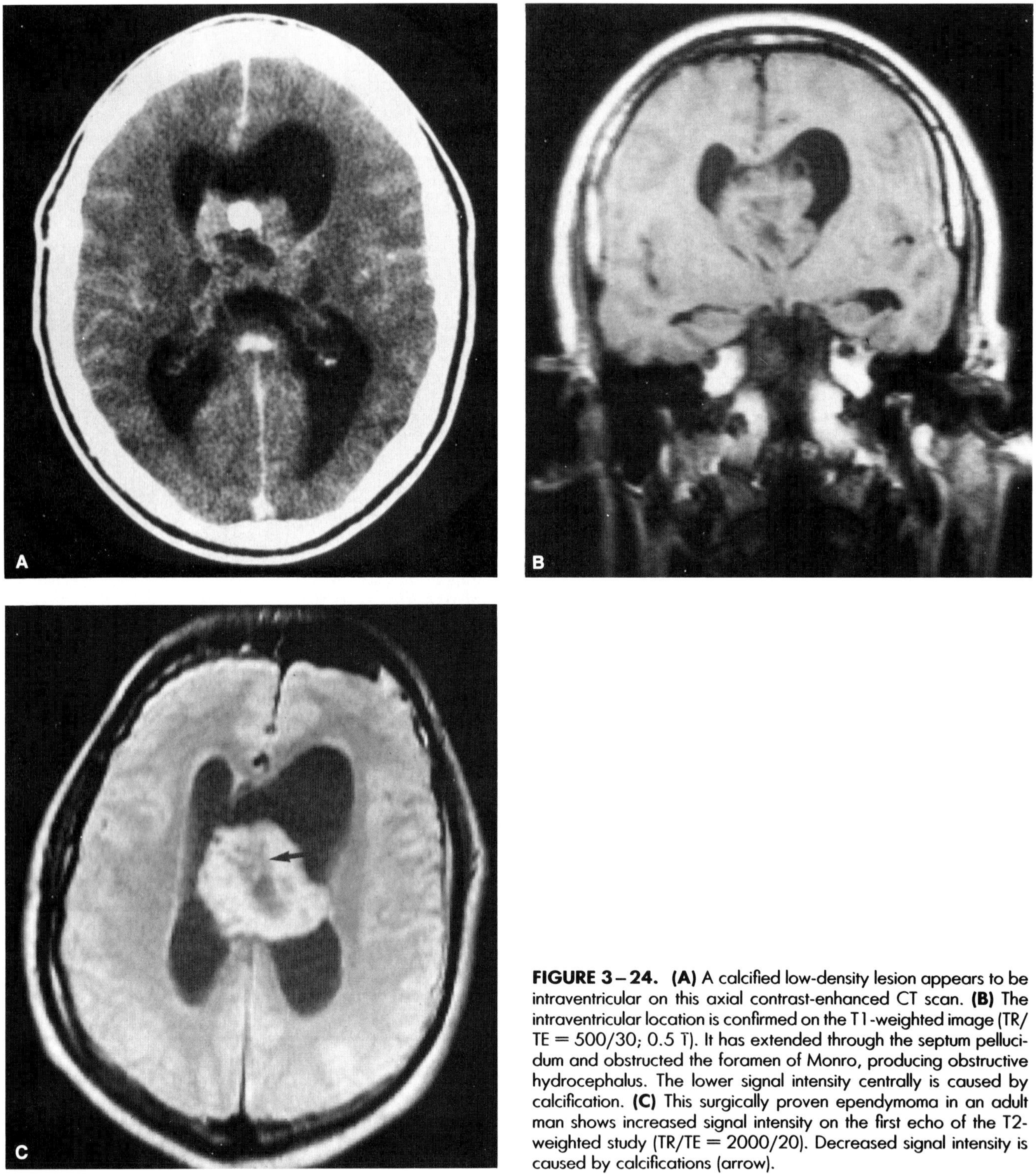

FIGURE 3–24. **(A)** A calcified low-density lesion appears to be intraventricular on this axial contrast-enhanced CT scan. **(B)** The intraventricular location is confirmed on the T1-weighted image (TR/TE = 500/30; 0.5 T). It has extended through the septum pellucidum and obstructed the foramen of Monro, producing obstructive hydrocephalus. The lower signal intensity centrally is caused by calcification. **(C)** This surgically proven ependymoma in an adult man shows increased signal intensity on the first echo of the T2-weighted study (TR/TE = 2000/20). Decreased signal intensity is caused by calcifications (arrow).

ential diagnosis must include other intraventricular tumors. The older age and intense enhancement may help in establishing the diagnosis.

Ependymomas

Ependymomas are derived from ependymal cells that line the ventricles or from cell rests in the adjacent periventricular white matter. In the adult, these tumors arise in the trigone of the lateral ventricle or near the foramen of Monro (Fig. 3–24).[28] They can grow through the septum pellucidum and involve both lateral ventricles.

Ependymomas occur more commonly in the posterior fossa in children, arising in the fourth ventricle (Fig. 3–25). These frequently extend through the for-

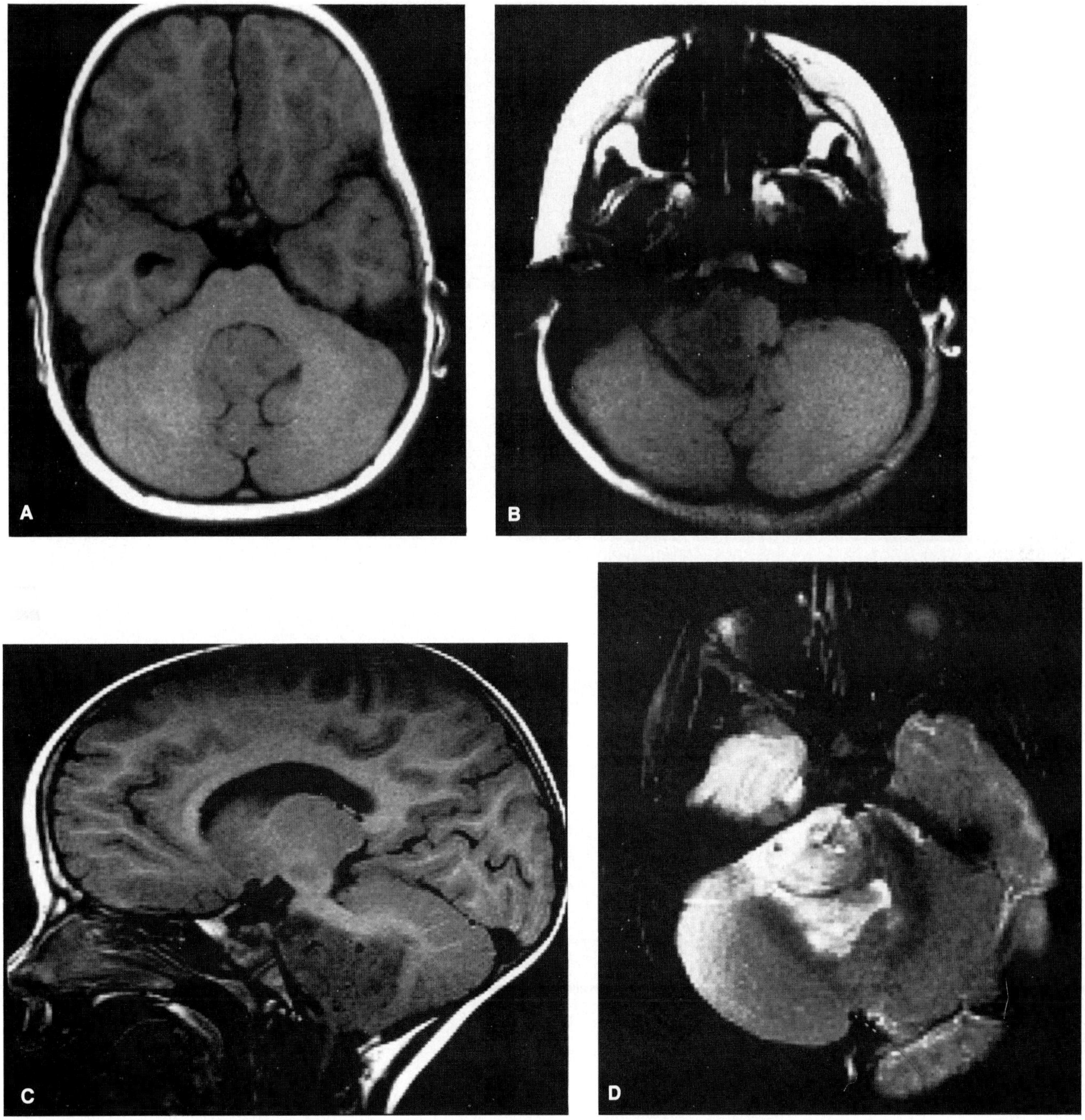

FIGURE 3–25. **(A)** The axial T1-weighted image (TR/TE = 700/17) shows a bulky, slightly lobulated ependymoma in the fourth ventricle. There is a halo of low signal intensity formed by the fourth ventricle anteriorly. **(B)** At a slightly lower anatomic level, the tumor extends into the right CP angle. Notice the displacement of the medulla to the left. **(C)** A sagittal T1-weighted image shows greater tumor mottling than the axial views. These areas of low signal intensity may be due to calcifications. **(D)** An increase in signal intensity occurs on the axial T2-weighted image (TR/TE = 3000/90). The extension into the CP angle is difficult to see, compared with the T1-weighted image. Slight mottling from tumor calcifications is evident.

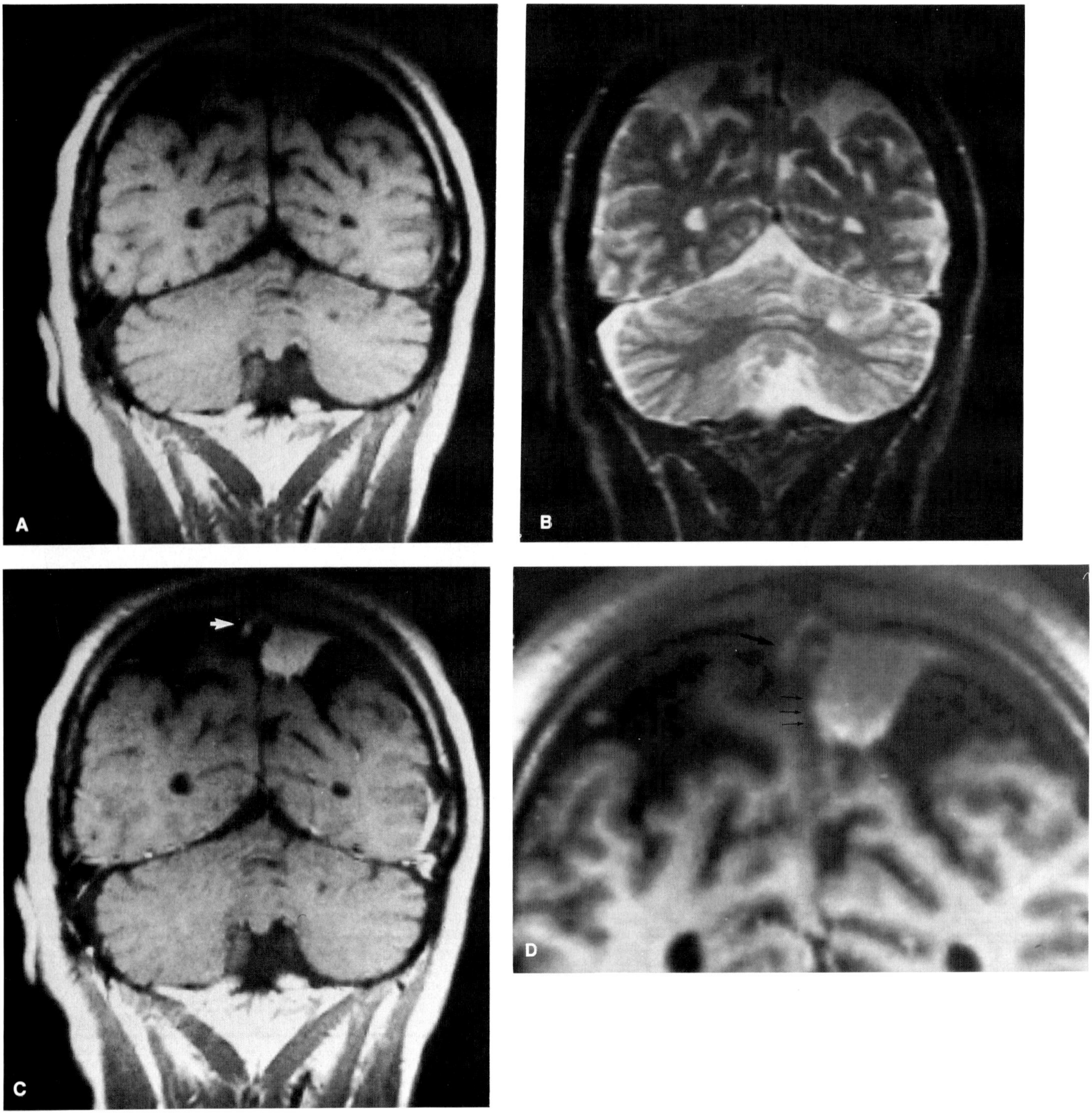

FIGURE 3–26. (A) There is a vague, soft tissue density in the left posterior parietal parasagittal region on this T1-weighted image (TR/TE = 700/17). **(B)** Due to the lack of a significant signal intensity change on the T2-weighted image (TR/TE = 3000/90), the abnormality could be mistaken for normal cortex with surrounding cortical loss. **(C)** With contrast enhancement (T1-weighted image), the diagnosis of a meningioma is possible. More importantly, there is extension across the midline, indicating invasion of the superior sagittal sinus (arrow). This finding was surgically documented. **(D)** A magnified view of this area is from a 3D FLASH examination (50°, TE = 8, TR = 40). The reformatted view more clearly shows the irregular margin of the sinus from its invasion (arrows) and the extension across the midline (large arrow).

amen of Luscha into the cerebellopontine angle, a feature that can be used in distinguishing them from other posterior fossa tumors, such as medulloblastoma and astrocytoma.[28]

Because of their intraventricular origin, seeding through the CSF pathways is common. The prognosis is poor with the occurrence of drop metastases. Hydrocephalus is a nearly uniform feature of this tumor, particularly of those occurring in the posterior fossa. Whether these tumors occur above or below the tentorium, they are usually calcified, and 50% may contain areas of cystic change.

MRI is helpful in confirming the intraventricular location, particularly if these tumors occur in the supratentorial ventricular system (Fig. 3–25). Ependymomas usually appear as large, bulky, soft tissue masses. If there is cystic change or calcification, the soft tissue mass will show focal areas of low signal intensity on T1-weighted images. An increase in signal intensity occurs on T2-weighted images (in both cystic and non-cystic regions). CT contrast enhancement is moderate and diffuse for supratentorial lesions and may be ring enhancing in the posterior fossa.[28] Similar enhancing changes should be true for MRI, but this awaits confirmation.

EXTRA-AXIAL AND CEREBELLOPONTINE ANGLE LESIONS

Meningiomas

Meningiomas are the most common extra-axial adult tumors, comprising 15 to 18% of all intracranial neoplasms. These tumors are more frequent in women between the ages of 40 and 70 years.[28] Their most frequent location is high over the convexity adjoining the superior sagittal sinus in its middle or anterior third. Other sites, in decreasing order of frequency, are the lateral convexity, sphenoid ridge, olfactory groove, suprasellar-parasellar region, and posterior fossa (i.e., petrous bone, clivus, foramen magnum). When these tumors are multiple or occur in childhood, they are usually associated with neurofibromatosis.[42,43]

Meningiomas are usually benign and slow-growing tumors that compress rather than invade the adjacent brain tissue. Occasionally, they exhibit aggressive changes by invading osseous structures and adjacent dural sinuses (Fig. 3–26). After these changes occur, complete resection may not be possible, and recurrences are more likely to occur.

Regardless of location, these lesions are usually broad-based on a bony or dural margin, producing imaging changes that are characteristic of extra-axial lesions: arcuate bowing of the white matter due to compression of the brain (Fig. 3–27); a low-signal-in-

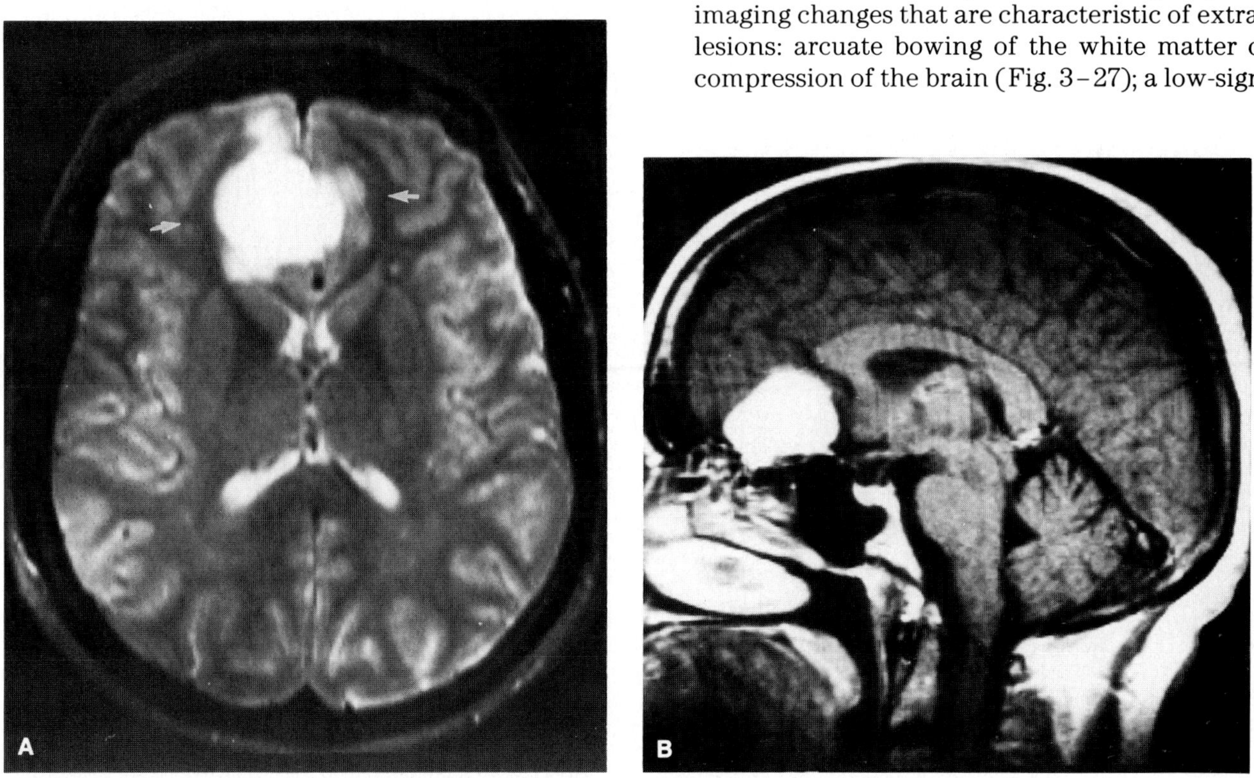

FIGURE 3–27. **(A)** This meningioma arising from the olfactory groove clearly shows the arcuate bowing of white matter (arrows). The tumor is unusual in the degree of signal intensity change on the T2-weighted image (TR/TE = 3000/90). This is usually less intense than glial tumors. **(B)** The origin of this tumor is more clearly shown on the sagittal postcontrast T1-weighted view in a patient who presented with anosmia.

tensity vascular rim caused by the circumferential displacement of pial vessels (Fig. 3-28); a CSF cleft that is more apparent on T2-weighted images (Fig. 3-29); and displacement of the low-intensity lateral dural margin, which occurs in lesions arising in the cavernous sinus (Fig. 3-30).[42-44]

Meningiomas are often highly vascular, with calcifications and cystic changes that produce an intrinsic tumor mottling (Fig. 3-31). These findings are more obvious at higher field strengths, perhaps due to the differences in magnetic susceptibility.[42-44] Meningiomas may have a variable amount of associated edema (Figs. 3-27, 3-29, 3-31, and 3-32). Occasionally the edema or edema cuff will be the only means of tumor identification on precontrast T2-weighted studies (Fig. 3-32).[44]

Meningiomas are classified into several histologic types, which probably explains their variability in signal intensity changes.[45] The signal intensity changes fail to follow those of other intracranial tumors, which show decreased signal intensity on T1-weighted images and increased signal intensity on T2-weighted images (Figs. 3-26 and 3-31). This is particularly true at field strengths between 0.5 and 1.0 T, at which only 10 to 50% of lesions can be identified on the basis of signal intensity changes.[42,43,46] Thus, a small or plaque-like lesion at the convexity or skull base may not be visualized. Until the development of Gd DTPA, the lack of detection of such lesions cast doubt on MRI as a primary imaging modality.

Contrast administration is necessary to overcome the variable signal intensity pattern. The enhancement is intense due to the lack of a BBB. A 180% enhancement has been quantitated in a small series of these tumors, representing one of the most intensely

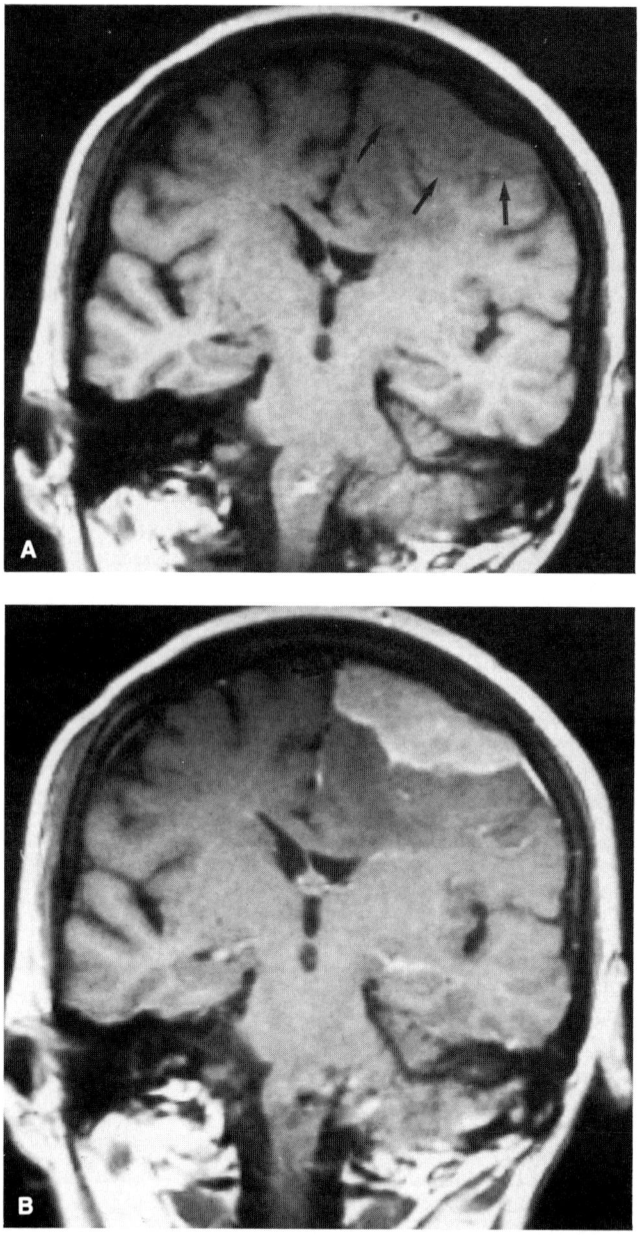

FIGURE 3-28. **(A)** A low-signal-intensity rim (arrows) marks the margin of this large anterior convexity meningioma on this coronal T1-weighted image (TR/TE = 700/20). **(B)** There is intense tumor enhancement on the postcontrast T1-weighted image. The surgically documented invasion of the sagittal sinus is better shown (arrow) after contrast.

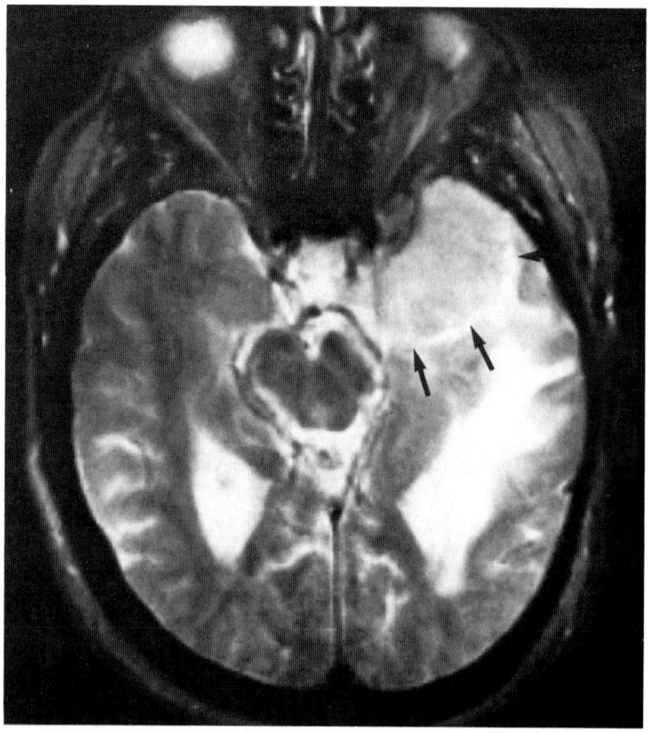

FIGURE 3-29. This large sphenoid wing meningioma is also shown in Figure 3-2. Although the CSF cleft (arrows) is better seen on this T2-weighted image (TR/TE = 3000/90), the vascular changes of cavernous sinus invasion and arterial encasement are better shown on the previous T1-weighted postcontrast images.

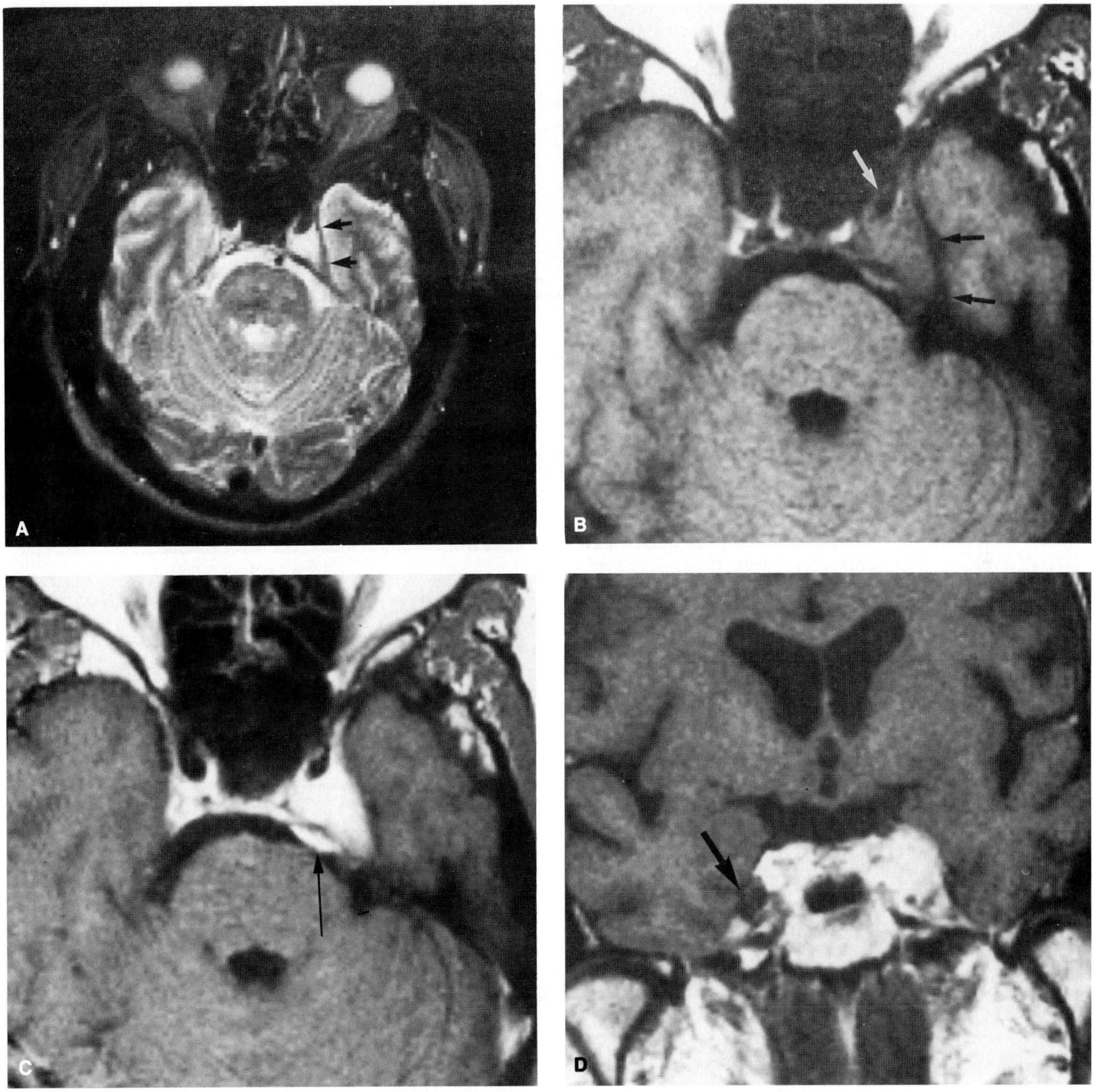

FIGURE 3–30. Cavernous sinus meningioma. **(A)** The T2-weighted sequence (TR/TE = 3000/90) shows an area of increased signal intensity in the left parasellar region. There is normally an area of increased signal intensity due to Meckel's cave or the normal space that surrounds the Gasserian ganglion of the CN V. The arrows mark the displaced lateral dural margin. **(B)** The 3-mm T1-weighted image (TR/TE = 700/17) clearly shows the cavernous sinus enlargement and displacement of the lateral dural line (arrows). The irregular contour of the slightly anteriorly displaced internal carotid artery is indicative of vascular encasement in this cavernous sinus meningioma (white arrow). **(C)** After contrast administration, the asymmetry of the cavernous sinuses is more obvious, as is the transdural extension (arrow) into the prepontine cistern. **(D)** The coronal plane helps in assessing the vascular changes and the CN involvement. The sagittal plane does not help in assessing these parasellar abnormalities. Notice the normal Meckel's cave on the right (arrow).

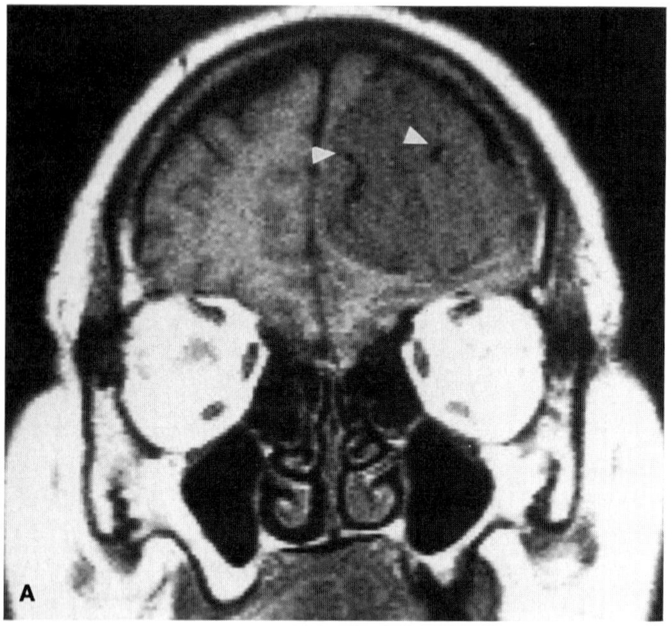

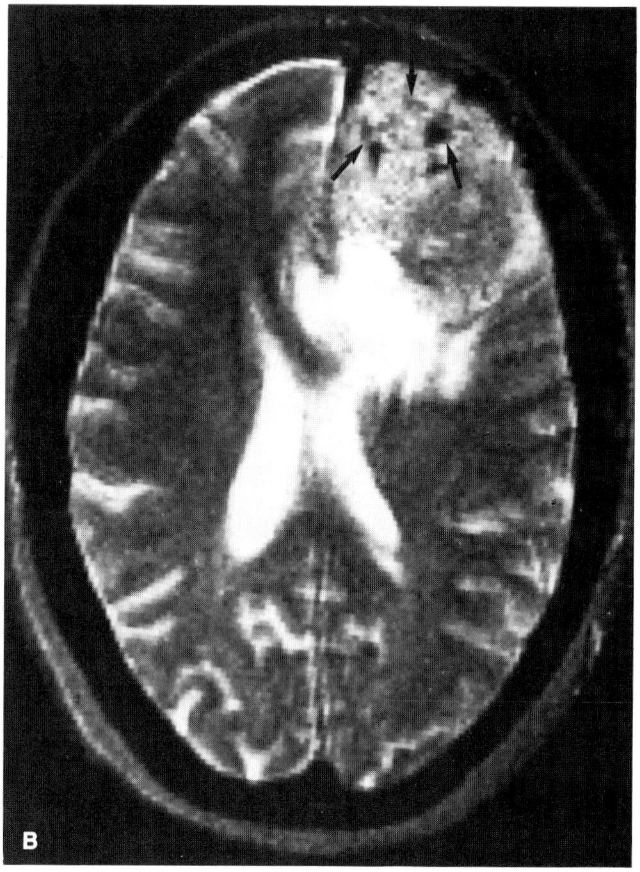

FIGURE 3-31. **(A)** On the coronal T1-weighted image (TR/TE = 700/17), the low-signal-intensity meningioma shows small punctate areas of even lower signal intensity (arrowheads). **(B)** The mottling (arrow) is more apparent on the T2-weighted image (TR/TE = 3000/90). This tumor was highly vascular by angiography and at surgery. The more irregular, higher-signal-intensity abnormality at the posterior aspect of the lesion is due to the moderate degree of associated edema.

enhancing intracranial abnormalities (Figs. 3-26 through 3-30, 3-32, and 3-33).[10] A more intensely enhancing rim occasionally occurs (Fig. 3-2).[12] Contrast administration aids visualization, accurate localization, and the assessment of secondary vascular changes (Figs. 3-26, 3-28 through 3-30, 3-32, and 3-33).

Meningiomas often invade adjacent dural sinuses (Figs. 3-26 and 3-28). Signs of dural sinus invasion on MR include an irregular contour to the signal void in the sinus created by flowing blood and an increased signal on T1-weighted images when the flow in the sinus is significantly slowed by the obstructing or nearly obstructing tumor.[44] In the latter case, phase imaging can assess slow flow and may eventually find greater clinical utility. Contrast agents better demonstrate the proximity of these lesions to the sagittal sinus (Figs. 3-26 and 3-28), the irregularity of the invaded sinuses, and tumor extending across the midline (Fig. 3-26).[43] MRI is more sensitive in the assessment of dural sinus invasion than CT or angiography.[44]

When meningiomas arise in the cavernous sinus or secondarily extend into this structure, encasement and displacement of the carotid artery is common (Figs. 3-2, 3-30, 3-32, and 3-33).[43,44] The evaluation of this type of vascular involvement is more accurate with MRI than with CT or angiography.[44] Angiographically, it may be difficult to determine if the change in vessel caliber is atherosclerotic or due to vascular encasement. With MRI, the encasement is seen as a soft tissue mass effect that narrows the caliber of the internal carotid artery and often displaces vessels.[44] Contrast enhancement accentuates this change (Figs. 3-30, 3-32, and 3-33).[43]

Contrast enhancement more clearly shows the enlargement of the cavernous sinus when meningiomas arise within or extend into it. The displaced lateral hypointense dural line also becomes more obvious. For small tumors and greater detail of involvement, 3-mm or less thin sections are necessary (Fig. 3-30).[43]

Plaque-like meningiomas represent a special and often clinically frustrating form of meningiomas. These may become rather extensive, with involvement of the tentorium, cavernous sinus, brain stem, and cranial nerve VIII. Transdural and subperiosteal spread may also occur. These have been called the "impossible meningiomas" because total resection is not possible, and recurrence and enlargement, albeit slow, is progressive (Fig. 3-33).

Although osseous changes are better detailed by CT, the multiplanar capability of MRI usually depicts

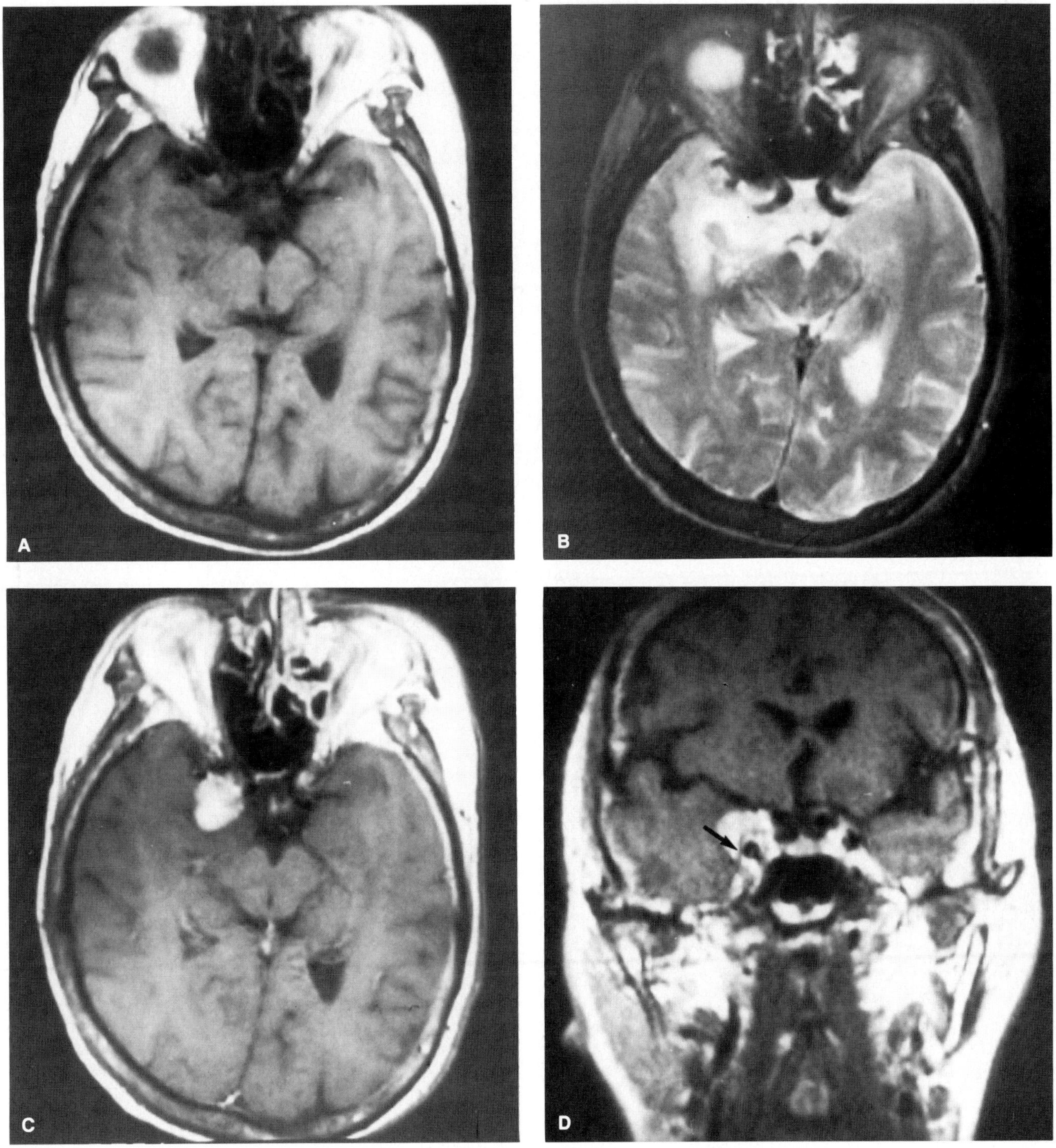

FIGURE 3–32. **(A)** The T1-weighted image (TR/TE = 700/20) shows a vague mass effect in the uncus of the right temporal lobe. **(B)** An increase in signal intensity occurs in the region on the T2-weighted image (TR/TE = 3000/90). The cause of the abnormality is not evident. **(C)** A focal area of intense enhancement made diagnosis of this parasellar meningioma possible. On T2-weighted images, this tumor showed no signal intensity changes, but was identified by the edema. **(D)** The 3-mm coronal postcontrast view shows more extensive change than suspected from the axial view. There is invasion of the cavernous sinus with displacement of the internal carotid artery (arrow). This illustrates the need for thinner sections or additional planes when a meningioma is in the parasellar region or adjacent to a venous sinus.

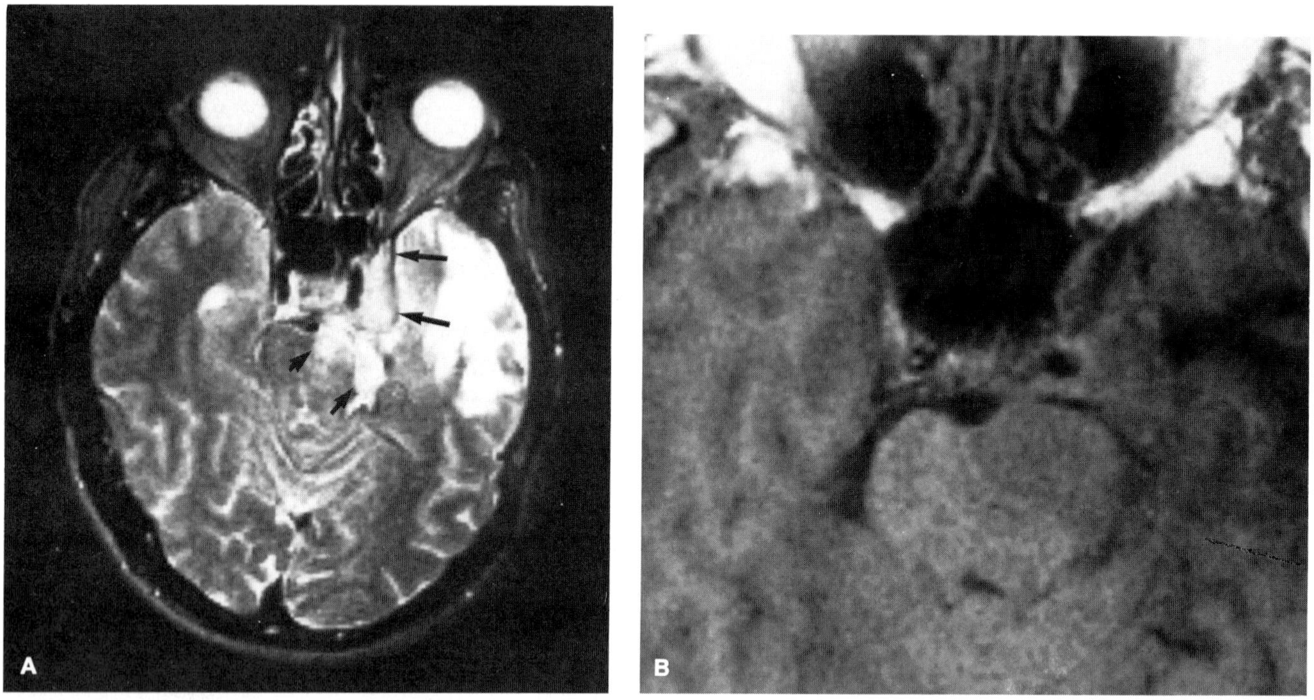

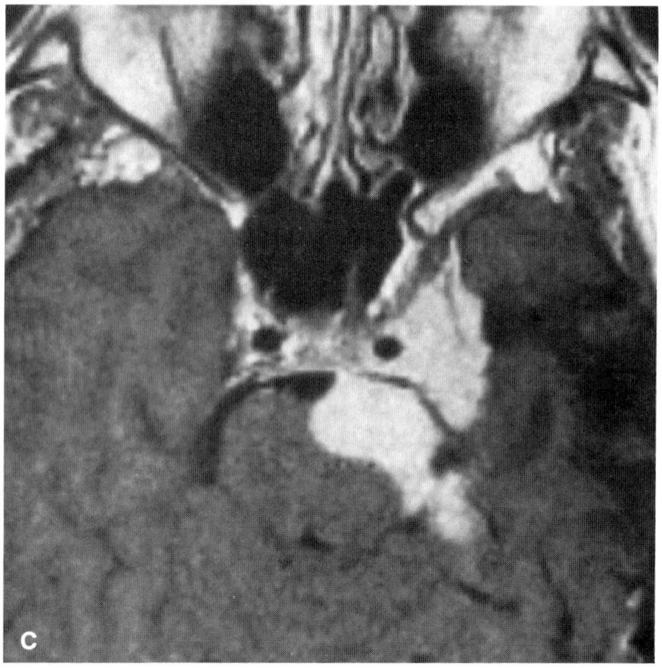

FIGURE 3–33. **(A)** There are multiple confluent areas of increased signal intensity on this T2-weighted image (TR/TE = 3000/90). The transdural extent of the recurrent tentorial meningioma is seen as a bright area that impresses the brain stem (short arrows). The low-signal-intensity dural line of the cavernous sinus is laterally displaced, indicating cavernous sinus invasion (longer arrows). Elsewhere, the tumor is difficult to distinguish from postsurgical encephalomalacia. **(B)** Despite the 3-mm slice thickness, the tumor and postoperative changes are difficult to assess. **(C)** After contrast agent administration, the full extent of this meningioma and differentiation of the mass from post-operative changes are clearly shown. Notice the encasement of the left cavernous carotid.

osseous changes that axial CT frequently misses (Figs. 3–34 and 3–35).[44] Calcifications are better shown by CT, but the enhancement and extra-axial localization rarely pose difficulty in diagnosis by MRI.

Meningiomas that occur in the CP angle are often difficult to differentiate from acoustic neuromas. Although en plaque meningiomas can involve the sheath of cranial nerve (CN) VIII, the smaller more focal tumors do not appear to do so (Figs. 3–36 and 3–37). Thus, the lack of enhancement of CN VIII favors the diagnosis of a meningioma.

Acoustic Neuromas

Acoustic neuromas are benign tumors that arise from the neurilemmal sheath of the vestibular division of the CN VIII. It is the most common benign extra-axial tumor of the posterior fossa. Patients are usually 40 to 60 years of age and have a unilateral sensorineural hearing loss and tinnitus. Larger tumors with brainstem involvement cause unsteadiness, ataxia, vertigo, and diminished corneal reflexes.[28,47]

MRI has rapidly supplanted other imaging tech-

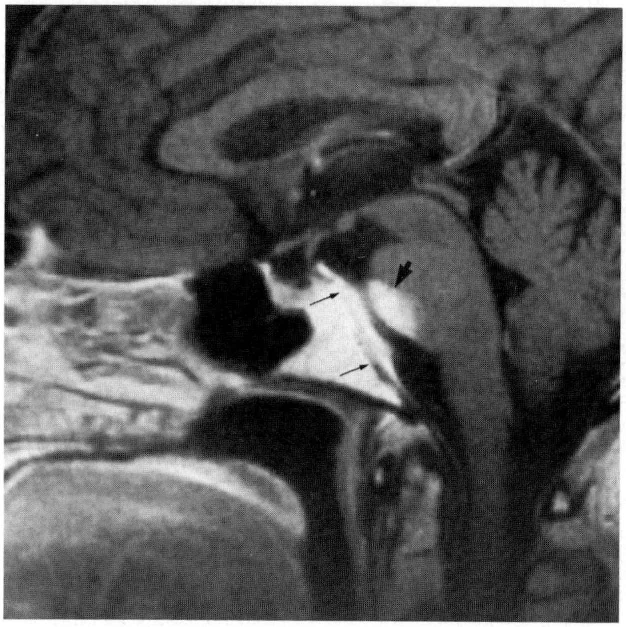

FIGURE 3–34. There is a low-signal-intensity line (arrows) that separates the clivus from an enhanced mass on this T1-weighted image (TR/TE = 700/17). The CT term for this abnormality is a lucent dural line indicating subperiosteal extension of tumor and is thought to be more common in, if not specific for, meningiomas. This patient had a large, recurrent tentorial meningioma. The enhancement over the pons (single arrow) is due to volume averaging. The osseous change could not be seen by CT.

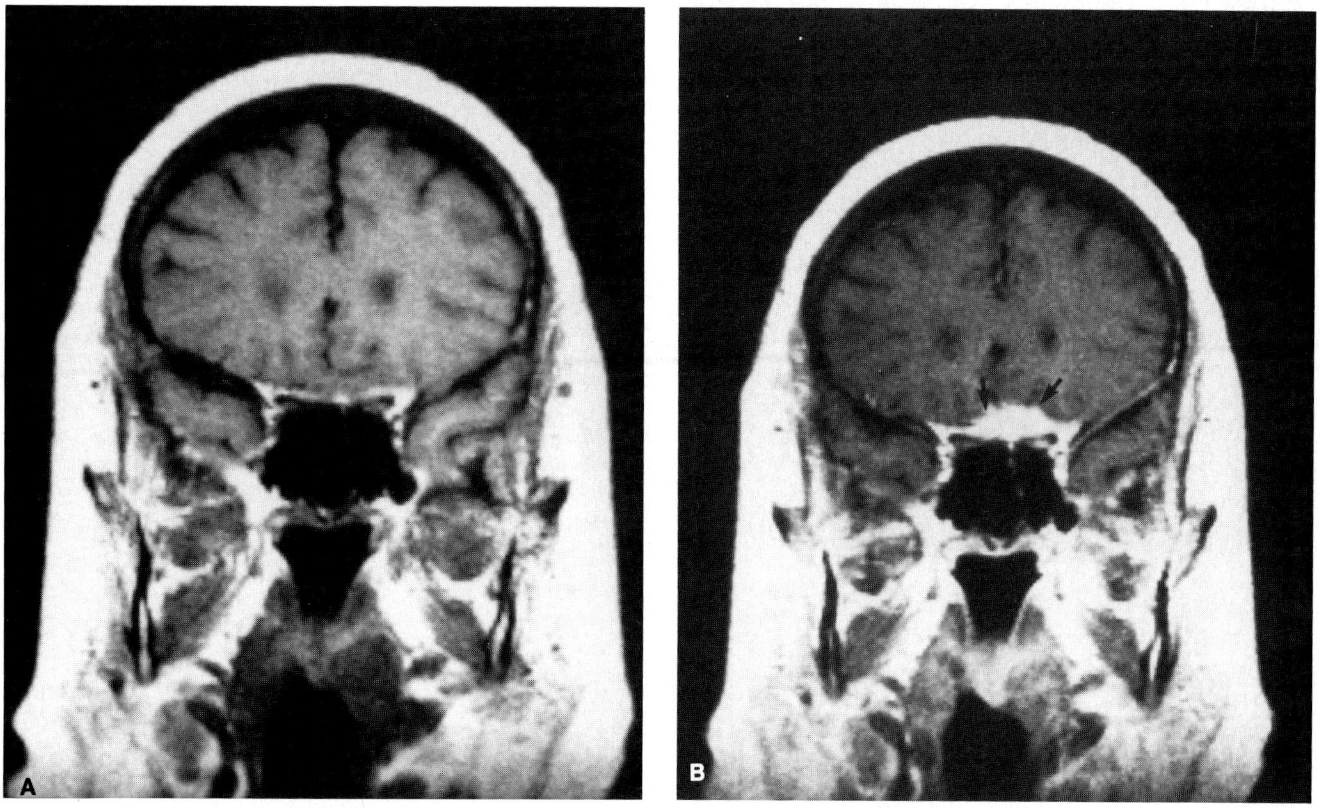

FIGURE 3–35. (A) The coronal T1-weighted image (TR/TE = 700/17) before contrast agent administration is normal in a patient with a planum sphenoidale meningioma. **(B)** The postcontrast study shows enhancement of the periosteal extension of the tumor (arrows). This change would be difficult to assess by CT, particularly in axial sections.

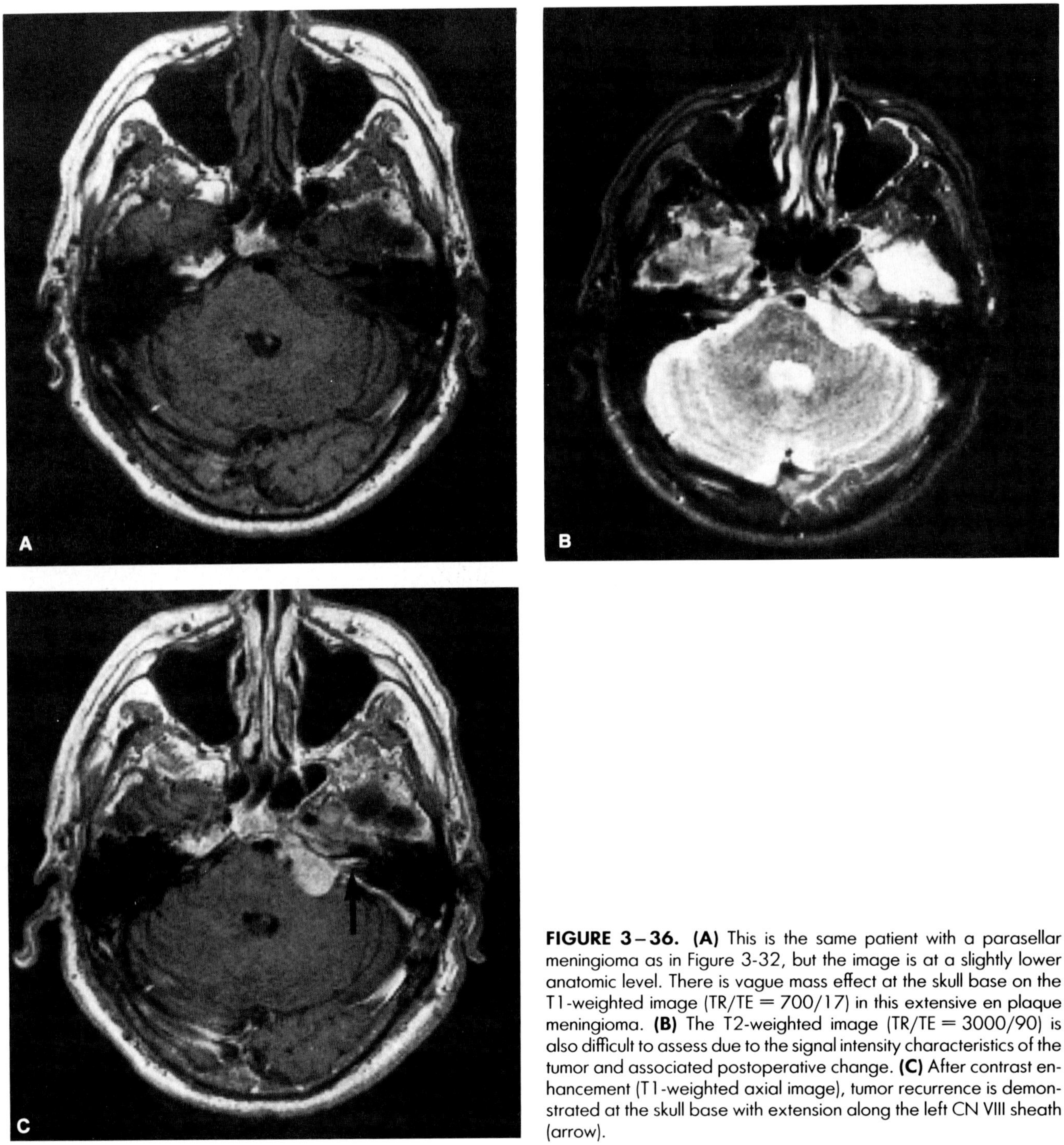

FIGURE 3–36. (A) This is the same patient with a parasellar meningioma as in Figure 3-32, but the image is at a slightly lower anatomic level. There is vague mass effect at the skull base on the T1-weighted image (TR/TE = 700/17) in this extensive en plaque meningioma. **(B)** The T2-weighted image (TR/TE = 3000/90) is also difficult to assess due to the signal intensity characteristics of the tumor and associated postoperative change. **(C)** After contrast enhancement (T1-weighted axial image), tumor recurrence is demonstrated at the skull base with extension along the left CN VIII sheath (arrow).

niques in evaluating these tumors, especially after the development of contrast agents. Polytomography, iophendylate cisternography, and air-contrast CT are former techniques that involved significant radiation and were often invasive, thereby adding to patient morbidity.[48]

With MRI, the lack of signal from the dense, bony structures allows direct and excellent visualization of CN VII and CN VIII and often their visualization as separate structures. Thin-section, high-resolution images are necessary for optimal evaluation.[47,49]

The normal CN VIII does not enhance; thus, enhancement in this region is abnormal.[47,49] Enhancement is caused by tissue vascularity, because the cap-

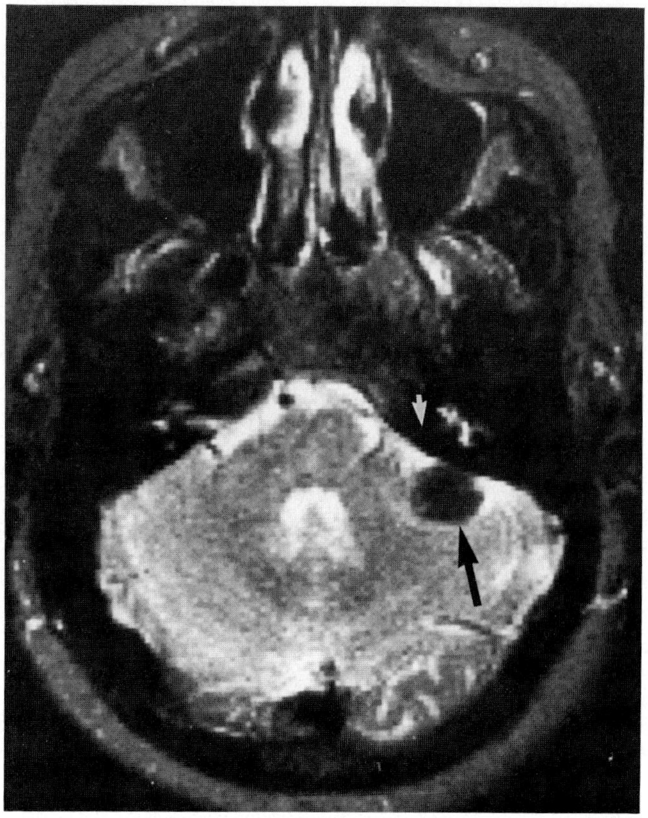

FIGURE 3–37. This T2-weighted image (TR/TE = 3000/90) shows a CP angle meningioma as a low-signal-intensity lesion (large arrow) that is separate from the left CN VIII (arrowhead). This lesion was densely calcified on CT.

illaries of these tumors do not exhibit a BBB.[12] The degree of enhancement (200–400%) is greater than for any other intracranial tumor.[10]

The typical changes described on sequences without contrast are enlargement of the nerve sheath on T1-weighted images, an extracanalicular soft tissue mass on T1-weighted images, and ISO-to-increased intensity of the nerve and mass on T2-weighted images (Fig. 3–38).[47,49] The extracanalicular tumor may show a variable or mixed signal intensity on both sequences if there is necrosis or hemorrhage. Contrast agents are quite accurate in demonstrating the degree of intracanalicular and extracanalicular involvement (Fig. 3–38).[47,49] More accurate knowledge of both intracanalicular and extracanalicular tumor extent is beneficial in planning surgery.[49]

The accurate assessment of these tumors requires both a precontrast and postcontrast examination, because MRI without contrast can produce both false negatives and false positives. In one series, the combination of these errors affected 10% of patients studied.[49] Thus, small intracanalicular tumors could be seen with contrast that went undetected without contrast (Fig. 3–39). More alarming is the prospect of suggesting a tumor on sequences without Gd DTPA when none can be found with enhancement. Occasionally the nerve may appear enlarged on T1-weighted images, or dural ectasia can produce a signal intensity on T2-weighted images that is indistinguishable from the signal intensity change of intracanalicular tumor (Fig. 3–40).[49]

Although T2-weighted sequences are diminishing in importance for evaluating acoustic tumors, there are abnormalities that may mimic CN VIII disease, and these are better visualized with this sequence. Some examples are multiple sclerosis, mastoiditis, and vascular brain stem compression.

A special word of caution is offered for evaluating postsurgical recurrence. In the translabyrinthine approach, the resected portion of the mastoid is often packed with an autologous graft that contains fat. This may superimpose the course of the CN VIII so that coronal imaging may be necessary to separate the enhancing recurrence from the increased signal in the graft. Dural enhancement may also occur after surgery, obscuring the area of interest in the axial plane. Coronal imaging may be necessary in this circumstance.[49]

Fast imaging with the 3D volume technique, with its T1-based contrast, is being used more often. For

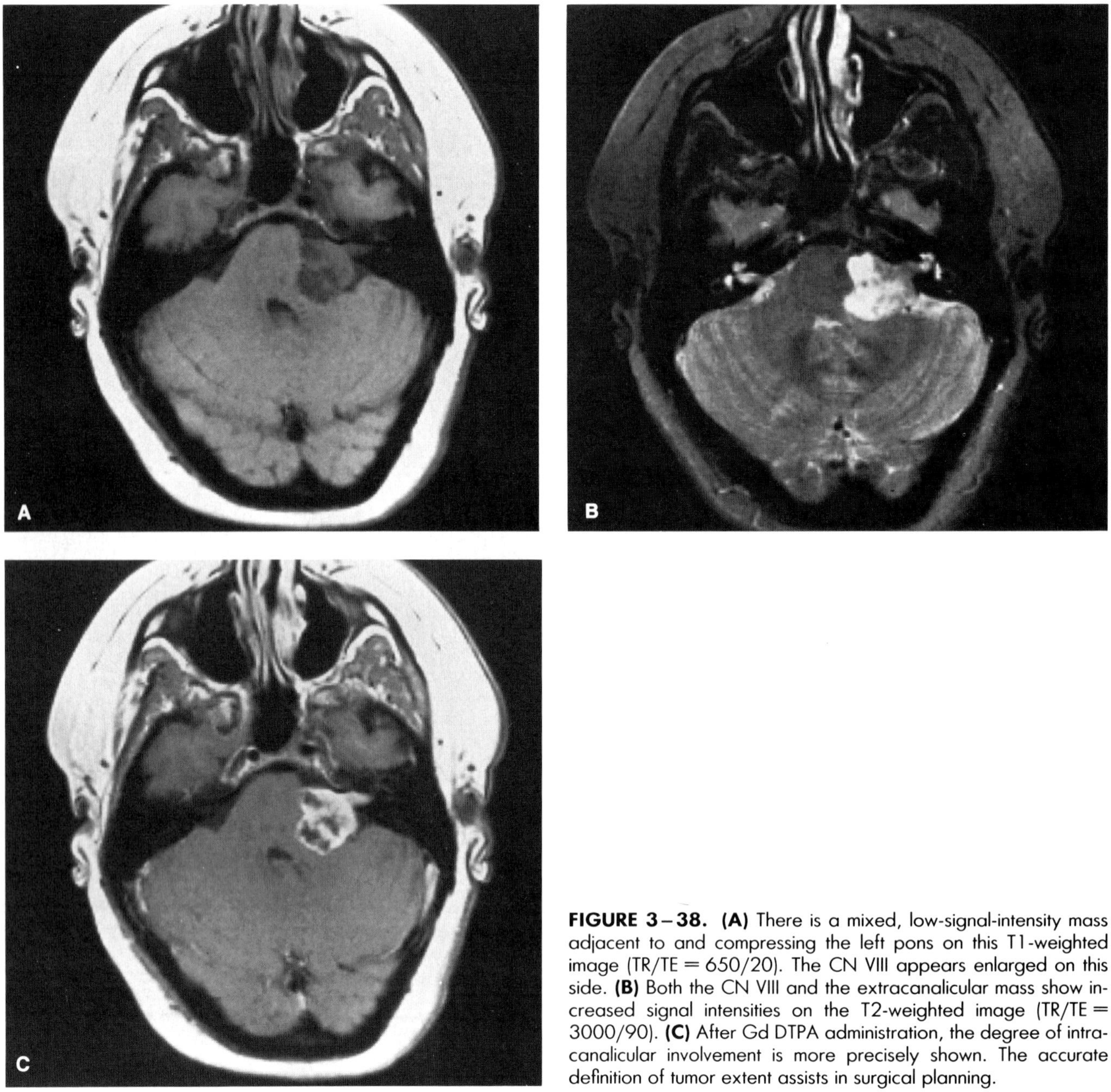

FIGURE 3–38. **(A)** There is a mixed, low-signal-intensity mass adjacent to and compressing the left pons on this T1-weighted image (TR/TE = 650/20). The CN VIII appears enlarged on this side. **(B)** Both the CN VIII and the extracanalicular mass show increased signal intensities on the T2-weighted image (TR/TE = 3000/90). **(C)** After Gd DTPA administration, the degree of intracanalicular involvement is more precisely shown. The accurate definition of tumor extent assists in surgical planning.

example, FLASH imaging with a flip angle of 50° may provide a time-efficient, thinner-section alternative to the more lengthy SE imaging technique in multiple planes. Reformatted images with this technique can show excellent detail of intracanalicular acoustic tumors in approximately 10 minutes of imaging time (Fig. 3–41).[49]

The benefits of contrast-enhanced MRI in the differential diagnosis of other extra-axial lesions has been discussed. Although en plaque meningiomas may occasionally involve the CN VIII sheath, small, more focal lesions do not appear to do so (Figs. 3–36 and 3–37).

Epidermoids

Epidermoids are also known as primary cholesteatomas. These tumors are thought to result from incomplete cleavage of the neural from the cutaneous ectoderm, with inclusions of epiblasts in the neural groove at the time of neural tube closure (3–5 weeks).[50] Midline abnormalities, such as those occur-

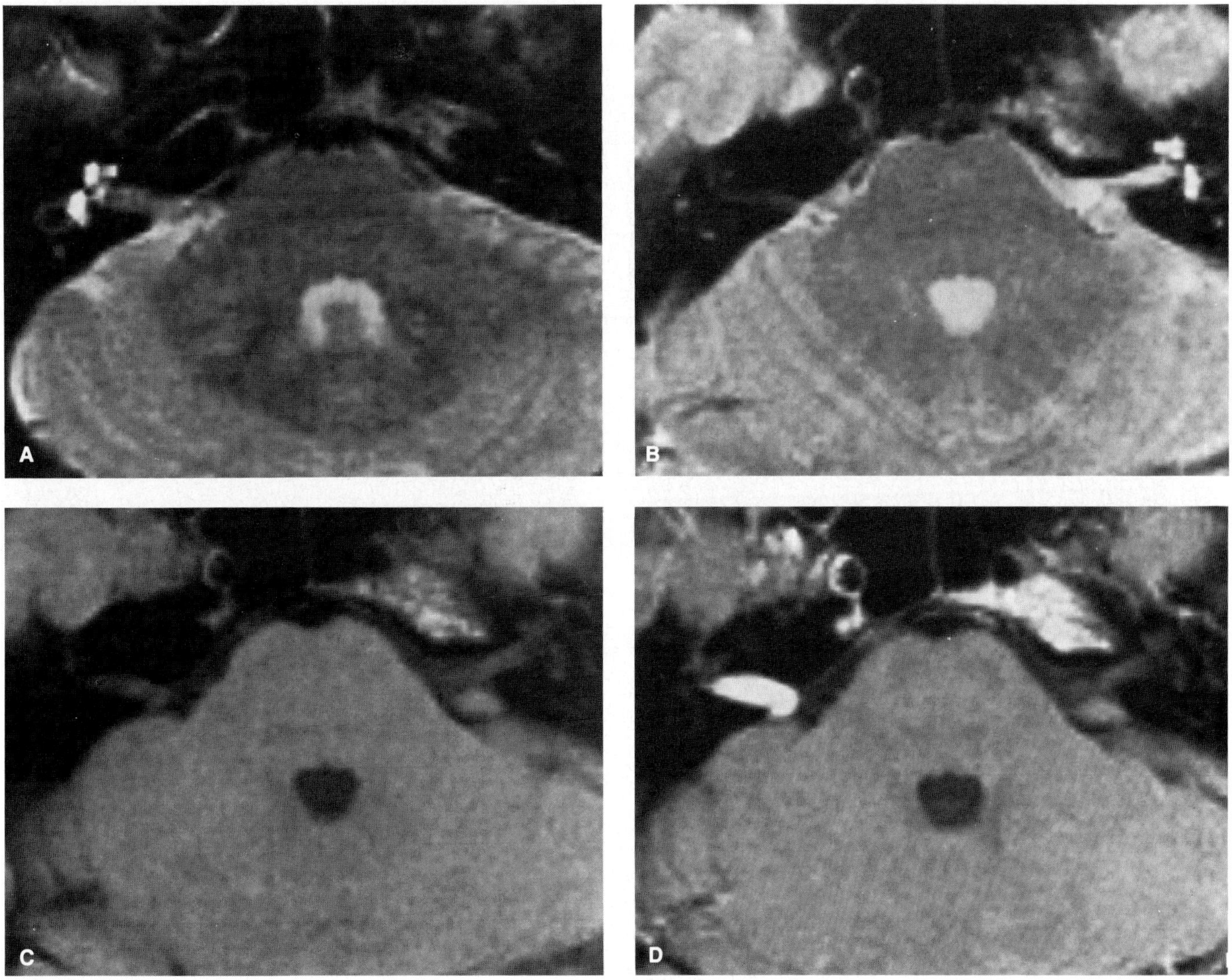

FIGURE 3–39. (A,B) T2-weighted axial images (TR/TE = 3000/90) of the right and left CN VIII appear normal, with no apparent difference in canal dimensions or abnormal signal intensity change. **(C)** The T1-weighted image before contrast agent administration shows no enlargement of either CN VIII. **(D)** The T1-weighted postcontrast axial image (TR/TE = 450/20) shows an intensely enhancing intracanalicular acoustic neuroma, on the right.

ring in the suprasellar and intraventricular regions, represent early gestational abnormalities. The more eccentrically positioned tumors, such as those occurring in the CP angle, represent a later gestational occurrence (Fig. 3–42).[28]

Epidermoids grow by desquamation of epithelial cells, which break down into keratin and cholesterol within the tumor capsule. These fatty elements are soft and pliable, and in the slow accumulation process, they conform to the shape of the subarachnoid space or ventricle.[50] Thus, the mass is fairly well demarcated, with compressive changes occurring late. These congenital tumors may not become symptomatic until patients are 25 to 30 years of age. Rupture occasionally produces a chemical meningitis.

As with other lipid tumors, their appearance on MR images depends on the type of fat and its physical state. Many contain cholesterol and show a prolongation of both T1 and T2 relaxation times. A difference in the fat content or physical state yields a brighter signal intensity on T1-weighted images. These tumors do not enhance; therefore, contrast administration adds little of diagnostic significance except to exclude other CP angle lesions that may show similar signal

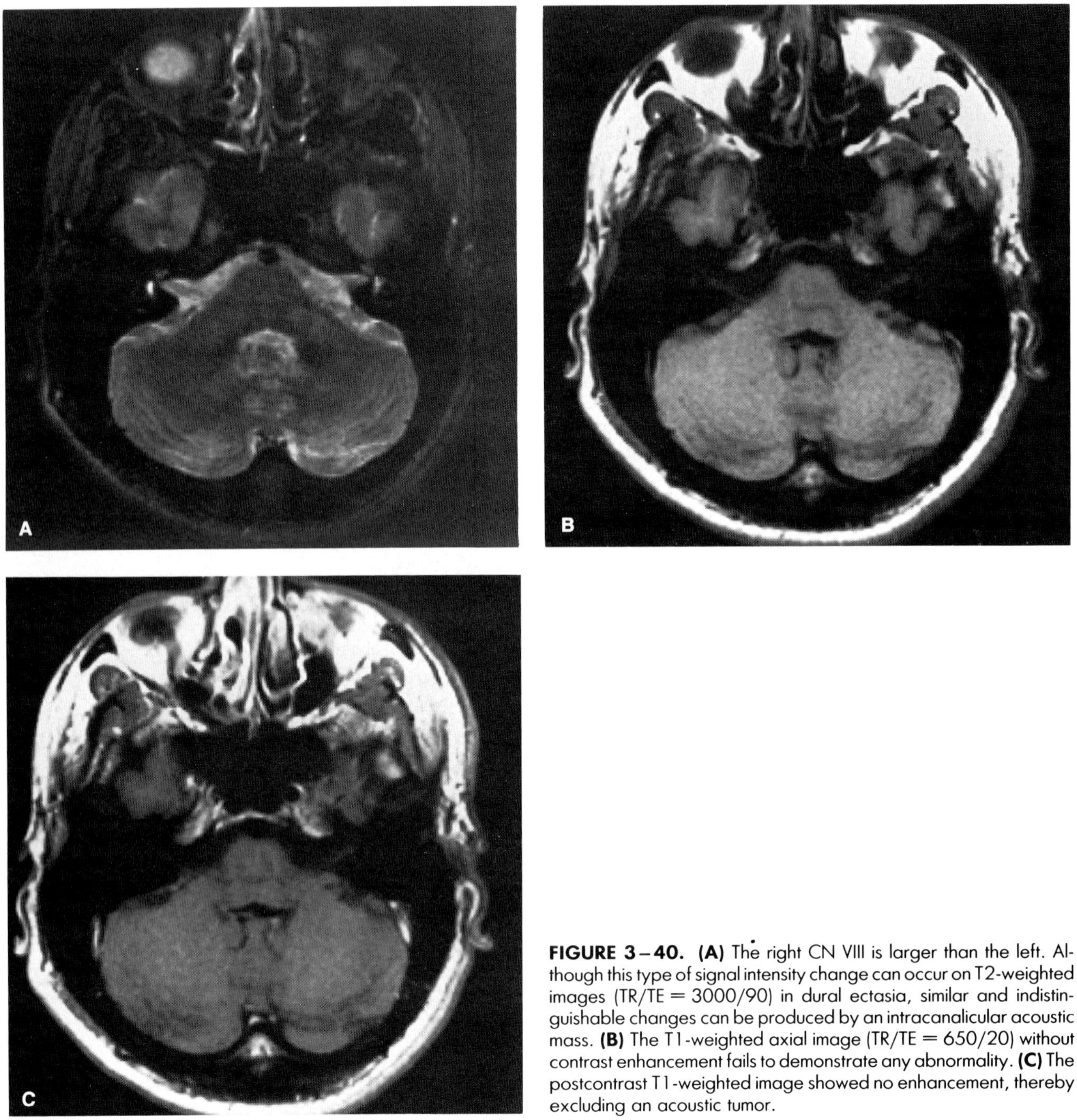

FIGURE 3–40. **(A)** The right CN VIII is larger than the left. Although this type of signal intensity change can occur on T2-weighted images (TR/TE = 3000/90) in dural ectasia, similar and indistinguishable changes can be produced by an intracanalicular acoustic mass. **(B)** The T1-weighted axial image (TR/TE = 650/20) without contrast enhancement fails to demonstrate any abnormality. **(C)** The postcontrast T1-weighted image showed no enhancement, thereby excluding an acoustic tumor.

intensity changes before contrast but enhance after contrast (i.e., meningiomas).

Dermoids

Dermoids are congenital tumors arising from inclusions of both the ectodermal and mesodermal germ layers at the time of neural tube closure. These tumors arise near the midline and are less common than epidermoids (Fig. 3–43).

Because there are ectodermal and mesodermal components, these tumors may contain fat, calcifications, hair follicles, and sebaceous and apocrine glandular elements.[28]

Dermoids containing a larger amount of fatty elements display a high signal intensity on T1-weighted images and a progressive decline in signal intensity with the first and second echoes of the T2-weighted sequences. Having a preserved BBB and little vascularity, these tumors do not enhance after contrast administration.

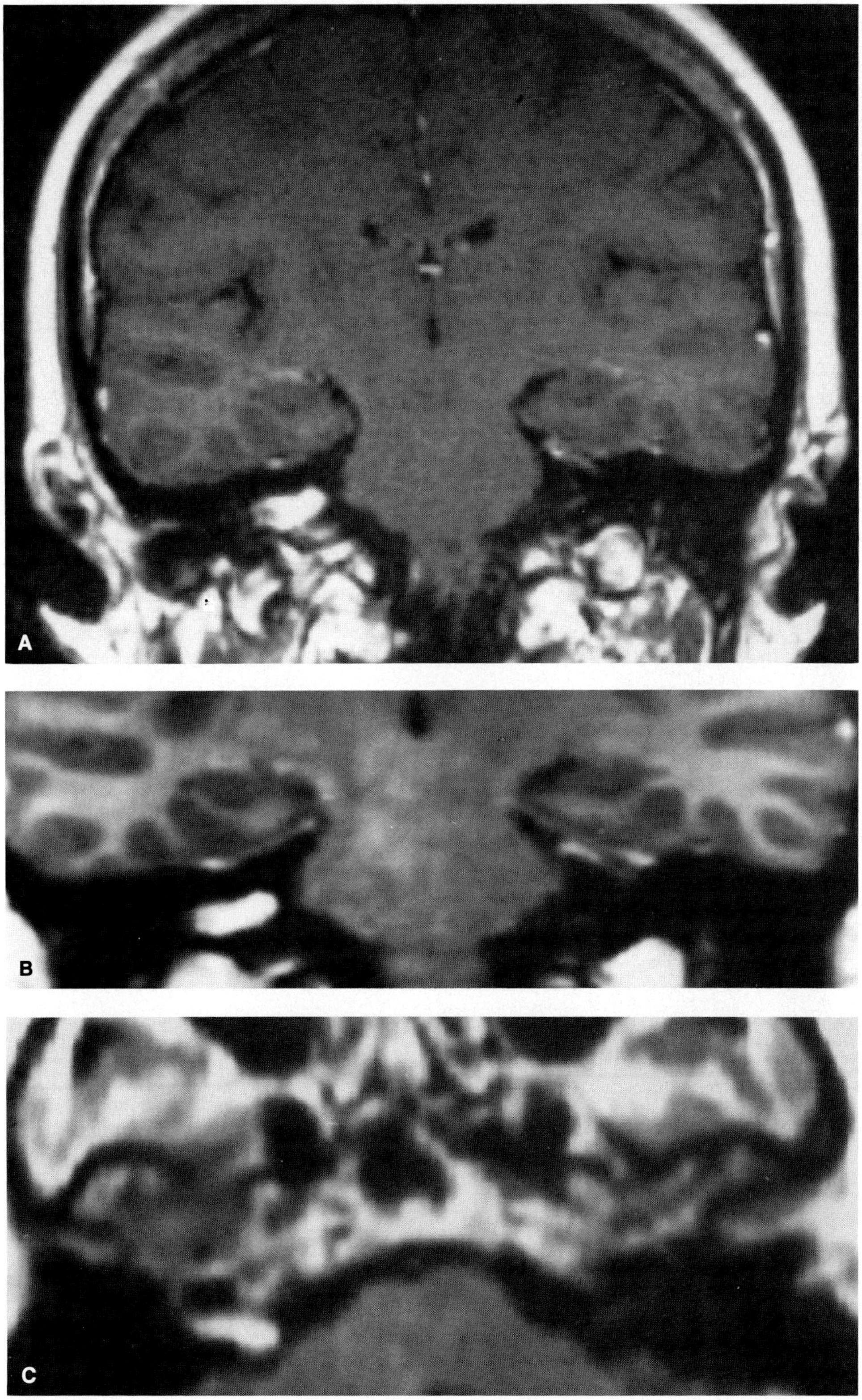

FIGURE 3–41. **(A)** A 3 mm coronal postcontrast T1-weighted spin-echo image (TR/TE = 650/20) shows an enhanced intracanalicular acoustic neuroma on the right. **(B)** The coronal reformatted section from a postcontrast 3D FLASH volume acquisition (50°, TE = 8, TR = 40) equally shows the abnormality. **(C)** This axial 1 mm section was also reformatted from the same 3D volume study. The imaging time for the volume study was 10 minutes. Axial and coronal images with spin-echo technique require 11 to 22 minutes, and the sections are not as thin as the reformatted views. The realized time savings can therefore be substantial.

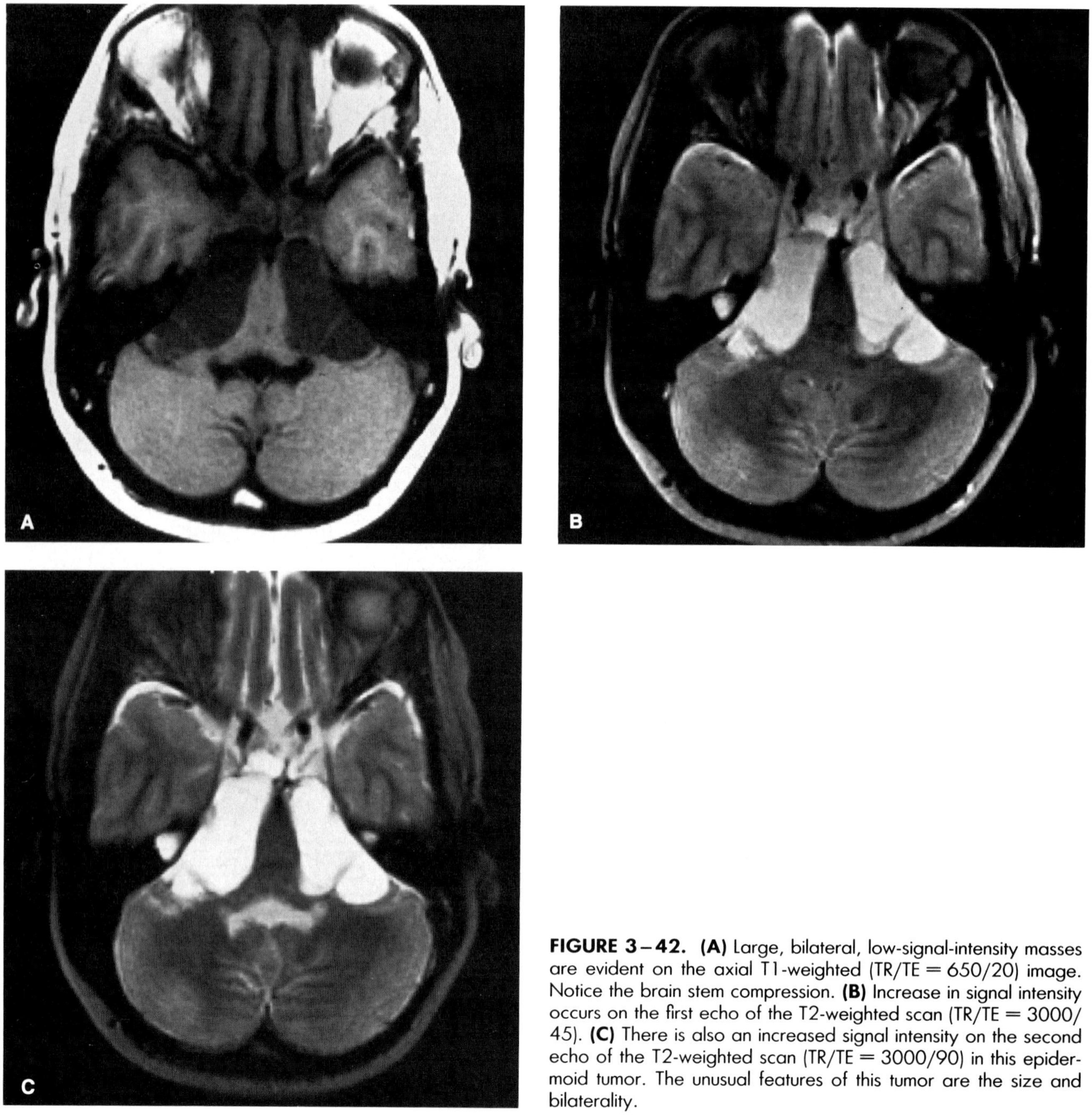

FIGURE 3–42. **(A)** Large, bilateral, low-signal-intensity masses are evident on the axial T1-weighted (TR/TE = 650/20) image. Notice the brain stem compression. **(B)** Increase in signal intensity occurs on the first echo of the T2-weighted scan (TR/TE = 3000/45). **(C)** There is also an increased signal intensity on the second echo of the T2-weighted scan (TR/TE = 3000/90) in this epidermoid tumor. The unusual features of this tumor are the size and bilaterality.

Arachnoid Cysts

Arachnoid cysts are benign congenital malformations. Their importance lies in the differentiation from other masses, including epidermoids, dermoids, subdural hygromas or hematomas, and some cystic tumors. These cysts most frequently occur in the midline or temporal regions, but they also occur in the posterior fossa, in the suprasellar region, in the quadrageminal plate region, and at the cerebral convexities.[28]

These masses are generated by a splitting of the arachnoid membrane. This space becomes filled with fluid that is usually clear but may be slightly xanthochromic. The margins of these lesions are sharp. The signal intensity changes usually parallel those of CSF, with low signal intensity on T1-weighted images and a high signal intensity on T2-weighted images (Fig. 3–44). No contrast enhancement occurs.

POSTERIOR FOSSA LESIONS

Since early clinical usage, MRI has shown its effectiveness in diagnosing posterior fossa lesions. The absence of bone streak artifacts and multiplanar imaging capa-

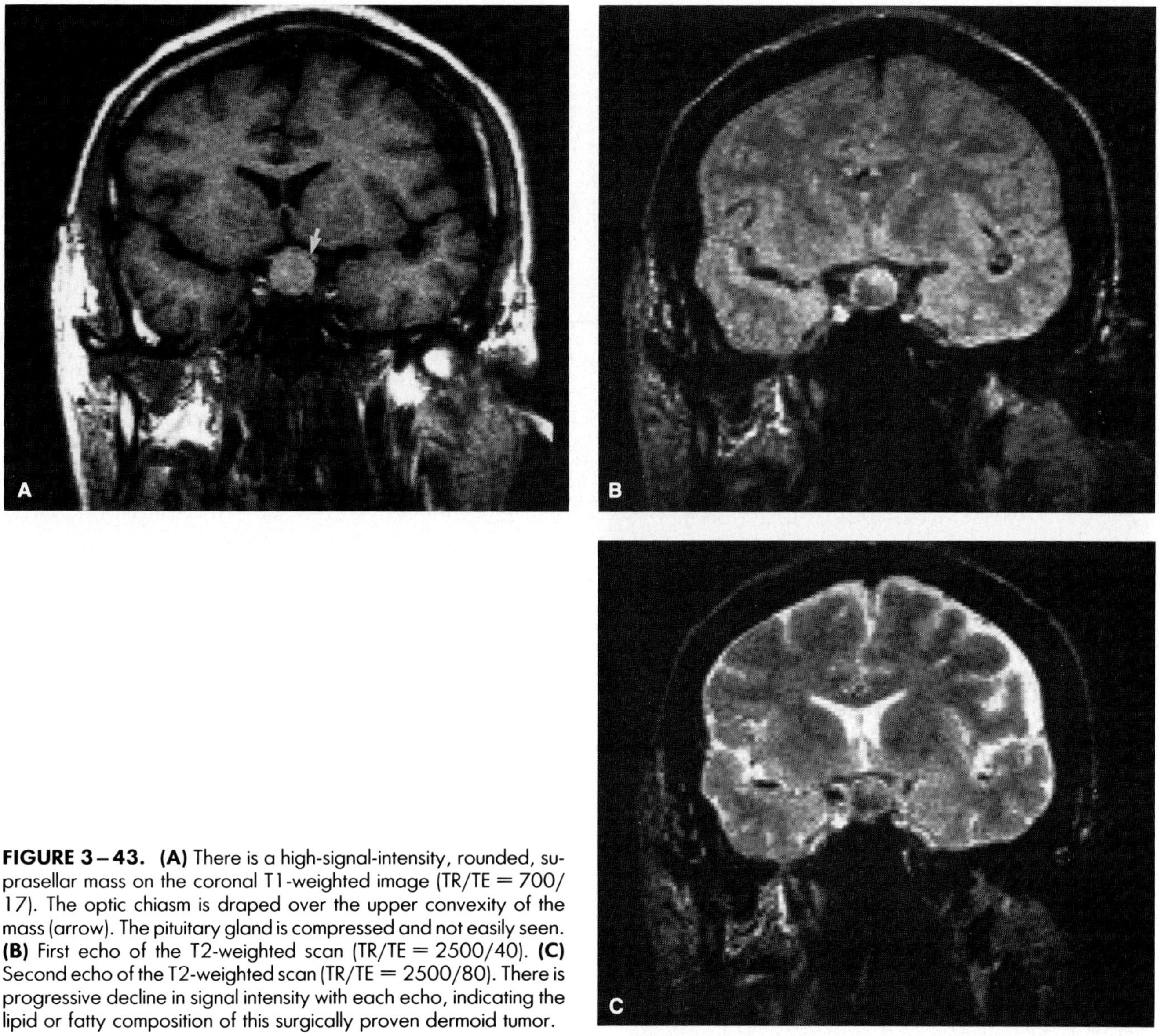

FIGURE 3–43. **(A)** There is a high-signal-intensity, rounded, suprasellar mass on the coronal T1-weighted image (TR/TE = 700/17). The optic chiasm is draped over the upper convexity of the mass (arrow). The pituitary gland is compressed and not easily seen. **(B)** First echo of the T2-weighted scan (TR/TE = 2500/40). **(C)** Second echo of the T2-weighted scan (TR/TE = 2500/80). There is progressive decline in signal intensity with each echo, indicating the lipid or fatty composition of this surgically proven dermoid tumor.

bilities are the two principal features that have accelerated diagnosis in this region.[51] The recent FDA approval and widespread availability of Gd DTPA has accelerated diagnosis by improved lesion localization and definition. For many of the less frequently occurring lesions, full evaluation awaits further clinical experience.

Ependymomas

These tumors frequently occur in the posterior fossa and are described in the section on Intraventricular Tumors.

Cystic Astrocytoma

Astrocytomas are one of the most common posterior fossa tumors and occur more commonly in children. Although these tumors may extend into the fourth ventricle, they usually arise in the cerebellar hemispheres. This is an important feature in the differential diagnosis of other posterior fossa tumors that occur in the midline, such as medulloblastomas and ependymomas.[28]

The cystic changes associated with these tumors are variable. Larger cysts may have a small peripheral nidus that shows focal enhancement. This type of enhancement may be difficult to identify by CT. In other astrocytomas, the cystic portion may appear multilocated, and the larger, solid portion may show nodular or ring enhancement (Fig. 3–3). The calcifications that occur in 20% of these tumors may be easier to detect with CT.

On T1-weighted images, a hemispheric mass with low-signal-intensity cystic changes is evident. An increase in signal intensity occurs on T2-weighted

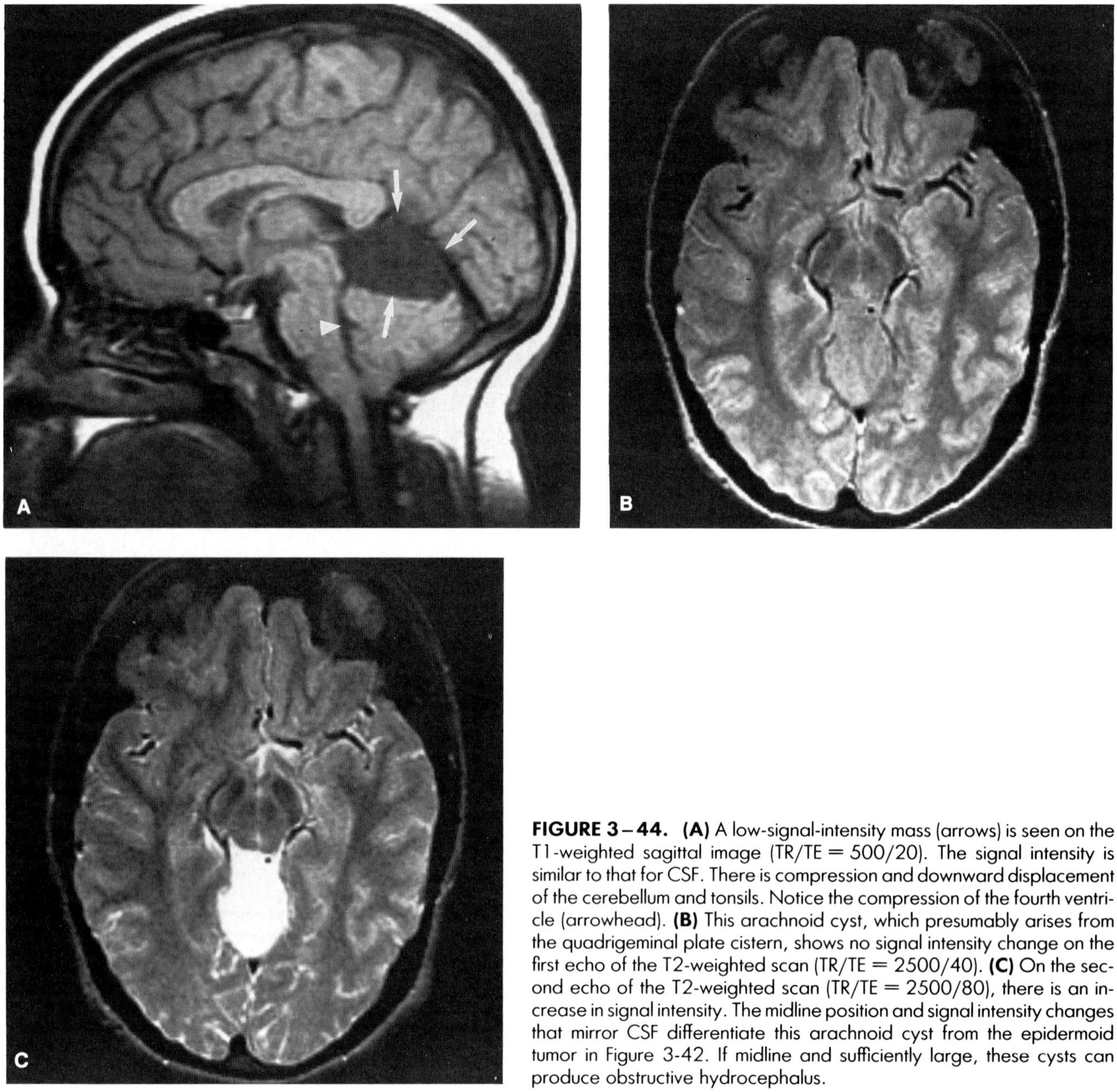

FIGURE 3–44. **(A)** A low-signal-intensity mass (arrows) is seen on the T1-weighted sagittal image (TR/TE = 500/20). The signal intensity is similar to that for CSF. There is compression and downward displacement of the cerebellum and tonsils. Notice the compression of the fourth ventricle (arrowhead). **(B)** This arachnoid cyst, which presumably arises from the quadrigeminal plate cistern, shows no signal intensity change on the first echo of the T2-weighted scan (TR/TE = 2500/40). **(C)** On the second echo of the T2-weighted scan (TR/TE = 2500/80), there is an increase in signal intensity. The midline position and signal intensity changes that mirror CSF differentiate this arachnoid cyst from the epidermoid tumor in Figure 3-42. If midline and sufficiently large, these cysts can produce obstructive hydrocephalus.

images, which may be slightly inhomogeneous due to the cystic change and calcifications (Fig. 3–3).

Brain Stem Gliomas

Brain stem gliomas usually affect older children and young adults. They are often suspected clinically before imaging studies are performed due to the anatomic structures involved. Symptoms include progressive cranial nerve palsies, extremity weakness, or respiratory difficulty.[28]

Gliomas in this location are more accurately assessed by MRI; they are frequently large when diagnosed by CT. A low-signal-intensity abnormality on T1-weighted images may be accompanied by areas of necrosis or cystic change, especially in more aggressive tumors. An increase in signal intensity occurs on T2-weighted images and, similar to intracranial

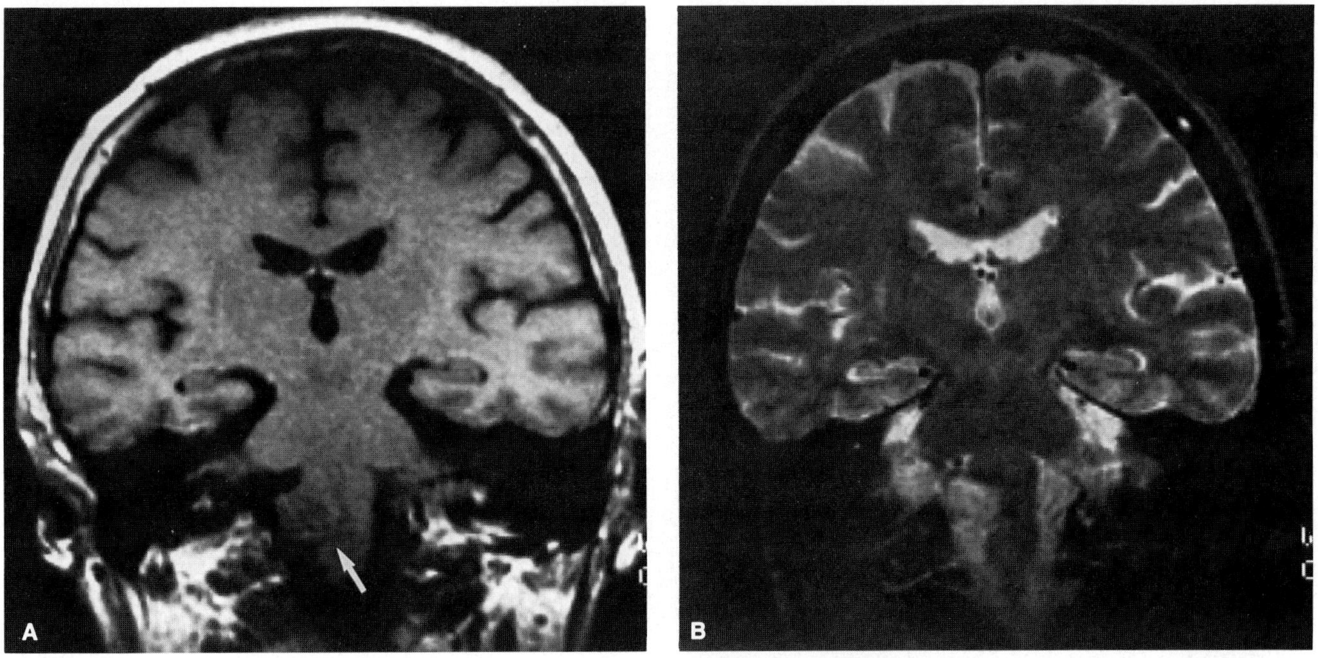

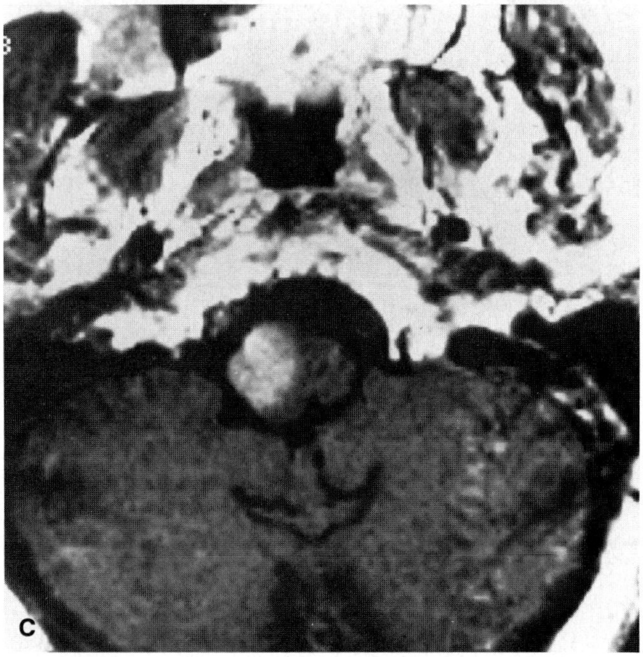

FIGURE 3–45. (A) There is an ill-defined soft tissue mass in the right medulla (arrow) on this T1-weighted coronal image (TR/TE = 450/20). **(B)** Although there is an increase in signal intensity on the T2-weighted image (TR/TE = 3000/90), this glioma is difficult to confirm because it lies adjacent to the bright signal of the CSF. **(C)** The axial postcontrast T1-weighted image is the most convincing for diagnosis of tumor. This clearly illustrates the hazard in totally relying on the T2-weighted image in tumor diagnosis, especially for masses adjacent to CSF spaces.

gliomas, may be the most convincing indication of a small existing tumor. Enhancement with Gd DTPA is variable but may provide essential localizing information in some strategically located abnormalities (Fig. 3–45).

Medulloblastomas

Medulloblastomas are one of the most common posterior fossa tumors in childhood, particularly young males. These embryonal tumors arise in the roof of the fourth ventricle or less commonly in the cerebellar hemispheres of older patients.[28] They are difficult to distinguish from ependymomas, unless the ependymoma extends into the CP angle, an abnormality easier to define by MRI. A soft tissue mass of slightly diminished signal intensity is seen on T1-weighted images. Increased signal intensity occurs on T2-weighted images. Precise enhancing characteristics with Gd DTPA await further investigations.

Hemangioblastomas

Hemangioblastomas are histologically benign neoplasms of vascular structures. They may occur at any age but are more frequent in young and middle-aged adults. They occur in association with von Hippel-Lindau disease.

Half of these tumors are cystic, and half are solid. A characteristic feature on CT scans is an enhancing mural nodule.[28] The cystic components of these lesions can be easily diagnosed by MRI as areas of T1 and T2 prolongation (Fig. 3–46). The enhancing mural nodule and rim of the cyst can be easily identified.

Because these tumors involve the cerebellar hemispheres (para median), the main differential diagnosis is a cystic astrocytoma. Cystic astrocytomas tend to be larger tumors and occur in a younger population.[28] Angiography has been regarded as the most sensitive and specific method for arriving at the diagnosis; whether MR is as sensitive in identifying the mural nodule that shows a characteristic angiographic stain awaits further experience.

Pituitary and Parasellar Region

The inherent advantages of MRI are used to the fullest extent in examining the pituitary and parasellar region. The direct multiplanar imaging capability provides greater accuracy and ease in examination than CT, which requires a change in patient orientation or time-consuming reformatted views from axial sections. The coronal plane in MR is also relatively unaffected by otherwise troublesome dental artifacts.

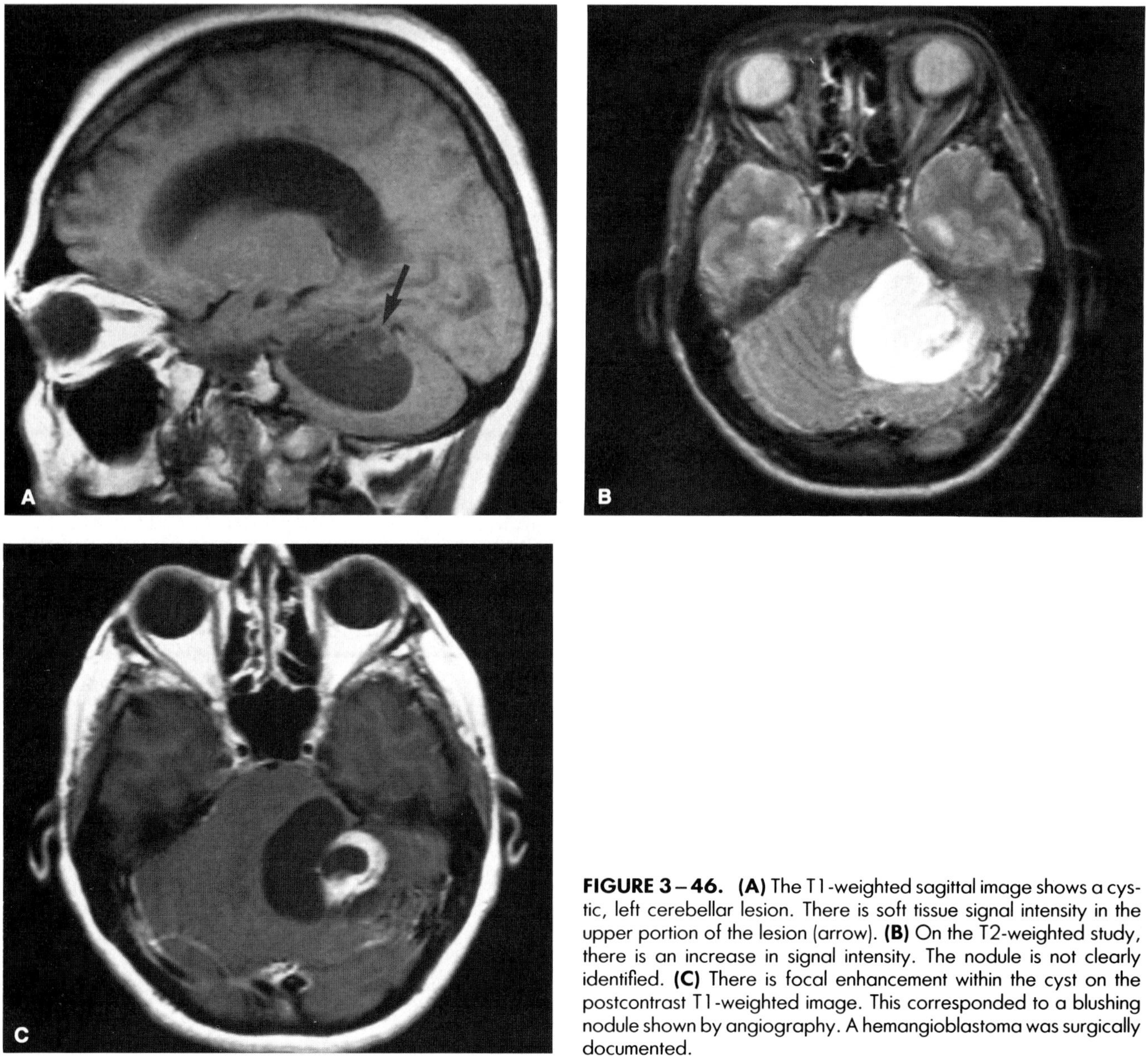

FIGURE 3–46. **(A)** The T1-weighted sagittal image shows a cystic, left cerebellar lesion. There is soft tissue signal intensity in the upper portion of the lesion (arrow). **(B)** On the T2-weighted study, there is an increase in signal intensity. The nodule is not clearly identified. **(C)** There is focal enhancement within the cyst on the postcontrast T1-weighted image. This corresponded to a blushing nodule shown by angiography. A hemangioblastoma was surgically documented.

The lack of ionizing radiation is another significant imaging advantage, because multiple or serial examinations may be required of younger patients with tumors that, although hormonally active, are predominantly benign. Patients with prolactin-secreting adenomas form one such group. Many studies may be necessary to evaluate recurrences after surgery or alteration in tumor size after bromocriptine therapy.

Perhaps the greatest assets of MRI are the lack of bone artifacts and superior resolution of soft tissue planes, which are important in imaging a small anatomic region situated in the dense skull base. This allows clearer distinction of the normal anatomic structures, particularly of the cavernous sinus with its internal carotid artery and cranial nerves. Also intrinsic abnormalities within the pituitary can be separated from extrinsic abnormalities. CT often has difficulty in such distinctions, as in the case of parasellar aneurysms that may mimic an intrasellar tumor. This abnormality is easily characterized by MRI (Fig. 3–47).

The identification and characterization of lesions in this region require 3-mm or less thin-section imaging. With further technologic developments, slice widths may be reduced; 3D imaging with the gradient-echo technique provides truly contiguous sections with slice widths as small as 1 mm.[52] Images generated with this technique can be reformatted in multiple planes, providing diagnostic quality images with excellent demonstration of the anatomy and abnormalities, particularly after contrast enhancement (Fig. 3–48). With this type of imaging, TEs must remain short (≤8 msec) or "blow-out" artifacts from

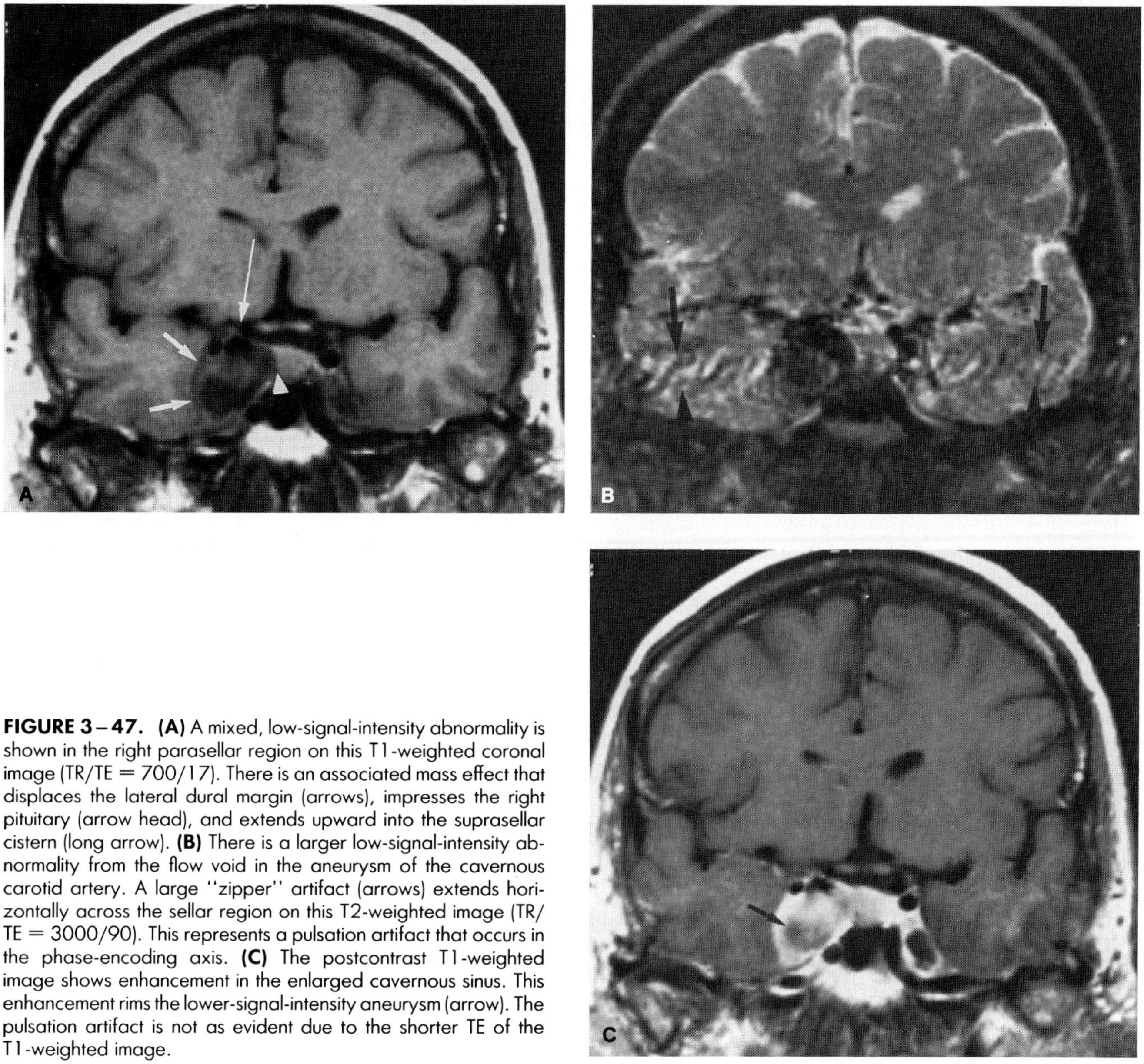

FIGURE 3–47. **(A)** A mixed, low-signal-intensity abnormality is shown in the right parasellar region on this T1-weighted coronal image (TR/TE = 700/17). There is an associated mass effect that displaces the lateral dural margin (arrows), impresses the right pituitary (arrow head), and extends upward into the suprasellar cistern (long arrow). **(B)** There is a larger low-signal-intensity abnormality from the flow void in the aneurysm of the cavernous carotid artery. A large "zipper" artifact (arrows) extends horizontally across the sellar region on this T2-weighted image (TR/TE = 3000/90). This represents a pulsation artifact that occurs in the phase-encoding axis. **(C)** The postcontrast T1-weighted image shows enhancement in the enlarged cavernous sinus. This enhancement rims the lower-signal-intensity aneurysm (arrow). The pulsation artifact is not as evident due to the shorter TE of the T1-weighted image.

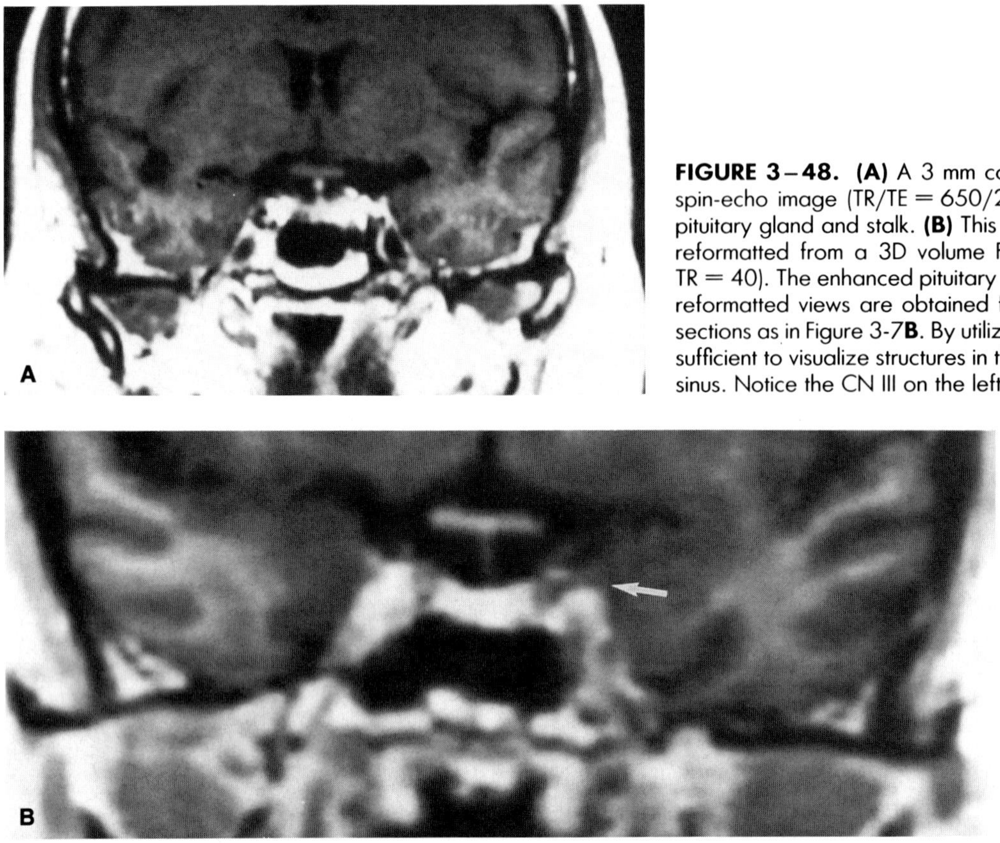

FIGURE 3–48. (A) A 3 mm coronal postcontrast T1-weighted spin-echo image (TR/TE = 650/20) shows a normally enhanced pituitary gland and stalk. **(B)** This postcontrast coronal image was reformatted from a 3D volume FLASH acquisition (50°, TE = 8, TR = 40). The enhanced pituitary gland is better seen because the reformatted views are obtained from 127 truly contiguous 1-mm sections as in Figure 3-7**B**. By utilizing a thinner section, resolution is sufficient to visualize structures in the contrast-enhanced cavernous sinus. Notice the CN III on the left (arrow).

magnetic susceptibility effects will obscure the gland.[52]

There is considerable CSF motion in the suprasellar cistern, necessitating T2-weighted images with cardiac gating or gradient suppression of CSF motion. Without these motion-suppression techniques, considerable dephasing artifacts may be superimposed on the pituitary, and areas of increased signal intensity may be obscured or falsely diagnosed. T2-weighted images are most useful in the characterization of areas of necrosis, cystic change, and areas of increased signal intensity on T1-weighted images.

Necrotic and cystic areas within pituitary tumors show decreased signal intensity on T1-weighted images, with cystic changes generally exhibiting smoother margins (Fig. 3–49). On T2-weighted images, there is increased signal intensity due to fluid or cellular debris.

Lesions that show increased signal intensity on T1-weighted images contain subacute hemorrhage or have a high lipid content, such as craniopharyngiomas or prolactinomas (Fig. 3–50). A hemorrhagic lesion (extracellular methemoglobin) shows an increase in signal intensity on T2-weighted images (Fig. 3–51), but a lesion with a high lipid content shows a decrease in signal intensity on T2-weighted images (Fig. 3–50). Those abnormalities that contain a combination of hemorrhage and fat show signal intensity changes of the major component. Lesions that show a balance of these two components have been described in other tumors.[53] These show decreased signal intensity on both T1-weighted and T2-weighted images.

With the exception of these changes, most pituitary abnormalities are characterized with T1-weighted images before and after contrast administration. Most current imaging protocols use precontrast thin-section T2-weighted coronal or sagittal images and T1-weighted sagittal and coronal images before and after contrast administration. With further experience, T2-weighted sequences may be shown to be noncontributory, unless there are signal intensity changes on the T1-weighted image that require further definition.

Pituitary and parasellar region abnormalities are similar to other extra-axial lesions in their lack of a BBB.[4,10,12] Abnormalities are identified by the greater enhancement of normal adjacent structures, as in the case of many microadenomas (Fig. 3–49), or because

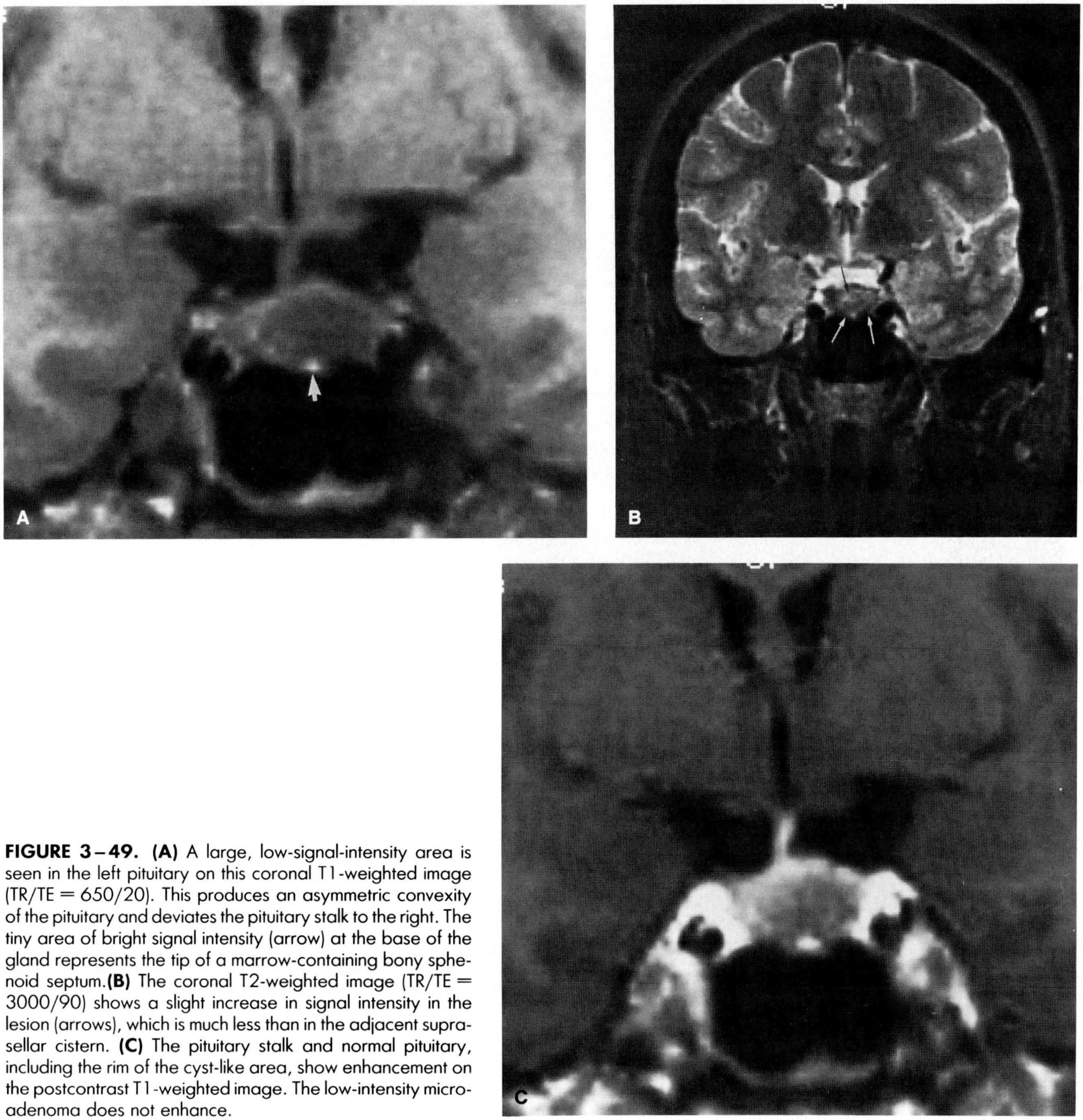

FIGURE 3–49. (A) A large, low-signal-intensity area is seen in the left pituitary on this coronal T1-weighted image (TR/TE = 650/20). This produces an asymmetric convexity of the pituitary and deviates the pituitary stalk to the right. The tiny area of bright signal intensity (arrow) at the base of the gland represents the tip of a marrow-containing bony sphenoid septum. **(B)** The coronal T2-weighted image (TR/TE = 3000/90) shows a slight increase in signal intensity in the lesion (arrows), which is much less than in the adjacent suprasellar cistern. **(C)** The pituitary stalk and normal pituitary, including the rim of the cyst-like area, show enhancement on the postcontrast T1-weighted image. The low-intensity microadenoma does not enhance.

the lesions that enhance do so due to inherent tumor vascularity, as in the case of macroadenomas (Fig. 3–52).

Normal Pituitary

The size of the normal pituitary gland can vary widely. The upper limit of normal is generally around 10 mm in height. During puberty and in the early child-bearing years, this may increase by several millimeters, and a gland of 12 mm may not be considered abnormal. The configuration also varies; the upper surface may be flat, concave, or convex in the midline (Figs. 3–53 and 3–54).[54]

T1-weighted images provide excellent anatomic definition. In the coronal plane, the pituitary is localized as a soft tissue signal intensity structure lying between the rounded areas of signal void from the

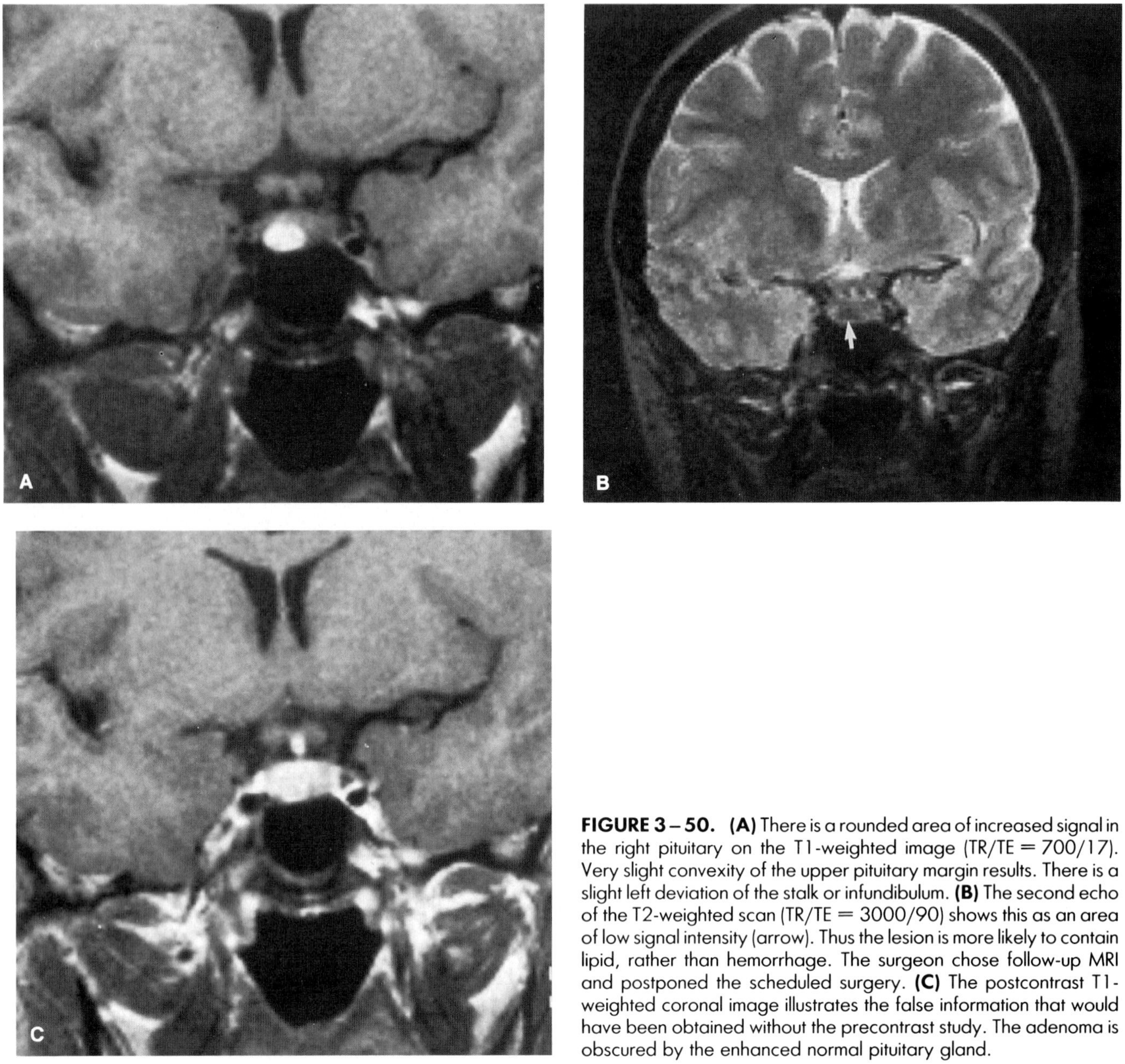

FIGURE 3–50. (A) There is a rounded area of increased signal in the right pituitary on the T1-weighted image (TR/TE = 700/17). Very slight convexity of the upper pituitary margin results. There is a slight left deviation of the stalk or infundibulum. **(B)** The second echo of the T2-weighted scan (TR/TE = 3000/90) shows this as an area of low signal intensity (arrow). Thus the lesion is more likely to contain lipid, rather than hemorrhage. The surgeon chose follow-up MRI and postponed the scheduled surgery. **(C)** The postcontrast T1-weighted coronal image illustrates the false information that would have been obtained without the precontrast study. The adenoma is obscured by the enhanced normal pituitary gland.

internal carotid arteries. The signal intensity of the gland is similar to the white matter of brain (Fig. 3–53). In the sagittal plane, the anterior and posterior lobes of the pituitary can be distinguished by high signal intensity in the posterior lobe.[55] This signal intensity change has been attributed to lipid metabolism of the posterior pituitary, and the degree depends on metabolic activity. This is separate from the fat in the marrow of the dorsum sellae. With higher field strengths, a chemical shift artifact may be interposed between the pituitary gland and bone marrow as a curvilinear area of low signal intensity (Fig. 3–54).[56] Frequently, there is a normal area of increased signal intensity on T1-weighted images that occurs at the base of the pituitary. This may be mistaken for an abnormality, such as a hemorrhagic microadenoma, but it actually represents fatty marrow in the upper extreme of a sphenoid sinus septum (Fig. 3–49).

The optic chiasm and pituitary stalk are outlined by the low-signal-intensity CSF in the suprasellar cistern on T1 weighted images. These structures are easy to identify in both the sagittal and coronal planes (Figs. 3–53 and 3–54). The coronal plane is more useful in assessing gland symmetry. The cavernous sinus, with the ICA, CN III through VI and lateral dural margin, is also easier to evaluate in the coronal plane (Fig.

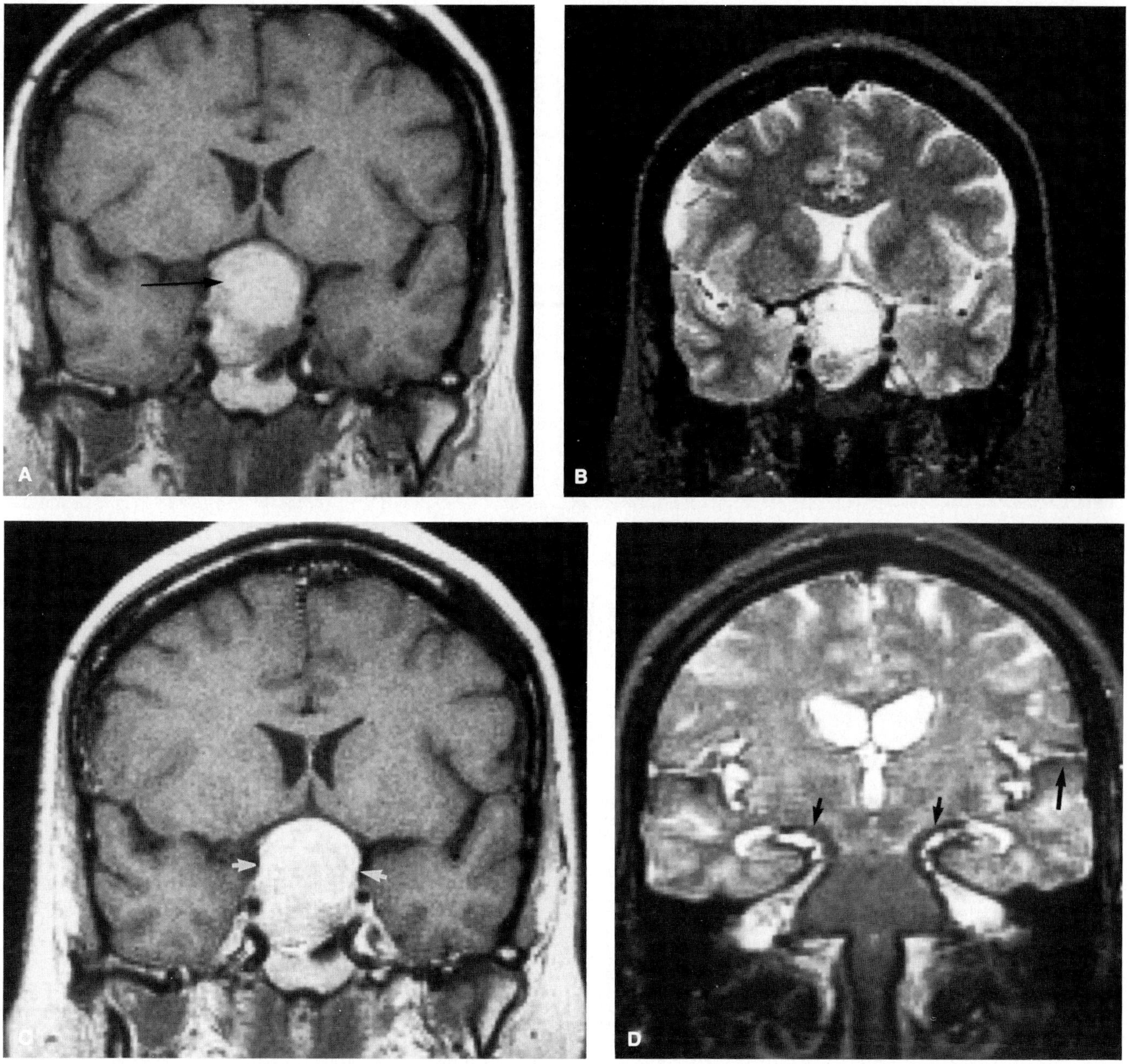

FIGURE 3–51. **(A)** There is a large macroadenoma of the pituitary, with draping of optic chiasm over the upper convexity of the mass. There is an increase in signal intensity in several areas, but it is most intense in the dome (arrow) of the mass (T1-weighted image). **(B)** Increase in signal intensity occurs in the same regions on the T2-weighted image (TR/TE = 3000/90). This is consistent with subacute hemorrhage, which was surgically documented. **(C)** The postcontrast T1-weighted image (TR/TE = 700/17) demonstrated enhancement, which obscures the underlying pathology. The smooth displacement of the carotid arteries that occurs in macroadenomas is better shown after enhancement (arrows). **(D)** This T2-weighted coronal image (TR/TE = 3000/90) was obtained from a pituitary study in another patient with pituitary apoplexy and subarachnoid hemorrhage several months before this scan. Notice the black or low-signal outlining the subarachnoid space. This represents superficial hemosiderin deposition from previous hemorrhage (arrows).

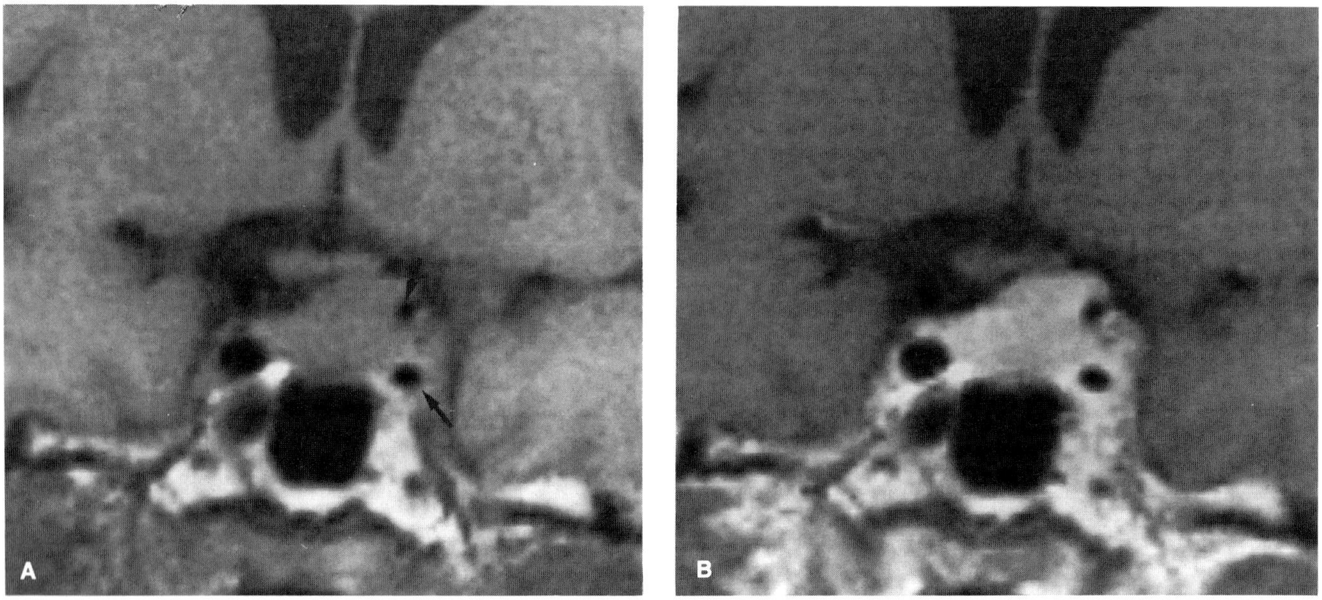

FIGURE 3–52. (A) A coronal precontrast T1-weighted image (TR/TE = 650/20) shows a macroadenoma of the pituitary. The upper margin abuts the optic chiasm on the left. There is lateral extension of the tumor into the left cavernous sinus, evident from the narrowing of the internal carotid artery and displacement (arrows). **(B)** There is diffuse enhancement of the macroadenoma on the postcontrast T1-weighted coronal scan. The arterial encasement is well defined. The thinning of the sellar floor and downward extension of the tumor into the sphenoid sinus are better seen with contrast enhancement.

3–53). The sagittal plane confirms the gland configuration and the anterior-posterior dimension of the sella turcica (Fig. 3–54).

On T2-weighted images, there is little or no signal intensity change within the gland, which remains isointense with white matter.[54] The CSF in the suprasellar cistern is bright. The low signal intensity of the lateral dural margin of the cavernous sinus is better defined than on T1-weighted images (Fig. 3–53B,C).

With MR contrast agents, the pituitary gland, stalk, and cavernous sinus show excellent enhancement. It is the intense enhancement of these normal structures that greatly facilitates the diagnosis of pituitary and parasellar pathology (Figs. 3–53D and 3–54C).

Prolactin-Secreting Microadenomas

Microadenomas are small (<10 mm) pituitary tumors that come to early clinical attention due to the secretion of prolactin, which produces symptoms of infertility, amenorrhea, and galactorrhea in women and galactorrhea and impotence in men. A clinically silent nonsecretory microadenoma called a null cell adenoma is found frequently at autopsy (22.5–45 %) and is being detected with increasing frequency by MRI.[57]

Prolactinomas produce some characteristic changes: focal asymmetric gland convexity, displacement of the pituitary stalk to the contralateral side, and an area of low signal intensity on T1 weighted scans, unless there is associated hemorrhage (Figs. 3–49 and 3–55). Any two of these changes may indicate a tumor.

T2-weighted sequences may show a microadenoma as an area of hypointensity, an area of increased signal intensity (Figs. 3–49 and 3–55), or an area of isointensity that can be surrounded by a rim of increased signal intensity. T2-weighted sequences are also useful in demonstrating sphenoid sinus septations before surgery.

With thin-section, high-resolution imaging, the evaluation of these tumors by MRI (without contrast) is more accurate than by CT. Studies comparing these imaging modalities were performed before the availability of MR contrast agents.[57]

Gd DTPA is useful in diagnosing microadenomas. The normal gland and stalk usually show more intense enhancement than an adenoma (Fig. 3–49). This pattern of enhancement appears to be more common than that in which there is greater enhancement of the microadenoma relative to the pituitary gland (Fig. 3–55). Another enhancement pattern occurs in

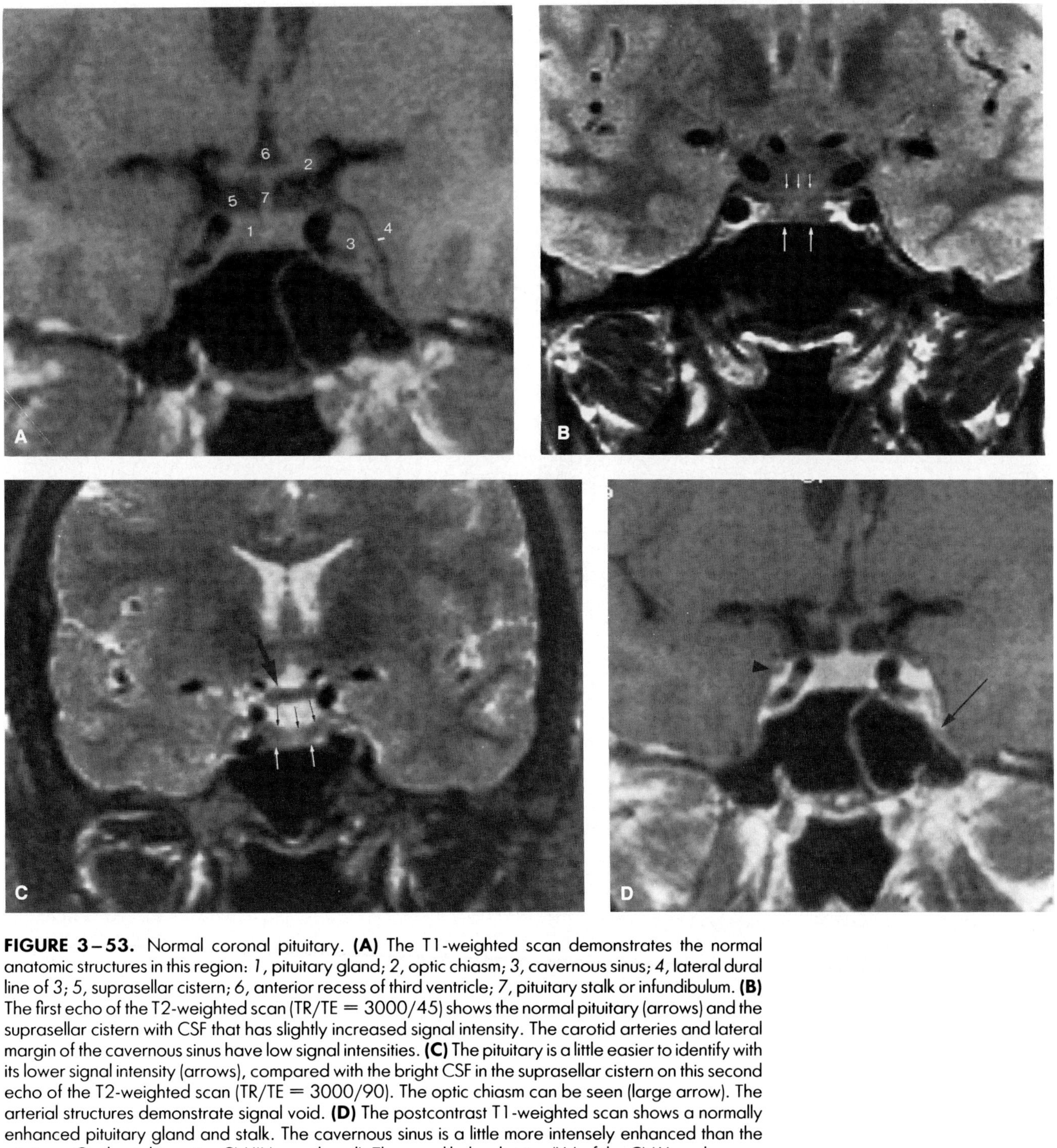

FIGURE 3–53. Normal coronal pituitary. **(A)** The T1-weighted scan demonstrates the normal anatomic structures in this region: *1*, pituitary gland; *2*, optic chiasm; *3*, cavernous sinus; *4*, lateral dural line of *3*; *5*, suprasellar cistern; *6*, anterior recess of third ventricle; *7*, pituitary stalk or infundibulum. **(B)** The first echo of the T2-weighted scan (TR/TE = 3000/45) shows the normal pituitary (arrows) and the suprasellar cistern with CSF that has slightly increased signal intensity. The carotid arteries and lateral margin of the cavernous sinus have low signal intensities. **(C)** The pituitary is a little easier to identify with its lower signal intensity (arrows), compared with the bright CSF in the suprasellar cistern on this second echo of the T2-weighted scan (TR/TE = 3000/90). The optic chiasm can be seen (large arrow). The arterial structures demonstrate signal void. **(D)** The postcontrast T1-weighted scan shows a normally enhanced pituitary gland and stalk. The cavernous sinus is a little more intensely enhanced than the pituitary. On the right, notice CN III (arrowhead). The mandibular division (V_3) of the CN V can be seen extending through the foramen ovale on the left (arrows).

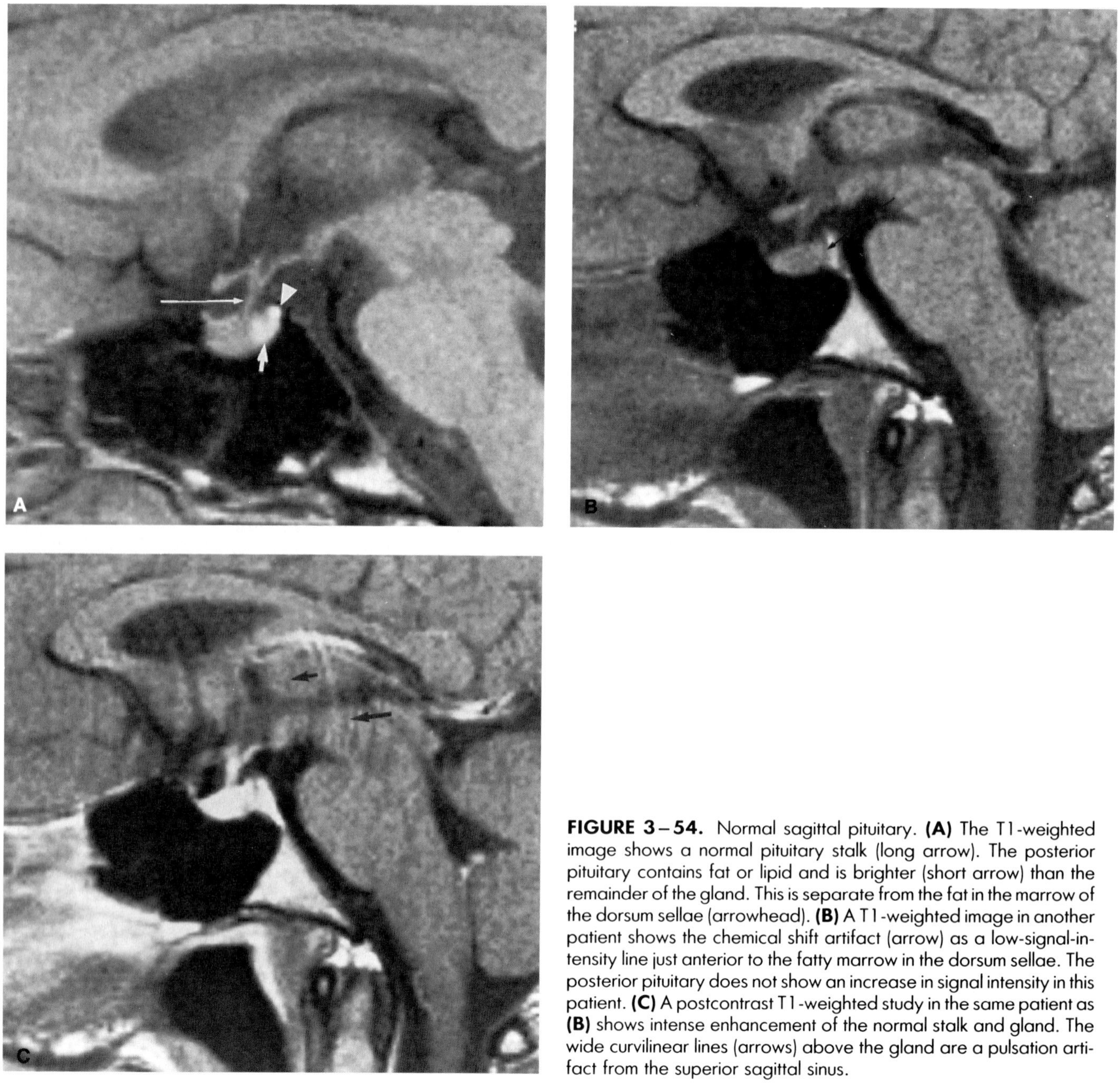

FIGURE 3–54. Normal sagittal pituitary. **(A)** The T1-weighted image shows a normal pituitary stalk (long arrow). The posterior pituitary contains fat or lipid and is brighter (short arrow) than the remainder of the gland. This is separate from the fat in the marrow of the dorsum sellae (arrowhead). **(B)** A T1-weighted image in another patient shows the chemical shift artifact (arrow) as a low-signal-intensity line just anterior to the fatty marrow in the dorsum sellae. The posterior pituitary does not show an increase in signal intensity in this patient. **(C)** A postcontrast T1-weighted study in the same patient as **(B)** shows intense enhancement of the normal stalk and gland. The wide curvilinear lines (arrows) above the gland are a pulsation artifact from the superior sagittal sinus.

some tumors that are isointense with the remainder of the gland before contrast and become hypointense after contrast (Fig. 3–56).

Cushing's Adenoma

Cushing syndrome is frequently (60%) caused by ACTH-producing adenomas of the pituitary. The remainder of these tumors arise in the adrenal glands or in ectopic sites, such as oat cell carcinomas of the lung. Most (97%) of the adrenal tumors are easily diagnosed by CT. However, the distinction of pituitary from ectopic adenomas is often difficult by imaging and clinical means.[58] Enhanced MR scans may be pivotal. These tumors show a wide spectrum of presentations on CT scans, perhaps more than any other pituitary-origin neoplasm. The emotional and physical changes (i.e., weight gain, hirsutism, moon facies) that occur because of excess cortisol production usually brings these tumors to clinical attention while they are still small, although large cystic tumors can also occur.[54]

The smaller adenomas may vary in size, attenua-

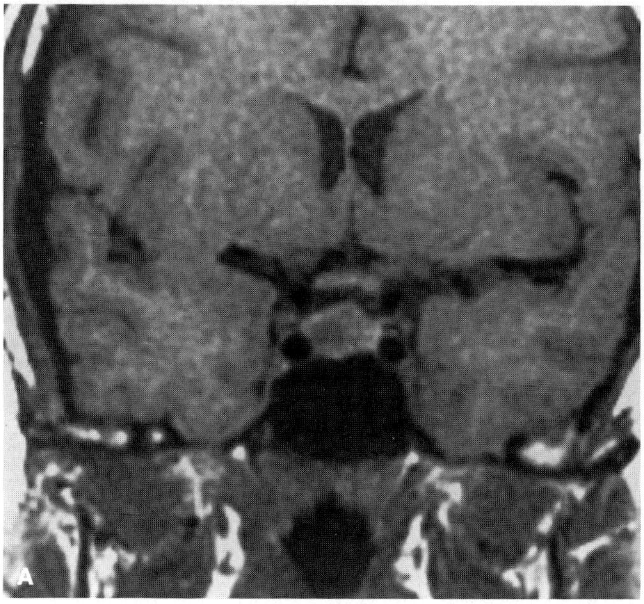

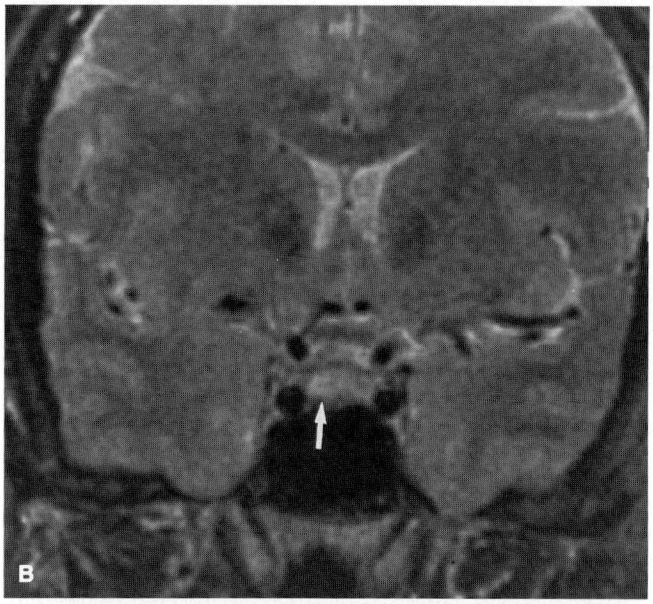

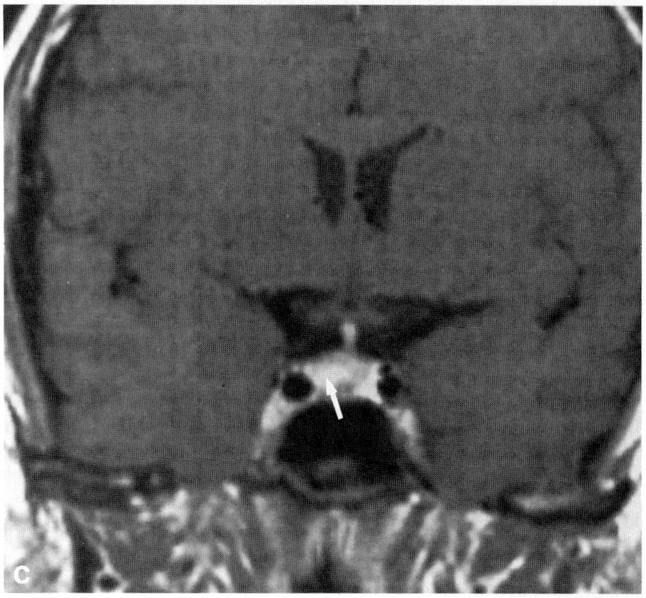

FIGURE 3–55. **(A)** There is a low-signal-intensity, large microadenoma in the right pituitary on this T1-weighted coronal image (TR/TE = 650/20). **(B)** The first echo of the T2-weighted scan shows the adenoma as an area of increased signal (arrow). **(C)** After contrast, a portion of the adenoma shows intense enhancement (arrow) on the T1-weighted image. This is a more unusual pattern because most adenomas remain hypointense after contrast, as in Figure 3-49.

tion characteristics, and degree of enhancement on CT. The most diagnostically troublesome feature is that as many as 70% are not identified because of their small size or lack of enhancement. The pre-surgical localization in these cases has relied on more invasive and technically difficult angiographic procedures, such as petrosal vein sampling.[54]

Due to the relative rarity of this tumor, MR studies to date are limited. Early investigations at low field strengths showed an 83% detection rate with MR contrast agents.[58] The tumors in this series showed an early relative hypointensity with respect to the normally enhancing pituitary gland (Fig. 3–56). This pattern was reversed with delayed imaging at 55 minutes after contrast injection, showing more intense enhancement of the adenoma and diminishing contrast in the pituitary. In a smaller series performed at 1.5 T using thin-section contrast-enhanced imaging, all the adenomas were identified, compared with 40% identified by CT. A target sign of enhancement was reported in the study.[59]

A detection rate of 80 to 100% by MRI represents significant strides in the diagnosis of this tumor. The accuracy and detection rate of MRI today for these tumors awaits further investigation because of many recent technical improvements.

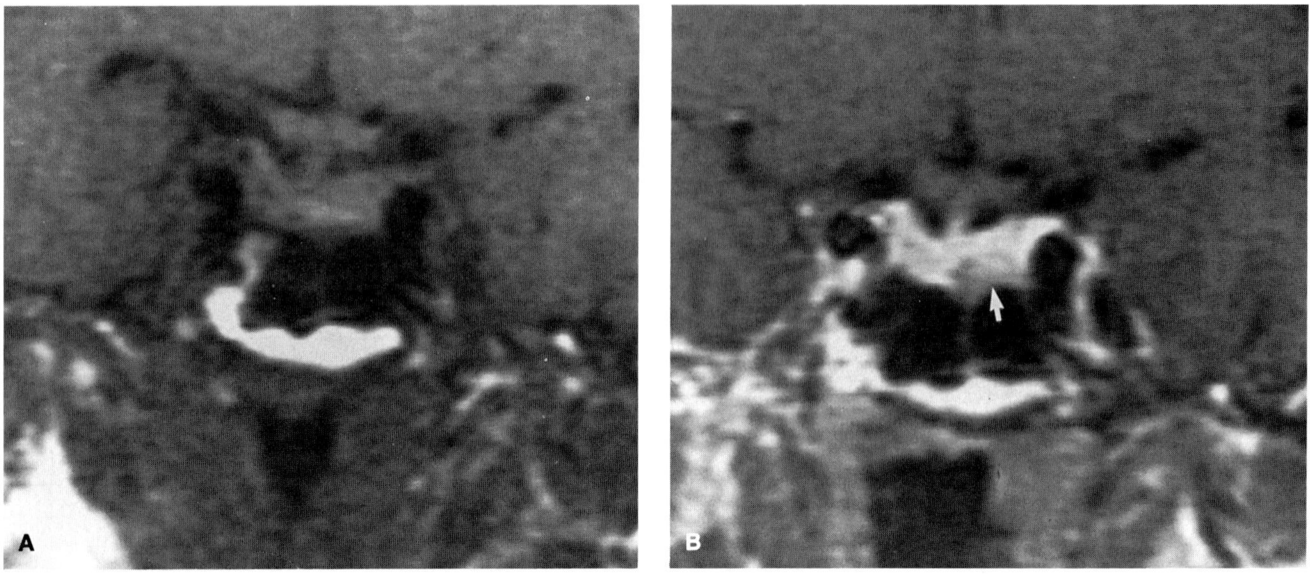

FIGURE 3–56. **(A)** The coronal precontrast T1-weighted image (TR/TE = 500/20) shows no significant abnormality in the pituitary signal intensity. **(B)** A diminished area of signal intensity is noted on the T1-weighted postcontrast image on the left side of the pituitary gland (arrow). The patient had clinical symptoms of Cushing's disease.

Growth Hormone Tumors

Adenomas producing human growth hormone (HGH) usually come to the attention of the clinician early in their course due to the marked alteration in the patient's body habitus. HGH adenomas are the least common of the microadenomas, and the descriptions of CT imaging changes vary. The enhancement patterns tend to be more heterogeneous and less consistently hypodense than prolactin-secreting adenomas and may occasionally go unrecognized.[60]

There are few MR descriptions of this tumor due to its relative rarity. The distinction from other types of hormonally active tumors may be difficult (Fig. 3–57), but MRI, particularly with contrast, offers advantages over CT for improved lesion detection, visualization, and characterization.

Macroadenomas

Large pituitary adenomas are rarely a diagnostic dilemma for CT or MRI. These bulky tumors are usually hormonally inactive, with only a few tumors secreting prolactin. Because of the superior resolution of soft tissue planes, MRI offers the advantage of clearer assessment of suprasellar or lateral temporal extension. The changes involving the cavernous sinus are often those of smooth displacement (Fig. 3–58), but some tumors may behave in a fashion similar to the prolactin-secreting microadenoma and invade the cavernous sinus (Fig. 3–52), with secondary changes that suggest arterial encasement.

These tumors are usually isointense with respect to white matter on T1-weighted images unless there is associated hemorrhage.[54,61] Subacute hemorrhage is better demonstrated by MRI than CT in most primary tumors. Pituitary hemorrhage appears to be more common than indicated by CT or clinical criteria. Smaller areas of pituitary hemorrhage may be accompanied by no more than a severe headache and may not proceed to more severe neurologic symptoms, as indicated by the term pituitary apoplexy (Fig. 3–51). Classically, pituitary apoplexy produces a sudden alteration in mental status occasionally accompanied by blindness due to hemorrhage into the optic chiasm. With MRI, smaller areas of hemorrhage are being recognized with less obvious clinical symptoms. The hemorrhage usually is confined within the tumor and is common after radiation therapy.

On T2-weighted images, macroadenomas generally show little signal intensity change unless there is associated necrosis (Fig. 3–58).[54] If there is significant necrosis or liquefaction, the macroadenoma may be confused with a craniopharyangioma, which usually shows an increased signal intensity on T2-weighted images. Macroadenomas more frequently produce a

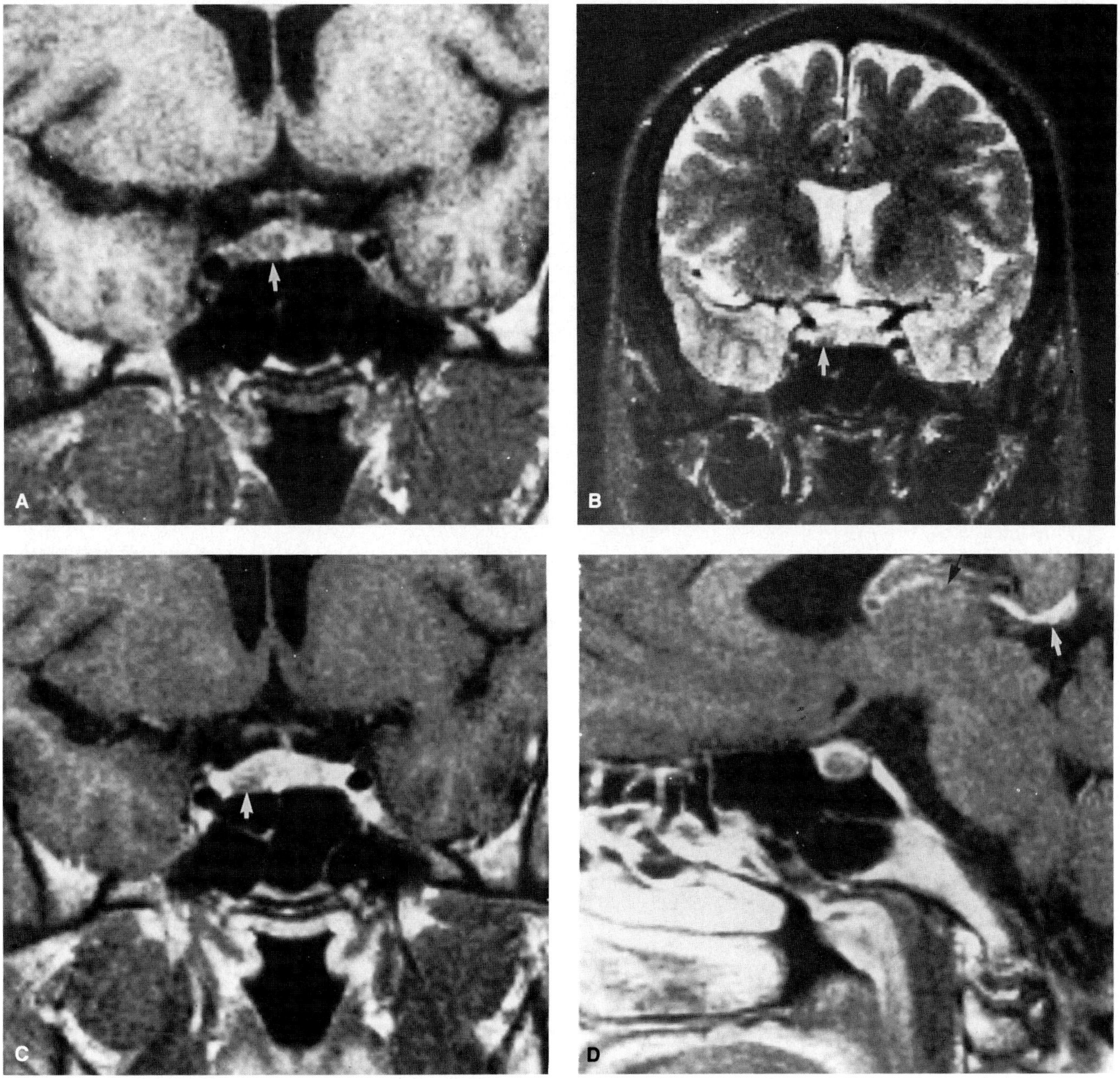

FIGURE 3–57. **(A)** There is a small area of slightly diminished signal intensity (arrow) in the right pituitary in this patient with elevated growth hormone assays. The gland shows a slight upward convexity on the right and deviation of the stalk to the left on this T1-weighted coronal image (TR/TE = 700/17). **(B)** The T2-weighted coronal image (TR/TE = 3000/90) shows the adenoma as an area of diminished signal intensity (arrow). **(C)** The normal pituitary gland intensely enhances after contrast administration. The adenoma does not enhance. **(D)** The lack of enhancement of the adenoma is better shown on the sagittal T1-weighted scan. Notice the enhancement in the internal cerebral vein (black arrow) and the great vein of Galen (white arrow).

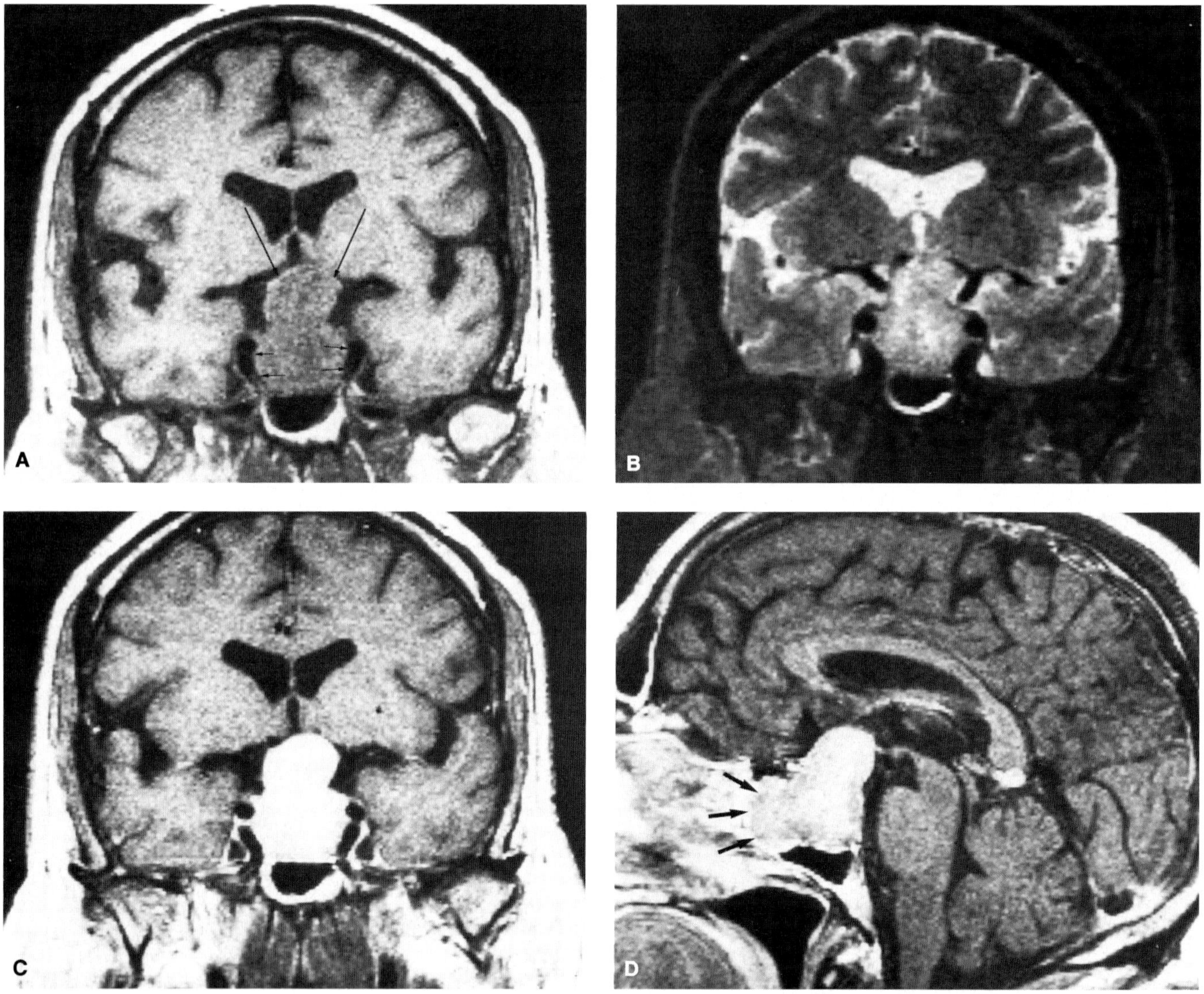

FIGURE 3–58. **(A)** There is a large, smoothly lobulated macroadenoma on the coronal T1-weighted image (TR/TE = 700/17). The optic chiasm is thin and draped over the lesion (long arrows). The carotid arteries show smooth lateral displacement (small arrows). **(B)** The tumor is mottled in signal intensity on the coronal T2-weighted image (TR/TE = 3000/90). There are no focal bright areas to suggest cystic or necrotic changes, which are not infrequent in these tumors. **(C)** The tumor demonstrates intense enhancement on the coronal post-contrast T1-weighted image. **(D)** The postcontrast sagittal image shows significant extension of the tumor into the sphenoid sinus (arrows).

greater degree of enlargement and expansion of the sella.

Contrast enhancement with Gd DTPA is usually excellent, unless there are areas of liquefaction or necrosis, which produces more patchy, less intense enhancement. Tumor margins are usually better seen with contrast. This may lead to demonstration of greater tumor extent than anticipated from the noncontrast exam.[62] The secondary changes involving the cavernous sinus are also a little easier to assess because the cavernous sinus enhances to a slightly greater extent (Fig. 3–58).

Craniopharyngioma

Craniopharyngiomas are benign, slow-growing tumors that arise from the epithelial rests of Rathke's pouch. There is a bimodal incidence peak occurring in children and young adults and in middle and older age groups. These tumors more commonly present in the suprasellar region.[62,63] As a result, the sella shows no enlargement. Occasionally, a component of the tumor may extend into the sella, and the sella may be slightly enlarged, but it does not attain the size of a pituitary-origin tumor of similar dimensions (Fig. 3–59).

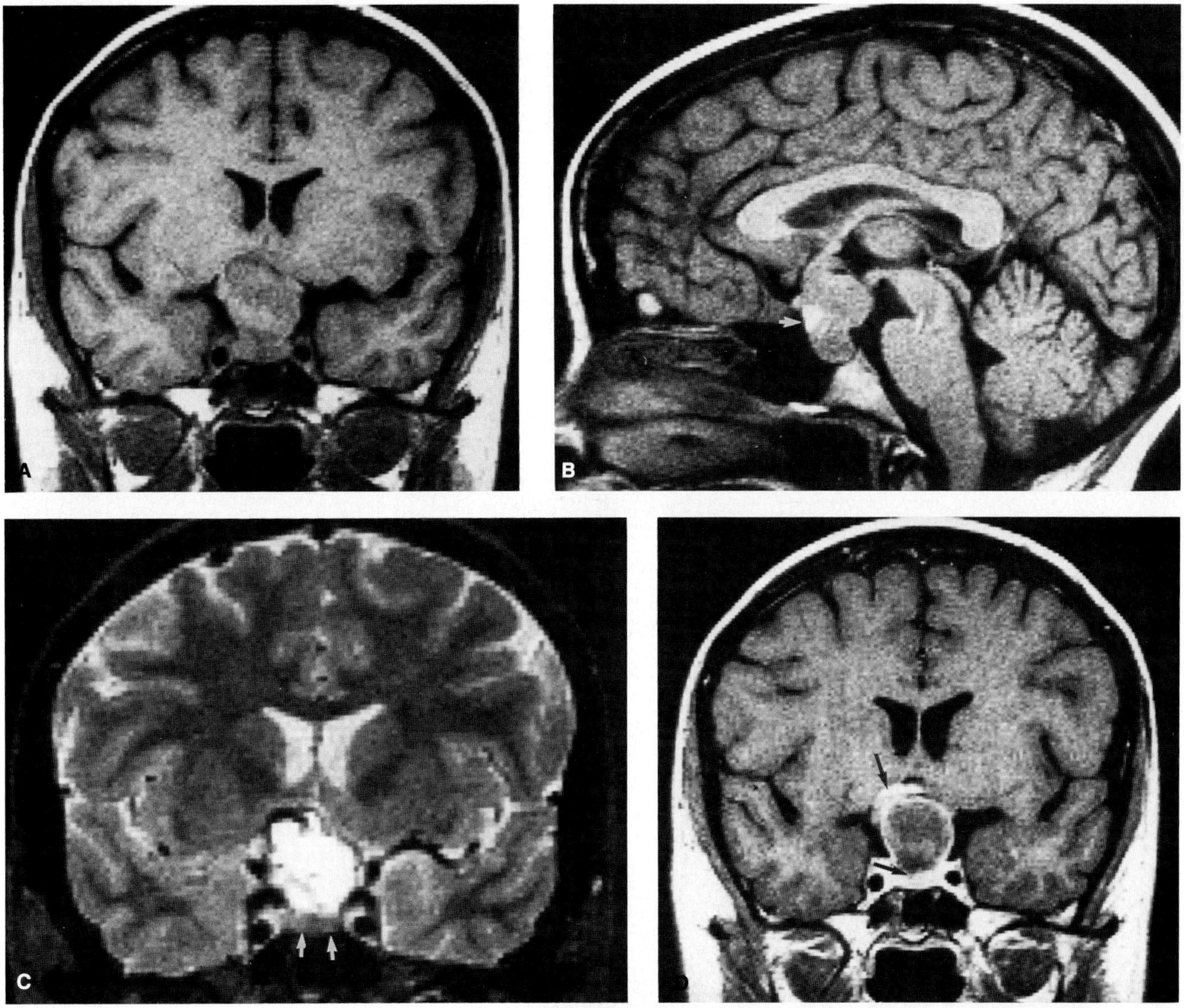

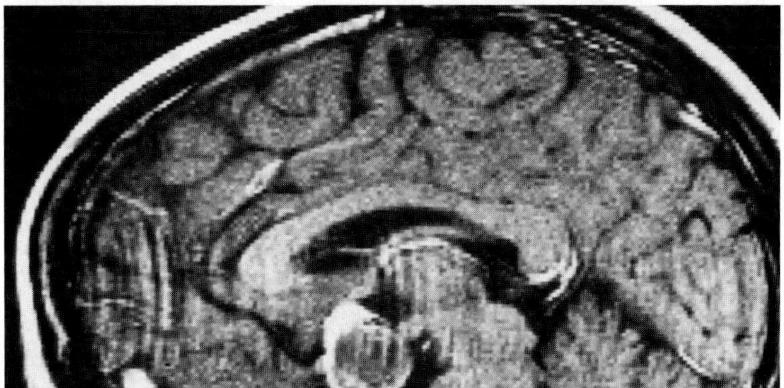

FIGURE 3–59. (A) There is a mottled-intensity suprasellar mass that extends upward and to the right on this coronal T1-weighted image (TR/TE = 700/17). **(B)** The sagittal image shows a high signal intensity region (arrow) that represents the more lipid component of the surgically proven craniopharyngioma. **(C)** The T2-weighted coronal image (TR/TE = 3000/90) shows typical, high signal intensity with a lobular tumor contour. Notice the different signals of the tumor and normal pituitary (arrows). **(D)** With enhancement of the tumor rim, the cystic component is accentuated. There is a small nodular area of enhancement along the upper rim (upper arrow). Notice the normally enhanced but slightly compressed pituitary (lower arrow). **(E)** The sagittal postcontrast study shows the cystic intrasellar extension, which is seen occasionally with craniopharyngiomas (arrows). The rim of enhanced tissue anterior to this cystic change is compressed normal pituitary. Notice the enhanced nodule and wide pulsation artifact.

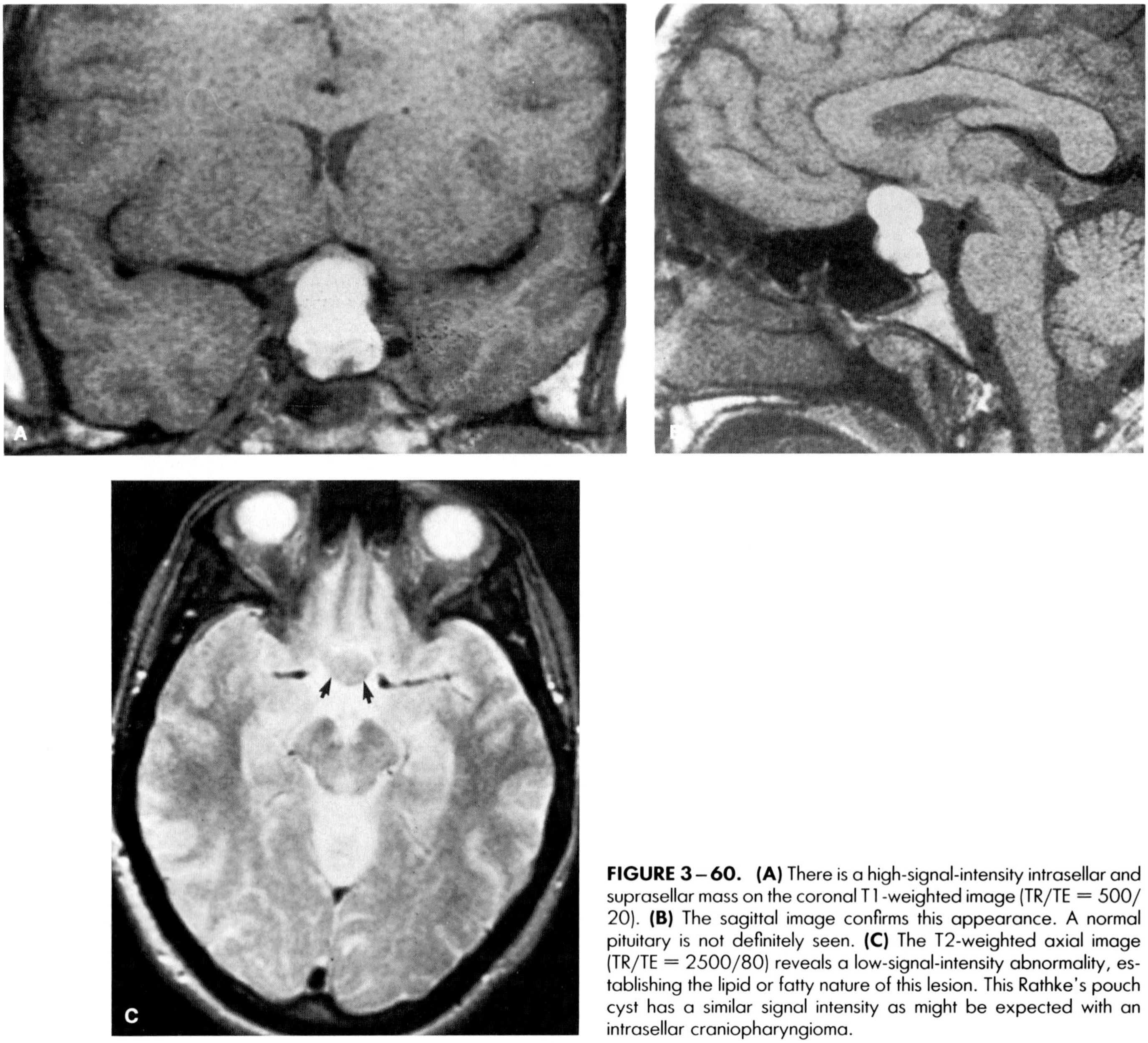

FIGURE 3–60. **(A)** There is a high-signal-intensity intrasellar and suprasellar mass on the coronal T1-weighted image (TR/TE = 500/20). **(B)** The sagittal image confirms this appearance. A normal pituitary is not definitely seen. **(C)** The T2-weighted axial image (TR/TE = 2500/80) reveals a low-signal-intensity abnormality, establishing the lipid or fatty nature of this lesion. This Rathke's pouch cyst has a similar signal intensity as might be expected with an intrasellar craniopharyngioma.

Rarely, these tumors may arise within the sella and be difficult to differentiate from Rathke's pouch cysts or prolactinomas on the basis of CT imaging changes (Fig. 3–60). Intrasellar craniopharyngiomas are generally smaller than those tumors that arise in the suprasellar region. They usually are accompanied by amenorrhea and galactorrhea due to low levels of prolactin.

On T1-weighted images, craniopharyngiomas are either low or high signal intensity. High-signal-intensity may be caused by either high cholesterol content or methemoglobin from previous hemorrhage.

There is usually a bright-signal-intensity change that occurs with these tumors on T2-weighted images. This is attributed to the protein or methemoglobin content which seems to predominate over the cholesterol component.[62] This occurs in both intrasellar and suprasellar tumors. The more diffuse increase in signal intensity may assist in differentiating these tumors from larger microadenomas with associated hemorrhage.

The suprasellar tumors may vary from smaller lobulated abnormalities to larger multicystic septated tumors. The margins are usually smooth and rounded. These tumors tend to be much larger and more calcified in pediatric patients. Although calcifications are not well visualized on spin-echo sequences, the rather characteristic bright signal intensity, along with the septations and lobulations, usually provides the diagnosis.

Enhancement with Gd DTPA is similar to CT enhancement.[54] An enhancing rim surrounds a low signal intensity or cystic abnormality (Fig. 3-59). There may be areas of nodular enhancement. If the enhancement is diffuse, it is usually less intense than other pituitary tumors. Delayed imaging by CT produces a more diffuse pattern. This should be the case for MR contrast enhancement, but this awaits confirmation.

Although the enhancing changes are not as characteristic or recognizable as those occurring on T2-weighted images, postcontrast MR studies clearly show the normally enhancing pituitary, establishing the suprasellar origin or partial intrasellar extension. With Gd DTPA, the suprasellar and lateral extension is better defined.[54] This is especially true in those tumors that may not be large enough to obliterate the suprasellar cistern. In this case, the signal intensity of the tumor blends with the signal intensity of the suprasellar cistern on T2-weighted studies.

Other Parasellar Tumors

MRI, especially if used in conjunction with contrast agents, has been particularly effective in visualizing and clearly localizing other parasellar lesions and in defining their relationship to important adjacent structures, such as the cavernous sinus, brain stem, and optic chiasm. These lesions include chordomas, hypothalamic gliomas, and meningiomas.[64] With the exception of the hypothalamic glioma, which shows variable enhancement, these tumors show excellent enhancement.

Because of their propensity for invading adjacent sinuses and encasing arterial structures, meningiomas produce special imaging problems, particularly in view of their variable delineation on T2-weighted images. In the parasellar region, these tumors generally require thin-section imaging for complete definition of involvement of the venous and arterial structures (Figs. 3-30 and 3-33). The other tumors may require the greater detail of imaging with thin sections because of the compact regional anatomy and proximity of crucial structures.

POSTOPERATIVE TUMOR EVALUATION

The evaluation of tumors that recur after surgery may be difficult by CT or MRI without contrast. Subtle mass effects and postsurgical encephalomalacia are difficult to assess (Fig. 3-61). Differentiation of encephalomalacia from edema associated with tumor recurrence is difficult or impossible on T2-weighted sequences because both cause an increase in signal intensity.[9]

T1-weighted images may show cystic, necrotic, or hemorrhagic involvement. There also may be degrees of mass effect or extension of low-signal-intensity changes into the corpus callosum that would be consistent with tumor recurrence (Fig. 3-6).

MRI enhancement with Gd DTPA is superior to CT contrast for diagnosing these abnormalities. One study demonstrated that 50% of postoperative tumor recurrences were primarily or more conclusively shown by MRI with contrast. This included definition of the tumor nidus and margin. MRI is being increasingly used in evaluating postoperative recurrences.[9]

The differentiation of tumor recurrence from radiation necrosis remains a diagnostic dilemma with MR, just as it is with CT. Whether significant differential features exist awaits investigation with a large series of patients, correlating dosages and radiation ports.

FURTHER APPLICATIONS

Further applications may include the labeling of antibodies with Gd for use as a tissue- or tumor-specific contrast agent. Experimental work has been performed with Gd-labeled antihuman T-cell monoclonal antibodies. This could have diagnostic clinical significance in the localization of CNS sanctuary sites of acute lymphoblastic and T-cell leukemia in childhood, allowing earlier therapy before presentation of neurologic symptoms. The possibility of developing other tissue-specific and tumor-specific compounds is an exciting prospect for more sophisticated and accurate diagnosis.[65]

ACKNOWLEDGEMENT

The authors thank Marjorie Hennessy for manuscript preparation and Mike Ciarmiello for his photographic illustrations.

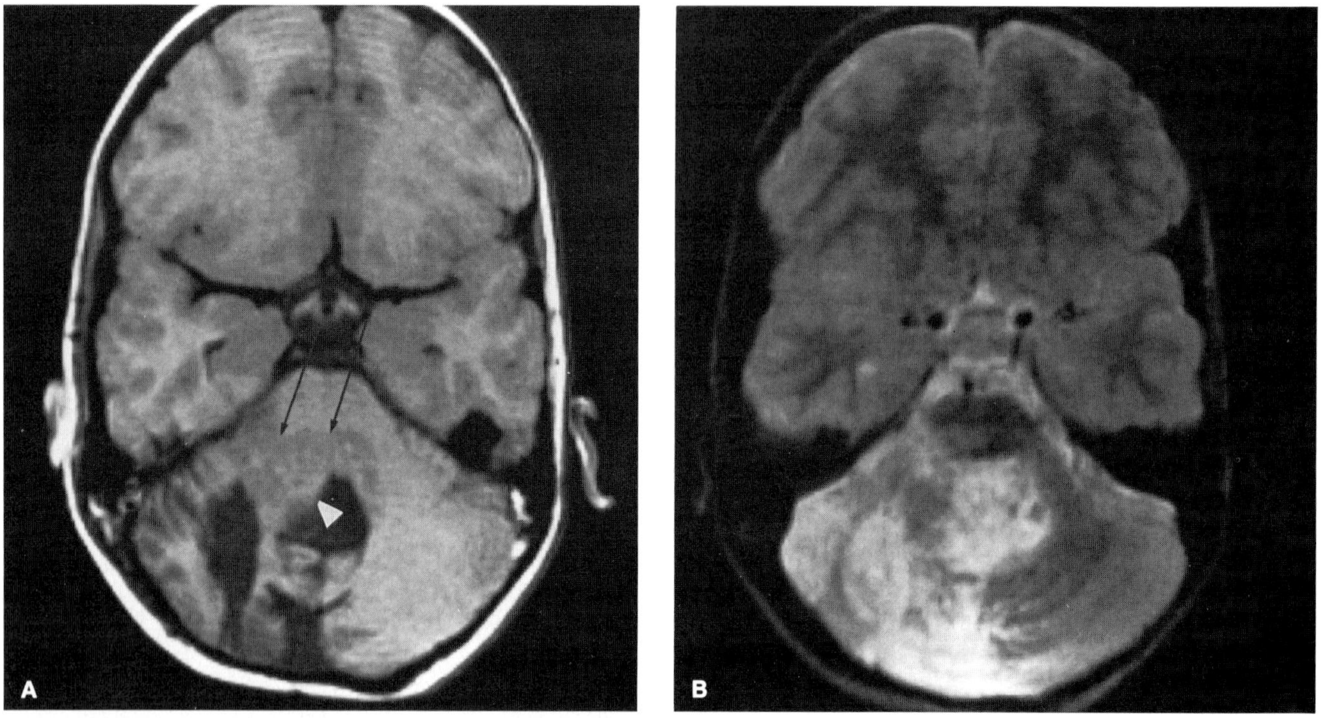

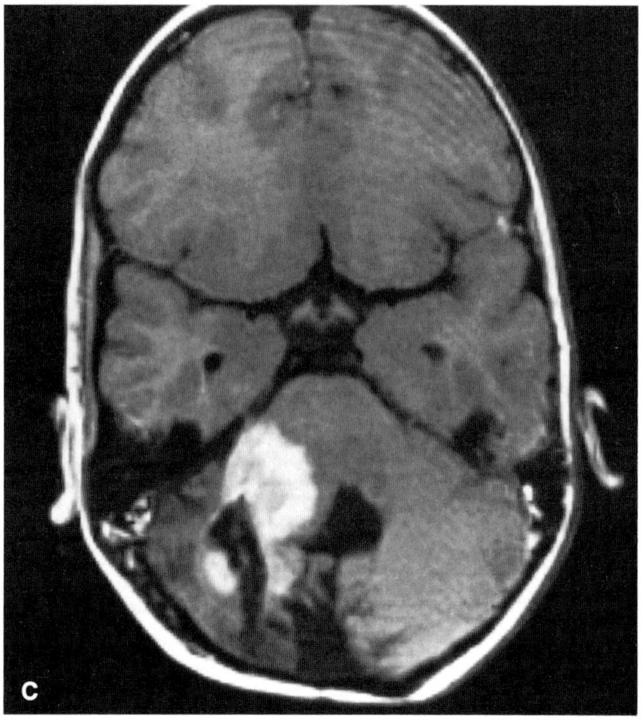

FIGURE 3–61. (A) The T1-weighted axial section (TR/TE = 650/20) shows an irregular area of low signal intensity in a postoperative cystic astrocytoma of the right cerebellum. There are vague areas of diminished signal intensity in the pons and brachium pontis (arrows). A slight mass effect effaces the fourth ventricle (arrowhead), which suggests tumor recurrence. **(B)** The T2-weighted image (TR/TE = 3000/90) is not helpful since postsurgical encephalomalacia and tumor have similar signal intensities. **(C)** The postcontrast T1-weighted image confirms the tumor recurrence, due to its enhancement, and shows a larger abnormality than would be suspected on the precontrast sequences.

REFERENCES

1. Brant-Zawadzki M, Badami JP, Mills C, et al. Primary intracranial tumor imaging: a comparison of magnetic resonance and CT. Radiology 1984;150:435.
2. Price AC, Runge VM, Allen JH, James AE, Jr. Primary glioma: diagnosis with magnetic resonance imaging. Comput Tomogr 1986;10:325.
3. Runge VM, Price AC, Kirshner HS, et al. The evaluation of multiple sclerosis by magnetic resonance imaging. AJR 1984;143:1015.
4. Felix R, Schorner W, Laniado M, et al. Brain tumors: MR imaging with gadolinium-DTPA. Radiology 1985;156:681.
5. Brant-Zawadzki M, Berry I, Asaki L, et al. Gd-DTPA in clinical MR of the brain: 1. Intraaxial lesions. AJR 1986;147:1223.
6. Brasch RC, Weinmann HJ, Wesby G: Contrast-enhanced NMR imaging: animal studies using gadolinium-DTPA complex. AJR 1984;142:625.
7. Weinmann HJ, Brasch RC, Press WR, Wesby GE. Characteristics of gadolinium-DTPA complex: a potential NMR contrast agent. AJR 1984;142:619.
8. Claussen C, Laniado M, Schorner W, et al. Gadolinium-DTPA in MR imaging of glioblastomas and intracranial metastases. AJNR 1985;6:669.
9. Price AC, Runge VM. Tumor imaging with Gd DTPA. In: Partain CL, ed. Magnetic resonance imaging. Philadelphia: WB Saunders, 1988.
10. Berger RK, Papke RA, Pojunas KW, et al. Benign extraaxial tumors: contrast enhancement with Gd DTPA. Radiology 1987;163:427.
11. Grossman RI, Gonzalez-Scarano F, Atlas S, et al. Multiple sclerosis: gadolinium enhancement in MR imaging. Radiology 1987;163:427.
12. Berry I, Brant-Zawadzki M, Asaki L, et al. Gd-DTPA in clinical MR of the brain: extraaxial lesions and normal structures. AJR 1986;147:1231.
13. Carr DN, Brown J, Bydder GM, et al. Gadolinium DTPA as a contrast agent in MRI: initial clinical experience in 20 patients. AJR 1984;143:215.
14. Lasser EC. Pretreatment with corticosteroids to prevent reactions to IV contrast materials: overview and implication. AJR 1988;150:257.
15. Lee DH, Fox AJ. Low-dose gadolinium enhancement—is it feasible? Presented at the 27th Annual Meeting of the American Society of Neuroradiology, March 1989, Orlando, FL.
16. Niendorf HP, Laniado M, Semmler W, et al. Dose administration of Gadolinium-DTPA in MR imaging of intracranial tumors. AJNR 1987;8:803.
17. Runge VM, Clanton JA, Price AC, et al. Evaluation of contrast enhanced MR imaging in a brain abscess model. AJNR 1985;6:139.
18. Butler AR, Passalagua AM, Berenstein A, Kricheff II. Contrast enhanced CT scan and radionuclide brain scan in supratentorial gliomas. AJR 1979;132:607.
19. Front D, Israel O, Kohn S, Nir I. The blood-tissue barrier of human brain tumors: correlation of scintigraphy and ultrastructure findings: concise communication. J Nucl Med 1984;25:461.
20. Butler AR, Horii SC, Krichiff II, et al. Computed tomography in astrocytomas: a statistical analysis of the parametria of malignancy and the positive contrast enhanced CT scan. Radiology 1978;129:433.
21. Runge VM, Price AC, Wehr CJ, et al. Contrast enhanced MRI: evaluation of a canine model of osmotic blood-brain-barrier disruption. Invest Radiol 1984;20:830.
22. Wolf GL, Joseph PM, Goldstein EJ. Optimal pulsing sequences for MR contrast agents. AJR 1986;147:367.
23. Price AC, Runge WM. Optimization of pulse sequences in Gd DTPA tumor enhanced MRI. In: Runge VM, Claussen C, Felix R, James AE, eds. Contrast agents in magnetic resonance imaging. New York: Excerpta Medica, 1986.
24. Runge VM, Wood ML, Kaufman D, Price AC. Gd DTPA future applications with advanced imaging techniques. Radiographics 1988;8:161.
25. Graif M, Bydder GM, Steiner RE, et al. Contrast-enhanced MR imaging of malignant brain tumors. AJNR 1985;6:855.
26. Runge VM, Wood ML, Kaufman DM: FLASH: Clinical three-dimensional magnetic resonance imaging. Radiographics 1988;8:947.
27. Schorner W, Laniado M, Niendorf HP, et al. Time-dependent changes in image contrast in brain tumors after Gd DTPA. AJNR 1986;7:1013.
28. Williams AL. Tumors. In: Williams AL, Haughton VM, eds. Cranial computed tomography: a comprehensive test. St. Louis: CV Mosby, 1985.
29. Drayer BP. Supratentorial tumors: MRI strategies. MRI Decisions 1987;1:3.
30. Johnsen PC, Hunt SJ, Drayer BP. Human cerebral gliomas: correlation of postmortem MR imaging on neuropathologic findings. Radiology 1988;170:211.
31. Runge VM, Schaible TF, Goldstein HA, et al. Gd DTPA—clinical efficacy. Radiographics 1988;8:147.
32. Lilja A, Bergstrom K, Spansare B, et al. Reliability of computed tomography in assessing histopathological features of malignant supratentorial gliomas. J Comput Assist Tomogr 1981;5:625.
33. Lee YY, Tassel PV. Intracranial oligodendrogliomas: imaging findings in 35 untreated cases. AJNR 1989;10:119.
34. Shuman WP, Griffin BR, Haynor DR, et al. The utility of MR in planning the radiation of oligodendrogliomas. AJR 1987;148:595.
35. Atlas SW, Grossman RI, Hackney DR, et al. Calcified intracranial lesions: detection with gradient-echo-acquisition rapid MR imaging. AJNR 1988;9:253.
36. Healy ME, Hesselink JR, Press GA, et al. Increased detection of intracranial metastases with intravenous Gd DTPA. Radiology 1987;165:619.
37. Russell EJ, Geremia GK, Johnson CE, et al. Multiple cerebral metastases: detectability with Gd DTPA-enhanced MR imaging. Radiology 1987;165:609.
38. Hayman LA, Evans RA, Hinck VC, et al. Delayed high dose contrast computed tomography: cranial neoplasms. Radiology 1980;136:677.
39. Sze G, Abramson A, Krol G, et al. Gadolinium-DTPA in the evaluation of intradural extramedullary spine disease. AJNR 1988;9:153.
40. Post MJD, Kursunoglu SJ, Hensley GT, et al. Cranial CT in acquired immunodeficiency syndrome: spectrum of disease and optimal contrast enhancement technique. AJR 1985;145:929.
41. Scotti G, Scialfa G, Landoni L. MR in the diagnosis of colloid cysts of the third ventricle. AJNR 1987;8:370.
42. Price AC, Runge V, Nelson KL. MR of meningiomas. MRI Decisions 1988;2:2.
43. Price AC, Runge VM, Nelson KL, et al. Gd-DTPA imaging of meningiomas. Radiology 1988;169:143.
44. Spagnoli MV, Goldberg HI, Grossman RI, et al. Intracranial meningiomas: high field strength MR imaging. Radiology 1986;161:369.
45. Elster AD, Venkata RC, Tucker NG, et al. Meningiomas: MR and histopathological features. Radiology 1989;170:857.
46. Zimmerman RD, Fleming CA, Saint-Louis LA, et al. Magnetic resonance imaging of meningiomas. AJNR 1985;6:149.
47. Nelson KL, Runge VM. Radiologic evaluation of acoustic neuromas. MRI Decisions 1987;1:31.
48. Pinto RS, Kircheff IJ, Bergeron RT, et al. Small acoustic neuromas: detection by high-resolution gas-CT cisternography. AJNR 1982;3:283.
49. Price AC, Runge VM, Carollo BR, et al. Contrast enhancement in the evaluation of cerebellopontine angle (CPA) lesions. Presented at the 27th Annual Meeting of the American Society of Neuroradiology, March 1989, Orlando, FL.
50. Yuk WTC, Barloon TJ, Jacoby CG, Schultz DH. MR of fourth-ventricular epidermoid tumors. AJNR 1988;9:794.
51. Randall CP, Collins AG, Young IR, et al. Nuclear magnetic

resonance imaging of the posterior fossa tumors. AJR 1983;141:489.

52. Price AC, Runge VM, Wood ML, Nelson KL. FLASH: Three-dimensional pituitary imaging with multiplanar reconstructions. Radiology 1988;169:520.

53. Dillon WP, Norman D, Newton T, et al. Intradural spinal cord-lesions: Gd-DTPA enhanced MR imaging. Radiology 1989;170:229.

54. Price AC, Runge VM, Allen JH. Pituitary and parasellar region. In: Partain CL, ed. Magnetic resonance imaging. Philadelphia: WB Saunders, 1988.

55. Sze G, Pardo F, Kucharczyk W, et al. The posterior pituitary gland: MR correlation with anatomy and function. Presented at the 25th Annual Meeting of the American Society of Neuroradiology, May 1987, New York, NY.

56. Mark L, Pech P, Daniels D, et al. The pituitary fossa: a correlative anatomic MR study. Radiology 1984;153:143.

57. Kulkarni MV, Lee KF, McArdle CB, et al. 1.5-T MR imaging of the pituitary microadenomas: technical considerations and CT correlation. AJNR 1988;9:5.

58. Saris SC, Patronas NJ, Doppman JL, et al. Cushing syndrome: pituitary CT scanning. Radiology 1987;162:775.

59. Khandhi A, Bello J, Hilal S, et al. Thin-section MR imaging of gadolinium enhanced pituitary microadenoma. Presented at the 6th Annual Meeting of the Society of Magnetic Resonance, August 1987, New York, NY.

60. Daniels DL. The sella and juxtasella region. In: Williams AL, Haughton VM, eds. Cranial computed tomography. St. Louis: CV Mosby, 1985.

61. Kucharczyk W, Davis DO, Kelly WM, et al. Pituitary adenomas: high resolution MR imaging at 1.5 T. Radiology 1986;161:761.

62. Pusey E, Kortman K, Flannigan B, et al. MR of craniopharyngioma: tumor delineation and characterization. AJR 1987;149:383.

63. Price AC, Runge VM, Allen JH, et al. Craniopharyngioma: correlation of high resolution CT and MRI. Presented at the 23rd Annual Meeting of the American Society of Neuroradiology, February 1985, New Orleans, LA.

64. Sze G, Ulchance LS, Brant-Zawadzki M, et al. Chordoma: MR imaging. Radiology 187;1988:166.

65. Kornguth SE, Turski PA, Perman WH, et al. Magnetic resonance imaging of gadolinium-labeled monoclonal antibody polymers directed at human T lymphocytes implanted in canine brain. J Neurosurg 1987;66:898.

4

Brain: Congenital

Stephen J. Robertson
Samuel M. Wolpert

Magnetic resonance imaging (MRI) has been established as an excellent modality for imaging structural abnormalities of the central nervous system associated with congenital anomalies. T1-weighted spin echo imaging precisely delineates the structural anatomy of the common congenital anomalies, with the T2-weighted spin echo image sequences only occasionally contributing information about the structural defects and their significant associated sequelae.[1] Contrast enhancement with Gd DTPA has little role in common congenital malformations, except for the tumors associated with the neurocutaneous syndromes, most commonly neurofibromatosis.

This chapter presents the MR features of common congenital malformations and reviews the recent literature concerning the normal myelination process within the brain.

NORMAL MYELINATION

MR offers a revolutionary tool for the radiologic evaluation of the patterns of myelination. Changes of myelination can be observed on T1-weighted and T2-weighted spin echo imaging to follow a predictable course. Myelination proceeds from the brain stem and ascends into the cerebrum and cerebellum. At birth, T1-weighted images should demonstrate myelination within the brain stem, middle cerebellar peduncles, cerebellar white matter, and the posterior limb of the internal capsule.[2] The appearance of normal white matter myelination on T1-weighted images is that of increased signal intensity or brightness in those areas that are myelinated. This corresponds to decreased water content, which is observed as increased signal intensity. T2-weighted images delineate these myelinated regions as areas of decreased signal intensity, reversing the pattern of intensities seen on T1-weighted images. This neonatal white matter pattern (in nonmyelinated brain) is the opposite of that seen with mature myelination (Fig. 4–1).[3]

The increased water content within the brain is the primary influence on the imaging characteristics of the neonatal brain. The increasing myelin constituent contributes less to the observed signal intensity. As myelination proceeds within the white matter, the signal intensity of water within brain is replaced with the mature adult pattern of higher signal intensity on T1-weighted images and lower signal intensity on T2-weighted images.[3] Barkovich, using imaging at 1.5 T, identified myelination changes earlier with T1-weighted imaging than T2-weighted imaging, because T1-weighted images are also influenced by the lipid component of the developing myelin sheaths. The T2-weighted images are dominated by the intense water signal. The contribution due to the lower signal intensity of myelin is negligible.[2]

Neonatal T2-weighted imaging demonstrates low intensity signal within the myelinated brain stem and cerebellar peduncles, but not within the cerebellar hemispheric white matter. The posterior limb of the internal capsule may also exhibit the adult pattern of replaced water signal intensity as myelination matures (Fig. 4–1). The variance in temporal maturation, as detected by T1-and T2-weighted imaging, reflects the predominant imaging effects of water on T2-weighted images. Myelination proceeds superiorly throughout the brain stem into the anterior limb of the internal capsule at 4 to 7 months (Fig. 4–2), and subsequently into the centrum semiovale by 7 to 11

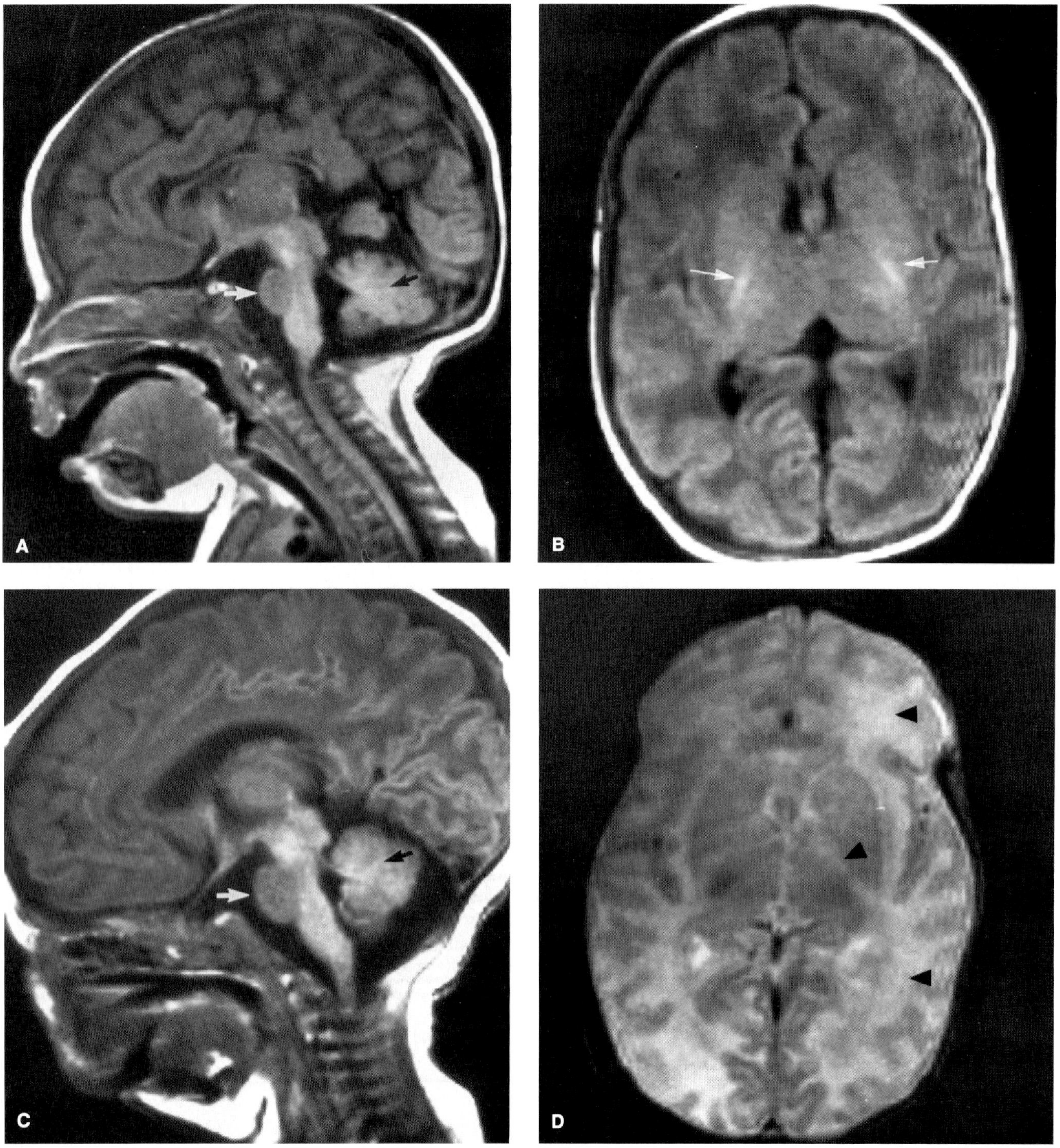

FIGURE 4–1. Normal neonatal myelination patterns in a 2-week-old girl and a 3-week-old boy. **(A)** Sagittal T1-weighted (TR/TE = 650/20), **(B)** axial T1-weighted (TR/TE = 650/20), **(C)** sagittal T1-weighted (TR/TE = 650/20), and **(D)** axial T2-weighted (TR/TE = 3000/90) images demonstrate the expected degree of maturation in the neonatal period. T1-weighted sequences demonstrate myelination as increased signal intensity within the brain stem, except for the belly of the pons (white arrow), and within the **(A,C)** cerebellar white matter (black arrow), **(B)** posterior limb of the internal capsule (small white arrows), and middle cerebellar peduncle. T2-weighted sequences image myelination as decreased signal intensity within the brain stem, and by 2 months, within the middle cerebellar peduncle and posterior portion of the posterior limb of the internal capsule. **(D)** The immature white matter appears as areas of high signal intensity (arrowheads).

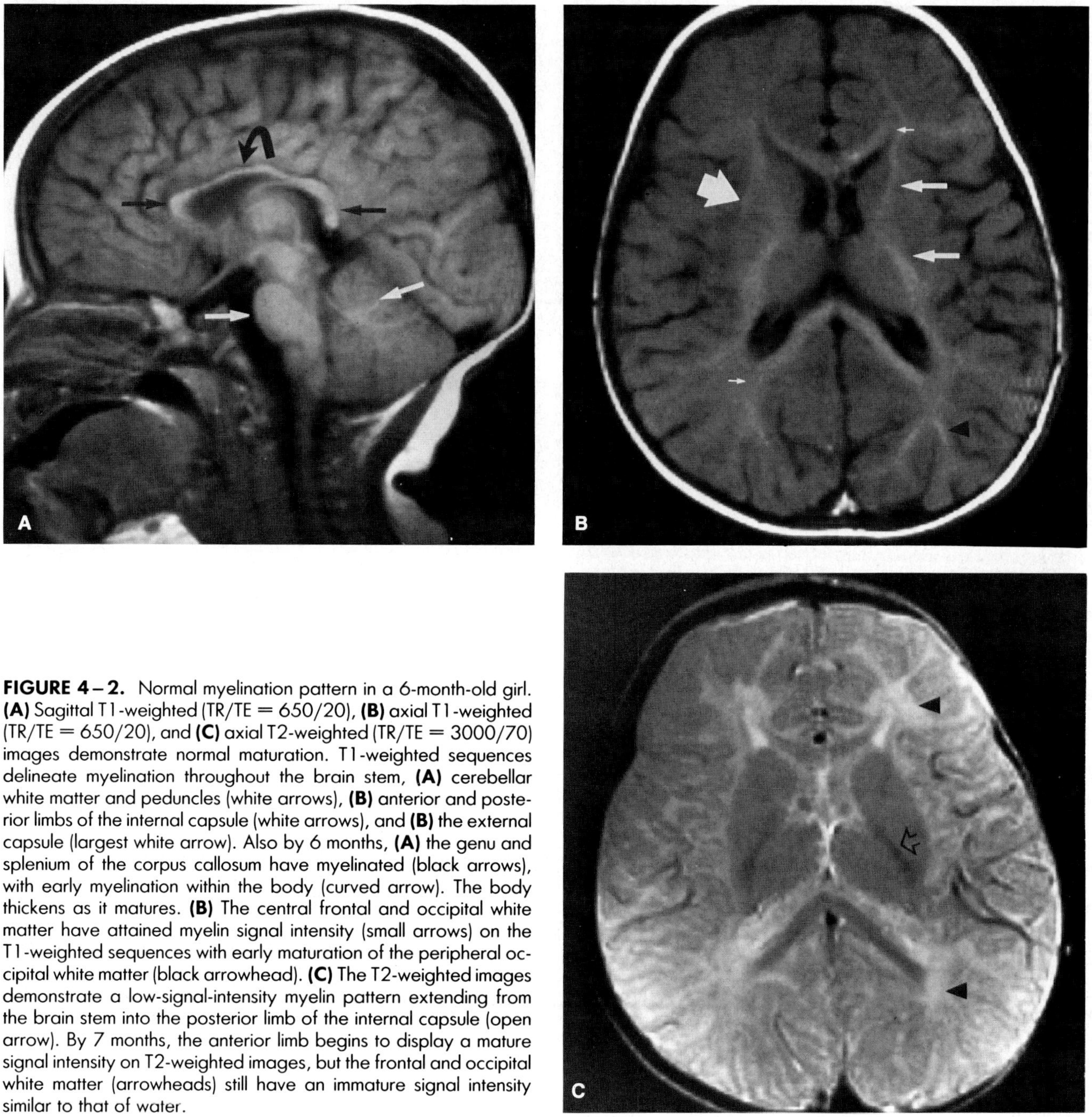

FIGURE 4–2. Normal myelination pattern in a 6-month-old girl. **(A)** Sagittal T1-weighted (TR/TE = 650/20), **(B)** axial T1-weighted (TR/TE = 650/20), and **(C)** axial T2-weighted (TR/TE = 3000/70) images demonstrate normal maturation. T1-weighted sequences delineate myelination throughout the brain stem, **(A)** cerebellar white matter and peduncles (white arrows), **(B)** anterior and posterior limbs of the internal capsule (white arrows), and **(B)** the external capsule (largest white arrow). Also by 6 months, **(A)** the genu and splenium of the corpus callosum have myelinated (black arrows), with early myelination within the body (curved arrow). The body thickens as it matures. **(B)** The central frontal and occipital white matter have attained myelin signal intensity (small arrows) on the T1-weighted sequences with early maturation of the peripheral occipital white matter (black arrowhead). **(C)** The T2-weighted images demonstrate a low-signal-intensity myelin pattern extending from the brain stem into the posterior limb of the internal capsule (open arrow). By 7 months, the anterior limb begins to display a mature signal intensity on T2-weighted images, but the frontal and occipital white matter (arrowheads) still have an immature signal intensity similar to that of water.

months (Fig. 4–3). Most periventricular white matter tracks are myelinated by 12 months.[2]

The splenium of the corpus callosum myelinates first at 6 months of age and at the genu at approximately 8 months of age, with the body of the corpus callosum thickening subsequently. Subcortical white matter myelination first appears within the occipital lobes posteriorly at approximately 9 months, then proceeds anteriorly into the frontal lobes at approximately 12 months. Peripheral arborization then occurs with visual thinning of the gray matter cortex thickness and approaches the adult pattern by approximately 18 months of age (Fig. 4–4).[2] Histologically, however, myelination proceeds into late adolescence.[3]

Dietrich described the myelination process as occurring in three broad stages on T2-weighted imaging using lower field strengths of 0.3 and 0.35 T.[4] The first is an infantile stage extending from the neonatal period to 6 months of age, in which the deep white matter of the cerebral hemispheres is more intense than the gray matter, a reversal of the adult pattern. The

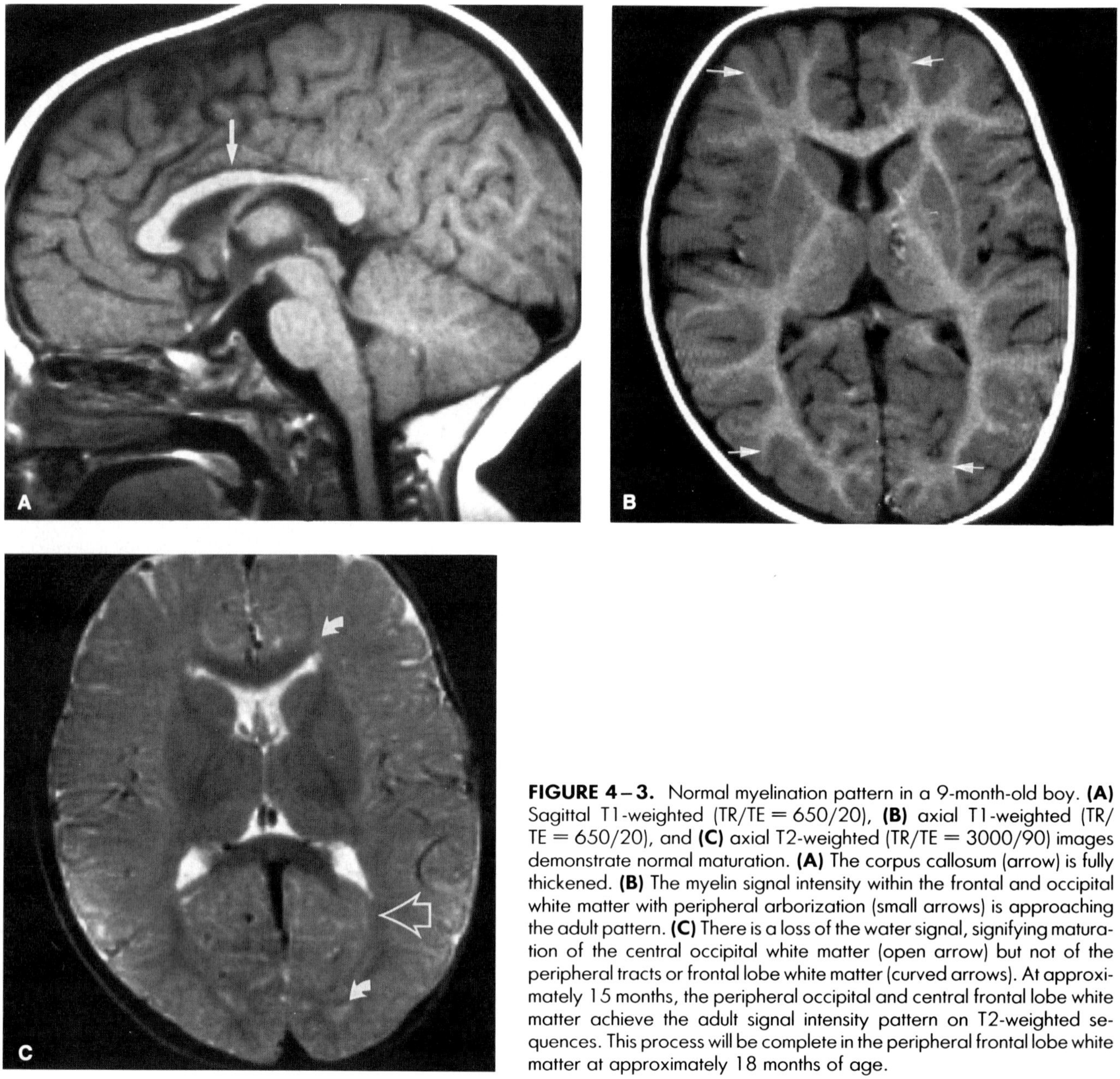

FIGURE 4–3. Normal myelination pattern in a 9-month-old boy. **(A)** Sagittal T1-weighted (TR/TE = 650/20), **(B)** axial T1-weighted (TR/TE = 650/20), and **(C)** axial T2-weighted (TR/TE = 3000/90) images demonstrate normal maturation. **(A)** The corpus callosum (arrow) is fully thickened. **(B)** The myelin signal intensity within the frontal and occipital white matter with peripheral arborization (small arrows) is approaching the adult pattern. **(C)** There is a loss of the water signal, signifying maturation of the central occipital white matter (open arrow) but not of the peripheral tracts or frontal lobe white matter (curved arrows). At approximately 15 months, the peripheral occipital and central frontal lobe white matter achieve the adult signal intensity pattern on T2-weighted sequences. This process will be complete in the peripheral frontal lobe white matter at approximately 18 months of age.

second is an isointense stage, in which these structures are isointense to gray matter on T2-weighted images from approximately 8 to 12 months of age. The third stage is the early adult pattern, in which gray matter is more intense than the deep white matter. This pattern appears at 10 to 12 months of age. In her series, if the infantile pattern persisted beyond 9 months of age, the radiographic abnormality correlated with developmental delay.[4]

In addition to myelination patterns, other features of immaturity can be observed. The relative ventricular size and width of the extra-axial cerebral spaces may appear differently in the neonate and in the older child. The normal ventricle-to-brain ratio in the neonatal period, as measured at the frontal horns, should be approximately 25 to 33% of the width of the brain. If the measurement is greater than 0.36, follow-up MRI can evaluate normal progression of maturation. The extra-axial spaces are less variable; the normal width over the convexities should be 4 mm. If the width is greater than 5 to 6 mm, repeat MRI is also prudent to exclude abnormalities.[5]

CHIARI MALFORMATIONS

Chiari I and Chiari II are commonly encountered entities in clinical practice. Chiari II malformations, because of the associated spinal anomalies and their sequelae, are frequently studied. The anatomic features

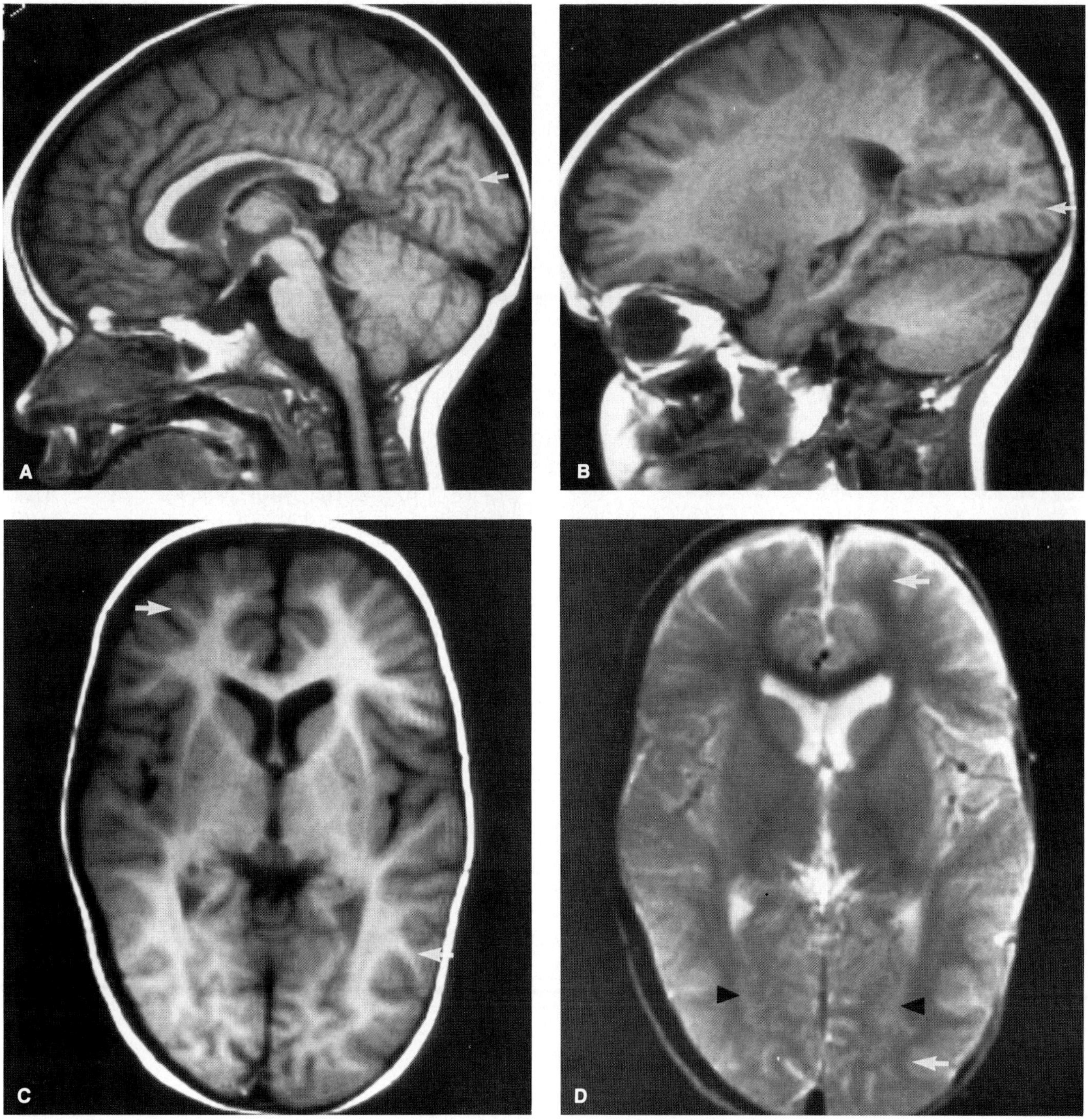

FIGURE 4–4. Normal myelination pattern in a 2-year-old girl. **(A,B)** Sagittal T1-weighted (TR/TE = 650/20), **(C)** axial T1-weighted (TR/TE = 650/20), and **(D)** axial T2-weighted (TR/TE = 3000/90) images demonstrate the normal adult pattern. Arborization of white matter into the periphery is complete on all sequences (white arrows). **(D)** T2-weighted images may demonstrate symmetrical, faint, high-intensity signals adjacent to the atria (black arrowheads) into early adolescence.

of these conditions are well delineated by MRI. Because Chiari I may present with clinical symptoms suggesting demyelination or neoplastic disease, MRI is the usual mode of examination. It is the easiest and most accurate method of diagnosis because of the anatomic detail that can be visualized within the posterior fossa and upper cervical canal.

Chiari I

Chiari I malformation is considered a hind brain dysgenesis. The primary characteristic of Chiari I is the abnormal cerebellar tonsil morphology and position, with associated sequelae. These are features of Chiari I:

1. Downward and posterior herniation of the cervicomedullary junction with variable amount of tissue below the foramen magnum. Two-thirds of cases with Chiari I have downward displacement of the tonsils inferior to C1. In up to 25% of the cases, the herniation reaches the C3 level. This rarely extends more inferiorly (Fig. 4-5).
2. The tonsillar edge is wedge-shaped, instead of globular as in Chiari II.
3. Absent or minute cisterna magna.
4. Syringohydromyelia in approximately 50% of cases, with variable extent within the cord, including possible involvement superiorly into the brain stem (Fig. 4-6).
5. Hydrocephalus in approximately 33 to 50% of the cases.[6]

Chiari I may also be associated with multiple bony anomalies involving the skull base and cervical spine. These anomalies include basilar impression, fusion of C1 to the occiput, fusion of C2 and C3, Klippel-Feil deformity, and spina bifida occulta.[1]

The primary features of Chiari I which separate it from Chiari II are the normal position of the fourth ventricle, absence of supratentorial structural anomalies, and no associated myelomeningocele, as in Chiari II.

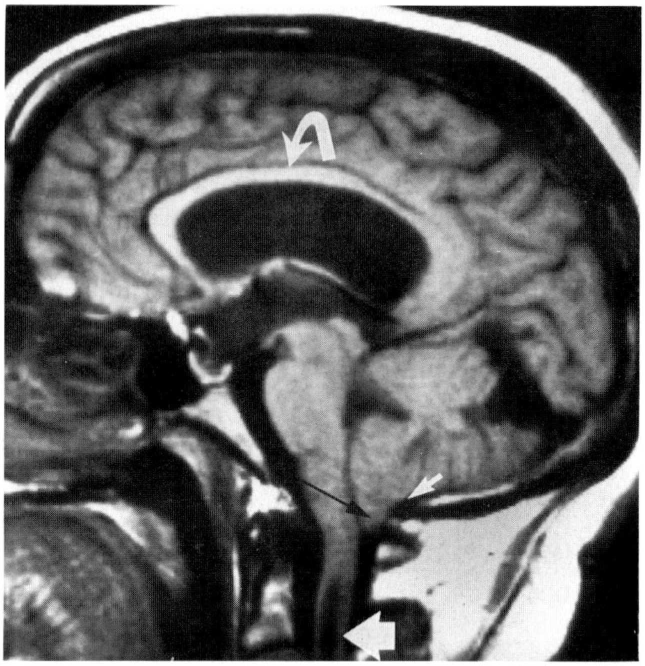

FIGURE 4-5. Chiari I malformation in a 38-year-old woman. A sagittal T1-weighted (TR/TE = 650/20) image demonstrates the abnormally low position of the cerebellar tonsils (black arrow), which approach the superior rim of C1. Notice the wedge-shaped tonsils within the upper cervical canal. The low position of the tonsils is confirmed by identification of the posterior margin of the foramen magnum (small white arrow). The low-signal-intensity cortical margin denoting the posterior rim may be difficult to identify, but proper localization of the posterior arch of C1 and the posterior rim will enable the correct diagnosis of Chiari I. A syrinx extends inferiorly from the level of the odontoid (large white arrowhead). Hydrocephalus and thinning of the corpus callosum (curved arrow) are associated with as many as 50% of Chiari I cases. The fourth ventricle is in its normal position.

Chiari II

Chiari II refers to a cerebral dysgenesis associated with a neural tube closure abnormality, specifically the myelomeningocele. Chiari II is associated with myelomeningoceles in almost 100% of the cases. Myelomeningoceles are the extreme form of spinal dysraphism, involving a midline defect of the posterior bony elements of the vertebral body, usually in the lumbosacral region. Although the muscle, fascia, and skin are usually also split along the midline, the meninges typically remain intact. The incidence of this sporadically appearing syndrome is approximately 3 per 1000 births.[7]

The infratentorial structural changes of Chiari II commonly seen with MRI (Fig. 4-7, 4-8) include:

1. Downward displacement of the cervical spinal cord.
2. Elongation of the brain stem, with the medulla inferiorly displaced into the cervical canal. The displaced medulla may fold over on itself behind the cervical spinal cord, forming a kink.
3. Inferiorly displaced fourth ventricle, which may be below the foramen magnum.
4. Enlarged foramen magnum.
5. Protrusion of the cerebellum through the foramen magnum to create a cerebellar peg with compressed inferior vermis.
6. Forward displacement of the cerebellum which can envelop the brain stem, with the anterior cerebellar components possibly surrounding the brain stem (Fig. 4-8).

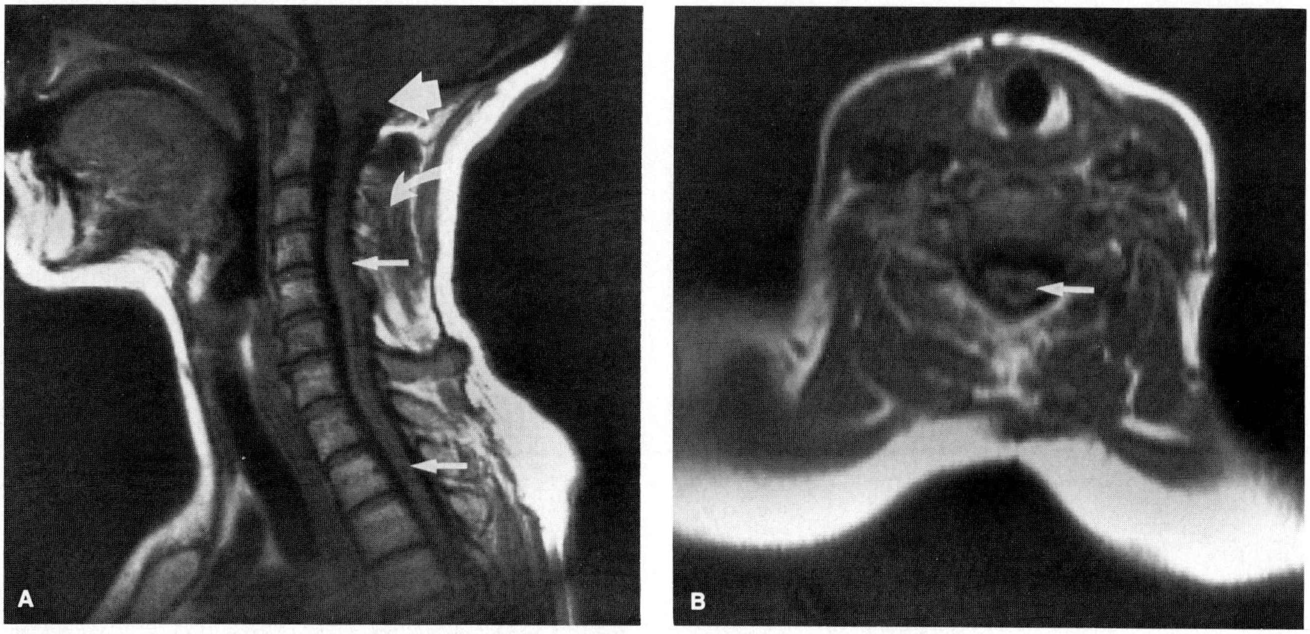

FIGURE 4–6. Chiari I malformation in a 42-year-old woman. **(A)** Sagittal T1-weighted (TR/TE = 650/20) and **(B)** axial T1-weighted (TR/TE = 650/20) images demonstrate a midcervical syrinx extending from C4 to T2 (small arrows). The axial image better defines the syrinx because there are no partial volume effects, emphasizing the value of multiplanar imaging. Notice the anomalous position of the cerebellar tonsils at C1 (arrowhead) and the postoperative midcervical laminectomies with soft tissue scarring (curved arrow).

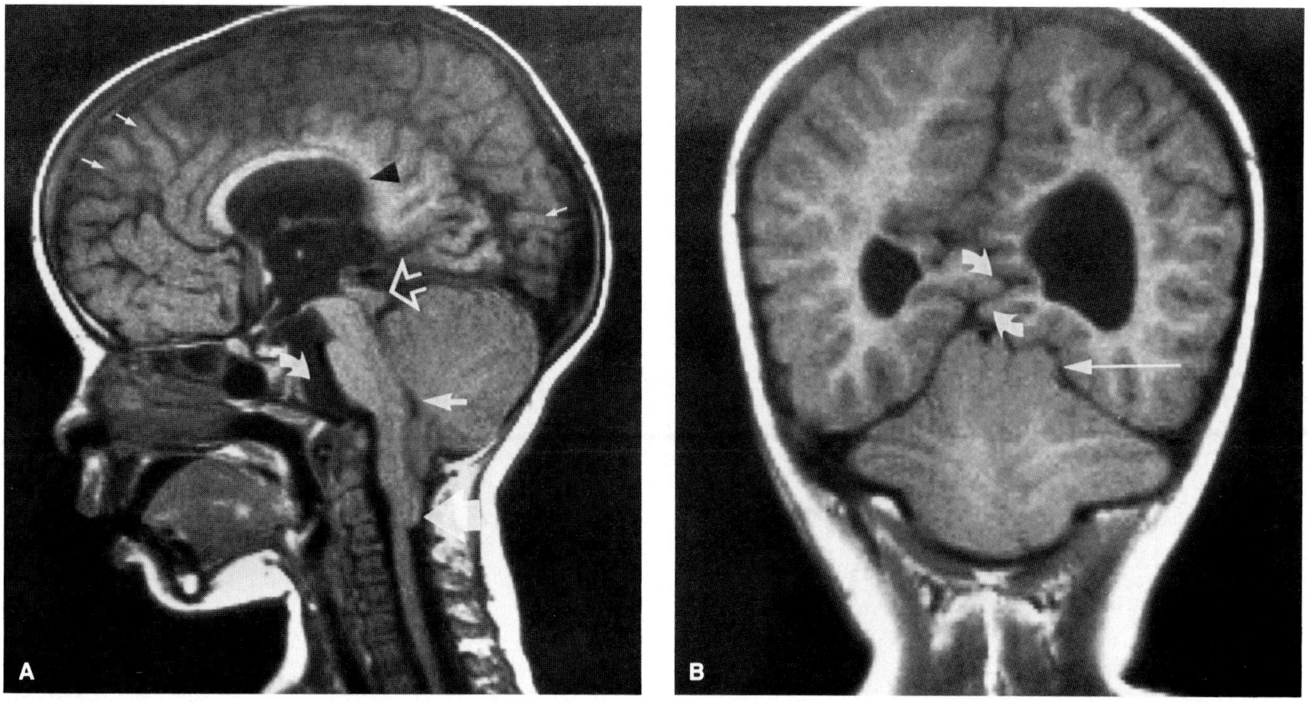

FIGURE 4–7. Chiari II malformation in a 3-year-old girl. **(A)** Sagittal T1-weighted (TR/TE = 650/20) and **(B)** coronal T1-weighted (TR/TE = 650/20) images demonstrate the sequelae of Chiari II. **(A)** The sagittal view defines the abnormally low fourth ventricle (white arrow) and kinking of the displaced medulla (white arrowhead), which characterize Chiari II. The foramen magnum is enlarged and the clivus is abnormally arched, expanding the prepontine cistern (white curved arrow). The clival deformity represents typical mesodermal bone changes. Other stigmata on the sagittal view include a beaked tectum (open arrow), dilatation of the third and lateral ventricles with hypogenesis of the posterior corpus callosum (black arrowhead), and multiple thin gyri or stenogyri (small white arrows). **(B)** The coronal view best demonstrates the widened tentorial incisura and "towering" cerebellum (long white arrow) and the interdigitating gyri due to fenestration of the falx (curved arrows).

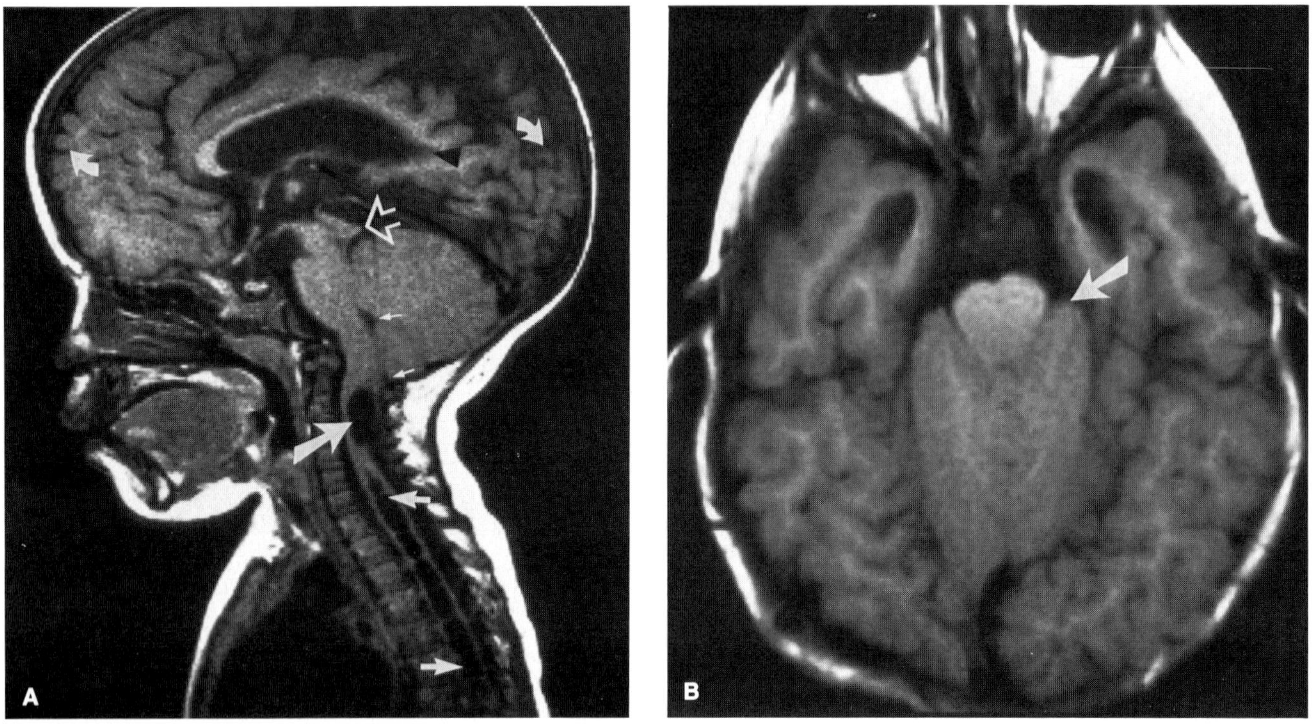

FIGURE 4–8. Chiari II malformation in a 1-year-old boy. **(A)** Sagittal T1-weighted (TR/TE = 650/20) and **(B)** axial T1-weighted (TR/TE = 650/20) images delineate features of Chiari II. **(A)** The sagittal view demonstrates extensive syringomyelia extending throughout the cervical and thoracic spinal cord (white arrows). There is a separate cavity within the inferiorly displaced medulla representing syringobulbia (large oblique arrow). Notice the characteristic low position of the fourth ventricle, approaching the foramen magnum (small white arrows), and a beaked tectum (open arrow), dilated third and lateral ventricles with hypogenetic posterior corpus callosum (black arrowhead), and stenogyria (curved arrows). **(B)** The axial view demonstrates cerebellar tissue extending anteriorly to envelop the lateral aspects of the brain stem (oblique arrow). The hemispheric tissue may completely surround the brain stem and abut ventrally in some cases.

7. Altered folia pattern over the superior surface of the cerebellum, with the folia running in an exaggerated anterior-posterior direction.
8. Wide tentorial incisura, creating the visual effect of a towering cerebellum with enlarged supracerebellar cerebrospinal fluid (CSF) spaces.
9. Mesodermal changes of the clivus and petrous ridges, altering their usual contour (Fig. 4–7).[8]

Features of Chiari II commonly identified on MRI in the upper midbrain and supratentorial structures include:

1. Fusion of the colliculi, creating a beaked or bulbous tectum.
2. A large massa intermedia.
3. Hydrocephalus with the frontal horns pointing inferiorly, large atria, and prominent suprapineal recess of the third ventricle.
4. Interdigitating gyri.
5. Thin, numerous gyri, called stenogyria.[8] (Not polymicrogyria, a pathologic term describing reduced cellular layers within the gyri.)
6. Agenesis of the corpus callosum in approximately 33% of the cases.
7. Large interhemispheric CSF space of variable size and configuration.

Myelomeningocele in Chiari II malformations are associated with syringohydromyelia in approximately 20 to 75% of the cases.[7]

COMMON CONGENITAL ANOMALIES OF THE POSTERIOR FOSSA

In addition to the Chiari malformations, there are other common congenital disorders affecting the posterior fossa. Dandy–Walker malformation, retrocerebellar arachnoid cyst, and cerebellar hypoplasia are syndromes of anomalous cerebellar organization that can be easily distinguished by MR imaging.

Dandy – Walker Malformation

The Dandy – Walker malformation is characterized by the absence of the inferior vermis, creating a large communication from the fourth ventricle posteriorly into a cyst-like structure, filling the posterior fossa. This cystic structure freely communicates with the fourth ventricle. The posterior fossa is usually expanded, with elevation of the torcula, but a few patients may have smaller CSF collections without posterior fossa expansion. The anomaly may be associated with obstruction at the foramen of Magendie or Luschka, possibly altering normal CSF flow (Fig. 4 – 9).[9] However, not all cases have obstructed foramina at autopsy, and in vivo demonstration of foraminal patency is difficult.

The observed structural anomalies are related to the embryologic dysgenesis and not to a permanent obstructive process. Hydrocephalus is usually present and is highly variable in severity. The severity of hydrocephalus is the most important prognostic factor. Other cerebral anomalies associated with Dandy – Walker malformation are agenesis of the corpus callosum, cortical heterotopias, polymicrogyria, and brainstem lipomas.[10]

Retrocerebellar arachnoid cysts have distinctive imaging features. The cysts often have an elevated torcula, but unlike the Dandy – Walker malformation, the inferior vermis is intact, and the CSF space anterior to the brain stem is usually compressed (Fig. 4 – 10).

Cerebellar or vermian hypoplasia is characterized by absence of vermial or cerebellar hemispheric tissue, with only residual, passive CSF spaces present. The cerebellar peduncles and brain stem are hypoplastic. Usually, only the most-anterior portions of the cerebellar hemispheres are present, and these cerebellar hemispheric remnants may be asymmetrical (Fig. 4 – 11). Therefore, the posterior fossa appears small, with a low torcula, little cerebellar tissue, small brainstem and cerebellar peduncles, and passive CSF filling the remainder of the fossa.

The literature also describes a Dandy – Walker variant in which the fourth ventricle and cyst are smaller than in the Dandy – Walker malformation. There is normal positioning of the torcula due to a patent foramen of Magendie, allowing for normal CSF dynamics. No large posterior fossa CSF collections expand the fossa and elevate the torcula.[11,12]

(text continues on page 188)

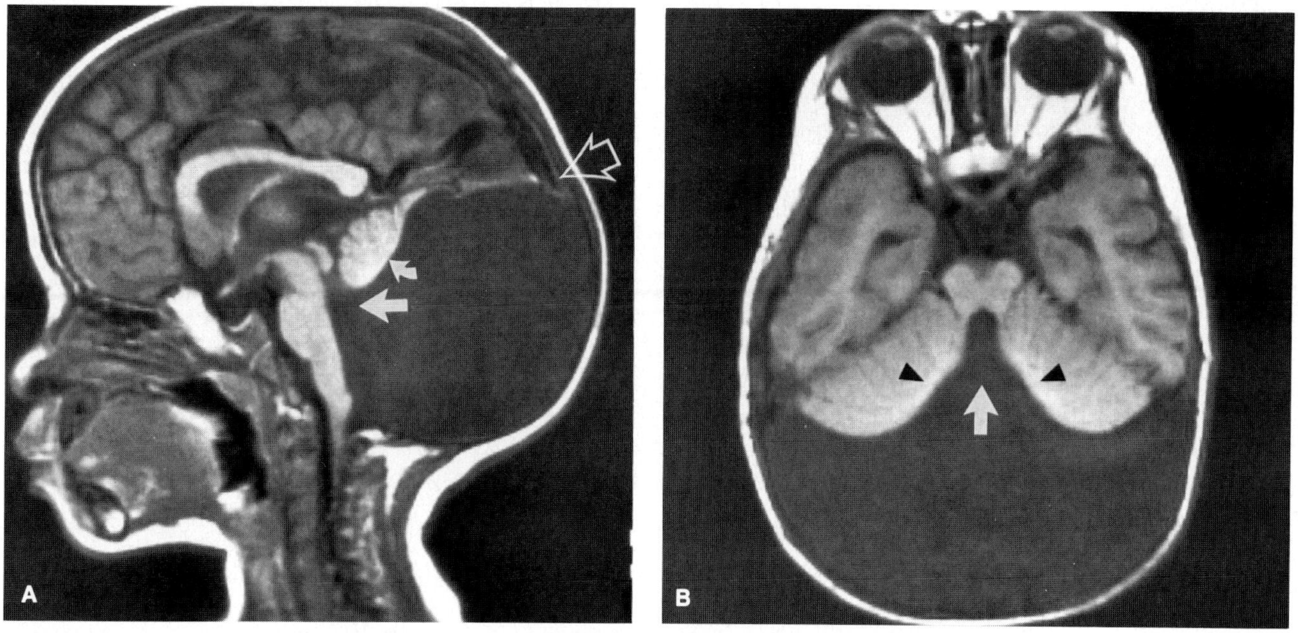

FIGURE 4 – 9. Dandy-Walker malformation in a 1-year-old boy. **(A)** Sagittal T1-weighted (TR/TE = 650/20) and **(B)** axial T1-weighted (TR/TE = 650/20) images demonstrate the classic features of the Dandy-Walker syndrome and separate it from other posterior fossa syndromes. No inferior vermis and a large communication from the fourth ventricle into a massive posterior fossa CSF collection characterizes the syndrome (large white arrows). The torcula is usually markedly elevated (open arrow). The superior vermis remains intact (curved arrow), and the cerebellar hemispheres, although compressed anteriorly, are mostly intact (black arrows).

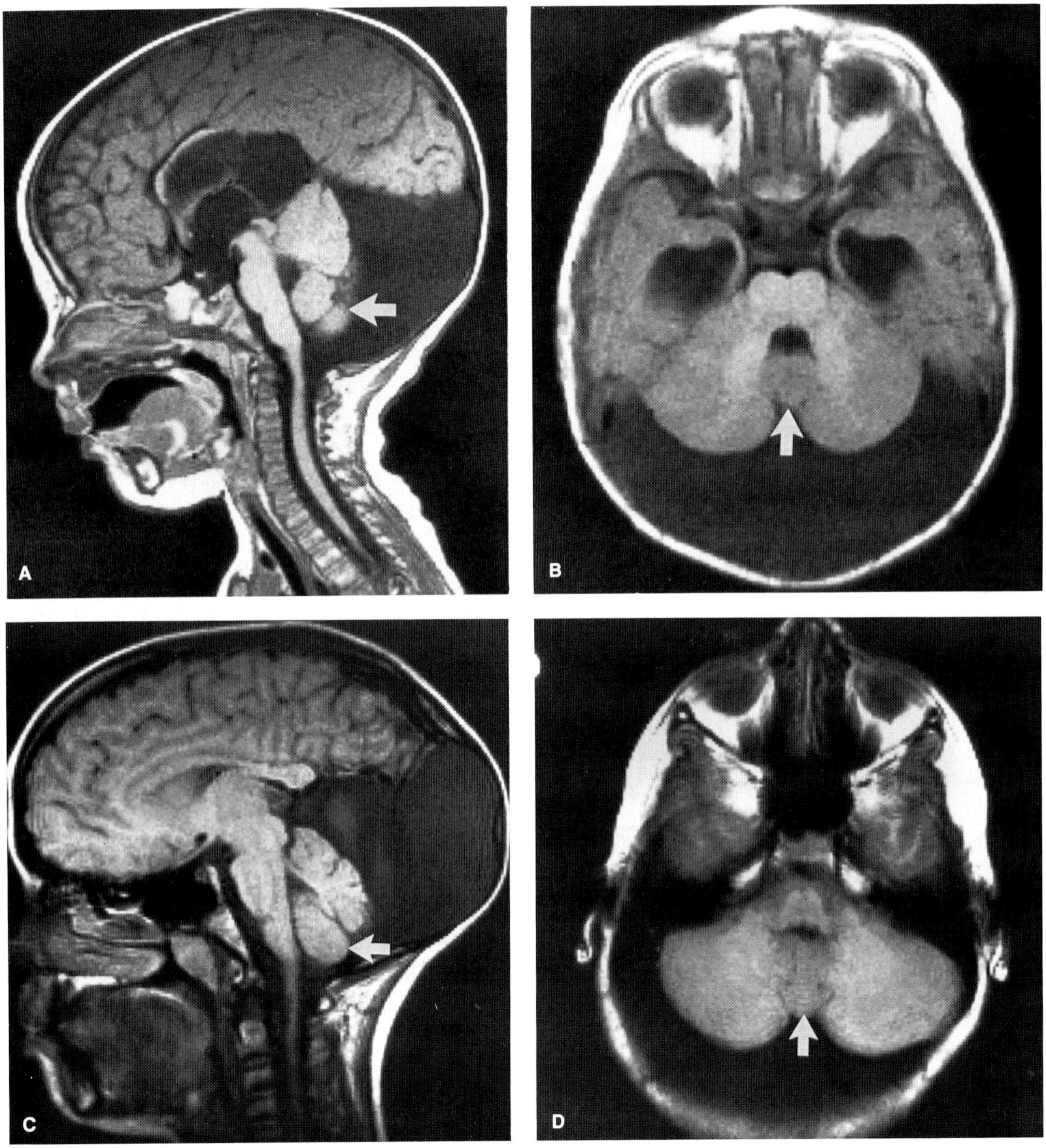

FIGURE 4–10. Retrocerebellar arachnoid cysts in 7- and 11-month-old boys. **(A,C)** Sagittal T1-weighted (TR/TE = 650/20) and **(B,D)** axial T1-weighted (TR/TE = 650/20) views demonstrate an intact inferior vermis (white arrows) and an intact cerebellum without agenesis. No direct communication exists from the fourth ventricle posteriorly into the CSF intensity structure or cyst, although there is normal communication through the foramen of Magendie. These features distinguish retrocerebellar arachnoid cysts from Dandy-Walker syndrome. Ten percent of arachnoid cysts occur in the posterior fossa, with 50 to 75% of the cysts occurring in the middle cranial fossa.

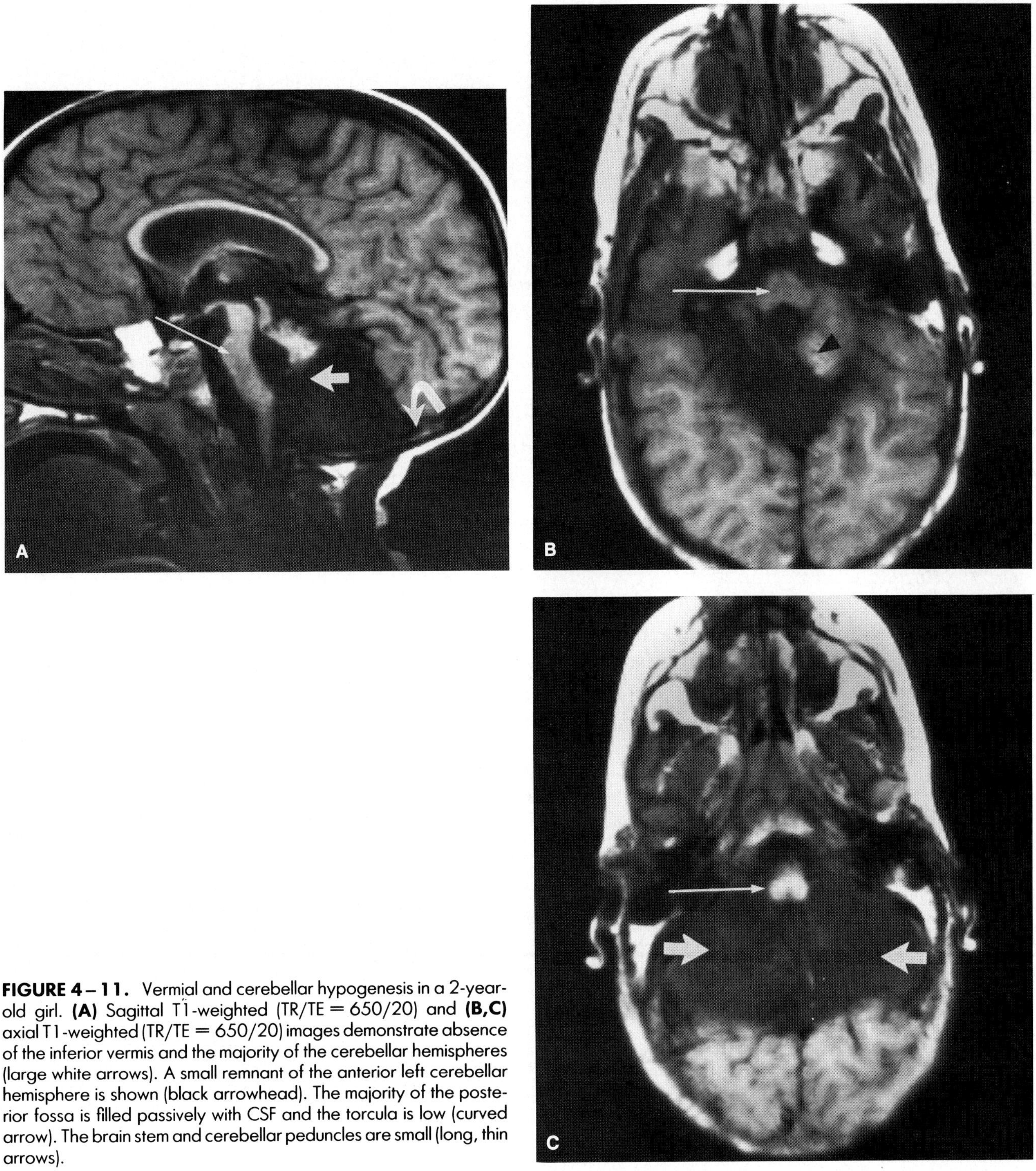

FIGURE 4–11. Vermial and cerebellar hypogenesis in a 2-year-old girl. **(A)** Sagittal T1-weighted (TR/TE = 650/20) and **(B,C)** axial T1-weighted (TR/TE = 650/20) images demonstrate absence of the inferior vermis and the majority of the cerebellar hemispheres (large white arrows). A small remnant of the anterior left cerebellar hemisphere is shown (black arrowhead). The majority of the posterior fossa is filled passively with CSF and the torcula is low (curved arrow). The brain stem and cerebellar peduncles are small (long, thin arrows).

DISORDERS OF CEREBRAL HEMISPHERIC ORGANIZATION

Agenesis of the Corpus Callosum

Agenesis of the corpus callosum is a common congenital anomaly that may be complete or partial. It may be associated with multiple anomalies of the limbic system, such as absence of the major commissures or the hippocampal and anterior commissures. The posterior commissure remains intact.[13]

The corpus callosum is composed of four parts. Progressing anteriorly to posteriorly, the rostrum, genu, body, and splenium can be identified. These structures form embryologically from the anterior rostral component to the posterior splenial component. This temporal sequence of formation explains the consistent absence of the more posterior elements in partial agenesis.[14,15] These are the associated features of agenesis of the corpus callosum (Fig. 4-12):

1. A large, high third ventricle.
2. Medially concave frontal horns and widely separated parallel lateral ventricles.
3. Radiating medial surface gyri due to the absent cingulate gyrus.
4. Enlarged, dysplastic, elevated anterior commissure.
5. Probst bundles, which are white matter bundles running along the medial wall of the lateral ventricle.
6. Rounded ventricular atria caused by the absence of the splenium and portions of the forceps major.
7. Heterotopic gray matter.
8. Wandering anterior cerebral artery.[14,15]

Agenesis of the corpus callosum is easy to identify on MR scans after myelination is complete. It is difficult to definitively diagnose complete agenesis of the corpus callosum before myelination, because the corpus callosum is extremely thin and difficult to visualize in the neonatal period. However, if the sulci on the medial surface of the brain radiate directly from the lateral ventricle, the diagnosis may be suggested even in the neonate. Eighty percent of cases of agenesis have other associated findings. The most common anomalies associated with agenesis are Chiari II malformation, Dandy-Walker malformation, holopros-

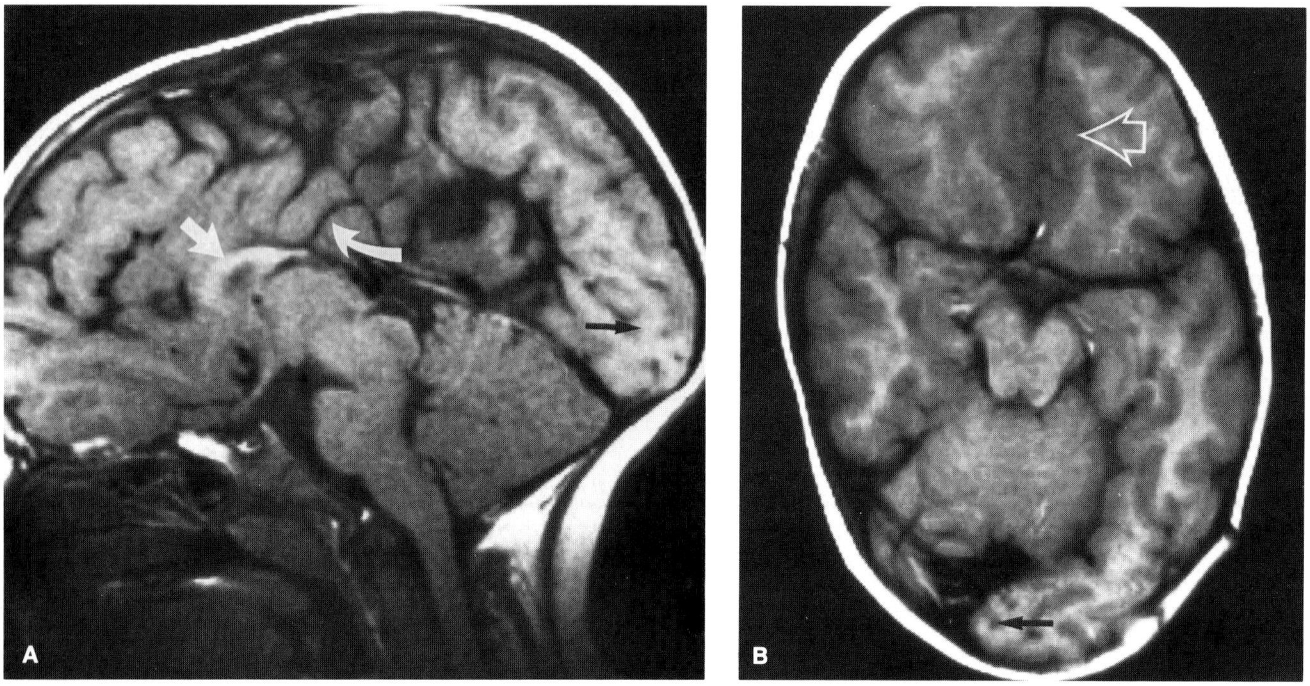

FIGURE 4-12. Partial agenesis of the corpus callosum in a 6-year-old boy. **(A)** Sagittal T1-weighted (TR/TE = 650/20) and **(B)** axial T1-weighted (TR/TE = 650/20) images demonstrate hypogenesis of the corpus callosum, with only the rostrum and genu remaining (white arrow). There is no cingulate gyrus, and the medial surface gyri radiate directly from the lateral ventricle (curved arrow). Other anomalies are commonly associated with agenesis or hypogenesis of the corpus callosum, and this patient demonstrates moderate asymmetry of the cerebral hemispheres, with the left hemisphere crossing the midline (black arrows). The axial view demonstrates thickened gray matter within the medial frontal lobes, suggesting pachygyria (open arrowhead).

encephaly, neuronal migration abnormalities, encephaloceles, and interhemispheric cysts.[14,15]

Lipomas

Intracranial lipomas are common anomalies seen in approximately 1 of 1000 persons. They are usually located midline within the interhemispheric fissure near the corpus callosum, but other common sites are the quadrigeminal plate cistern, tuber cinereum, and cerebello-pontine (CP) angle. Less common sites include the base of the cerebrum, the cerebellum, the brainstem, roots of the cranial nerves, ventral aspect of the midbrain, and the choroid plexus of the lateral ventricles. These lipomata arise from the pia and appear to insinuate into adjacent neural structures (Fig. 4–13).[16] If associated with agenesis of the corpus callosum, MRI demonstrates a fat-intensity mass within the interhemispheric fissure, at the site of the absent corpus callosum, most commonly at the genu. Ap-

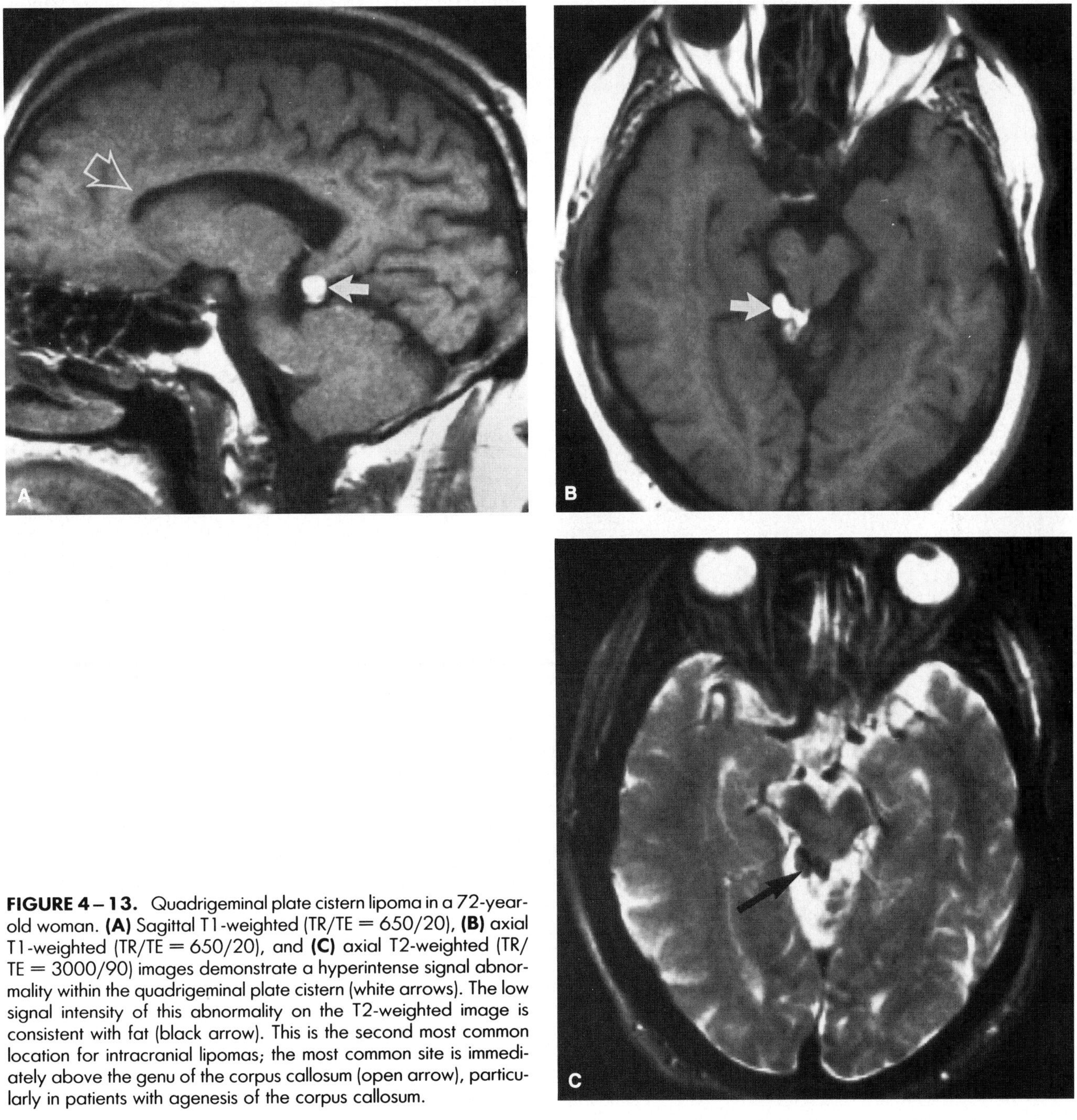

FIGURE 4–13. Quadrigeminal plate cistern lipoma in a 72-year-old woman. **(A)** Sagittal T1-weighted (TR/TE = 650/20), **(B)** axial T1-weighted (TR/TE = 650/20), and **(C)** axial T2-weighted (TR/TE = 3000/90) images demonstrate a hyperintense signal abnormality within the quadrigeminal plate cistern (white arrows). The low signal intensity of this abnormality on the T2-weighted image is consistent with fat (black arrow). This is the second most common location for intracranial lipomas; the most common site is immediately above the genu of the corpus callosum (open arrow), particularly in patients with agenesis of the corpus callosum.

proximately 50% of these cases have associated hypoplasia of the corpus callosum. Calcifications may be present but are not readily identified on MRI.[17]

Holoprosencephaly

Holoprosencephaly is a dysgenesis of cerebral hemisphere formation characterized by failure of hemispheric or thalamic separation. Fifty-five percent of these cases are associated with chromosomal abnormalities, with an incidence of 1 per 5000 to 1 per 16,000. Up to 16% of the cases recognized initially by fetal ultrasound as hydrocephalus are discovered after birth to be holoprosencephaly.[18]

This disorder includes the three classic gradations of allobar, semilobar, and lobar holoprosencephaly, with the allobar form being the most severe. These are the classic features of the severe allobar form:

1. Absent falx and interhemispheric fissure.
2. Fused thalami with absent third ventricle.
3. Horseshoe-shaped monoventricle.
4. Absent superior sagittal, inferior sagittal, and straight sinuses, as well as absence of the internal cerebral veins.

The allobar form may also have a large "dorsal cyst" or "sac," which is a CSF-intensity collection representing ballooning of the membranous roof of the third ventricle posteriorly. The corpus callosum is absent. Partial formation of the interhemispheric fissure and falx, with rudimentary differentiation of the occipital and temporal lobes and respective ventricular horns, comprise the semilobar form. Rudimentary corpus callosum formation and cleavage of the thalami to form a third ventricle are present (Fig. 4-14).

A nearly complete fissure and falx, with only a small area of frontal lobe fusion with well-formed occipital and temporal lobes, comprise the lobar form of holoprosencephaly. The thalami, third ventricle and corpus callosum appear normal or nearly normal.[19]

NEURONAL MIGRATION ANOMALIES

The migrational anomalies are a varied group of entities caused by abnormal migration of the embryologic neuroblasts, which are arrested along their normal course from the ventricular germinal matrix to the cortical periphery. The primitive neuroblasts nor-

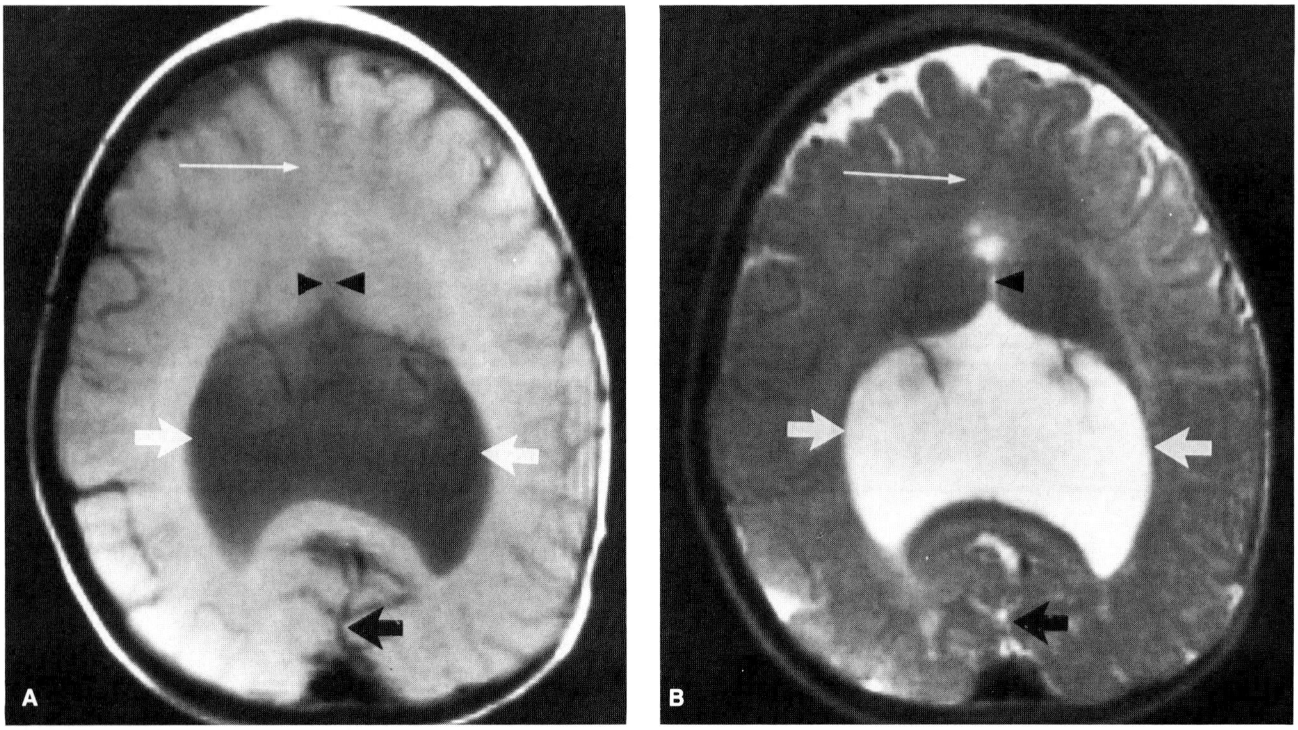

FIGURE 4-14. Semilobar holoprosencephaly in a 9-month-old boy. **(A)** Axial T1-weighted (TR/TE = 650/20) and **(B)** T2-weighted (TR/TE = 3000/90) images demonstrate a single bat-wing-shaped monoventricle characteristic of holoprosencephaly (white arrows). Anomalous thalami abut each other anteriorly (black arrowheads), and the gray and white matter of the frontal lobes is fused (long, thin arrows). There is partial falx formation posteriorly and early separation of the occipital horns denoting rudimentary lobe differentiation (black arrows). Rudimentary temporal horn differentiation (not shown) classified this as the semilobar form of holoprosencephaly.

mally ascend along radial glial cells during the third and fifth gestational months. If this cellular migration is prevented, abnormal cortical structures result. The entities included in this group are agyria and pachygyria, schizencephaly, gray matter heterotopia, polymicrogyria, and unilateral megaloencephaly.[20]

Agyria and Pachygyria

Agyria and pachygyria represent a spectrum of cortical malformations, with agyria being the most severe form. Lissencephaly is a term often used for agyria when gyral formation is very rudimentary, creating the appearance of a "smooth brain." Agyria and pachygyria describe regions of cortical brain that have diminished gyral formation, creating thick, broad gyri. The ratio of the gray matter to white matter is reversed; thus, the gray matter cortex is broad. The corpus callosum is thinned due to abnormal white matter migration, and the brain stem is small due to failure of the corticospinal tract formation. There is a band of increased signal intensity in the periphery of the cortex on T2-weighted images, which is called the cell-sparse layer. This band of abnormal signal intensity may represent the level of gestational insult, and it is theorized that normal migration is impaired at this cellular layer (Fig. 4–15).[20]

Schizencephaly

Schizencephaly is a disorder of cell migration within a segment of the brain, creating a cleft lined by gray matter traversing the hemisphere from the cortex to the ventricles (Fig. 4–16). These may be unilateral or bilateral; the bilateral clefts are associated with severe clinical impairment. Covering the gray-matter-lined cleft is a "pial-ependymal" seam, representing fusion of the pial lining of the brain and the ventricular ependyma. The clefts are always situated at the precentral or postcentral gyri and have abnormal gyral patterns surrounding the clefts, such as stenogyria or gray matter heterotopia. These clefts may be gaping or "open," or the clefts may be "closed," with only a gray matter seam extending from the peripheral cortex to the ventricular level. The identification of gray matter lining the cleft is a primary feature, which separates this abnormality from porencephaly or other acquired destructive lesions of the brain, which

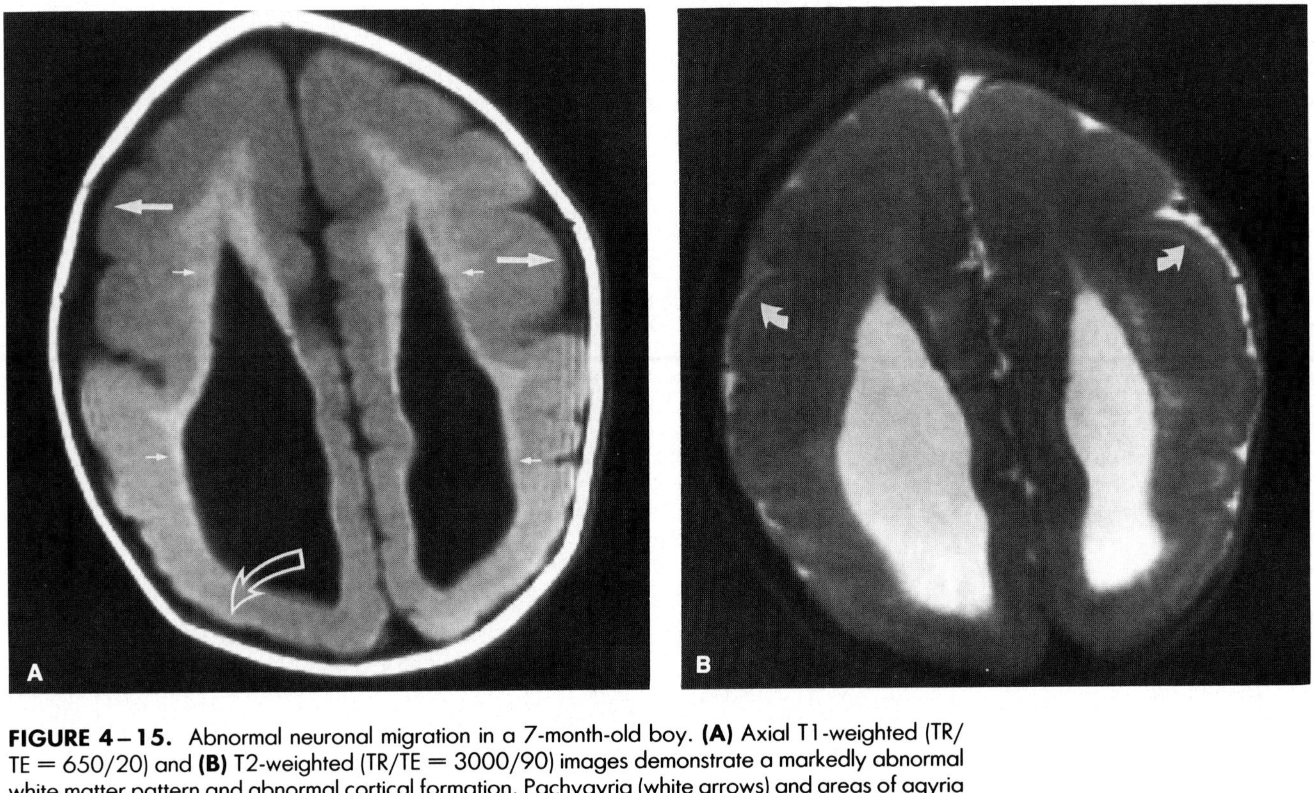

FIGURE 4–15. Abnormal neuronal migration in a 7-month-old boy. **(A)** Axial T1-weighted (TR/TE = 650/20) and **(B)** T2-weighted (TR/TE = 3000/90) images demonstrate a markedly abnormal white matter pattern and abnormal cortical formation. Pachygyria (white arrows) and areas of agyria (open curved arrow) create an abnormal cortical surface. The gray matter cortex is thickened, consistent with failure of the white matter to arborize peripherally. The white matter is characterized by thin, smooth, abnormal bands surrounding the dilated ventricles (small arrows). The T2-weighted axial image demonstrates a linear band of increased signal intensity under the cortex that probably represents the cell-sparse cellular layer or level of neuronal migrational insult (white curved arrows).

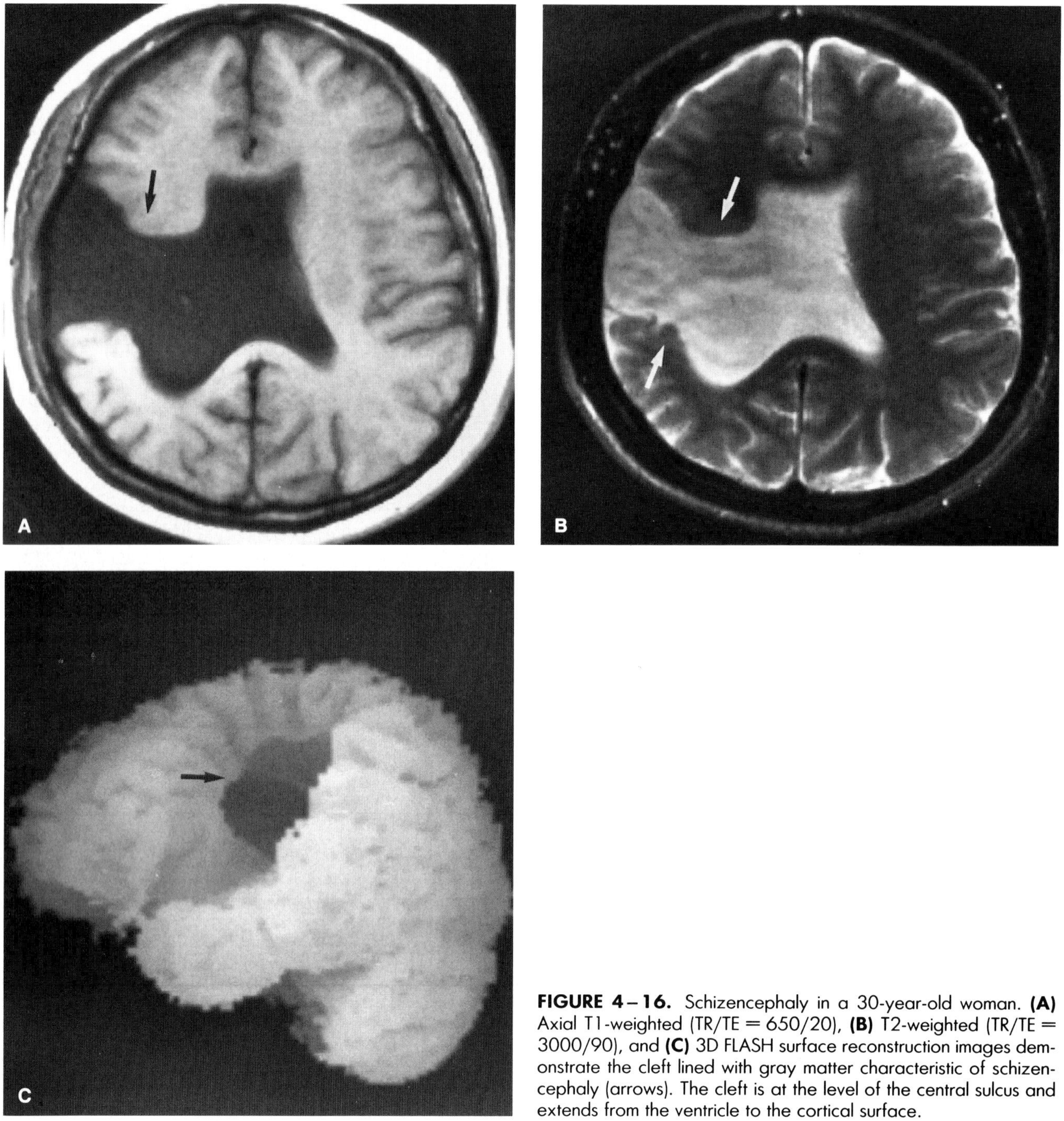

FIGURE 4–16. Schizencephaly in a 30-year-old woman. **(A)** Axial T1-weighted (TR/TE = 650/20), **(B)** T2-weighted (TR/TE = 3000/90), and **(C)** 3D FLASH surface reconstruction images demonstrate the cleft lined with gray matter characteristic of schizencephaly (arrows). The cleft is at the level of the central sulcus and extends from the ventricle to the cortical surface.

is important due to the genetic ramifications, as 5% to 20% of schizencephaly cases have siblings with other brain anomalies.[21]

Heterotopic Gray Matter

Heterotopic gray matter represents collections of neurons of varying size in aberrant locations, which appear between the subependymal zone at the ventricular level to the peripheral cortex. This may be an isolated asymptomatic lesion or may be associated with other anomalies, such as Chiari II or neuronal migration anomalies.[20] Sequences enhancing the gray-white matter distinction, such as heavily T1-weighted inversion recovery scans, best delineate these lesions.

Polymicrogyria

Polymicrogyria is an anomaly characterized by excessive cerebral convolutions, increased cortical thickness, and abnormal cellular histology. The abnormality is commonly associated with schizencephaly. The stenogyria of Chiari II is not a type of polymicrogyria, because the normal cellular layers are present. With polymicrogyria, four instead of the normal six histologic layers are present. The four-layered cortex is composed of the marginal, outer cellular, cell-sparse, and inner cellular layers.[20]

MRI of stenogyria demonstrates multiple thinned gyri, but polymicrogyria is identified by a thickened cortex without detectable gyri and with decreased adjacent underlying white matter. The gyri are not detected with MR imaging in polymicrogyria due to the excessive infolding and crowding of the gray matter. The infolding and cell layer deficiency can be detected only by histologic analysis.

Unilateral Megalencephaly

Unilateral megalencephaly is a rare anomaly of the brain characterized by overgrowth of part or all of a cerebral hemisphere, with distorted, thickened cortex and ipsilateral ventricular dilatation. Abnormal signal intensity within the centrum semiovale represents areas of decreased myelination that are detected on MR images due to increased water content. This is characterized by the prolonged T1 and T2 relaxation times of white matter. Due to the intractable seizures associated with this disorder, all areas of abnormal hemispheric tissue should be delineated to permit complete surgical resection.[20]

NEUROCUTANEOUS SYNDROMES OR PHAKOMATOSES

The neurocutaneous syndromes refer to a group of disorders that are dysplasias or neoplasias of tissues primarily derived from the embryonic ectoderm. These congenital disorders may also affect the embryonic mesoderm and endoderm. The more common syndromes in this group are Von Recklinghausen's neurofibromatosis, tuberous sclerosis, von Hippel–Lindau syndrome, and Sturge–Weber syndrome.

Neurofibromatosis

Neurofibromatosis is an autosomal dominant disorder of neuroectodermal and mesodermal tissues in which the Schwann cell is the primary abnormal element within the central nervous system (CNS).[22] The incidence of neurofibromatosis is approximately 1 in 3000 births.[23] Two main subclassifications exist. The first group is the classic Von Recklinghausen's neurofibromatosis with multiple CNS, cutaneous, and osseous lesions. The second group, or neurofibromatosis II, is an entity in which bilateral acoustic neuromas occur without other associated sequelae.

The central nervous system (CNS) manifestations of neurofibromatosis include neoplasms, such as schwannomas, meningiomas, and gliomas (Fig. 4–17). The gliomas most commonly involve the optic chiasm, but may also involve the brain stem, hypothalamus, and spinal cord (Fig. 4–18). Hamartomatous or dysplastic changes are seen by MR imaging within, most commonly, the basal ganglia, but also within the midbrain, cerebellum, and subcortical white matter (Fig. 4–19). These lesions can best be identified as areas of increased signal intensity on T2-weighted spin echo sequences. A rim-like pattern of increased signal intensity may be identified on T1-weighted images due to the central hypointensity, which correlates to the area of increased signal intensity on T2-weighted images (Fig. 4–20). These commonly visualized lesions have been described patho-

(text continues on page 196)

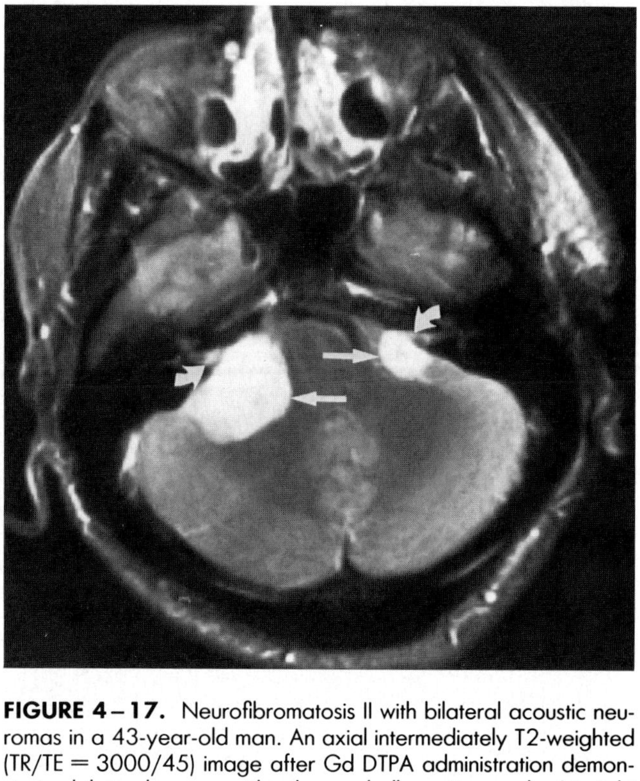

FIGURE 4–17. Neurofibromatosis II with bilateral acoustic neuromas in a 43-year-old man. An axial intermediately T2-weighted (TR/TE = 3000/45) image after Gd DTPA administration demonstrates bilateral masses within the cerebellopontine angles (straight arrows). The enhanced tumor extends bilaterally into the internal auditory canals, consistent with the diagnosis of acoustic neuroma (curved arrows). Bilateral acoustic neuromas commonly signify neurofibromatosis.

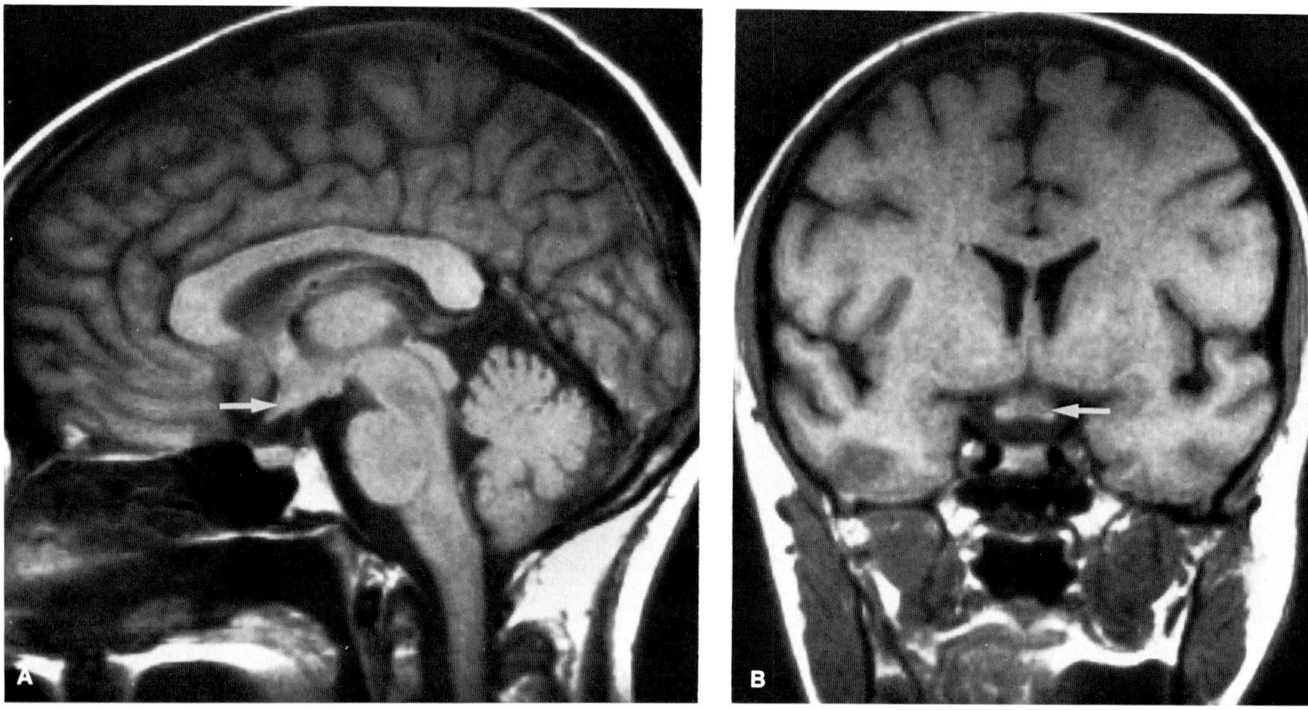

FIGURE 4–18. Neurofibromatosis with enlarged optic chiasm and optic tracts in a 34-year-old woman. **(A)** Sagittal T1-weighted (TR/TE = 650/20) and **(B)** coronal T1-weighted (TR/TE = 650/20) images demonstrate a thickened optic chiasm (arrows). No signal abnormality or enhancement with Gd DTPA was seen. Many neurofibromatosis patients with enlarged optic nerves, chiasm, or tracts do not demonstrate abnormal signal intensity or enhancement. These lesions may represent slowly growing gliomas or hamartomas.

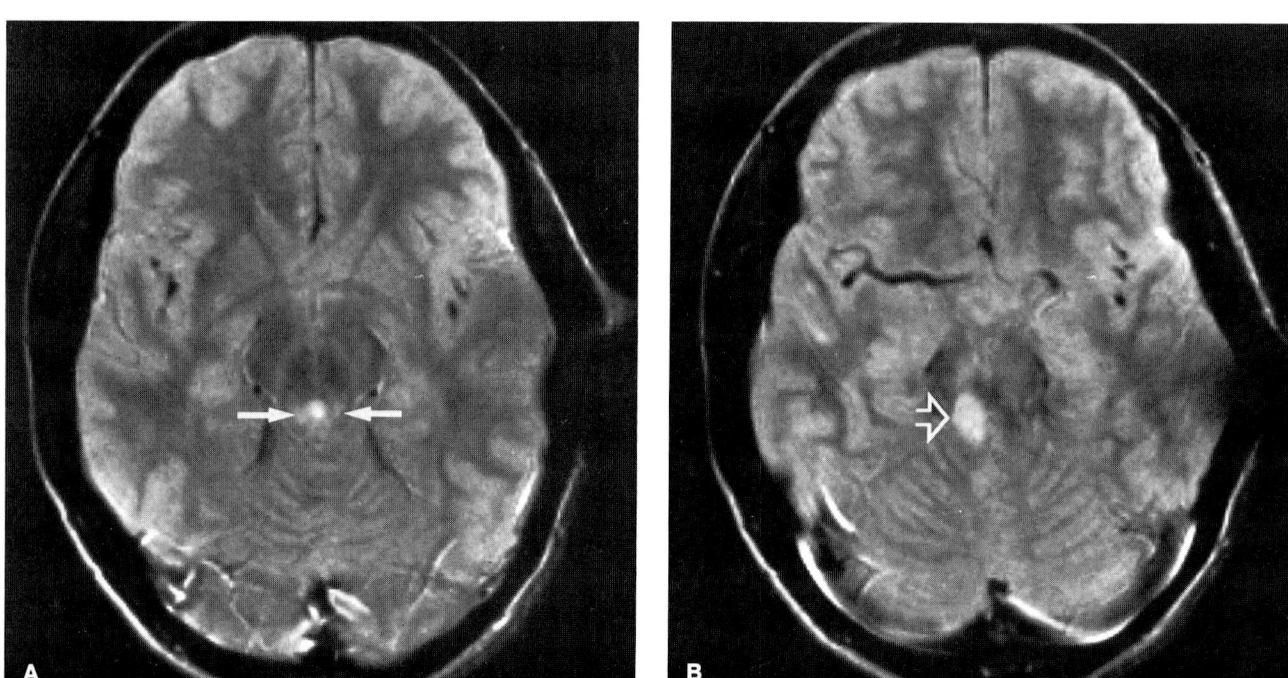

FIGURE 4–19. Neurofibromatosis with midbrain and periaqueductal hamartomas in a 16-year-old girl. **(A,B)** Axial T2-weighted (TR/TE = 3000/45) images demonstrate areas of increased signal intensity in the periaqueductal white matter (arrows) and right posterior midbrain (open arrow), which are common secondary locations of hamartomatous growth. However, gliomas can have a similar appearance and may arise in this location.

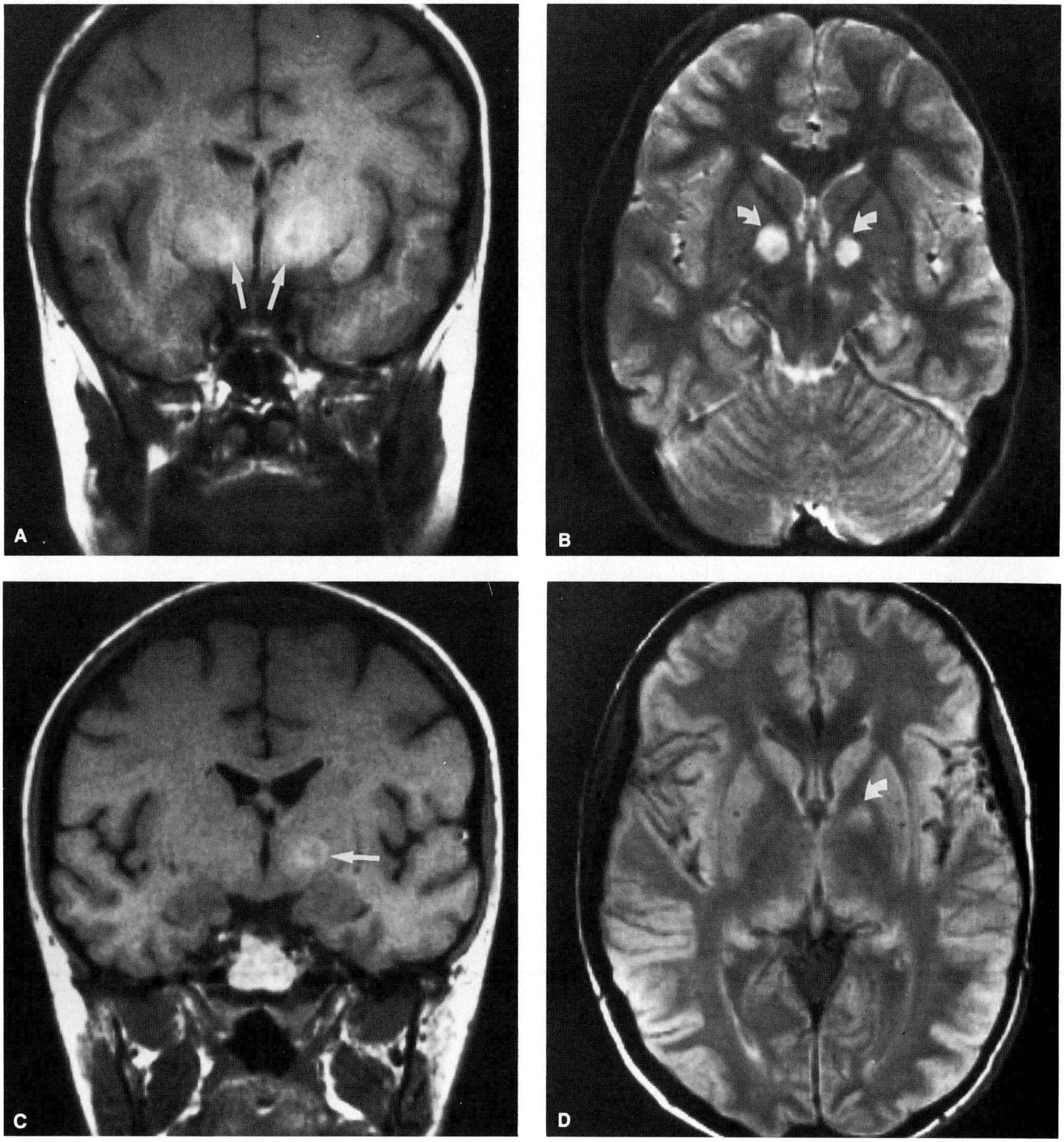

FIGURE 4–20. Neurofibromatosis with hamartomatous lesions in a 10-year-old girl and 34-year-old woman. **(A,C)** Coronal T1-weighted (TR/TE = 650/20) and **(B,D)** axial T2-weighted (TR/TE = 3000/90 and TR/TE = 3000/45) images demonstrate the hamartomatous or dysplastic abnormalities within the basal ganglia. On the T1-weighted images, a rim-like area of increased signal intensity is shown (straight arrows). On the T2-weighted images, the lesions are of diffusely increased signal intensity (curved arrows). These lesions may be unilateral **(C)** or bilateral **(A)** and are most commonly centered at the globus pallidus.

logically as atypical glial cell rests, subependymal glial nodules, ependymal ectopias, intramedullary schwannosis, and meningoangiomatous malformations. Some of the lesions involving the optic chiasm may be hamartomatous because many do not progress over time as expected with gliomas. The chiasm may be enlarged without a signal intensity abnormality, suggesting a more benign lesion.[22]

Many cutaneous and osseous abnormalities are associated with neurofibromatosis. The more common sequelae include cutaneous neurofibromas, cafe-au-lait spots, axillary freckling, kyphoscoliosis, tibial pseudoarthrosis, ribbon ribs, and posterior scalloping of the vertebral bodies.[24]

Tuberous Sclerosis

Tuberous sclerosis is an autosomal dominant disorder with hamartomatous lesions in multiple organs. The classic clinical triad of tuberous sclerosis is seizures, mental retardation, and facial adenoma sebaceum. The hamartomatous lesions within the CNS include subependymal nodules, cortical tubers, and white matter clusters of heterotopic giant cells. Rarely, a subependymal nodule may form a giant cell astrocytoma, which usually rises at the foramen of Monro and can be identified as an enlarging mass. The subependymal nodules are identified along the ventricular wall and have decreased signal intensity, not the increased signal intensity of astrocytomas seen on T2-weighted spin echo images.[25] The white matter lesions display increased signal intensity on T2-weighted spin echo images and probably correspond to clusters of heterotopic giant cells, which are histologically demonstrated (Fig. 4-21).[26] These heterotopic giant cells also compose the cortical tubers and subependymal nodules. The cortical tubers have an imaging pattern similar to pachygyria in that the cortical lesions appear as broad, thickened gray matter. These tubers may also have increased signal intensity on T2-weighted images. Hamartomas may involve many other organs, commonly the kidneys, skin, and orbit. The classic renal lesion is the angiomyolipoma, which is diagnosed by identification of fat within the renal mass.

Von Hippel-Lindau

Von Hippel-Lindau or CNS angiomatosis is an autosomal dominant disorder of the vascular elements within multiple organ systems. In the CNS, von Hippel-Lindau presents as vascular tumors. These lesions are hemangioblastomas located in the cerebellum or spinal cord, only rarely involving the supratentorial brain. These commonly appear as fluid-filled cystic structures of various sizes, with mural tumor nodules that are highly vascularized. The tumor may rarely appear as a solid lesion (Fig. 4-22).[26]

Angiography demonstrates two basic patterns: a densely staining nodule or an abnormal tangle of vessels. Both types may have a central lucency, and both may have enlarged feeding arteries and draining veins.[27] Malignant tumors may also involve the retina, kidney, adrenal gland, and pancreas. The retinal lesions are hemangioblastomas, but the malignancies involving the kidney and pancreas are carcinomas. The rarely associated adrenal tumors are pheochromocytomas.

Sturge-Weber

Sturge-Weber or encephalotrigeminal angiomatosis is a sporadic disorder characterized by a facial cutaneous vascular nevus within the first and second divisions of the trigeminal nerve and an ipsilateral leptomeningeal angiomatosis involving the parietal and occipital lobes. The cutaneous lesion is a capillary angioma, and the leptomeningeal lesion contains thin-walled venous structures confined to the pia mater.[26] MR imaging, like CT, demonstrates hemiatrophy of the involved cerebral hemisphere, but can better identify patchy, parenchymal increased signal on T2-weighted spin echo images. These abnormal areas probably represent regions of gliosis and demyelination, which are presumably caused by ischemic damage from the overlying angiomatous lesion in the pia mater. The gyriform calcifications that are readily identified on CT are not as well seen on MRI. Angiomas may also appear in many other organs in patients with the Sturge-Weber syndrome.[28]

CONCLUSION

Multiplanar T1-weighted spin echo imaging provides precise anatomic detail that is superior to other imaging modalities. This information permits accurate differential diagnosis of the common congenital anomalies. Multiple planes should be used to completely delineate the structural defects and possible sequelae. T2-weighted spin echo imaging and contrast enhancement with Gd DTPA are extremely important for diagnosing enhancing neoplasms associated with the neurocutaneous syndromes. T1-weighted and T2-weighted spin echo imaging also chronicles the normal myelination process, making possible early diagnosis of dysmyelinating and demyelinating diseases.

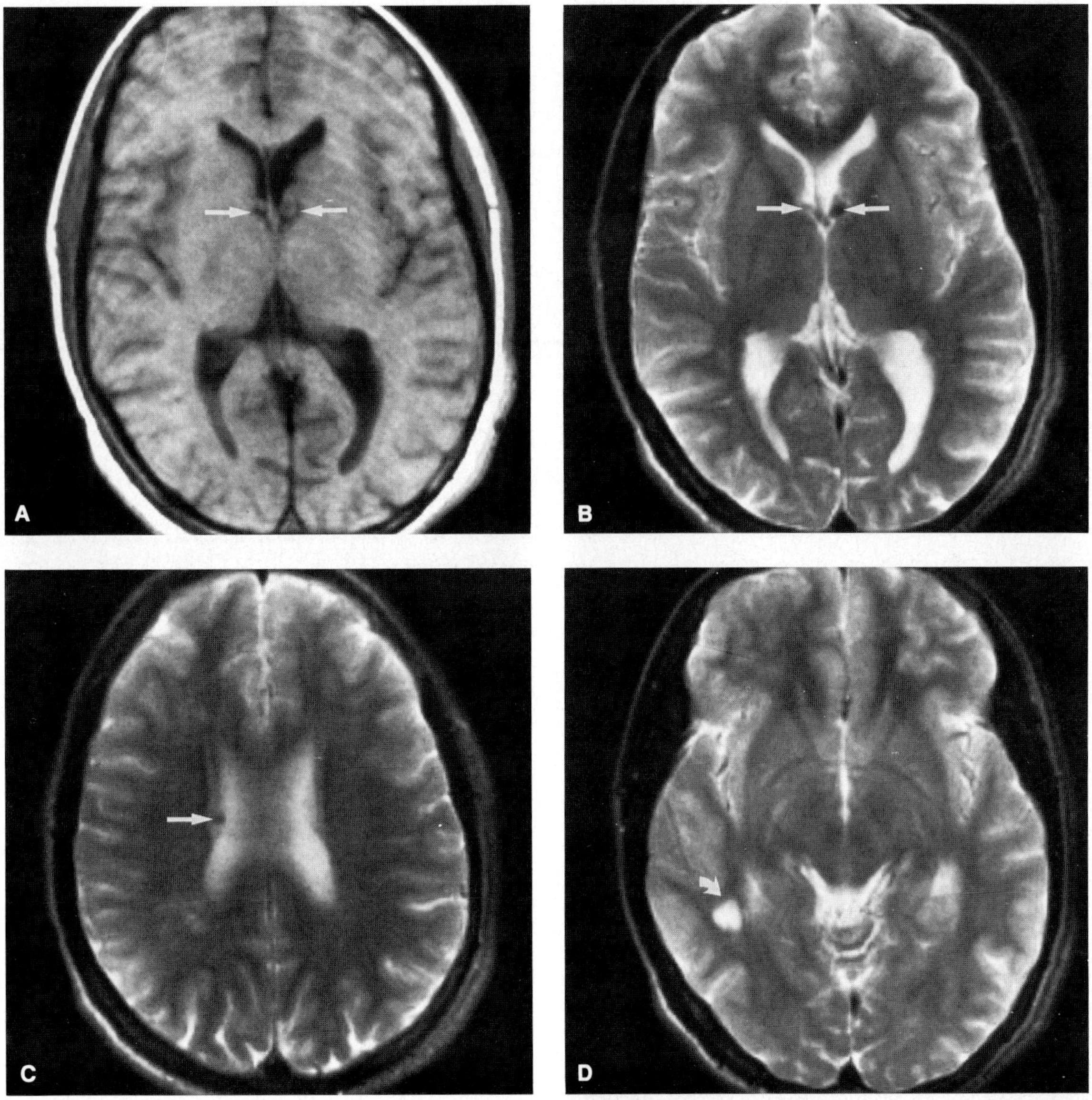

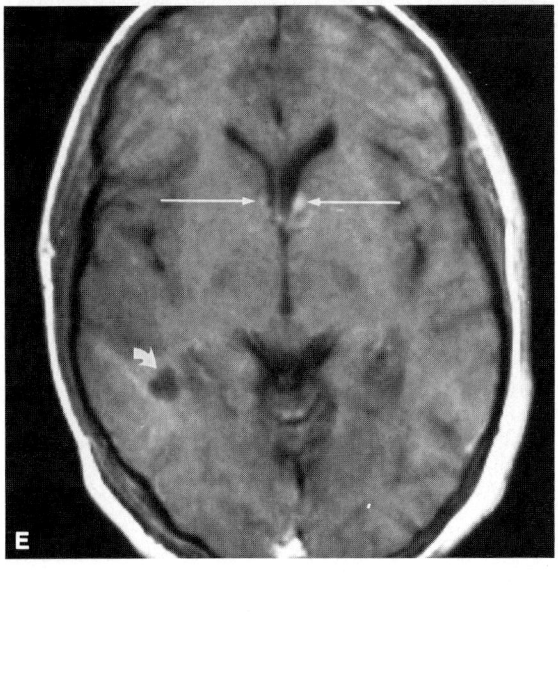

FIGURE 4–21. Tuberous sclerosis in a 15-year-old boy. **(A)** Axial T1-weighted (TR/TE = 650/20), **(B,C,D)** axial T2-weighted (TR/TE = 3000/90), and **(E)** axial post-Gd DTPA T1-weighted (TR/TE = 650/20) images demonstrate the typical features of tuberous sclerosis. **(A,B,C)** The periventricular subependymal nodules along the lateral ventricles and at the foramen of Monro are of low signal intensity on T1- and T2-weighted sequences (straight arrows). These signal characteristics are presumably due to mineral deposition and correspond to the CT findings of calcified periventricular nodules. **(D,E)** A presumed white matter cluster of heterotopic giant cells is identified within the white matter tracts of the right parietal lobe, characterized by high signal intensity on the T2-weighted image and decreased signal intensity on the T1-weighted image (curved arrows). This lesion does not enhance with Gd DTPA, but the subependymal nodules at the foramen of Monro do (long, thin arrows), possibly due to the formation of a giant cell subependymal astrocytoma. If enlarging, enhancing masses impinge into the ventricles, the diagnosis of giant cell astrocytoma is likely. Follow-up evaluation is needed to monitor these subependymal nodules to detect evolving malignancy.

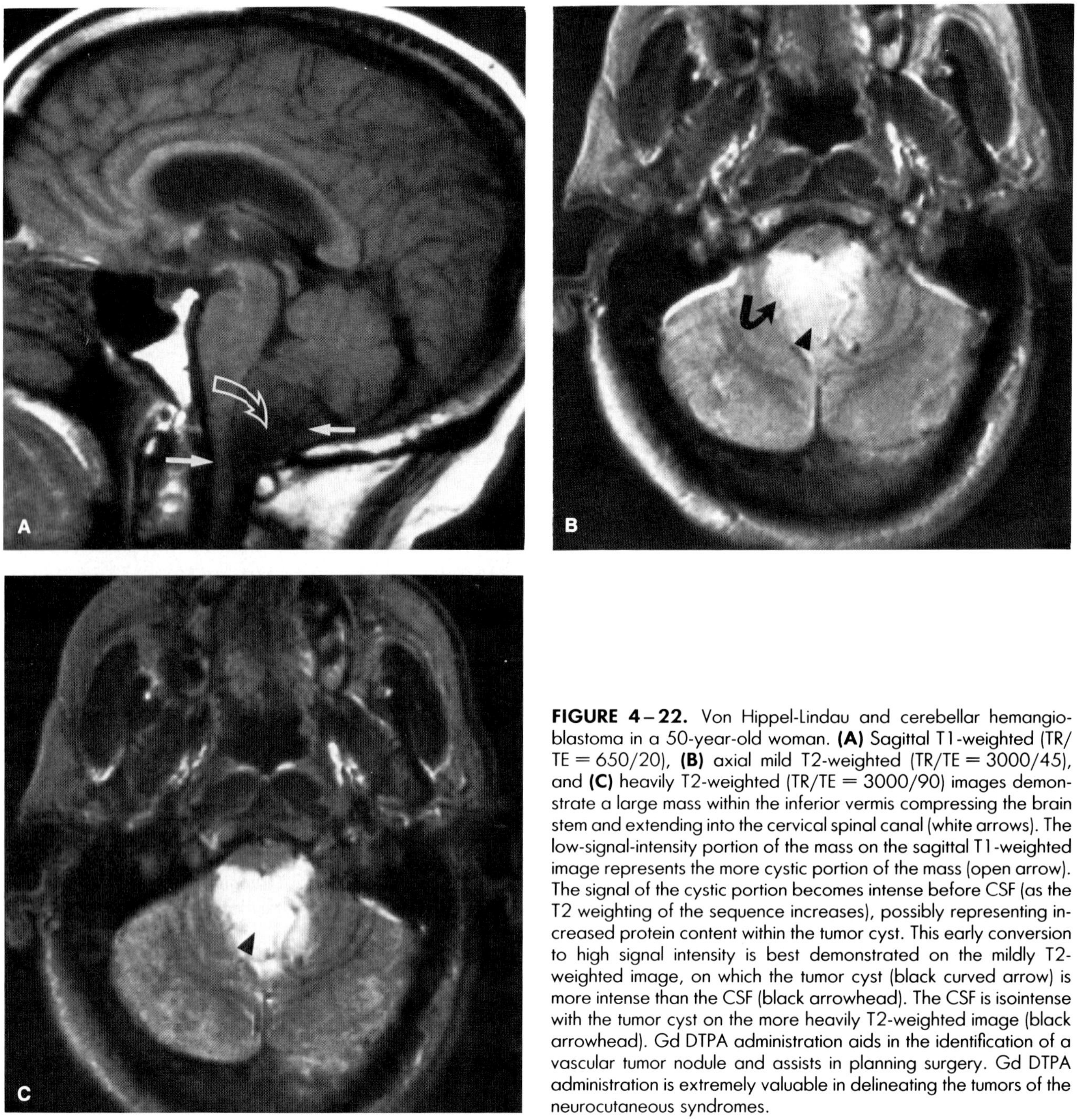

FIGURE 4–22. Von Hippel-Lindau and cerebellar hemangioblastoma in a 50-year-old woman. **(A)** Sagittal T1-weighted (TR/TE = 650/20), **(B)** axial mild T2-weighted (TR/TE = 3000/45), and **(C)** heavily T2-weighted (TR/TE = 3000/90) images demonstrate a large mass within the inferior vermis compressing the brain stem and extending into the cervical spinal canal (white arrows). The low-signal-intensity portion of the mass on the sagittal T1-weighted image represents the more cystic portion of the mass (open arrow). The signal of the cystic portion becomes intense before CSF (as the T2 weighting of the sequence increases), possibly representing increased protein content within the tumor cyst. This early conversion to high signal intensity is best demonstrated on the mildly T2-weighted image, on which the tumor cyst (black curved arrow) is more intense than the CSF (black arrowhead). The CSF is isointense with the tumor cyst on the more heavily T2-weighted image (black arrowhead). Gd DTPA administration aids in the identification of a vascular tumor nodule and assists in planning surgery. Gd DTPA administration is extremely valuable in delineating the tumors of the neurocutaneous syndromes.

REFERENCES

1. Nadich TP, Zimmerman RA. Common congenital malformations of the brain. In: Brant-Zawadzki M, Norman D, eds. Magnetic resonance imaging of the central nervous system. New York: Raven Press, 1987;131.
2. Barkovich AJ, Kjos BO, Jackson DE, et al. Normal maturation of the neonatal and infant brain: MR imaging at 1.5 T. Radiology 1988;166:173.
3. Holland BA, Haas DK, Norman D, et al. MRI of normal brain maturation. AJNR 1986;7:201.
4. Dietrich RB, Bradley WG, La Ragoza EJ. MR evaluation of early myelination patterns in normal and developmentally delayed infants. AJNR 1988;9:69.
5. McArdle CB, Richardson CJ, Nicholas SA, et al. Developmental features of the neonatal brain: MR imaging. Part II. Ventricular size and extracerebral space. Radiology 1987;162:230.
6. Spinos E, Laster DW, Moody DM, et al. MR evaluation of Chiari I malformations at 0.15 T. AJNR 1985;6:203.
7. Naidich TP, McLone DG, Fulling KH. The Chiari II malformation: Part IV. The hindbrain deformity. Neuroradiology 1983;25:179.
8. Wolpert SM, Anderson M, Scott RM. Chiari II malformation: MR imaging evaluation. AJNR 1987;8:783.
9. Naidich TP, Radkowski MA, Bernstein RA, et al. Congenital

malformation of the posterior fossa. In: Taveras JM, Ferucci JT, eds. Radiology. Philadelphia: JB Lippincott, 1986, Ch. 67:1.

10. Gardner E, O'Rahilly R, Prolo D. The Dandy-Walker and Arnold-Chiari malformation. Clinical, developmental and teratological considerations. Arch Neurol 1975;32:393.

11. Harwood-Nash DC, Fitz CR. Congenital malformations of the brain. In: Neuroradiology in infants and children. St. Louis: CV Mosby, 1978:998.

12. Raybaud T. Cystic malformations of the posterior fossa: abnormalities associated with the development of the roof of the fourth ventricle and adjacent meningeal structures. J Neuroradiol 1982;9:103.

13. Kendall BE. Dysgenesis of the corpus callosum. Neuroradiology 1983;25:239.

14. Atlas SW, Zimmerman RA, Bilaniuk LT, et al. Corpus callosum and limbic system: neuroanatomic MR evaluation of developmental anomalies. Radiology 1986;160:355.

15. Barkovich AJ, Norman D. Anomalies of the corpus callosum: correlation with further anomalies of the brain. AJNR 1988;9:493.

16. Faerber EN, Wolpert SM. The value of computed tomography in the diagnosis of intracranial lipomata. JCAT 1978;2:292.

17. Weinstein MA, Maseryk TJ, Modic MT, et al. Magnetic resonance of fatty CNS tumors. Presented at the 22nd Annual Meeting of the ASNR, June 1984, Boston, MA.

18. Fitz OR. Holoprosencephaly and related entities. Neuroradiology 1983;25:225.

19. Byrd SE, Naidich TP. Common congenital brain anomalies. In: Lee SH, Zimmerman RA, eds. Imaging in neuroradiology. Part I. Philadelphia, WB Saunders, 1988:755.

20. Barkovich AJ, Chuang SH, Norman D. MR of neuronal migration anomalies. AJNR 1987;8:1009.

21. Barkovich AJ, Norman D. MR imaging of schizencephaly. AJNR 1988;9:297.

22. Bognano JR, Edwards MK, Lee TA, et al. Cranial MR imaging in neurofibromatosis. AJNR 1988;9:461.

23. Crowe FW, Schull WJ, Neel JU, et al. A clinical, pathological, and genetic study of multiple neurofibromatosis. Springfield, IL: Charles C. Thomas, 1956.

24. Braffman BH, Bilaniuk LT, Zimmerman RA. The CNS manifestations of the phakomatoses on MR. In: Lee SH, Zimmerman RA, eds. Imaging in neuroradiology. Part I. Philadelphia: WB Saunders, 1988:773.

25. McMurdo SK, Moore SG, Brant-Zadwadski M, et al. MR imaging and intracranial tuberous sclerosis. AJNR 1987;8:77.

26. DeRecondo S, Haguemav M. Neuropathologic survey of the phakomatoses and allied disorders. In: Vinken PS, Gruy GW, eds. The phakomatoses: handbook of clinical neurology. Amsterdam: North Holland, 1972:19.

27. Wolpert SM. The neuroradiology of hemangioblastomas and the cerebellum. AJR 1970;110:56.

28. Bilaniuk LT, Zimmerman RA, Hochman M, et al. MR of the Sturge-Weber syndrome. AJNR 1987;8:945.

5

Cervical Spine

Ann C. Price
Gregory V. Babigian

There is a seemingly endless number of operator-selected magnetic resonance imaging (MRI) parameters. The most important of these include echo time (TE), relaxation time (TR), averages, matrix size, zoom factor or field of view, and mechanisms to suppress motion. Incorrect combinations of these parameters cause artifacts, poor image quality, and a complicated, frustrating examination. Fortunately, there is no single or right way to perform a study, and many different approaches may accomplish the same goal. However, to enjoy such latitude, a physician must have a thorough understanding of the abnormality to be demonstrated and the MR imager's capabilities, particularly the most recent software modifications. Many software modifications add quality and efficiency, but others impose unacceptable limitations in time, restrict the number of slices acquired, or adversely affect factors of resolution.

The study must be accomplished in an acceptable period of time, 1 hour or less for both patient comfort and examination cost. Many patients with spine complaints are not able to remain still for prolonged periods due to pain or discomfort. The use of analgesics, opiates, or tranquilizers appropriate to the patient's level of pain or anxiety can reward the examiner with a more cooperative, immobile patient. The high cost of MR equipment and continued stress on medical cost containment are practical reasons for time-efficient studies.

This chapter provides some guidelines for imaging a spectrum of commonly encountered disease processes of the cervical spine. These guidelines are intended to provide a high-quality diagnostic examination while optimizing the time of acquisition. Although the imaging parameters are for a 1.0-T imager, they can be applied with knowledge of another imaging systems' capabilities.

TECHNICAL CONSIDERATIONS

The cervical spine presents some unique imaging challenges for MRI. It is an anatomically compact region with a complex bone and joint anatomy and orientation. Also, there is rapidly pulsating cerebrospinal fluid (CSF). Due to these complexities, relevant detail of technical factors is an important component of these imaging guidelines. A technically limited study may lead to difficulties in the interpretation and raise more questions than it answers.

The parameters that optimize the signal-to-noise ratio (SNR) and, ultimately, the image quality must be appreciated by the individual performing the study.

Surface Coils

Routine imaging of the spine became possible only after the development of local or surface coils, which receive (i.e., receiver coil) the radio-frequency (RF) signal from a volume of tissue determined by the size of the coil. The threefold to fivefold increase in the SNR produces higher quality images.

Some manufacturers have a selection of coil sizes. The highest SNR and, consequently, the best images are obtained from the smallest coil that will cover the desired area. Larger coils receive noise from outside the region of interest, thereby decreasing the SNR. The smaller coil, with its higher SNR, requires fewer averages or excitations, and imaging time can be reduced.[1]

Surface coils for cervical spine imaging have many configurations, including the Helmholtz coil, posterior only coil, and contour coil. The majority of the images in this chapter were obtained with the Helmholtz coil. If properly applied and meticulously tuned, this coil generally provides high-quality images. One problem area is in the very lordotic cervical spine, where the major area of interest is displaced from the center of the coil. The sagittal images can appear "noisy" and be further degraded by wrap-around artifacts (Fig. 5-1). This problem can be partially offset by increasing the number of averages. Axial images may be even noisier than sagittal images depending upon the selection of pulse sequence and slice thickness.

Slice Thickness

Because the cervical spine is anatomically a small area of interest, thin-section imaging is necessary for evaluation. Sections no greater than 4 mm should be used in the sagittal plane. Slice widths of 3 mm or less are optimal. In children, true contiguous 3 mm images, obtained by interleaving, may be necessary if the cord is not to be missed. Axial sections should be 3 to 5 mm for a routine or survey study. Thin-section imaging requires extra averages or excitations in much the same fashion that thin-section CT requires additional peak kilovoltage (kVp) or current (mA) to produce images that are not "grainy" or lacking in definition. These are costly in time.

A gap between images is used to prevent image degradation by the "cross-talk" that results from the sinusoidal configuration or profile of the pulse. These tapered ends partially excite the tissue peripheral to the intended margin. On T2-weighted images, the partial excitation reduces the time for longitudinal recovery, introducing T1 contrast. Many manufacturers have software programs for improving the pulse profile to a more nearly optimal rectangular shape. These may have limitations, such as a minimum TE or slice thickness.

An acceptable gap is 1.0 to 1.5 mm (~30%). Truly contiguous slices can be obtained by interleaving. This is accomplished by obtaining two separate acquisitions that have a 100% gap. Interleaving will obviously take more time because there are two acquired data sets and two separate computer inputs by the technologist with some imagers. These will also have less SNR than a slightly longer TR single acquisition series with an appropriate gap. For instance, an interleaved acquisition with a TR of 0.5 seconds will have less SNR than a single acquisition with a TR of 0.7 seconds and an appropriate gap. Obviously, interleaving is feasible only with T1-weighted or shorter TR sequences.

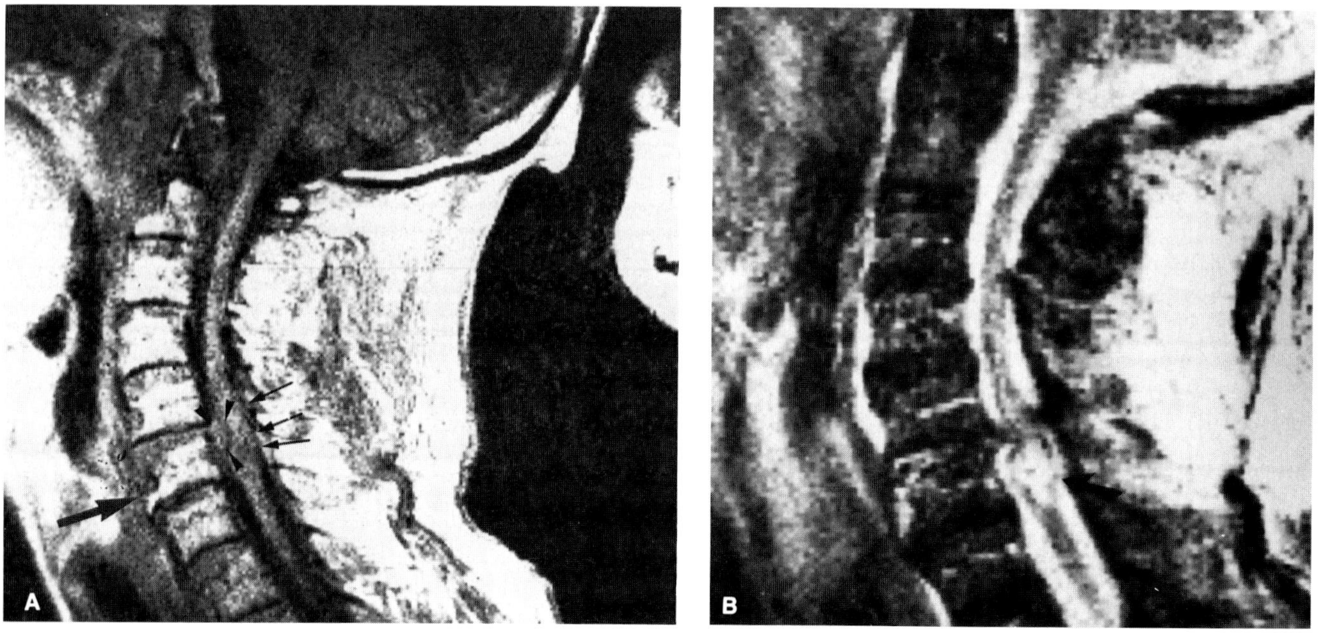

FIGURE 5-1. (A) The degree of lordotic spine curvature in this case results in a wrap-around artifact with the chin projecting posterior to the occiput. This contributes to the "noisy" appearance of the image. There is a posttraumatic C5-6 herniated disc (arrowheads) and a C6 vertebral body fracture (large arrow). Slight focal cord widening is seen (small arrows) on this T1-weighted image (TR/TE = 500/17). **(B)** A cord contusion is confirmed on the T2-weighted image (TR/TE = 3000/90) as an area of increased signal intensity (arrow). The low-signal-intensity herniated disc, degenerative change, and posterior ridging are clearly outlined by the bright CSF. The use of gradient moment nulling results in a sharp cord-CSF interface.

CSF Motion

The motion of the cerebrospinal fluid (CSF) further complicates cervical spine imaging. This to and fro motion occurs with each heartbeat. Although not of the same magnitude as blood, the degree of CSF motion can cause considerable dephasing artifacts. CSF motion is an imaging consideration to the level of the conus. With longer TR or T2-weighted sequences, the low-signal-intensity dephasing artifacts are more apparent. Without mechanisms to suppress motion, these are often of such magnitude that an arteriovenous malformation (AVM) may be falsely suspected (Fig. 5-2).

There are many mechanisms for dealing with CSF motion. These are more efficient than using sequences that take advantage of even-echo rephasing or switching the phase and frequency encoding gradients. Cardiac gating is one method that will effectively inhibit the motion artifact from CSF pulsations. The drawback of cardiac gating is that the TR is related to the heart rate. Thus, the TR may not be as long as desired or may be inconsistent from patient to patient. More importantly, the application of the gating device is technically more difficult, and the gating leads may occasionally become detached so that the examination has to be repeated.

An easier method of dealing with motion artifact is using flow-compensation or motion-suppressing sequences (gradient moment nulling), which apply computer-manipulated gradients to suppress motion (Fig. 5-1B). The technical involvement and their related errors are lessened. Limitations with these sequences, which vary depending upon the specific imager employed, include field of view, number of echoes, and lengthening of the minimum TE which can be achieved.

Gradient-motion-suppressing techniques (gradient moment nulling) are quite effective in the sagittal plane at 1.0 T (Figs. 5-1B and 5-3B); however, they are generally poor in the axial plane for the entire spine. These are especially ineffective in the cervical spine, where CSF velocity is rapid. If T2-weighted axial images are necessary, then cardiac gating is required to obtain a diagnostic image. For most abnormalities that have been evaluated with sagittal T2-weighted images, axial gradient-echo or T1-weighted images are usually adequate. At higher field strengths (1.5 T), CSF pulsation artifacts may be of such magnitude that cardiac gating or a combination of cardiac gating and flow compensation (gradient moment nulling) are necessary to suppress CSF motion.

Another effective and time-efficient method of dealing with CSF motion is the use of gradient echo (GRE) imaging. This type of imaging has many different designations, depending on the manufacturer: FISP, FLASH, or GRASS. It differs from spin echo (SE) imaging by the lack of the 180° pulse. The echoes are produced by gradients. The manner in which these gradients are applied determines the expected contrast (i.e., T1 or T2). FISP is commonly employed to achieve T2-weighted contrast, while FLASH can be used to generate T1-weighted contrast. In general, at low flip angles of 10 to 20° and TRs greater than 200 msec, FISP and FLASH images have a similar appearance. This is referred to as "CSF imaging" or the "CSF

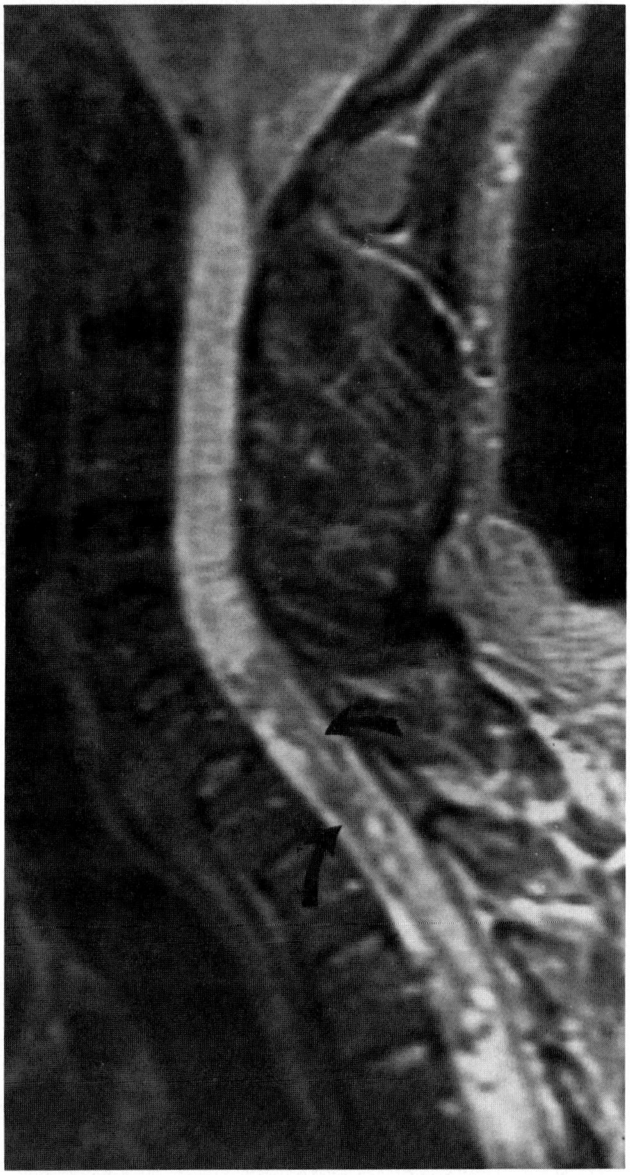

FIGURE 5-2. A high-signal-intensity cord tumor is poorly defined on this T2-weighted image (TR/TE = 2400/60). The margins of the cord, tumor, and CSF are poorly defined. CSF motion has also resulted in a long low signal-dephasing artifact (arrows). Compare with the sharper definition of the small cord contusion in Figure 5-1B.

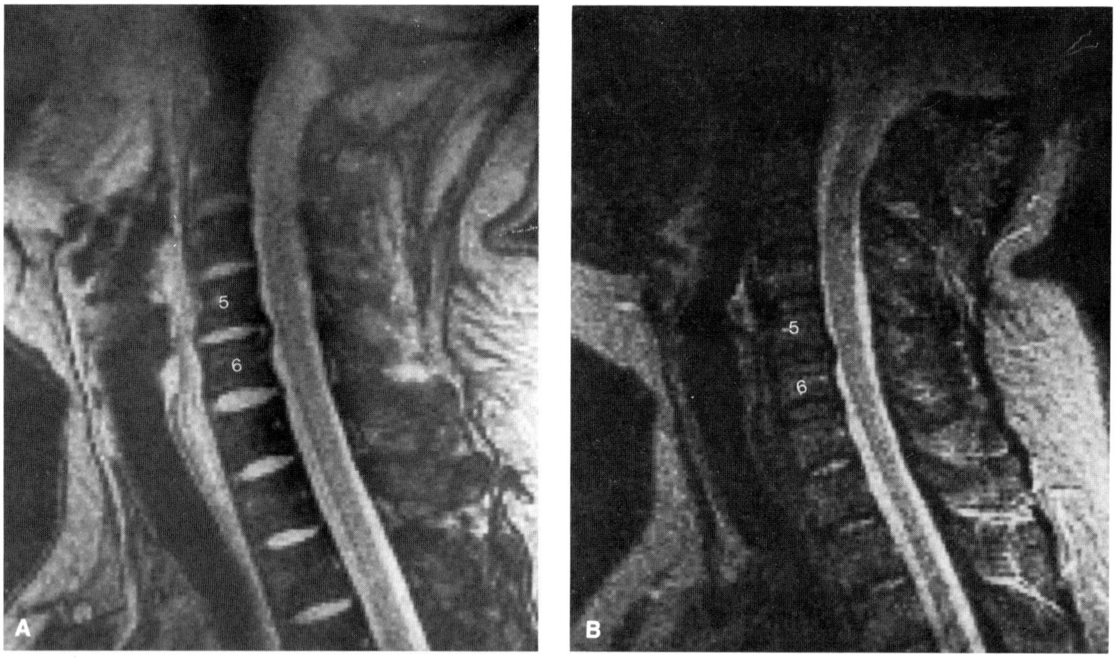

FIGURE 5–3. **(A)** A disc bulge is demonstrated at C5-6 by the bright CSF on this FLASH-10 (TR/TE = 200/11) sequence. The cord is low signal intensity on this 5-mm section, and the discs show increased signal intensity. **(B)** The 3-mm T2-weighted sequence (TR/TE = 3000/90) obtained with gradient moment nulling shows the disc bulge and cord similar to the GRE **(A)**. The discs do not appear as bright because desiccation is more accurately shown with this technique. The spin echo exam required 9.4 minutes more to acquire than the FLASH image.

myelographic effect" due to the bright signal intensity of CSF (Fig. 5–3A). TRs are short (200–700 msec), as are the TEs (10–15 msec), so that SNR is excellent for the TR. Because the TRs are quite brief, the images will appear noisy and usually require 4 to 8 averages. Short TEs and imaging times act to lessen motion artifact.

Imaging Guidelines

Perhaps the single most important formula for planning efficient SE imaging is this:

$$\text{Imaging Time} = \text{TR} \times \text{Matrix size} \times \text{Averages}$$

In this formula, TR = repetition time, and matrix size = number of phase-encoding steps. Software options that minimize artifacts (i.e., presaturation pulses) may alter this formula slightly by increasing the time above that calculated. This formula is also altered by mechanisms that minimize wrap-around artifacts, such as an extended matrix (in the phase-encoding direction).

Matrix

Because the cervical spine is small and anatomically compact, the 256 × 256 matrix produces the highest quality images. The 192 × 256 matrix produces adequate images, but further reduction in matrix size (128 × 256) produces images with poor resolution and significant truncation artifacts.

Zoom Factor or Field of View

Most of the illustrations in this chapter were obtained with a field of view (FOV) of 270 to 250 mm, depending on the desired area of coverage. The zoom factor (ZF) is related to the FOV by a simple conversion factor. The default or standard FOV for a coil (300 mm in the spine) is divided by the user-selected FOV to give the ZF.

$$\frac{300}{250} = 1.2$$

Thus, a ZF of 1.2 converts to a FOV of 250 mm. The difference between a 270 mm and 250 mm FOV (1.1 versus 1.2 zoom factor) usually has little effect on image quality so that additional averages are not required. Further decrease in the FOV may require additional averages, which leads to a longer examination.

The pixel dimension has considerable effect on resolution according to the formula:

$$\text{Pixel diameter} = \frac{\text{FOV}}{\text{Matrix size}}$$

For those who have greater matrix and FOV options, the reader is referred to an excellent discussion of the relationships of these factors to SNR, image quality, and acquisition time in Chapter 13 and other reference sources.[1]

Averages

Although some manufacturers offer a wide choice (e.g. 1 to 256 by increments of 1) and even fractional (e.g. 0.5) averages or number of excitations (NEX), averages are often limited to powers of 2 (e.g. 1, 2, 4, 8, 16, 32, etc.). Because slice widths are thin (3–5 mm), averages for SE sequences will generally be 2 to 4.

Averages increase the SNR by a factor equivalent to the $\sqrt{\text{averages}}$. Thus, doubling the averages in the previous imaging time formula doubles the imaging time, with only a 41% increase in the SNR.[1] Selecting the number of averages must be carefully assessed in terms of overall time for imaging in the uncooperative patient. Too many averages may actually decrease image quality as the result of motion.

TR

In choosing the TR, it is important to consider the area or levels to be covered while remaining within the limits of T1-weighted or T2-weighted imaging parameters. Increasing the TR increases the SNR, but this is not geometric; doubling the TR does not double the SNR. For a T1-weighted sagittal sequence, a TR of 700 msec should provide an adequate number of 3-mm-wide slices (including gap) to extend from pedicle to pedicle. Using the 256^2 matrix and 2 averages, the imaging time (IT) will be

$$\text{IT} = \frac{0.7 \times 256 \times 2}{60} = 5.97 \text{ minutes}$$

These images will have a higher SNR and shorter imaging time than interleaved sections with these values:

$$\text{IT} = \frac{0.5 \times 256 \times 2}{60} = 4.26 \text{ minutes}$$

Two interleaved sets therefore require 8.52 minutes.

An alternative for a high-quality study is to use a 3-mm slice with a gap (1–1.5 mm), increase the averages to 4, and use a TR of 0.6:

$$\text{IT} = \frac{0.6 \times 256 \times 4}{60} = 10.2 \text{ minutes}$$

Carefully observing the images with several different TRs (0.5–0.7 seconds) and varying the number of averages will provide the user with optimal images for personal preference and diagnostic purposes.

The TR selected for T2-weighted sequences usually provides ample slices to cover the cervical spine in the sagittal plane. The imaging time will be one crucial factor in selection. A TR of 2.5 seconds (2500 msec) usually requires 2 averages, while a TR of 3.0 seconds (3000 msec) often has sufficient SNR with one average, resulting in a considerable difference in imaging time:

$$\text{IT} = \frac{2.5 \times 256 \times 2}{60} = 24.3 \text{ minutes}$$

$$\text{IT} = \frac{3.0 \times 256 \times 1}{60} = 12.8 \text{ minutes}$$

For T2-weighted images, the TR must be long enough to extend beyond the CSF "cross-over" point. Before that point, the cord and CSF will be the same signal intensity so that certain intrinsic cord lesions cannot be visualized (Fig. 5–4). This point varies with field strength, so that a longer TR is required at 1.5 T than at 0.5 T. A longer TE (≥100 msec) can be used to generate T2-weighted images while retaining a lower TR (1500–2000 msec). Longer TEs, however, produce noiser images due to a reduction in SNR.

TE

The TE should be as short as possible to maximize the SNR. For T1-weighted spin echo sequences, this is 10

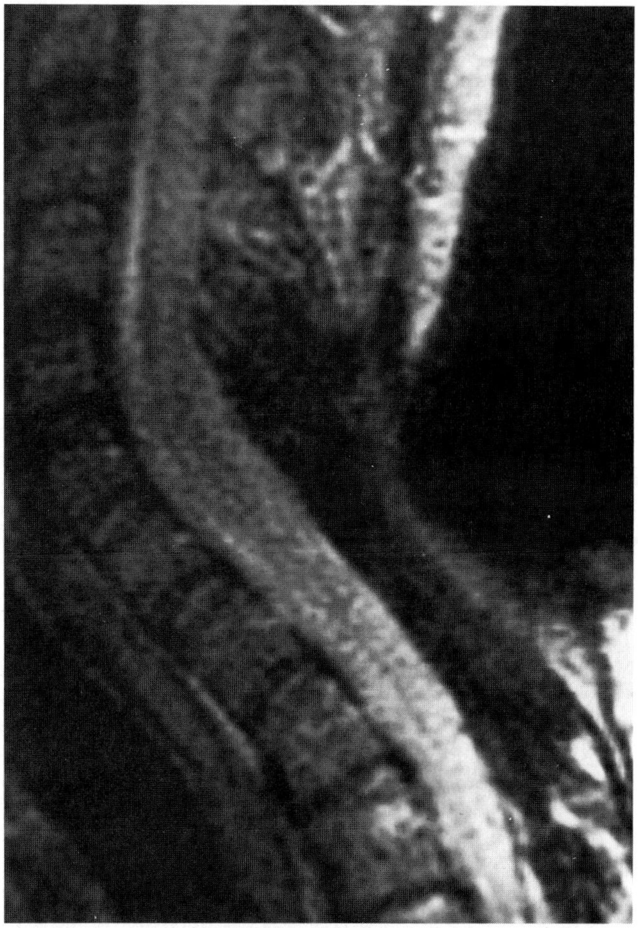

FIGURE 5–4. In this sagittal image (TR/TE = 1500/60), the cord is poorly defined, and the tumor in this patient shown in Figure 5–2 cannot be seen. For direct visualization of most intrinsic cord lesions, and in order to obtain a sharp cord–CSF interface, a longer TR is required which will result in greater T2 weighting. Motion-suppression techniques must also be used.

to 20 msec. Further decrease in TE can produce unacceptable pulsation artifacts. Increasing the TE produces noisier images and fewer slices. If gradient motion suppression is used with T2-weighted images, the TE selections may be predefined or limited.

T1-Weighted Sequences

To obtain T1-weighted sequences, a maximum TR should not be exceeded. This increases with field strength due to prolongation of T1. At 1.0 T, this TR is approximately 0.7 seconds. Each manufacturer supplies suggested guidelines for obtaining sequences that are best for assessing normal anatomy.

The normal cord has a signal intensity similar to muscle on T1-weighted images. It is tube-shaped and has a normal widening at C5, where the brachial plexus arises. The cord is almost centrally positioned in the subarachnoid space with low-signal-intensity CSF both anterior and posterior (Fig. 5-5).

Due to the relative lack of mobile hydrogen protons, osseous structures have diminished signal intensity. This is particularly true for cortical bone, which has virtually no signal. The vertebral end plates are an example of cortical bone. The end plate above the disc generally appears thicker due to a chemical shift artifact, which occurs in the frequency-encoding direction (Fig. 5-5). Although this should appear worse at high field strengths, in practice, the difference may be difficult to assess.

The very-low-signal-intensity cortical end plates provide a frame for the cancellous bone, which is similar in signal intensity to muscle due to its fat and marrow content (Fig. 5-5). Small, round spots of bright signal intensity are commonly seen. These are attributed to fatty replacement of the blood-forming elements in the marrow and are more frequent in the aging patient or after radiation therapy (Fig. 5-6). These bright areas become less intense on T2-weighted images, behaving in the same fashion as other fatty changes or structures. Situated between the very-low-signal-intensity end plates is the intervertebral disc. The intensity of the disc on T1-weighted images is slightly less than for cancellous bone (Fig. 5-5).

T1-weighted sequences are necessary for evaluating low-signal-intensity changes that occur in tumors, cysts, and syrinxes; to evaluate high-signal-intensity changes that occur in subacute hemorrhage, lipomas, and pantopaque; and to demonstrate contrast enhancement.

T1-weighted axial images can be obtained if additional information about the cord is desired. Because the subarachnoid space is relatively wide, and there is little epidural fat in the cervical spine, inherent contrast is low. Therefore, the axial evaluation of disc disease and degenerative change is complicated (Fig. 5-7). Small discs may be overlooked due to the width of the subarachnoid space with its low-signal-intensity CSF. Degenerative changes also produce low signal intensities, so they readily blend with and are obscured by the low-signal-intensity subarachnoid space. Indirect visualization may occur if the degenerative change has enough mass effect to abut or compress the cord.

For these reasons, GRE imaging with its CSF myelographic effect has gained wide acceptance.

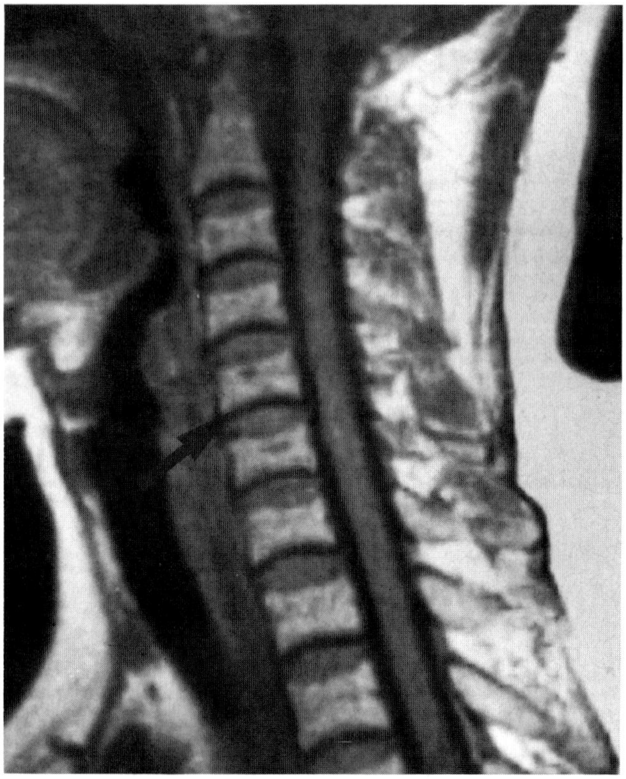

FIGURE 5-5. This sagittal T1-weighted image (TR/TE = 700/17) shows a normal cervical spine. The soft tissue signal intensity of the cord is outlined by the low-signal-intensity CSF. The slightly wider vertebral end-plate cephalad to the disc (arrow) is a chemical shift artifact.

FIGURE 5-6. **(A)** A medulloblastoma was resected in this patient 13 years ago. Radiation therapy has been administered in the past for known drop metastases. There is a bright signal intensity of the vertebral bodies on this sagittal T1-weighted image (TR/TE = 700/17) beginning at C6. This was the upper level of the previous radiation therapy port. There are areas of cord enlargement with irregular areas of low signal intensity (arrows). **(B)** On the T2-weighted sagittal image (TR/TE = 3000/90), the vertebral bodies show a decrease in signal intensity consistent with fatty marrow replacement. There is a rather diffuse increase in signal intensity in the abnormal cord. **(C,D)** Sagittal T1-weighted images after Gd DTPA administration show plaque-like areas of meningeal enhancement (small arrows) with larger areas of cord enhancement. These areas coincide with the cord enlargement (large arrows) and are consistent with tumor invasion of the cord. ▶

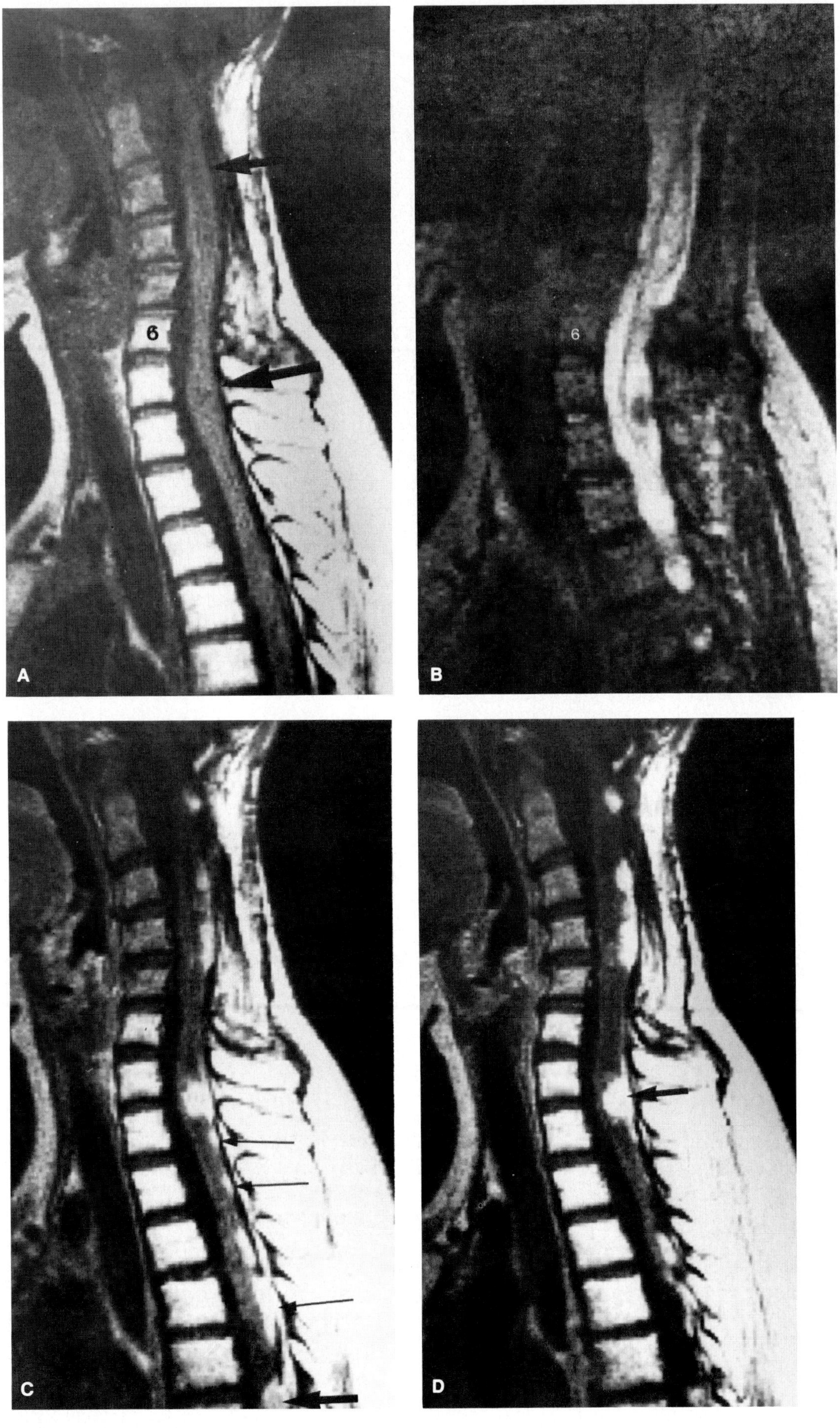

FIGURE 5–6.

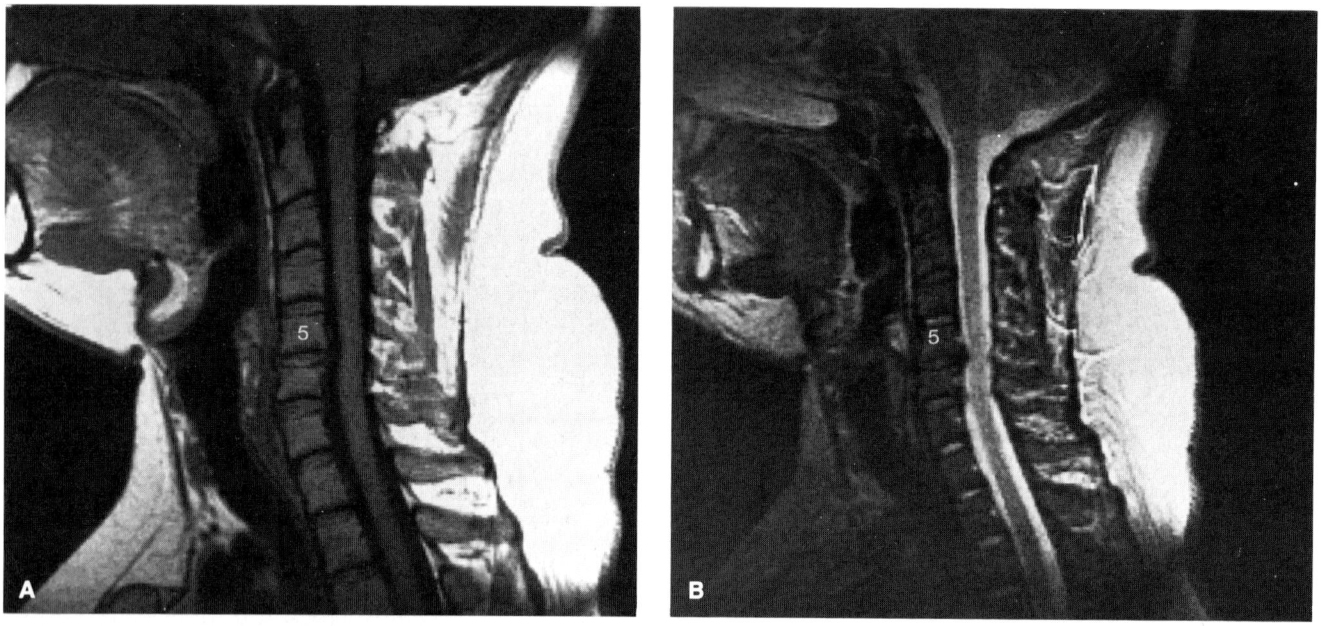

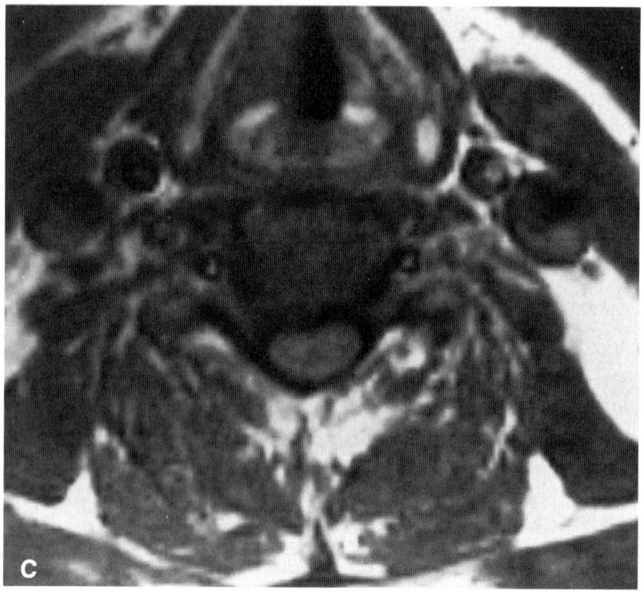

FIGURE 5–7. **(A)** The T1-weighted (TR/TE = 450/20) sagittal section shows a C5-6 disc bulge. **(B)** The degree of disc bulge and associated degenerative change are much better shown with the T2-weighted image (TR/TE = 3000/90). Cord impingement is evident. There is a lesser degree of degenerative change at C6-7 anteriorly and posteriorly. **(C)** The abnormality can be lateralized to the right on the axial T1-weighted image (TR/TE = 450/20) due to the slight cord effacement. Without the secondary cord change, the degeneration would be difficult to assess because it is similar in signal intensity to CSF.

Gradient Echo

GRE sequences are used in the sagittal and axial planes for the sharp contrast between the low-signal-intensity cord and the high-signal-intensity CSF (Fig. 5-3A). This provides the assets of a myelogram but in a noninvasive manner. These sequences are excellent for evaluating disc herniations, hypertrophic change (without myelopathy), epidural tumors, and other epidural changes that may impinge the thecal sac, extrinsically compress the cord, and narrow the spinal canal. They are time efficient, which decreases the study time, minimizes motion artifact, and ultimately increases throughput.

These sequences are not true T2-weighted sequences, but are referred to as T2*. This is due to a greater effect of magnet inhomogeneity, magnetic susceptibility, and chemical shift between fat and water. These effects are largely removed by the rephasing 180° pulse in SE imaging. Thus, in looking for multiple sclerosis plaques, intramedullary cord tumors, post-traumatic or degenerative myelopathy, or bony inflammatory changes, a true T2-weighted sequence must be obtained. The GRE sequence may not show the abnormality or may not accurately demonstrate its extent.

Low flip angles (LFA) are used for cervical spine imaging ($<20°$) for both FISP and FLASH, which may have slice, TE, and FOV limitations. As with SE imaging, increasing the TE decreases the SNR and decreases the number of slices. Flip angles and TR also affect the SNR. Increasing the flip angle increases the SNR; however, increasing the flip angle too much produces poor image quality because the higher the ratio of the flip angle to the TR, the greater the T1 contrast. This has two practical effects on imaging: there is decrease in contrast between the cord and CSF in both sagittal and axial planes (Fig. 5-8), and the high-signal-intensity CSF becomes more inhomogenous, with signal loss about the cord and anterior nerve root as it enters the lateral recess (Fig. 5-9). Both lead to difficulty in assessing the presence of disc herniations and their relationships to the cord. If these problems occur, the TR can be increased while maintaining the flip angle, or the flip angle can be lowered while maintaining the TR.

Increasing the TR increases the SNR. The main effect is that a longer TR allows a higher flip angle.[2] Similar to SE imaging, increasing the TR increases the exam time and, if too long, has little advantage over SE imaging.

The flip angles for sagittal and axial images do not need to be equal. In the sagittal plane, CSF may reach its peak at a smaller flip angle than in the axial plane. Thus a sagittal examination may be performed with a flip angle of 10 to 12°, while a 12 to 15° flip angle could be used for axial imaging.[2] The sagittal GRE (flip angle 10°, TR = 0.2, TE = 11, averages = 4) images produce a 73% time conservation compared with true T2-weighted sequences. The bony structures on GRE sagittal imaging are much lower in signal intensity than the spinal cord. The normal disc has a relatively high signal intensity but not as bright as CSF (Fig. 5-3A).

Axial GRE sequences, properly performed, contain as much or more diagnostic information than a postmyelogram CT scan (Fig. 5-10). Truly contiguous 5-mm slices obtained by interleaving will cover C3-4 to C6-7 in most patients (TR = 200 msec, flip angle 10-15°, matrix = 256^2, and averages = 8). Each set requires 6.8 minutes of imaging time, for total of 13.6 minutes. If the clinical history is more specific, thinner (3-4 mm) sections that cover slightly less area may be preferred.

The osseous structures in the axial plane are quite low in signal intensity, normally lower than the cord. The gray matter is often seen as an H- or butterfly-shaped area of bright signal within the spinal cord (Fig. 5-10). Separate white matter tracts cannot be distinguished. Minor, nonpathologic disc bulges have a slightly higher signal intensity than that of bone. The dorsal and ventral nerve roots, which exit from the spinal cord anterolaterally through the neural foramina, can usually be seen (Fig. 5-10). They exit in a dural root sleeve that is occasionally appreciated with coronal GRE imaging. The dorsal root ganglion, a widening of the dorsal root, is commonly visualized. Fat, which is lower in signal intensity than the CSF, fills the remainder of the neural foramina. The dural mar-

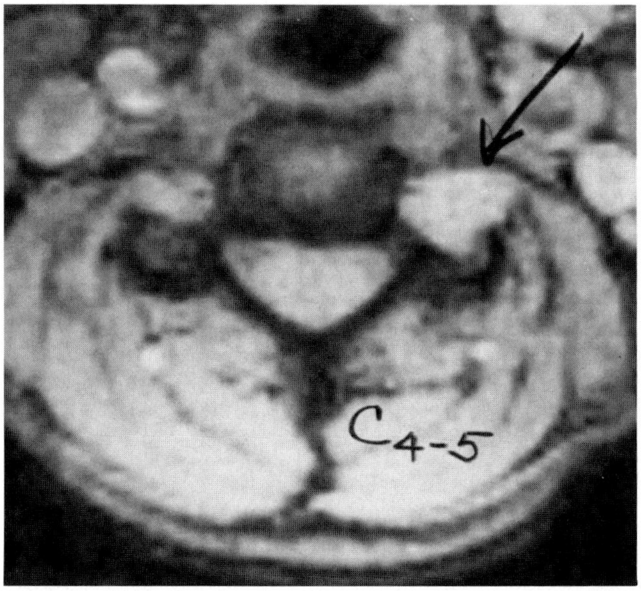

FIGURE 5-8. This axial FISP image (30°, TR/TE = 500/11) shows no differentiation between the cord and CSF. The neurofibroma in the left neural foramen (arrow) shows an increase in signal intensity in this patient with known neurofibromatosis.

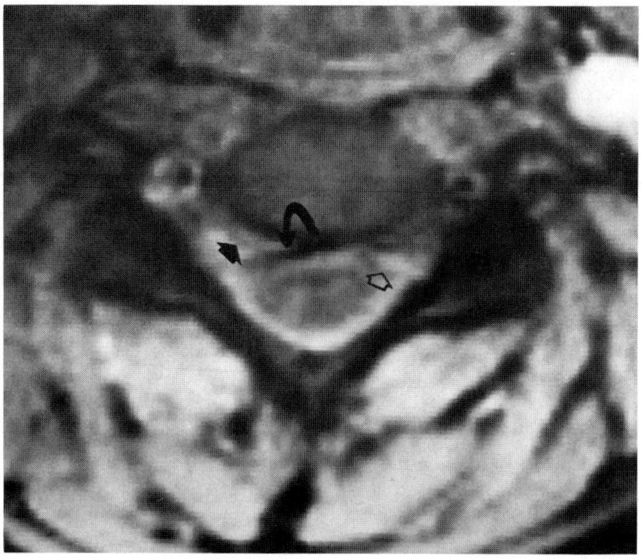

FIGURE 5-9. This FISP-20 (TR/TE = 200/11) shows a signal dropout (curved arrow) that partially obscures the margins of the disc herniation (closed arrow) on the right. The cord is slightly rotated. There is also signal loss on the left, near the exiting nerve root (open arrow). The bright signal intensity of the CSF is preserved in the remainder of the subarachnoid space.

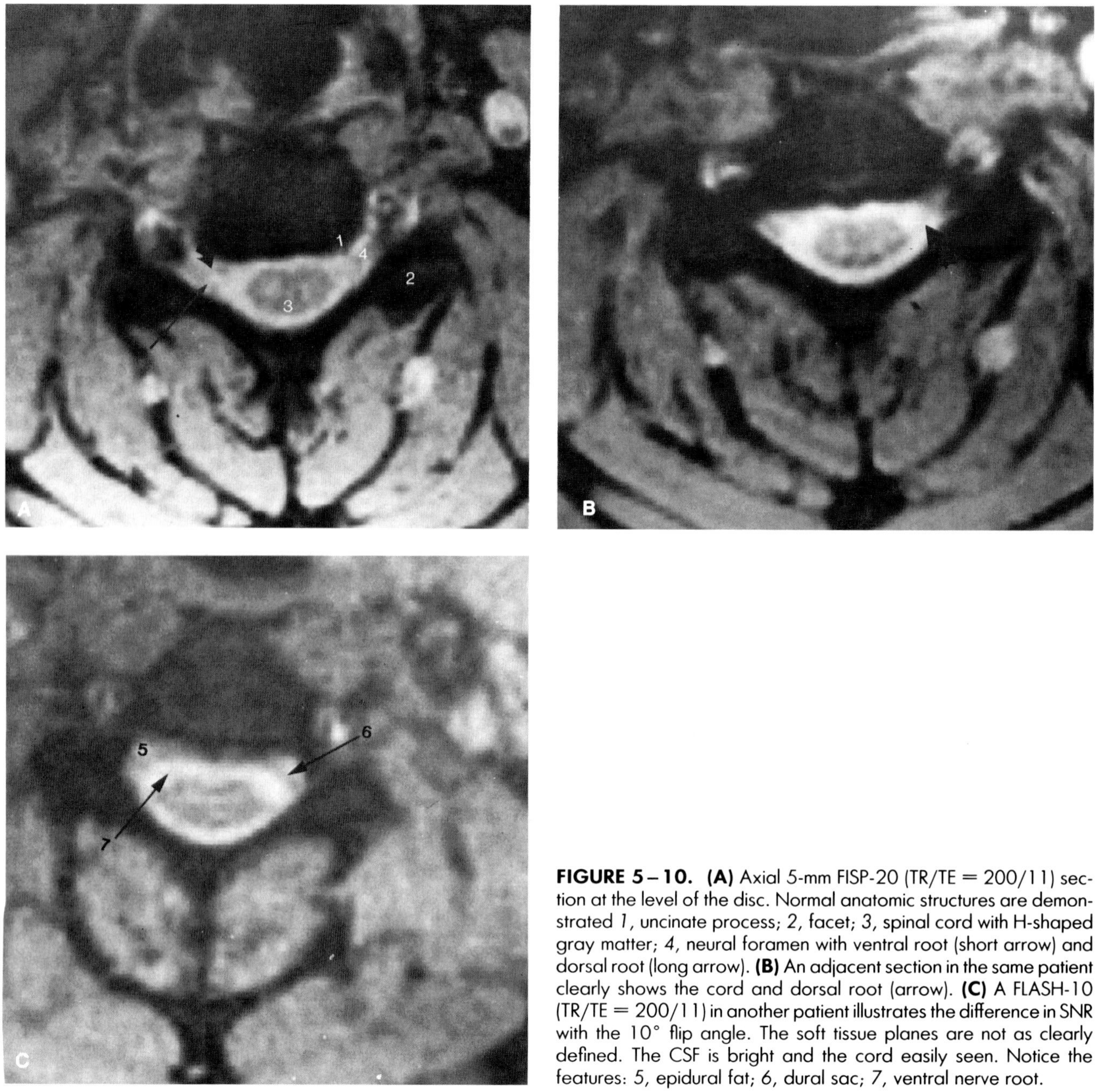

FIGURE 5–10. **(A)** Axial 5-mm FISP-20 (TR/TE = 200/11) section at the level of the disc. Normal anatomic structures are demonstrated *1*, uncinate process; *2*, facet; *3*, spinal cord with H-shaped gray matter; *4*, neural foramen with ventral root (short arrow) and dorsal root (long arrow). **(B)** An adjacent section in the same patient clearly shows the cord and dorsal root (arrow). **(C)** A FLASH-10 (TR/TE = 200/11) in another patient illustrates the difference in SNR with the 10° flip angle. The soft tissue planes are not as clearly defined. The CSF is bright and the cord easily seen. Notice the features: *5*, epidural fat; *6*, dural sac; *7*, ventral nerve root.

gin can be seen as a low-signal-intensity structure separating CSF from epidural fat (Fig. 5–10C). The epidural space also contains connective tissue and vascular structures. The epidural veins, if seen, appear as small oval areas of bright signal intensity on GRE imaging.

T2-Weighted Sequences

T2-weighted sequences may be preferred by clinicians without significant time constraints. Motion-compensation sequences must be used to avoid dephasing artifacts. Gradient-motion compensation (gradient moment nulling) produces excellent sagittal images (Figs. 5–1B, 5–3B, 5–6B, and 5–7B) but is not as effective in the axial plane.

A good rule of thumb is that GRE is diagnostic for abnormalities extrinsic to the cord, such as herniated discs, hypertrophic change without myelopathy, and epidural extension from bony metastases. There are exceptions to this rule. GRE does not always accurately differentiate discogenic sclerosis from interspace infections with adjacent osteomyelitis. GRE may not accurately predict degenerative changes within the disc (Fig. 5–3), and GRE is not as accurate in the assessment of bony metastases. The clinical relevance of these findings in assessment of patients with degenerative disc disease is uncertain. As previously stated, any suspected intrinsic cord abnormality requires T2-weighted sequences (Figs. 5-1B and 5-6B).

T2-weighted sequences also provide a myelogram effect, so that the CSF is bright in contrast to the lower-signal-intensity cord. Normal disc is also bright, with the posterior aspect bordered by the low signal intensity of the annulus fibrosis (Figs. 5-3B and 5-6B). The osseous structures are low signal intensity, with little distinction between cortical and cancellous bone. This occurs because the fatty content of the cancellous bone diminishes in signal intensity on T2-weighted sequences. The appearance of anatomic structures in the axial plane is similar to that described for GRE imaging.

Contraindications

The contraindications for cervical spine imaging are few. The general exclusions of pacemakers, aneurysm clips, and intraocular foreign bodies apply to spine imaging. Some indwelling catheters (i.e., epidural catheters) may be ferromagnetic, and consultation with the referring physician may be necessary. Claustrophobic or uncooperative patients may not be suitable candidates, as well as those on external life support devices.

DEGENERATIVE DISEASES

Herniated intervertebral discs and degenerative changes are the most frequent reasons for an MR study of the spine. It has rapidly become the modality of choice in the initial evaluation of these processes because multiple levels are evaluated noninvasively. This differs from CT, which requires intrathecal contrast for a thorough examination, provides limited coverage (2-3 levels) with ionizing radiation, costs more to perform, and carries the risk of contrast morbidity.

Herniated Disc

Herniated discs, particularly the laterally herniated discs, are not encountered as frequently in the cervical spine as in the lumbar spine due to the reinforcement or support provided by the uncinate processes. A typical protocol for this evaluation includes a sagittal T1-weighted sequence and a sagittal and axial low flip angle GRE sequence (LFAGRE). These sequences require 23 to 27 minutes of imaging time, depending on the selection of TR and averages. If a sagittal T2-weighted sequence is chosen, the imaging time will be 33 to 37 minutes.

On T1-weighted sagittal images, the herniated disc extends beyond the vertebral body. When significant extrusion is present, the disc may extend downward and posteriorly, impinging the cord (Figs. 5-11 and 5-12). The degenerated disc may have a mottled appearance with patchy areas of low signal intensity because of desiccation or aging.

Even though the disc and CSF are bright on the LFAGRE sagittal image, it is usually easy to identify the disc impressing the thecal sac in much the same fashion as myelographic identification. The posterior aspect of the disc may be slightly dark due to degeneration or outlined by the low signal of the annulus and posterior ligament (Fig. 5-3A). Disc mottling caused by desiccation is more apparent on GRE and T2-weighted images (Fig. 5-3).

The herniated disc on axial GRE images is slightly higher in signal intensity than the bony structures and can be easily distinguished from CSF as it impinges the thecal sac or exiting nerve root (Figs. 5-11B, 5-12B, and 5-13B). Although the disc may be identified in the sagittal plane, axial images serve five important functions: lateralization of the disc or abnormality (Figs. 5-11B, 5-12B, and 5-13B); evaluation of the neural foramina and lateral recesses (Figs. 5-12B and 5-13B); evaluation of existing bony changes (Fig. 5-14); soft tissue (i.e., ligamentum flavum) hypertrophy; and evaluation of any cord effects, such as compression, rotation or displacement (Figs. 5-11B and 5-12B). These are basic imaging principles that apply to the evaluation of disc and degenerative changes and to other spinal abnormalities as well.

Osseous Changes

With the uncinate process bordering the neural foramen anteromedially and the facet joints posterolaterally, it is easy to see how osseous spurs could impress the exiting nerve root and produce a radiculopathy (Figs. 5-10, 5-14B, and 5-15). Facet disease does not usually approach the degree that occurs in the lumbar spine due to the vast difference in weight support required of the two regions.

Hypertrophic change can occasionally produce radicular symptoms similar to a herniated disc (Fig. 5-14B). These have often been referred to as "hard" discs. Hypertrophic change with bulging or herniated discs may be difficult to separate by MRI. When a patient with a radiculopathy has a normal MR image, plain films may help in evaluating the hypertrophic change. Occasionally, a CT scan with intrathecal contrast may be needed. The thinner sections and greater

(text continues on page 214)

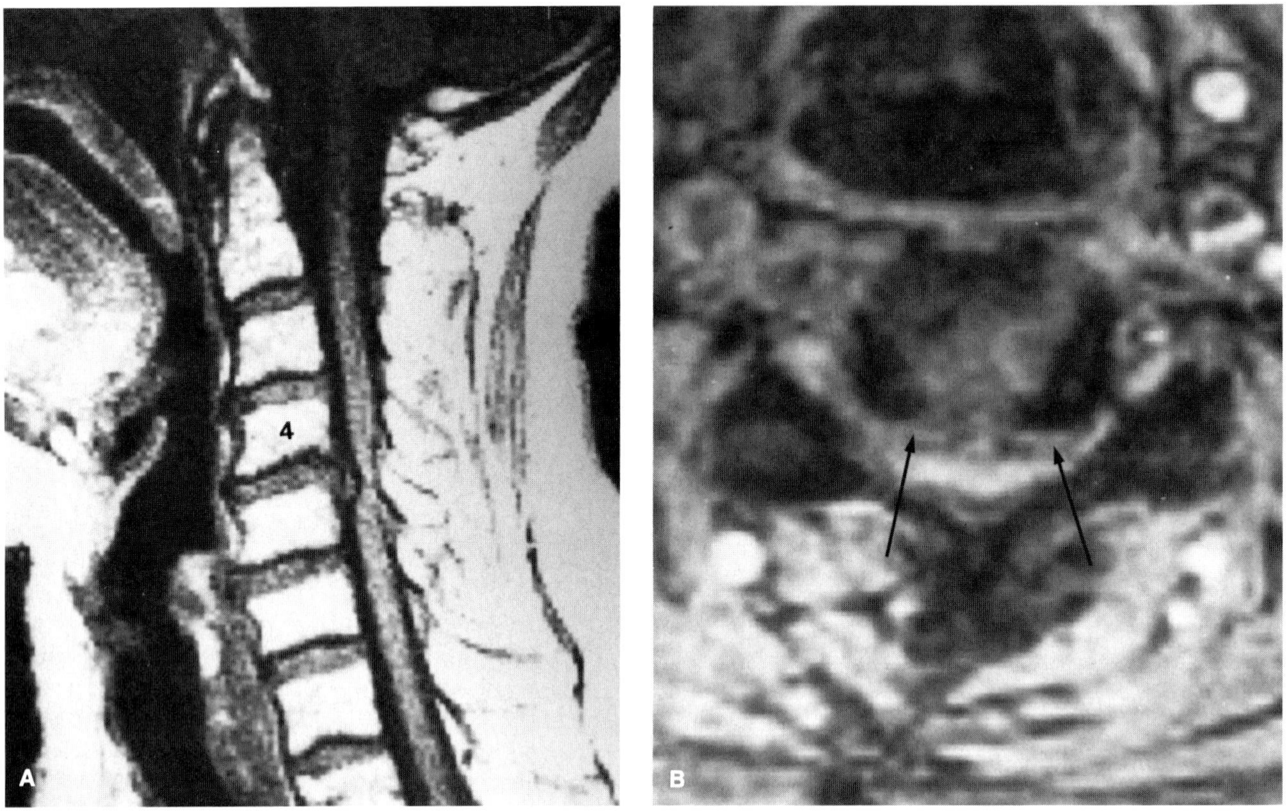

FIGURE 5–11. (A) There is a herniated disc at C4-5 on the sagittal T1-weighted sequence. This disc has a slightly mottled density, extends downward, and impinges the cord. **(B)** The axial FLASH-10 image (TR/TE = 200/11) shows a severely herniated disc, which has a slightly higher signal than the osseous structures (arrows). A dephasing, low-signal-intensity artifact exaggerates the size of the disc. Exaggeration and the obliteration of the cord are not unusual findings in discs with this degree of herniation.

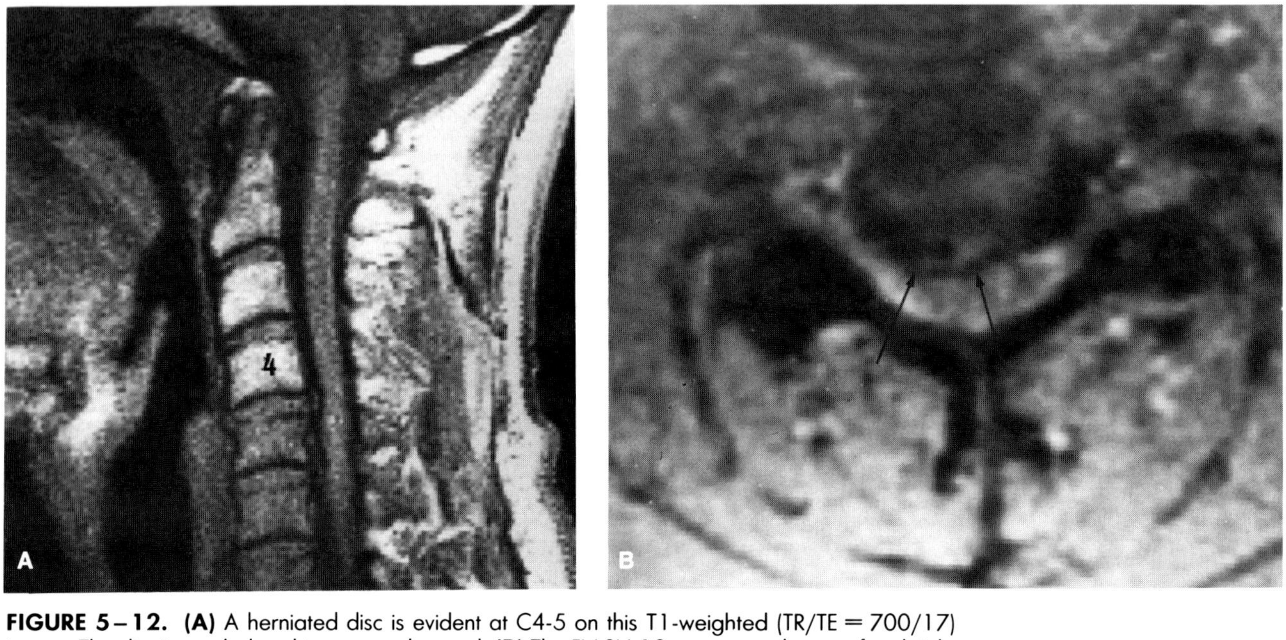

FIGURE 5–12. (A) A herniated disc is evident at C4-5 on this T1-weighted (TR/TE = 700/17) image. The disc is mottled and impresses the cord. **(B)** The FLASH-10 sequence shows a focal right herniation (arrows). The disc signal intensity is slightly higher than the adjacent osseous structures. The disc impresses the cord and obliterates the exiting nerve root.

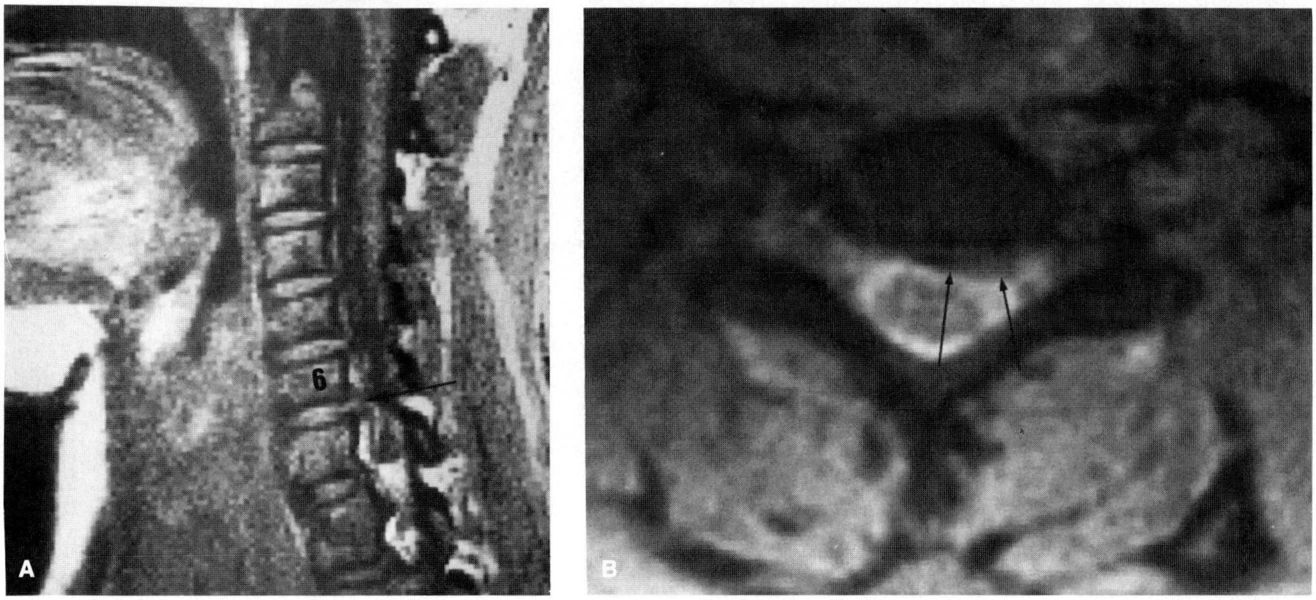

FIGURE 5–13. (A) This sagittal T1-weighted image (TR/TE = 700/17) was obtained to the left of midline. The herniated disc (arrow) is not as well seen as in the axial section. **(B)** On the axial FLASH-10 (TR/TE = 200/11), the disc is small but is focally herniated on the left (arrows).

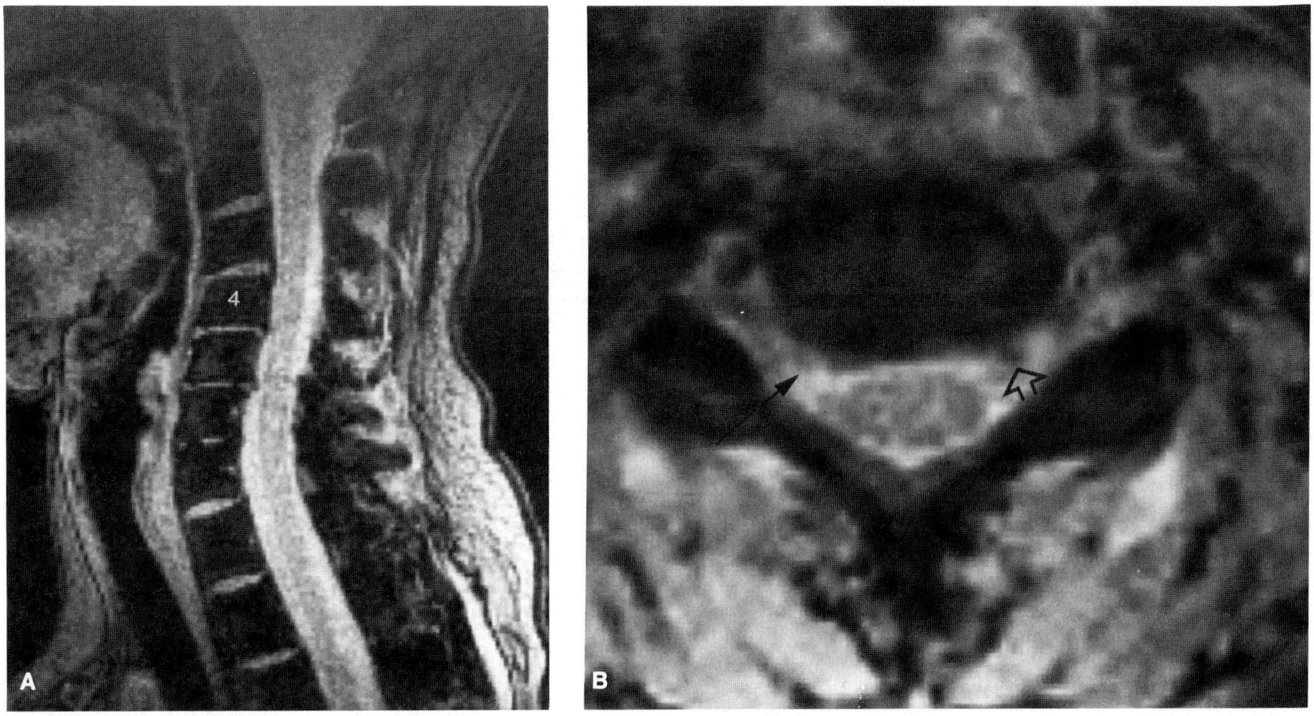

FIGURE 5–14. (A) Degenerative changes are evident on this FLASH-10 sagittal section. These are mild at C4-5 and C5-6, with associated neural canal narrowing. **(B)** Focal lateral hypertrophic change is seen on the right in this patient with a radiculopathy. The spur extends to the ventral root (arrow). This lateralizing change was better seen in the axial plane. Minimal signal dropout is seen around the ventral root on the left (open arrow).

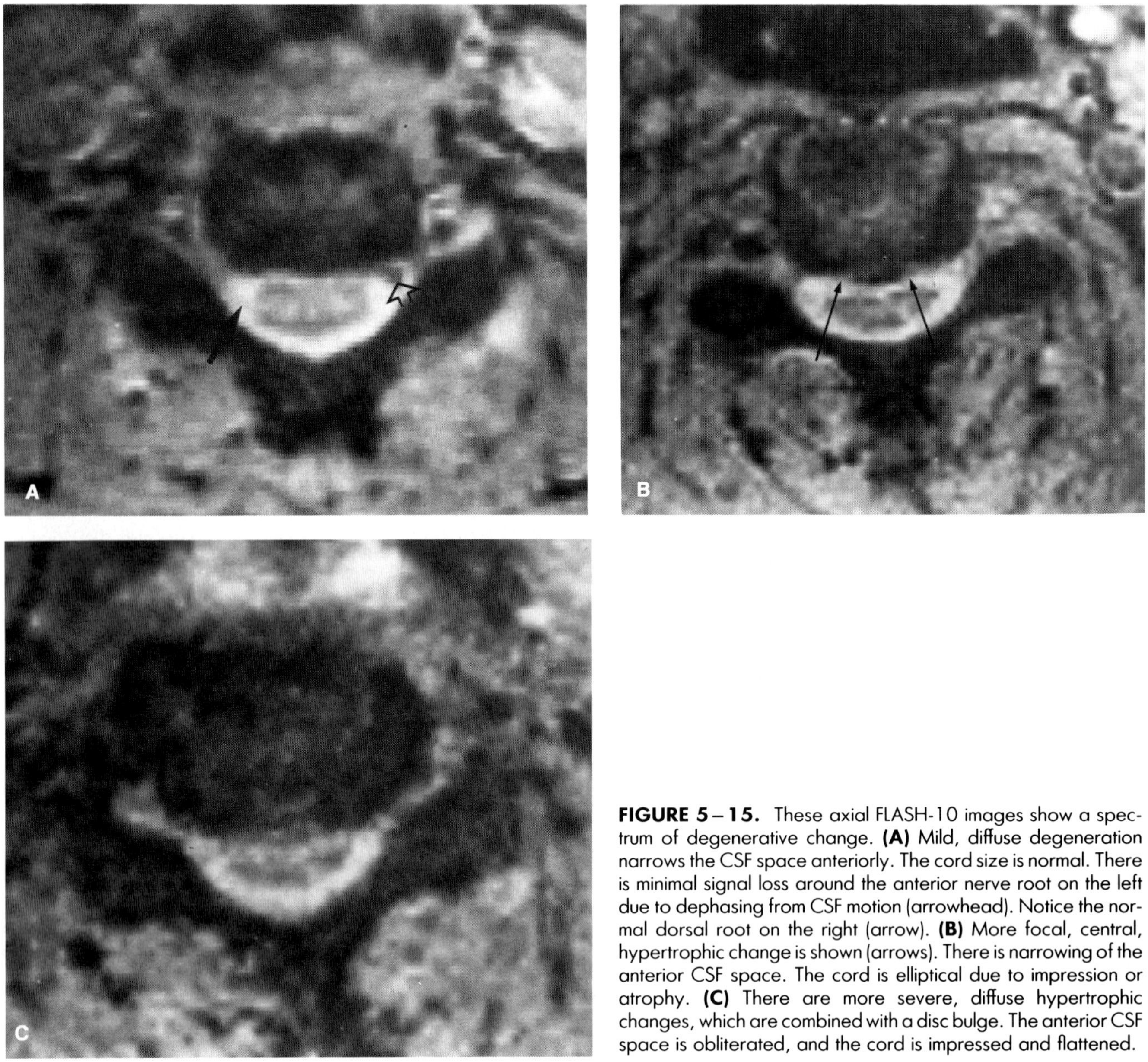

FIGURE 5 – 15. These axial FLASH-10 images show a spectrum of degenerative change. **(A)** Mild, diffuse degeneration narrows the CSF space anteriorly. The cord size is normal. There is minimal signal loss around the anterior nerve root on the left due to dephasing from CSF motion (arrowhead). Notice the normal dorsal root on the right (arrow). **(B)** More focal, central, hypertrophic change is shown (arrows). There is narrowing of the anterior CSF space. The cord is elliptical due to impression or atrophy. **(C)** There are more severe, diffuse hypertrophic changes, which are combined with a disc bulge. The anterior CSF space is obliterated, and the cord is impressed and flattened.

bone detail available with CT may be required for diagnosis.

More severe degenerative changes are frequently found in the aging patient. The spectrum of abnormalities includes disc degeneration with disc space narrowing and annular bulges, posterior vertebral body and uncinate process osteophytes, facet hypertrophy, thickening and buckling of the ligamentum flavum, and thickening and calcification of the posterior longitudinal ligament (Figs. 5-1B, 5-3B, and 5-14A). The discs and vertebral bodies have a mottled appearance on sagittal T1-weighted sequences due to this degenerative change. Bright spots from fatty degeneration may be present. The ridging of the spine and narrowing of the subarachnoid space are then clearly outlined by the myelographic effect of sagittal GRE sequences or T2-weighted sequences.

The axial GRE study is used to confirm the decrease in size of the canal and anterior subarachnoid space and to evaluate the secondary cord changes (Figs. 5-14B and 5-15). The separation of disc abnormality and osteophyte may be difficult in this plane, because the lower signal intensity of the osteophyte obscures the bulging disc. Referring to the T1-weighted sagittal image may help in some cases.

Myelopathy

When degenerative changes become severe, compression of the cord occurs, producing diffuse neurologic symptoms. Occasionally, areas of increased signal intensity can be identified on T2-weighted sequences (Fig. 5-16). This is a type of chronic posttraumatic change. The protocol for evaluation includes T1-weighted and T2-weighted sagittal sequences. A GRE axial examination can evaluate the bony, soft tissue, and cord changes. Additional evaluation with axial T2-weighted (gated) images provides little additional diagnostic information and lengthens the imaging time. Severe or chronic degenerative changes or disc compression may produce a syrinx (Fig. 5-17).

Syringomyelia and Hydromyelia

Syringomyelia and hydromyelia are cystic changes of the cord. Hydromyelia represents a dilatation of the central canal which communicates with the fourth ventricle. Ependymal cells line the cavity. Syringomyelia is a cavity within the cord that is eccentric to the central canal and may or may not communicate with it.[3] Numerous theories have been proposed with regards to etiology, but none have been uniformly accepted. Altered CSF dynamics with obstruction to CSF flow have a role in pathogenesis and are implicated in many cases.

Hydromyelia is frequently associated with Arnold-Chiari I malformations. The extension of the tonsils below the foramen magnum presumably obstructs the subarachnoid space, with dilatation of the central canal (Figs. 5-18 and 5-19). These abnormalities vary in size, and they may have a septated appearance if very large (Fig. 5-19). These cavities may extend to the level of the conus. For complete evaluation, the most inferior extent of the abnormality must be visualized. A syrinx that presents in the cervical spine may have its true cause in the thoracic or lumbar regions (i.e., tethered cord) (Fig. 5-20). T1-weighted sagittal images with a larger coil can localize the level and extent of abnormality and should be followed by a more detailed examination with the appropriate-size coil.

Hydromyelic dilatation of the cord may be found in other congenital abnormalities, such as the Dandy-Walker syndrome, Arnold-Chiari II malformations, spine malformations (e.g., scoliosis and dysraphism), tethered cord, and diastematomyelia. This type of dil-

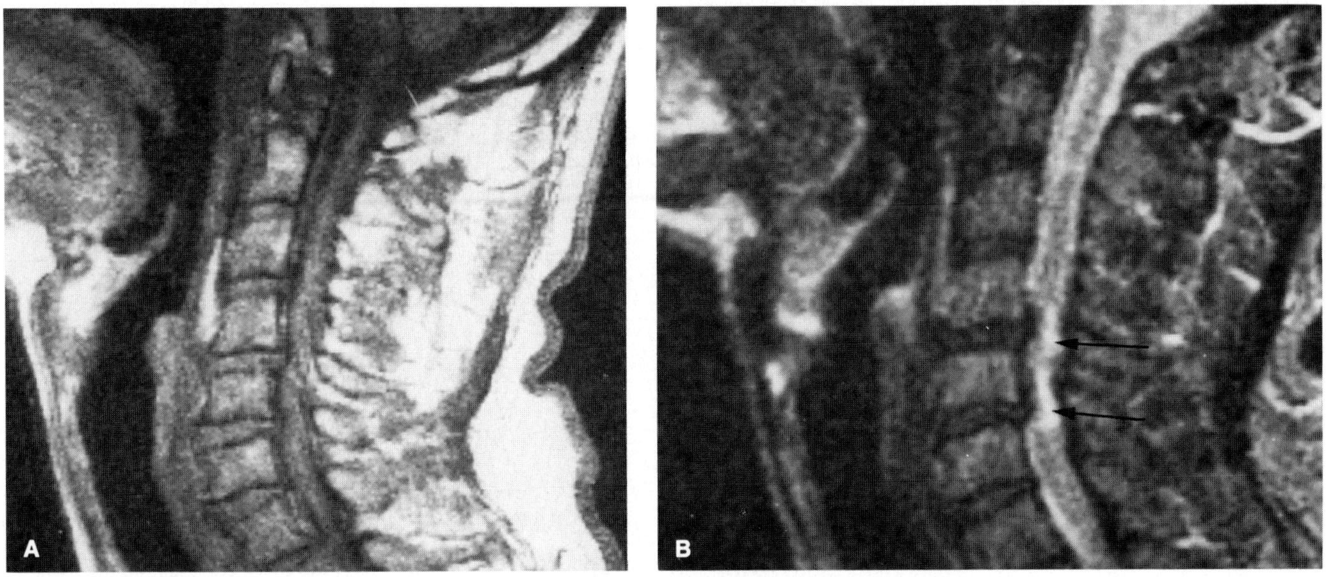

FIGURE 5-16. **(A)** Sagittal T1-weighted image (TR/TE = 700/17) of an elderly patient. There are many levels of disc bulge, degenerative change, and narrowing of the spinal canal. **(B)** The sagittal T2-weighted (TR/TE = 3000/90) image confirms the disc bulges and better demonstrates the degenerative change and neural canal narrowing. The increase in signal intensity (arrows) within the cord is consistent with cord injury in this patient with pain and myelopathy.

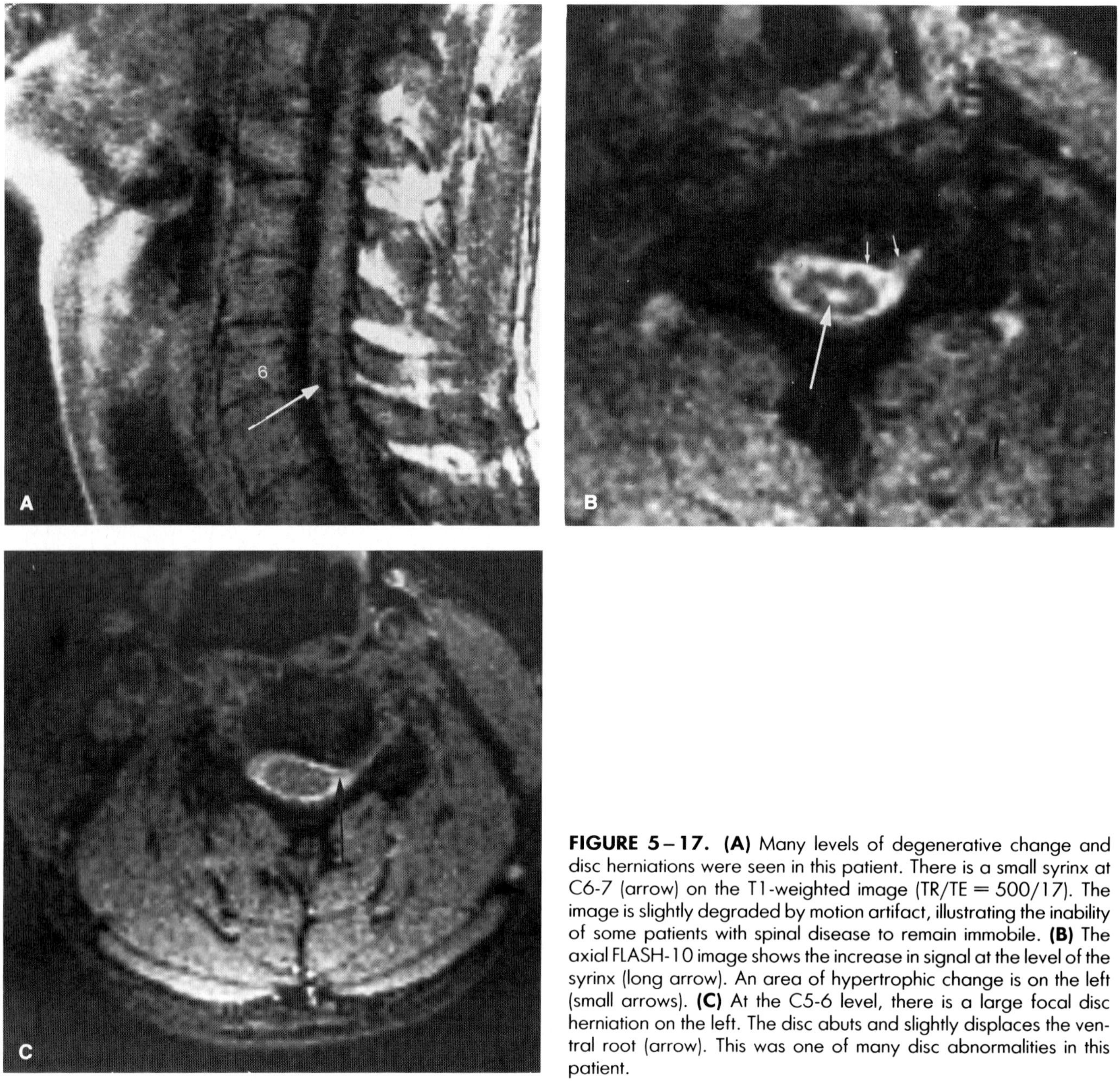

FIGURE 5–17. **(A)** Many levels of degenerative change and disc herniations were seen in this patient. There is a small syrinx at C6-7 (arrow) on the T1-weighted image (TR/TE = 500/17). The image is slightly degraded by motion artifact, illustrating the inability of some patients with spinal disease to remain immobile. **(B)** The axial FLASH-10 image shows the increase in signal at the level of the syrinx (long arrow). An area of hypertrophic change is on the left (small arrows). **(C)** At the C5-6 level, there is a large focal disc herniation on the left. The disc abuts and slightly displaces the ventral root (arrow). This was one of many disc abnormalities in this patient.

atation can also occur after trauma and inflammatory processes (e.g., meningitis).

Syringomyelia may occur after trauma, surgery, or vascular insults. There is usually a several-year interval between incident and presentation, and neurologic decline typically occurs after an asymptomatic interval.

MRI is the most sensitive modality for demonstration of these abnormalities, but their differentiation may be difficult. As a result, many abnormalities are lumped together under the term syringohydromyelia. A more appropriate use of clinical terminology would be to designate the lesion as a syrinx, followed by the presumed or diagnosed cause (i.e., syrinx, posttraumatic or syrinx secondary to a tethered cord).

A thin, dark line may occasionally be seen in the

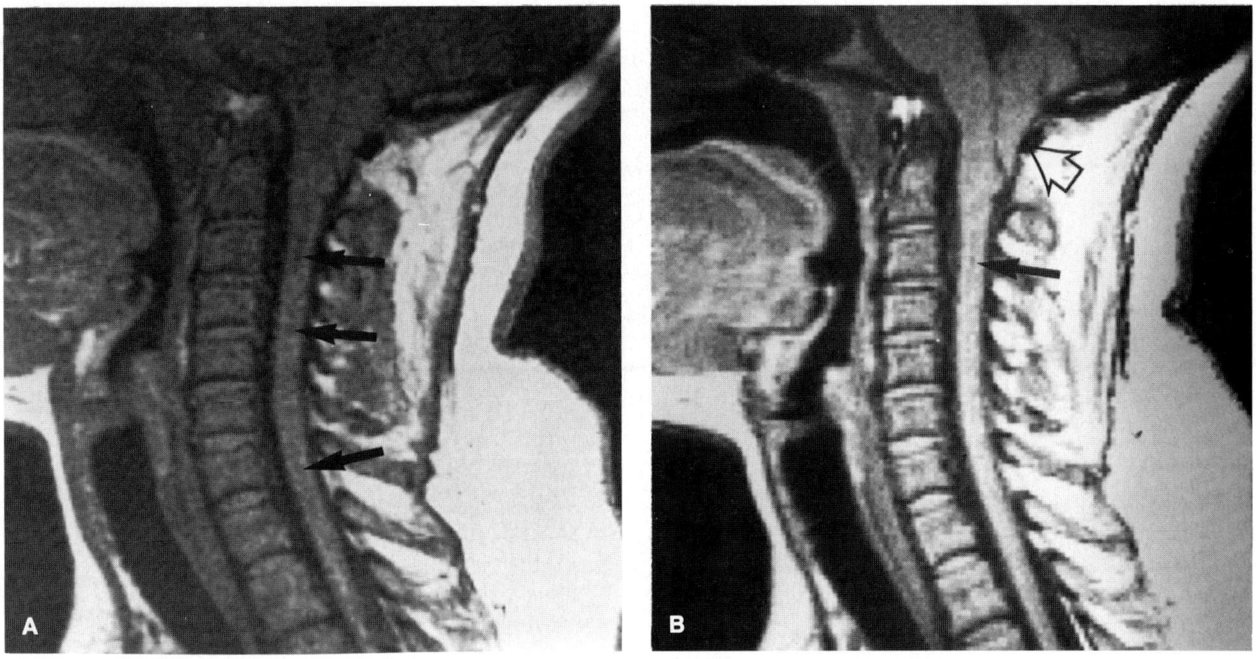

FIGURE 5–21. (A) This 3-mm T1-weighted image (TR/TE = 500/17) was obtained as an interleaved study with two averages. Notice the long, linear, low-signal-intensity abnormality within the cord (arrows). Because the patient has an Arnold Chiari I malformation, it is important to document the presence of a syrinx. **(B)** A second T1-weighted acquisition (TR/TE = 700/17) was performed and four averages were used to obtain this 3-mm image. The truncation artifact has been removed. The remaining linear, low-signal-intensity abnormality (arrow) requires observation for the development of a clinically significant syrinx. The tonsillar ectopia is better seen on this view (open arrow). Axial sections (not shown) are also commonly employed to confirm or rule out the presence of a syrinx.

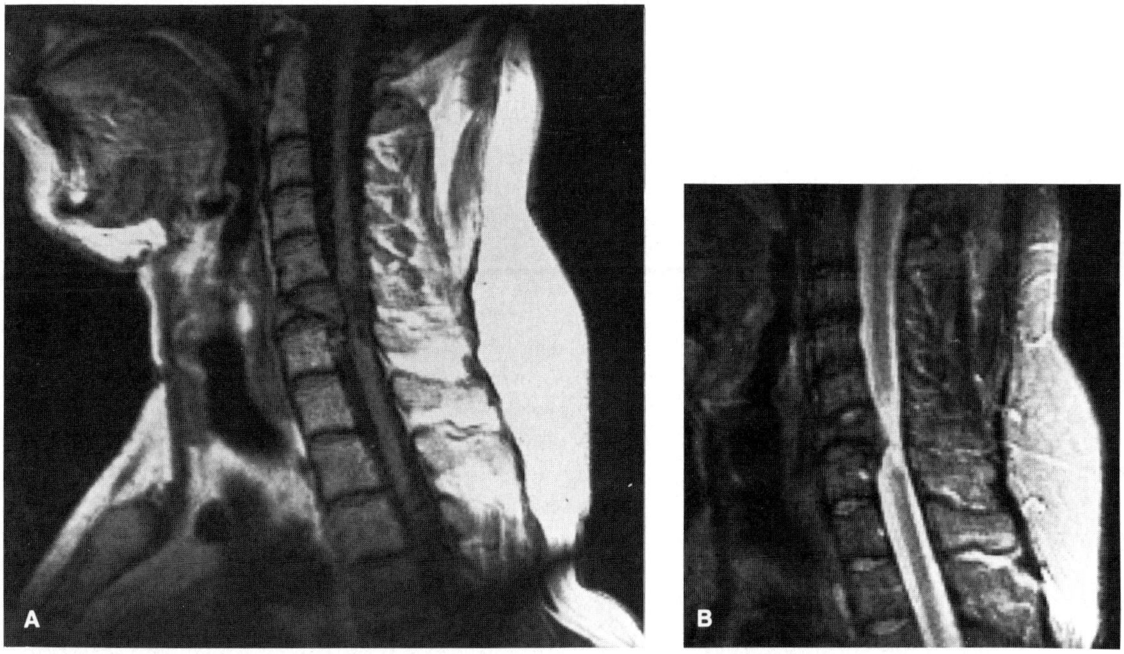

FIGURE 5–22. (A) The sagittal T1-weighted image (TR/TE = 650/20) shows a fracture of the C6 vertebral body. There is a retropulsed portion of the vertebral body extending into the canal, impinging the cord. A small "slit-like" syrinx involves the cord at this level. **(B)** The T2-weighted image (TR/TE = 3000/90) shows an increase in signal intensity that is larger and not as sharply defined as in the previous image. This is consistent with gliosis.

prove to be an efficient and easily interpreted method for assessing cavity motion.[7]

NEOPLASIA

Metastases are the most common neoplasia involving the spine. These are usually blood-borne and first involve the vertebral bodies. The neural canal is encroached on by pathologic osseous destruction and associated neoplastic epidural mass. On T1-weighted images, the involved vertebral body shows diminished signal intensity, with sparing of the intervertebral disc. The narrowing of the anterior subarachnoid space and secondary cord impingement is usually apparent. On T2-weighted and GRE images, the myelographic effect makes the extradural changes and cord effacement or displacement more apparent. The bone metastases usually demonstrate an increase in signal intensity. Axial GRE (LFA) can lateralize the change (Fig. 5-23).

Bony metastases are more efficiently surveyed with a nuclear medicine study, allowing a more detailed MR study at the proper level with greater speed. Usually, these patients present emergently with symptoms of a cord block. A larger coil, such as a body coil, may first be used to localize the abnormality, followed by imaging with the appropriate-size coil at the level or levels of interest. T1-weighted sagittal images and GRE (LFA) sagittal and axial sequences will provide ample detail (Fig. 5-23).

Contrast agents used in epidural neoplastic disease have been less rewarding and produced more variable results than in other tumor imaging. Its role may be an adjunctive one, mainly used in indicating more suitable biopsy sites, monitoring therapy, and differentiating disc from epidural tumor.[8] The introduction of new contrast media that can be administered at higher doses may result in more widespread use in bony neoplastic disease.

Meticulous attention to precise location and extent are very important to the neurosurgeon and radiation therapist. "What level is the lesion?" is one of the most important questions to be answered. MRI has several advantages over myelography, which can often be tedious and time consuming in the very ill patient with metastatic disease. These advantages include the demonstration of multiple osseous lesions, multiple levels of possible cord block that could be missed with myelography, and paravertebral tumor extension.[9] Significant morbidity can be avoided in a patient who is already quite ill.

Therapy can also be monitored with MRI. After radiation therapy, the vertebral bodies often become quite intense (T1-weighted images). This has been attributed to fatty marrow replacement and is a fairly accurate indicator of the area included in the radiation port (Fig. 5-6).

Intramedullary Neoplasms

Gliomas are the most common tumors, representing 90% of intramedullary cord neoplasms. These include the astrocytoma, glioblastoma, and ependymoma. No specific imaging characteristics separate these tumors. Tumor location and patient age may provide some guidelines. Ependymomas account for 60% of these tumors and are more common at the conus, followed in frequency by those in the cervical region. Astocytomas are more common in pediatric patients, occurring at the cervico-thoracic junction (Fig. 5-20).[10] Rather extensive tumors of this type are not infrequent in this age group.

MRI is the imaging modality of choice and is generally quite accurate, except in those cases that may simulate a syrinx or in those tumors that may have an associated nonneoplastic cyst. The cord is nearly always enlarged. This enlargement may be focal in small tumors (Fig. 5-24). An inhomogenous signal usually present on T1-weighted images is due to the associated cystic or necrotic change. These cysts may show an intensity slightly greater than CSF on T1-weighted images due to fluid stasis and elevated protein content (Figs. 5-20 and 5-25). Smoothly marginated cysts have been described at the extremes of the lesion. On T2-weighted images, the solid and cystic portion of the lesion show increased signal intensity (Fig. 5-25).

Cord tumors are visualized better with contrast agents (Figs. 5-20, 5-24, and 5-25). This provides greater accuracy in assessment and a higher level of diagnostic confidence, especially in cases that mimic a benign syrinx or have an associated benign syrinx (Fig. 5-20). A recent study showed that 4 of 15 cord tumors were missed without contrast. In these cases, the tumor was small, and focal areas of enlargement were obscured by volume averaging from sections that were too thick. Some tumors may be isointense on T1-weighted and T2-weighted images due to a combination of protein and serosanguineous fluid. In these cases, enhancement provides the only clue to their existence.

Because all portions of a cord tumor may not enhance, a sagittal T2-weighted sequence is needed with a T1-weighted sagittal sequence before and after contrast (Fig. 5-25). Axial postcontrast scans provide additional information but may not be as crucial as other sequences (Fig. 5-24). Contrast agents also are used to monitor the progress of therapy. Baseline examinations before and after contrast administration are advocated to exclude associated abnormalities (i.e.,

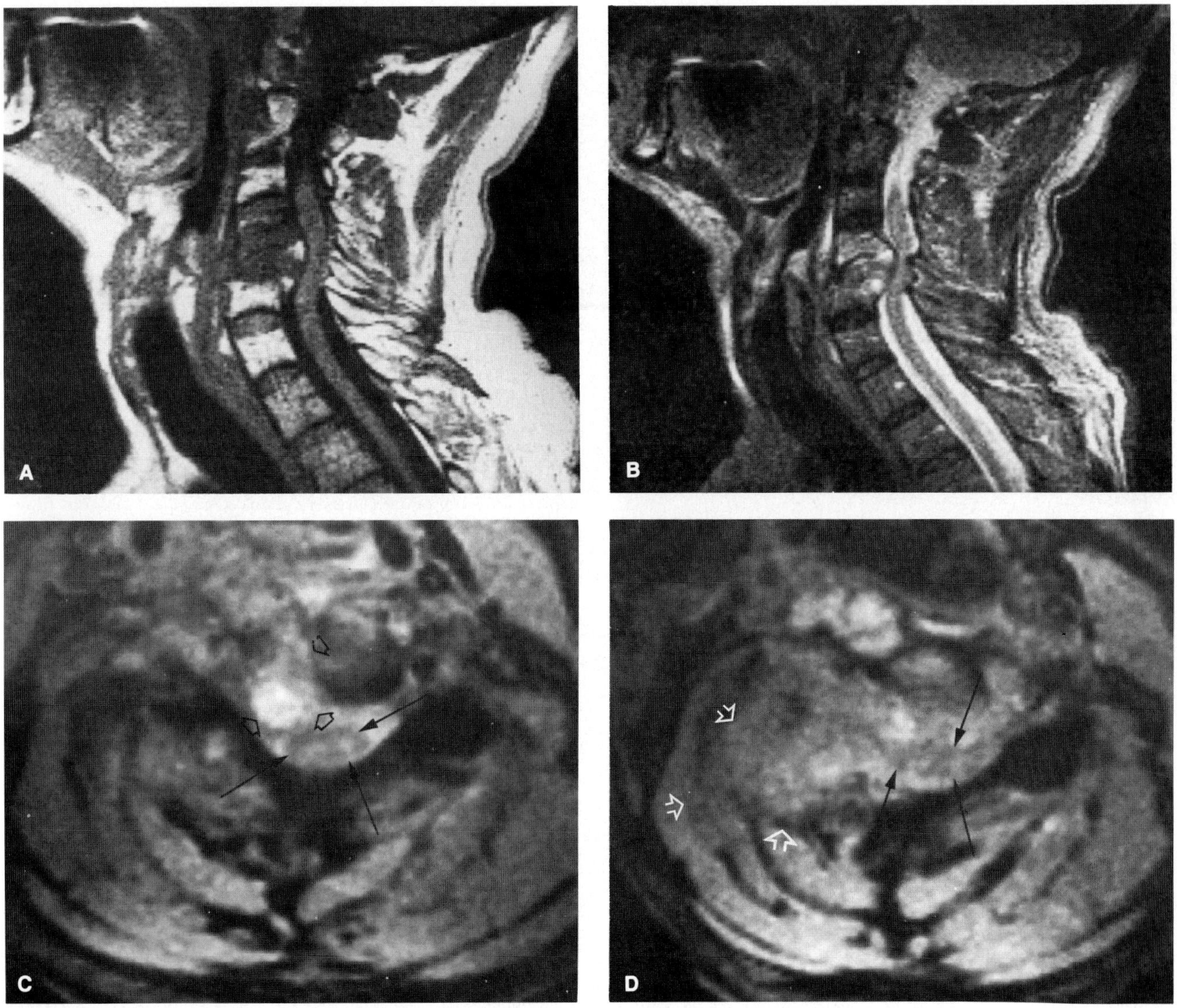

FIGURE 5–23. **(A)** There is metastatic involvement of the C4 and C5 vertebral bodies. An epidural neoplastic bone and soft tissue mass extends into the neural canal and compresses the cord. There is mixed signal intensity of the vertebral bodies on this T1-weighted image (TR/TE = 500/17). **(B)** The metastatic bony involvement shows an increase in signal intensity on the T2-weighted image (TR/TE = 3000/90). The degenerative posterior ridging and its role in cord compression are better shown with this or a GRE sequence. **(C)** An axial FLASH-10 image shows the cord compression (arrows) by neoplastic tissue. The bone and soft tissue components of the neoplastic process are not clearly separated or demarcated. This mass widens the neural foramina and destroys the vertebral body (open arrows). There is an ill-defined anterior soft tissue component. **(D)** At a slightly different level, greater cord compression (arrows) results from the epidural neoplastic disease. There is destruction of the vertebral body and posterior elements on the right. A large paravertebral mass is evident (open arrowheads).

hemorrhage). Follow-up studies can be obtained as a post-contrast examination in the absence of sudden neurologic decline or clinical circumstance that raises the question of cord hemorrhage.

Other intramedullary tumors include hemangioblastomas and metastases. Hemangioblastomas are uncommon cord tumors (2.5%) with one-third occurring in patients with von Hippel–Lindau disease. Even if associated with this syndrome, they are usually solitary lesions (90%) in the cord, and 60% of these lesions are cystic. Hemangioblastoma may simulate an AVM with serpiginous areas of signal void that, on T2-weighted images, have interspersed areas of increased signal intensity and a large draining dorsal

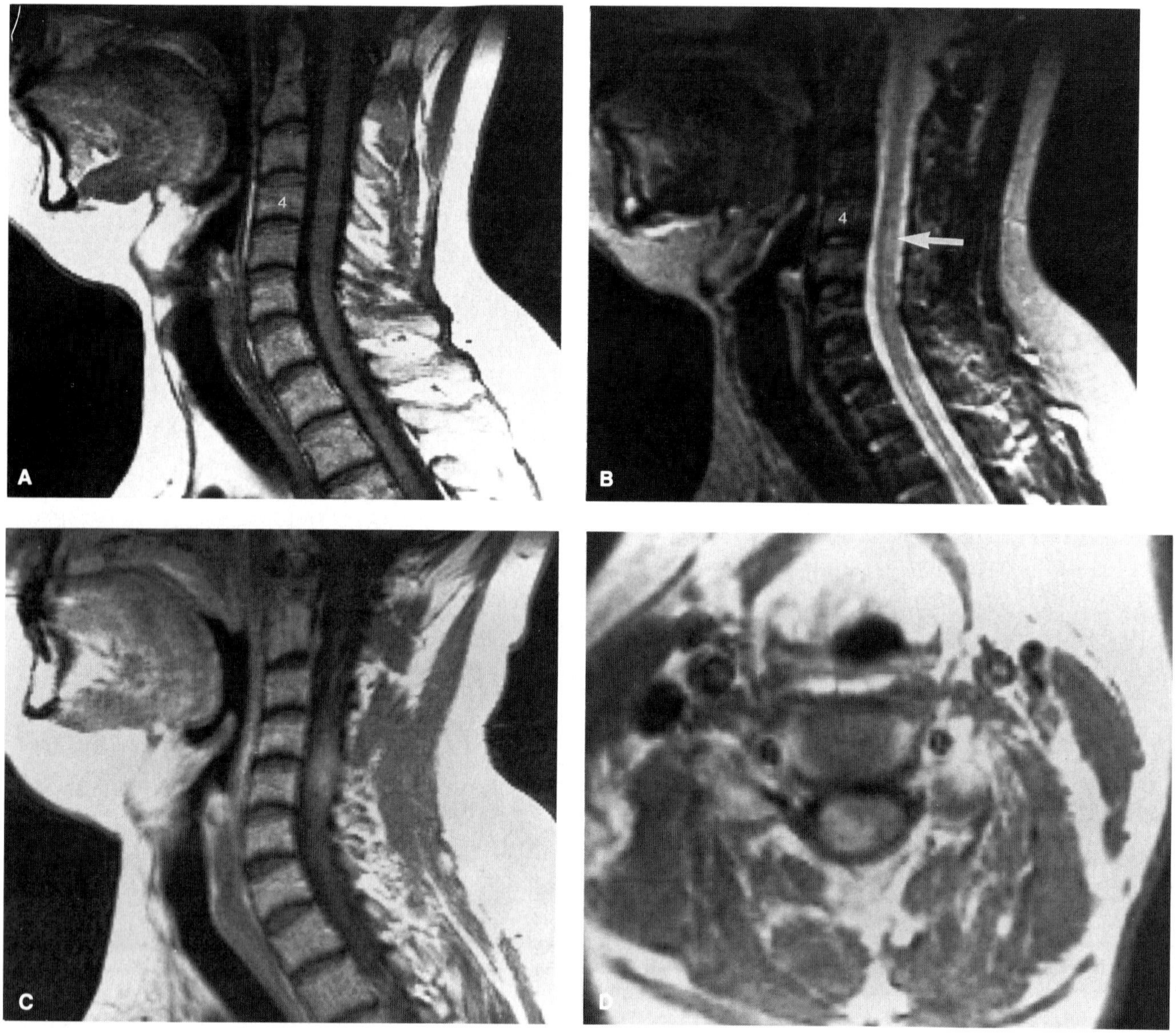

FIGURE 5–24. (A) The sagittal T1-weighted image (TR/TE = 450/20) shows only vague enlargement of the cord at C4-C5. **(B)** A small area of increased signal intensity occurs at this level on the T2-weighted image (arrow). **(C)** After contrast enhancement, this astrocytoma (presumptive diagnosis) is much more confidently diagnosed and appears larger than would be suspected from the previous T2-weighted image. **(D)** An axial postcontrast T1-weighted image (TR/TE = 650/20) confirms the cord enlargement and tumor enhancement. The abnormality lateralizes to the right.

vein. These findings and the associated cystic change will usually differentiate hemangioblastomas from AVMs.[10]

Intramedullary cord metastases of central nervous system (CNS) origin spread or seed by CSF pathways. These are often referred to as "drop metastases." Tumors that arise in or are adjacent to the ventricles are the most frequent sources. These include medulloblastoma, ependymoma, and astrocytoma. These tumors first produce leptomeningeal changes, which are followed by direct invasion of the cord. The demonstration of these changes is optimized by the use of contrast agents (Fig. 5–6). Leptomeningeal changes can be accurately demonstrated and assessed only with contrast.[12]

Intramedullary metastases of nonneurogenic origin are uncommon (1%), and 50% of these occur in carcinoma of the lung, with breast the second most common cause. Lymphoma, melanoma, and colorectal carcinoma are among other reported primaries.[13] These tumors should be sought in patients with bowel and bladder symptoms in whom no cord block can be

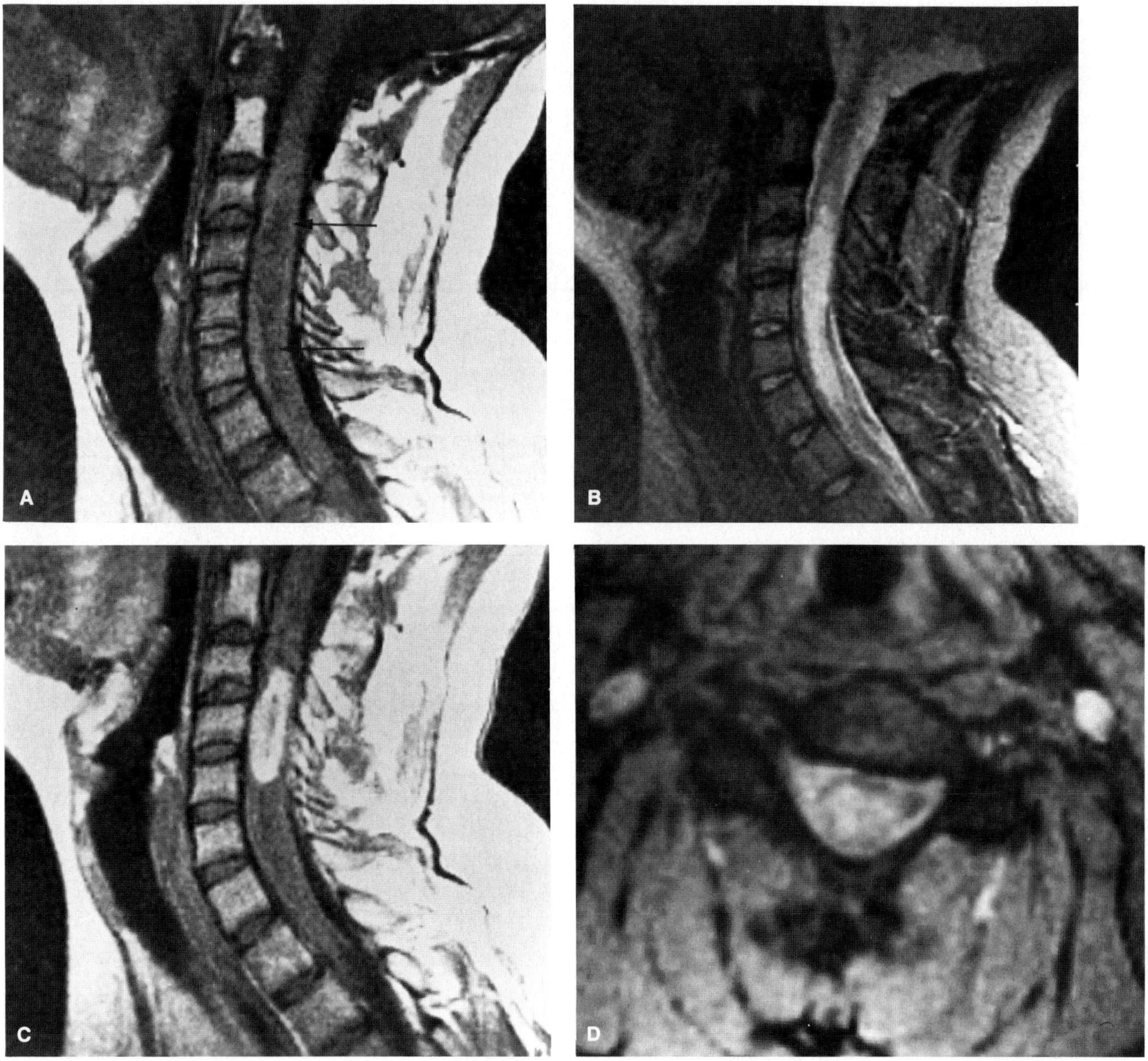

FIGURE 5–25. **(A)** There is an elongated area of low signal intensity within the cord on this T1-weighted (TR/TE = 700/17) image (arrows). The margins of this syrinx-like abnormality are irregular, and the density is greater than CSF. The cord is diffusely enlarged. **(B)** On the T2-weighted image (TR/TE = 3000/90), there is an increase in signal intensity. It extends over a larger area of the cord than the enhancement in the next image. **(C)** There is enhancement in this astrocytoma after contrast administration (T1-weighted image). **(D)** The precontrast axial FISP-20 image shows increased signal within the cord at the level of the tumor. This abnormal signal intensity within the cord is due to the cystic and necrotic changes. The cord enlargement and expansion are greater on the right.

demonstrated. Contrast-enhanced MRI should be beneficial in diagnosing this abnormality and in distinguishing it from leptomeningeal carcinomatosis, another cause for myelopathy in the cancer patient. Differential diagnosis of the cause of cord expansion must include multiple sclerosis, transverse myelitis, infarction, and AVM. History may be helpful in cord infarction, because it has a sudden onset.

Extramedullary Neoplasms

Neurofibromas and meningiomas account for 55% of spine neoplasms and are second in frequency to metastases. Meningiomas are more frequent in the middle-age female, occurring in the thoracic and cervical spine, particularly at the anterior foramen magnum. Most of these are easily identified as soft tissue masses anterior to the spinal cord and may have a similar intensity on both T1-weighted and T2-weighted images. A contrast-enhanced MR examination is often necessary if small lesions are not to be overlooked. These are readily identified by their bright or intense enhancement (Fig. 5–26).

Neurofibromas usually occur in patients with neurofibromatosis. These dumbbell-shaped lesions arise laterally to the cord in the neural foramen and may be both intradural and extradural. Both coronal and axial sections are useful in demonstrating the neuroforaminal origin (Fig. 5–27).

On T1-weighted images, the tumors are almost the same intensity as the cord. Due to a greater water content than meningiomas, neurofibromas generally show an increase in signal intensity on T2-weighted and GRE sequences (Fig. 5–8). These enhance almost as intensely as meningiomas.

In the clinical situation, the physician is often faced with finding the exact level(s) of the neurofibroma(s) in a patient with neurofibromatosis. The most efficient approach is performing precontrast and postcontrast T1-weighted sagittal and coronal views for localization, followed by postcontrast axials at the level of the abnormality. Coronal T2-weighted images can be used to localize the neurofibroma as an area of

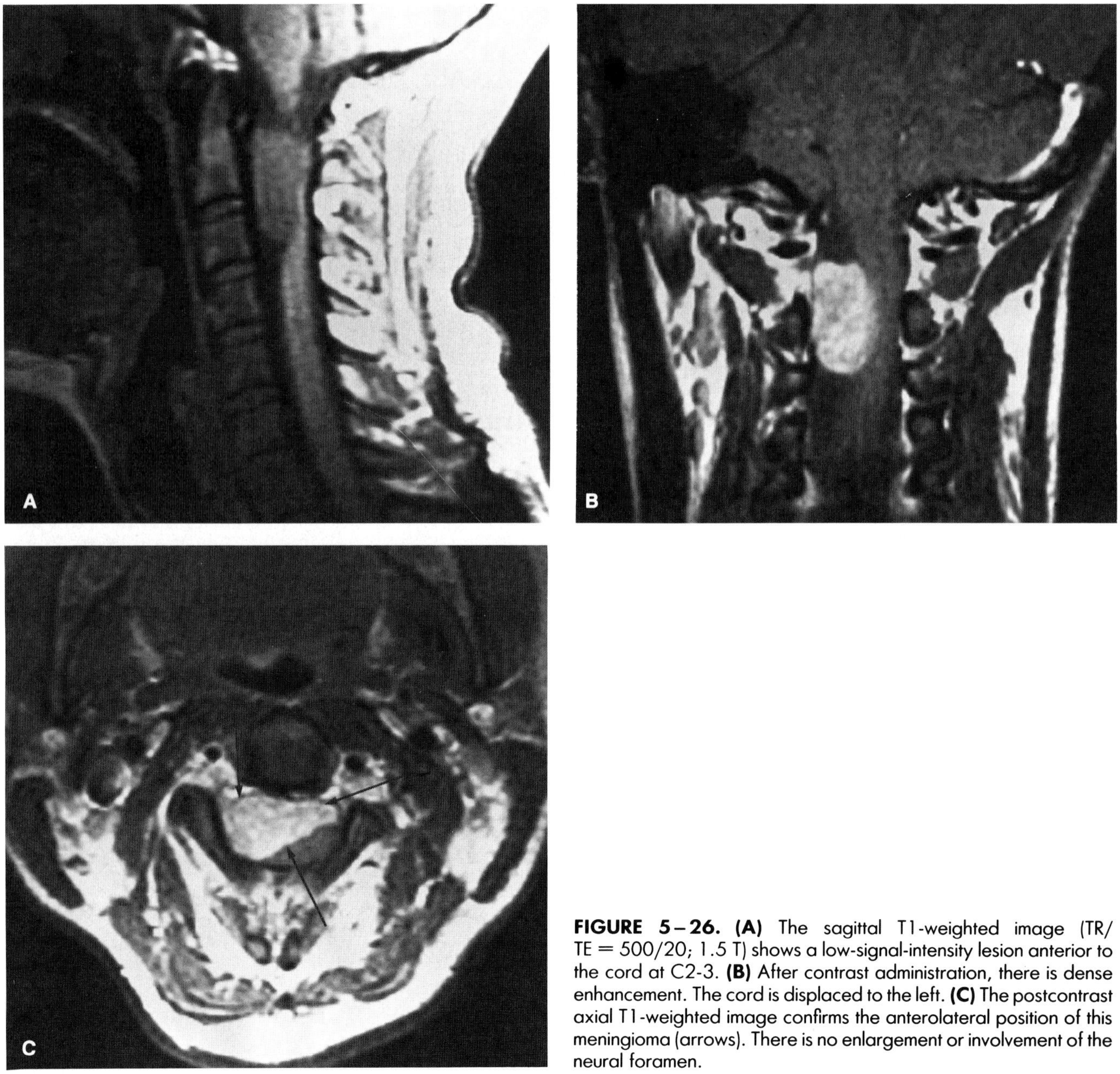

FIGURE 5–26. (A) The sagittal T1-weighted image (TR/TE = 500/20; 1.5 T) shows a low-signal-intensity lesion anterior to the cord at C2-3. **(B)** After contrast administration, there is dense enhancement. The cord is displaced to the left. **(C)** The postcontrast axial T1-weighted image confirms the anterolateral position of this meningioma (arrows). There is no enlargement or involvement of the neural foramen.

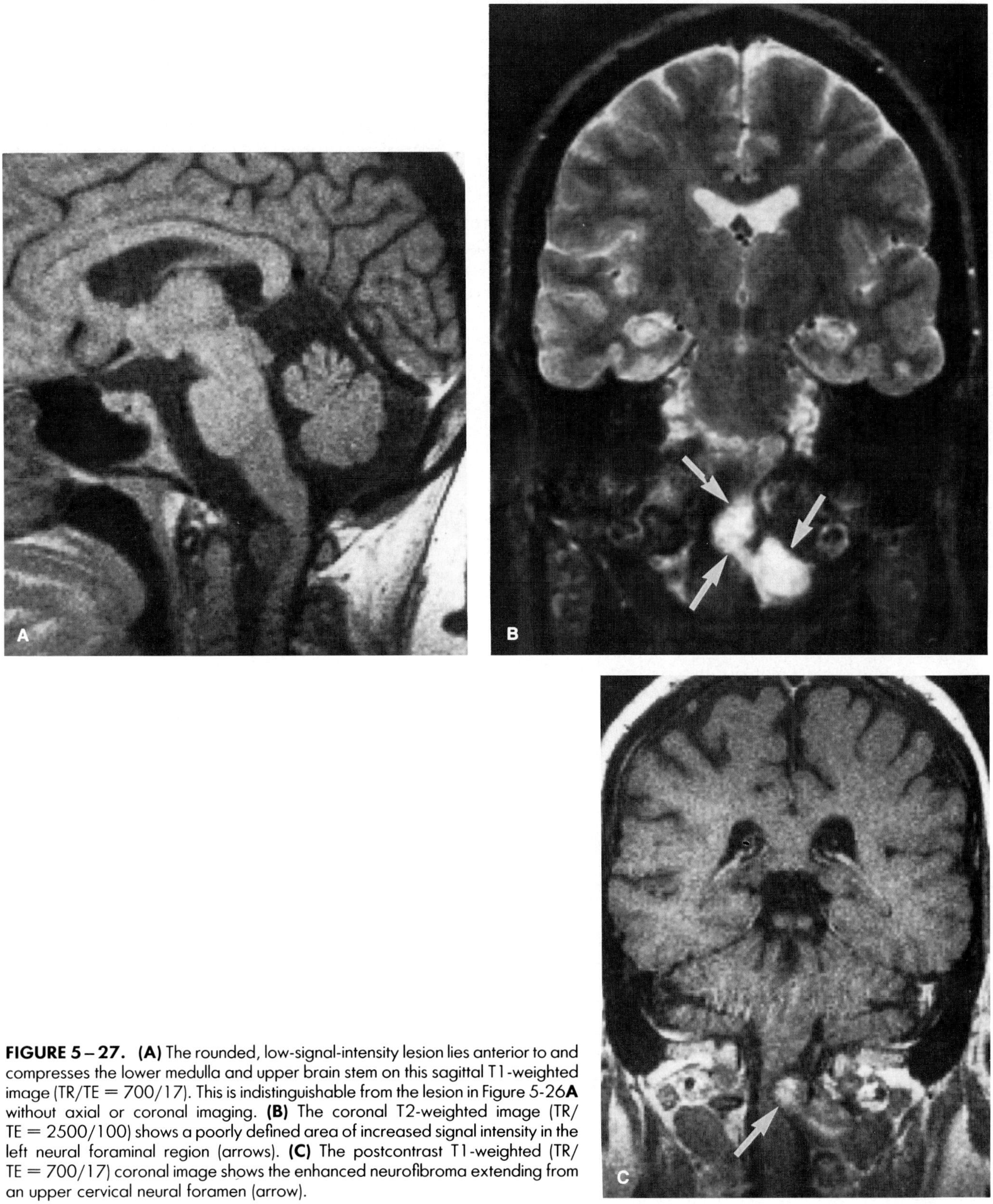

FIGURE 5–27. **(A)** The rounded, low-signal-intensity lesion lies anterior to and compresses the lower medulla and upper brain stem on this sagittal T1-weighted image (TR/TE = 700/17). This is indistinguishable from the lesion in Figure 5-26**A** without axial or coronal imaging. **(B)** The coronal T2-weighted image (TR/TE = 2500/100) shows a poorly defined area of increased signal intensity in the left neural foraminal region (arrows). **(C)** The postcontrast T1-weighted (TR/TE = 700/17) coronal image shows the enhanced neurofibroma extending from an upper cervical neural foramen (arrow).

increased signal intensity bordering the spinal canal. This second method of localization is time-consuming and may not be as accurate.

TRAUMA

MRI is the only imaging modality that simultaneously offers direct information about the status of the spinal cord and malalignment or fracture of the vertebral bodies, the degree of cord compression, the existence of disc herniation, and neural and soft tissue changes (Fig. 5-1). An MR study is safer and simpler than myelography in patients who must be handled with care if their neurologic deficit is not to be worsened and who are difficult to manage due to quadriplegia or quadriparesis.

Patients in ferromagnetic halo frames, on external life supports, or who are uncooperative due to a severe head injury may not be candidates for an MR study. Greater detail of osseous injury or stability may require more conventional radiologic examination, such as plain films, tomography, or CT. Graphite halo frames that are compatible with MRI are now available. If coil tuning is a problem, check that ferromagnetic screws have not been substituted for the graphite ones.

Hemorrhage may occur within the cord in severe neck trauma and is thought to have a less favorable clinical outcome than cord contusion or edema.[14] These can be distinguished because hemorrhage has a decreased signal in its acute phase on T1-weighted images and increased signal in its subacute phase. On T2-weighted images the signal intensity can be increased during both phases (see Chapter 2). Edema or contusion may be difficult to visualize or show ill-defined low-signal-intensity changes on T1-weighted images and have an increased signal intensity on T2-weighted images (Fig. 5-1).

Assessment of surgically correctable abnormalities, such as disc herniations and subdural or epidural hematomas, is important. By doing this, a complete quadriplegic may be converted to an incomplete quadriplegic, so that the patient may be able to participate in his daily care. The protocol for examination should include T1-weighted and T2-weighted sagittal images. Sagittal GRE (LFA) images may not be adequate in evaluating the true extent of cord injury. GRE imaging with higher flip angles has been suggested for accurate evaluation of hemorrhage and hemorrhagic lesions due to its sensitivity to magnetic susceptibility effects.[15] This awaits further investigation. T1-weighted or GRE (LFA) axials can be used if there are abnormalities (i.e., discs that need to be lateralized).

MRI is also the modality of choice in evaluating chronic cord trauma (Fig. 5-22). After a relatively stable postinjury course, the patient may show a neurologic decline. This has been called posttraumatic progressive myelopathy (PTPM). It can be caused by myelomalacia and cysts. This is an important distinction, because myelomalacia does not require and is not improved by therapy. When cysts are large, surgical intervention may produce clinical improvement. CT after intrathecal contrast is not accurate in separating these entities.

Myelomalacia may be due to direct trauma or ischemia, and it may appear at or away from the site of trauma. It is accompanied by microcystic changes, gliosis, and arachnoiditis. On T1-weighted images, areas of myelomalacia show decreased signal intensity. Increased signal intensity occurs on T2-weighted images, but these changes are not as intense or bright as CSF on long TE images.[16]

There are many theories of cyst origin, one of which is breakdown of an area of myelomalacia.[16] Most cysts closely mimic the behavior of CSF, except for an occasional one that has an elevated protein content.

PTPM changes may occur in degenerative disc disease and severe osseous degeneration, particularly after mild trauma and occasionally after surgery (Fig. 5-28). After laminectomies, pseudomeningoceles and apparent areas of cord tethering are not uncommon.

INFLAMMATORY DISEASE

Hematogenous infections with discitis, osteomyelitis, and epidural abscess are more common in the lumbar and lower thoracic spine, where low-grade inflammatory changes may be difficult to distinguish from discogenic sclerosis (Fig. 5-29).[17] See Chapter 7 for a more detailed discussion.

Vertebral body changes may occur after discectomy that are similar to osteomyelitis (i.e., decreased signal on T1 and increased on T2-weighted sequences). After discectomy, the disc remains low signal intensity, but in discitis, the disc usually increases in signal intensity. Frank discitis and osteomyelitis may occasionally occur after surgery.

Epidural therapy is currently used for control of acute or chronic pain. Occasionally, an epidural abscess results, but most epidural abscesses occur in conjunction with vertebral osteomyelitis and discitis (Fig. 5-29). Some epidural catheters are ferromagnetic. Careful history before the MR study is necessary if neurologic symptoms or decline as the result of catheter movement are to be avoided.

Contrast agents have an important role in leptomeningeal inflammatory change due to the dense enhancement of the meninges and dura.[18] Administra-

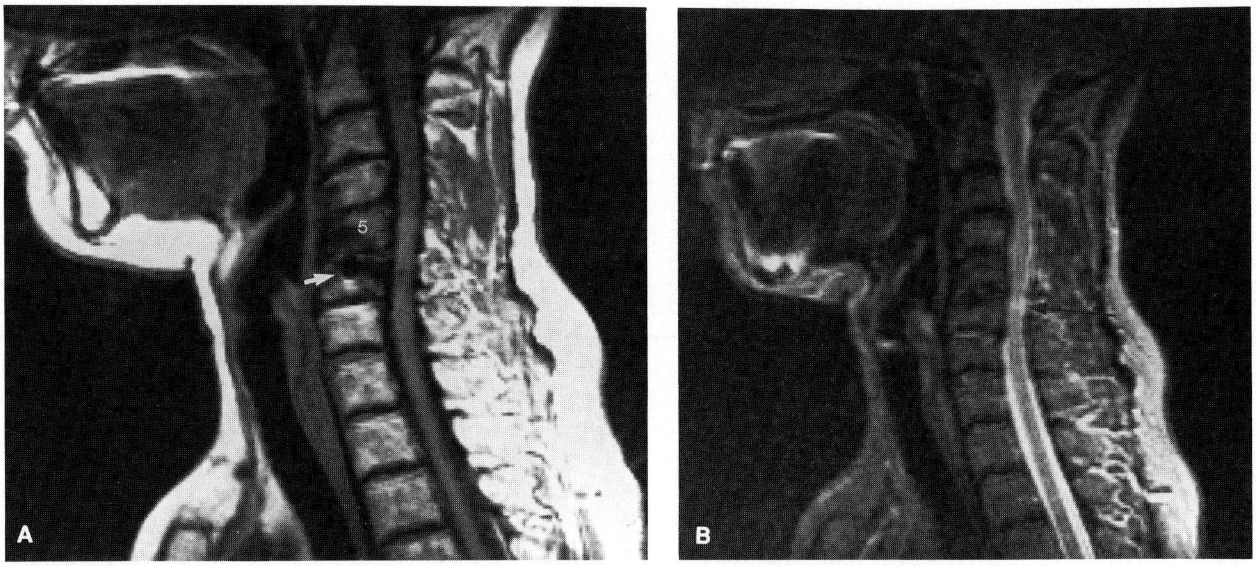

FIGURE 5 – 28. (A) Low-signal-intensity change involves the C5, the C6, and the anterior margin of C4.Small metal artifacts represent tiny fragments from the surgical drill (arrow). These usually cannot be seen on plain films. There is a questionable low-signal-intensity change within the cord, but no cystic abnormality is seen. **(B)** The T2-weighted sequence (TR/TE = 3000/90) shows a postsurgical change in the signal intensity of the cord in a patient with symptoms of a myelopathy (arrow).

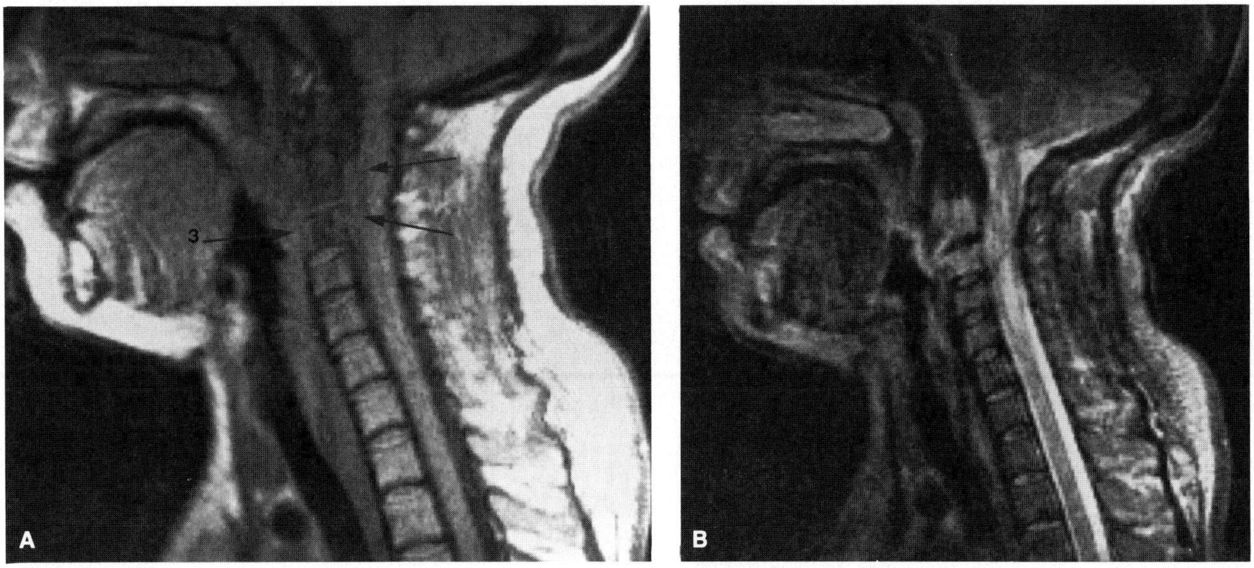

FIGURE 5 – 29. (A) There is slight decrease in signal intensity of the C2 and C3 vertebral bodies on this T1-weighted image (TR/TE = 450/20). The disc is also decreased in signal intensity, and there is an ill-defined epidural mass obliterating the anterior cord margin. In most interspace infections, there is greater destruction of the disc and end plates. **(B)** On the T2-weighted image (TR/TE = 3000/90), there is slight increased signal intensity in the vertebral bodies and epidural mass, which was an abscess at surgery. There is also an increase in signal intensity of the cord, which presumably represents inflammation.

tion in epidural inflammatory disease has not been studied in depth. An epidural abscess can only be diagnosed in many cases following IV contrast injection.

A suggested protocol for imaging of inflammatory processes includes T1-weighted and T2-weighted sagittal images and axial GRE (LFA) or T1-weighted images. If contrast agents are administered, T1-weighted images are required.

DEMYELINATING DISEASE

Multiple sclerosis (MS) is the most common demyelinating disease involving the cord. It is easier to demonstrate in the cervical cord because this portion of the cord is normally larger. MS plaques are often difficult to demonstrate even with optimal techniques and known intracranial disease of moderate severity. Thus, the lack of demonstration does not exclude cord disease (Fig. 5–30).

The plaques appear as areas of increased signal intensity on T2-weighted images and may be better demonstrated in the coronal plane. No signal intensity change is identified on T1-weighted images. An active plaque may enhance with contrast (Fig. 5–30). Similar to intracranial MS plaques, only a few may show enhancement even when multiple plaques are shown on the T2-weighted study. Intracranial enhancement has been correlated with the most acute or active plaques. Occasionally, the cord may be widened and the presence of a tumor may be questioned. An MR examination of the head may help the differential diagnosis, as does correlation with clinical and laboratory data.

Cord MS may occur without intracranial lesions. If this occurs in association with optic neuritis, it is known as De Vic's syndrome. The incidence of occur-

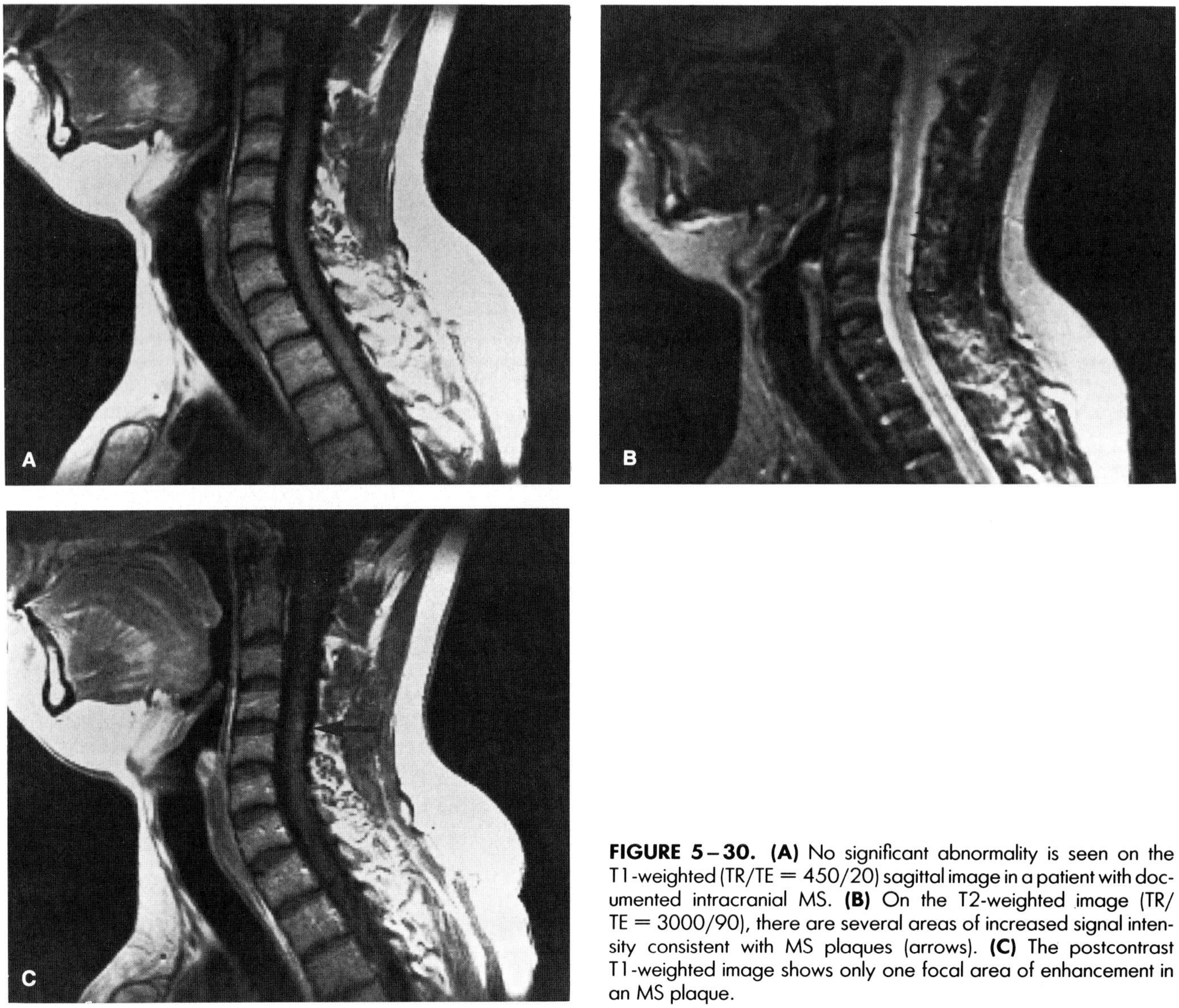

FIGURE 5–30. **(A)** No significant abnormality is seen on the T1-weighted (TR/TE = 450/20) sagittal image in a patient with documented intracranial MS. **(B)** On the T2-weighted image (TR/TE = 3000/90), there are several areas of increased signal intensity consistent with MS plaques (arrows). **(C)** The postcontrast T1-weighted image shows only one focal area of enhancement in an MS plaque.

rence of cord MS without intracranial lesions is unknown.

A protocol for examination should include T1-weighted sagittal images, T2-weighted sagittal or coronal sections, and T1-weighted sagittal images after contrast if the patient has acute cord symptomatology. GRE (LFA) sequences cannot be substituted for the more accurate T2-weighted images.

CONGENITAL ABNORMALITIES

There are many congenital spine abnormalities that usually involve all or large portions of the spinal axis. MRI is uniquely suited for their evaluation due to the number of spine levels covered and the superior anatomic detail demonstrated.

The most common and most frequently overlooked cervical spine anomaly is the Arnold–Chiari I malformation, in which the cerebellar tonsils are classically pointed and displaced into the upper cervical spine. There is no displacement of the fourth ventricle or the posterior fossa structures (Figs. 5–18, 5–19, and 5–20).[19] Tonsillar displacement or tonsillar ectopia is assessed by drawing a line from the tip of the clivus to the tip of the foramen magnum. Displacement greater than 2 mm is regarded as clinically significant.[19] The displaced tonsils produce abnormal CSF dynamics that may ultimately result in a syrinx.

In Arnold–Chiari II, further displacement of the tonsils is accompanied by downward displacement of the brainstem, fourth ventricle, and cerebellum. This is accompanied by other CNS malformations, such as partial agenesis of the corpus callosum, hydrocephalus, and myelomeningoceles.[20]

The Arnold–Chiari III malformation is a more severe anomaly, with further downward displacement of the posterior fossa structures, which extend through a cervical spina bifida forming a cervical encephalocele. This rare anomaly is easily seen on physical examination.[19]

Other spine anomalies, such as bony abnormalities, dysraphism, diastematomyelia, and tethered cord, may present elsewhere with secondary cervical spine manifestations (e.g., syrinx). Scoliosis may be the clinical presentation in many of these abnormalities (Fig. 5–20). In a scoliosis evaluation, it is these abnormalities and an occasional glioma that the referring physician wishes to exclude before definitive therapy (i.e., rod placement). If spine curvatures are severe, coronal imaging may be the only plane that will visualize the cord in its entirety (Fig. 5–31).

The visualization of most congenital abnormalities requires T1-weighted images in the sagittal, coronal, and possibly axial planes for adequate demonstration of the altered anatomy. T2-weighted images are needed only if there are cord symptoms or cord abnormalities (i.e., syrinx) that require further clarification, such as exclusion of an underlying tumor.

CRANIOVERTEBRAL JUNCTION ABNORMALITIES

Craniovertebral (CV) junction abnormalities deserve special consideration because the symptoms are so diverse that they mimic many other neurologic entities, including MS. The diversity in clinical presentation is due to the compression or impingement of adjacent anatomic structures. Symptoms include brain

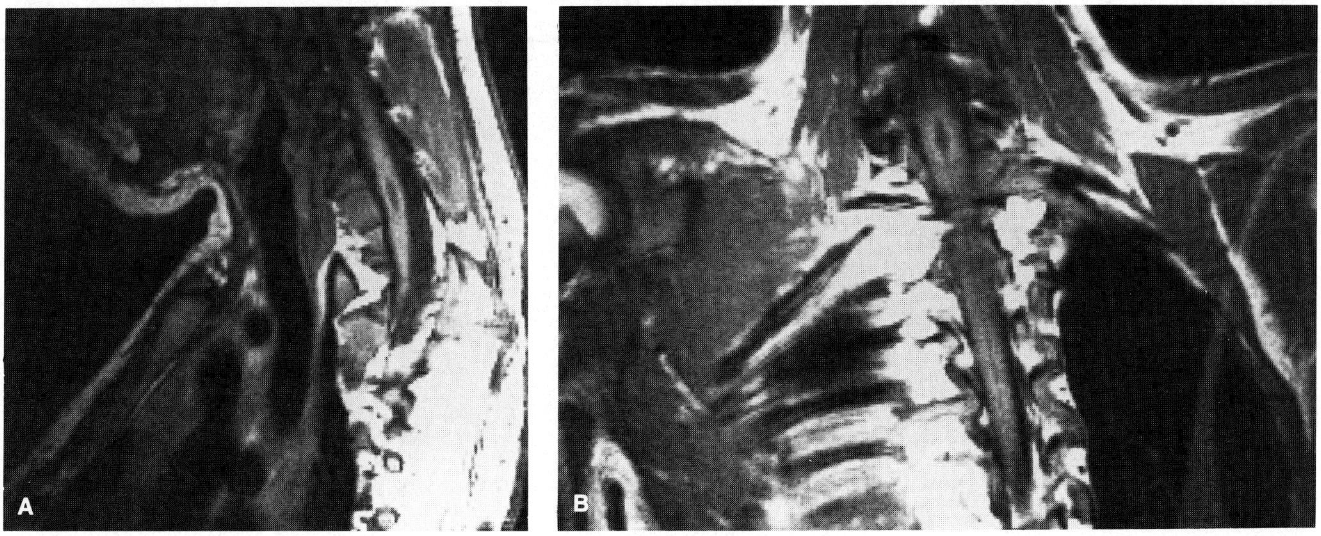

FIGURE 5–31. **(A)** There is a small focal syrinx that is presumably related to the severity of the long-standing scoliosis. The cord is difficult to visualize in its entirety on this T1-weighted sagittal image. **(B)** Both the cord and syrinx are better seen in the coronal plane.

stem compression (e.g., vertigo, facial pain), cerebellar signs (e.g., nystagmus, ataxia), compression of the pyramidal tracts of the anterior medulla (e.g., spastic paraparesis), and compression of the posterior columns of the cord (e.g., proprioception and vibratory difficulty). If these abnormalities are not to be missed, sagittal T1-weighted SE imaging is required for evaluating any cranial complaint.

A number of causes have been presented, including the Arnold-Chiari malformations (Figs. 5-18, 5-19, and 5-21), meningiomas (Fig. 5-26), and neurofibromas (Fig. 5-27). Osseous changes can produce similar symptoms, including congenital dysplasia (Fig. 5-32) and benign hypertrophic changes that may have a soft tissue fibrotic component and are referred to as pseudotumors (Fig. 5-33).

Late sequelae of rheumatoid arthritis may produce craniovertebral junction abnormalities (Fig. 5-34). This connective tissue disease with its inflammatory component may show a mass or pannus at the CV junction, seen as an indenting soft tissue mass on T1-weighted images.[22] As with hypertrophic change, this will be more apparent on CSF images, because there is a low-signal-intensity component that can be obscured on T1-weighted images by the low-signal-intensity CSF (Fig. 5-33). GRE (LFA) images are usually adequate in these cases. Axial imaging in this and other osseous abnormalities will rarely reflect the severity of the upper cord or lower brain stem compression (Figs. 5-32 through 5-34).

ARTERIOVENOUS MALFORMATIONS

AVMs or AV fistulas are usually easily identified as serpiginous areas of signal void. The veins are usually larger than the arteries. These may bleed, producing areas of hemorrhage. Hemorrhage often ablates these abnormalities. The result is a low-signal-intensity abnormality because of hemosiderin deposition, the final stage of hemoglobin degradation. Contrast may help distinguish hemosiderin from a small malformation, with enhancement of the venous side of the malformation on spin echo imaging.

CONCLUSION

The MRI user must be aware that this technology is rapidly changing and that today's guidelines may be altered by these changes. For example, fast scanning with GRE technique and volume imaging (Fig. 5-35) may soon replace CT as the modality of choice for focal radiculopathy.

A continued self-education program of software updates and usage is necessary. Although an applications scientist is often not at your disposal to teach basic MR principles, he or she can serve as an excellent source in acquainting you with the capabilities of your imager's software programs. Most of all, personal knowledge and input are mandatory for generating images that maximize clinical diagnosis.

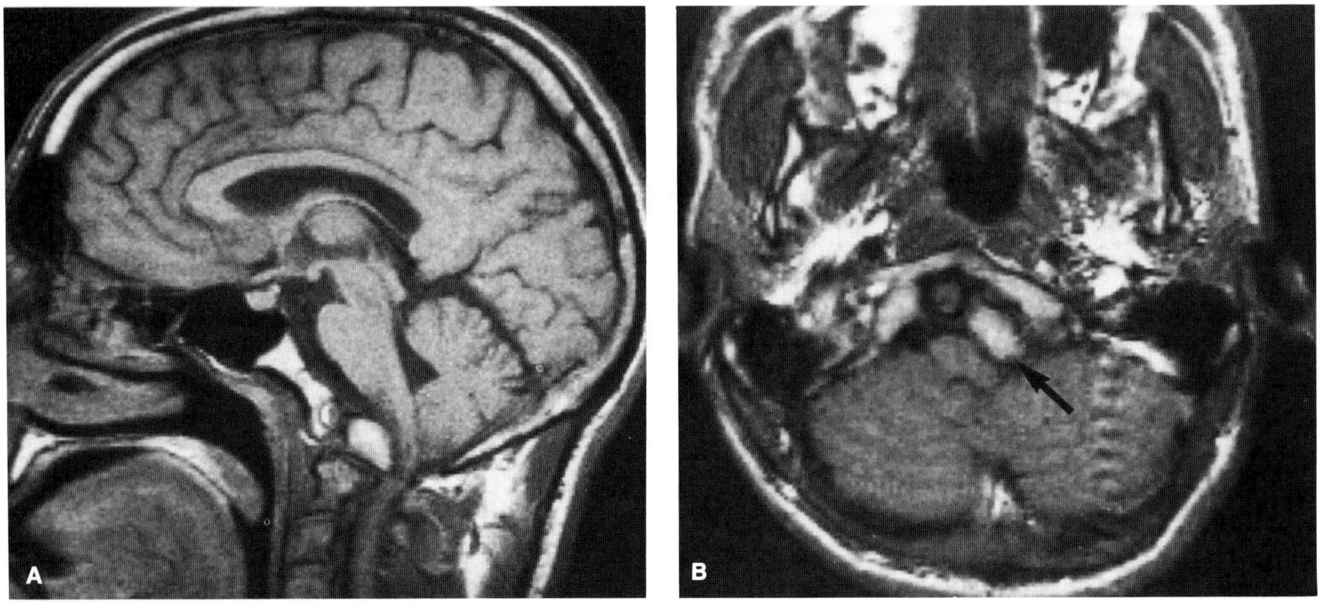

FIGURE 5-32. (A) This sagittal T1-weighted image (TR/TE = 700/17) shows an abnormal articulation between the skull base and C1. This compresses the medulla and upper cervical cord. **(B)** The axial view lateralized the abnormality to the left (arrow) but does not show the severity of compression of the medulla as shown in the sagittal plane.

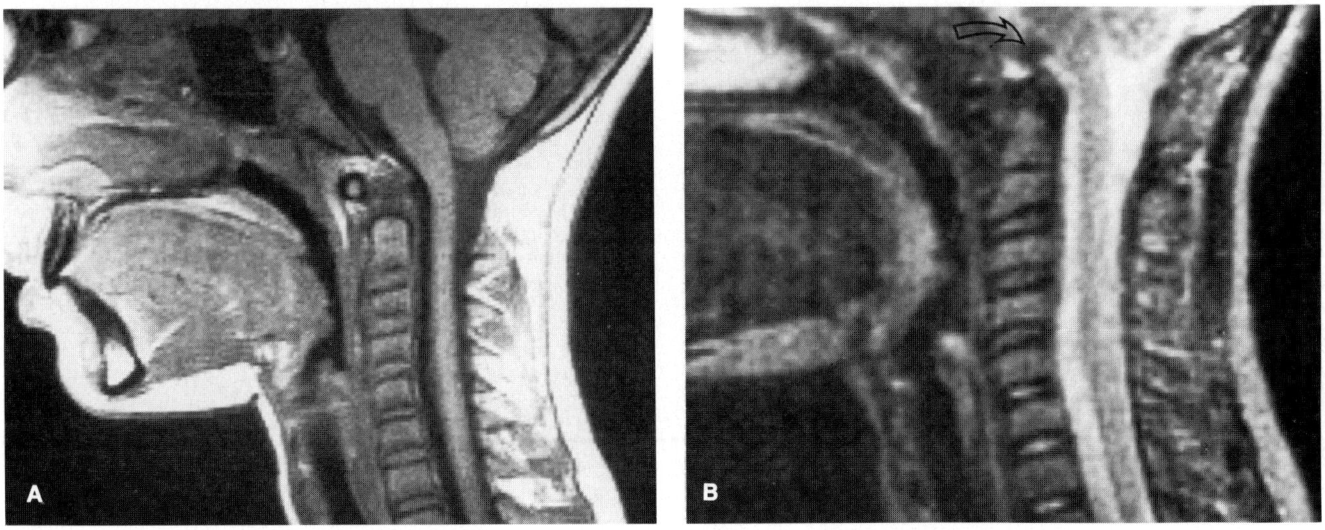

FIGURE 5–33. (A) This T1-weighted image shows proliferative changes at the craniovertebral junction. **(B)** The degree of impingement of the medulla (arrow) is better shown on the T2-weighted sequence. The osseous proliferation requires CSF imaging for adequate assessment.

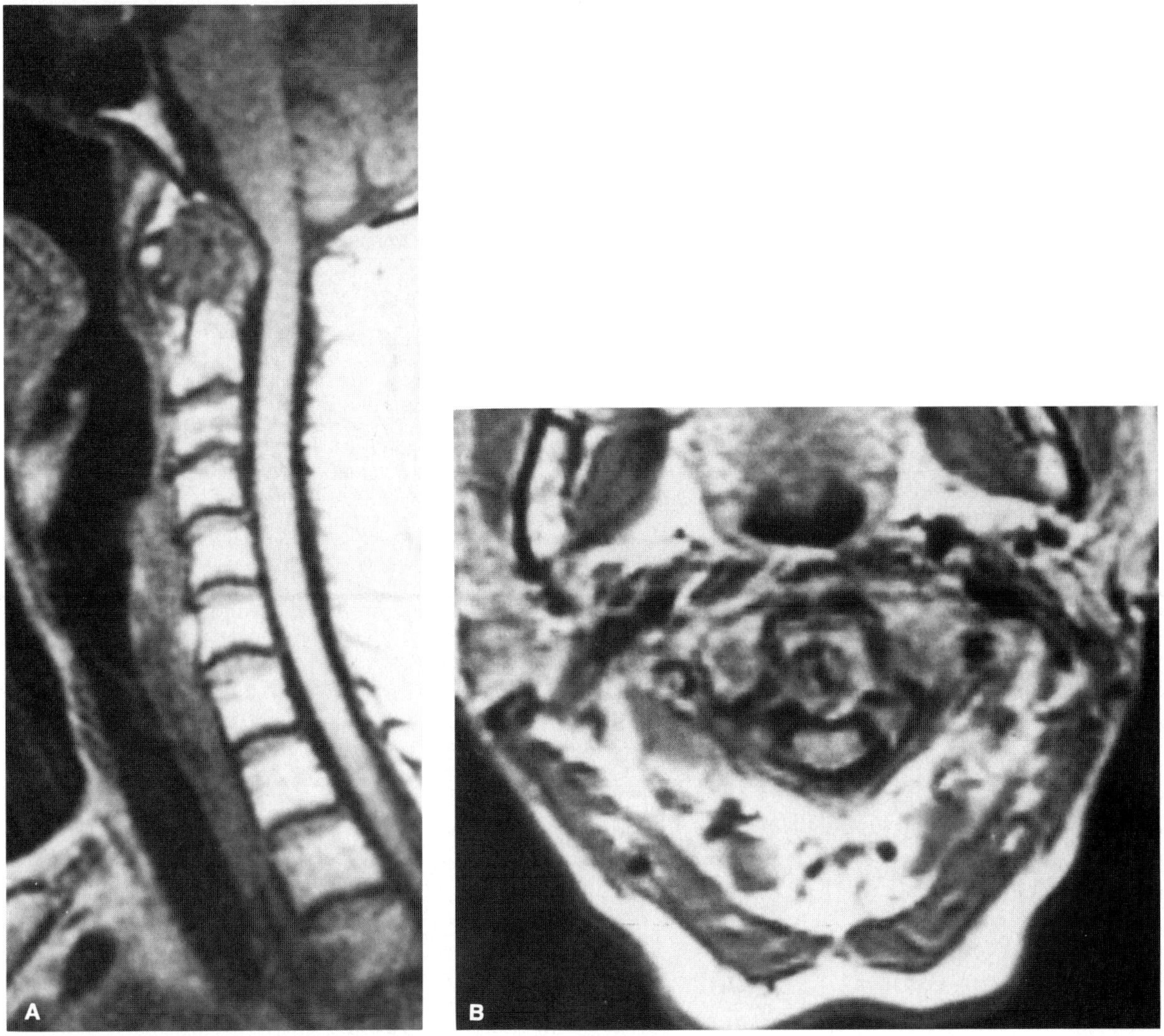

FIGURE 5–34. (A) There is a large pannus impressing the medulla and upper cervical cord on this T1-weighted image in a patient with rheumatoid arthritis. **(B)** The axial image fails to demonstrate the severity of the compression, stressing the need for sagittal imaging in routine head examinations.

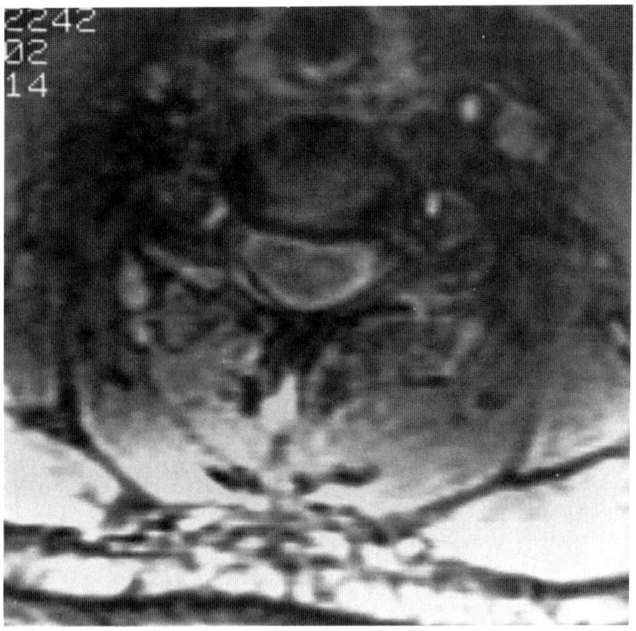

FIGURE 5–35. An axial section from a 3D volume collection that yielded 26 truly contiguous 3-mm sections in 13.4 minutes. There is excellent differentiation between the cord and CSF. The H-shaped gray matter of the cord is nicely demonstrated in this normal volunteer.

ACKNOWLEDGMENT

The authors thank Marjorie Hennessy, whose help in manuscript preparation was invaluable and deeply appreciated.

REFERENCES

1. Kjos BO, Norman D. Strategies for efficient imaging of the lumbar spine. In: Brant-Zawadzki M, Norman D, eds. Magnetic resonance imaging of the central nervous system. New York: Raven Press, 1987.
2. Enzmann DR, Rubin JB. Cervical spine: MR imaging with a partial flip angle, gradient-refocused pulse sequence. Radiology 1988;166:467.
3. Batnitzky S, Price HI, Caughan MJ, et al. The radiology of syringohydromyelia. Radiographics 1983;3:585.
4. Bronskill MJ, McVeigh ER, Kucharczyk W, Henkelman RM. Syrinx-like artifacts on MR images of the spinal cord. Radiology 1988;166:485.
5. Williams AL, Haughton VM, Pojunas KW, et al. Differentiation of intramedullary neoplasms and cysts by MR. AJR 1987;149:159.
6. Enzmann DR, O'Donohue J, Rubin JB. CSF pulsations within nonneoplastic spinal cord cysts. AJR 1987;149:149.
7. Atlas SW, Mark AS, Fram EK. Aqueductal stenosis: evaluation with gradient-echo rapid MR imaging. Radiology 1988;169:449.
8. Sze G, Krol G, Zimmerman RD, Deck MDF. Malignant extradural spinal tumors: MR imaging with Gd DTPA. Radiology 1988;167:217.
9. Smoker WRK, Godersky JC, Knutzon RK. The role of MR imaging in evaluating metastatic spinal disease. AJR 1987;149:1241.
10. Norman D. The spine. In: Brant-Zawadzki M, Norman D, eds. Magnetic resonance imaging of the central nervous system. New York: Raven Press, 1987.
11. Dillon WP, Norman D, Newton TH, et al. Intradural spinal cord lesions: Gd-DTPA-enhanced MR imaging. Radiology 1989;170:229.
12. Sze G, Abramson A, Krol G, et al. Gadolinium-DTPA in the evaluation of intradural extramedullary spinal disease. AJR 1988;150:911.
13. Post MJD, Quencer RM, Green BA, et al. Intramedullary spinal cord metastases, mainly of nonneurogenic origin. AJR 1987;148:1015.
14. Kulkarni MV, McArdle C, Kopanicky D, et al. Acute spinal cord injury: MR imaging at 1.5 T. Radiology 1987;164:837.
15. Atlas SW, Mark AS, Grossman RJ, Gomori JM. Intracranial hemorrhage: Gradient-echo MR imaging at 1.5 T, comparison with spin-echo imaging and clinical application. Radiology 1988;168:803.
16. Gebarski SS, Maynard FW, Gabrielsen TO, et al. Posttraumatic progressive myelopathy. Radiology 1985;157:357.
17. Price AC, Allen JH, Eggers FM, et al. Intervertebral disc space infection: CT changes. Radiology 1983;149:725.
18. Matthews VP, Kuharik MA, Edwards MK, et al. Gd-DTPA-enhanced MR imaging of experimental bacterial meningitis: evaluation and comparison with CT. AJNR 1988;9:1045.
19. Barkovich AJ, Wippold FJ, Sherman JL, Citrin CM. Significance of cerebellar tonsillar position on MR. AJNR 1986;7:795.
20. Wolpert SM, Anderson M, Scott RM, et al. Chiari II malformation: MR imaging evaluation. AJR 1987;149:1033.
21. Sze G, Brant-Zawadzki M, Wilson CB, et al. Pseudotumor of the craniovertebral junction associated with chronic subluxation: MR imaging studies. Radiology 1986;161:391.
22. Bundschuh C, Modic MT, Kearney F, et al. Rheumatoid arthritis of the cervical spine: surface coil MR imaging. AJR 1988;151:181.

6

Thoracic Spine

Kevin L. Nelson
Val M. Runge

Magnetic resonance imaging (MRI) is now considered by many to represent the primary imaging modality for evaluation of the thoracic spine.[1] MRI should be the initial imaging modality employed in most instances because it is noninvasive, uses no ionizing radiation, and has multiplanar imaging capabilities, providing images with excellent soft tissue detail. Although it is the best first test for many indications, plain films, myelography, and computed tomography (CT) will continue to be used as complementary studies because they provide additional valuable information in many instances.

The development and improvement of surface coil technology have been major factors in the advancement of MRI to its current stature in thoracic spine imaging.[2,3] Surface coils allow smaller fields of view with increased signal-to-noise ratios (SNR) and better spatial resolution than body coil images. Introduction of improved motion compensation techniques and other refinements in pulse sequences have helped to significantly reduce distracting motion artifacts from cerebrospinal fluid (CSF) and venous pulsations. Gradient-echo imaging is another evolving technique that may find significant clinical use in thoracic spine MRI.[4] The clinical introduction of gadolinium DTPA (Gd DTPA) has improved lesion detection and depiction in the thoracic spine.[5]

This chapter discusses techniques for obtaining diagnostic images of the thoracic spine and reviews the MR appearance of commonly encountered thoracic spine abnormalities.

THORACIC SPINE IMAGING TECHNIQUES

Although surface coils improve definition of lesions by allowing smaller fields of view, they may not be sufficient because the entire spinal axis is not included on high-resolution surface coil images. A simple solution to this problem is to obtain, for anatomic reference, an initial sagittal body coil scout image, including one end of the spinal column. These body coil images can then be correlated with the high-resolution surface coil images for easy reference in accurately determining the level of an abnormality. By using a short TR and short TE (TR/TE = 200–300/15–30 msecs), one data acquisition, 128 phase-encoding steps, and 5-mm-thick contiguous slices, a multislice survey of the spine can be obtained in less than 1 minute of imaging time. The entire cervical or lumbar spine must be included on these body coil images so levels in the spine can be accurately determined by counting either from the cephalad or caudad end of the spinal axis.

A rectangular surface coil is most commonly used for high-resolution thoracic spine MRI. In most patients, the rectangular surface coil provides coverage of the entire thoracic spine in the sagittal plane; circular surface coils find greater utility in the cervical spine. Although a rectangular surface coil does not provide the depth of penetration achieved with a circular surface coil, this usually is not a problem in thoracic spine imaging.

The initial pulse sequence preferred with the surface coil is a T1-weighted sagittal spin echo sequence (relaxation time [TR]/echo time [TE] = 400–600/10–30 msec, 3–5-mm-thick slices, and 1–1.5-mm interslice gap). A matrix with either 192 or 256 phase-encoding steps and two to four data acquisitions is employed for high-resolution images obtained in 3 to 10 minutes.

These images provide excellent morphologic detail of the thoracic spine. (Fig. 6–1A). The spinal cord is well-defined in the spinal canal, because it is of intermediate signal intensity surrounded by low-signal-intensity CSF. The vertebral bodies contain high-signal-intensity marrow fat and are surrounded by cortical

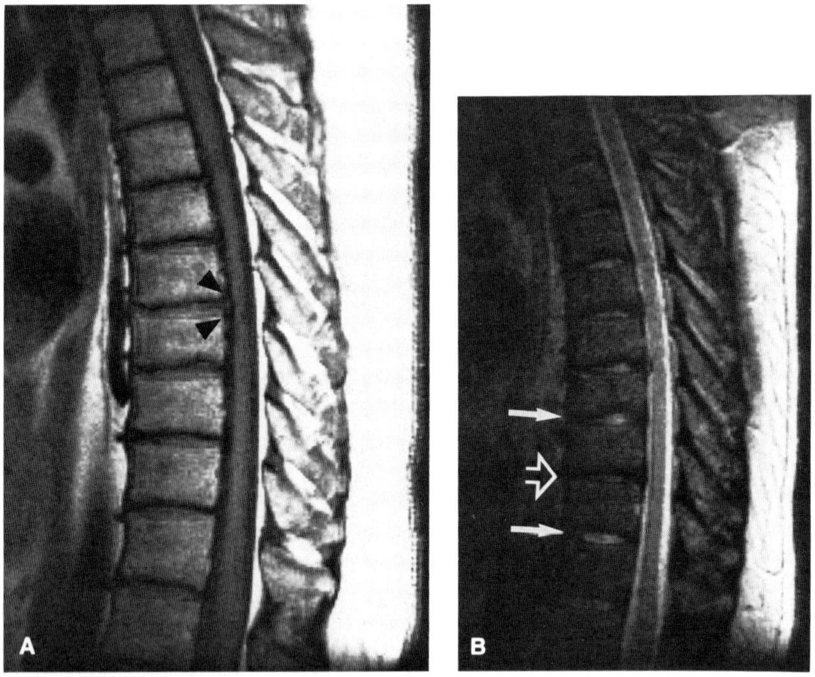

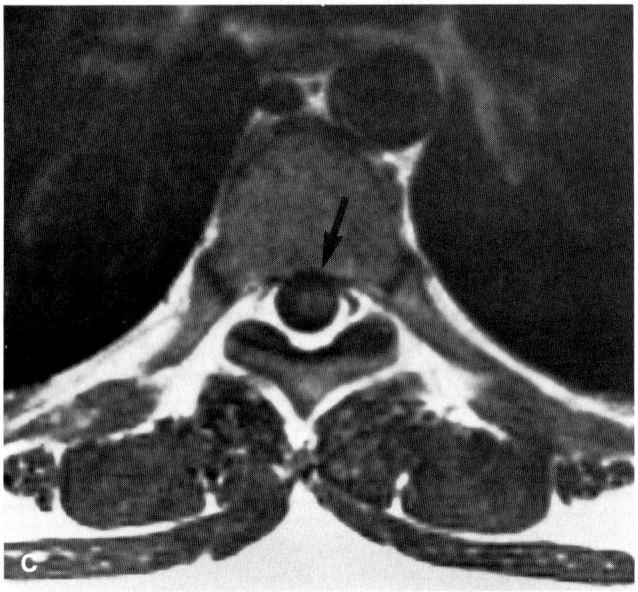

FIGURE 6–1. Normal thoracic spine. **(A)** Sagittal T1-weighted (TR/TE = 450/20), **(B)** T2-weighted (TR/TE = 2600/90), and **(C)** axial T1-weighted (TR/TE = 450/20), spin echo images. The intermediate-signal-intensity thoracic spinal cord is well defined within the spinal canal by surrounding low- and high-signal-intensity CSF on T1- and T2-weighted images, respectively. The normal fat-containing bone marrow in the thoracic vertebral bodies is of slightly increased signal intensity on the T1-weighted image, decreasing in signal intensity on the T2-weighted image, which is typical of fat. The normally hydrated nucleus pulposus and inner fibers of the annulus fibrosis display increased signal intensity (closed arrows) on the T2-weighted image. There is slightly decreased signal intensity of the nucleus pulposus of the T9-10 intervertebral disc (open arrow), indicating mild dehydration secondary to early degenerative disc disease. On the sagittal T1- and T2-weighted images, a subtle thoracic intervertebral disc herniation can be seen (black arrowheads) at the T8-9 level. The disc herniation is accentuated on the T2-weighted image due to turbulent CSF flow around it in the subarachnoid space. The axial T1-weighted image **(C)** shows the normal appearance of the symmetric thoracic spinal cord (arrow) within the spinal canal surrounded by low-signal-intensity CSF.

bone, which produces no signal. The intervertebral discs are of intermediate signal intensity, similar to the spinal cord.

The next pulse sequence commonly employed is a double-echo sagittal multislice spin echo sequence to obtain both proton density and T2-weighted images. A long TR/intermediate TE sequence (TR/TE = 2000–3000/30–50 msec) provides proton-density-weighted images. The second echo of this sequence uses a long TE (50–120 msec), providing T2-weighted images. A 4- to 5-mm slice is chosen, depending on the amount of SNR available with a 1-mm interslice gap. A matrix with 256 phase-encoding steps, one data-set acquisition, and low bandwidth to increase SNR usually provide excellent quality proton density and T2-weighted images. If adequate SNR can not be obtained with this technique, an alternative is to use 128 phase-encoding steps and two data-set acquisitions (or other variations between these two extremes). Although more SNR is present with this technique, the spatial resolution of the images is lower. Both techniques have approximate imaging times of 10 to 12 minutes.

It is particularly important when obtaining T2-weighted images in the thoracic spine to employ a motion-compensation technique to minimize CSF and venous pulsations on the images. Gradient moment nulling is the most commonly recommended technique.[6] Cardiac or pulse gating may also be used alone or in conjunction with gradient moment nulling.[7,8] Presaturation pulses can eliminate artifact from motion of the anterior chest wall, heart, and to a lesser extent, the thoracic aorta.[9,10] These techniques are discussed in greater depth in Chapter 13.

Proton density and T2-weighted pulse sequences provide images in which the signal intensity of CSF is greater than on T1-weighted images (Fig. 6–1B). The lower-signal-intensity spinal cord is usually well-visualized within the CSF if adequate motion compensation techniques are used. As in the brain, most spinal cord abnormalities possess a prolonged T2 relaxation time, producing increased signal intensity on these pulse sequences. The fat within the vertebral body marrow, due to its shorter T2 relaxation time, is depicted with lower signal intensity than on T1-weighted images. The nucleus pulposus of the intervertebral discs and inner fibers of the annulus fibrosis display increased signal intensity compared with the lower-signal-intensity outer fibers of the annulus fibrosis.

A third pulse sequence is recommended in the axial plane through the region of interest or level of a suspected abnormality defined on the sagittal images. Most commonly, the pulse sequence employed is a short TR/short TE sequence, providing T1-weighted images (Fig. 6–1C). A 3- to 5-mm slice is used with a matrix of 192 or 256 phase-encoding steps for high-resolution images. Generally four data acquisitions are recommended for adequate SNR.

Potential alternatives exist for decreasing the amount of scanning time to tolerable limits. A shorter TR may be employed to proportionally decrease the total imaging time, but a shorter TR decreases SNR and provides fewer images in a multislice sequence. Another alternative is to decrease the number of data-set acquisitions from four to two. This decreases the imaging time by half but causes a 40% loss of SNR. Decreasing the number of data acquisitions may be useful in obtaining diagnostic images of uncooperative patients. Although a larger number of data acquisitions helps to average motion artifacts, decreasing the total scan time by halving the number of acquisitions often provides the best images of these patients. Another alternative to decreasing scan time is to use a matrix with 128 phase-encoding steps. Although this decreases the imaging time by half and increases SNR in the images, the major disadvantage is a decrease in spatial resolution.

Axial proton density or T2-weighted images are preferred in some cases. The pulse sequence parameters used are the same as those outlined for the sagittal plane. These images can more clearly define a tumor or a demyelinating plaque within the spinal cord of patients with multiple sclerosis. Because the CSF has increased signal intensity on these pulse sequences, the CSF-extradural interface can be evaluated effectively (e.g., in a thoracic disc herniation). The major disadvantage of these images are the long imaging times required.

A final alternative is the use of gradient-echo images. These images are generated through the use of partial tip angles instead of an initial 90° radio frequency (RF) pulse. Refocussing is done through the use of the MR gradient coils in the scanner. By changing the tip angle and TR, various degrees of contrast can be achieved in thoracic spine imaging.

The primary value of gradient-echo images is their ability to produce a myelogram-like image by increasing the CSF signal intensity. This allows evaluation of the CSF-extradural interface with shorter imaging times than required for T2-weighted spin echo images. Gradient-echo scans obtained in a 2D-mode can be completed in 1 to 2 minutes of scanning time.

Future applications of gradient-echo images will include their use in 3D-modes, whereby thin-section (1–2 mm) images can be obtained.[11] This allows computer-assisted reformations in multiple projections from scans obtained in a single plane.

The pharmacokinetic effects of Gd DTPA and its ability to more clearly depict spine abnormalities are outlined in Chapter 15 and other sources.[12,13] Contrast-enhanced images have been very useful for more clearly defining abnormalities, such as spinal cord tumors or epidural fibrosis, in the postoperative spine.[14,15] Gd DTPA causes shortening of both T1 and T2 relaxation times. A shortening of T1 relaxation times produces increased signal intensity on conventional T1-weighted spin echo images. Therefore, a heavily T1-weighted pulse sequence is used for contrast-enhanced MRI.

Many alternatives exist for obtaining MR images of the thoracic spine and for decreasing the total scan time, and guidelines are offered for what are felt to be the most acceptable techniques.[16,17] Personal preferences and optimal techniques with different scanners are significant factors when deciding upon a particular pulse sequence and the parameters used for that sequence.

THORACIC SPINE PATHOLOGY

Neoplasms

Intramedullary Tumor

The most common intramedullary tumor to involve the thoracic spinal cord is a glioma. Most of these gliomas are low-grade astrocytomas (Fig. 6–2). These lesions tend to diffusely infiltrate the spinal cord and

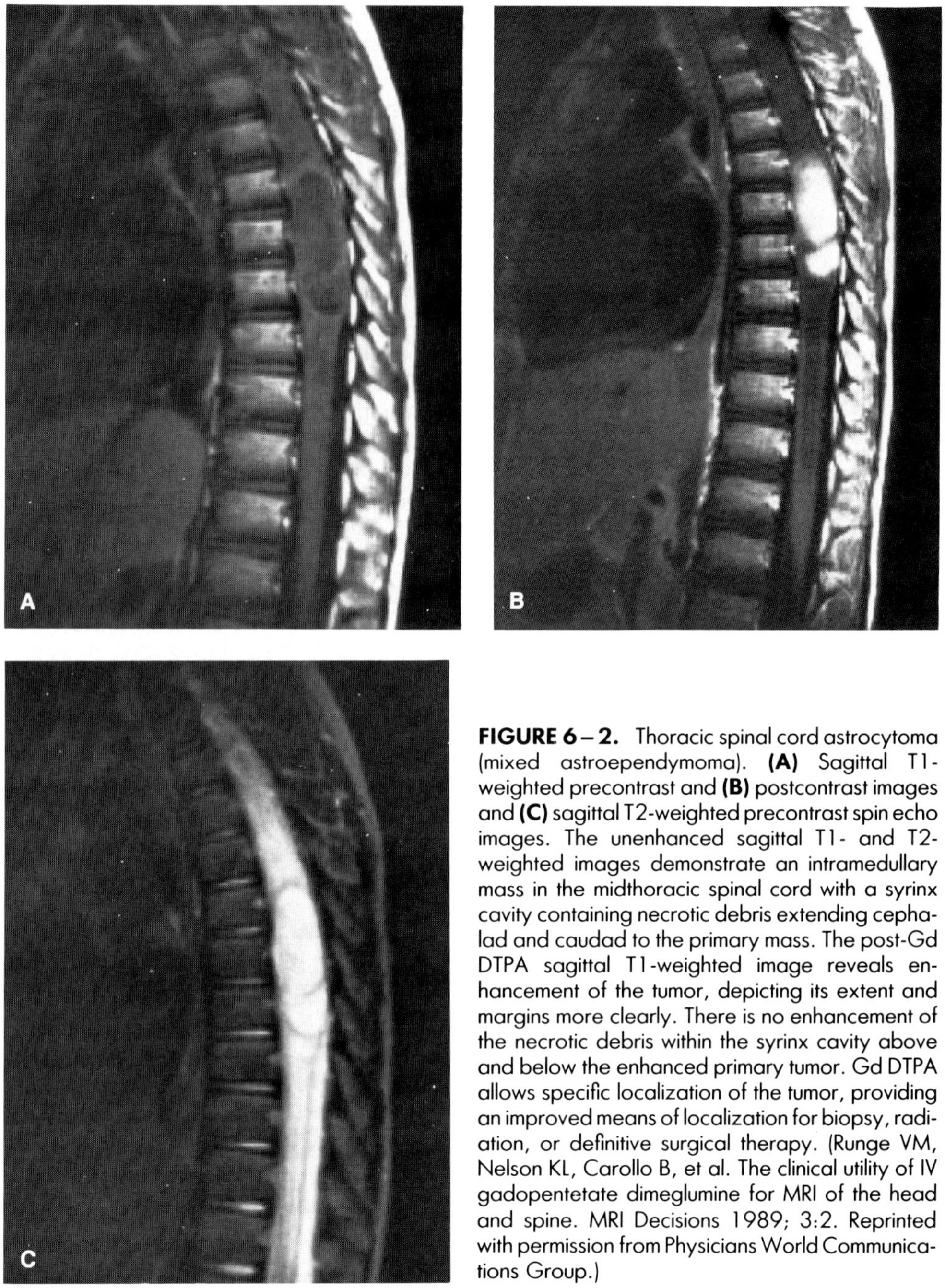

FIGURE 6–2. Thoracic spinal cord astrocytoma (mixed astroependymoma). **(A)** Sagittal T1-weighted precontrast and **(B)** postcontrast images and **(C)** sagittal T2-weighted precontrast spin echo images. The unenhanced sagittal T1- and T2-weighted images demonstrate an intramedullary mass in the midthoracic spinal cord with a syrinx cavity containing necrotic debris extending cephalad and caudad to the primary mass. The post-Gd DTPA sagittal T1-weighted image reveals enhancement of the tumor, depicting its extent and margins more clearly. There is no enhancement of the necrotic debris within the syrinx cavity above and below the enhanced primary tumor. Gd DTPA allows specific localization of the tumor, providing an improved means of localization for biopsy, radiation, or definitive surgical therapy. (Runge VM, Nelson KL, Carollo B, et al. The clinical utility of IV gadopentetate dimeglumine for MRI of the head and spine. MRI Decisions 1989; 3:2. Reprinted with permission from Physicians World Communications Group.)

have poorly defined margins. On T1-weighted spin echo images, there is usually fusiform enlargement of the spinal cord over one or more segments.[18] The tumor is usually isointense or has decreased signal intensity compared with the normal spinal cord. On T2-weighted images, tumor usually displays increased signal intensity, as does surrounding edema in the spinal cord.[19,20] Enhancement with Gd DTPA may vary and depends on the integrity of the blood–spinal-cord barrier. Although most spinal cord astrocytomas are low-grade tumors, they usually enhance with Gd DTPA.[21]

One of the more useful aspects of contrast enhancement with Gd DTPA is its ability to differentiate benign syringomyelia from neoplastic cavitation within a tumor.[21,22] Although not extensively studied, a benign syrinx typically does not enhance, whereas neoplastic cavities usually do display some enhancement, generally within their walls.[21–23] Gd DTPA may also be useful for separating tumor from edema, although studies have not been performed to confirm this, particularly for astrocytomas. The ability to make this differentiation would be critical for planning surgery or radiation therapy.

Ependymomas occur throughout the thoracic spinal cord, including the conus medullaris and the filum terminale.[24] These tumors cause spinal cord enlargement and are usually fairly well-defined. They are isointense or have decreased signal intensity on T1-weighted images compared with the normal spinal cord. On T2-weighted images increased signal intensity usually can be recognized within the tumor. Ependymomas commonly enhance after Gd DTPA administration.[22] There may be only peripheral enhancement early following injection with more homogenous enhancement on delayed images, or there may be intense, uniform enhancement early in the course after injection.[22]

Less common intramedullary tumors involving the thoracic spinal cord include hemangioblastomas. These tumors most commonly occur in patients with von Hippel–Lindau disease.[25] They may be multiple throughout the spinal cord and associated with hemangioblastomas occurring in the posterior fossa.

Arteriovenous malformations (AVM) may occur in an intramedullary location within the spinal cord (Figs. 6–3 and 6–4).[26,27] Hemorrhage, and in particular hemosiderin deposition, is commonly present. Ser-

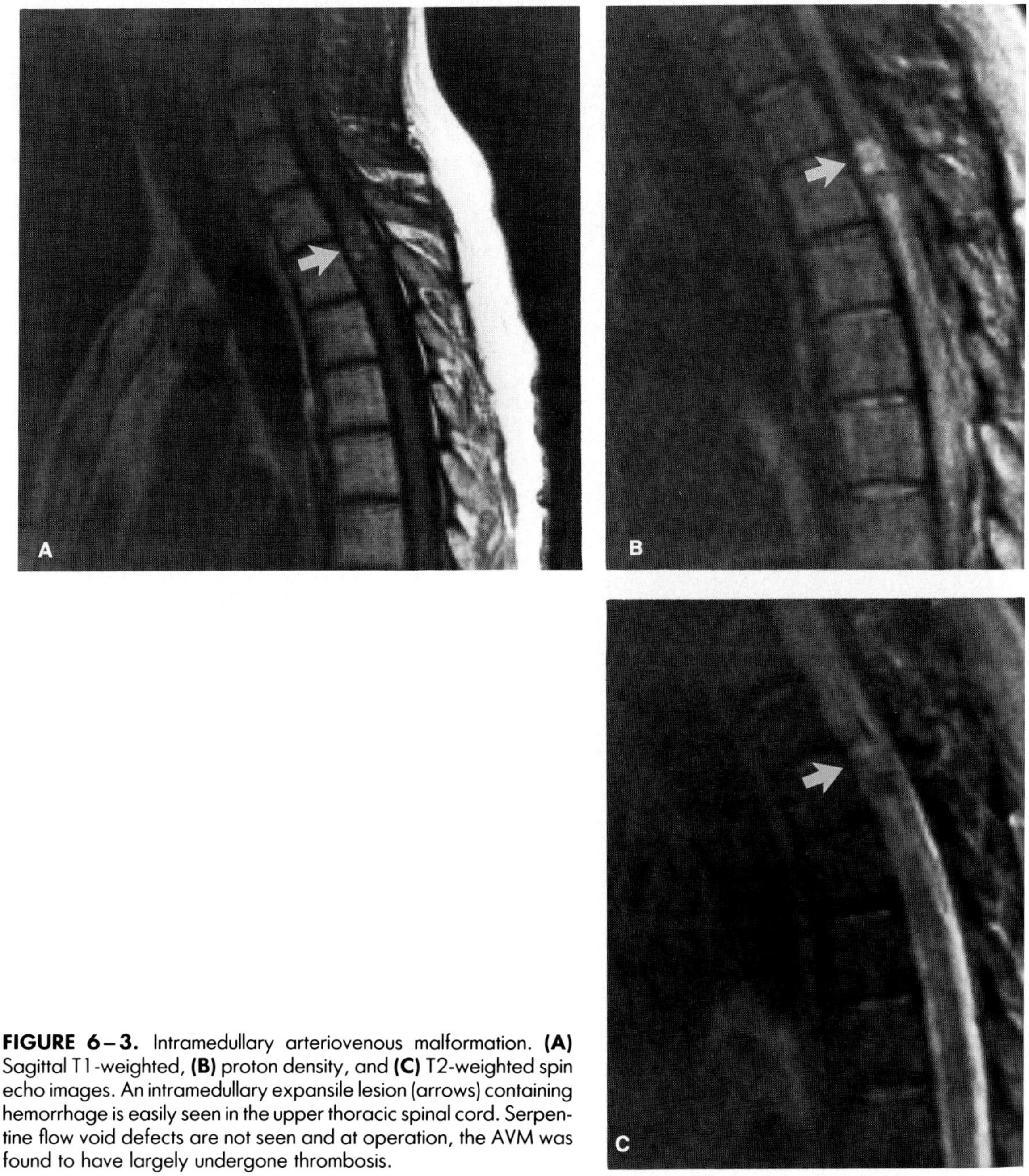

FIGURE 6–3. Intramedullary arteriovenous malformation. **(A)** Sagittal T1-weighted, **(B)** proton density, and **(C)** T2-weighted spin echo images. An intramedullary expansile lesion (arrows) containing hemorrhage is easily seen in the upper thoracic spinal cord. Serpentine flow void defects are not seen and at operation, the AVM was found to have largely undergone thrombosis.

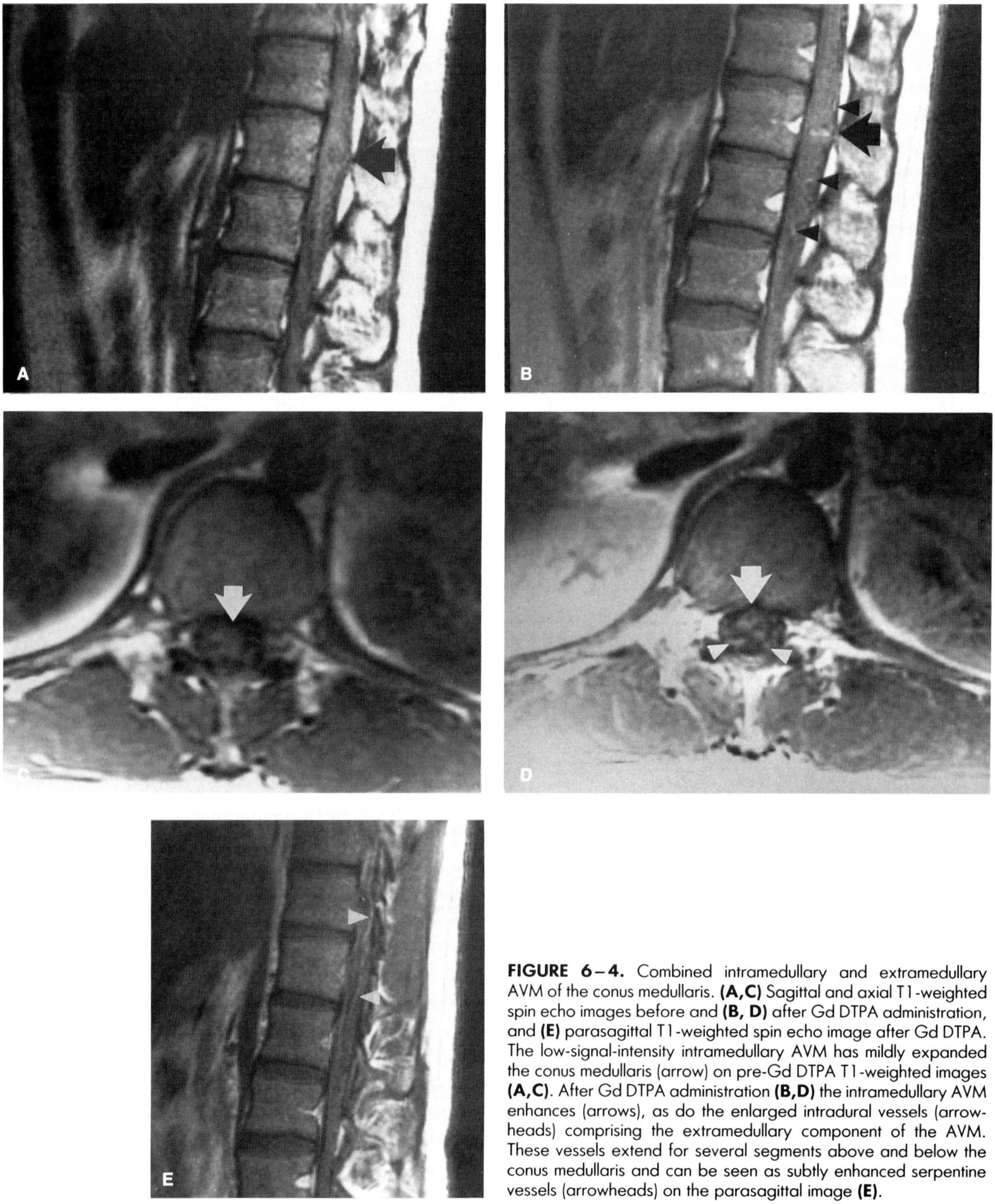

FIGURE 6–4. Combined intramedullary and extramedullary AVM of the conus medullaris. **(A,C)** Sagittal and axial T1-weighted spin echo images before and **(B, D)** after Gd DTPA administration, and **(E)** parasagittal T1-weighted spin echo image after Gd DTPA. The low-signal-intensity intramedullary AVM has mildly expanded the conus medullaris (arrow) on pre-Gd DTPA T1-weighted images **(A,C)**. After Gd DTPA administration **(B,D)** the intramedullary AVM enhances (arrows), as do the enlarged intradural vessels (arrowheads) comprising the extramedullary component of the AVM. These vessels extend for several segments above and below the conus medullaris and can be seen as subtly enhanced serpentine vessels (arrowheads) on the parasagittal image **(E)**.

pentine flow void defects may be seen within the lesion. Extramedullary components cause subtle scalloping of the spinal cord secondary to enlarged vessels.

Metastases can occur in the spinal cord.[28,29] This can be due to direct seeding of the spinal cord or represent drop metastases from a primary intracranial neoplasm, with direct extension into the spinal cord. Metastatic disease commonly enhances with Gd DTPA.

Intradural-Extramedullary Tumor

The most common tumors occurring in this location in the thoracic spine are benign meningiomas and nerve sheath tumors. MRI is a noninvasive means of evaluating these tumors.

Meningiomas usually occur in middle-aged female patients and are benign, slow-growing tumors. While most commonly present in an intradural-extramedullary location, extradural extension of tumor can occur, and a purely extradural meningioma may be encountered occasionally. Their appearance on MRI is variable, similar to extra-axial meningiomas seen in the brain (Fig. 6–5).[21,22] Generally these tumors are isointense with the normal spinal cord on T1-weighted images, making them difficult to appreciate if small. A subtle soft tissue mass may be recognized with mass effect upon the spinal cord. Meningiomas have variable signal intensity characteristics on T2-weighted images, but in the thoracic spine, they are often intermediate or low signal intensity surrounded by the high-signal-intensity CSF. Meningiomas typically show uniform homogenous contrast enhancement with Gd DTPA unless central necrosis is present.[21,22] This allows improved depiction of the enhancing tumor against the low-signal-intensity CSF on T1-weighted images.

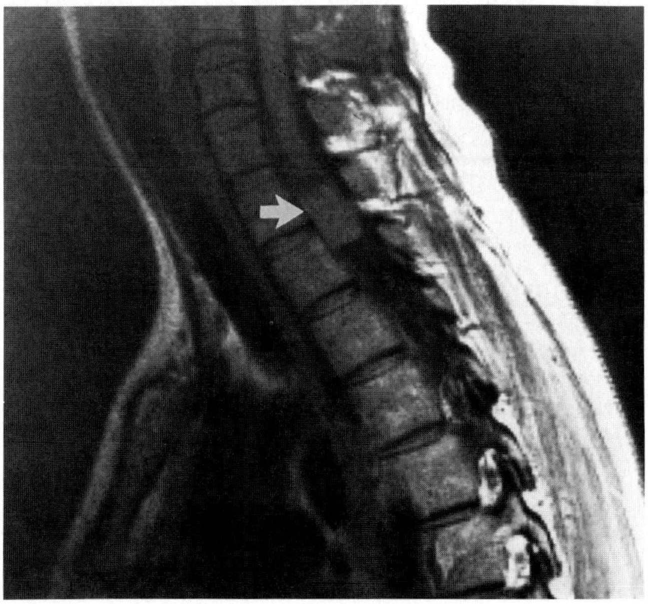

FIGURE 6–5. Meningioma on a sagittal T1-weighted spin echo image. A well-defined intradural extramedullary soft tissue mass (arrow) has isointense signal characteristics compared with the normal spinal cord.

Nerve sheath tumors are most commonly seen in the thoracic spine, usually in younger adult patients. Schwannomas are solitary lesions, but neurofibromas occur in multiples in patients with neurofibromatosis (Fig. 6–6). They are slow-growing lesions and may extend into the neuroforamina, causing bone erosion and expansion of the neuroforamina, a finding often recognized on plain films.

Nerve sheath tumors can be well-defined on MRI. On T1-weighted images, the tumors are usually recognized as isointense soft tissue masses, which may displace the spinal cord.[29,30] They generally have increased signal intensity on T2-weighted images. Lateral meningoceles can occur in patients with neurofibromatosis and can be distinguished from a neurofibroma by signal intensity characteristics (Fig. 6–7). Nerve sheath tumors almost always show contrast enhancement after Gd DTPA administration.[22] This allows improved detection and depiction of these tumors, particularly of smaller neurofibromas in patients with von Recklinhausen's disease.

Drop metastases are the third most common type of intradural-extramedullary tumors in the thoracic spine. They generally originate from intracranial neoplasms, most commonly glioblastomas, medulloblastomas, and ependymomas. On unenhanced images, they may be seen as small nodular masses within the subarachnoid space or as spinal cord expansion after direct invasion from the subarachnoid space. Their intense contrast enhancement after Gd DTPA administration accounts for the greater sensitivity of MRI compared with CT or myelography.[32]

Dural or radiculomeningeal vascular malformations may be recognized when enlarged extramedullary-intradural vascular channels produce scalloping of the spinal cord.[33,34] This may be subtle and go unrecognized unless carefully evaluated. It has been shown that Gd DTPA may enhance the intradural medullary slow-flowing veins, increasing the conspicuity of these lesions (Fig. 6–4).[22] T2-weighted images may reveal abnormal increased signal intensity within the spinal cord caused by ischemia or infarction from chronic venous hypertension.[22] Although MRI may be useful in helping to separate these lesions from an intramedullary process, angiography will continue to play a role in defining the primary vessels supplying the malformation and showing the full extent of the lesion.

Iophendylate (Pantopaque), an oil-soluble myelographic contrast agent, presents a typical appearance

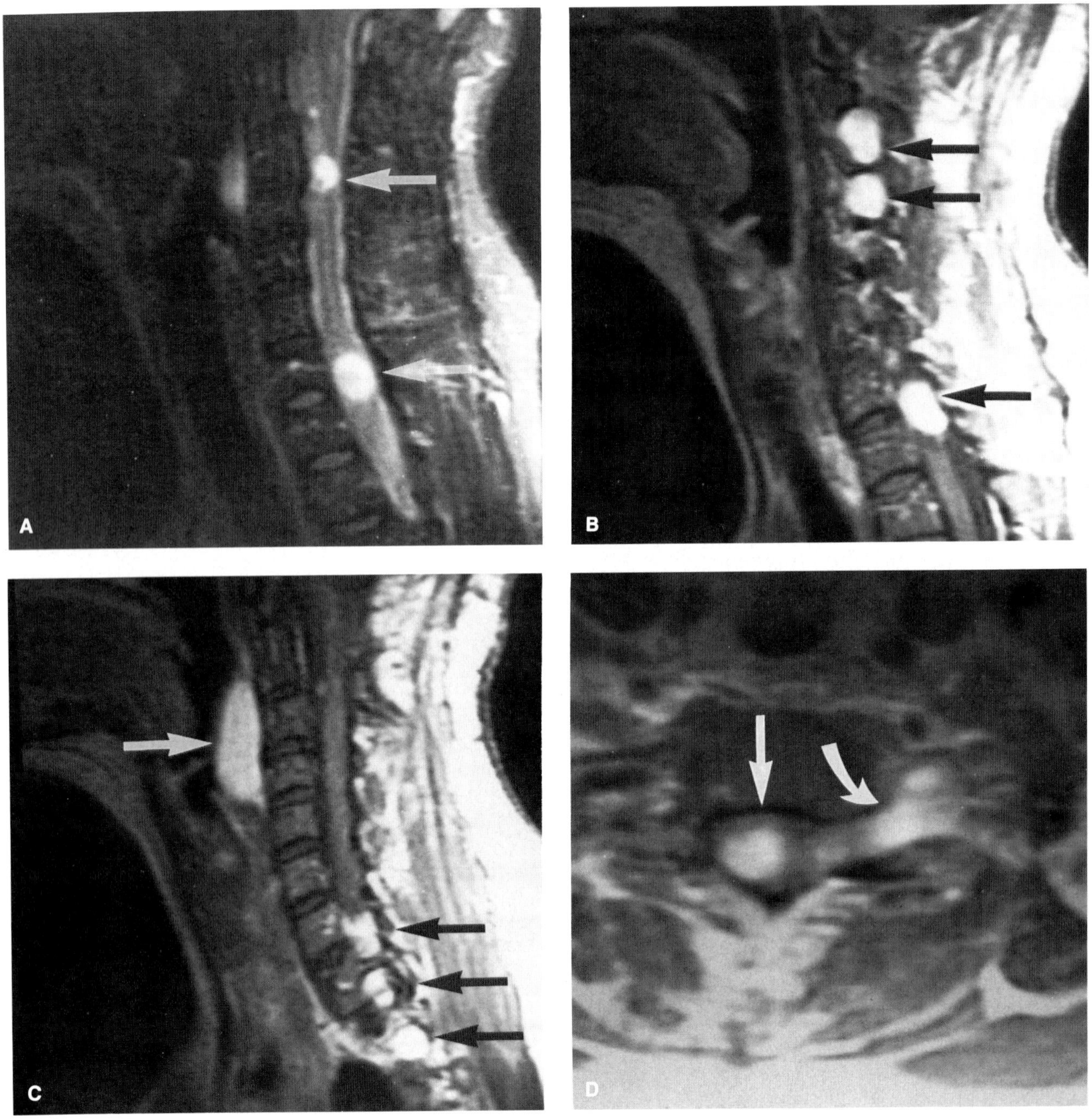

FIGURE 6–6. Neurofibromatosis on **(A)** sagittal T2-weighted, and post-Gd DTPA **(B,C)** T1-weighted parasagittal, and **(D)** axial spin echo images. Two extramedullary intradural high-signal-intensity neurofibromas (arrows) are seen in the cervical and upper thoracic spine on the midline sagittal T2-weighted image. **(B,C)** Parasagittal Gd-DTPA-enhanced T1-weighted images show multiple enhancing neurofibromas (black arrows) in the neuroforamina of the cervical and thoracic spine. Notice the enhanced prevertebral soft tissue mass, presumed to be a soft tissue neurofibroma (white arrow). **(D)** Axial Gd-DTPA enhanced T1-weighted image at the T1-2 intervertebral disc space. There is an enhancing intradural extramedullary neurofibroma (arrow) and a second extradural neurofibroma (curved arrow) in the left neuroforamen at this level. (Courtesy Dr. W. Benton Copple, Immanuel Hospital, Omaha, NE)

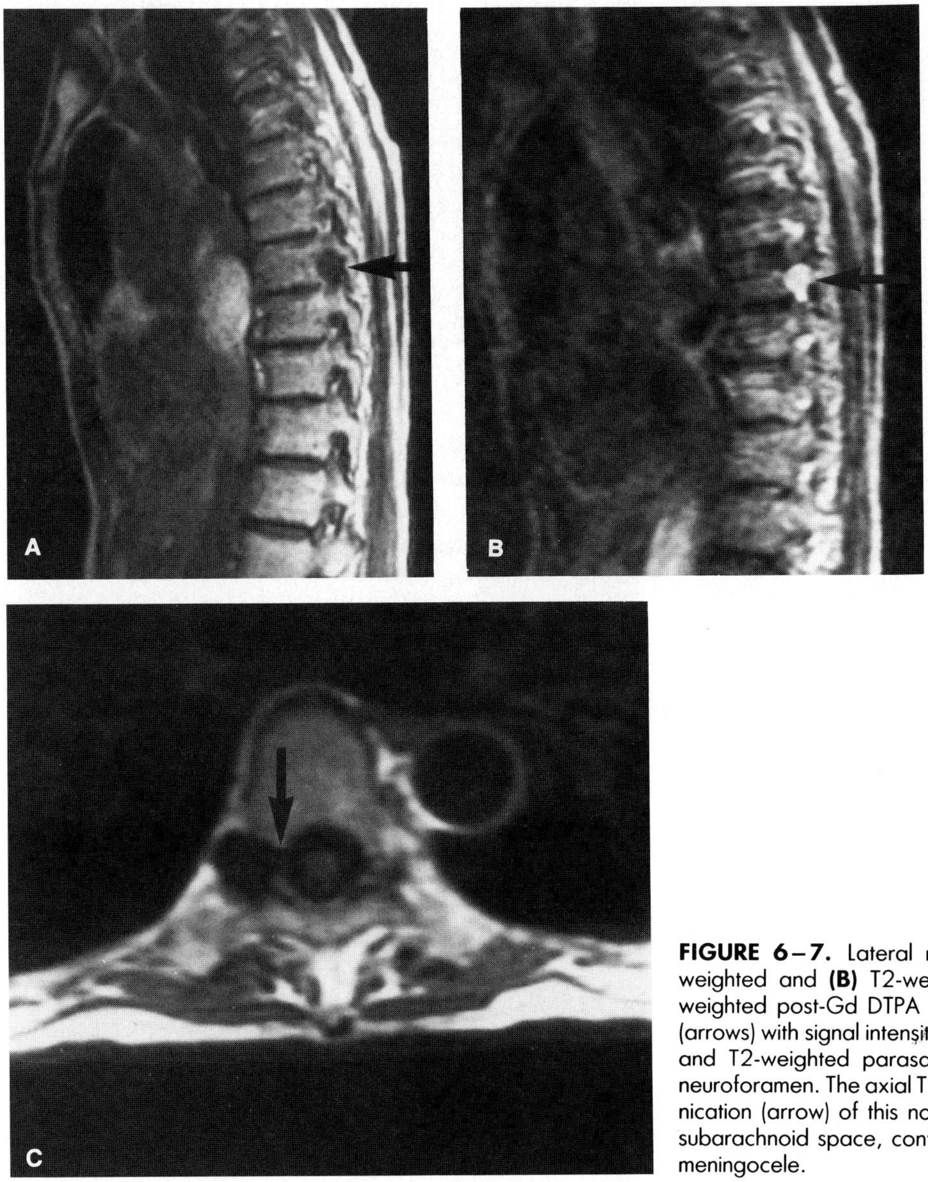

FIGURE 6–7. Lateral meningocele. **(A)** Right parasagittal T1-weighted and **(B)** T2-weighted spin echo images; **(C)** axial T1-weighted post-Gd DTPA spin echo image. There is a cystic mass (arrows) with signal intensity characteristics similar to CSF on both T1- and T2-weighted parasagittal images expanding the right T7-8 neuroforamen. The axial T1-weighted image demonstrates a communication (arrow) of this nonenhancing cystic mass with the thoracic subarachnoid space, confirming the diagnosis of a lateral thoracic meningocele.

on MR images and should not be mistaken for a pathologic process (Fig. 6–8).[35] On T1-weighted images, it displays high signal intensity due to its lipid content. On T2-weighted images, iophendylate appears as an area of low signal intensity and is well-visualized due to surrounding high-signal-intensity CSF in the subarachnoid space.

Extradural Tumor

As in other areas of the spine, the most common extradural tumor involving the thoracic spine is metastatic disease. Although single metastatic lesions can occur in the thoracic spine, multiple metastatic foci can commonly be delineated and help to confirm the diagnosis.

On T1-weighted images, metastases are recognized as low-signal-intensity lesions replacing the normal high-signal-intensity fat-containing bone marrow (Fig. 6–9). Proton density and T2-weighted images generally show the metastatic foci to be of increased signal intensity, although this varies (Fig. 6–10). Extradural soft tissue components can be well-defined with MRI. Collapse of the vertebral body and retropulsion of vertebral body fragments into the spinal canal may be demonstrated (Fig. 6–11). These fragments can compress the thoracic spinal cord and produce high-signal-intensity edema within the spinal cord on T2-weighted images.

Differentiation of metastatic compression fractures from benign osteoporotic compression fractures may be difficult with MRI in the acute stages.[36] Both lesions will show low signal intensity on T1-weighted images and generally increased signal intensity on

(text continues on page 244)

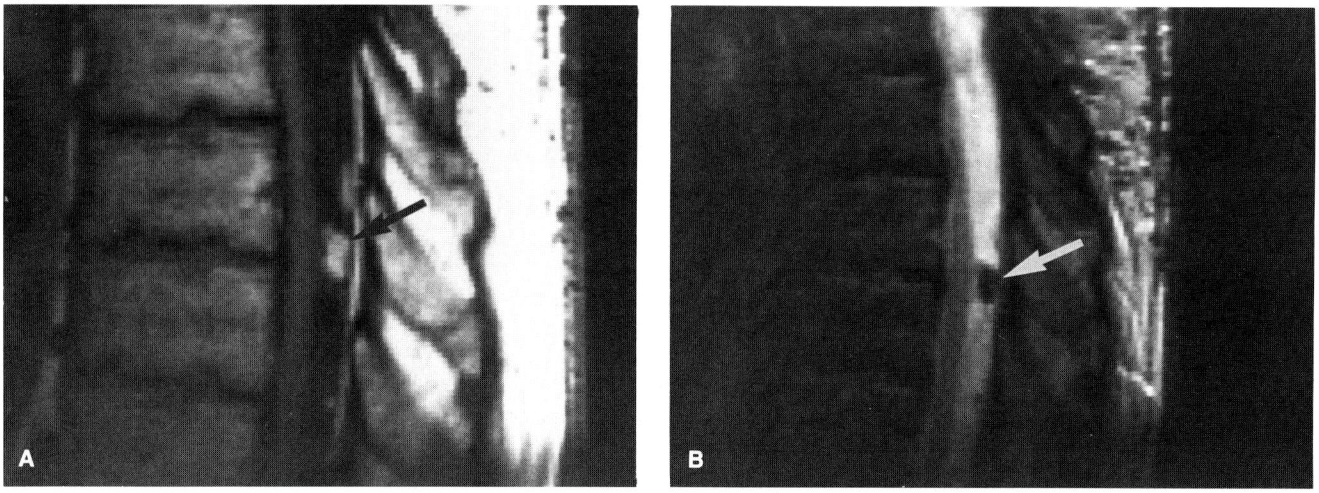

FIGURE 6–8. Iophendylate (Pantopaque). **(A)** Sagittal T1-weighted and **(B)** T2-weighted spin echo images. The oil-containing myelographic contrast agent, iophendylate (arrows), is seen as a high-intensity signal on the T1-weighted image and low-intensity signal on the T2-weighted image, which is typical of a lipid-containing substance.

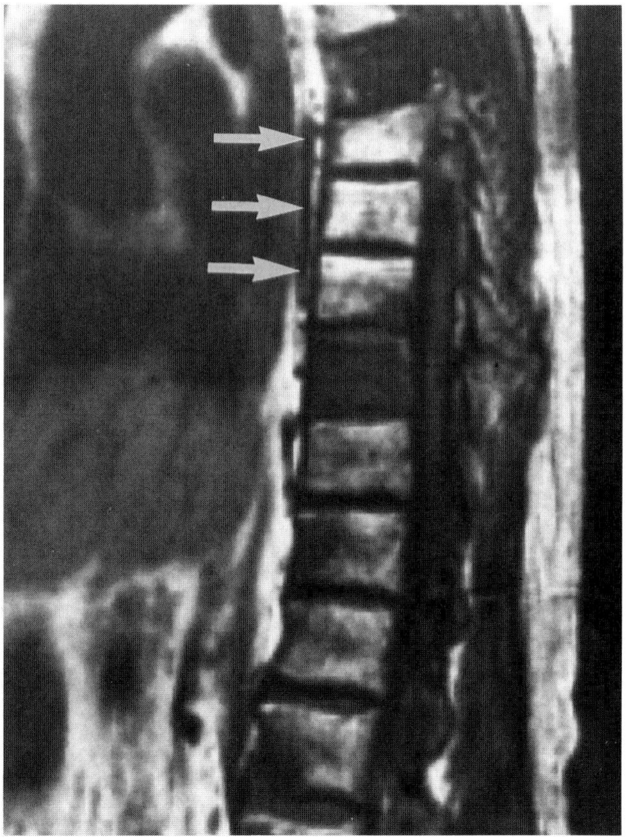

FIGURE 6–9. Thoracic spine metastases from carcinoma of the lung. Sagittal T1-weighted image reveals multiple low-signal-intensity metastatic lesions throughout the thoracic spine, replacing the normal high-signal-intensity fat-containing bone marrow. There is abnormally increased signal intensity in the bone marrow of several of the upper thoracic vertebral bodies (arrows) due to previous radiation therapy. This signal intensity pattern occurs due to fatty replacement of normal hematopoietic elements in the irradiated bone marrow.

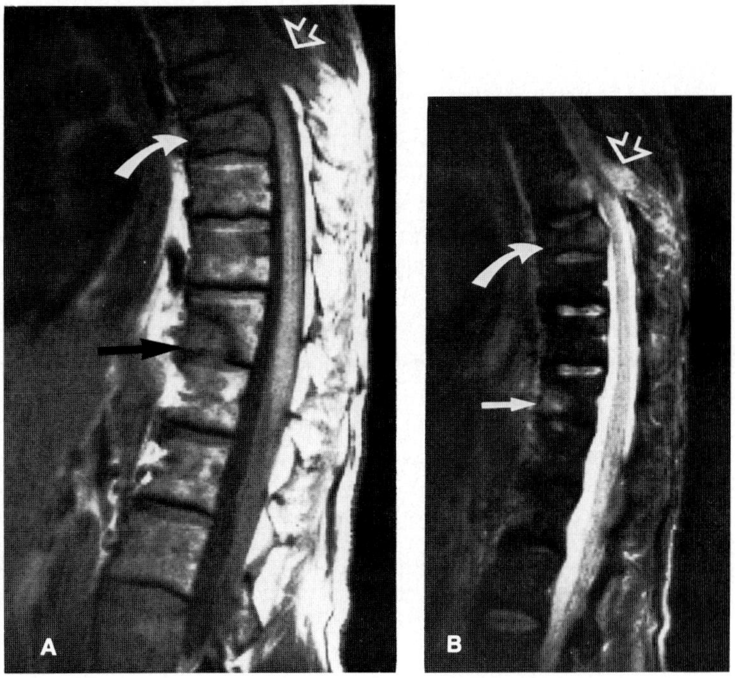

FIGURE 6–10. Metastatic colon cancer. **(A)** Sagittal T1-weighted and **(B)** T2-weighted spin echo images. Metastatic lesions are seen throughout the thoracic spine (closed arrows), with a metastatic compression fracture of T9 (curved arrow). Typical of metastatic disease, these lesions are of decreased signal intensity on T1-weighted images and increased signal intensity on T2-weighted images. There is metastatic involvement of T8 and its posterior elements (open arrow), causing compression of the spinal cord anteriorly and posteriorly.

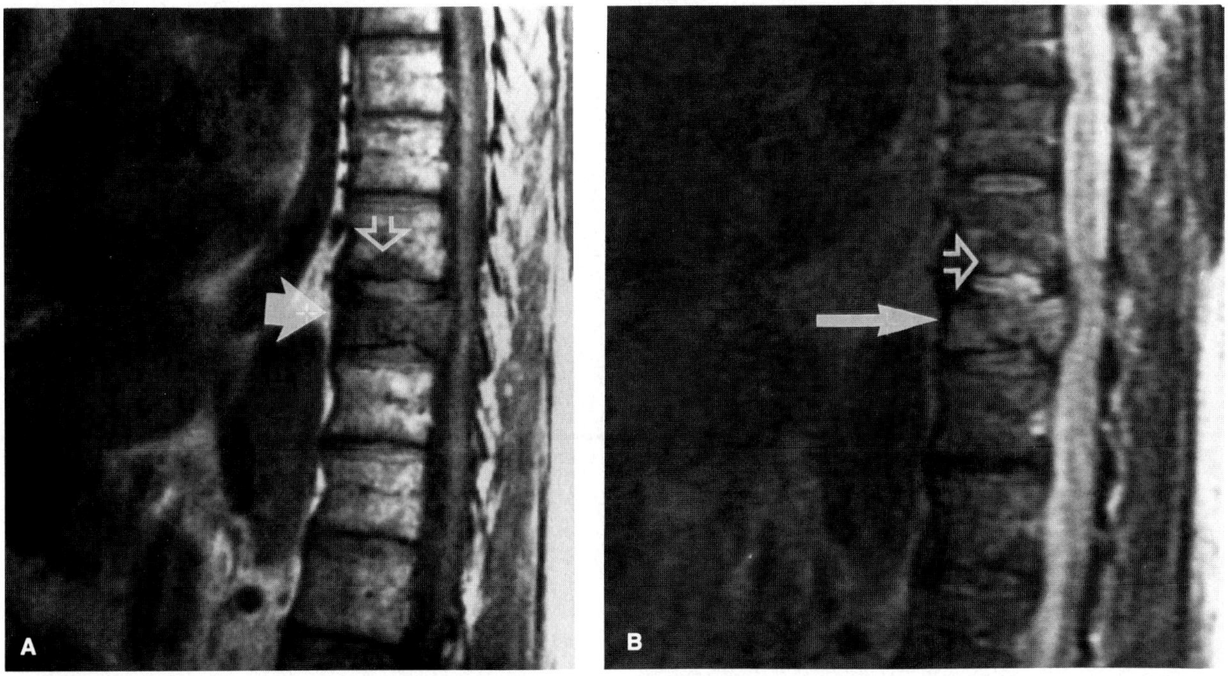

FIGURE 6–11. Thoracic spine metastases, with spinal cord compression, from carcinoma of the breast. **(A)** Sagittal T1-weighted and **(B)** T2-weighted images reveal a metastatic lesion involving the entire T8 vertebral body, with low signal intensity on T1-weighted images and increased signal intensity on T2-weighted images. A compression fracture has developed with retropulsion of the vertebral body posteriorly, causing anterior compression of the spinal cord. There is also metastatic involvement of the inferior end-plate of T7 (open arrow), with signal intensity characteristics similar to the T8 lesion. Notice the preservation of the normal signal intensity of the T7-8 intervertebral disc, indicating there is no involvement of the disc by the metastatic lesion. Metastatic disease of the spine typically respects the intervertebral disc, which is usually involved by infection.

T2-weighted images in the acute phase after fracture. If additional low-signal-intensity lesions are seen on T1-weighted images in other areas of the spine, the diagnosis of metastatic disease is suggested. On follow-up imaging, most metastatic compression fractures continue to display increased signal intensity on T2-weighted images, because they are infiltrated with a tumor having long T2 relaxation times.[37] Exceptions to this do occur, and all lesions must be carefully evaluated (Fig. 6-12). By contrast, benign osteoporotic compression fractures typically develop low signal intensity on the T2-weighted images as edema and hemorrhage resolve after the acute phase (Fig. 6-13).[37] Early studies suggest that Gd DTPA may be useful in this differentiation because metastatic tumor in bone shows contrast enhancement, but benign osteoporotic compression fractures do not (Fig. 6-14).[37] Although radionuclide bone scanning and myelography remain important screening modalities for metastatic disease, it is now felt that MRI is the best means of evaluating the patient with possible spinal cord compression caused by metastatic disease.

Most metastatic disease involving the thoracic spine originates from primary carcinoma of the lung, breast, prostate, or kidney in adult patients. In the spine, lymphoma most commonly presents with epidural disease but may also diffusely infiltrate the bone marrow.[38]

Primary tumors of the thoracic spine usually have a similar appearance to metastatic disease on MRI and may be difficult to differentiate.[39] Typically primary tumors of the spine involve only one level, helping to separate them from metastases. Like metastatic disease, primary tumors of the spine commonly display low signal intensity on T1-weighted images and, although variable, are usually of increased signal intensity on T2-weighted images. The best-known exceptions to this rule are vertebral body hemangiomas. These benign tumors consistently show increased signal intensity on T1-weighted images, probably due to fat, and also have increased signal intensity on T2-weighted images within the more cellular components of the tumor.[40] Plain films are often useful for confirming these findings by showing the character-

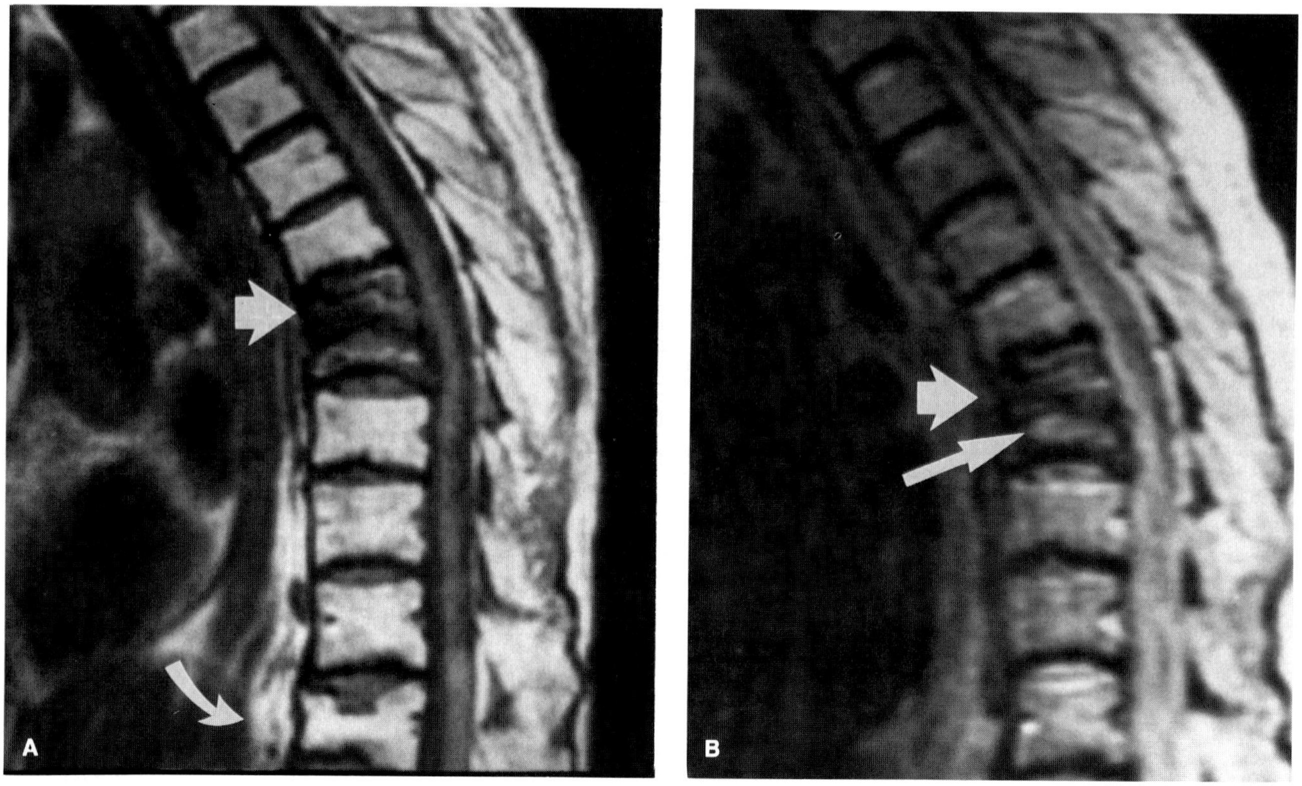

FIGURE 6–12. Thoracic spine metastases from carcinoma of the breast. **(A)** Sagittal T1-weighted and **(B)** T2-weighted spin echo images. There is abnormal low signal intensity on both images in the compression fractures of T7 and T8 (short arrows) without cord compression. Some increased signal intensity is seen in the metastatic tumor infiltrating the superior end-plate of T8 (long arrow) on the T2-weighted image. There is a chronic, anterior osteoporotic compression fracture of T12 (curved arrow), with normal signal intensity on the T1-weighted image. Typically, metastatic lesions of the spine have some increased signal intensity on T2-weighted images, but as in this case, a lack of signal change may cause difficulty in differentiating tumors from acute osteoporotic compression fractures.

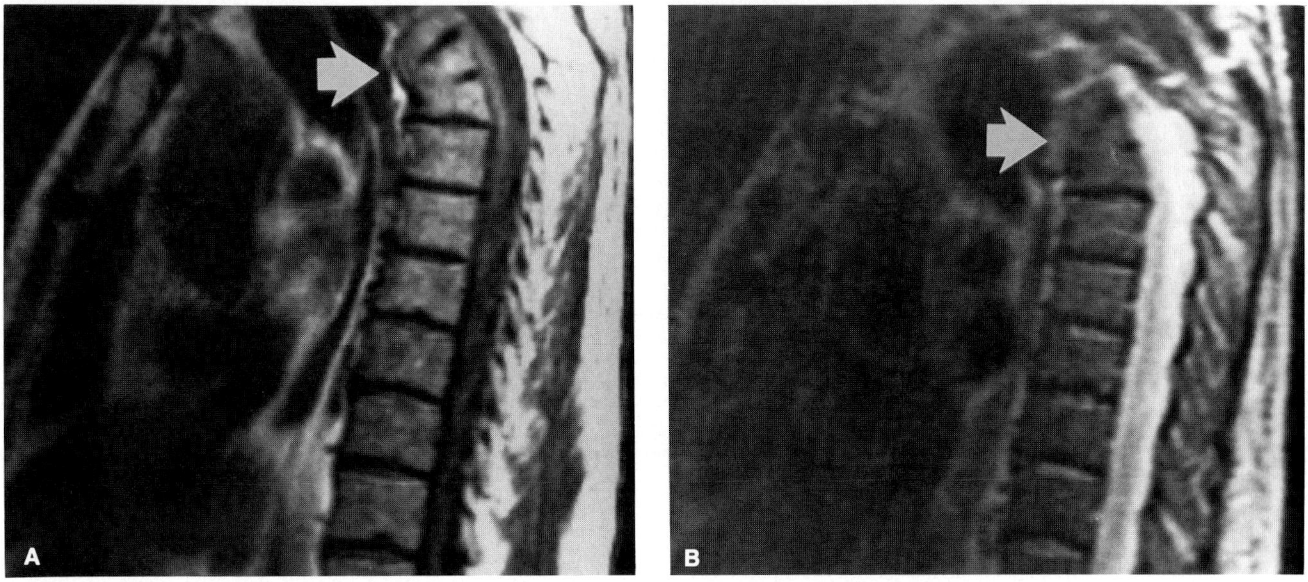

FIGURE 6–13. Osteoporotic compression fractures. **(A)** Sagittal T1-weighted and **(B)** T2-weighted images. There are anterior compression fractures of T3 through T5 (arrow), with signal intensity characteristics similar to the other normal thoracic vertebral bodies on both T1- and T2-weighted images. These normal-signal-intensity characteristics and lack of abnormal-signal-intensity lesions in other areas of the thoracic spine indicate that the compression fractures are caused by osteoporosis and not metastatic disease.

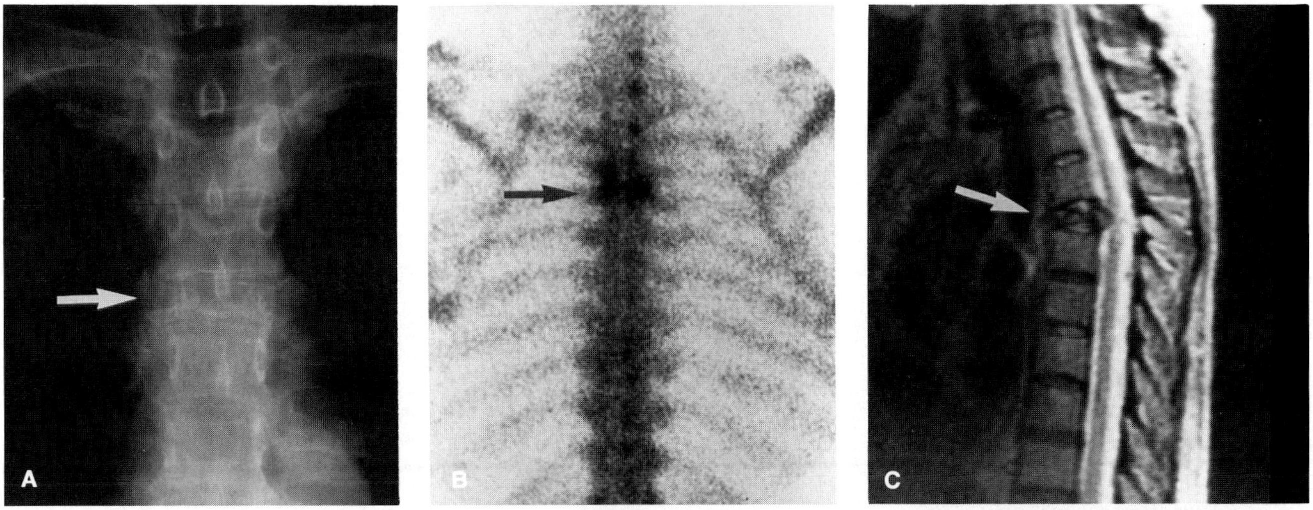

FIGURE 6–14. Metastatic breast carcinoma with spinal cord compression. **(A)** AP radiograph of thoracic spine, **(B)** radionuclide bone scan, **(C)** sagittal T2-weighted spin echo image, **(D,E)** sagittal T1-weighted spin echo images before and after Gd DTPA administration. Radiograph of the thoracic spine reveals a compression fracture (arrow) of T4, which displays an abnormal, increased accumulation of ^{99m}Tc methylene diphosphonate (arrow) on the radionuclide bone scan. Unenhanced sagittal T1- and T2-weighted images **(C,D)** show decreased and increased signal intensity, respectively, within the T4 compression fracture (arrows). There is retropulsion of a vertebral fracture fragment posteriorly, compressing the thoracic spinal cord. After Gd DTPA administration **(E)**, the compression fracture fragments are enhanced, suggesting the fracture is due to metastatic disease (subsequently proven by biopsy), rather than representing a benign osteoporotic compression fracture.

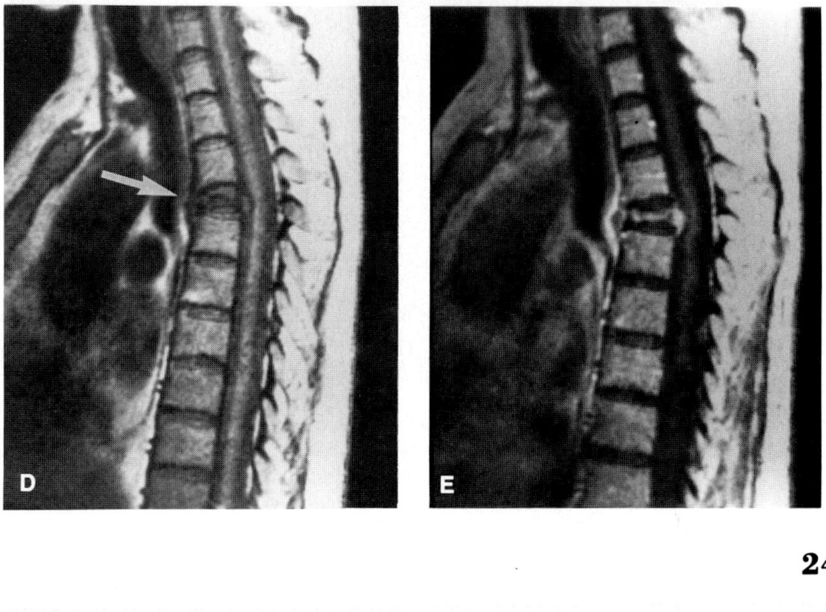

istic coarse striations of the vertebral body hemangioma.

Aneurysmal bone cysts have a characteristic appearance on MRI.[41] Cystic cavities in these tumors showing various stages of hemorrhage may be seen, with occasional fluid–fluid levels noted.

Focal fat deposition occurs commonly in the axial bone marrow. It is seen as focal high signal intensity on T1-weighted images, with decreased signal intensity on T2-weighted images paralleling the signal intensity of fat (Fig. 6–15).[42] The importance of focal fat deposition is that it must be recognized for its benign nature and not confused with metastatic disease or a small vertebral body hemangioma.

Occasionally extradural components of a meningioma or nerve sheath tumors may be seen, but most commonly these tumors occupy an intradural location (Fig. 6–6D).

Gd DTPA has been used in evaluating extradural disease. Tumor involving the vertebral bodies can be easily recognized on unenhanced T1-weighted images as low-signal-intensity lesions contrasted against the high-signal-intensity fat-containing bone marrow. Gd DTPA enhances the tumor, which can obscure metastatic lesion confined to bone.[43] However, Gd DTPA is extremely useful for defining epidural tumor outside the confines of the vertebral body because the conspicuity of the enhancing epidural tumor is increased against the low-signal-intensity CSF and surrounding paraspinous musculature.[43]

Inflammation

Infections involving the thoracic spine may present different appearances on MRI, depending upon the age of the patient and the type of infecting organism. Most pathogens involve the spine after hematogenous spread. The disc is a relatively vascular structure in the pediatric patient, and bacteria tend to initially involve the disc itself and spread to the adjacent vertebral body end-plates. With aging, the disc loses some of this vascularity and pathogens that are spread hematogenously tend to lodge in small vessels of the vertebral body end-plates and then invade the disc. Ultimately, in pyogenic infections, the appearance is similar in both age groups, with narrowing of the disc space and involvement of both vertebral body end-plate margins next to the involved disc.

Early studies have shown MRI to be as accurate and sensitive as radionuclide scans in the diagnosis of vertebral osteomyelitis.[44] Early infections involving the disc may show a decreased signal intensity within the disc on T1-weighted images and poor definition of the margin between the disc and the adjacent vertebral body end-plates. Very early in the course of infection there may be no or minimal increased signal intensity

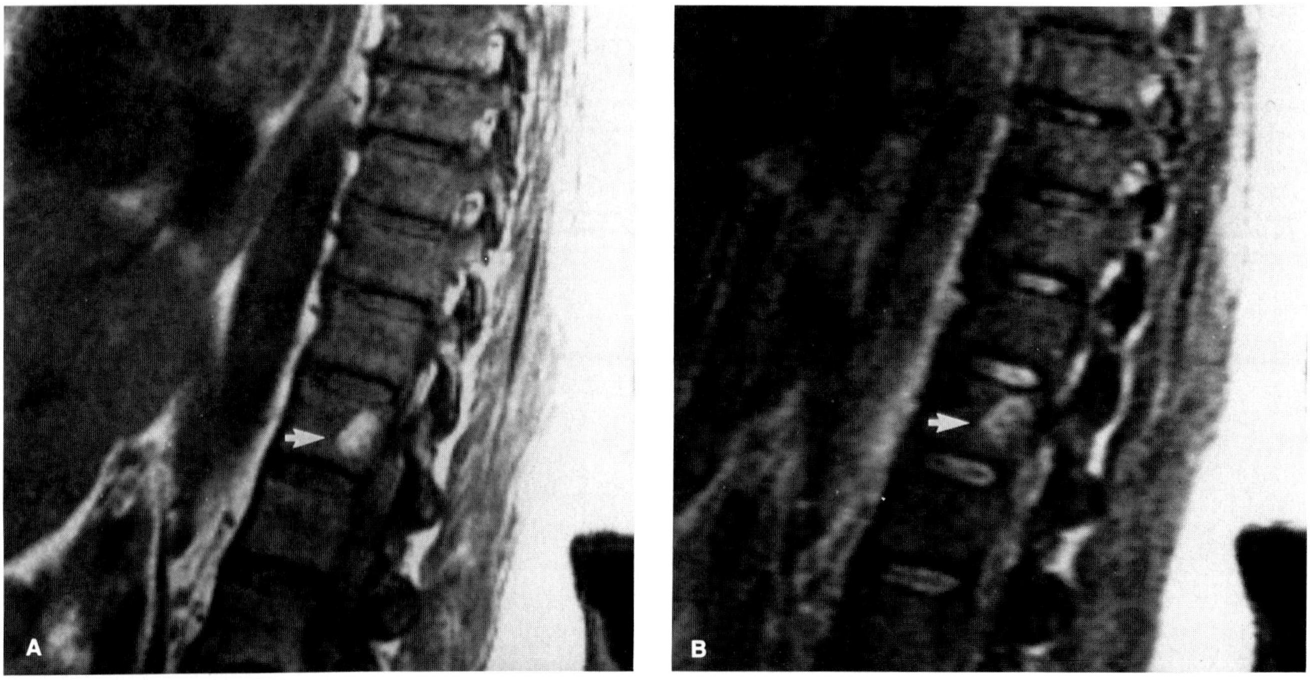

FIGURE 6–15. Focal fat deposition. **(A)** Sagittal T1-weighted and **(B)** T2-weighted spin echo images. **(A)** A high-signal-intensity area (arrow) is observed in the posterior aspect of T12 on the T1-weighted image. **(B)** The signal intensity of this area decreases (arrow) on the T2-weighted image, characteristic of focal fat deposition in the axial bone marrow.

in the disc on T2-weighted images. Generally, some increased signal intensity is recognized, and there may also be an abnormal configuration of the disc (Fig. 6–16). It is therefore critical to obtain T2-weighted images in cases of suspected osteomyelitis.

The increased signal intensity eventually involves the infected portions of the vertebral body in the end-plates. This abnormal signal on T2-weighted images can be recognized even after initiation of appropriate antibiotic therapy. The amount of time required for the high signal intensity to return to a more normal appearance during antibiotic therapy has not been studied. Usually radionuclide scans with ^{67}Ga show an earlier response to appropriate antibiotic therapy than MRI, indicating successful treatment.[45] Eventually, the MRI signal intensity decreases, assuming a more normal appearance on T2-weighted images. The chronic sequela of a narrowed disc space with decreased signal intensity on T2-weighted images and irregularity of the vertebral body end-plate margins is eventually seen. Therefore, monitoring of resolving discitis or vertebral body osteomyelitis is perhaps best accomplished by following the decrease in signal intensity on T2-weighted images.[45]

The major complication feared with thoracic vertebral osteomyelitis is the development of an epidural abscess. This may occur secondary to direct extension of the osteomyelitis into the epidural tissues and often must be surgically drained. If they become large enough, the abscess can cause spinal cord compression and produce paraplegia. Although the MRI appearance of epidural abscesses has not been extensively described, they probably are best evaluated by MRI (Fig. 6–17). When large enough to result in spinal cord compression, they are easily recognized. If the epidural abscess is small, it may be unrecognized, due to the difficulty in differentiation from surrounding CSF, which can demonstrate similar signal intensity characteristics on both T1-weighted and T2-weighted images.[45]

Tumor may also occasionally present a problem in the differential diagnosis of spine infections. Usually, the disc is involved in infection, but tumor remains confined to the vertebral body, rarely involving the disc itself. Degeneration of a thoracic disc produces decreased signal intensity within the disc on T2-weighted images without vertebral body end-plate involvement. Infection usually involves both the disc and vertebral body end-plates, with increased signal intensity on T2-weighted images.

Tuberculous spondylitis may also be confused with tumor, because tuberculous spondylitis tends to involve several vertebral bodies and often produces extradural masses. This produces an appearance very similar to metastatic disease. The clinical history and cultures are often the only bases for a correct diagnosis.

The use of paramagnetic contrast agents to study

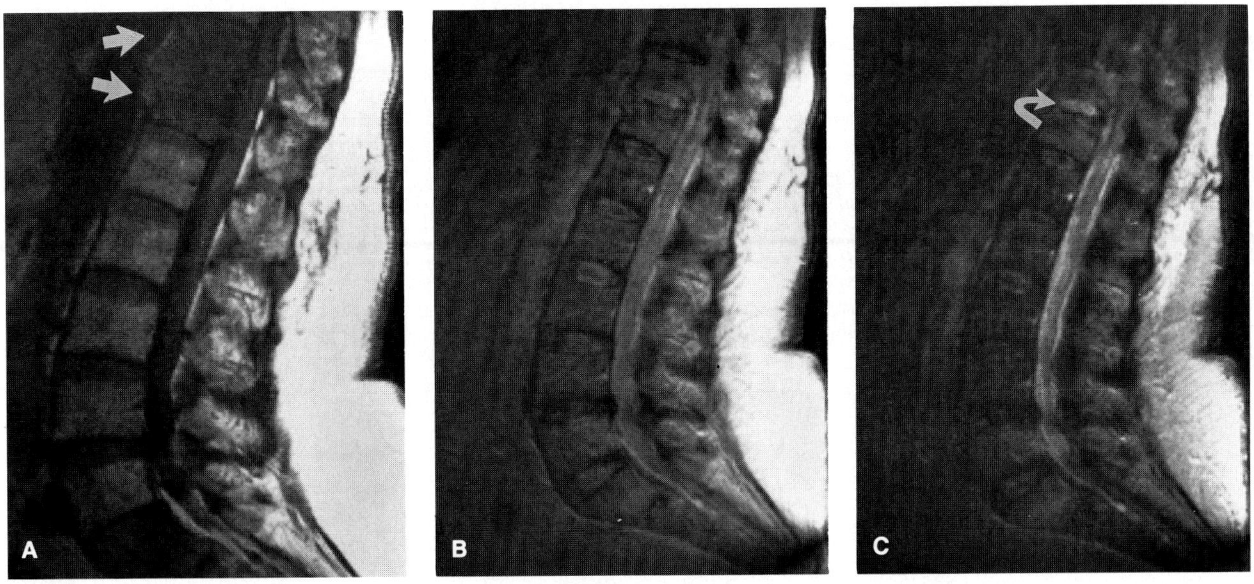

FIGURE 6–16. Vertebral osteomyelitis and discitis. **(A)** Sagittal T1-weighted, **(B)** proton density, and **(C)** T2-weighted spin echo images. The T1-weighted image shows a diffuse low-intensity signal involving the T11 and T12 vertebral bodies (closed arrows) and the interposed intervertebral disc. The involved vertebral bodies have diffuse increased signal intensity on both proton density and T2-weighted images, with the interposed intervertebral disc displaying dramatically abnormal increased signal intensity (curved arrow) compared with the normal intervertebral discs. Although not entirely specific, the morphologic pattern and signal intensity characteristics, as in this case of *Staphylococcus aureus* osteomyelitis, strongly suggest acute infection.

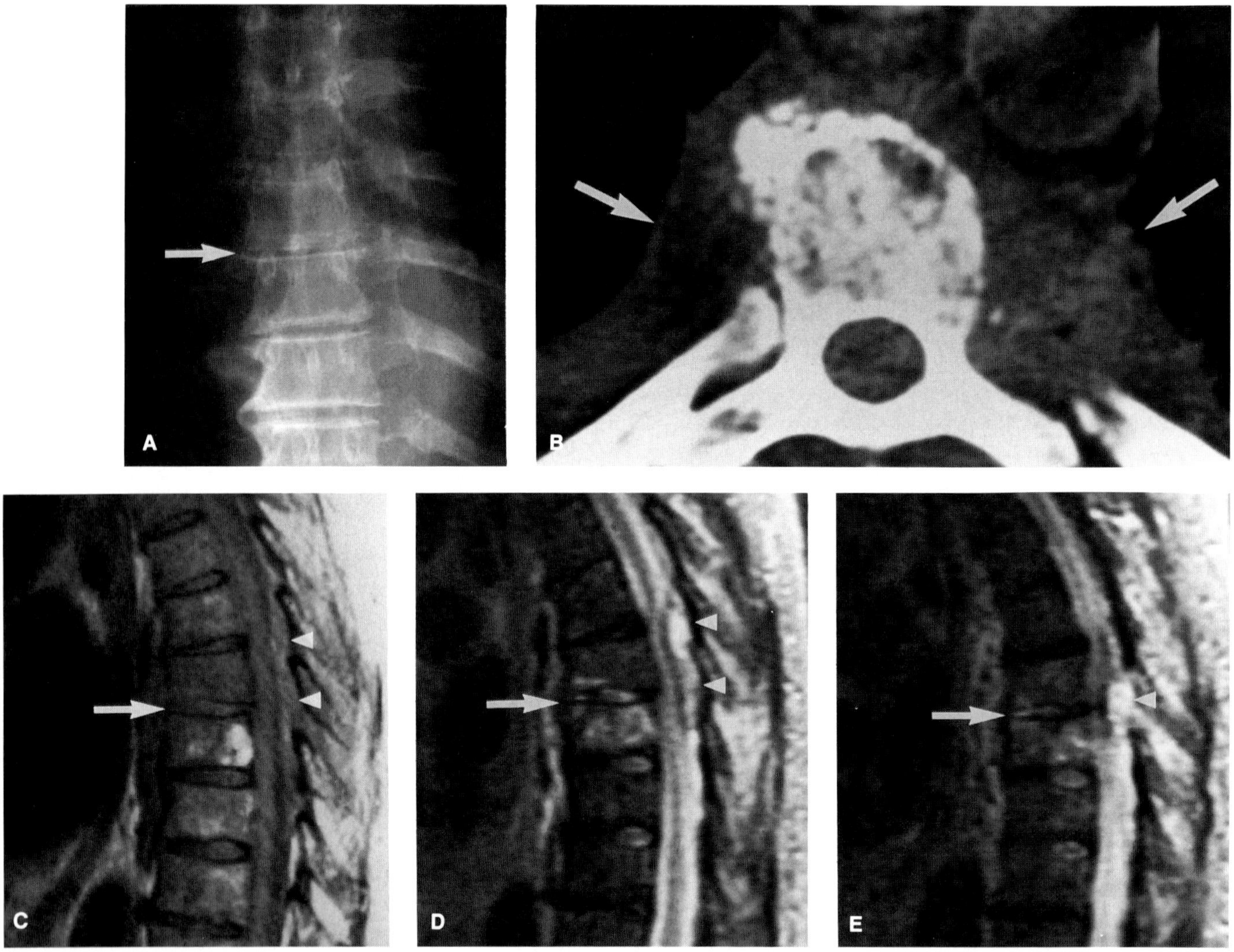

FIGURE 6–17. Discitis and vertebral osteomyelitis with epidural abscess. **(A)** AP radiograph of the thoracic spine, **(B)** axial CT, **(C)** sagittal T1-weighted, **(D)** midline sagittal, and **(E)** parasagittal T2-weighted spin echo images. Radiograph of the thoracic spine reveals only minimal narrowing of the T7-8 intervertebral disc space (arrow). Bone destruction of the T8 vertebral body and bilateral paravertebral soft tissue inflammatory masses (arrows), caused by *Staphylococcus aureus* infection, are seen on the CT image. The involved T7 and T8 vertebral bodies and their interposed intervertebral disc (arrow) display abnormally decreased and increased signal intensities on T1- and T2-weighted images, respectively. The high signal intensity on the T1-weighted image in the posterior aspect of T8 represents focal fat deposition in the bone marrow. A large epidural abscess (arrowheads) is seen posteriorly on the T1- and T2-weighted images with an abnormal high signal intensity.

infections of the spine has not been evaluated extensively. In one instance, Gd DTPA was useful for more clearly demonstrating communication of a paravertebral abscess with the spinal column.[46] Gd DTPA may be useful in certain instances of vertebral osteomyelitis, particularly in demonstrating epidural components of infection.

Syringohydromyelia

Intramedullary cystic cavities involving the spinal cord have been classically separated into two entities. Hydromyelia is cystic dilation of the central canal, which is lined with ependyma and filled with CSF. Syringomyelia represents dilated cystic cavities in the spinal cord, which are lined with glial cells and filled with CSF. Because these represent two distinct pathologic entities, which may appear similar on MRI, intramedullary cystic cavities of the spinal cord are perhaps best called syringohydromyelia. There are congenital and acquired syrinx cavities in the spinal cord.[46] The primary role of MRI is to define the extent of involvement of the spinal cord by the syrinx cavity and to exclude the possibility of an underlying tumor. Congenital anomalies, such as Chiari malformations involving the brain, or post-traumatic changes may be easily defined by MR imaging.

MRI has supplanted other imaging modalities for evaluating a patient presenting with myelopathy. When a syrinx cavity is discovered, it is usually best demonstrated on T1-weighted images in the sagittal plane.[48] Care must be taken not to confuse truncation artifacts with a small syrinx cavity.[49] Axial T1-weighted images can confirm suspicous findings on sagittal images. The size and extent of the syrinx cavity must be demonstrated, and the entire spinal cord may need to be imaged, because an underlying intramedullary tumor must be excluded as the cause of the syrinx cavity.

An uncomplicated syrinx cavity shows smooth margins containing low-signal-intensity fluid on both sagittal and axial T1-weighted images.[48] T2-weighted images show the fluid within the cystic cavity to behave like CSF, with high signal. Generally, no intramedullary high signal intensity is seen adjacent to the syrinx cavity, although it has been recently recognized that reactive gliosis may occur in the adjacent spinal cord. In some cases, septations in the syrinx cavity can be seen, giving the appearance of multiple separate cavities. These may be more prominent after shunting of the syrinx cavity at one level. In the vast majority of cases, all of these cavities are interconnected. After surgical treatment of syringohydromyelia, MRI provides the best means for evaluating the extent of collapse of the syrinx cavity.

Great difficulty has been encountered in differentiating a complicated simple syrinx from neoplastic cavities.[18,50] Paramagnetic contrast agents may prove useful in clarifying this problem. Although not extensively studied, enhancement in a syrinx cavity probably indicates neoplasia.[21] Areas of enhancement should undergo more extensive follow-up or biopsy.

Trauma

In the acutely injured patient, thoracic spine trauma is best evaluated by plain films and CT. Most acutely injured patients are unable to cooperate for the relatively long imaging times required for a diagnostic MRI examination. The patient requiring stabilization devices containing ferromagnetic material or ventilatory support with a respirator cannot undergo MRI. More effort is being devoted to develop nonferromagnetic MRI-compatible traction and stabilization devices and respirators.[51,52]

MRI is best suited for evaluating patients who are in stable condition and in the subacute or late stages after trauma for posttraumatic complications.[53,54] Compression fractures of the vertebral bodies and displacement of fracture fragments can be seen with MRI.[55,56] Ligamentous injuries can occasionally be recognized as high signal intensities on T2-weighted images, disrupting the normal intermediate-signal-intensity spinal ligaments. The signal intensity of fracture fragments depends on their age and the presence of hemorrhage. Usually, acute vertebral body fractures are seen as having isointense or decreased signal intensity on T1-weighted images and increased signal intensity on T2-weighted images, although this can vary.[53] Old fractures have decreased signal intensity on both T1-weighted and T2-weighted images, although fatty replacement within the fracture fragments can occasionally be seen as high signal intensity on T1-weighted images, with decreasing intensity on T2-weighted images characteristic of fat. Complications, including spinal canal compromise and possible compression of the thoracic spinal cord, can be quickly and efficiently evaluated by MRI.[57] Spinal cord edema and hematomyelia can be recognized.[58] More appropriate decisions with regards to patient management can be made if MRI is included in evaluating thoracic spine trauma.

The evaluation of posttraumatic progressive myelopathy or increasingly severe back pain in the posttraumatic patient is best done with MRI.[59] Diagnosis of a posttraumatic syrinx is important since surgical correction can prevent progressive neurologic deterioration. Myelomalacia can be confused with a posttraumatic syrinx on delayed myelographic CT images. These two entities can be differentiated by MRI.

Degenerative Disc Disease

Thoracic intervertebral discs are subject to degenerative changes in a fashion similar to intervertebral discs elsewhere in the spine. As in the cervical and lumbar regions, the earliest recognizable finding on MRI of disc degeneration is the loss of the normal high signal intensity from the nucleus pulposus on T2-weighted images. Loss of disc-space height, secondary reactive changes in the vertebral body marrow, and osteophyte formation can also be identified. Asymptomatic herniation of thoracic discs, once thought to be relatively uncommon, is becoming more routinely recognized on MRI.[60] These are most commonly seen in the lower thoracic spine.

MRI provides a rapid, noninvasive means of surveying the thoracic spine in a patient with suspected disc herniation. Disc herniations can be identified before they have progressed to impinge the thoracic spinal cord. As in other areas of the spine, a herniated thoracic disc can usually be identified by its intermediate signal intensity on T1-weighted images (Fig. 6-18). Axial images are the best means for defining the extent of cord compression. T2-weighted images show the herniated disc as intermediate or low signal intensity surrounded by high-signal-intensity CSF. Turbulent CSF flow around the herniated disc in the subarachnoid space may accentuate the size of the herniated disc on T2-weighted images (Fig. 6-1B).

As in the cervical and lumbar spine, osteophytes secondary to degenerative disease may be confused with a disc herniation. Careful attention to the morphologic appearance of the abnormality can distinguish these two entities.

Multiple Sclerosis

MRI using T2-weighted pulse sequences sensitively demonstrates multiple sclerosis (MS) plaques in the brain. MS plaques in the cervical spinal cord have also been demonstrated using a head coil.[61] Most MS plaques recognized in the spinal cord have an elongated, linear appearance. They usually cannot be seen on T1-weighted images. Their characteristic high signal intensity, due to prolongation of T2 and increased proton density, leads to ready recognition on T2-weighted images in the thoracic spine. It is critical that some type of motion-compensation sequence be employed on T2-weighted images. Gradient moment nulling, pulse, or ECG gating are recommended to decrease motion artifacts and allow detection of small MS plaques in the spinal cord. Active MS plaques in the brain display contrast enhancement after administration of Gd DTPA.[62] Although not extensively evaluated, Gd DTPA will probably be useful for increasing the conspicuity of active MS plaques in the spinal cord.

Transverse Myelitis

Transverse myelitis has many causes. This disease may be caused by excessive doses of radiation to the spinal cord and present months after cessation of radiation therapy. The spinal cord usually shows fusiform enlargement on T1-weighted images, with some decreased signal intensity within the involved segment of the spinal cord. Often the best indication of previous radiation therapy to the spine is the characteristic high signal intensity seen within the marrow of the irradiated vertebral bodies (Fig. 6-9). Sharply demarcated boundaries correspond to the radiation therapy treatment portals employed. These changes

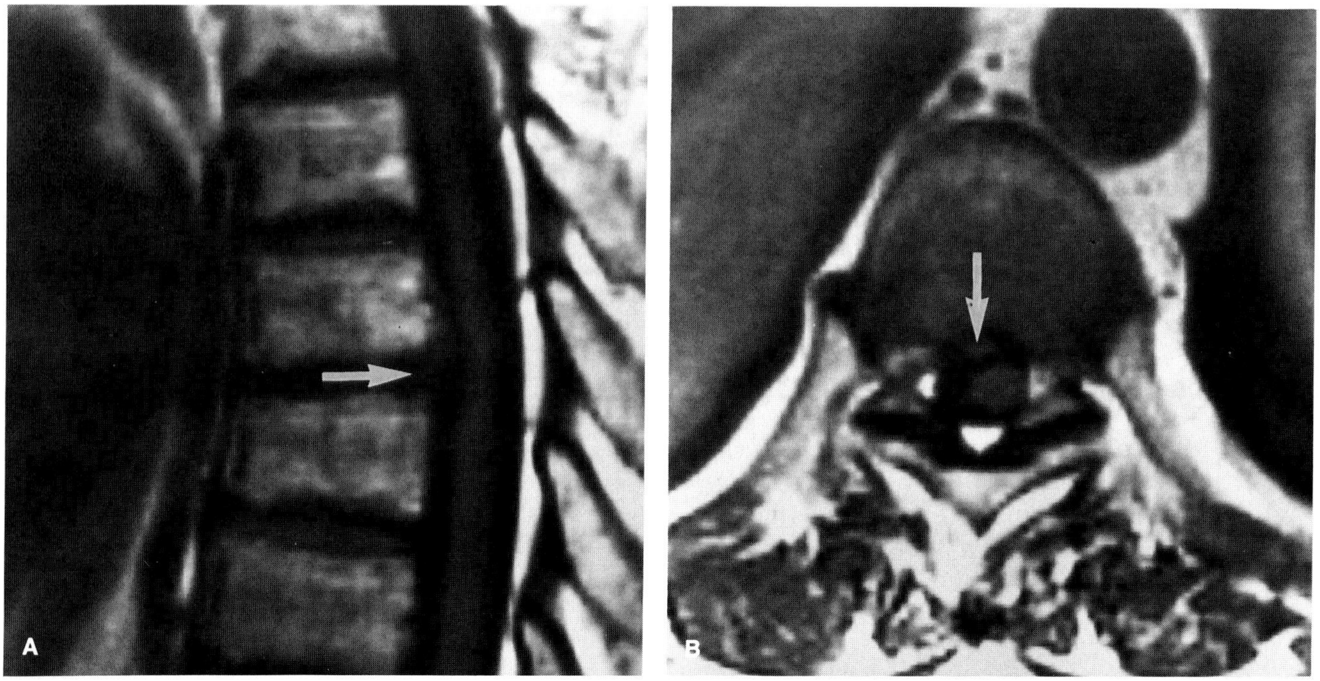

FIGURE 6-18. Thoracic disc herniation. **(A)** Sagittal and **(B)** axial T1-weighted spin echo images. The intermediate-signal-intensity herniated thoracic disc (arrows) is identified. Effacement of the anterolateral aspect of the spinal cord is best appreciated on the axial image. Axial images often provide the most accurate depiction of the amount of mass effect upon the thoracic spinal cord from a herniated disc.

are due to replacement of normal hematopoietic elements by fat.[63] On T2-weighted images, the portion of the spinal cord affected by transverse myelitis is seen as high signal intensity and is fusiform. This appearance is similar to that of an infiltrating, low-grade, noncystic neoplasm like an astrocytoma. The portion of the spinal cord affected by transverse myelitis may enhance after Gd DTPA administration.[21]

Congenital Anomalies

The most commonly encountered congenital anomaly seen in thoracic spine MRI is a tethered spinal cord in which the conus medullaris is in an abnormally low position. A tethered cord may be associated with other congenital anomalies, including a meningocele or myelomeningocele. A lipomyelomeningocele occurs when a lipoma develops distally, adjacent to the neural placode, and is recognized by its high signal intensity on T1-weighted images. Syringohydromyelia may be associated with a tethered cord and is easily recognized on MRI.

Embryonal tumors can present in the thoracic spine and are best evaluated with MRI. Dermoids, teratomas, epidermoids, and lipomas can be recognized on MRI and are often associated with spinal dysraphism (Fig. 6–19). These tumors have a variety of appearances on T1-weighted and T2-weighted images depending upon the type of tissue present. Lipomas display high signal intensity on T1-weighted images, and decreased signal intensity on T2-weighted images. They most commonly occur in an intradural-extramedullary location, although intramedullary lipomas can be seen.

Diastematomyelia occurs most often in the lower thoracic spine and can be recognized when a sagittal cleft, which may be bony or fibrous, develops, splitting the spinal cord (Fig. 6–20). The two hemicords may be asymmetric and are occasionally associated with hydromyelia.[64] When diastematomyelia occurs in the thoracic spine, commonly two hemicords exist for one or two vertebral body segments and reunite below the cleft. They may occasionally continue as two separate cords into the lumbar region. Diastematomyelia is often associated with other forms of spinal dysraphism, including myelomeningocele or lipomyelomeningocele, lipomas, and other bone or soft tissue abnormalities. Diastematomyelia is best evaluated through the use of MRI after initial plain films.[65]

Scoliosis can be evaluated with MRI to exclude the possibility of an underlying tumor, although the vast majority of cases are idiopathic in nature. Coronal T1-weighted images are often helpful in these cases in addition to routine sagittal and axial images.

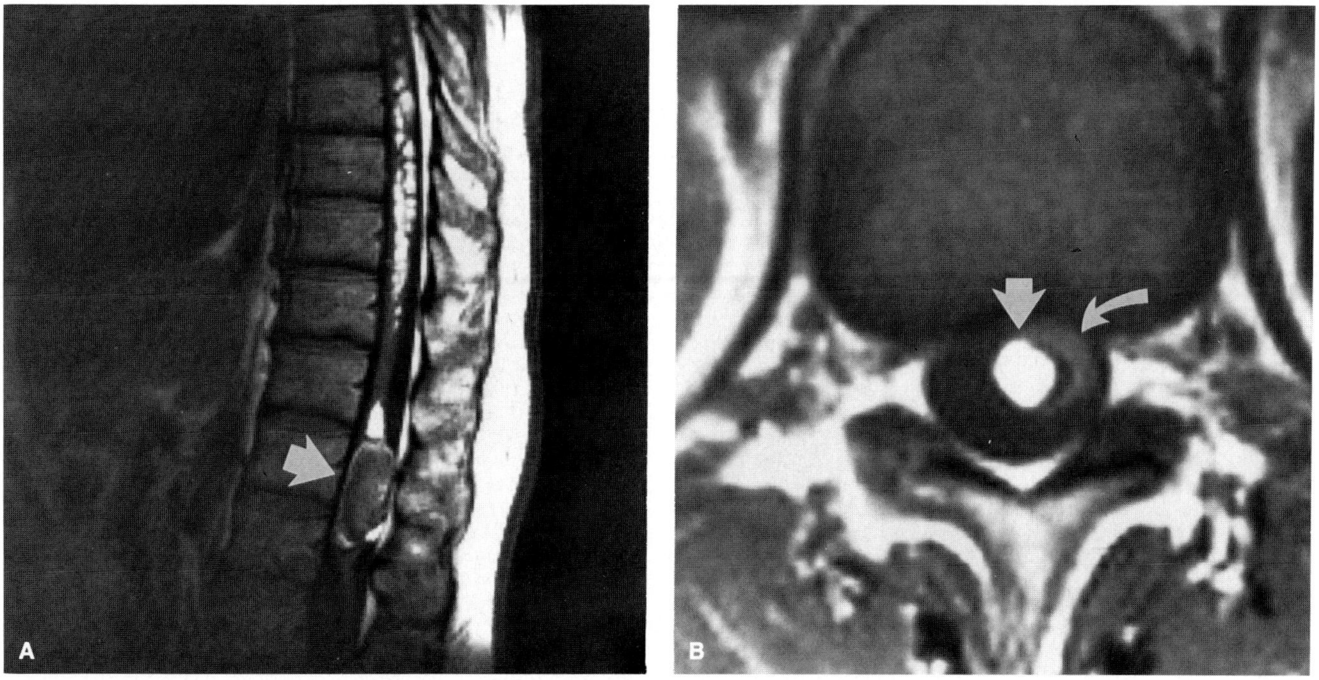

FIGURE 6–19. Intramedullary dermoid tumor with lipomatous infiltration of the thoracic spinal cord. **(A)** Sagittal and **(B)** axial T1-weighted spin echo images (no contrast has been administered). A large intramedullary dermoid tumor (arrow) is seen within the conus medullaris. Diffuse lipomatous infiltration of the thoracic spinal cord cephalad to the dermoid tumor is seen as high signal intensity. The axial image **(B)** confirms an intramedullary location of this lipoma (arrow) within the intermediate-signal-intensity spinal cord (curved arrow).

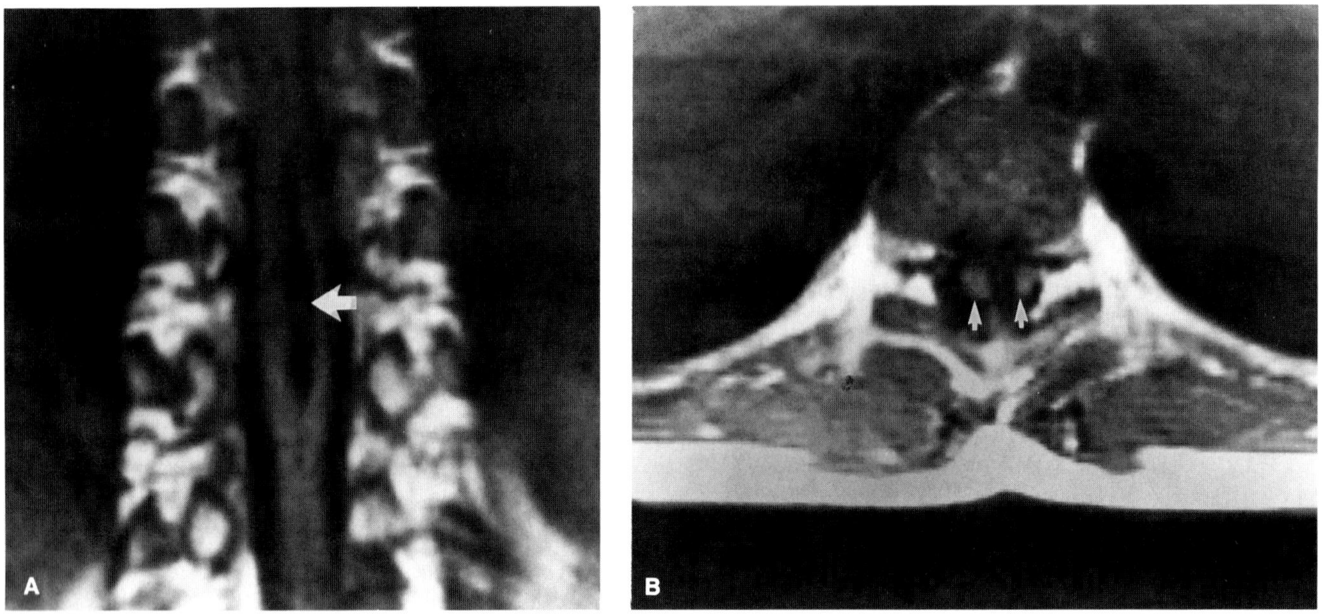

FIGURE 6–20. Diastematomyelia. **(A)** Coronal and **(B)** axial T1-weighted spin echo images. A bony septa, identified on plain films, is also identified on the coronal image (arrow), splitting the spinal cord over two thoracic segments. The two hemicords (arrows) are seen on the axial image. (Traill MT, Runge VM, Wolpert SM: Dysraphism: MRI strategies. MRI Decisions 1989; 2:2. Reprinted with permission from Physicians World Communications Group)

MRI is the best imaging modality for evaluating congenital anomalies in pediatric patients.[66] Although plain films should always be obtained to help define bony spinal anatomy, MRI allows complete evaluation of both the complex bone and soft tissue anatomy in these patients. The multiplanar imaging capabilities and lack of ionizing radiation are important advantages for the pediatric patient.

REFERENCES

1. Haughton VM. MR imaging of the spine. Radiology 1988;166:297.
2. Edelman RR, Shoukimas GM, Stark DD, et al. High resolution surface coil imaging of lumbar disc disease. AJR 1985;144:1123.
3. Berger PE, Atkinson D, Wilson WJ, Wiltse JL. High resolution surface coil magnetic resonance imaging of the spine; normal and pathologic anatomy. Radiographics 1986;6:573.
4. Mills TC, Ortendahl DA, Hylton NM. Partial flip angle MR imaging. Radiology 1987;162:531.
5. Valk J. Gd-DTPA in MR of spinal lesions. AJR 1988;150:1163.
6. Haacke EM, Lenz GW. Improving MR image quality in the presence of motion by using rephasing gradients. AJR 1987;148:1251.
7. Rubin JB, Enzmann DR. Optimizing conventional MR imaging of the spine. Radiology 1987;163:777.
8. Enzmann DR, Rubin JB, Wright A. Use of cerebrospinal fluid gating to improve T2-weighted images. I. The spinal cord. Radiology 1988;166:225.
9. Edelman RR, Atkinson DJ, Silver MS, et al. FRODO pulse sequences: a new means of eliminating motion, flow, and wraparound artifacts. Radiology 1988;166:235.
10. Felmlee JP, Ehman RL. Spatial presaturation: a method for suppressing flow artifacts and improving depiction of vascular anatomy in MR imaging. Radiology 1987;164:559.
11. Runge VM, Wood ML, Kaufman DM, et al. FLASH: clinical three-dimensional magnetic resonance imaging. Radiographics 1988;8:947.
12. Engelstad BL, Wolf GL. Contrast agents. In: Stark DD, Bradley WB, eds. Magnetic resonance imaging. St. Louis: CV Mosby, 1988.
13. Nelson KL, Runge VM. Basic principles of paramagnetic contrast media. In: Runge VM, ed. Enhanced magnetic resonance imaging. St. Louis: CV Mosby, 1989.
14. Weinmann H-J, Brasch RC, Press WR, Wesbey GE. Characterizations of gadolinium DTPA complex: a potential NMR contrast agent. AJR 1984;142:619.
15. Nelson KL, Modic MT. Enhanced magnetic resonance imaging of the spine. In: Runge VM, ed. Enhanced magnetic resonance imaging. St. Louis: CV Mosby, 1989.
16. Bradley WG, Tsuruda JS. MR sequence parameter optimization: an algorithmic approach. AJR 1987;149:815.
17. Hyman RA, Gorey MT. Imaging strategies for MR of the spine. Radiol Clin North Am 1988;26:505.
18. Scotti G, Scialfa G, Colombo N, et al. Magnetic resonance diagnosis of intramedullary tumors of the spinal cord. Neuroradiology 1987;29:130.
19. Goy AMC, Pinto RS, Raghavendra BN, et al. Intramedullary spinal cord tumors: MR imaging, with emphasis on associated cysts. Radiology 1986;161:381.
20. Carsin M, Gandon Y, Rolland Y, et al. MRI of the spinal cord: intramedullary tumours. J Neuroradiol 1987;14:337.
21. Sze G, Bravo S, Krol G. Spinal lesions: quantitative and qualitative temporal evolution of gadopentetate demeglumine enhancement in MR imaging. Radiology 1989;170:849.
22. Dillion WP, Norman D, Newton TH, et al. Intradural spinal cord lesions: Gd-DTPA-enhanced MR imaging. Radiology 1989;170:229.
23. Slasky BS, Bydder GM, Niendorf HP, et al. MR imaging with gadolinium-DTPA in the differentiation of tumor, syrinx and cyst of the spinal cord. JCAT 1987;11:845.
24. Wagle WA, Jaufman B, Mincy JE. Intradural extramedullary ependymoma: MR-pathologic correlation. JCAT 1988;12:705.
25. Sato Y, Waziri M, Smith W, et al. Hipple-Lindau disease: MR imaging. Radiology 1988;166:241.

26. Dormont D, Assouline E, Gelbert F, et al. MRI study of spinal arteriovenous malformations. J Neuroradiol 1987;14:351.
27. Minami S, Sagoh T, Nishimura K, et al. Spinal arteriovenous malformation: MR imaging. Radiology 1988;169:109.
28. Post MJD, Quencer RM, Green BA, et al. Intramedullary spinal cord metastases, mainly of nonneurogenic origin. AJNR 1987;8:339.
29. Costigan DA, Winkelman MD. Intramedullary spinal cord metastases. Clinicopathological study of 13 cases. [Abstract] Radiology 1986;158:285.
30. Lewis TT, Kingsley DPE. Magnetic resonance imaging of multiple spinal neurofibromata-neurofibromatosis. Neuroradiology 1987;29:562.
31. Burk DL Jr, Brunberg JA, Kanal E, et al. Spinal and paraspinal neurofibromatosis: surface coil MR imaging at 1.5 T. Radiology 1987;162:797.
32. Sze G, Abramson A, Krol G, et al. Gadolinium-DTPA in the evaluation of intradural extramedullary spinal disease. AJNR 1988;9:153.
33. Dormont D, Assouline E, Gelbert F, et al. MRI study of spinal arteriovenous malformations. J Neuroradiol 1987;14:351.
34. Masaryk TJ, Ross JS, Modic MT, et al. Radiculomeningeal vascular malformations of the spine: MR imaging. Radiology 1987;164:845.
35. Hackney DB, Grossman RI, Zimmerman RA, et al. MR characteristics of iophendylate (Pantopaque). JCAT 1986;10:401.
36. Li KC, Poon PY. Sensitivity and specificity of MRI in detecting malignant spinal cord compression and in distinguishing malignant from benign compression fractures of vertebrae. Magn Reson Imaging 1988;6:547.
37. Dooms G, Maldaque B, Malghem J, et al. MR differential diagnosis between benign and malignant vertebral collapses. Radiology 1988;169:65.
38. Holtas SL, Kido DK, Simon JH. MR imaging of spinal lymphoma. J Comput Assist Tomogr 1986;10:111.
39. Bloem JL, Bluemm RG, Taminian AHM, et al. Magnetic resonance imaging of primary malignant bone tumors. Radiographics 1987;7:425.
40. Ross JL, Masaryk TJ, Modic MT, et al. Vertebral hemangiomas: MR imaging. Radiology 1987;165:165.
41. Hudson TM: Fluid levels in aneurysmal bone cysts: a CT feature. AJR 1984;142:1001.
42. Hajek PC, Baker LL, Goobar JE, et al. Focal fat deposition in axial bone marrow: MR characteristics. Radiology 1987;162:245.
43. Sze G, Krol G, Zimmerman RD, Deck MDF. Malignant extradural spinal tumors: MR imaging with Gd-DTPA. Radiology 1988;167:217.
44. Modic MT, Feiglin DH, Piraino DW, et al. Vertebral osteomyelitis: assessment using MR. Radiology 1985;157:157.
45. Masaryk TJ, Modic MT. Lumbar spine. In: Stark DD, Bradley WB, eds. Magnetic resonance imaging. St. Louis: CV Mosby, 1988.
46. de Roos A, van Persijn van Meerten Els L, Bloem JL, et al. MRI of tuberculous spondylosis. AJR 1986;146:79.
47. Aubin ML, Baleriaux D, Cosnard G, et al. MRI in syringomyelia of congenital, infectious, traumatic or idiopathic origin: a study of 142 cases. J Neuroradiol 1987;14:313.
48. Houang MTW, Stern M, Brew B, et al. Magnetic resonance imaging (MRI) appearances of syringohydromyelia. Australas Radiol 1988;32:172.
49. Kucharczyk W, Henkelman RM. Syrinx-like artifacts on MR images of the spinal cord. Radiology 1988;166:485.
50. Williams AL, Haughton VM, Pojunas KW, et al. Differentiation of intramedullary neoplasms and cysts by MR. AJNR 1987; 8:527.
51. Mirvis SE, Borg U, Belzberg H. MR imaging of ventilator-dependent patients: preliminary experience. AJR 1987;149:845.
52. Hedlund LW, Deitz J, Nassar R, et al. Ventilator for magnetic resonance imaging. Invest Radiol 1986;21:18.
53. Tarr RW. MR imaging of recent spinal trauma. J Comput Assist Tomogr 1987;11:412.
54. Mcardle CB, Crofford MJ, Mirfakhrace M, et al. Surface coil MR of spinal trauma: preliminary experience. AJNR 1986;7:885.
55. Larsson E-M, Holtas S, Cronqvist S. Emergency magnetic resonance imaging of patients with spinal cord symptoms. Acta Radiol 1988;29:69.
56. Chakeres DW, Flickinger F, Bresnahan JC, et al. MR imaging of acute spinal cord trauma. AJNR 1987;8:5.
57. Quencer RM, Beasley RE, Cammisa FJ, et al. MR in nonpenetrating spine injuries: use in clinical management. AJNR 1988;9:1001.
58. Hackney DB, Asato R, Joseph PM, et al. Hemorrhage and edema in acute spinal cord compression: demonstration by MR imaging. Radiology 1986;161:387.
59. Gebarski SS, Gebarski KS, Bowerman RA, Silver TM. Posttraumatic progressive myelopathy. Radiology 1985;157:379.
60. Ross JS, Perez-Reyes N, Masaryk TJ, et al. Thoracic disk herniation: MR imaging. Radiology 1987;165:511.
61. Maravilla KR, Weinreb JC, Suss RA, et al. Magnetic resonance demonstration of multiple sclerosis plaques in the cervical cord. AJR 1985;144:381.
62. Grossman RI, Braffman BH, Brorson JR, et al. Multiple sclerosis; serial study of gadolinium-enhanced MR imaging. Radiology 1988;169:117.
63. Ramsey RG, Zacharias CE. MR imaging of the spine after radiation therapy: easily recognizable effects. AJR 1985;144:1131.
64. Sclesinger AE, Naidich TP, Quencer RM. Concurrent hydromyelia and diastematomyelia. AJNR 1986;7:473.
65. Hans JS, Benson JE, Kaufman B, et al. Demonstration of diastematomyelia and associated abnormalities with MR imaging. AJNR 1985;6:215.
66. Barnes PD, Lester PD, Yamanashi WS, et al. Magnetic resonance imaging in infants and children with spinal dysraphism. AJNR 1986;7:465.

7

Lumbar Spine

Kevin L. Nelson
Val M. Runge

Magnetic resonance imaging (MRI) has progressed to become a major modality in the radiologic evaluation of lumbar spine disease. MRI is a versatile means of imaging the lumbar spine, allowing simultaneous visualization of all the lumbar vertebral bodies and posterior elements, intervertebral discs, subarachnoid space, and traversing lumbar nerves. The conus medullaris can be evaluated on routine sagittal images, allowing a number of pathologic conditions to be excluded. The multiplanar imaging capabilities and lack of ionizing radiation are additional advantages over computed tomography (CT) and myelography. Recent technologic advancements, including the development of improved surface coils, allow thin-section images approaching that of CT to be obtained. These surface coils allow sufficient signal-to-noise ratios (SNR) in smaller voxel elements, thereby improving spatial resolution.[1,2] Many authorities now use MRI first for evaluating patients presenting with symptoms suggesting lumbar spine abnormalities.[3]

This chapter discusses current MRI techniques and effective imaging strategies for obtaining diagnostic scans. Common pathologic entities involving the lumbar spine and their appearance on MR images are reviewed.

MRI TECHNIQUES

There are many other operator-dependent parameters besides scan plane thickness to consider in MRI. Relaxation time (TR), echo time (TE), matrix size, number of data acquisitions, and interslice gap must be considered with conventional spin echo techniques. Radio-frequency (RF) tip angle is a technical factor that may be altered when obtaining gradient echo images of the lumbar spine.[4]

Variation in scan techniques occur among institutions performing MRI examinations of the lumbar spine. Most of these variations are based on the personal preference of the radiologist interpreting the exam and to some extent on the operating magnetic field strength and surface coils being used. The primary premise for obtaining diagnostic images of the lumbar spine is to use the thinnest sections achievable while maintaining adequate SNR. In addition to improved surface coils for spine imaging, other technical developments, such as low bandwidth techniques, have improved SNR. Although an improved SNR is realized with low bandwidths, a disadvantage is the increased chemical shift artifact encountered.

The initial scan commonly used is a short TR/short TE (400–600 msec/10–30 msec) sequence in the sagittal plane. Generally, a 256 × 256 matrix is used with four data-set acquisitions to obtain high-resolution images with adequate SNR. Although the scan time for this sequence can be decreased by half when using a 128 matrix, there will be a corresponding loss of resolution with the larger voxel elements. The use of 192 phase-encoding steps is another alternative that usually provides adequate SNR images while decreasing scanning time and maintaining resolution. Alternatively, decreasing the number of data acquisitions by half to two causes the pulse sequence to be completed in half the time, but there will be a 40% loss of SNR, producing lower-quality images. A third alternative to decreasing the scan time is to use as short a TR as possible, which will decrease the imaging time proportionally. However, a shorter TR also yields lower SNR in the images and fewer images in the multislice sequence.

Whatever TR is chosen, a sufficient number of sections are needed in the sagittal plane to provide images from one set of neuroforamina to the other.

Adequate coverage depends to some extent on the scan plane thickness that is chosen. With most equipment used today a slice thickness of 3 to 5 mm is employed for adequate SNR images. This allows a TR of 400 to 500 milliseconds to be used, providing a sufficient number of images in the sagittal plane. Small abnormalities can be missed with this scan thickness due to partial volume averaging. Optimally, a 1- to 2-mm scan thickness is desirable to decrease or eliminate partial volume averaging effects. Unfortunately, this cannot be routinely obtained with conventional spin echo techniques used today because adequate signal is usually not present in these thin-section images. With further developments and improvements in three-dimensional gradient-echo imaging techniques, the promise of true thin-section contiguous images may be realized. These techniques have been studied mostly in the cervical spine region and have not been refined for routine use in imaging the lumbar spine.[5,6]

A rectangular surface coil is usually chosen for lumbar spine imaging to allow the flexibility of greater coverage in the cranio-caudad direction, although circular surface coils are suitable alternatives. The field of view (FOV) chosen for the initial T1-weighted sagittal scan should include the entire lumbar spine and superior portion of the sacrum. The conus medullaris should also be included on these images. As a rule, if a FOV is chosen to encompass this anatomy, adequate signal is usually not a critical factor affecting the images. If a smaller FOV is chosen, including only the lower lumbar spine, there is less SNR in the images. This occurs because the voxel elements are smaller in size, decreasing SNR. Therefore, decreasing the FOV can dramatically decrease image quality.

These multiple-imaging parameters and their effects on image quality must be carefully considered in choosing a protocol for lumbar spine imaging. Guidelines may be offered, but personal preferences influence the trade-offs chosen when deciding upon a particular protocol over another. As in other radiologic imaging modalities, high image quality is preferred with MRI while maintaining adequate throughput and cost effectiveness.

The initial T1-weighted multislice pulse sequence obtained in the sagittal plane provides excellent morphologic detail of the lumbar spine and allows subsequent scans in other planes to be accurately localized. The normal anatomy on these images (Fig. 7-1A) includes the lumbar vertebral bodies and posterior elements, which contain high-signal-intensity fat in the marrow. Cortical bone is represented by a signal void, and the surrounding ligamentous structures and intervertebral discs are of intermediate signal intensity. Epidural fat is of high signal intensity and is easily seen on parasagittal images within the neuroforamina, which also contain the lower-signal-intensity exiting nerve root directly beneath the lumbar vertebral body pedicle. The cerebral spinal fluid (CSF) in the thecal sac is of low signal intensity and contains the intermediate-signal-intensity conus medullaris and traversing lumbar nerves.

The second set of images usually obtained consists of a multiecho pulse sequence in the sagittal plane. The first echo uses a long TR/intermediate TE (2000–3000 msec/30–50 msec). This provides proton density weighted images if a TE of 30 to 40 msec is chosen or mild T2-weighting if a longer TE of 40 to 50 msec is selected. The second echo uses the same long TR of 2000 to 3000 milliseconds but a longer TE, varying from 50 to 120 msec. The longer TEs provide heavily T2-weighted images in this pulse sequence. In order to obtain proton density and T2-weighted images with adequate SNR, a thicker slice (> 3 mm) may be required. By using a rectangular or 128 matrix in the phase-encoding direction, increased SNR is realized due to the larger voxel elements. This allows two data acquisitions to be employed, which also increases the SNR in the images.

Long TR/intermediate or long TE pulse sequences are critically affected by motion. Even the simple use of a physical restraint over the abdomen decreases respiratory motion from the anterior abdominal wall. When obtaining proton density and T2-weighted images of the lumbar spine, it is critical that some type of motion-compensation technique be employed to minimize motion artifacts from CSF and venous pulsations. In most instances, gradient moment nulling is recommended to minimize these motion artifacts. However, cardiac gating is a viable alternative and may be used alone or in conjunction with gradient moment nulling for even greater effectiveness.[7-11] Presaturation pulses have also been used in lumbar spine imaging to help eliminate motion artifacts from the abdominal wall and vascular structures in the abdomen. Presaturation pulses generally find greater utility in imaging the thoracic and cervical spine.[12]

The normal anatomy seen on proton density and T2-weighted images (Fig. 7-1B,C) includes the nucleus pulposus and the inner fibers of the annulus fibrosis. They display increased signal intensity due to their increased water content; the outer fibers of the annulus fibrosis are of low signal intensity. A central intranuclear cleft of decreased signal intensity is normally present in the nucleus pulposus on T2-weighted images. This is presumed to be secondary to the presence of fibrous tissue and becomes more prominent with age.[13,14] Dense cortical bone is represented by a signal void, and the spinal ligamentous structures are intermediate in signal intensity, analogous to T1-weighted images. Normal marrow within the verte-

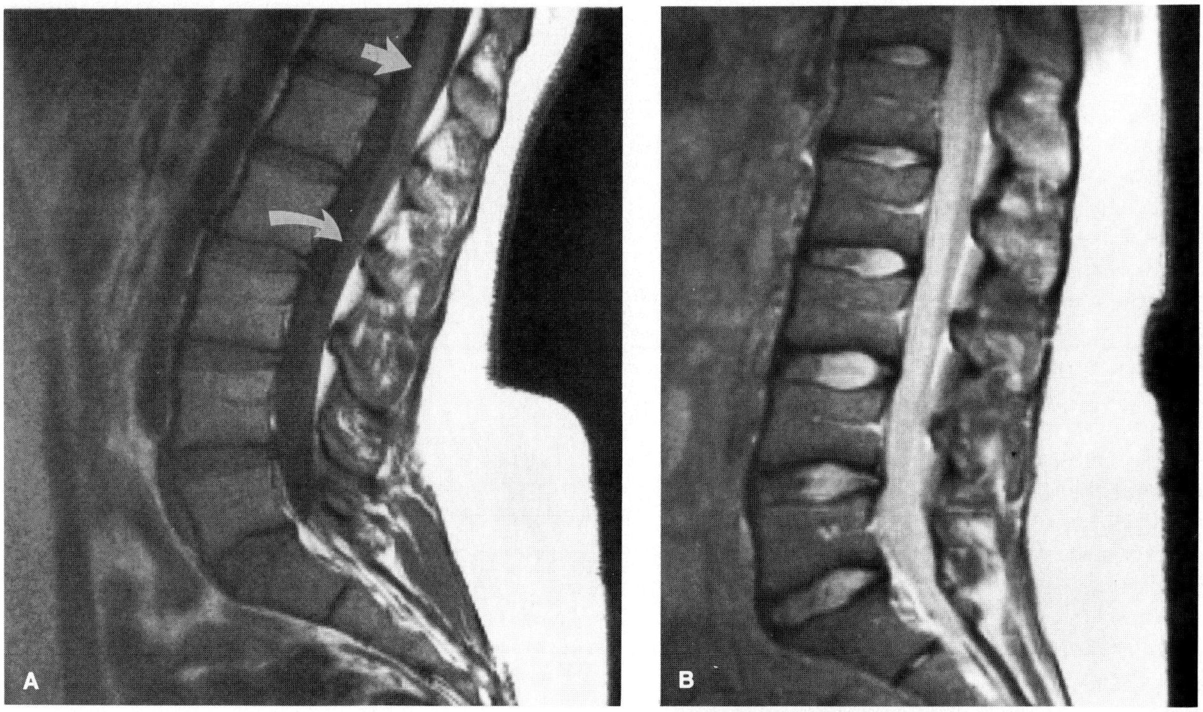

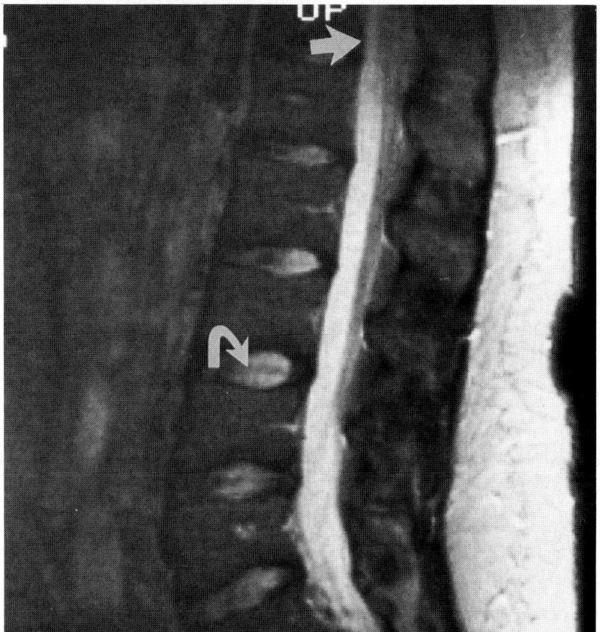

FIGURE 7–1. (A) Normal sagittal T1-weighted (TR/TE=450/20) spin echo image of the lumbar spine. The lumbar vertebral bodies are of slightly higher signal intensity than the intervertebral discs due to fat within the bone marrow. The conus medullaris (arrow), well defined at the T12-L1 level, is of intermediate signal intensity and is surrounded by low-signal-intensity CSF. Because the patient is supine, the traversing intermediate-signal-intensity lumbar nerves (curved arrow) lie posteriorly in the dependent portion of the lumbar subarachnoid space. Normal lumbar spine on **(B)** proton density (TR/TE=3000/45) and **(C)** T2-weighted (TR/TE=3000/90) spin echo images of another patient. The high-signal-intensity intervertebral discs are identified due to the high water content of the nucleus pulposus and inner fibers of the annulus fibrosis in the normal nondesiccated intervertebral disc. The central intranuclear cleft (curved arrow) is seen as decreased signal intensity within the disc and is probably due to fibrous tissue. The normal fat-containing bone marrow is of lower signal intensity on these images than on the T1-weighted images. The CSF displays increased signal intensity, allowing the CSF-extradural interface to be evaluated. The intermediate-signal-intensity conus medullaris (arrow) and traversing lumbar nerves are seen.

bral body loses some of its signal because it contains fat with its shorter T2 relaxation time. Because the T2 relaxation time of CSF is long, it displays increased signal intensity on both proton density and T2-weighted images. This produces a myelogram-like effect, useful in evaluating the CSF-extradural interface.

The intermediate-signal-intensity conus medullaris is usually easily seen and can be assessed for tumor or other intramedullary abnormalities displaying long T2 relaxation times. These are seen as abnormal areas of increased signal intensity. Often the intermediate-signal-intensity traversing lumbar nerves can be visualized within the high-signal-intensity CSF in the thecal sac.

A third pulse sequence is usually recommended in

an orthogonal plane. The axial plane is most often chosen because it is useful in evaluation of the posterior bony elements, intervertebral discs, and vertebral bodies (Fig. 7–2). It is also useful for correlation with CT in which axial images are the routine. Although controversy does exist about the type of pulse sequence to use, most authorities recommend a short TR/short TE sequence (400–600 msec/10–30 msec), providing T1-weighted images that yield excellent morphologic detail of the lumbar spine. As for sagittal T1-weighted images of the lumbar spine, a 3- to 5-mm slice is used for adequate signal, with 192 or 256 phase-encoding steps in the matrix for high-resolution images. Two to four data acquisitions are used, depending on the image quality desired.

The FOV must be large enough to provide adequate SNR in the images. Some magnification of the images may be done after acquisition of the data to obtain more aesthetically pleasing images and to improve ease of interpretation. This is probably preferred to using a smaller FOV for the scans because a significant penalty in signal loss is incurred with small FOVs.

Many MR scanners can angle the axial scan planes with respect to the discs at multiple levels when evaluating potential disc herniations. Although this decreases slightly the number of images acquired in the multislice sequence, it is recommended for evaluating potential disc herniations.

Often the imaging time in the axial plane can be decreased somewhat with T1-weighted images if the TR is decreased to 400 milliseconds. This however allows a more limited number of axial images. These images usually provide enough signal, despite the shorter TR, to be diagnostic. The primary disadvantage is that, due to the limited number of slices (because of the short TR) the L3-4 intervertebral disc may be covered with only one axial image or not at all. Many authorities believe that axial images in the lumbar spine should cover at least the last three lumbar intervertebral discs in order to exclude the rare L3-4 herniated nucleus pulposus. This level can usually be evaluated adequately on the initial T1-weighted sagittal images unless a true lateral herniated L3-4 disc is present. Lateral disc herniations can be missed with sagittal images alone.

An alternative pulse sequence for axial images is a long or intermediate TR/intermediate TE (2000–3000 msec or 1000–2000 msec/30–50 msec), providing proton density weighted images. The long TR used in these pulse sequences allows more slices to be obtained in the multislice sequence, covering a greater number of disc-space levels. Angulation of the scan planes with respect to the discs is recommended if it can be done. Because the CSF becomes intermediate in signal intensity on these images, there is some advantage with this pulse sequence in evaluating herniated discs because the CSF-extradural interface is easily seen. Sometimes herniation of a nondesiccated nucleus pulposus may be more easily appreciated on proton density images than on T1-weighted images, because a high-signal-intensity pedicle of the herniated nucleus pulposus can be visualized in contiguity with the parent disc on these axial images. One of the primary disadvantages of the proton density images is the increased imaging time necessitated by the long TR.

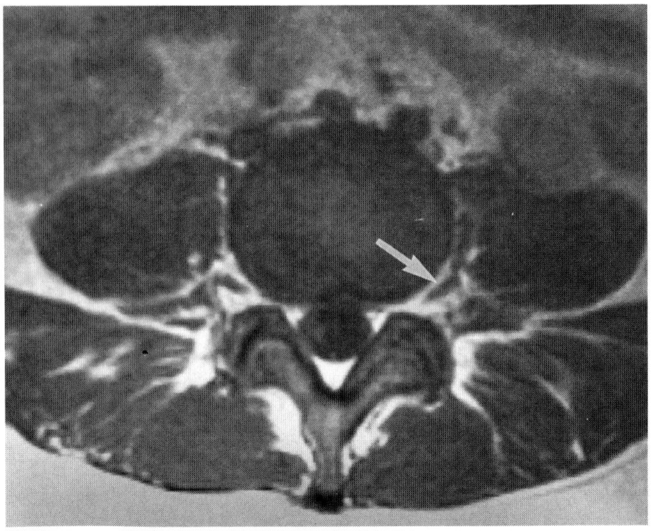

FIGURE 7–2. Normal L4-5 intervertebral disc. Axial T1-weighted spin echo image. The disc is seen as an intermediate-intensity signal against the low-signal-intensity CSF within the thecal sac. The exiting intermediate-signal-intensity L4 nerve root (arrow) is surrounded by high-signal-intensity epidural fat in the neuroforamina.

Rarely, an additional scan in the coronal plane may be chosen to better depict an abnormality. This may be useful for more clearly defining paraspinal abnormalities, such as a neurofibroma, and their relationship to the spinal axis. For most lumbar spine abnormalities, the combination of sagittal and axial images provides sufficient data for characterization.

Fast imaging techniques are being explored as possible alternatives to conventional spin echo scans. A number of different types of gradient-echo imaging techniques are available, depending on the MR scanner being used. GRASS, FLASH, FISP, and CE-FAST are examples. In contrast to conventional spin echo sequences, in which an initial RF pulse produces a proton tip angle of 90°, gradient-echo images use an initial RF pulse to create a proton tip angle of less than 90°. Unlike the 180° refocussing pulse used in spin echo sequences, the protons are refocussed with the gradient coils of the MR scanner. Gradient echo images may be employed in a 2D mode in which several images are obtained in 1 to 2 minutes of scan time. Gradient-echo images obtained in a 2D mode were used initially for the lumbar spine but have fallen into disfavor with many people and now are most commonly used in the cervical spine.[5,6] Alternatively, 3D acquisitions are being investigated for use in lumbar spine imaging. Thin-section (1–2 mm) high-resolution truly contiguous images can be obtained in one plane with approximately 10 minutes of scanning time (Fig. 7–3). Using computer-assisted reformations, scans obtained in one plane may be reconstructed into a multitude of other planes, including curved and oblique projections, providing greater imaging flexibility.[15]

The primary value of gradient-echo images is their ability to display CSF in the lumbar subarachnoid space as white and in a shorter amount of imaging time than is required for T2-weighted spin echo images. This provides a myelogram-like effect, with short scan times allowing effective evaluation of the CSF-extradural interface. Although initial inspection of some gradient-echo images in the lumbar spine suggest they may be similar to T2-weighted images, they represent a different type of contrast, referred to as T2*. The magnitude of abnormal signal intensity seen on gradient-echo images may not be as impressive as on T2-weighted spin echo images. An example of this decreased contrast with gradient-echo images is the dehydrated lumbar disc seen in early degenerative disc disease. Compared with conventional T2-weighted spin echo images, a desiccated lumbar disc is not as easily recognized on gradient-echo images as having decreased signal intensity. Gradient-echo images are also much more sensitive to magnetic susceptibility. This is detrimental because a small ferromagnetic metal fragment can produce an extremely large signal loss. It can be advantageous in detecting hemorrhage in the conus medullaris or elsewhere in the lumbar spine. The decrease in signal intensity caused by hemosiderin deposition is accentuated on gradient echo images due to magnetic susceptibility. A hemorrhage may thus become more obvious on gradient-echo images if hemosiderin is present.

PARAMAGNETIC CONTRAST MEDIA

The use of paramagnetic contrast media in defining certain abnormalities of the spine has been well-documented.[16–18] Gadolinium DTPA (gadopentetate dimeglumine, Gd DTPA) is currently the only clinically available intravenous MR contrast medium, although many others are undergoing evaluation.[19–22] Gd DTPA possesses seven unpaired electrons in its outer orbital shells.[23–25] The paramagnetic effect of the gadolinium ion produces alteration of the local magnetic environment, enhancing proton relaxation and shortening T1 and T2 relaxation times.

With conventional spin echo techniques, T1 shortening produces increased signal intensity on T1-weighted images. T2 shortening produces an undesirable effect of decreased signal intensity on T2-weighted images. At currently used clinical doses of 0.1 mmol/kg of Gd DTPA, the predominate effect is T1 shortening. Therefore, heavily T1-weighted images are used with paramagnetic metallochelates such as Gd DTPA to visualize contrast enhancement.

Gd DTPA has been useful in the lumbar spine for evaluating intramedullary disease involving the conus medullaris and intradural-extramedullary tumor and in differentiating recurrent disc herniation from epidural fibrosis in the post operative lumbar spine.[16,18,26,27] The use of paramagnetic contrast agents has shown less than favorable results for evaluating extradural disease limited to the bony spine.[28] Extradural soft tissue extension from the bone and epidural metastatic deposits are more clearly defined with Gd DTPA enhancement than tumor confined only to the bone. Generally the most diagnostic images are obtained immediately or within 30 minutes after injection of Gd DTPA.

LUMBAR SPINE ABNORMALITIES

Degenerative Disc Disease

Degenerative disc disease represents a spectrum of changes involving the lumbar intervertebral discs and occurs to some extent in all individuals. It is not a well-understood process and may begin early in life; no specific causes have been defined. A significant component of the general population develop low back pain sometime during their lives for which medical attention is sought. The majority of these patients have had muscular strain. It is estimated that 10% have herniated lumbar discs.[29] The patient may present with a unilateral radiculopathy suggesting a lumbar disc herniation. This knowledge is useful for the radiologist in order to direct attention during the radiologic evaluation to the specific disc level suggested clinically. However, discrepancies between the clinical and radiologic interpretations can occur. This can be attributed to migration of a free disc fragment or anatomic variability in the position of nerve roots in the spinal canal.

The vast majority of degenerative lumbar disc disease occurs at the L4-5 and L5-S1 levels because the greatest mechanical stresses occur at these levels. Approximately 90 to 95% of lumbar disc herniations occur at these two levels, with 5 to 7% involving the L3-4 intervertebral disc.[30,31] The majority of herniations of the nucleus pulposus occur in the posterolat-

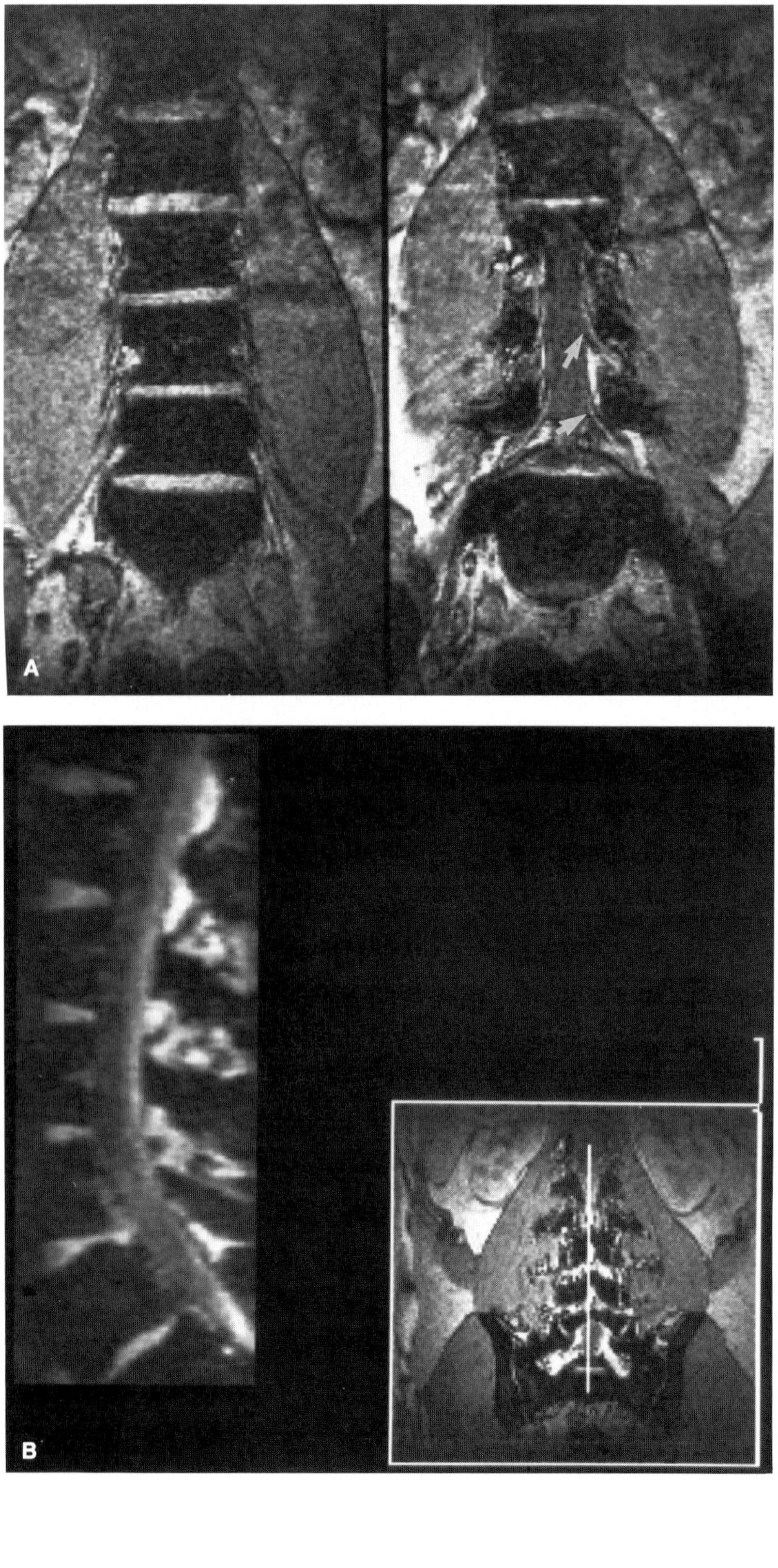

FIGURE 7–3. 3D FLASH gradient echo images of the normal lumbar spine. **(A)** Coronal 2-mm images chosen at two widely separate levels in the lumbar spine. The intervertebral discs are of high signal intensity. The bone marrow in the vertebral bodies is of decreased signal intensity because the magnetic susceptibility of normal hematopoietic elements is accentuated on gradient echo images. Exiting nerves from the thecal sac (arrows) are demonstrated. Computer-assisted reformation of midline sagittal **(B)** and axial **(C)** images were obtained from the original coronal data set, as indicated by the cursors. Images may be reformatted into oblique or curved planes from the original coronal data set if desired.

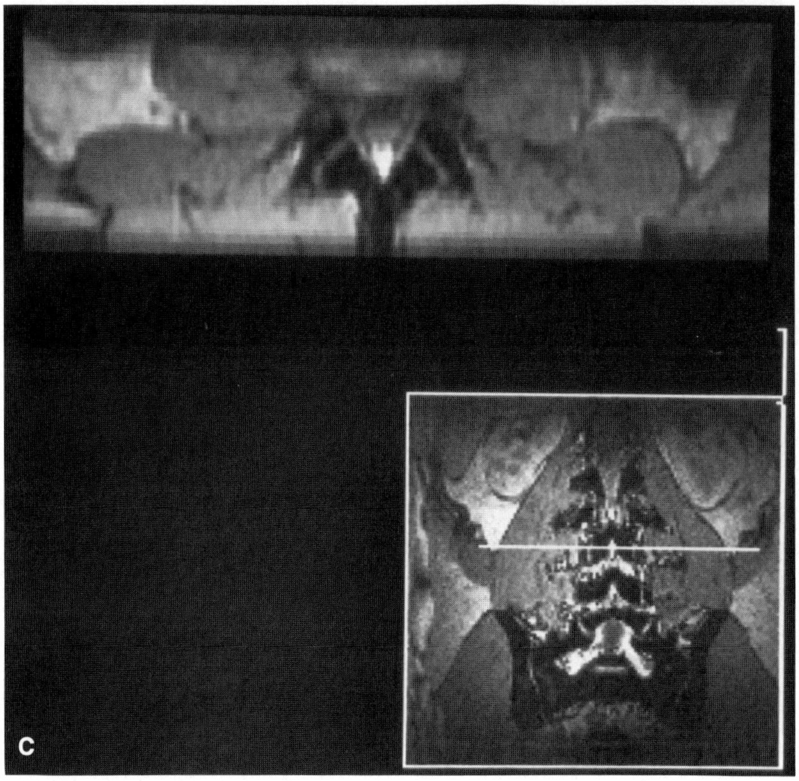

FIGURE 7–3. (Continued)

eral direction, which may compress an exiting nerve root, resulting in a localizing unilateral radiculopathy (Fig. 7–4). Although the strong posterior longitudinal ligament may be helpful in confining central disc herniations, they do occur more commonly than was once thought (Fig. 7–5). Lateral herniations of the nucleus pulposus are the most uncommon type (Fig. 7–6).[32]

The major indication for MRI examinations of the lumbar spine is for evaluation of potential disc herniations. Compared with myelography, CT, and post-myelography CT, MRI appears to be as accurate in detecting the presence of disc herniation.[1,33] Although MRI may be the best first test, it is often a complimentary study and combined with CT, accuracy in diagnosing lumbar disc herniations is definitely improved.[34]

Although there is some variability among radiologists in using the classification system for disc degeneration and herniation, a generally accepted scheme based on surgical criteria has been adopted for MR imaging.[35,36] The normal intervertebral disc on MR images can be separated into two components. In young patients, the central portion of the nucleus pulposus represents a semifluid mass with a high water content, which gradually decreases with age.[37] The normal nondesiccated disc is recognized as an area of high signal intensity on T2-weighted images, representing increased water content within the central portion of the nucleus pulposus and inner annulus fibrosis. The concentric lower-signal-intensity ring of the outer annulus fibrosis encases the nucleus pulposus and inner annulus fibrosis and unites the vertebral bodies. The earliest recognizable change of disc degeneration observed on T2-weighted images is the loss of the normal high signal intensity from the nucleus pulposus and inner annulus fibrosis due to desiccation (Fig. 7–7).[1] This causes poor differentiation of the outer fibers of the annulus fibrosis from the nucleus pulposus and inner annulus fibrosis fibers. A vacuum disc phenomenon caused by accumulation of nitrogen gas within the disc also can be recognized on MR images as a linear area of decreased signal intensity.[38]

As disc degeneration progresses, there is usually narrowing of the disc space. A bulging disc is defined

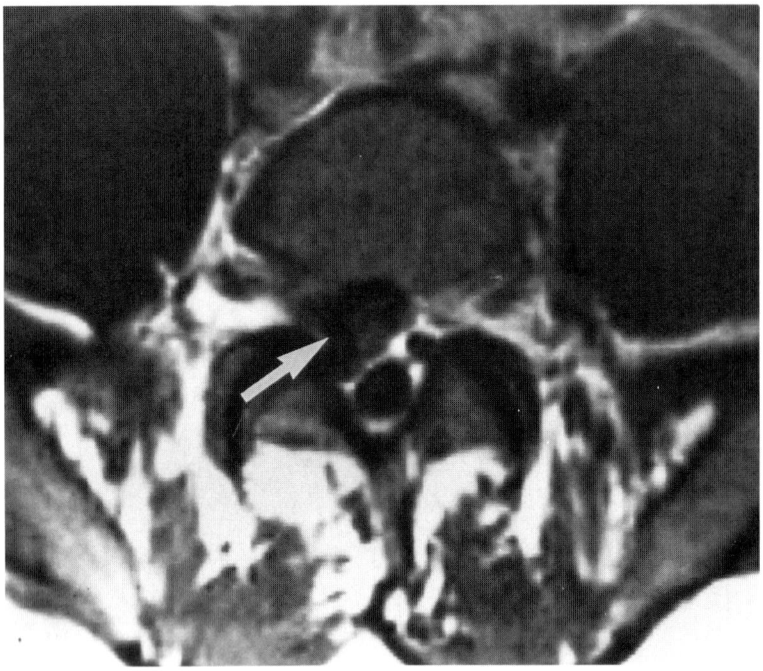

FIGURE 7–4. Posterolateral disc herniation. Axial T1-weighted spin echo image reveals posterolateral herniation of the disc (arrow). This is the most common direction of herniation of a lumbar intervertebral disc.

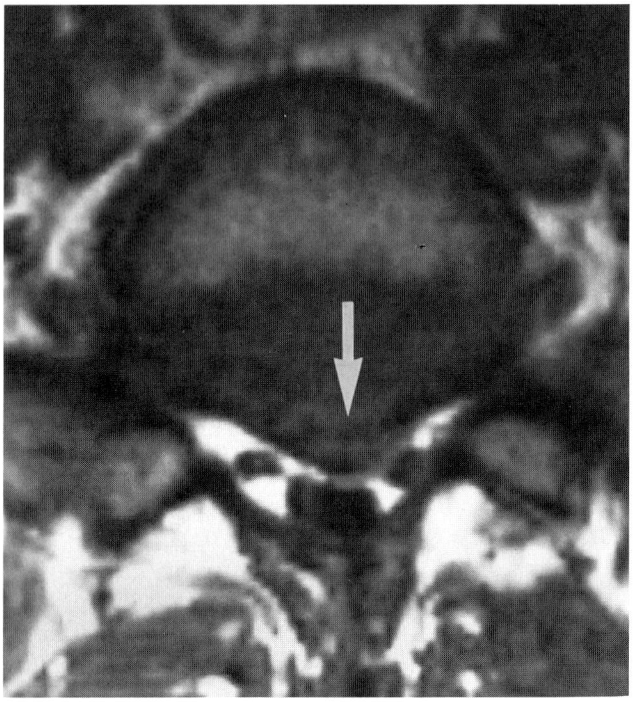

FIGURE 7–5. Central disc herniation. Axial T1-weighted spin echo image through the L5-S1 intervertebral disc shows a central posterior herniation of the disc (arrow).

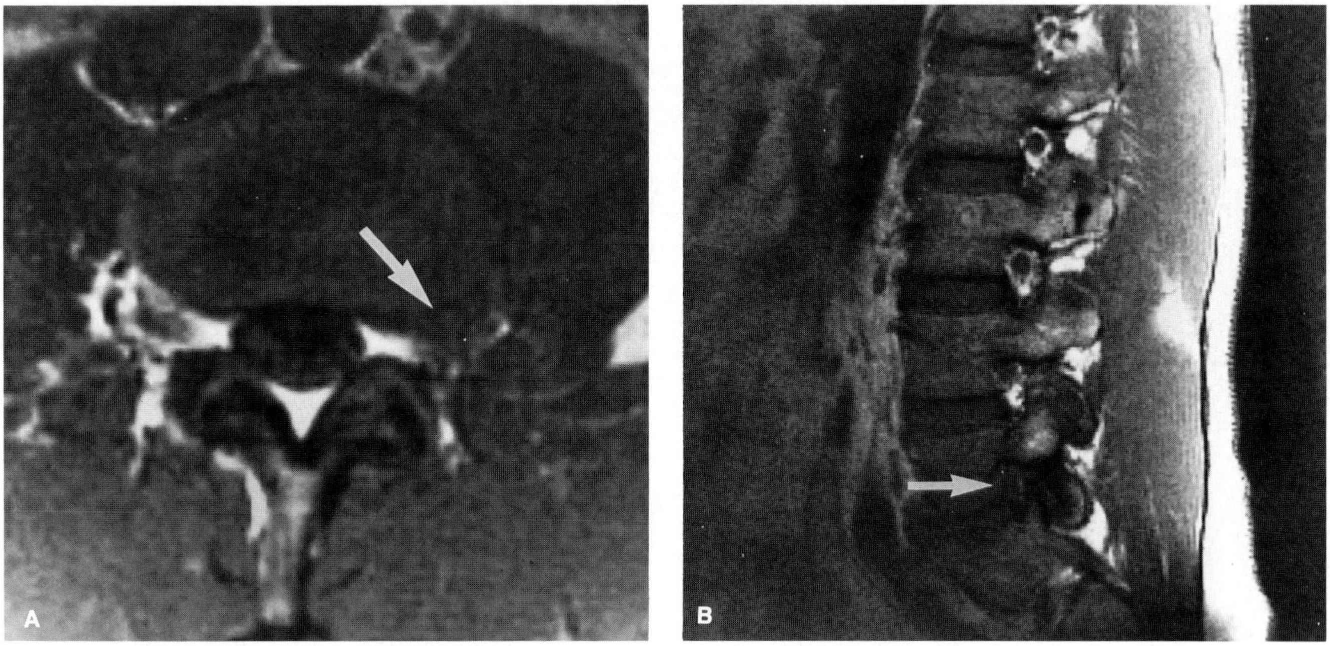

FIGURE 7–6. Lateral disc herniation. **(A)** Axial and **(B)** parasagittal spin echo images reveal a left lateral herniation of the L4-5 disc (arrow), compressing the exiting nerve root and obliterating the surrounding epidural fat in the neuroforamen.

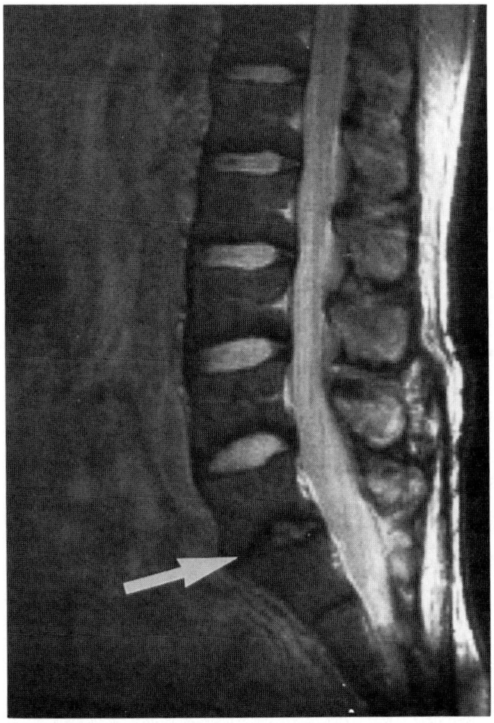

FIGURE 7–7. Early degenerative disc disease. Sagittal T2-weighted spin echo image of the lumbar spine shows a decrease in the normal high signal intensity from the L5-S1 intervertebral disc (arrow) and narrowing of the disc space. This is due to dehydration of the normally high water content of the nucleus pulposus. Notice the normal high signal intensity of the other lumbar intervertebral discs.

as concentric extension of the disc margins beyond the vertebral body end-plates (Fig. 7–8). The annulus fibrosis remains intact, confining the nucleus pulposus in a bulging disc. Disc prolapse occurs when nuclear material extends through a defect in the annulus fibrosis but remains in contact with the parent nucleus pulposus (Fig. 7–9). Several low-signal-intensity fibers of the outer annulus can be visualized on T2-weighted images as confining the nuclear material. Disc extrusion occurs after the nucleus pulposus has completely herniated through the annulus fibrosis, producing a recognizable high-intensity-signal pedicle on T2-weighted images (Fig. 7–10). A sequestered disc is identified if there is no longer contiguity between the herniated nuclear material and the parent disc (Fig. 7–11). The sequestered disc may migrate as a free fragment away from the original disc level and come to rest anterior or posterior to the posterior longitudinal ligament (Fig. 7–12).

Most disc herniations are seen in discs that are degenerated. T1-weighted images reveal the herniated nuclear material as isointense with the signal of the normal parent disc. T2-weighted sequences reveal most herniated nuclear material as an area of decreased signal intensity, although nondesiccated disc herniations can be seen as increased signal intensity like the parent disc. Sequestered discs are unique in that, in addition to being low to intermediate in signal

(text continues on page 266)

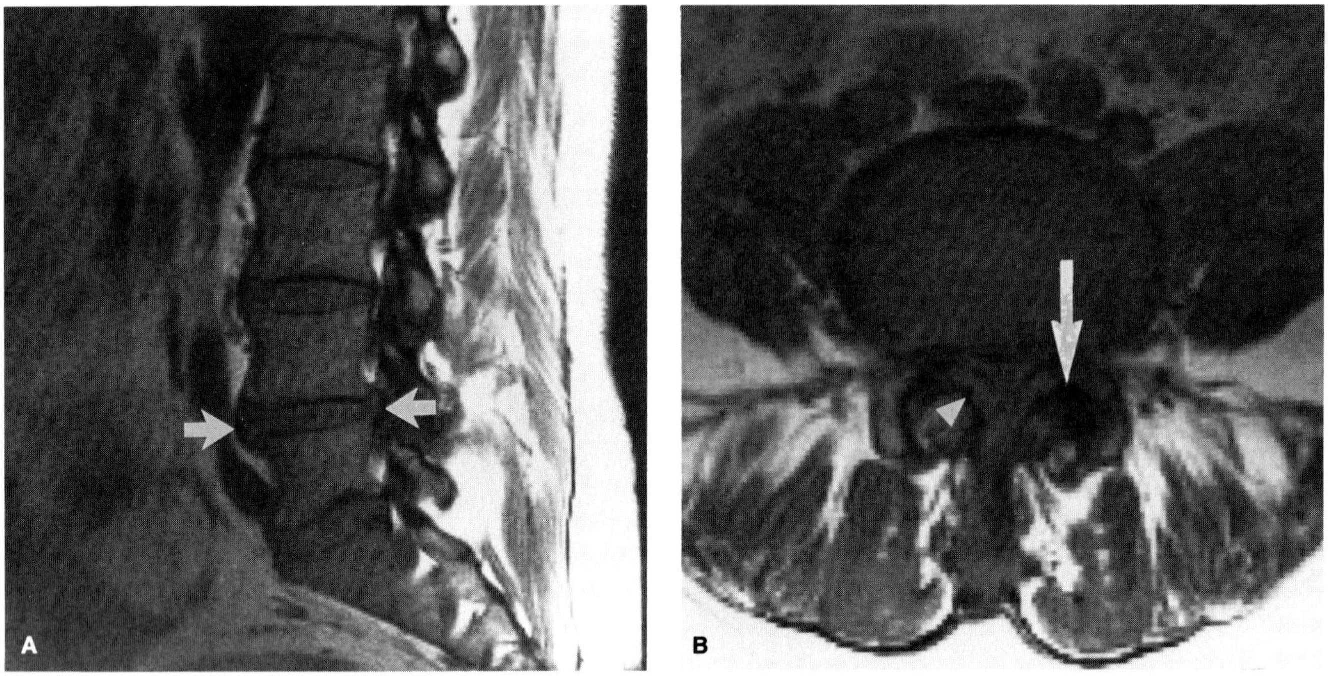

FIGURE 7–8. Diffuse disc bulging complicating central spinal canal stenosis. **(A)** Sagittal T1-weighted spin echo image shows diffuse anterior and posterior bulging of the L4-5 intervertebral disc (arrows). **(B)** Axial T1-weighted spin-echo image displays the associated degenerative change in the facet joints (arrow) and mild hypertrophy of the ligamentum flavum (arrowhead), resulting in central spinal canal stenosis. The associated bulging of the disc into the spinal canal further compounds the degree of spinal canal stenosis.

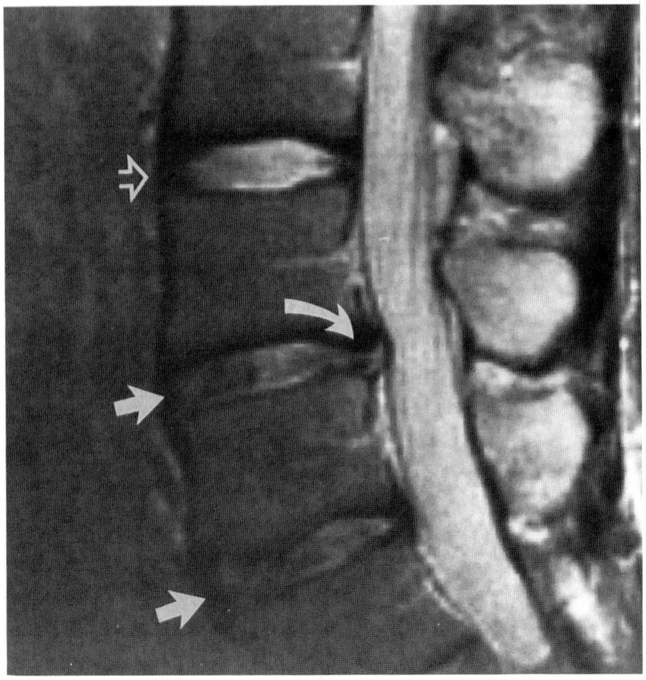

FIGURE 7–9. Disc prolapse. Sagittal T2-weighted spin echo image reveals the posterior extension of a portion of the high-signal-intensity L4-5 nucleus pulposus (curved arrow). Several low-signal-intensity fibers of the outer annulus fibrosis confine the herniated nucleus pulposus. The signal intensity of the nucleus pulposus of the dehydrated L4-5 and L5-S1 intervertebral discs (closed arrows) is lower than for the normal L3-4 intervertebral disc (open arrow).

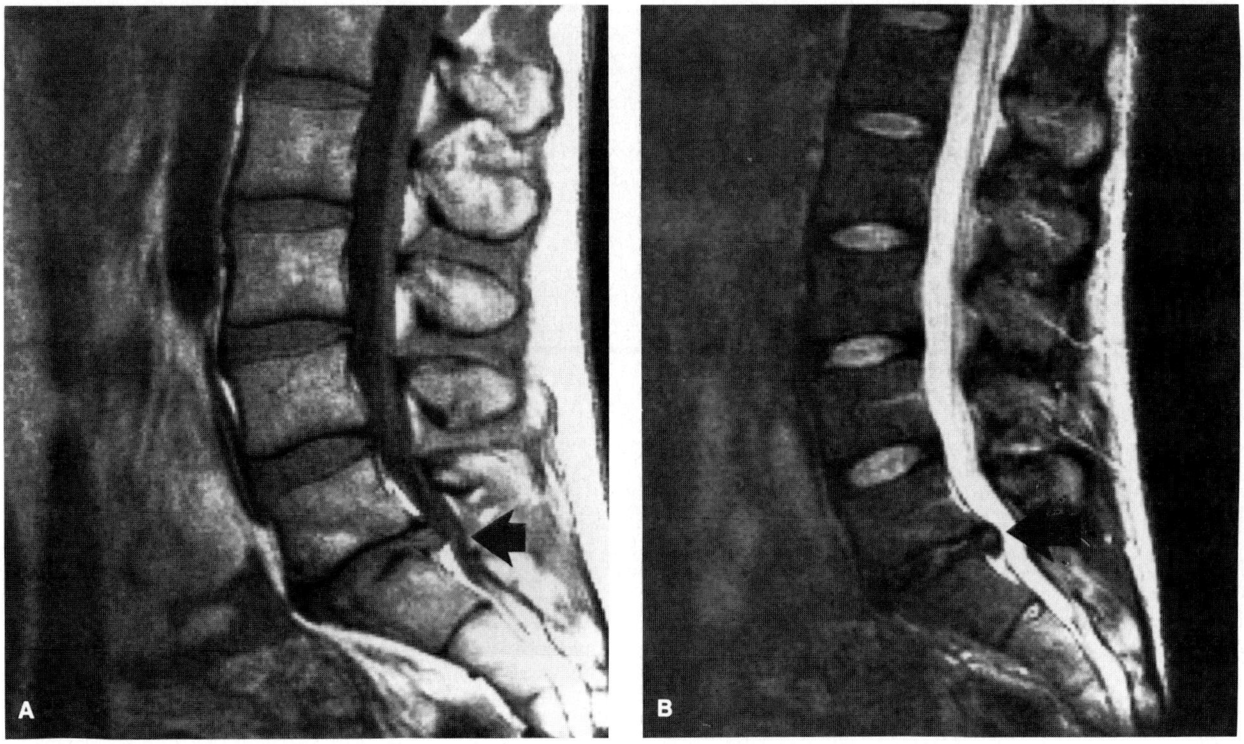

FIGURE 7–10. Disc extrusion. **(A)** Sagittal T1-weighted and **(B)** T2-weighted spin echo images show posterior herniation of the L5-S1 nucleus pulposus centrally (arrows). There has been complete herniation through the annulus fibrosis, with a pedicle connecting the extruded nuclear material to the parent disc.

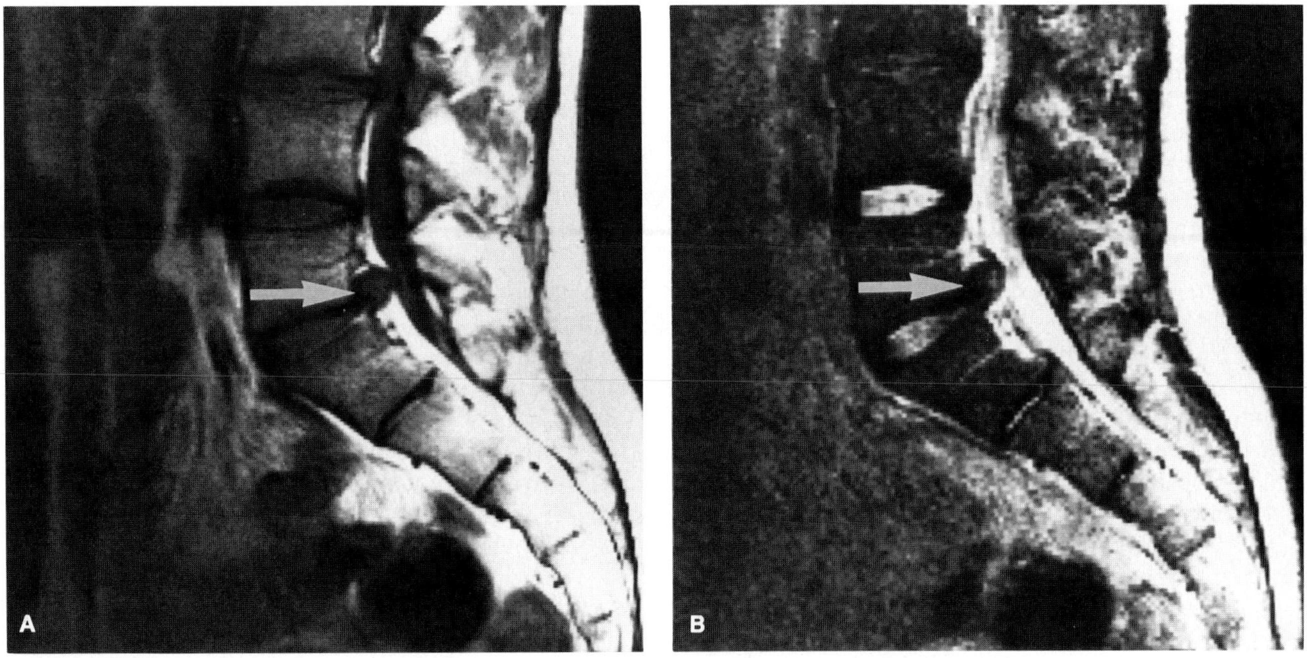

FIGURE 7–11. Sequestered disc with migration of a free fragment. **(A)** Sagittal T1-weighted and **(B)** T2-weighted spin echo images reveal herniation of the L5-S1 nucleus pulposus, which has migrated superiorly from the disc of origin (arrow). Notice the high signal intensity within the migrated, sequestered fragment on the T2-weighted image.

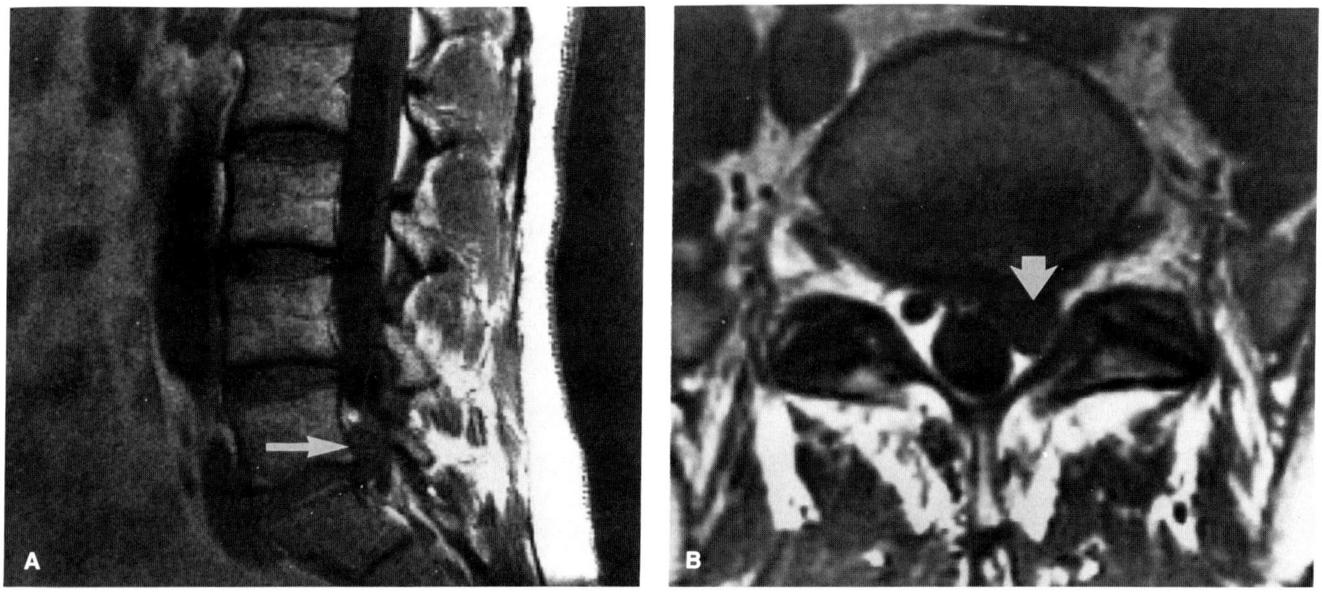

FIGURE 7–12. Migrated free disc fragment. **(A)** Sagittal T1-weighted spin echo image shows superior migration of a free fragment of the herniated L5-S1 disc (arrow). **(B)** Axial T1-weighted spin echo image shows posterior displacement of the traversing left L5 nerve root (arrow) by the fragment.

intensity on T1-weighted images, they possess increased signal intensity on T2-weighted images (Fig. 7–11B).[36]

In addition to careful evaluation of the lumbar intervertebral discs, several lower thoracic intervertebral discs can be evaluated simultaneously on the sagittal images. As more experience is gathered in MRI of the lumbar spine, more asymptomatic thoracic disc herniations are being recognized.[39] For patients presenting with symptoms suggesting lesions involving the conus medullaris, in addition to evaluating possible intramedullary disease, the thoracic intervertebral discs must be closely scrutinized for herniation producing extradural mass effect.

Degenerative changes occurring in the intervertebral disc increase the stresses on the end-plates of the adjacent vertebral bodies. Signal intensity changes involving the vertebral body marrow adjacent to the end-plates have been observed.[40] Modic and colleagues have investigated these changes on spin echo images and classified them based on comparison with normal vertebral body marrow.[41] Type I changes showed decreased signal intensity on T1-weighted images and increased signal intensity on T2-weighted images, which histologically represented fibrovascular replacement of normal marrow. Type II changes showed increased signal intensity on T1-weighted images and isointense or increased signal intensity on T2-weighted images, which correlated histologically with yellow marrow replacement of normal hematopoietic elements in the marrow (Fig. 7–13). Type I changes are not as commonly observed as Type II changes. Type I changes tend to convert to Type II changes with time; Type II changes tend to remain stable. Vertebral marrow signal intensity changes occur with increasing frequency with age and are associated with degenerative disc disease. The clinical importance of these findings is that these changes are always associated with degenerative disc disease and can be separated from changes caused by malignancy or vertebral osteomyelitis.[41]

Spinal Stenosis

Degenerative changes in the posterior spinal structures can be produced by abnormal stresses. Stress can cause abnormal narrowing and hypertrophy of the facet joints, thinning of the articular cartilage of the facet joints, and hypertrophy of the ligamentum flavum. Osteophyte formation along the vertebral end-plate margins can also be observed. One or more of these features can cause central and lateral recess spinal stenosis or foraminal stenosis.

Combined with an increased potential for disc herniation, the problem of spinal canal stenosis can be further compounded (Fig. 7–8). Secondary degenerative changes in the posterior spinal structures can be visualized on MR images of the lumbar spine.[42] Sclerotic osteophytes protruding into the spinal canal from the vertebral end-plates or hypertrophied facet joints may be difficult to differentiate from a desiccated disc herniation or hypertrophied spinal ligaments because they all possess low signal intensity. By comparison, osteophytes, which contain fatty marrow, can usually be distinguished by their high-signal-intensity fat on T1-weighted images and surrounding signal void from

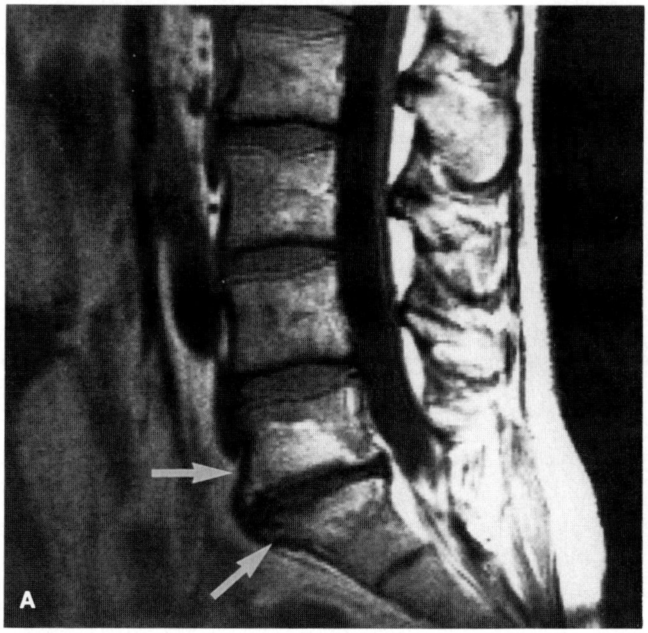

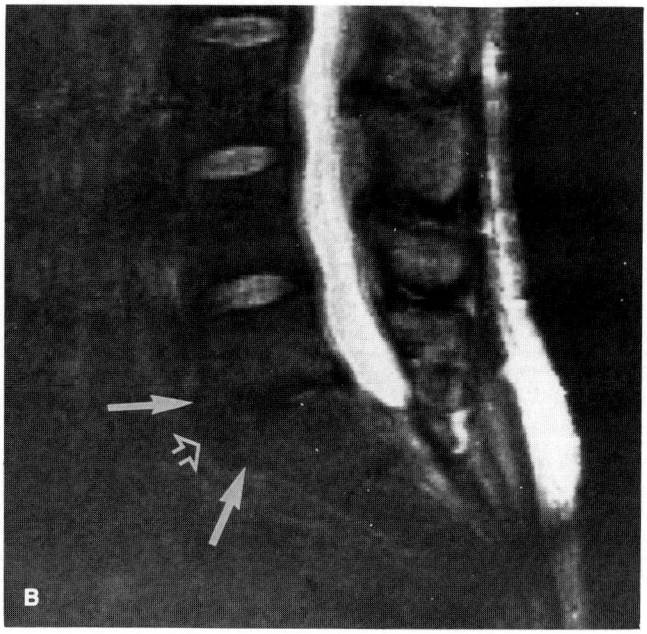

FIGURE 7–13. Type II bone marrow changes. **(A)** Sagittal T1-weighted and **(B)** T2-weighted spin echo images. The nucleus pulposus of the L5-S1 intervertebral disc is dehydrated, manifested as low signal intensity (open arrow) on the T2-weighted image. The disc space is narrowed, and reactive end-plate changes (closed arrows) in the vertebral bone marrow adjacent to the disc are seen with increased and decreased signal intensity, respectively, on T1- and T2-weighted images. This represents secondary marrow changes seen with progressive disc degeneration and increasing stresses placed upon the vertebral body end-plates. Type II changes are the most commonly encountered vertebral body marrow changes in degenerative disc disease, and they tend to remain stable.

the cortical bone. Close inspection of a suspected osteophyte often reveals its cortical margins, represented by signal void, contiguous with those of the normal vertebral body or facet joint, confirming the diagnosis.

The ligamentum flavum is visualized on axial images as an intermediate-signal-intensity structure on both T1-weighted and T2-weighted images. The ligamentum flavum on gradient-echo images is usually exquisitely defined. Normally, the ligamentum flavum is 5 mm thick in the axial plane.[42] If hypertrophied, it can easily be seen on MR images or CT scans and can be confirmed on parasagittal images. Thinning of the articular cartilage is difficult to measure accurately on MR images due to variable obliquity on axial images and chemical shift artifacts. Calcification in spinal ligaments and herniated discs (which produces signal void) may also be difficult to appreciate.[38]

Postoperative Lumbar Spine

Patients who have undergone previous lumbar spine surgery, most commonly for disc herniation or spinal canal stenosis, often present with recurrent low back pain, suggesting the failed back surgery syndrome (FBSS). This occurs in 10 to 40% of patients and can have several causes, including recurrent or persistent disc herniation (12–16%), epidural fibrosis (6–8%), arachnoiditis (6–16%), and lateral (58%) or central (7–14%) spinal stenosis.[43] The differentiation of recurrent or persistent disc herniation from epidural fibrosis is important, because reoperation of recurrent or persistent disc herniation usually alleviates the patient's symptoms, but reoperation of epidural fibrosis usually has poor surgical results.

In a prospective evaluation of MR imaging to differentiate epidural fibrosis from recurrent disc herniation, there was an 86% agreement between MR scans and surgical findings.[44] In this study, scar displayed isointense or hypointense signal on T1-weighted sequences and hyperintense signal on T2-weighted sequences compared with the normal annulus. Free disc fragments displayed a slightly hyperintense signal on T1-weighted scans compared with scar, but they were hyperintense on T2-weighted images, similar to scar. Prolapsed or extruded disc fragments were hypointense or isointense compared with the annulus on both T1-weighted and T2-weighted sequences. The morphology, epidural location, and presence or absence of mass effect were also important features in distinguishing scar from recurrent disc herniation.

Although MRI is superior to unenhanced CT in differentiating scar from recurrent disc herniation, it is equal to or slightly more accurate than contrast-enhanced CT.[44-47] Because the pharmacokinetic properties of Gd DTPA and iodinated contrast agents are similar and the sensitivity for visualization of contrast enhancement is greater on MRI than CT, it was theorized that the sensitivity of contrast-enhanced MRI would be even greater.[48] Initial evaluations of Gd DTPA-enhanced MR imaging in the postoperative lumbar spine have been favorable.[16,27]

Using T1-weighted spin echo images, epidural fibrosis consistently enhances after Gd DTPA injection on immediate postinjection images and displays more homogenous enhancement on delayed images. Enhancement of the curettage site along the native disc margins is often seen. Epidural fibrosis may have mass effect on the thecal sac and encase traversing lumbar nerve roots (Fig. 7-14). Margins of the parent disc can show enhancement, reflecting fibrovascular changes along the disc margins produced by degeneration. By comparison, the recurrent or herniated disc demonstrates no enhancement on immediate postinjection images but may show slight enhancement on delayed images (Fig. 7-15). Peridiscal fibrosis surrounding a recurrent disc herniation, called a "wrapped disc," can be observed.[16] The immediate postinjection images, usually in the axial plane, are the most valuable in evaluating the postoperative lumbar spine with contrast-enhanced MRI.

The differences in the time course of enhancement between scar and disc have been attributed to differences in vascularity.[16] Scar is more vascular than a herniated disc and enhances soon after Gd DTPA injection. Herniated disc does not show enhancement on immediate postinjection images, but diffusion of Gd DTPA into the disc from surrounding, more vascular tissue can enhance the disc on delayed images. Although contrast enhancement may not be warranted in every postoperative lumbar spine case, it can identify those postoperative patients with recurrent disc herniation who can benefit from repeat operations.

Arachnoiditis

The many causes of arachnoiditis include infection, trauma, previous surgery, and intrathecal administration of drugs, anesthetic agents, or oil-soluble myelographic contrast media. Arachnoiditis represents a spectrum of inflammatory changes involving the lumbar nerves. Ultimately a fibrinous exudate covers them, adhering the nerves to each other and to the thecal sac.[49] Although typical findings on myelography and CT have been described, the appearance of lumbar arachnoiditis on MRI has not been as extensively evaluated.[50] Ross and colleagues have described the various MR appearances of lumbar arachnoiditis.[51] These studies showed that axial T1-weighted images are useful in separating lumbar arachnoiditis into three groups. Type I arachnoiditis represents early, mild changes, manifested as clumping of nerves

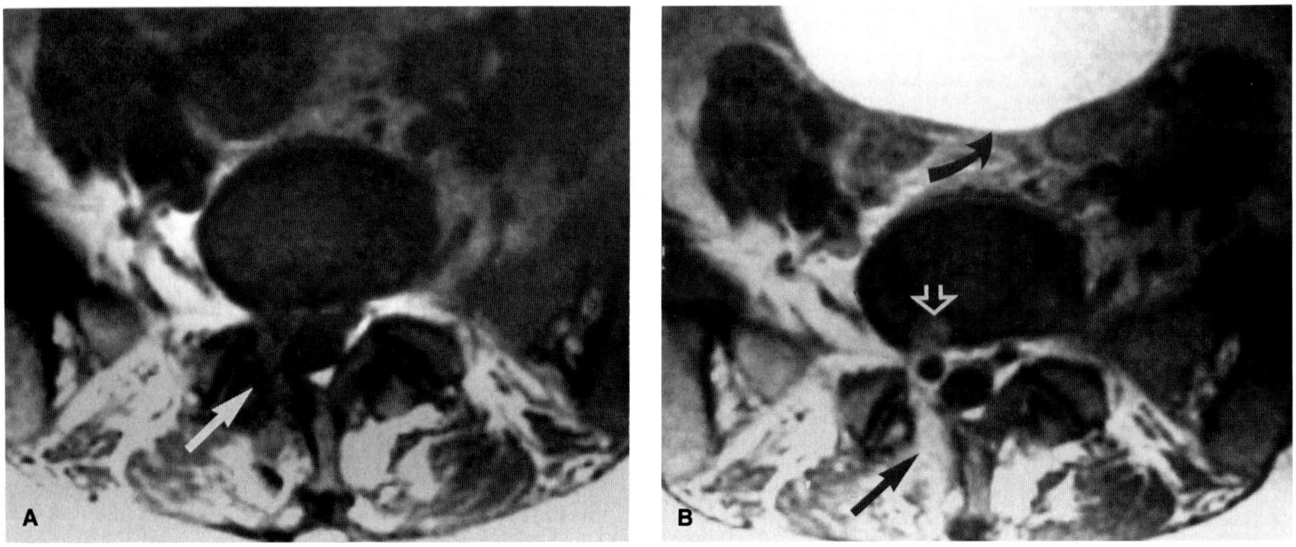

FIGURE 7-14. Postoperative epidural fibrosis. **(A)** Axial T1-weighted spin echo image at the L4-5 level shows a soft tissue mass extending anteriorly from the laminectomy site (arrow), obliterating the normal high-signal-intensity epidural fat. The traversing low-signal-intensity right L5 nerve root is difficult to define. **(B)** After Gd DTPA administration, a repeat axial T1-weighted spin echo image shows enhancement of the epidural fibrosis (straight black arrow), which is now well defined, encasing the low-signal-intensity traversing L5 nerve root on the right. Enhancement of the surgical curettage site (open white arrow) along the native disc margin is present. Notice the high-intensity accumulation of Gd DTPA (curved black arrow) within the urinary bladder after renal excretion.

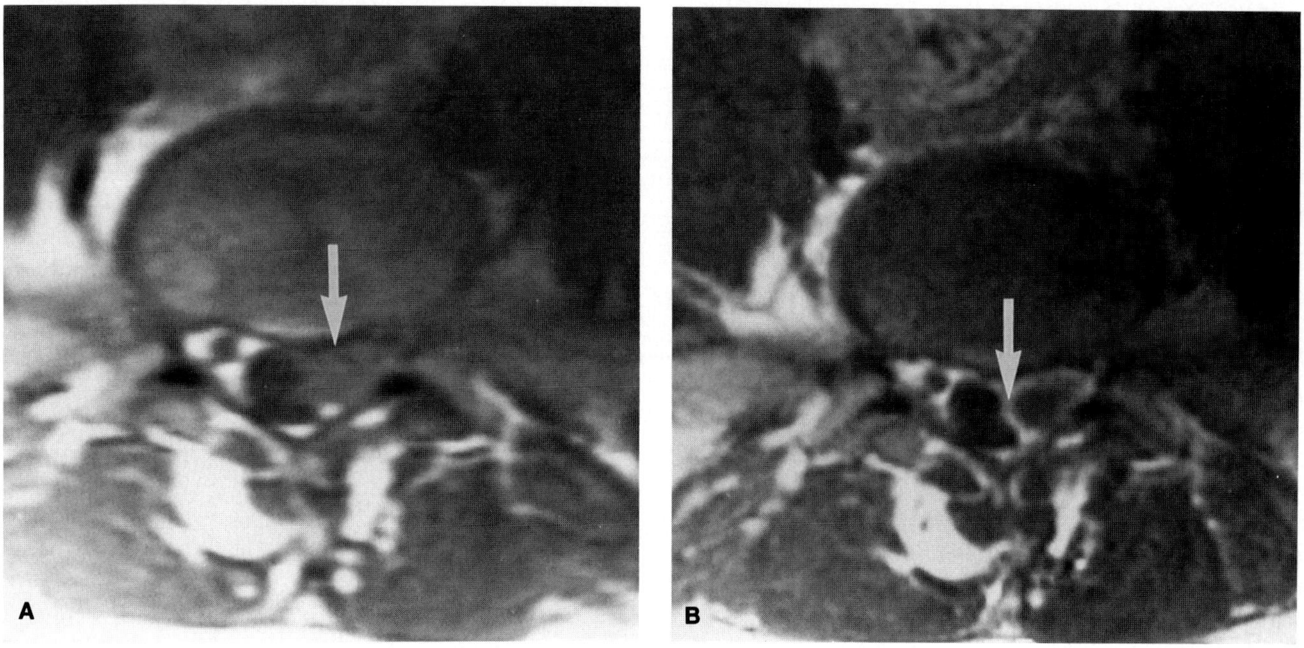

FIGURE 7–15. Recurrent disc herniation. **(A)** Before and **(B)** after Gd DTPA administration, axial T1-weighted spin echo images. A recurrent disc herniation of the L4-5 intervertebral disc of intermediate signal intensity (arrow) is seen on the unenhanced image. The recurrent disc herniation does not enhance after Gd DTPA administration, but surrounding peridiscal fibrosis (arrow) does.

centrally within the thecal sac. Type II lumbar arachnoiditis shows peripheral clumping of nerves, producing an "empty thecal sac" appearance. In the most severe form, Type III, the lumbar subarachnoid space may be obliterated by a soft tissue mass and may be difficult to distinguish from tumor. The use of Gd DTPA in evaluating arachnoiditis has received limited study, but some degree of enhancement should be expected.[52]

Chemonucleolysis

Treatment of lumbar disc herniations with chemonucleation, as an alternative to laminectomy, has been performed for several years. The therapy-induced changes in the lumbar intervertebral disc have been described (Fig. 7–16).[53] Treatment accelerates the degenerative process of the lumbar intervertebral disc. The intervertebral disc space becomes narrowed, with decreased signal intensity in the nucleus pulposus on T2-weighted images. Vertebral body bone marrow changes adjacent to the end-plates are also commonly observed.

Infection

MRI is extremely useful in the diagnosis of vertebral osteomyelitis and discitis. It is considered the imaging modality of choice for these entities and usually obviates the need for myelography or CT. In a study by

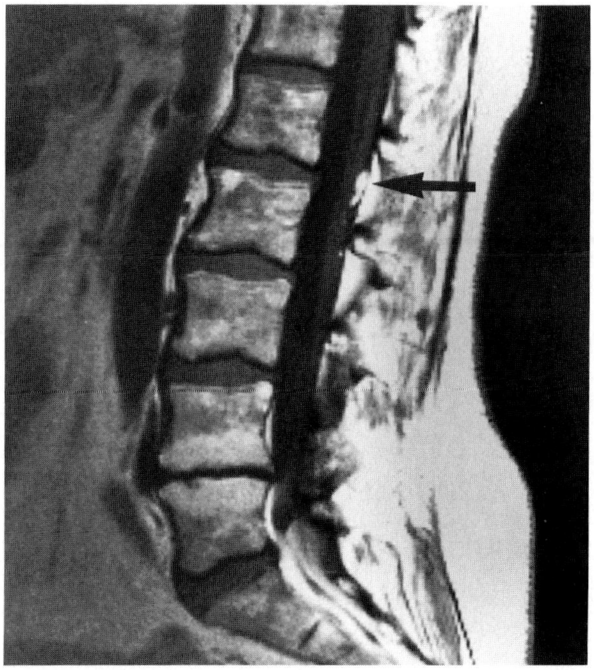

FIGURE 7–16. Chemonucleation changes. Sagittal T1-weighted spin echo image shows the reduced height of the L4-5 intervertebral disc space with high signal intensity in the adjacent vertebral body bone marrow. Notice the small amount of high-signal-intensity iophendylate (arrow) from a previous myelogram within the subarachnoid space.

Modic and colleagues, MRI had a sensitivity of 96%, a specificity of 92%, and an accuracy of 94% in diagnosing vertebral osteomyelitis.[54] MRI also proved to be more specific than nuclear medicine studies in these patients. MRI allowed earlier detection, improved specificity in the diagnosis of infection of the spine, and provided additional anatomic information about epidural extension and involvement of the thecal sac and surrounding neural elements.

Acute infection involving the vertebral body or disc presents as decreased signal intensity on T1-weighted images, with narrowing of the disc space and an indistinct margin between the disc and vertebral body end-plates. Increased signal intensity is seen on T2-weighted images in the region of the disc and involved vertebral body (Fig. 7–17). Follow-up of patients undergoing antibiotic therapy for discitis or vertebral osteomyelitis is best accomplished with MRI.[54] The resolution of infection is accompanied by a return to normal or near normal signal intensity on both T1-weighted and T2-weighted images.

Epidural abscesses have fewer characteristic findings on MRI than osteomyelitis or discitis.[55] MRI is probably the best imaging modality for evaluating the patient with epidural abscess, although this needs confirmation. Signal intensity changes with epidural abscesses are variable, and they may not always display increased signal intensity on T2-weighted images. False-negative results may be obtained if only MRI is used because the signal characteristics of some epidural abscesses may be similar to CSF and go unrecognized.

The role of paramagnetic contrast media in defining infections of the spine has not been investigated extensively. In one instance, Gd DTPA was useful in defining the communication of the vertebral and paravertebral components of inflammation.[56] Enhancement of inflammatory components is expected due to increased vascularity, and Gd DTPA may be very useful in defining inflammatory processes in the spine and in their follow-up evaluation during antibiotic therapy.

Tumor

Extradural Tumor

The most common extradural tumors affecting the lumbar spine are metastases. Lung, breast, and prostate are the most common primary malignancies to metastasize to the spine. Lymphoma and leukemia can infiltrate the bone marrow of the vertebral bodies and posterior elements, in addition to their more common presentation with involvement of the epidural space (Fig. 7–18).

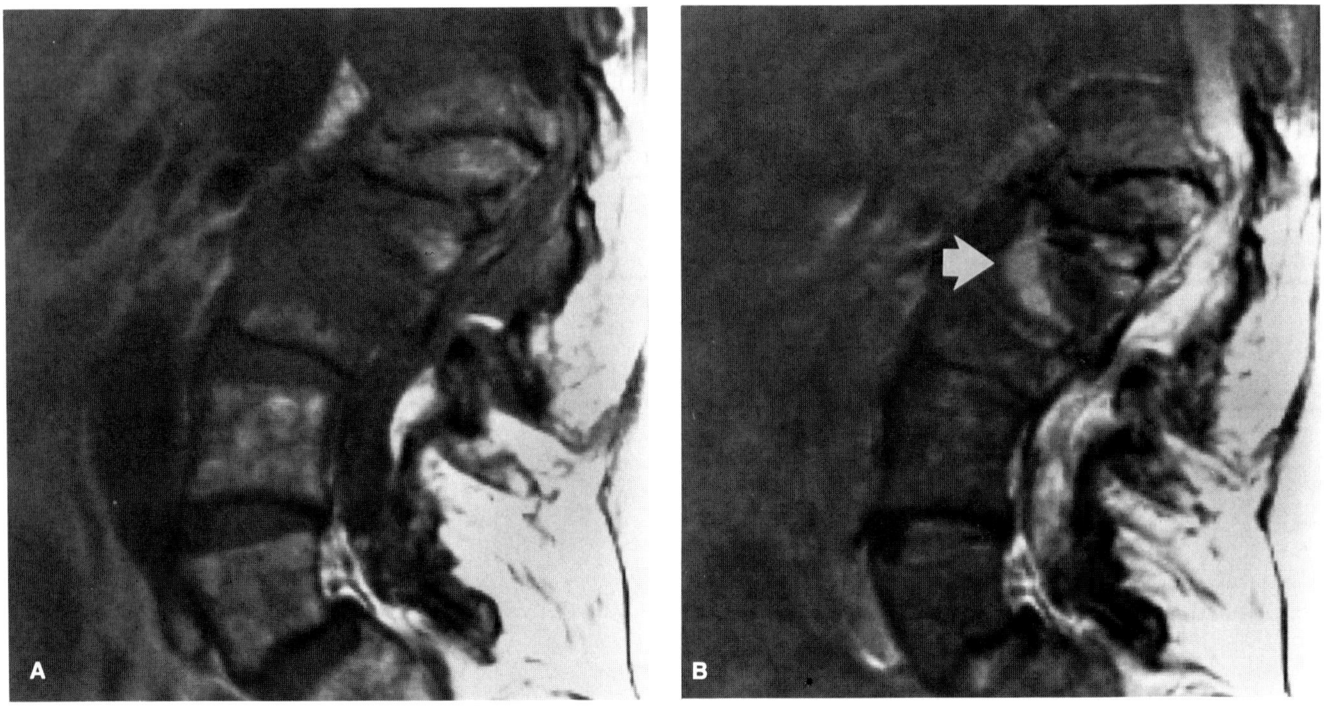

FIGURE 7–17. Vertebral osteomyelitis in a patient with history of old trauma and multiple compression fractures who presented with fever and back pain in this region. **(A)** Sagittal T1-weighted spin echo image shows the old fractures in the upper lumbar spine, with resultant deformity. **(B)** Sagittal T2-weighted image reveals the abnormal increased signal intensity within one of the vertebral bodies (arrow), which was subsequently proven to be acute osteomyelitis.

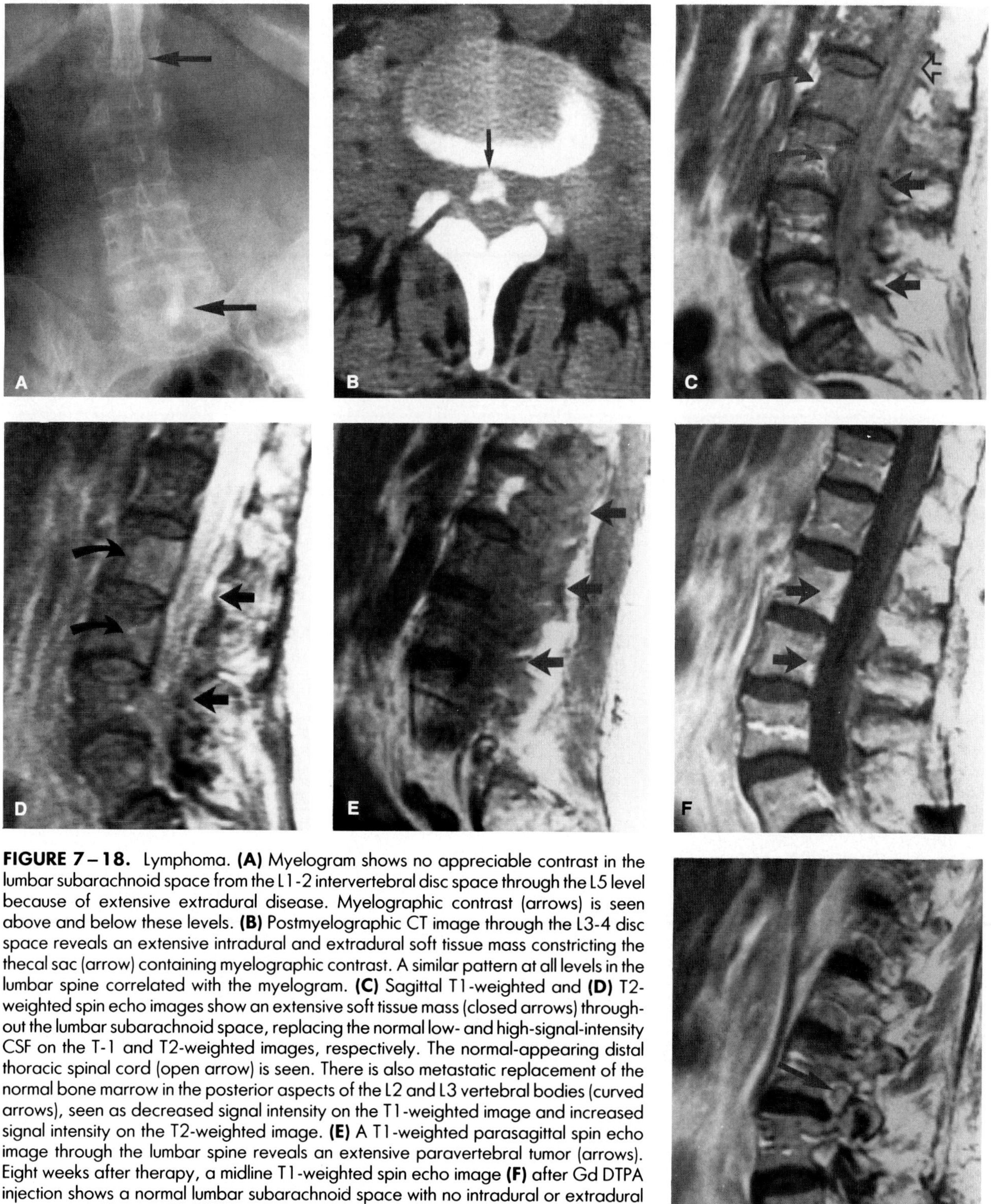

FIGURE 7–18. Lymphoma. **(A)** Myelogram shows no appreciable contrast in the lumbar subarachnoid space from the L1-2 intervertebral disc space through the L5 level because of extensive extradural disease. Myelographic contrast (arrows) is seen above and below these levels. **(B)** Postmyelographic CT image through the L3-4 disc space reveals an extensive intradural and extradural soft tissue mass constricting the thecal sac (arrow) containing myelographic contrast. A similar pattern at all levels in the lumbar spine correlated with the myelogram. **(C)** Sagittal T1-weighted and **(D)** T2-weighted spin echo images show an extensive soft tissue mass (closed arrows) throughout the lumbar subarachnoid space, replacing the normal low- and high-signal-intensity CSF on the T-1 and T2-weighted images, respectively. The normal-appearing distal thoracic spinal cord (open arrow) is seen. There is also metastatic replacement of the normal bone marrow in the posterior aspects of the L2 and L3 vertebral bodies (curved arrows), seen as decreased signal intensity on the T1-weighted image and increased signal intensity on the T2-weighted image. **(E)** A T1-weighted parasagittal spin echo image through the lumbar spine reveals an extensive paravertebral tumor (arrows). Eight weeks after therapy, a midline T1-weighted spin echo image **(F)** after Gd DTPA injection shows a normal lumbar subarachnoid space with no intradural or extradural tumor outside the vertebral bodies. Enhancing tumor is still seen in the L2 and, to a lesser extent, the L3 vertebral bodies (arrows). **(G)** A parasagittal T1-weighted spin echo image after Gd DTPA administration shows normal lumbar neuroforamina with no tumor. Epidural fat surrounds the enhanced L3 dorsal root ganglion (arrow). Enhancement of the dorsal root ganglion is a normal finding on postcontrast images.

Although single bone metastases do occur, multiplicity of lesions is the key to the diagnosis (Figs. 7–19 and 7–20). Metastatic deposits within the spine are usually easily appreciated on unenhanced images. Metastatic lesions typically produce decreased signal intensity on T1-weighted images and can be easily recognized due to their contrast against the normal high-signal-intensity fat-containing bone marrow. On T2-weighted images, metastases usually display increased signal intensity due to their long T2 relaxation times, although this can vary (Figs. 7–21 and 7–22).

Primary extradural tumors of the lumbar spine are usually single, isolated lesions and present an appearance on MRI similar to metastatic disease, with one exception.[57] Vertebral hemangiomas commonly have short T1 and long T2 relaxation times, producing increased signal intensity on both T1-weighted and T2-weighted sequences.[58] Benign deposition of fat within the axial bone marrow can also be seen and should not be confused with tumor because it displays increased signal intensity on T1-weighted images, which decreases on more heavily T2-weighted images typical of lipomatous tissue.[59] Aneurysmal bone cysts have displayed characteristic cystic appearances with different signal intensities on T1-weighted and T2-weighted images due to various stages of hemorrhage within the lesion.[60,61] With these exceptions, most primary tumors of the lumbar spine display low signal intensity on T1-weighted images and variable, increased signal intensity on T2-weighted images.

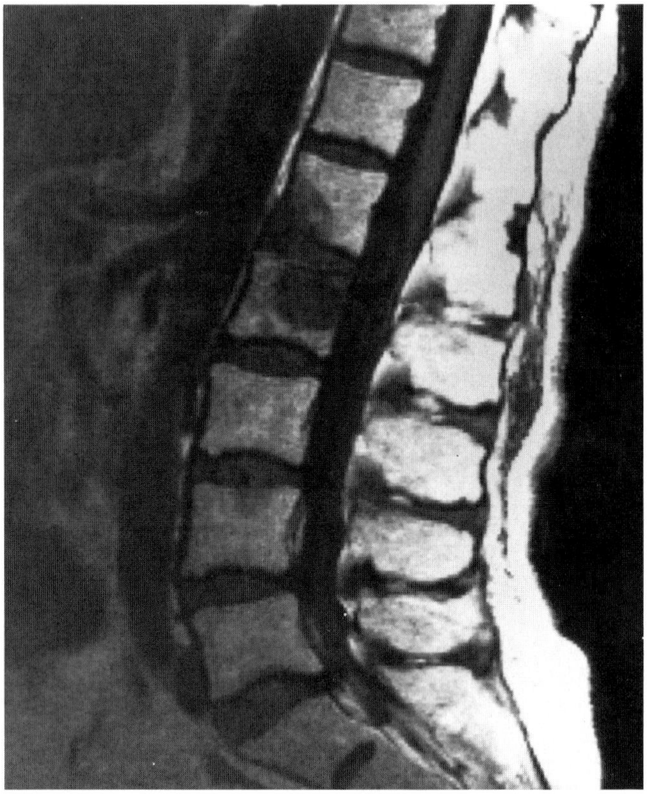

FIGURE 7–19. Malignant melanoma metastases. Sagittal T1-weighted spin echo image. Multiple low-signal-intensity metastatic deposits are seen within the vertebral bodies. These are depicted with high contrast relative to the adjacent normal high-signal-intensity fat-containing marrow.

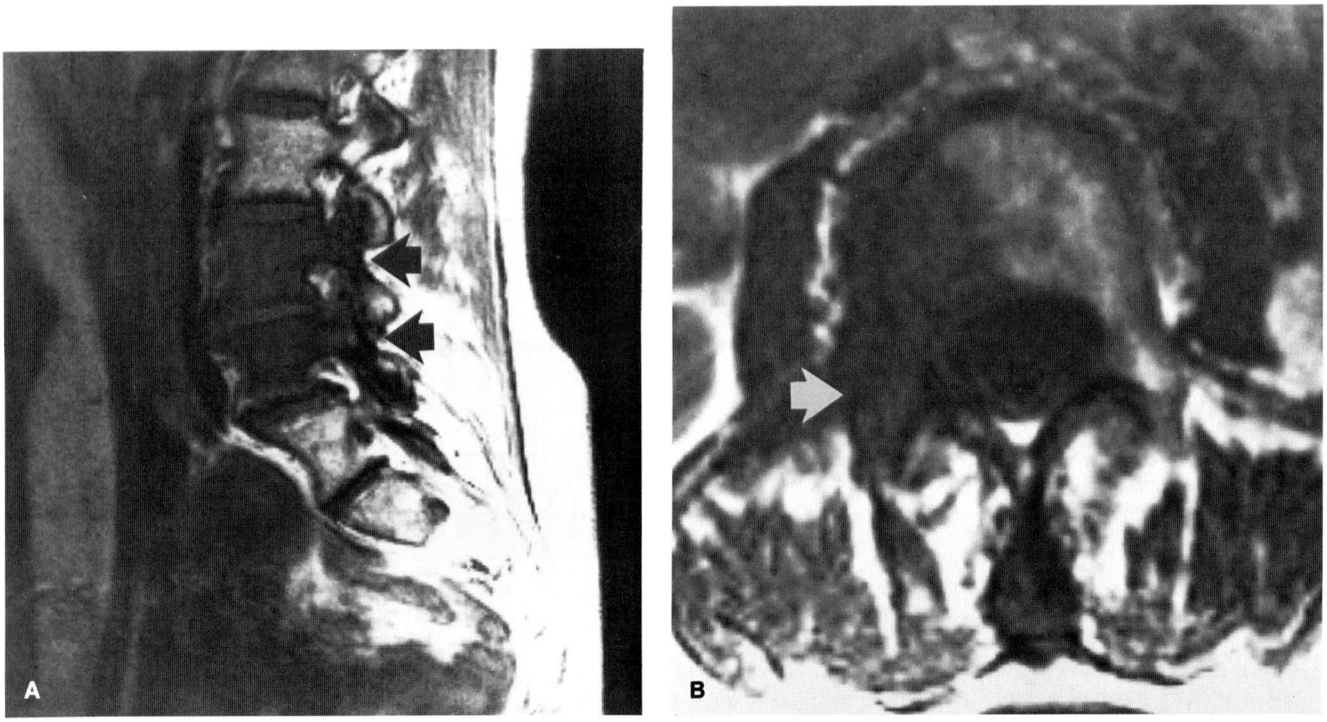

FIGURE 7–20. Breast metastases. **(A)** Sagittal and **(B)** axial T1-weighted spin echo images show the low-signal-intensity metastatic lesions replacing the normal high-signal-intensity marrow in the vertebral bodies with extension of tumor into the pedicles (arrows).

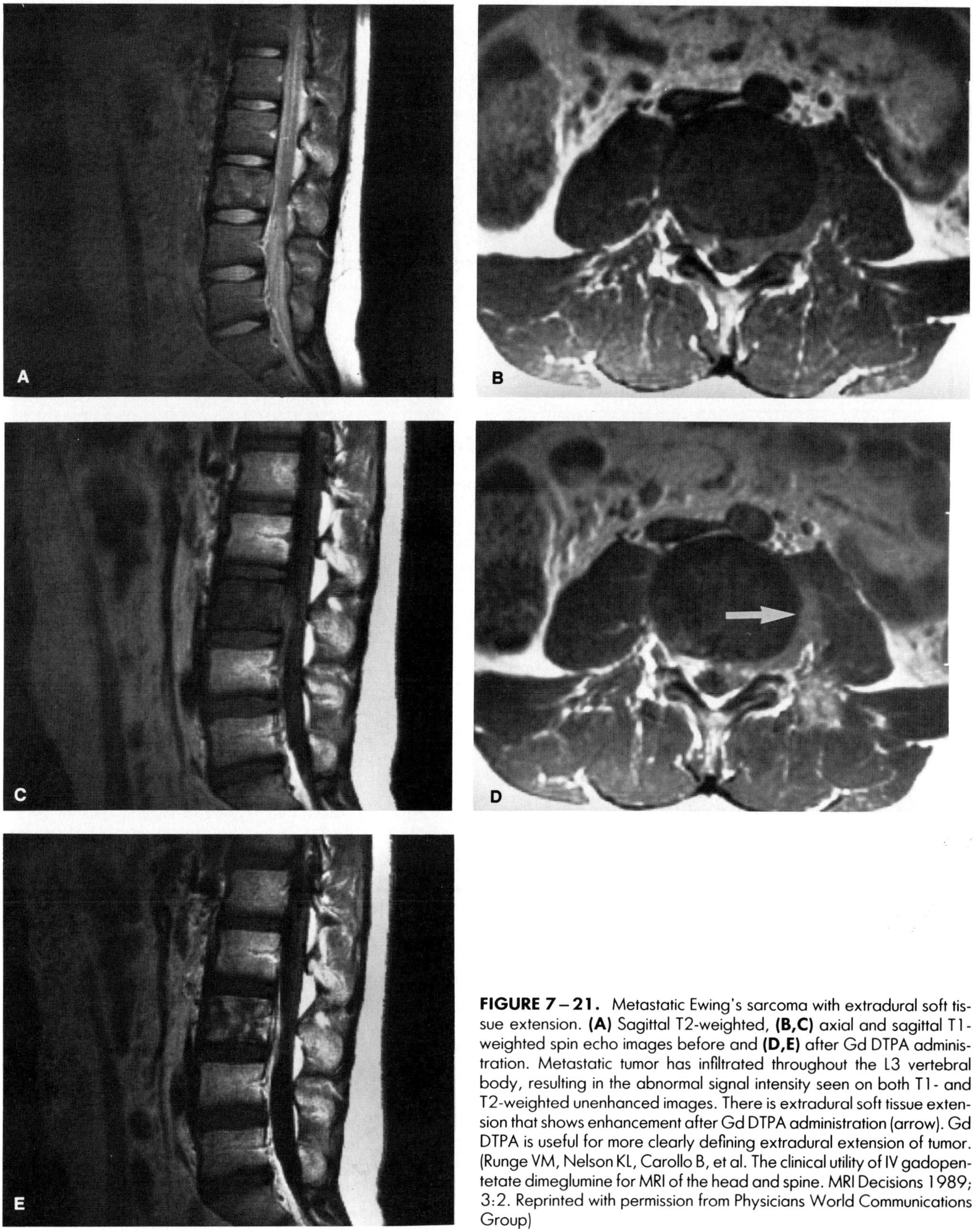

FIGURE 7–21. Metastatic Ewing's sarcoma with extradural soft tissue extension. **(A)** Sagittal T2-weighted, **(B,C)** axial and sagittal T1-weighted spin echo images before and **(D,E)** after Gd DTPA administration. Metastatic tumor has infiltrated throughout the L3 vertebral body, resulting in the abnormal signal intensity seen on both T1- and T2-weighted unenhanced images. There is extradural soft tissue extension that shows enhancement after Gd DTPA administration (arrow). Gd DTPA is useful for more clearly defining extradural extension of tumor. (Runge VM, Nelson KL, Carollo B, et al. The clinical utility of IV gadopentetate dimeglumine for MRI of the head and spine. MRI Decisions 1989; 3:2. Reprinted with permission from Physicians World Communications Group)

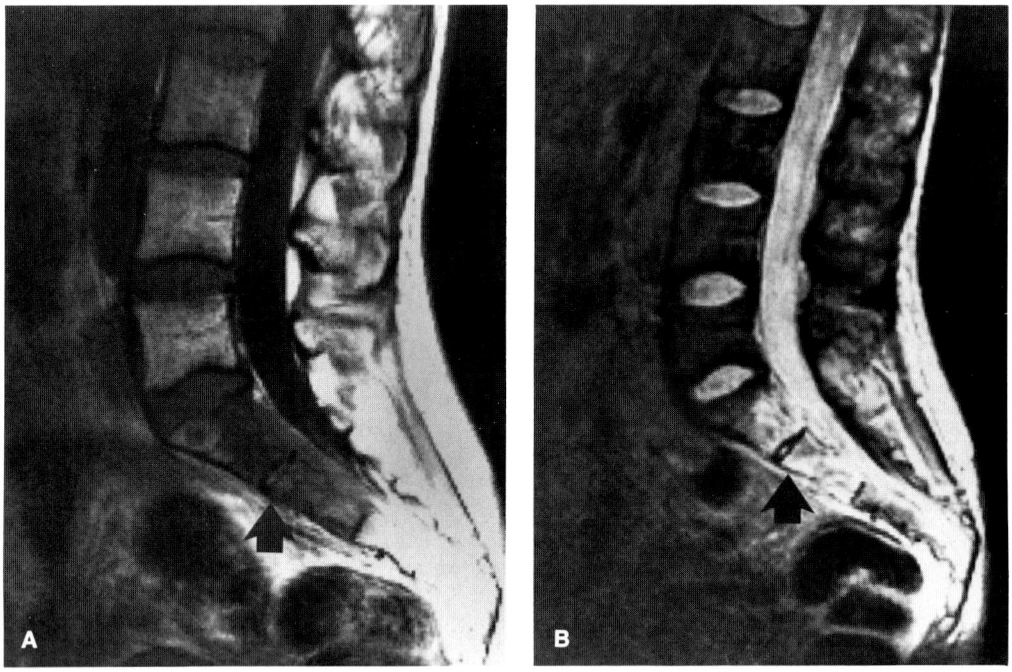

FIGURE 7–22. Metastatic Ewing's sarcoma. **(A)** Sagittal T1-weighted spin echo image shows low-signal-intensity metastatic disease involving the S1 and S2 vertebral bodies (arrow), which on the T2-weighted image **(B)** displays increased signal intensity (arrow).

Initial studies of the use of paramagnetic contrast agents have proven to be less than favorable for evaluating extradural disease limited to the bony spine. These low-signal-intensity tumors are easily demonstrated on unenhanced T1-weighted images because the tumor is contrasted against the high-signal-intensity, fat-containing, normal bone marrow. After injection of Gd DTPA, these tumors enhance and can be obscured because they display a signal intensity similar to that of normal bone marrow. Extradural soft tissue extension from bone metastases and epidural metastatic deposits may be more clearly defined by contrast enhancement, which increases their conspicuity against the normal lower-signal-intensity CSF on T1-weighted sequences (Fig. 7–21). Extension of tumor into the spinal canal therefore can be more clearly defined on Gd DTPA-enhanced images.

Extramedullary-Intradural Tumor

In the lumbar spine the most common tumors encountered in this compartment are drop metastases from intracranial neoplasms, such as gliomas, medulloblastomas, and ependymomas. Other primary malignancies of nonneurogenic origin may metastasize to the subarachnoid space.[63] Lymphoma and leukemia can also infiltrate the subarachnoid space.

These metastatic deposits usually present as nodular, well-defined masses against normal CSF within the subarachnoid space on T1-weighted images. These tumors are usually more difficult to define on T2-weighted images because both the tumor and normal CSF have long T2 relaxation times, allowing the tumor to blend with the normal high-signal-intensity CSF. Gd DTPA has been very useful in defining these tumors.[28] They generally show intense contrast enhancement on the T1-weighted sequences, becoming well-defined against the low-signal-intensity CSF. Contrast-enhanced MRI has shown greater sensitivity for detection of subarachnoid metastases than myelography or CT.[28]

The most common benign lesions in this location are the nerve sheath tumors. They include primarily neurofibromas, paragangliomas, neurolemmomas, and schwannomas. Most neurofibromas occur in multiple locations in the spine of patients with neurofibromatosis. These tumors often present as soft tissue masses in an intradural-extramedullary location although extradural extension does occur.[62,64] They usually are fairly well-defined on T1-weighted images due to their intermediate signal intensity, compared with the lower-signal-intensity CSF. They typically display increased signal intensity on T2-weighted

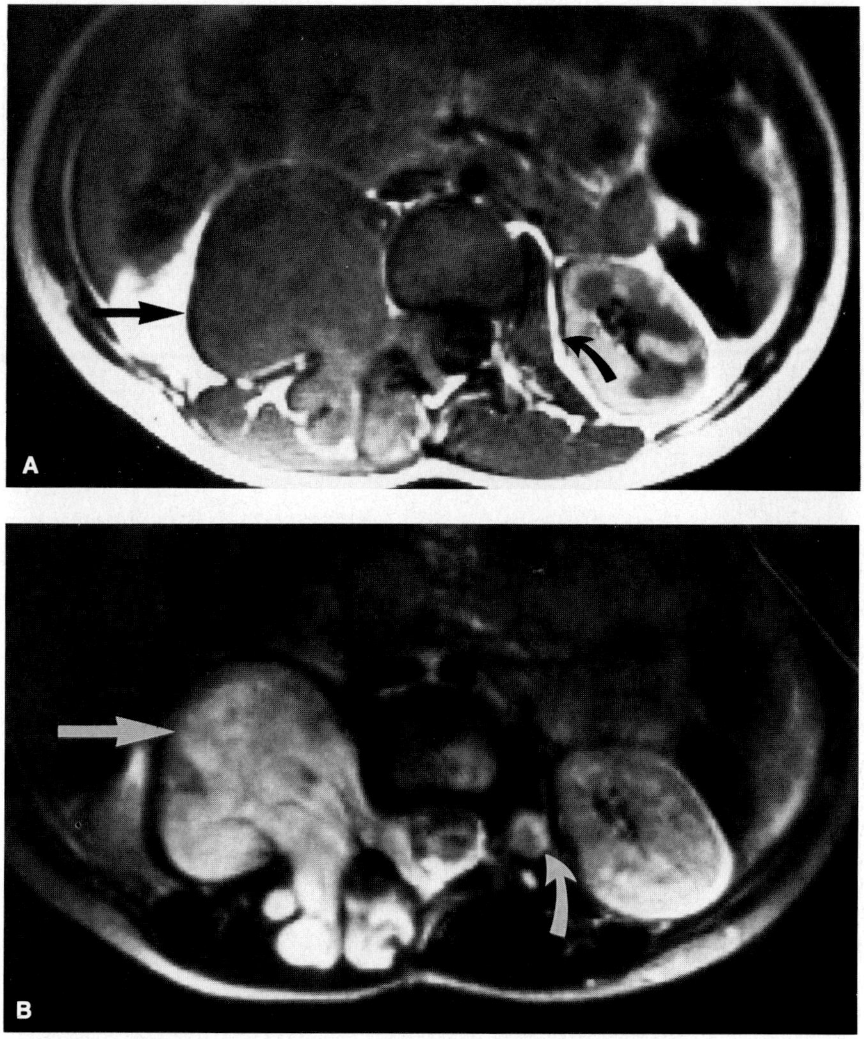

FIGURE 7–23. Paragangliomas. **(A)** Axial T1-weighted and **(B)** T2-weighted spin echo images reveal a large, primarily extradural tumor on the right (straight arrows) with a smaller left sided tumor (curved arrows). These lesions are particularly well defined on the T2-weighted image due to their prolonged T2 relaxation time.

images (Figs. 7–23 to 7–25). Most nerve sheath tumors show contrast enhancement with Gd DTPA, dramatically increasing their conspicuity in most instances (Fig. 7–26).

Meningiomas may occur rarely in the lumbar spine. They are most commonly seen in middle-aged female patients. Meningiomas usually display isointense signal characteristics on T1-weighted images, compared with normal neural tissue. Their appearance on T2-weighted images varies, although the majority display some increase in signal intensity. Like intracranial meningiomas, these tumors in the spine show excellent enhancement with paramagnetic contrast agents.

Other tumors which may be encountered in this anatomic location include developmental tumors, such as lipomas, teratomas, dermoids, and epidermoids. Most of these tumors are associated with spinal dysraphic states. Although the MR appearance of these tumors can be variable as a group, lipomas are an exception in that they consistently display in-

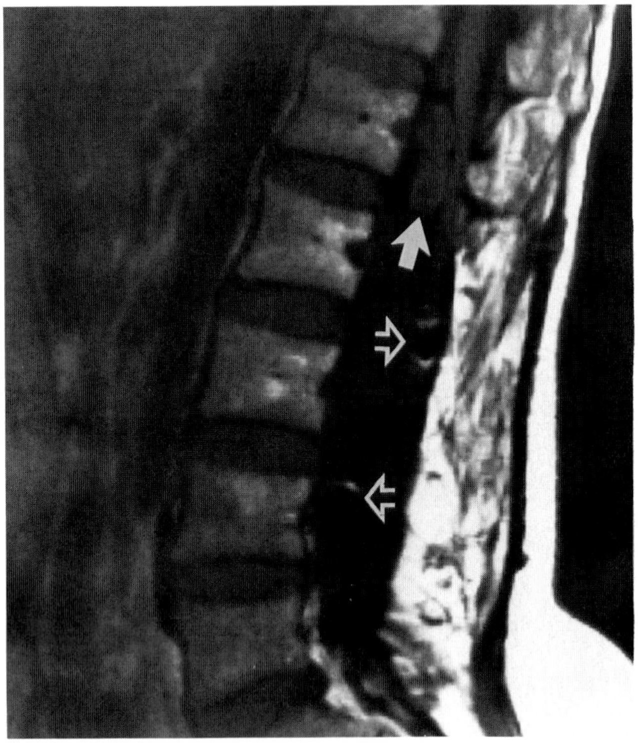

FIGURE 7–24. Schwannomas. Sagittal T1-weighted spin echo image. Three well-defined schwannomas (closed arrow) are seen in an intradural extramedullary location anterior to the conus medullaris. Areas of signal void inferiorly within the lumbar subarachnoid space (open arrows) represent small metallic artifacts from a previous surgical resection of schwannomas involving the lumbar nerves.

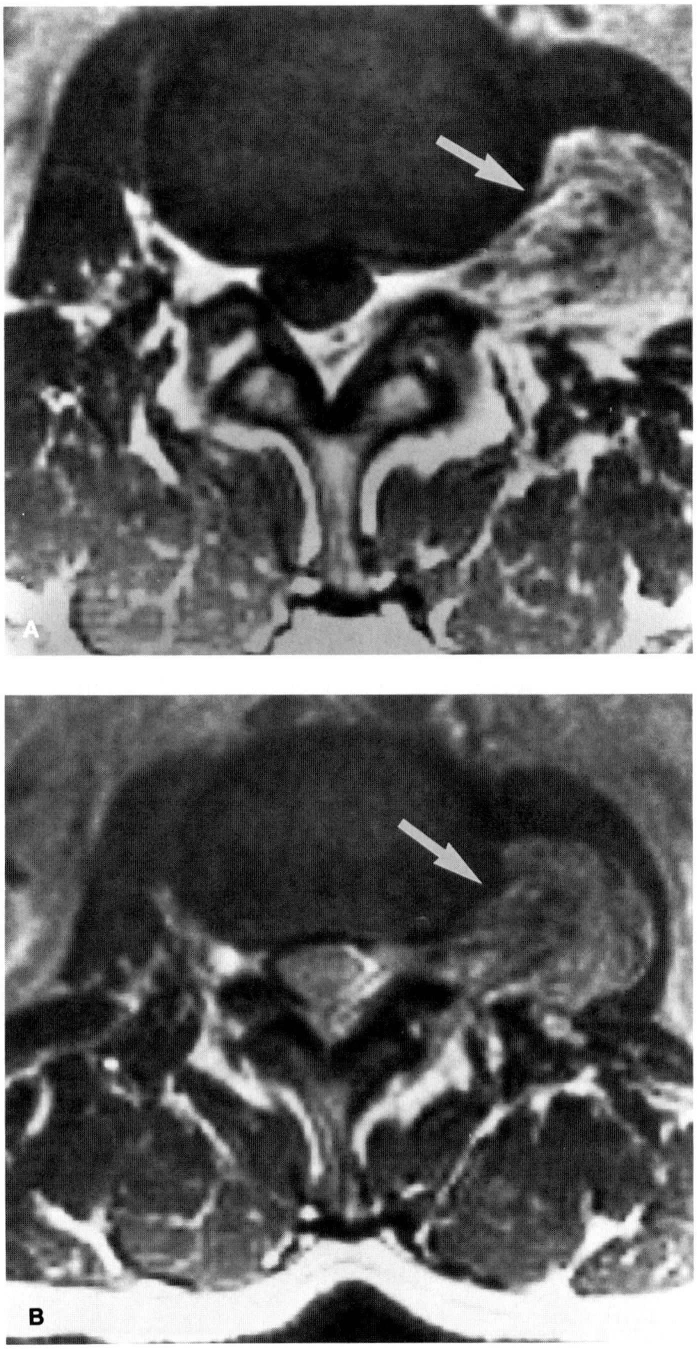

FIGURE 7–25. Liposarcoma. **(A)** Axial T1-weighted and **(B)** T2-weighted spin echo images show a fat-containing extradural tumor extending into the left L3-4 neuroforamen (arrow) and infiltrating the left psoas muscle.

creased signal intensity on T1-weighted images, which decreases with T2-weighted sequences.[65] Occasionally, lipomatous infiltration of the filum terminale can be incidently recognized (Fig. 7–27). This is rarely clinically significant, although it must be correlated with the patient's clinical presentation.

Intramedullary Tumor

Although generally not an indication for lumbar spine MRI, intramedullary disease of the conus medullaris is occasionally identified. MRI is the best way to study lesions of the conus medullaris. The most common intramedullary neoplasms occurring in the conus

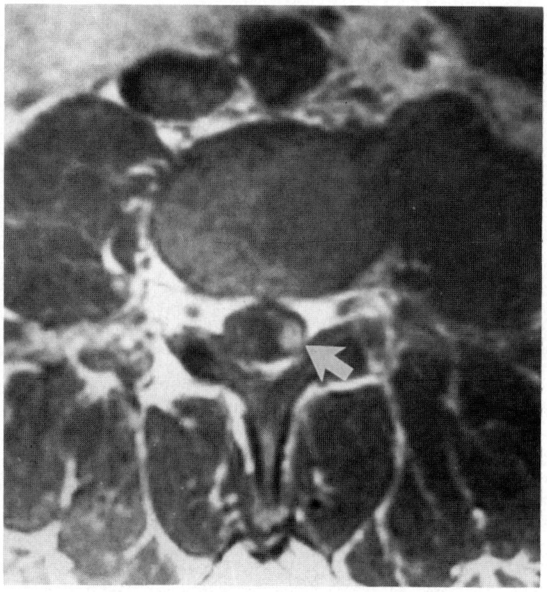

FIGURE 7–26. Neurolemmoma. Axial T1-weighted spin echo image after Gd DTPA enhancement. The contrast-enhanced neurolemmoma (arrow) originating from a lumbar nerve is well defined in the subarachnoid space. Almost all nerve sheath tumors display enhancement, increasing their conspicuity against the surrounding normal low-signal-intensity CSF.

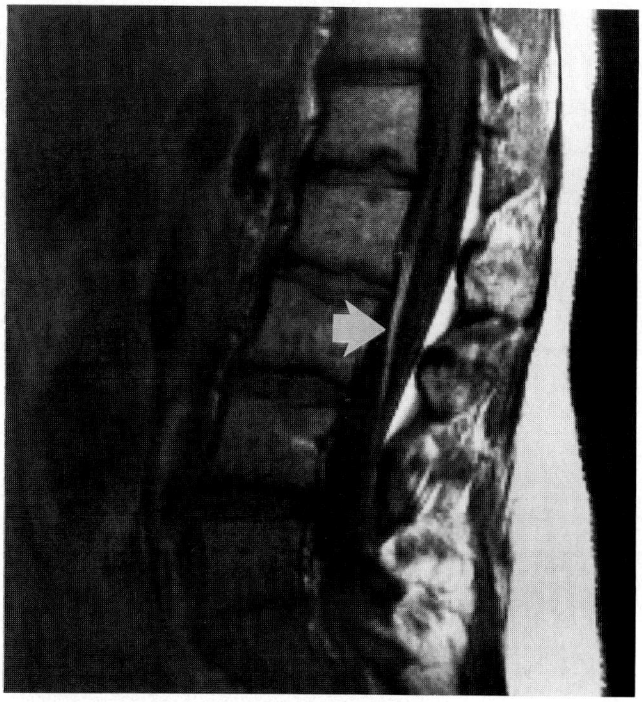

FIGURE 7–27. Lipomatous infiltration of the filum terminale. Sagittal T1-weighted spin echo image shows high-signal-intensity lipomatous infiltration (arrow) of the filum terminale.

medullaris are ependymomas, which can also involve the filum terminale (Fig. 7–28).[66] These tumors may enlarge to fill the lumbar subarachnoid space and cause posterior vertebral body scalloping (Fig. 7–29). Often cystic components can be recognized within the tumor. These tumors are usually amenable to surgery and radiation therapy.

Gliomas in the spinal cord are most commonly low-grade astrocytomas. They can be recognized by their expansion of the conus medullaris on T1-weighted images, and they usually have increased signal intensity on T2-weighted images. Syrinx cavities may accompany the tumor.

Although uncommon, hemangioblastomas can occur in the spinal cord and are most often associated with von Hippel-Lindau disease. Usually multiple in the spinal cord, these tumors are associated with intracranial hemangioblastomas occuring in the posterior fossa.

Paramagnetic contrast agents are beneficial in assessing intramedullary spinal cord tumors. They may allow the separation of tumor from edema, better define tumor extent, and differentiate a benign simple syrinx cavity from neoplastic cavitation.[67,68] This is useful for planning a surgical approach or defining radiation therapy portals.

Trauma

MRI is usually not employed for the initial examination in the posttraumatic patient with a suspected lumbar spine abnormality. Difficulties include the inability to image patients in critical condition who require ventilatory support or stabilization devices containing ferromagnetic metal. It is often impossible for these patients to cooperate during the long imaging times required for a diagnostic MRI examination. Plain film radiography and CT are the modalities of choice for defining fractures, dislocations, and displacement of cortical bone fragments in acutely traumatized patients.

If these patients can be safely imaged, MRI is able to provide excellent morphologic detail of the fracture fragments.[69] The multiplanar imaging capabilities allow demonstration of the relationship between fracture fragments and the conus medullaris or their positions within the spinal canal. Acute fractures of the vertebral body typically display isointense or de-

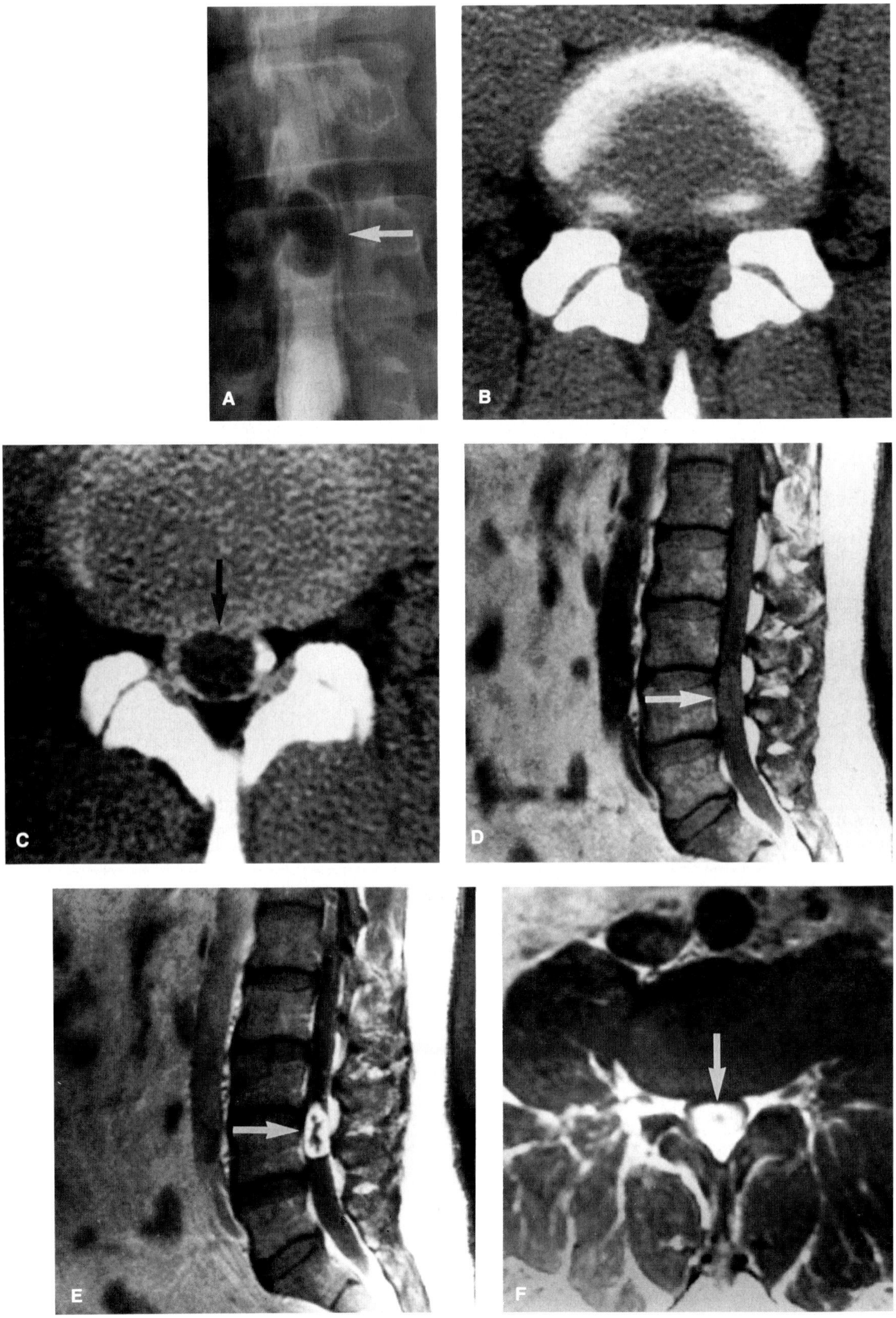

FIGURE 7–28.

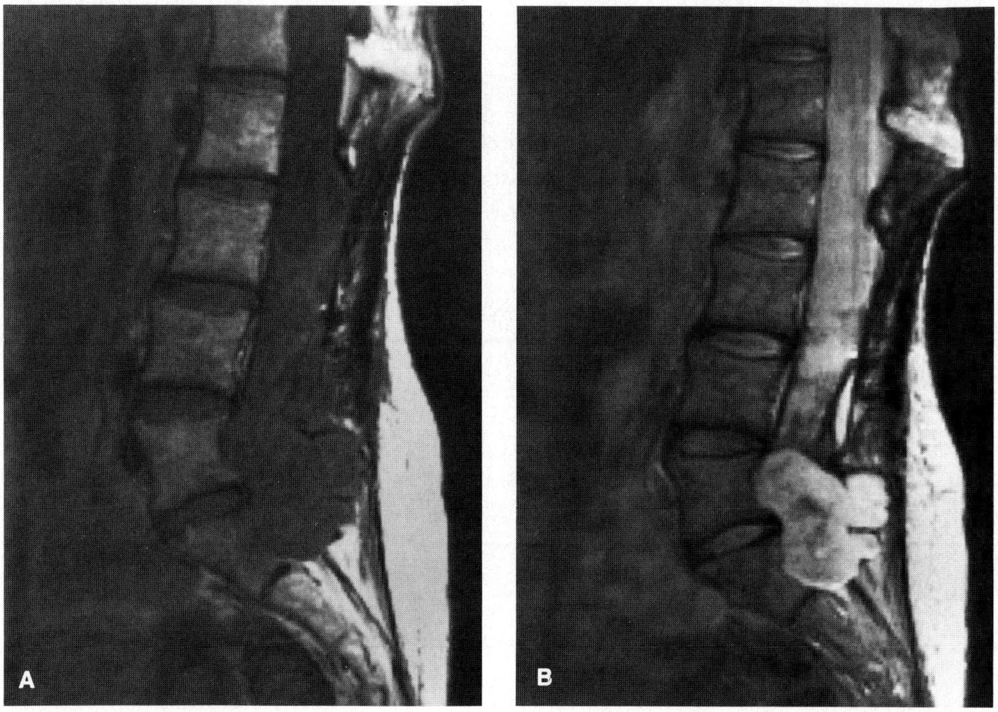

FIGURE 7–29. Ependymoma. **(A)** Sagittal T1-weighted and **(B)** T2-weighted spin echo images show a large mass filling the lumbar subarachnoid space inferiorly from the L3 level, with posterior scalloping of the L5 and S1 vertebral bodies.

creased signal intensity characteristics on T1-weighted images and increased signal intensity on T2-weighted images.[70] These findings are attributed to hemorrhage and edema. Old fractures typically display low signal intensity on both T1-weighted and T2-weighted sequences.

In the subacute stages of spine trauma, persistent pain may be caused by disc herniation and epidural hematoma formation. MRI can confirm disc herniation associated with spine fractures and epidural hematomas, thereby obviating the need for myelography.[71]

In elderly patients presenting with trauma, which may be minimal, it may be very difficult to differentiate an osteoporotic compression fracture from a metastatic compression fracture. Both osteoporotic and metastatic compression fractures display low signal intensities on T1-weighted images, and separation of the two entities can not be accomplished with T1-weighted or T2-weighted images.[72] By defining other hypointense foci of metastatic disease in other noncollapsed vertebral bodies, the diagnosis of metastatic disease can be suggested. Gd DTPA is useful for differentiation, because metastatic compression fractures display contrast enhancement, but osteoporotic compression fractures do not. Follow-up examinations are useful. Osteoporotic compression fractures eventually assume a more normal signal intensity compared with normal bone marrow, but metastatic compression fractures continue to display abnormal low signal intensity on T1-weighted images.

The evaluation of posttraumatic myelopathy is best accomplished with MRI.[73] Posttraumatic cysts or myelomalacia can be easily recognized within the

◀ **FIGURE 7–28.** Ependymoma of the filum terminale. **(A)** Myelogram, **(B,C)** axial CT images before and after injection of intrathecal contrast at the level of the L3-4 intervertebral disc. A large intradural tumor (arrow) is seen in the lumbar subarachnoid space on the myelogram. The tumor cannot be seen on the premyelogram CT image, because it has attenuation characteristics similar to that of the normal CSF in the lumbar subarachnoid space. The postmyelogram CT image at the same level defines the low attenuation tumor (arrow) because it is outlined by the surrounding myelographic contrast agent within the subarachnoid space. **(D)** Sagittal precontrast, **(E)** sagittal postcontrast and **(F)** axial postcontrast T1-weighted spin echo images. Before Gd DTPA administration, the slightly increased signal intensity tumor (arrow) can be seen in the lumbar subarachnoid space. After Gd DTPA, the tumor shows marked peripheral enhancement (arrows) and central nonenhancement. The conspicuity of many intradural tumors, such as ependymomas, is increased with the use of Gd DTPA.

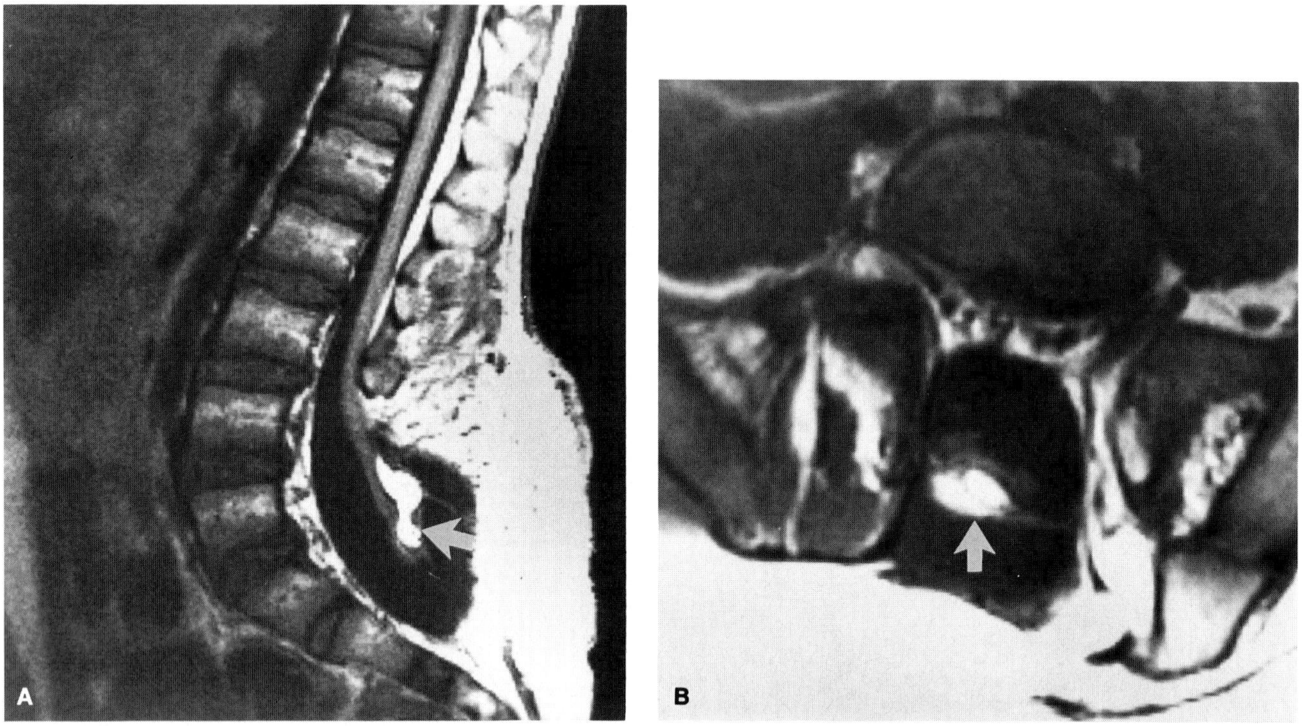

FIGURE 7–30. Postoperative lipomyelomeningocele. **(A)** Sagittal and **(B)** axial T1-weighted spin echo images show a large lipoma (arrow) adjacent to the neural placode posteriorly. (Traill MT, Runge VM, Wolpert SM. Dysraphism: MRI strategies. MRI Decisions 1989; 2:2. Reprinted with permission from Physicians World Communications Group)

conus medullaris. In the acute or subacute stage, MRI can also demonstrate contusion of the conus or hematomyelia.[74] In the chronic stages, hemosiderin can be recognized.

Spinal Dysraphism

Spinal dysraphism represents a spectrum of congenital disorders caused by a failure of fusion of midline mesenchymal, bone, and neural structures. There is universally a defect in the bony spine. Spina bifida occulta is the most benign form of spinal dysraphism.

More severe forms of spinal dysraphism can occur. Meningoceles are formed as a protrusion of the dura and arachnoid tissue through the bony defect in the spine to the skin surface. Myeloceles contain neural elements extending through the defect to the skin surface. Myelomeningoceles protrude outisde the skin surface, with dilatation of the underlying subarachnoid space. In myeloceles and myelomeningoceles, the dysraphic spinal cord is exposed to the skin surface as a neural plaque. The dorsal and ventral nerve roots originate from the ventral surface of the plaque. A lipomyelomeningocele occurs if a lipoma develops dorsal to the surface of the neural plaque (Fig. 7–30).

In these disorders the distal spinal cord is usually in an abnormally low location, tethered to the neural plaque (Fig. 7–31). In tethered cord syndrome, there

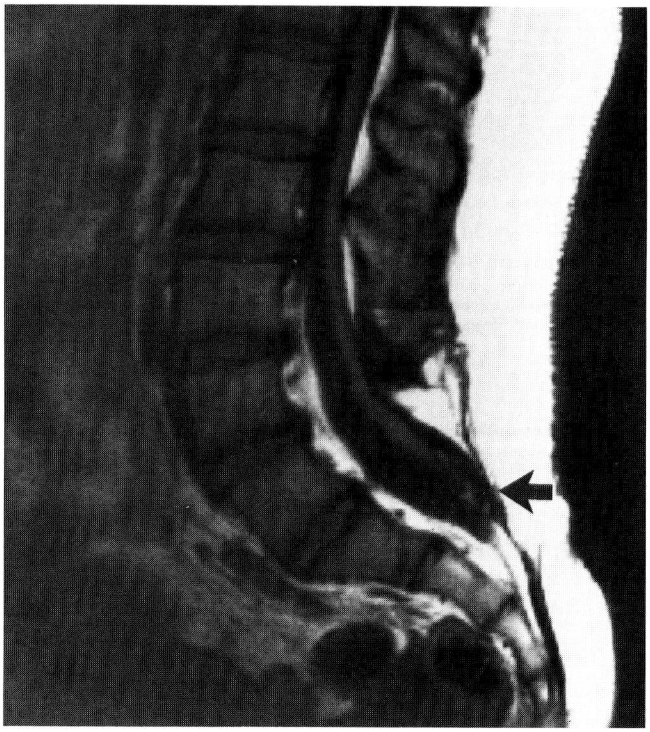

FIGURE 7–31. Tethered spinal cord with small lipoma. Sagittal T1-weighted spin echo image. There is a tethered spinal cord, with lipomatous infiltration distally (arrow) at the site of tethering seen as high signal intensity. (Trail MT, Runge VM, Wolpert SM. Dysraphism: MRI strategies. MRI Decisions 1989; 2:2. Reprinted with permission from Physicians World Communications Group)

is an abnormally low conus medullaris due to a thickened filum; it is not associated with any of the other described abnormalities.

Diastematomyelia is a form of spinal dysraphism. It occurs as a sagittal bony or fibrous cleft, over one or, less commonly, two segments. This produces two asymmetric hemicords, which usually reunite below the cleft (Fig. 7–32). Myeloschisis is cleavage of the spinal cord; diplomyelia is an almost perfect duplication of the spinal cord. Usually diastematomyelia is associated with a tethered spinal cord, myelomeningocele, or lipomyelomeningocele. Uncommon spinal dysraphic states include lipomyeloschisis, dorsal dermal sinus, spinal lipomas, and sacral agenesis. Scoliosis and vertebral body abnormalities, including congenital block vertebrae or hemivertebrae, can usually be defined with MRI.

Although plain films should always be obtained to define bony anatomy, MRI is now the best means for evaluating spinal dysraphism.[75] Its multiplanar imaging capabilities allow excellent morphologic detail of abnormal neural and soft tissue anatomy. The exami-

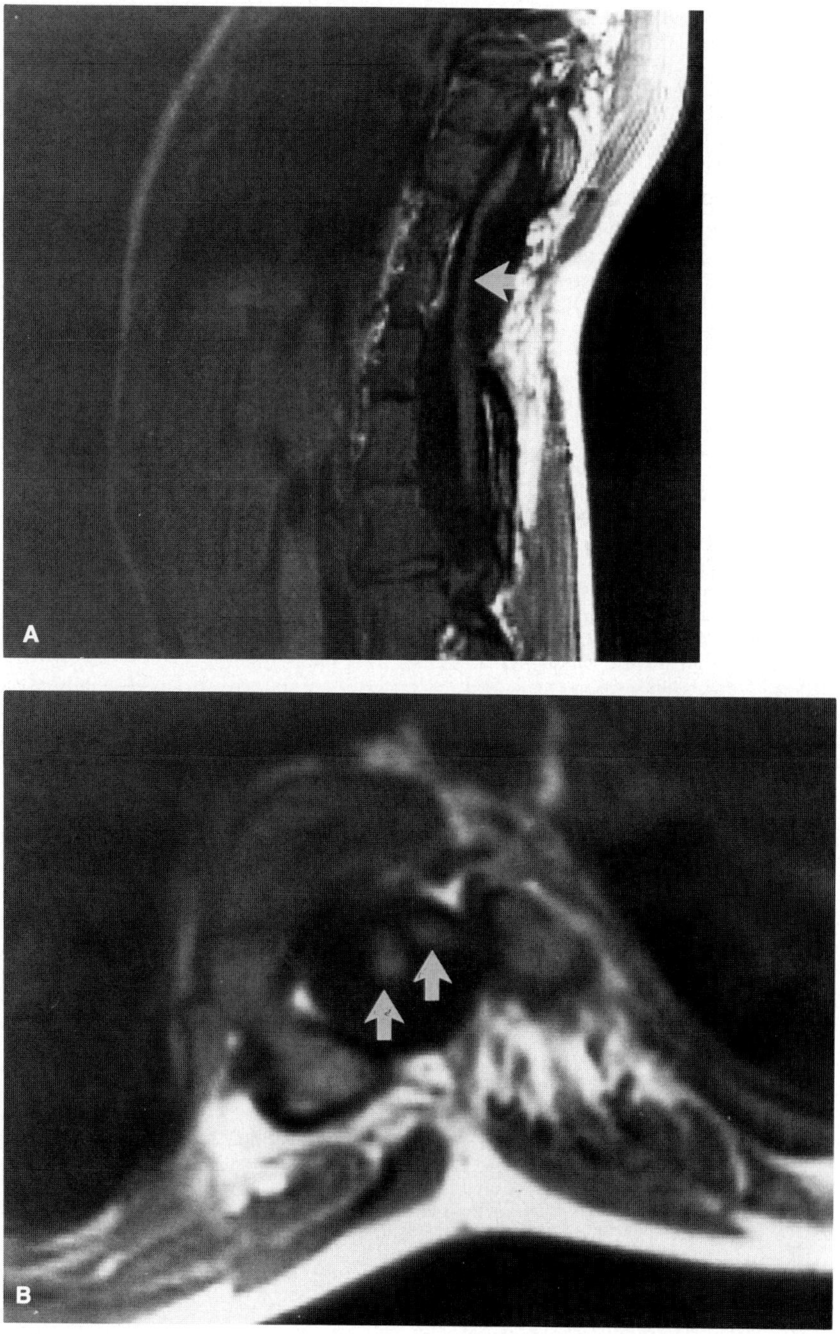

FIGURE 7–32. Diastematomyelia. **(A)** Sagittal T1-weighted spin echo image through one of the two hemicords (arrow). **(B)** Axial T1-weighted image reveals the two hemicords (arrows) within the spinal canal.

nation is less hazardous than water-soluble myelography and lacks ionizing radiation, which is an important consideration in pediatric patients.[76]

REFERENCES

1. Edelman RR, Shoukimas GM, Stark DD, et al. High resolution surface coil imaging of lumbar disc disease. AJR 1985;144:1123.
2. Berger PE, Atkinson D, Wilson WJ, Wiltse JL. High resolution surface coil magnetic resonance imaging of the spine: normal and pathologic anatomy. Radiographics 1986;6:573.
3. Haughton VM. MR imaging of the spine. Radiology 1988;166:297.
4. Mills TC, Ortendahl DA, Hylton NM. Partial flip angle MR imaging. Radiology 1987;162:531.
5. Enzmann DR, Rubin JB. Cervical spine: MR imaging with a partial flip angle gradient refocused pulse sequence. I. General considerations and disc disease. Radiology 1988;166:467.
6. Enzmann DR, Rubin JB. Cervical spine: MR imaging with a partial flip angle gradient refocused pulse sequence. II. Spinal cord disease. Radiology 1988;166:473.
7. Rubin JB, Enzmann DR, Wright A. CSF-gated MR imaging of the spine: theory and clinical implementation. Radiology 1984;163:784.
8. Haacke EM, Lenz GW. Improving MR image quality in the presence of motion by using rephasing gradients. AJR 1987;148:1251.
9. Rubin JB, Enzmann DR. Optimizing conventional MR imaging of the spine. Radiology 1987;163:777.
10. Enzmann DR, Rubin JB, Wright A. Use of cerebrospinal fluid gating to improve T2-weighted images. I. The spinal cord. Radiology 1987;162:763.
11. Rubin JB, Wright A, Enzmann DR. Lumbar spine: motion compensation for cerebrospinal fluid on MR imaging. Radiology 1988;166:225.
12. Edelman RR, Atkinson DJ, Silver MS, et al. FRODO pulse sequences: a new means of eliminating motion, flow, and wraparound artifacts. Radiology 1988;166:231.
13. Aguila LA, Piraino DW, Modic MT, et al. Intranuclear cleft of the intervertebral disk: magnetic resonance imaging. Radiology 1985;155:155.
14. Pech P, Haughton VM. Lumbar intervertebral disk: correlative MR and anatomic study. Radiology 1985;156:699.
15. Runge VM, Wood ML, Kaufman D, Price AC: Gd DTPA: future applications with advanced imaging techniques. Radiographics 1988;8:161.
16. Hueftle MG, Modic MT, Ross JS, et al. Lumbar spine: postoperative MR imaging with Gd-DTPA. Radiology 1988;167:817.
17. Valk J. Gd-DTPA in MR of spinal lesions. AJR 1988;150:1163.
18. Sze G, Abramson A, Krol G, et al. Gadolinium DTPA in the evaluation of intradural extramedullary spinal disease. AJNR 1988;9:153.
19. Knop RH, Frank JA, Dwyer AJ, et al. Gadolinium cryptelates as MR contrast agents. J Comput Assist Tomogr 1987;11:35.
20. Bousquet JC, Saini S, Stark DD, et al. Gd DOTA: characterization of a new paramagnetic complex. Radiology 1988;166:693.
21. Runge VM, Jacobson S, Wood ML, et al. MR imaging of rat brain glioma: Gd DTPA versus Gd DOTA. Radiology 1988;166:835.
22. Magerstadt M, Gansow OA, Brechbiel MW, et al. Gd (DOTA): an alternative to Gd (DTPA) as a T1,2 relaxation agent for NMR imaging or spectroscopy. Magn Reson Med 1986;3:808.
23. Weinmann H-J, Brasch RC, Press WR, Wesbey GE. Characterizations of gadolinium DTPA complex: a potential NMR contrast agent. AJR 1984;142:619.
24. Engelstad BL, Wolf GL. Contrast agents. In: Stark DD, Bradley WB, eds. Magnetic resonance imaging. St. Louis: CV Mosby, 1988.
25. Nelson KL, Runge VM. Basic principles of paramagnetic contrast media. In: Runge VM, ed. Enhanced magnetic resonance imaging. St. Louis; CV Mosby, 1989.
26. Sze G, Krol G, Zimmerman RD, et al. Intramedullary disease of the spine: diagnosis using gadolinium-DTPA-enhanced MR imaging. AJNR 1988;9:847.
27. Nelson KL, Runge VM, Pacetti M. Differentiation of recurrent disc herniation from epidural fibrosis in the postoperative lumbar spine with Gd DTPA enhanced MRI. Presented at the Sixth Annual Meeting of the Society of Magnetic Resonance Imaging, February/March 1988, Boston, MA.
28. Sze G, Krol G, Zimmerman RD, Deck MDF. Malignant extradural spinal tumors: MR imaging with Gd-DTPA. Radiology 1988;167:217.
29. Stauffer RN: Orthopedic surgery. JAMA 1984;252:2237.
30. Peterson HO, Kieffer SA. Radiology of intervertebral disk disease. Semin Roentgenol 1972;7:260.
31. Hudgins WR. The predictive value of myelography in the diagnosis of ruptured lumbar discs. J Neurosurg 1970;32:152.
32. Williams AL, Haughton VM, Daniels DL, et al. CT recognition of lateral lumbar disk herniation. AJNR 1982;139:245.
33. Modic MT, Masaryk TJ, Boumphrey F, et al. Lumbar herniated disc disease and canal stenosis: prospective evaluation by surface coil MR, CT and myelography. AJNR 1986;7:709.
34. Maravilla KR, Lash HP, Weinreb JC, et al. Magnetic resonance imaging of the lumbar spine with CT correlation. AJNR 1985;6:237.
35. Bosaco SJ, Berman AT. Surgical management of lumbar disc disease. Radiol Clin North Am 1983;21:377.
36. Masaryk TJ, Ross JS, Modic MT. High-resolution MR imaging of sequestered lumbar intervertebral disks. AJR 1988;150:1155.
37. Lipson SJ, Muir H. Experimental disc degeneration: morphologic and proteoglycan changes over time. Arthritis Rheum 1981;24:12.
38. Grenier N, Grossman RI, Scheibler ML, et al. Degenerative lumbar disk disease: pitfalls and usefulness of MR imaging in detection of vacuum phenomenon. Radiology 1987;164:861.
39. Ross JS, Perez-Reyes N, Masaryk TJ, et al. Thoracic disk herniation: MR imaging. Radiology 1987;165:511.
40. deRoos A, Kressel H, Spritzer C, et al. MR imaging of marrow changes adjacent to end plates in degenerative lumbar disk disease. AJR 1987;149:531.
41. Modic MT, Steinberg PM, Ross JS, et al. Degenerative disk disease: assessment of changes in vertebral body marrow with MR imaging. Radiology 1988;166:193.
42. Grenier N, Kressel HY, Sachiebler ML, et al. Normal and degenerative posterior spinal structures: MR imaging. Radiology 1987;165:517.
43. Burton CV, Kirkaldy-Willis WH, Yong-Hing K, Heithoff KB. Cause of failure of surgery on the lumbar spine. Clin Orthop 1981;157:191.
44. Bundschuh CV, Modic MT, Ross JS, et al. Epidural fibrosis and recurrent disk herniation in the lumbar spine; MR imaging assessment. AJR 1988;150:923.
45. Ross JS, Masaryk TJ, Modic MT, et al. Lumbar spine: post-operative assessment with surface-coil MR imaging. Radiology 1987;164:851.
46. Teplick JG, Haskin ME. Intravenous contrast enhanced CT of the postoperative lumbar spine. AJR 1984;143:845.
47. Braun IF, et al. Contrast enhancement in CT differentiation between recurrent disk herniation and postoperative scar: prospective study. AJR 1985;145:785.
48. Runge VM. Gd DTPA: an I.V. contrast agent for clinical MRI. Nucl Med Biol 1988;15:37.
49. Quiles M, Marchisello PJ, Tsairis R, et al. Lumbar adhesive arachnoiditis, etiologic and pathologic aspects. Spine 1978;3:45.
50. Quencer RM, Tenner M, Rothman L. The postoperative myelogram. Radiology 1977;123:667.
51. Ross JS, Masaryk TJ, Modic MT, et al. MR imaging of lumbar arachnoiditis. AJNR 1988;8:885.
52. Ross JS: Gadolinium DTPA imaging of the lumbar spine. Presented at the Sixth Annual Meeting of the Society of Magnetic Resonance Imaging, February/March 1988, Boston, MA.
53. Huckman MS, Clark JW, McNeil TW, et al. Chemonucleation and changes observed on lumbar MR scan: preliminary report. 1987;AJNR 8:1.

54. Modic MT, Feiglin DH, Piraino DW, et al. Vertebral osteomyelitis: assessment using MR. Radiology 1985;157:157.
55. Masaryk TJ, Modic MT. Lumbar spine. In: Stark DD, Bradley WB, eds. Magnetic resonance imaging. St. Louis: CV Mosby, 1988.
56. de Roos A, van Persijn van Meerten Els L, Bloem JL, et al. MRI of tuberculous spondylosis. AJR 1986;146:79.
57. Bloem JL, Bluemm RG, Taminian AHM, et al. Magnetic resonance imaging of primary malignant bone tumors. Radiographics 1987;7:425.
58. Ross JS, Masaryk TJ, Modic MT, et al. Vertebral hemangiomas: MR imaging. Radiology 1987;165:165.
59. Hajek PC, Baker LL, Goobar JE, et al. Focal fat deposition in axial bone marrow: MR characteristics. Radiology 1987;162:245.
60. Hudson TM. Fluid levels in aneurysmal bone cysts: a CT feature. AJR 1984;142:1001.
61. Beltran J, Simon DC, Levy M, et al. Aneurysmal bone cysts: MR imaging at 1.5 T. Radiology 1986;158:689.
62. Scotti G, Scaialfa G, Colombo N, et al. MR imaging of intradural extramedullary tumors of the cervical spine. J Comput Assist Tomogr 1985;9:1037.
63. Post MJD, Quencer RM, Green BA, et al. Intramedullary spinal cord metastases, mainly of non-neurogenic origin. AJNR 1987;8:339.
64. Burk DL Jr, Brunberg JA, Kanal E, et al. Spinal and paraspinal neurofibromatosis: distinction from benign tumors using imaging techniques. AJR 1987;149:1059.
65. Thomas JE, Miller RH. Lipomatous tumors of the spinal canal. Mayo Clin Proc 1973;48:393.
66. Wagle WA, Jaufman B, Mincy JE. Intradural extramedullary ependymoma: MR-pathologic correlation. J Compt Assist Tomogr 1988;12:705.
67. Solomon RA, Stein BM. Unusual spinal cord enlargement related to intramedullary hemangioblastoma. J Neurosurg 1970;33:676.
68. Nelson KL, Modic MT. Enhanced magnetic resonance imaging of the spine. In: Runge VM, ed. Enhanced magnetic resonance imaging. St. Louis: CV Mosby, 1989.
69. Tarr RW. MR imaging of recent spinal trauma. J Comput Assist Tomogr 1987;11:412.
70. McArdle CB, Crofford MJ, Mirfakhrace M, et al. Surface coil MR of spinal trauma: preliminary experience. AJNR 1986;7:885.
71. Quencer RM, Beasley RE, Cammisa FJ, et al. MR in nonpenetrating spine injuries: use in clinical management. AJNR 1988;9:1001.
72. Dooms G, Maldaque B, Malghem J, et al. MR differential diagnosis between benign and malignant vertebral collapses. Radiology 1988;169:65.
73. Gebarski SS, Gebarski KS, Bowerman RA, Silver TM. Posttraumatic progressive myelopathy. Radiology 1985;157:379.
74. Hackney DB, Asato R, Joseph PM, et al. Hemorrhage and edema in acute spinal cord compression: demonstration by MR imaging. Radiology 1986;161:387.
75. Barnes PD, Lester PD, Yamanashi WS, et al. Magnetic resonance imaging in infants and children with spinal dysraphism. AJNR 1986;7:465.
76. Davis PC, Hoffman JC Jr, Ball TI, et al. Spinal abnormalities in pediatric patients: MR imaging findings compared with clinical, myelographic and surgical findings. Radiology 1988;166:679.

8 Neck, Oropharynx, and Nasopharynx

E. Kent Yucel
Barbara L. Carter

The technical considerations applicable to head and neck magnetic resonance imaging (MRI) are similar to those involved in nonneurologic imaging of other areas of the body: maximizing the signal-to-noise ratio (SNR) within an acceptable imaging time, optimizing contrast among abnormalities, fat, and muscle, and achieving satisfactory resolution. The parameters that must be selected by the operator for each examination are coil, pulse sequences, imaging plane(s), slice thickness, number of acquisitions, and matrix size.

The oropharynx and nasopharynx, paranasal sinuses, salivary glands, and facial bones are usually imaged with a standard head coil. However, to maximize SNR, the smallest-diameter cylindrical coil that can be fitted to a given patient's head and will provide an adequate field of view should be used. Coils with quadrature detection may soon provide superior SNRs.

As in all MR imaging, the choice of pulse sequences is crucial in determining the diagnostic quality of the examination. MRI of the head and neck has been performed almost entirely with spin echo sequences. Use of both heavily T1-weighted and T2-weighted sequences is essential in the examination of this region. To attain adequate T1 weighting, a repetition time (TR) of less than 700 msec should be used with the shortest echo time (TE) attainable (15–25 msec). For adequate T2 weighting, a TR of 2000 to 3000 msec should be used. A longer TR is necessary with higher-field-strength magnets to achieve comparable T2 weighting, due to the prolongation of T1 times. With a long TR, two echoes are routinely obtained. A short TE (30 msec) produces a proton density image, which possesses a relatively high SNR, but relatively little contrast. If an intermediate TE (40–50 msec) is used, the relatively high SNR is maintained, but the addition of slight T2 weighting increases image contrast and facilitates comparison with the more heavily T2-weighted image.

For a heavily T2-weighted image (in which the intensity of most abnormalities exceeds that of fat), a TE of 70 to 100 is necessary. This image will have the lowest SNR, but often the highest contrast between pathologic and normal tissue. For high contrast, it is necessary that the TR and TE be long enough to invert the signal intensities of fat and pathologic tissue. Otherwise, the fat and abnormality may be indistinguishable on a sequence with intermediate TR and TE.

These two kinds of sequences are complementary. The short TR, short TE, T1-weighted sequence provides essentially anatomic information and is useful in analyzing the architectural distortion of tissues, disruption of fat planes, mass effect, and adenopathy. The T2-weighted image provides high contrast between pathologic and normal tissues, providing precise localization of the pathologic process. The actual signal characteristics of most pathologic tissues are nonspecific, with the exceptions of cystic and lipomatous lesions.

Optimal slice thickness varies with the kind of abnormality being examined, but a 5-mm thickness (20–30% gap) is usually suitable for evaluating this anatomic region. The number of acquisitions and matrix size to be used will vary with the technical capabilities of the scanner and coil. As T1-weighted images are obtained for anatomic information, a 256 × 256 matrix with two acquisitions is usually necessary to obtain the requisite spatial resolution and SNR characteristics. With the T2-weighted sequence, fine resolution is relatively less crucial, but obtaining adequate SNR becomes more difficult within a reasonable imaging time. For these reasons, a reduced matrix (256 × 128 or 256 × 192) with one to two signal acquisitions may be suitable. Especially with high-field-strength magnets, a motion-compensating technique, such as gradient moment nulling, may help eliminate artifacts from respiratory and vascular motion.

An initial imaging plane must be chosen which can be used as a localizer for the remainder of the examination. The sagittal plane with one data acquisition and relatively thick slices is usually the most convenient. In general, the axial plane is the most informative single plane, and images in this plane are obtained in most examinations of the oropharynx and nasopharynx, salivary glands, and neck. Images in the coronal and sagittal planes are helpful adjuncts, and at least one of these additional planes is used in most examinations. The sagittal plane is most helpful in evaluating midline lesions, and the "localizer" image may be tailored for this purpose by choosing a thinner slice (4–5 mm) with two acquisitions. Four acquisitions may be necessary if a slice thickness of 3 mm or less is selected. The coronal plane is useful for evaluating laterally located abnormalities and side-to-side symmetry. To facilitate interpretation, both T1-weighted and T2-weighted images should be obtained in one of the planes, typically the axial. One or both of the adjunctive planes may then be obtained using a single pulse sequence. Because strictly anatomic information is usually desired from these supplementary planes, a T1-weighted image offers the highest spatial resolution and SNR.

NOSE AND NASOPHARYNX

MRI has great use in evaluating mass lesions of the nose and nasopharynx.[1-3] The indications for an MRI examination of this region are basically fourfold: suspicion of an occult nasopharyngeal carcinoma, documenting the extent of deep invasion by a known nasopharyngeal carcinoma, evaluation of large, benign lesions, and assessment of a deep, parapharyngeal lesion inaccessible to direct visualization. Metastatic adenopathy can be evaluated with an accuracy comparable to CT. The relationship of tumor to vessels and any intracranial extension can be assessed with a greater degree of accuracy than contrast-enhanced CT; the multiplanar imaging capabilities of MRI are especially helpful for this. The degree of bone invasion (e.g., the skull base) can be estimated but remains slightly inferior to CT.

Nasopharyngeal Carcinoma

The clinical findings that may prompt suspicion of occult squamous cell carcinoma include palpable cervical lymph node metastasis, usually involving the deep cervical chain; nasal obstruction or epistaxis; cranial nerve symptoms, commonly from cranial nerves 9, 10, 11, and 12 and more unusually 2, 3, 4, and 6; and unilateral serous otitis media.[4] Rarely, trismus may occur after invasion of the pterygoid muscles.

The nasopharynx is a difficult area to examine clinically, and small lesions may easily be missed. Adults usually have a thin layer of adenoidal and mucosal tissue lining the posterior and lateral walls of the nasopharynx, just superficial to the longus capitis and colli muscles and the pharyngeal constrictors. This tissue layer is slightly higher in signal intensity than the adjacent muscles on T1-weighted images and much higher in intensity on T2-weighted images. The signal characteristics of nasopharyngeal tumors are often similar to this band of tissue. Signs of early nasopharyngeal carcinoma include obliteration of the lateral pharyngeal recess (located posterior on axial and superior on coronal images to the torus tubarius and orifice of the eustachian tube) and infiltration of the fat planes around the lateral tensor and medial levator palatini muscles, which mark the medial boundary of the parapharyngeal space. Subtle asymmetries of the superficial pharyngeal tissue layer are frequently identified in normal patients.

In more advanced cases, an obvious soft tissue mass may be seen in the nasopharynx (Fig. 8–1), with possible extension into the parapharyngeal space fat. Invasion of the skull base, cavernous sinus, foramen ovale, jugular foramen, carotid canal, maxillary, ethmoid, and sphenoid sinuses, nose, pterygopalatine fossa, and orbits should be assessed in every case. Displacement of the carotid artery and jugular vein is easily evaluated by MRI, especially with sagittal and coronal images. A flow void within vessels, even on a single imaging plane, reliably indicates vascular patency. However, vascular occlusion may at times be difficult to distinguish from flow-related artifacts by standard spin echo MRI. Phase images and gradient-echo scans may be helpful in making this distinction.

Bone destruction can be visualized on MRI. It appears as a replacement of signal void from cortical bone (or cortical bone and air in the case of the petrous portion of the temporal bone) with intermediate- or high-signal-intensity soft tissue. Bone-marrow-containing cancellous bone, such as the clivus, exhibits replacement of normal high-signal marrow fat with intermediate-signal material on T1-weighted images. On T2-weighted images, one may see intermediate- or high-signal-intensity material infiltrating the low-signal-intensity marrow, although T1-weighted images are better for visualizing most cases of marrow invasion. MRI is usually adequate for assessing bony involvement, although CT may be necessary in some cases for evaluating fine bony detail. There is no doubt that MRI is superior to CT in assessing intracranial extension of tumor.

The nodal groups typically involved by nasopharyngeal carcinoma are the lateral retropharyngeal nodes (the node of Rouviere is the highest of these), the jugular group, including the jugulodigastric node, and the spinal accessory group in the posterior triangle deep to the sternocleidomastoid muscle. Imaging evaluation is especially important in the last group, because these nodes are relatively inaccessible to clinical evaluation. Involvement of upper cervical nodes is common, but mid- and lower-cervical-node metastases may also occur. Among all head and neck neoplasms, nasopharyngeal carcinoma has the highest incidence of contralateral nodal metastasis (i.e., up to 33% of cases). As in other parts of the body, the signal characteristics of nodes do not establish the presence of metastases, and reliance must be placed on node size, with a diameter of 1.0 to 1.5 cm (and greater) usually considered suspicious.[5] Use of size criteria for nodes carries a penalty in sensitivity and specificity: microscopic involvement is missed and postinflammatory nodal enlargement is mistaken for metastatic disease. The larger and more numerous the nodes are, the more likely they are to actually represent metastatic involvement. Necrosis within a node of any size, identified as a central area with a signal intensity similar to fluid, identifies likely metastatic involvement.

Fluid in obstructed ethmoid and sphenoid sinuses and in the mastoid air cells due to obstruction of the eustachian tube can be recognized by its homogeneous appearance and very high intensity on T2-weighted images and low intensity on T1-weighted images.[6] Unusual, malignant lesions, such as esthesioneuroblastoma, lymphoma, rhabdomyosarcoma, and minor salivary gland tumors, cannot be distinguished by their MR characteristics alone. In such cases, anatomic and clinical data, such as the origin of esthesioneuroblastoma in the upper nasal cavity and the occurrence of rhabdomyosarcoma in pediatric patients, are necessary in differential diagnosis.

Benign Lesions

Inverted papilloma is an aggressive lesion that arises in the nares, expanding the nasal cavity and invading the adjacent maxillary and ethmoid sinuses. These lesions may recur after resection, and there is a known association with squamous cell carcinoma, either at presentation (Fig. 8-2) or with recurrences. The signal characteristics of this lesion are nonspecific, and CT may help in assessing the precise degree of bony destruction.

Nasopharyngeal angiofibroma, the most common benign tumor of the nasopharynx, is seen in young male patients presenting with nasal obstruction or epistaxis. This tumor is thought to arise from the posterolateral wall of the nasal cavity and nasopharynx and may spread extensively via foramina and fissures of the skull base. Extension into the pterygopalatine fossa via the sphenopalatine foramen with anterior bowing of the posterior wall of the maxillary sinus is characteristic. There may be involvement of the sphenoid and ethmoid sinuses, infratemporal fossa, and orbit.

Documentation of the extent of this lesion by axial imaging is crucial in management. In particular, intracranial extension greatly complicates surgical management and must be carefully evaluated. MRI is superior to CT in this regard due to the lack of artifact from dental fillings, the availability of high-resolution coronal and sagittal imaging, and exquisite lesion contrast relative to the brain, extracranial fat and muscle. This lesion may exhibit characteristic signal voids on MR imaging.[7] This appearance, in association with the clinical findings and typical anatomic involvement, should allow specific diagnosis by MRI. These tumors exhibit marked enhancement with Gd DTPA, which can help evaluate the full extent of these infiltrating lesions (Fig. 8-3).

Noninvasive diagnosis is important because surgeons prefer not to biopsy these highly vascular masses. Angiography is still required for preoperative evaluation.

Nasal polyps are hyperplastic lesions secondary to allergenic stimuli, and they may become large enough to deform the nasal septum. Antrochoanal polyps have a typical appearance, arising in the maxillary antrum and extending into the posterior nasopharyngeal airway (Fig. 8-4). There may be an associated deformity of bone. An unusual lesion occurring in the nasopharynx is the Tornwaldt's cyst, a well-defined, rounded structure in the midline of the posterior nasopharynx. As is typical for a cystic lesion, it shows

(text continues on page 292)

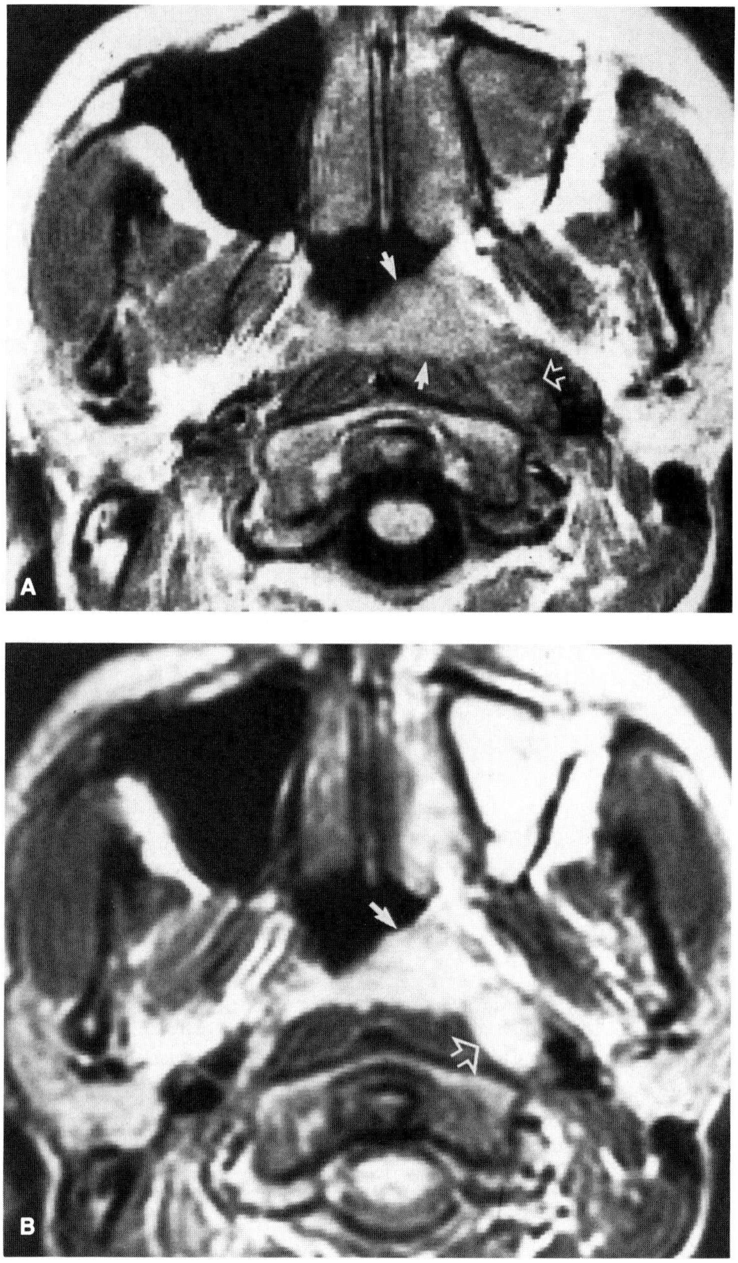

FIGURE 8–1. Squamous cell carcinoma of the nasopharynx and associated sinusitis. **(A)** T1-weighted, **(B)** proton density, **(C)** T2-weighted axial, and **(D)** T1-weighted coronal images of the nasopharynx. There is a left nasopharyngeal mass (arrows) involving the adjacent longus capitis muscles. The signal intensity of the tumor increases on T2-weighted images, but it remains lower than that of the associated left maxillary sinusitis. Tumor has spread to the left node of Rouviere (open arrow). (Carter BL. Nasopharynx and infratemporal fossa: pathologic findings. In: Valvassori GE, Buckingham RA, Carter BL, et al. Head and neck imaging. New York: Thieme, 1988).

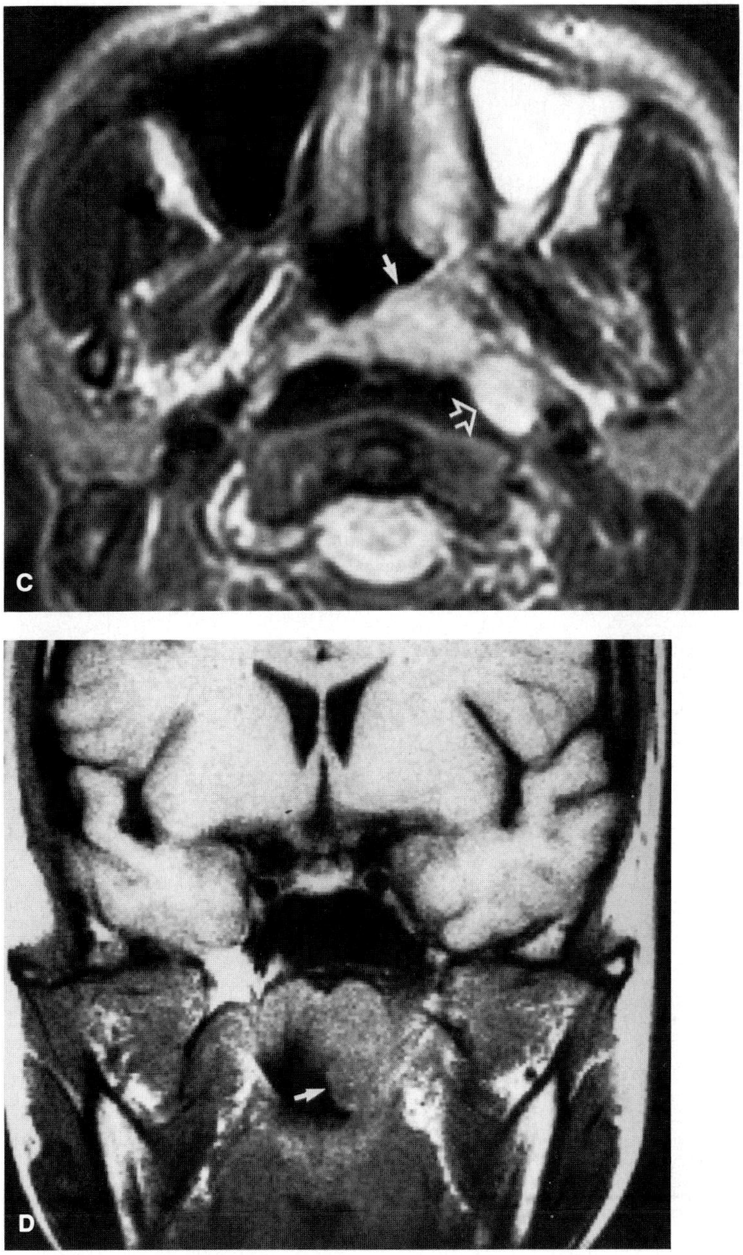

FIGURE 8–1. (Continued)

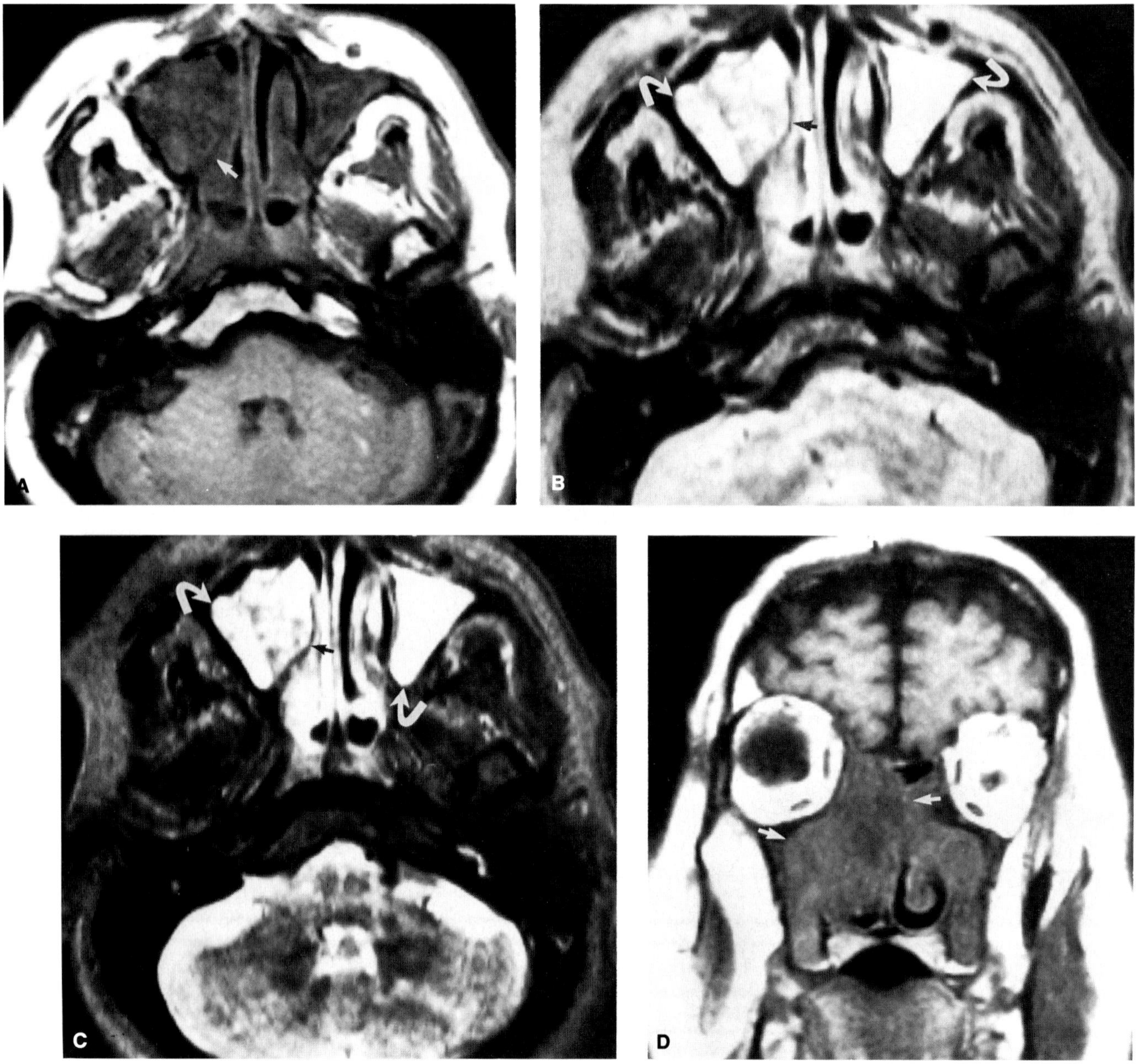

FIGURE 8–2. Inverted papilloma with carcinoma. **(A)** T1-weighted, **(B)** proton density, **(C)** T2-weighted axial, and **(D)** T1-weighted coronal images through the nose and maxillary sinuses. There is a mass (arrows) involving the right maxillary antrum and nasal cavity, which is of mixed signal intensity on the T2-weighted sequence and of low signal on the T1-weighted sequences. The mass can be easily differentiated from the higher-signal-intensity secretions (curved arrows) in both maxillary sinuses on the T2-weighted images.

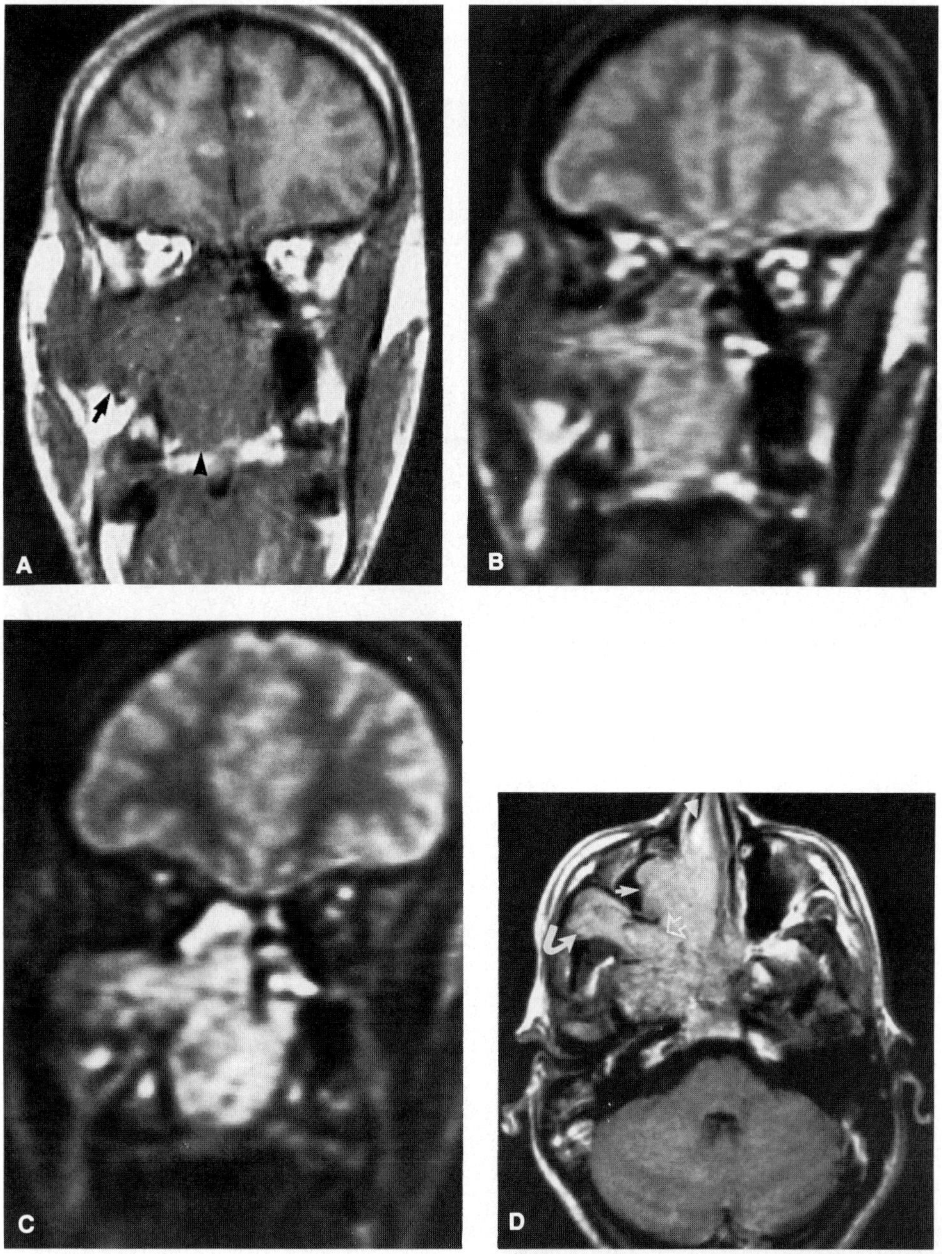

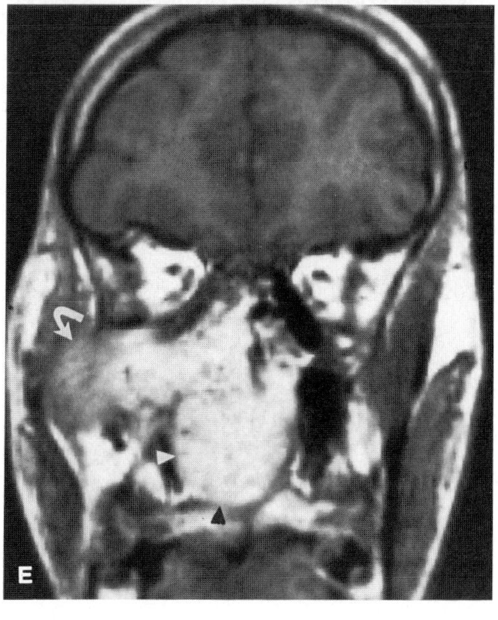

FIGURE 8–3. Juvenile angiofibroma. **(A)** T1-weighted, **(B)** proton density, and **(C)** T2-weighted coronal images before administration of Gd DTPA. **(D)** T1-weighted axial and **(E)** coronal images after Gd DTPA. A large mass involves the nasal cavity (arrowhead), right maxillary antrum (arrow), pterygopalatine fossa (open arrow), and infratemporal fossa (curved arrow). Characteristic foci of signal void within the mass are seen on the T2-weighted image, representing blood vessels and areas of fibrosis. The mass exhibits marked, homogeneous enhancement with Gd DTPA, allowing clear delineation of tumor extent.

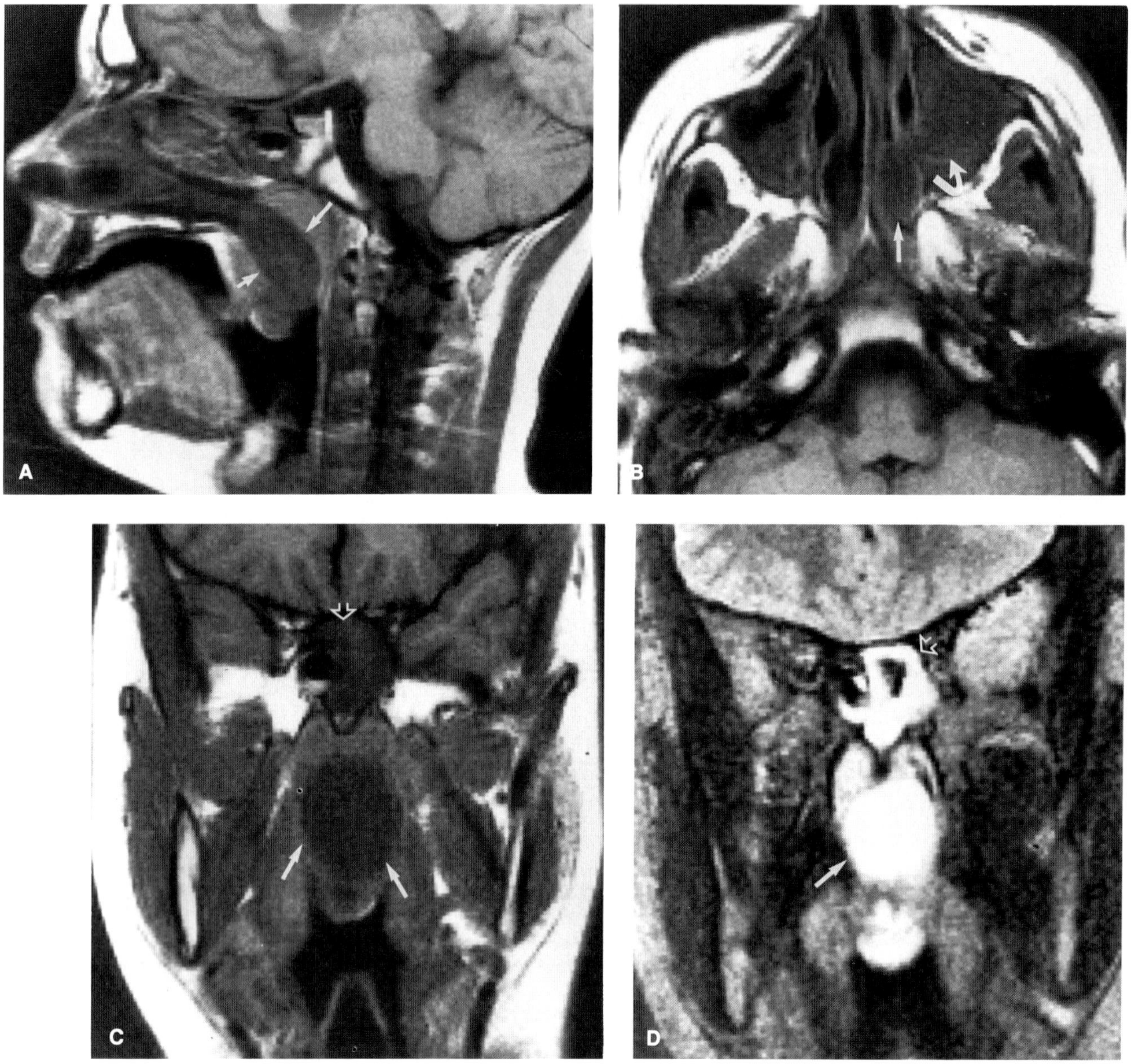

FIGURE 8–4. Antrochoanal polyp. **(A)** T1-weighted sagittal, **(B)** axial, and **(C)** coronal images; **(D)** T2-weighted coronal image of the nasopharynx. There is a polypoid soft tissue mass (arrow) originating in the left maxillary sinus (curved arrow) and filling the nasopharyngeal airway. Retained secretions in the sphenoid sinus (open arrow) have similar signal characteristics: low on T1-weighted and bright on T2-weighted images.

very high, homogeneous signal intensity on T2-weighted images (Fig. 8–5).

Parapharyngeal Space

The parapharyngeal space is marginated by the pharyngobasilar fascia, medially; the mandible and pterygoid muscles, laterally; the prevertebral fascia, posteriorly; and the pterygoid plates, anteriorly.[8,9] It may be further subdivided into prestyloid and poststyloid (or carotid sheath) spaces. Masses in this space may develop insidiously because this is a relatively silent area clinically. The most common lesions of this space include neural tumors (e.g., schwannomas and neurofibromas), paragangliomas (e.g., glomus jugulare and

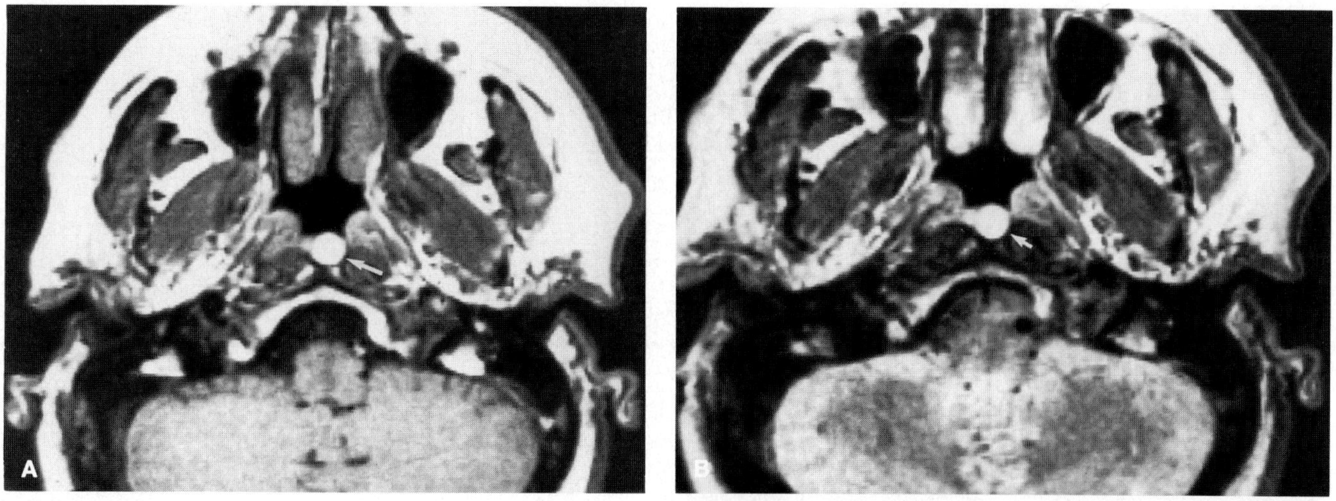

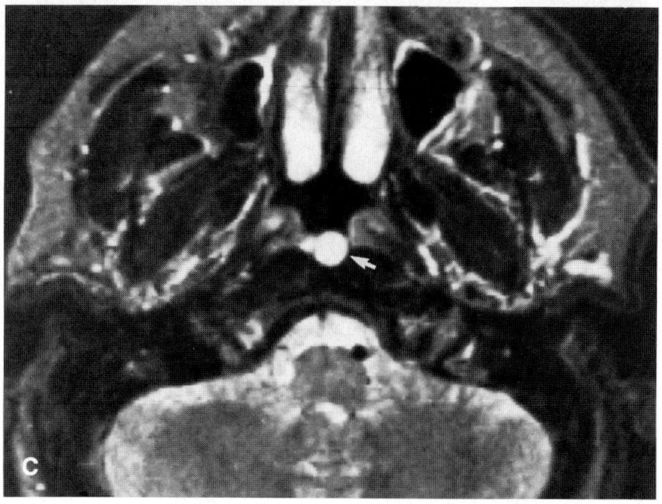

FIGURE 8–5. Presumed Tornwaldt's cyst. **(A)** T1-weighted, **(B)** proton density, and **(C)** T2-weighted axial images of the nasopharynx. There is a small, rounded, well-defined soft tissue structure (arrow) in the nasopharynx near the midline. The high signal on T1-weighted images may be due to high protein content of the cyst fluid.

vagale tumors), and benign or malignant salivary gland tumors, which may arise from the deep portion of the parotid gland or from minor salivary glands in the parapharyngeal space (Figs. 8–6 through 8–10). Less common lesions are lymphoma, metastases, congenital second branchial cleft cysts, and mesenchymal tumors, such as lipoma, liposarcoma, rhabdomyosarcoma, hemangioma, and hemangiopericytoma.

MRI facilitates the precise diagnosis of glomus tumors, because these lesions may exhibit characteristic foci of low signal intensity on both T1-weighted and T2-weighted sequences, probably due to a combination of flow void from vessels and foci of fibrosis.[10,11] These low-signal areas are easily seen on T2-weighted images, because they contrast with the high signal from the bulk of the tumor and from foci of flow-related enhancement in vessels. Glomus and neural tumors arise within the carotid sheath and tend to anteriorly displace the carotid artery and may posteriorly displace the internal jugular vein. Salivary gland tumors, arising in the prestyloid space, posteriorly displace the carotid artery and jugular vein.

Distinguishing between tumors of parotid and extraparotid origin in the prestyloid space is important for surgery. This may be accomplished by assessing the status of the parapharyngeal fat plane. If the fat plane is displaced medially or obliterated, tumor originating from the deep portion of the parotid is likely. If displaced laterally, clearly separating the lesion from the deep lobe of the parotid gland, an extraparotid origin may be assumed.

Infectious processes may extend into the parapharyngeal space from the petrous bone or tonsils. These are characterized by infiltration of the parapharyn-

(text continues on page 296)

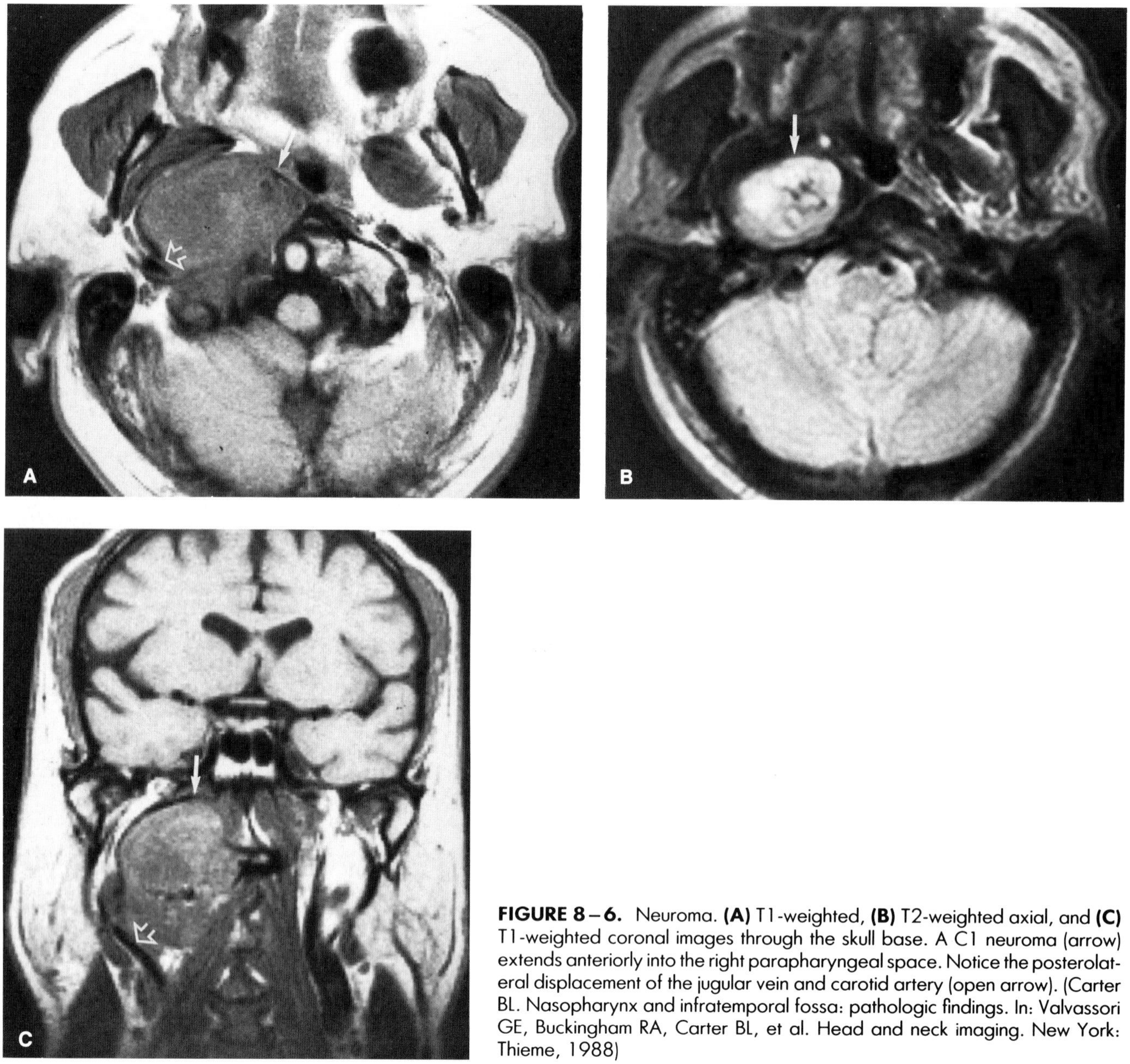

FIGURE 8–6. Neuroma. **(A)** T1-weighted, **(B)** T2-weighted axial, and **(C)** T1-weighted coronal images through the skull base. A C1 neuroma (arrow) extends anteriorly into the right parapharyngeal space. Notice the posterolateral displacement of the jugular vein and carotid artery (open arrow). (Carter BL. Nasopharynx and infratemporal fossa: pathologic findings. In: Valvassori GE, Buckingham RA, Carter BL, et al. Head and neck imaging. New York: Thieme, 1988)

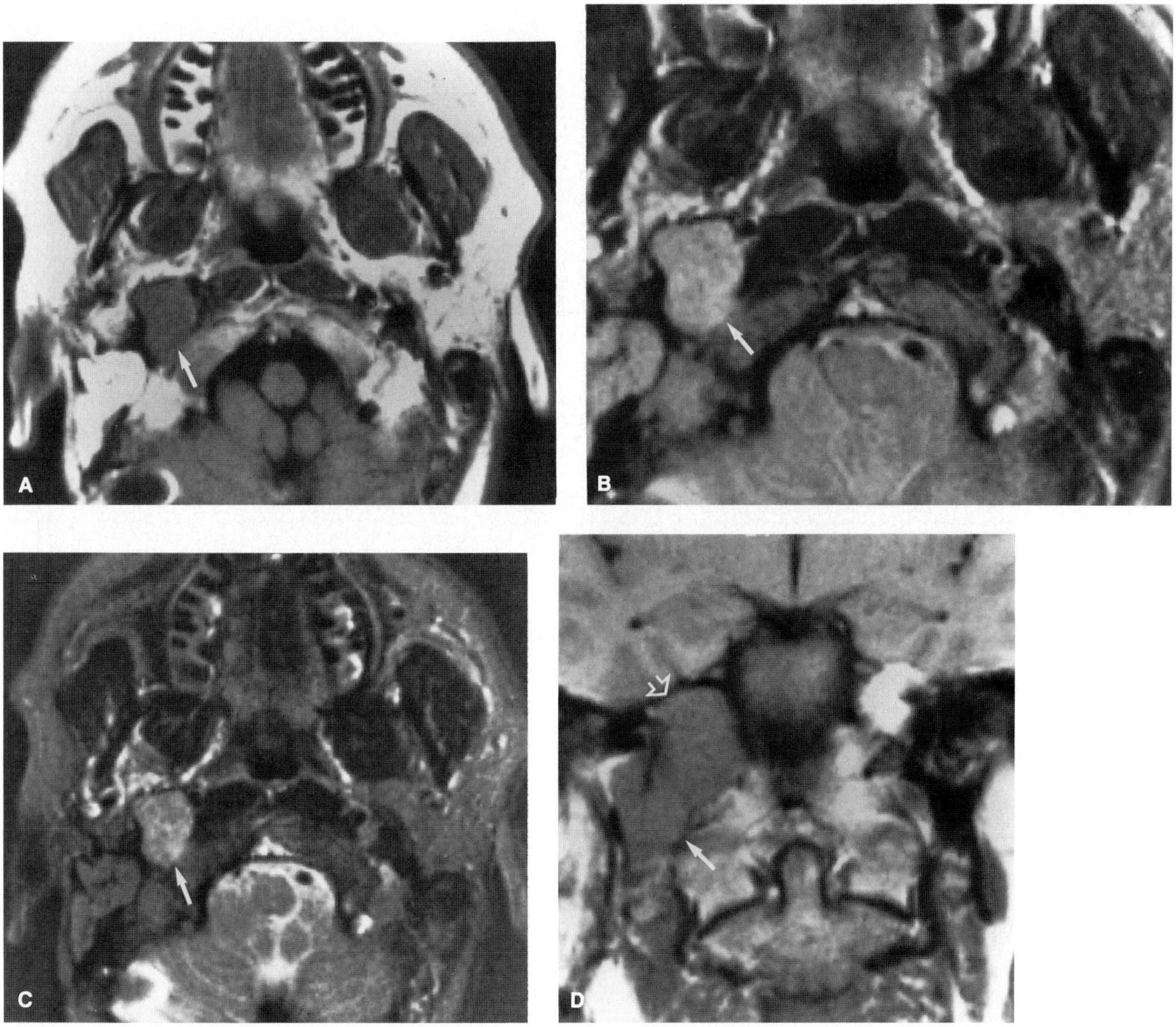

FIGURE 8–7. Glomus jugulare tumor. **(A)** T1-weighted, **(B)** proton density, **(C)** T2-weighted axial, and **(D)** T1-weighted coronal images through the skull base. Notice the characteristic inhomogeneity of signal of the tumor on the T2-weighted images. The tumor (arrow) extends through the jugular fossa (open arrow) to below the skull base.

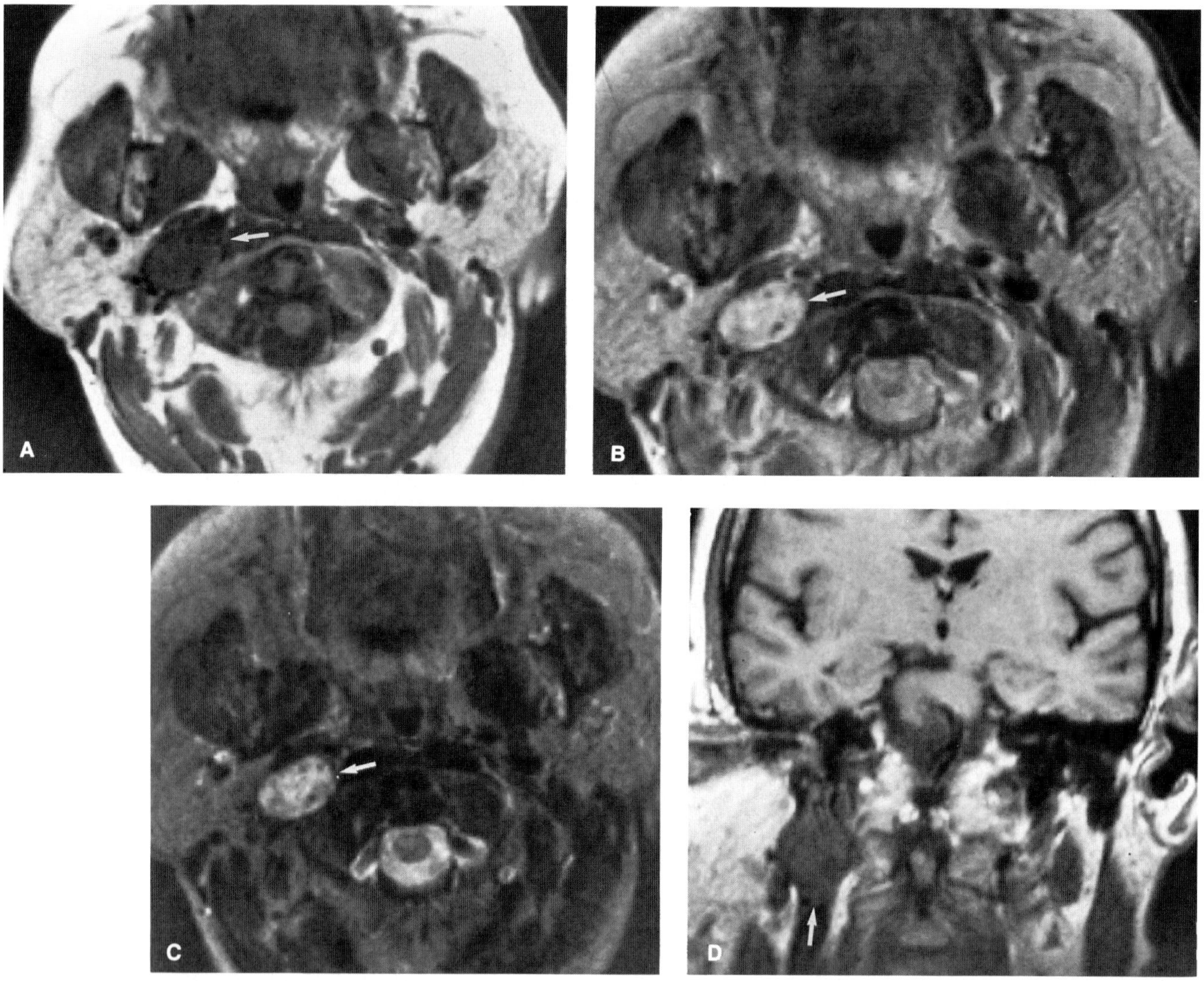

FIGURE 8–8. Glomus jugulare tumor. **(A)** T1-weighted, **(B)** proton density, **(C)** T2-weighted axial, and **(D)** T1-weighted coronal images through the skull base. The T2-weighted images demonstrate the classic salt and pepper appearance due to blood vessels and areas of fibrosis within the tumor (arrow). The coronal images show the tumor to be within the lumen of the internal jugular vein.

geal tissue planes by high-signal-intensity material on T2-weighted images. Frank abscess formation may be identified by a localized collection exhibiting the signal characteristics of fluid.

OROPHARYNX

Squamous Cell Carcinoma

This is the most common oral and oropharyngeal condition referred for MRI evaluation (Figs. 8–11 and 8–12).[12] Oropharyngeal carcinoma may be relatively occult clinically. It can present initially with referred pain distant to the oral cavity (e.g., otalgia) or with metastatic cervical adenopathy. More commonly, the lesion will be diagnosed by the referring clinician in the course of an evaluation of an oral mass or localized pain or by the dentist during a routine oral examination or an examination for ill-fitting dentures. An evaluation of the extent of disease may then be requested. Local submucosal invasion of lesions of the tongue, tongue base, and floor of the mouth may be quite deceiving clinically, and MRI can accurately assess the degree of local involvement or midline spread, a very important factor in deciding whether a lesion is resectable.

The likelihood of widespread disease depends on

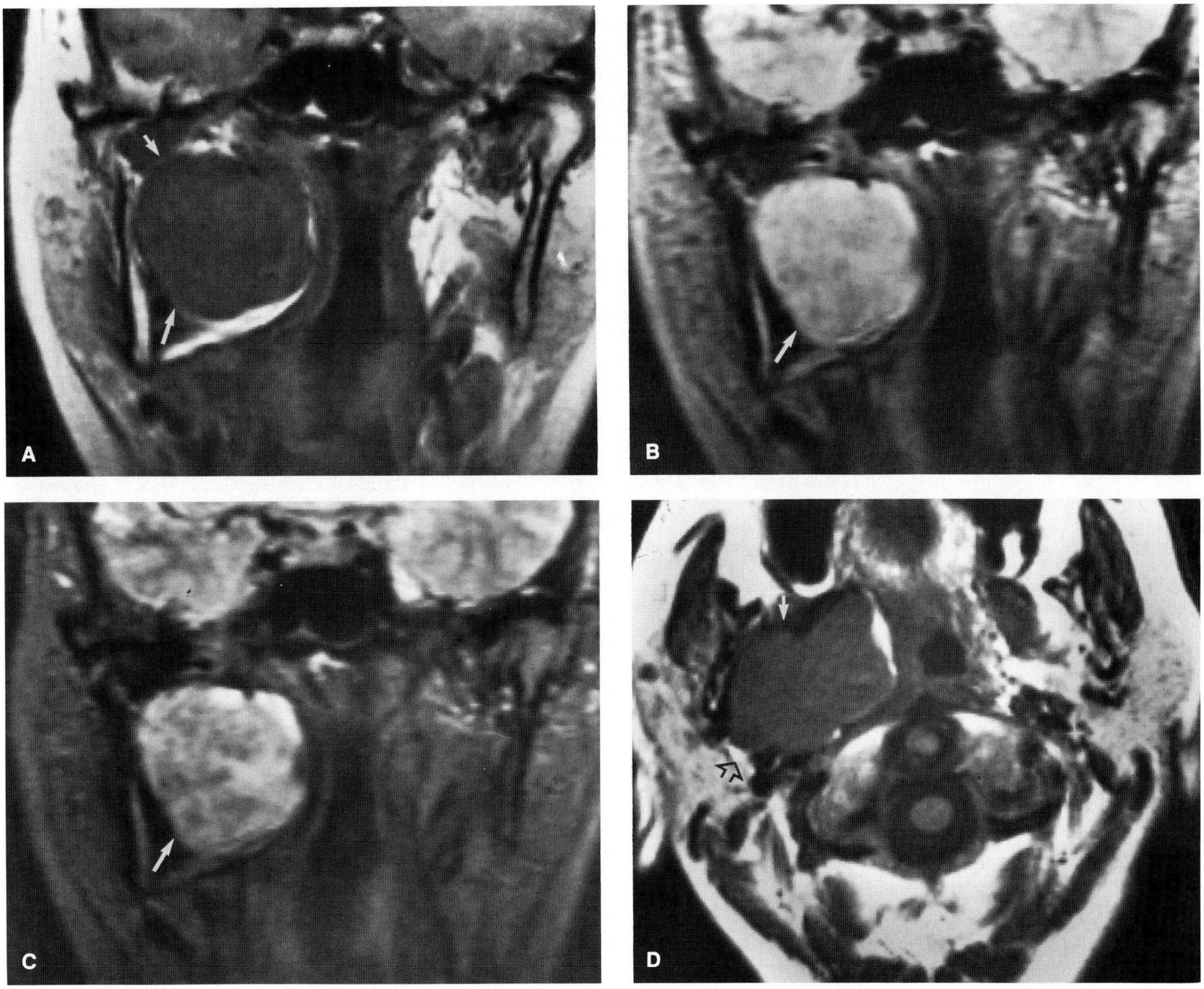

FIGURE 8–9. Parapharyngeal pleomorphic adenoma arising from a minor salivary gland. **(A)** T1-weighted, **(B)** proton density, **(C)** T2-weighted coronal, **(D)** T1-weighted axial images through the nasopharynx. On the T1-weighted axial image, clear fat planes (open arrow) separate the tumor (arrow) both from the nasopharyngeal mucosa and from the parotid gland, indicating an origin from the parapharyngeal space. Notice the characteristic posterior displacement of the carotid artery and jugular vein.

the anatomic site of origin of oropharyngeal carcinoma. More than 75% of lesions of the tonsillar regions and base of the tongue and more than 40% of lesions of the retromolar trigone and soft palate exhibit metastatic adenopathy at presentation. Adenopathy most commonly affects the submandibular and high anterior cervical chain, later extending to the middle and lower anterior cervical and posterior triangle nodes. Contralateral adenopathy is commonly seen (20–30%) with lesions arising in midline structures, such as the soft palate and tongue base. Thus, imaging of oropharyngeal carcinoma has multiple roles similar to those in the nasopharynx: searching for an occult primary lesion, evaluating the extent of local invasion of a lesion diagnosed clinically, evaluating regional nodes, and assessing involvement of adjacent blood vessels.

MRI has a distinct advantage over CT in the evaluation of the oropharynx. The image is not as severely degraded by dental amalgam, although local field dis-

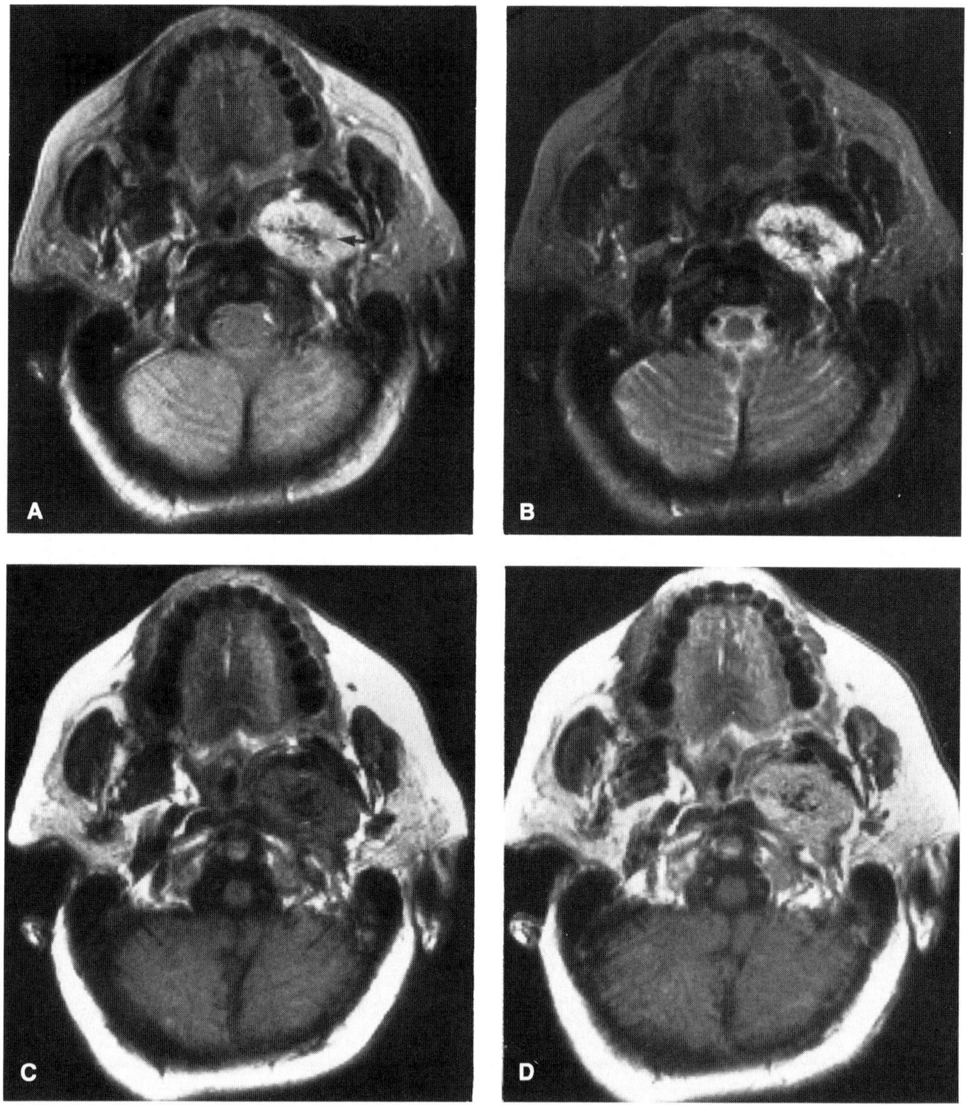

FIGURE 8–10. Glomus vagale tumor. **(A,B)** Moderately and heavily T2-weighted images and **(C,D)** pre- and post-Gd DPTA T1-weighted images. A smoothly marginated mass is identified in the left parapharyngeal space, which enhances after contrast. Foci of low signal intensity (arrow) represent a combination of fibrosis and vessel flow voids.

tortions may occur. The additional imaging planes offered by MRI can be very useful in the oral cavity and oropharynx. Lesions of the tongue, floor of the mouth, and palate are often best defined in the coronal plane. The sagittal plane is the least useful for anatomic definition, although it may help in evaluating midline lesions.

The signal characteristics of oropharyngeal carcinoma are nonspecific: low or intermediate signal on T1-weighted and intermediate or high signal on T2-weighted images, and both types of images are necessary for complete evaluation. Oropharyngeal carcinoma may exhibit submucosal spread in all directions from the site of the primary tumor, and the precise extent of involvement must be assessed for the purposes of radiation or surgical therapy. Extensive invasion of the tongue is common with lesions of tongue base and floor of mouth, and the extent of tongue involvement is especially important for assessing the morbidity of surgical resection. Lesions of the retromolar trigone, palate, tonsil, and posterior oropharynx may extend into the pterygopalatine fossa, pterygoid muscles, and parapharyngeal space. Invasion of adjacent bony structures, such as the mandible, max-

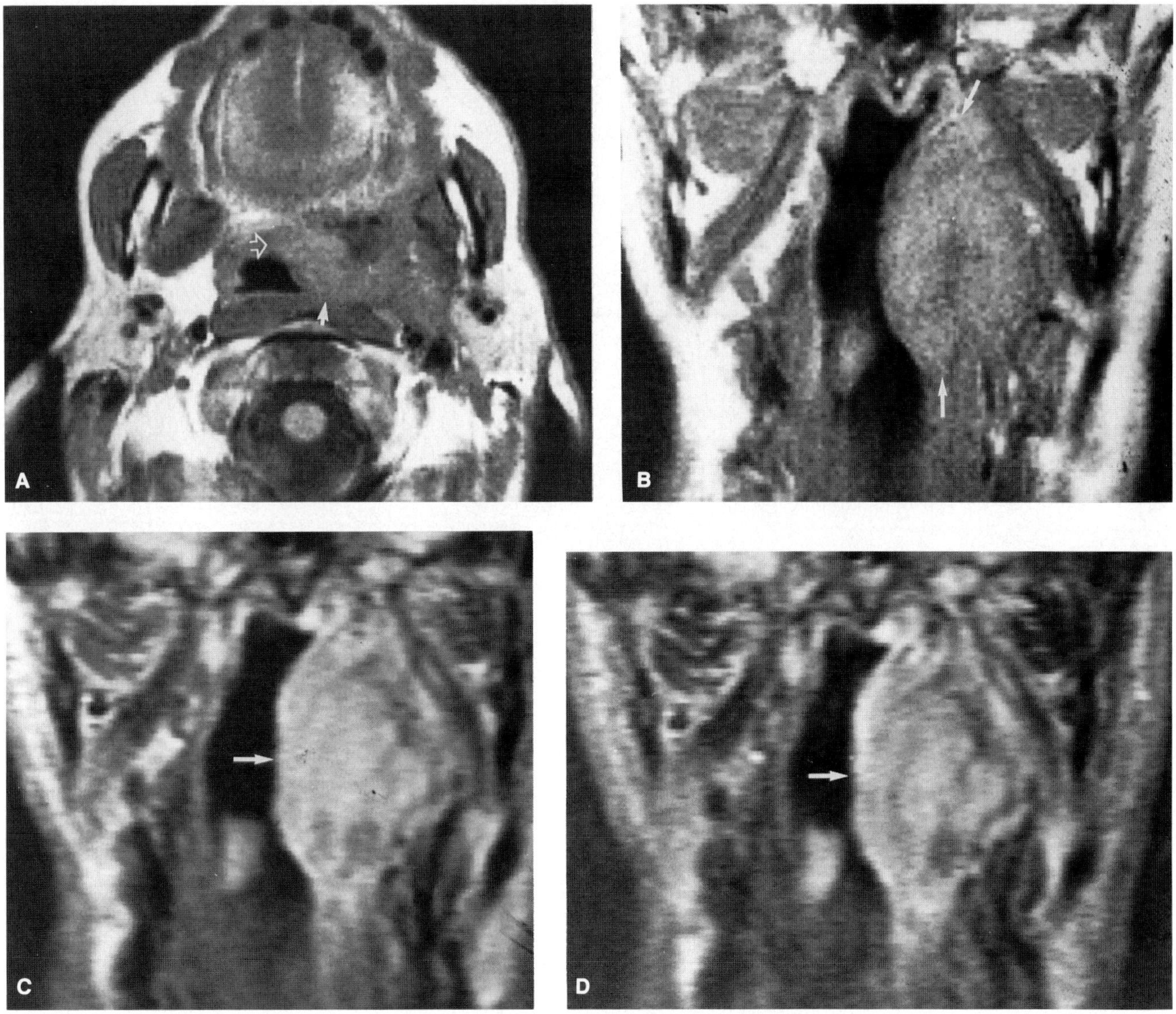

FIGURE 8 – 11. Squamous cell carcinoma of the tonsil. **(A)** T1-weighted axial, **(B)** T1-weighted, **(C)** proton density, and **(D)** T2-weighted coronal images of the oropharynx. A large mass (arrow) with extensive, deep invasion into the parapharyngeal space replaces the left tonsil. There is invasion of the soft palate (open arrow), which approaches the midline.

illa, and skull base, can be assessed by discontinuity of the cortical signal void and loss of normal high signal of the marrow fat on T1-weighted images. The coronal plane is especially helpful in assessing bony involvement of the maxilla and skull base. Superficial tumor, as in the nasopharynx, may be impossible to identify or to differentiate from normal asymmetry, but this is not a serious limitation, because it is usually apparent clinically.

Examination of the posttreatment patient is complicated by the resulting architectural distortion and fibrosis. CT has not shown great reliability in distinguishing fibrosis from recurrent tumor. There is preliminary evidence that MRI may help by demonstrating high signal intensity from recurrent tumor on T2-weighted images, while fibrosis tends to remain isointense with muscle (Figs. 8 – 13 and 8 – 14).[13] However, edema, infection, and inflammatory adenopathy may also demonstrate increased signal on T2-weighted images, reducing the specificity of this finding. Squamous cell carcinoma does demonstrate enhancement with Gd DTPA (Fig. 8 – 15), and this may aid in distinguishing recurrent tumor from scar.[14]

(text continues on page 304)

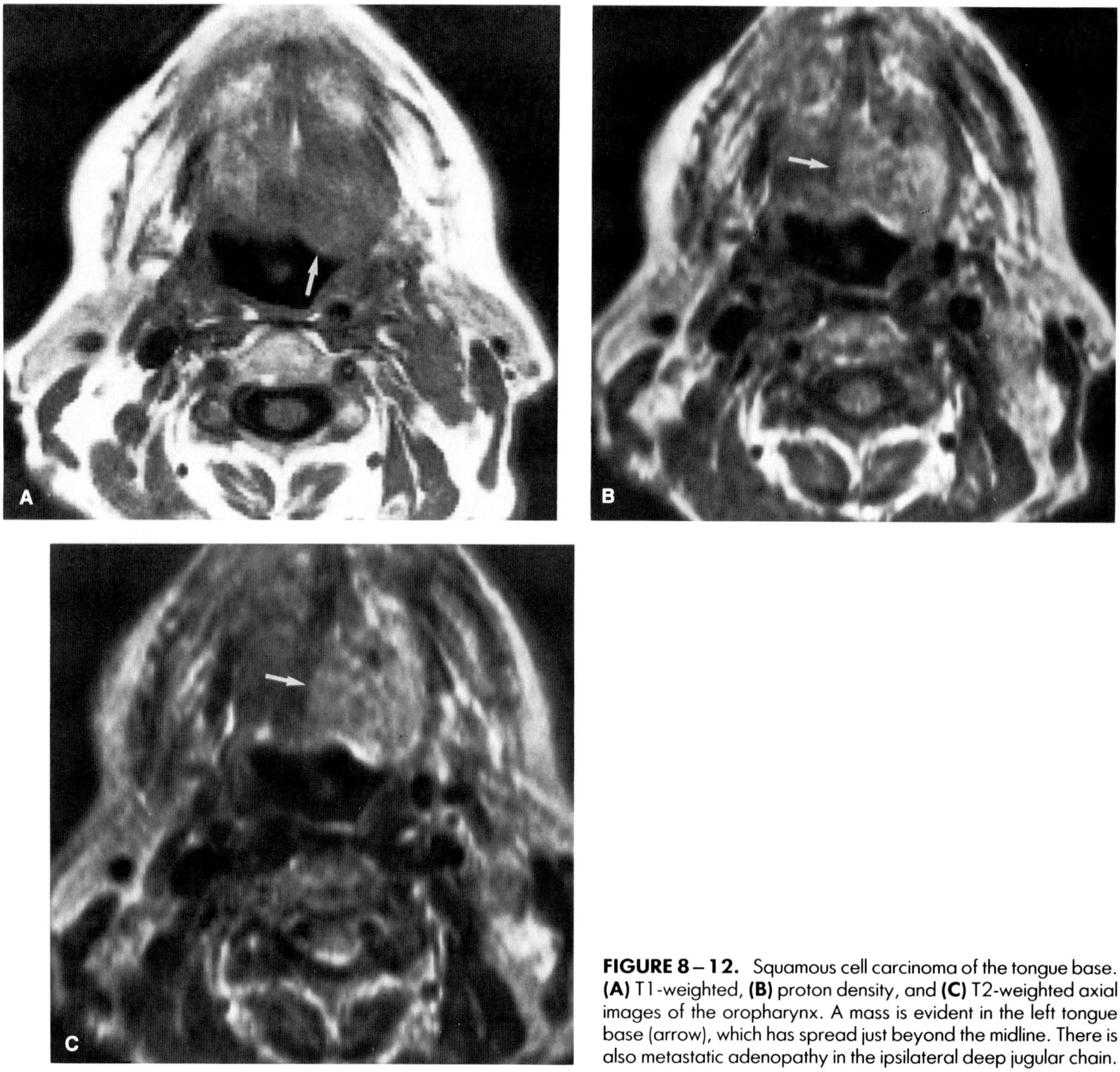

FIGURE 8–12. Squamous cell carcinoma of the tongue base. **(A)** T1-weighted, **(B)** proton density, and **(C)** T2-weighted axial images of the oropharynx. A mass is evident in the left tongue base (arrow), which has spread just beyond the midline. There is also metastatic adenopathy in the ipsilateral deep jugular chain.

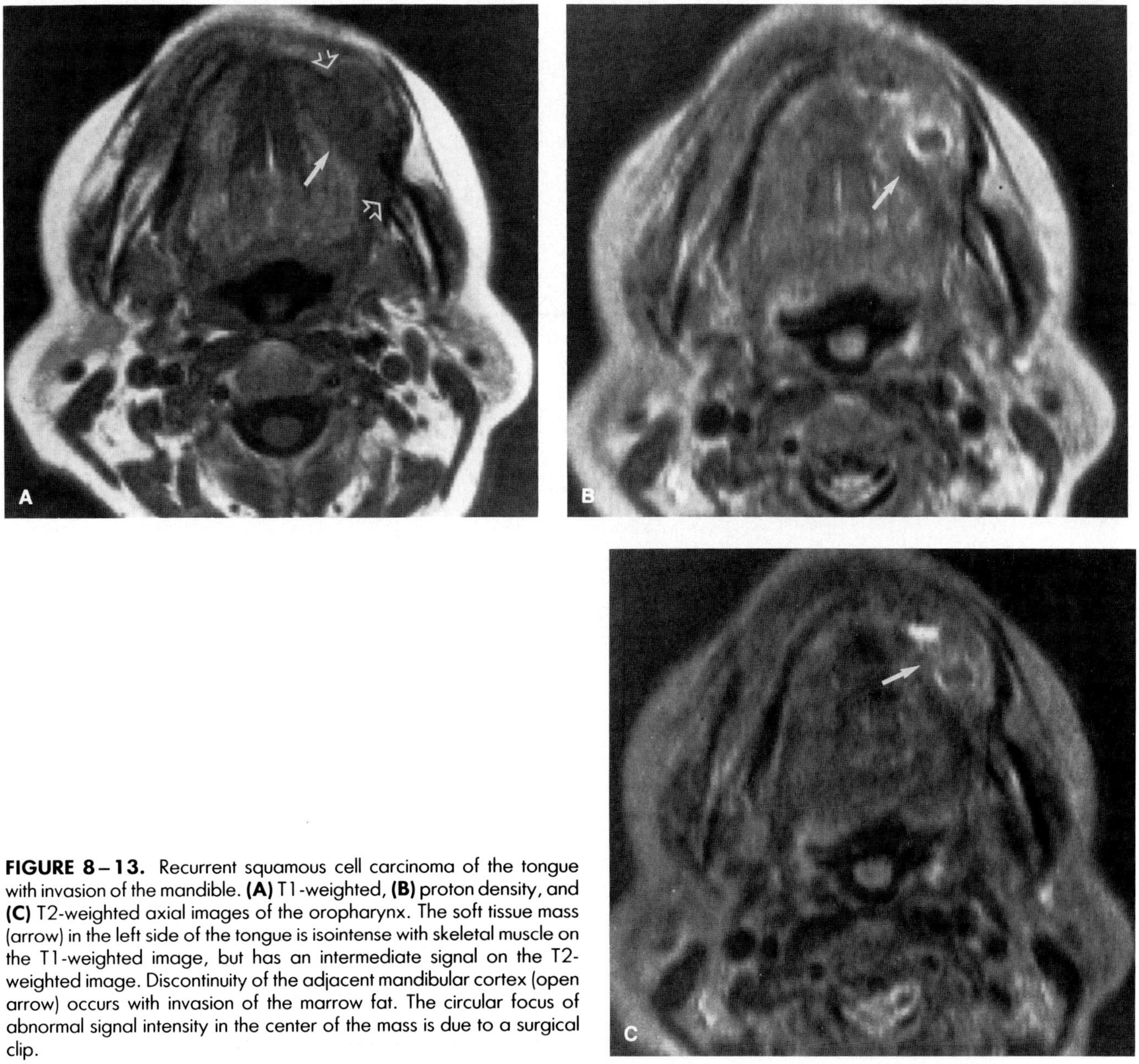

FIGURE 8–13. Recurrent squamous cell carcinoma of the tongue with invasion of the mandible. **(A)** T1-weighted, **(B)** proton density, and **(C)** T2-weighted axial images of the oropharynx. The soft tissue mass (arrow) in the left side of the tongue is isointense with skeletal muscle on the T1-weighted image, but has an intermediate signal on the T2-weighted image. Discontinuity of the adjacent mandibular cortex (open arrow) occurs with invasion of the marrow fat. The circular focus of abnormal signal intensity in the center of the mass is due to a surgical clip.

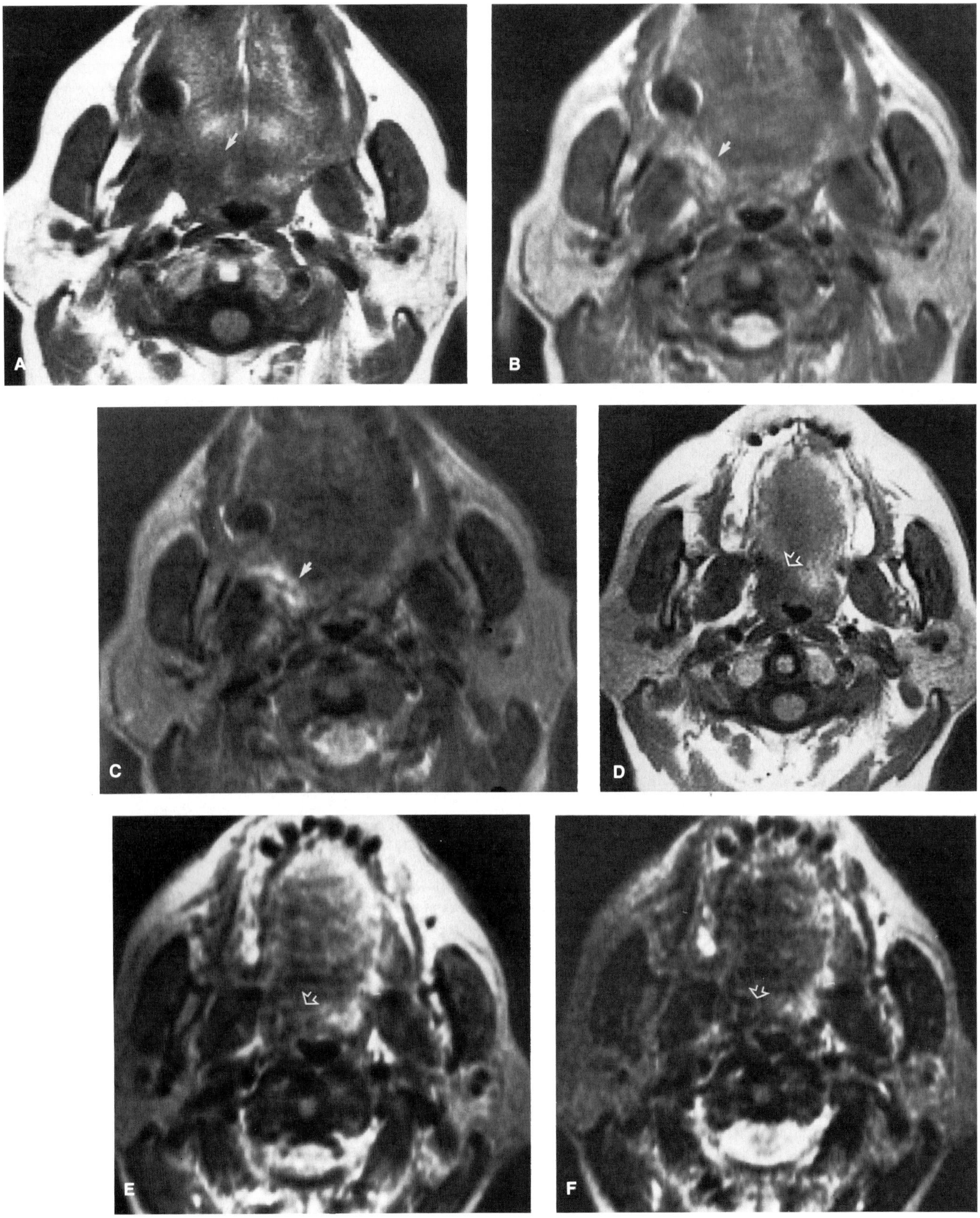

FIGURE 8–14. Carcinoma of the tonsil with postoperative fibrosis on follow-up examination. **(A)** T1-weighted, **(B)** proton density, and **(C)** T2-weighted axial images of the oropharynx show a small tumor (arrow) with a typical intermediate signal on T1-weighted and a bright signal on T2-weighted images. **(D)** T1-weighted, **(E)** proton density, and **(F)** T2-weighted axial images from a follow-up examination after surgery reveal a persistent mass (open arrow) in the area of the original tumor on T1-weighted images. This area remains isointense with muscle on T2-weighted images and biopsy confirmed fibrosis.

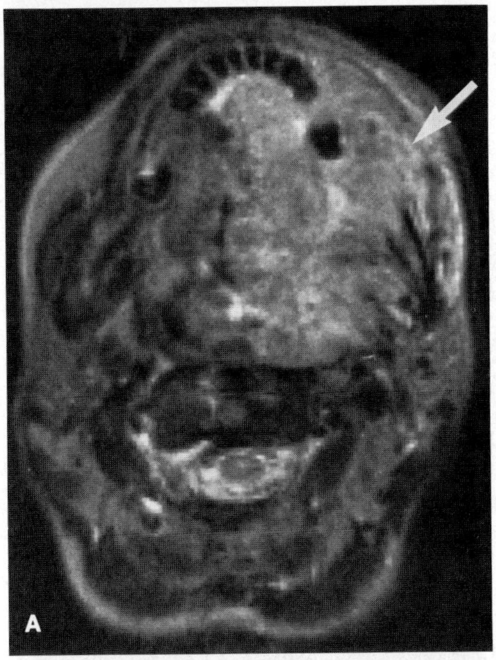

FIGURE 8–15. Squamous cell carcinoma of the left oropharynx. **(A)** T2-weighted, **(B,C)** T1-weighted, and **(D,E)** postcontrast T1-weighted images. Images from two anatomic levels are illustrated before and after contrast agent administration. A large multilobulated soft tissue mass is demonstrated with extensive destruction of the mandible (closed arrow). There is marked enhancement of the lesion after Gd DPTA administration. Peripheral enhancement of an enlarged jugulodigastric node (open arrow) is consistent with neoplastic involvement and central necrosis.

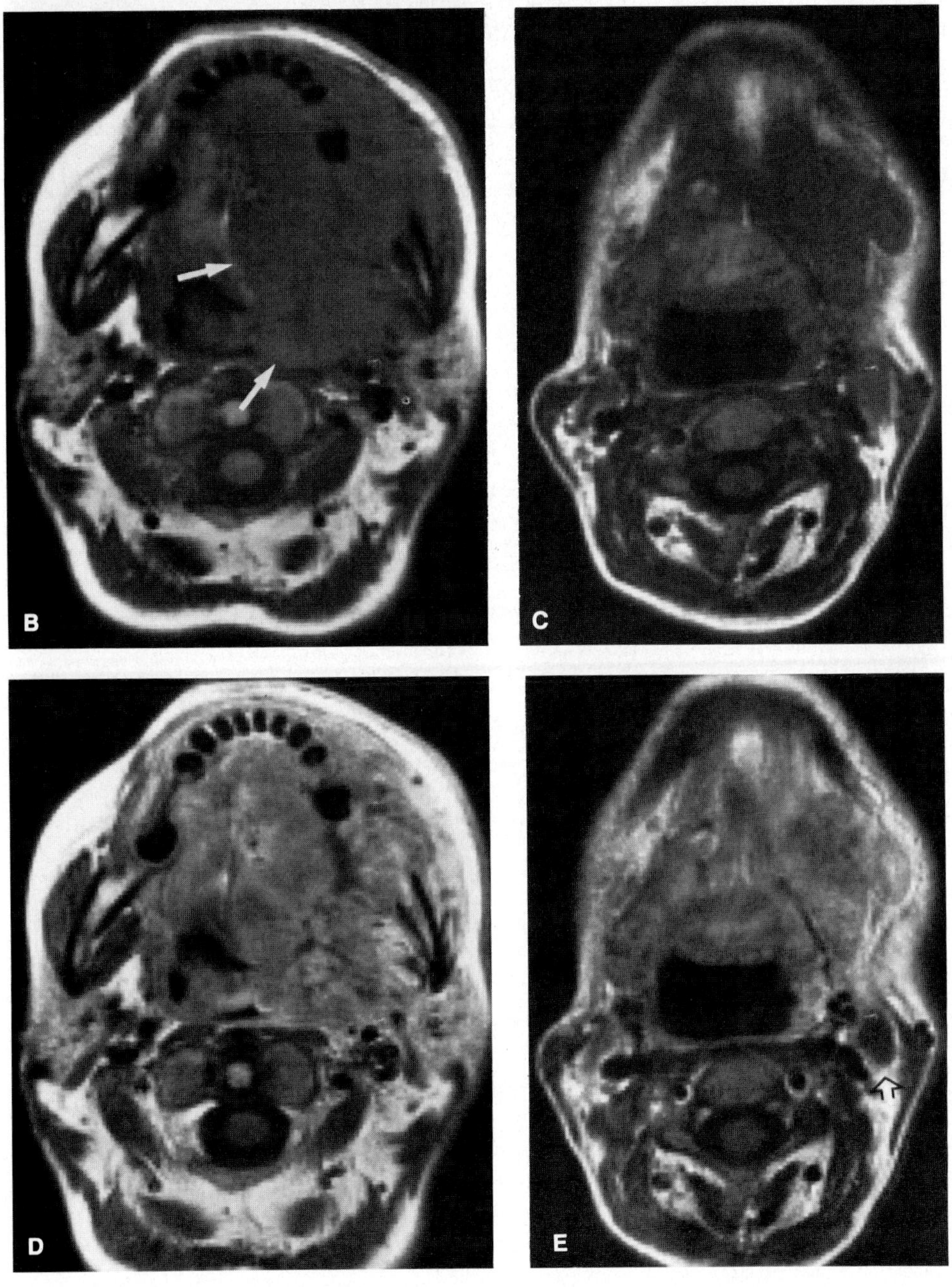

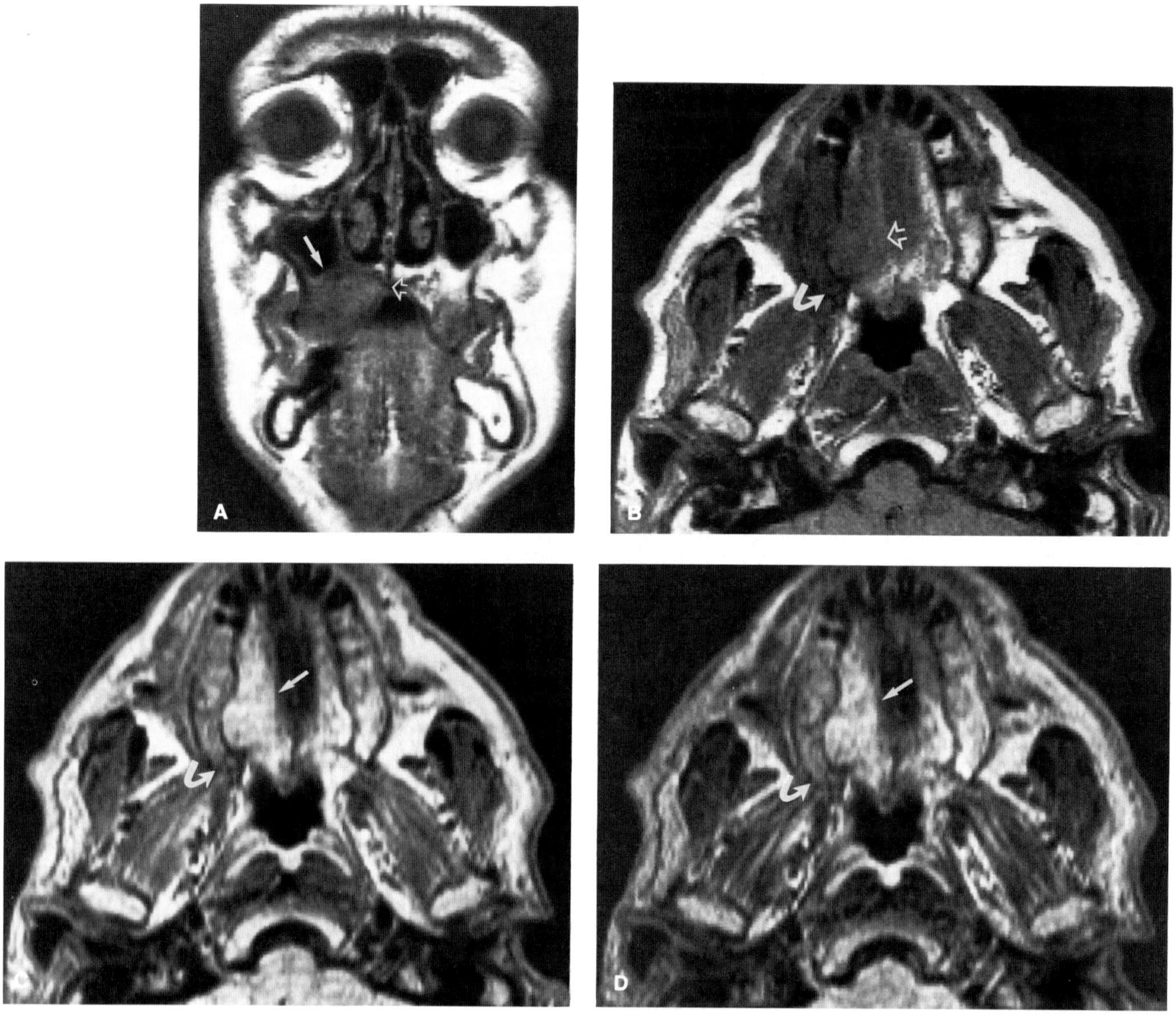

FIGURE 8–16. Adenoid cystic carcinoma of the alveolar ridge and palate. **(A)** T1-weighted coronal, **(B)** T1-weighted, **(C)** proton density, and **(D)** T2-weighted axial images show a mass (arrow) originating in the right maxillary alveolus and invading the palate. The mass exhibits increased signal intensity on the T2-weighted image, characteristic of these lesions. The tumor extends medially to the midline (open arrow) and posterolaterally under the buccinator muscle to the pterygopalatine fossa (curved arrow). (Carter BL. Tumors of the paranasal sinuses and nasal cavity. In: Valvassori GE, Buckingham RA, Carter BL, et al. Head and neck imaging. New York: Thieme, 1988)

Minor Salivary Gland Tumors

The sublingual glands in the floor of the mouth rarely give rise to tumors, although 80% of those occurring are malignant (Figs. 8–16 and 8–17). The more common site of origin of oral salivary gland tumors is the minor salivary glands, scattered throughout the mouth and oropharynx, but most numerous in the hard and soft palate. Approximately 40% of these tumors are benign (i.e., preponderantly of the benign mixed type), and 60% are malignant (i.e., adenoid cystic carcinoma, adenocarcinoma, and mucoepidermoid carcinoma being the most frequent types).[15] The salivary gland tumors typically present as smooth, rounded masses without ulceration, unlike the ulcerated, exophytic appearance of typical squamous cell carcinomas. Although irregular local extension is characteristic of the malignant tumors, with the adenoid cystic variety typically invading along neural pathways, the benign and malignant types cannot be reliably distinguished on the basis of imaging alone. The MR signal characteristics of all these tumors are

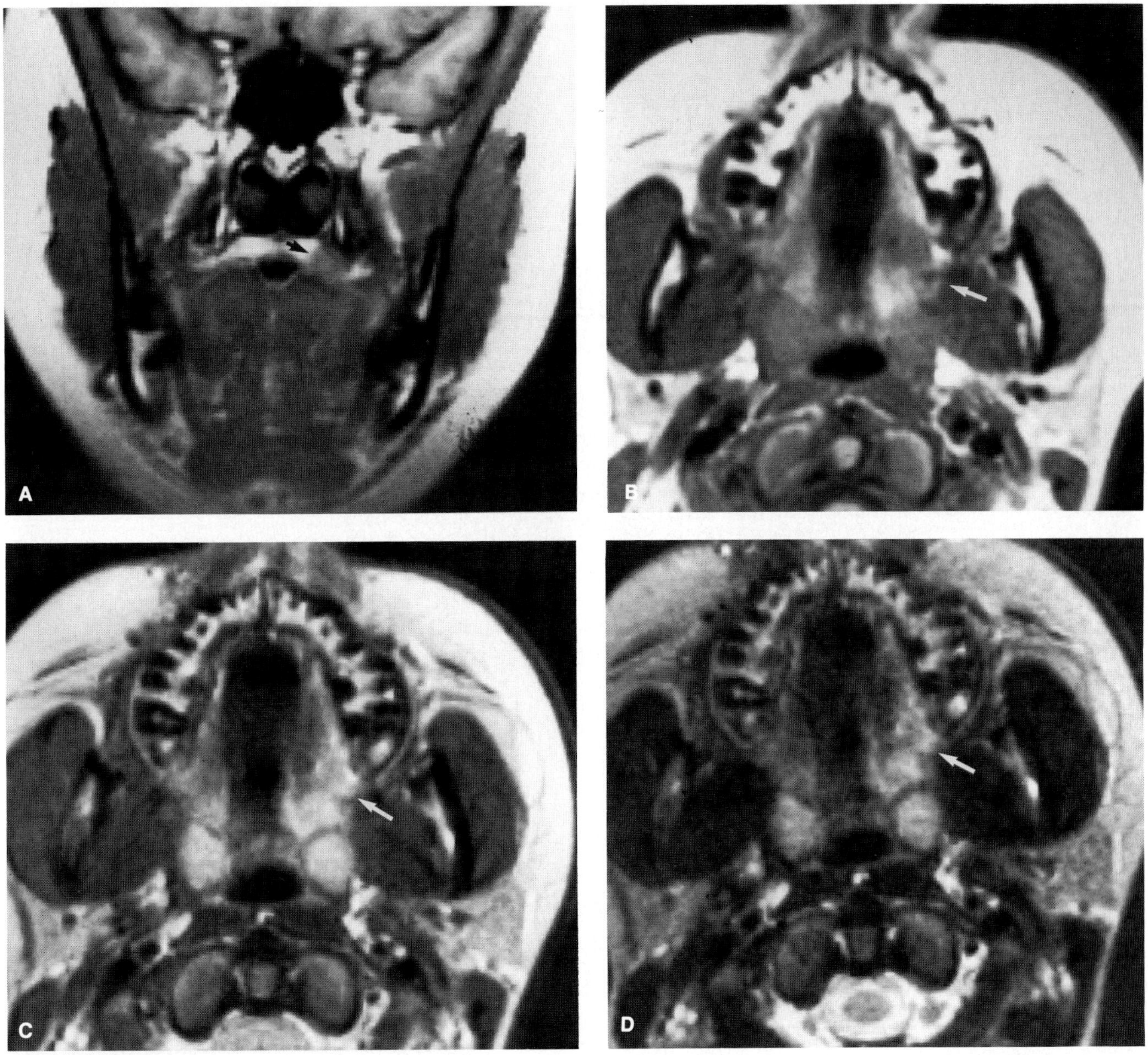

FIGURE 8–17. Mucoepidermoid carcinoma of the palate. **(A)** T1-weighted coronal, **(B)** T1-weighted, **(C)** proton density, and **(D)** T2-weighted axial images. There is a small mass (arrow) replacing the fat in the soft palate. Like most palatine lesions, this mass is easiest to appreciate in the coronal plane. The mass exhibits only a moderately increased signal on T2-weighted images.

nonspecific. Although these lesions tend to have a higher signal intensity than squamous cell carcinomas on T2-weighted images, in our experience, there is a significant amount of overlap, and this differentiation cannot be made reliably on the basis of signal intensity alone.[6]

Miscellaneous Benign Lesions

Benign cystic lesions of the mouth and oropharynx are commonly encountered, and MR may be requested to evaluate their nature and extent. Cystic lesions may arise from mucus extravasation from salivary ducts, from partial obstruction of salivary ducts with resulting cystic dilatation, from epithelial inclusions (i.e., lymphoepithelial cyst), or from cystic dilatation of thyroglossal duct remnants in the base of the tongue (i.e., thyroglossal duct cyst). All of these lesions may be expected to show the characteristic signs of cysts on MRI (Fig. 8–18): low intensity on T1-weighted images, although higher intensities are seen if the fluid contents are hemorrhagic or proteina-

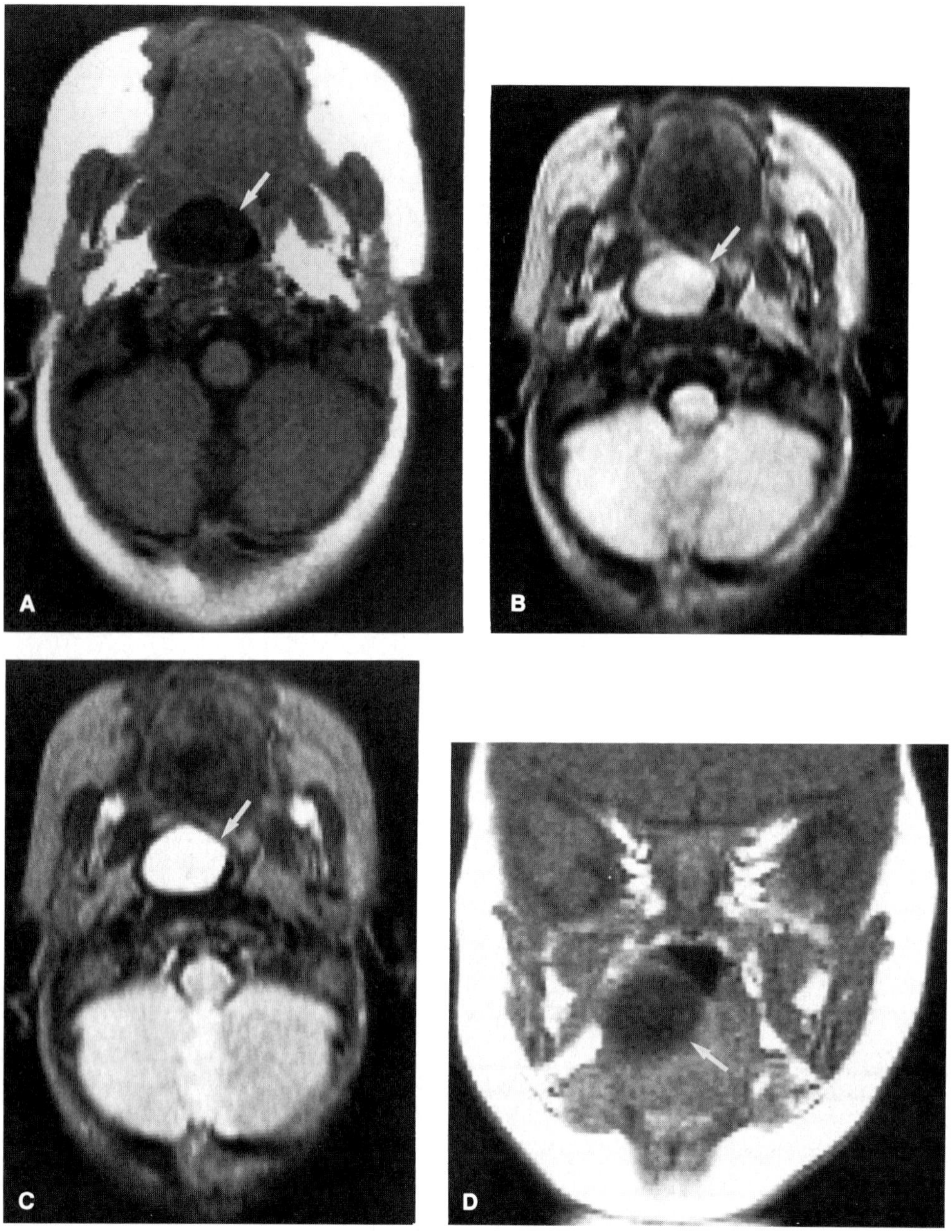

FIGURE 8–18. Oropharyngeal cyst in an infant, probable branchial cleft origin. **(A)** T1-weighted, **(B)** proton density, **(C)** T2-weighted axial, and **(D)** T1-weighted coronal images through the oropharynx. The cyst (arrow) demonstrates the typical signal characteristics of simple fluid, with well-defined, smoothly marginated borders.

ceous, and very high, homogeneous signal intensity on T2-weighted images, on which cyst contents should equal the signal intensity of CSF.

A characteristic cystic lesion in the mouth is the ranula (Fig. 8–19), which represents either a mucocele or mucus retention cyst of the sublingual glands. The mucus retention type, or simple ranula, presents as a smooth, fluctuant mass in the floor of the mouth and may be easily excised or marsupialized. The mucocele type, or plunging ranula, represents mucus extravasation from a sublingual duct and may exhibit extensive spread through the floor of the mouth to the submental area and even to the neck. Surgical treatment in this case is much more difficult, and MRI may help determine the extent of involvement of these lesions.

A variety of miscellaneous benign lesions may be seen. Lingual hemangiomas exhibit the signal characteristics of hemangiomas elsewhere in the body; low or intermediate signal intensity on T1-weighted and very high signal intensity on T2-weighted images (Fig. 8–20). Infections and abscesses in the tonsillar fossa or floor of the mouth show variable low intensity on T1-weighted images and high intensity on T2-weighted images, depending on the degree of liquefaction.

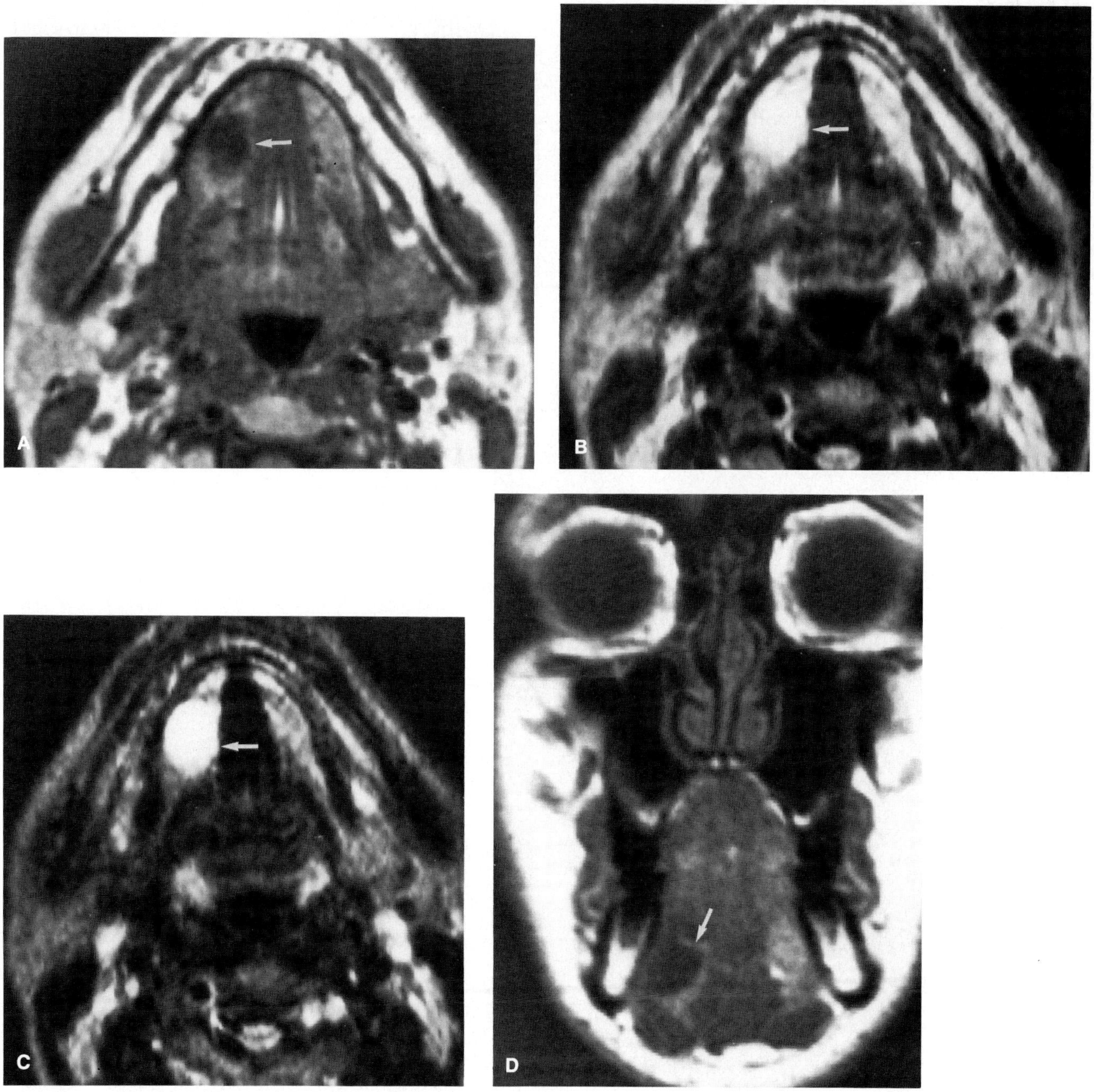

FIGURE 8–19. Ranula. **(A)** T1-weighted, **(B)** proton density, **(C)** T2-weighted axial, and **(D)** T1-weighted coronal images. There is a rounded lesion (arrow) in the right sublingual region that exhibits fluid signal intensity on all sequences.

MAJOR SALIVARY GLANDS

The major salivary glands include the parotid and submandibular glands. The sublingual glands were discussed with the oropharynx. By far the leading indication for MRI examination of the major salivary glands is the evaluation of the location and extent of mass lesions.[3,16–18] Chronic inflammatory diseases of the salivary glands remain the domain of sialography and, to a lesser extent, CT. Typically, 5-mm slices are obtained through the gland of interest. Although axial images usually supply most of the necessary information, coronal images often help in evaluating the salivary glands and surrounding structures.

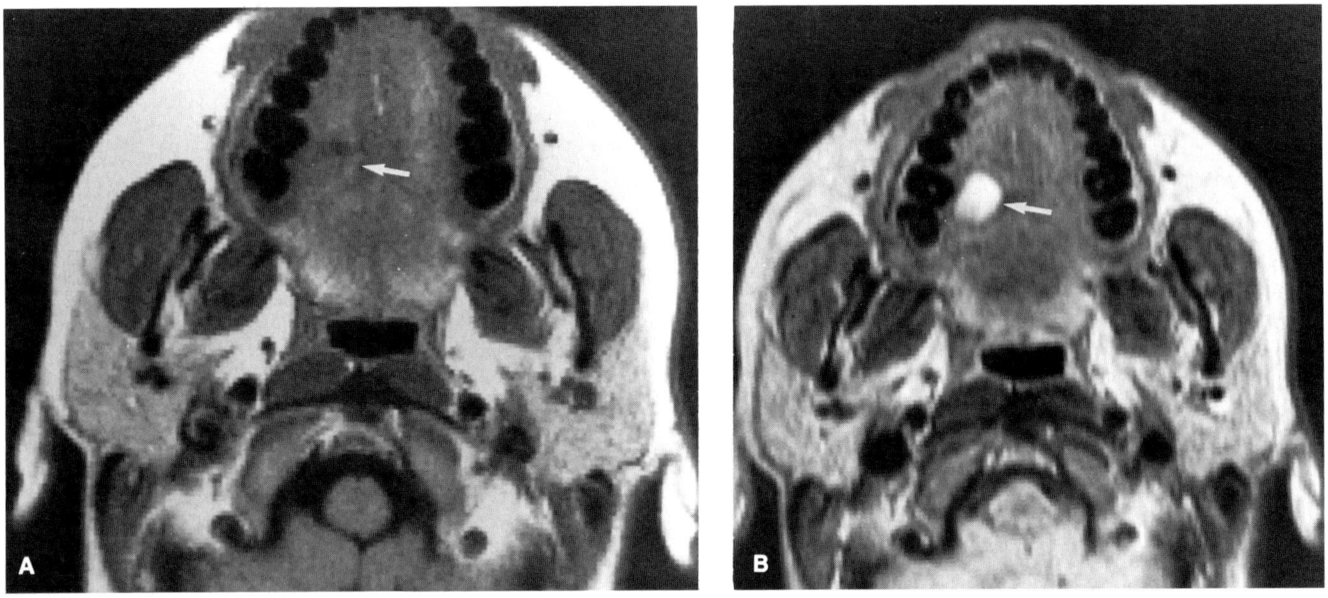

FIGURE 8–20. Hemangioma of the tongue. **(A)** T1-weighted and **(B)** T2-weighted axial images through the tongue. The hemangioma (arrow) exhibits a characteristic very bright signal on T2-weighted images.

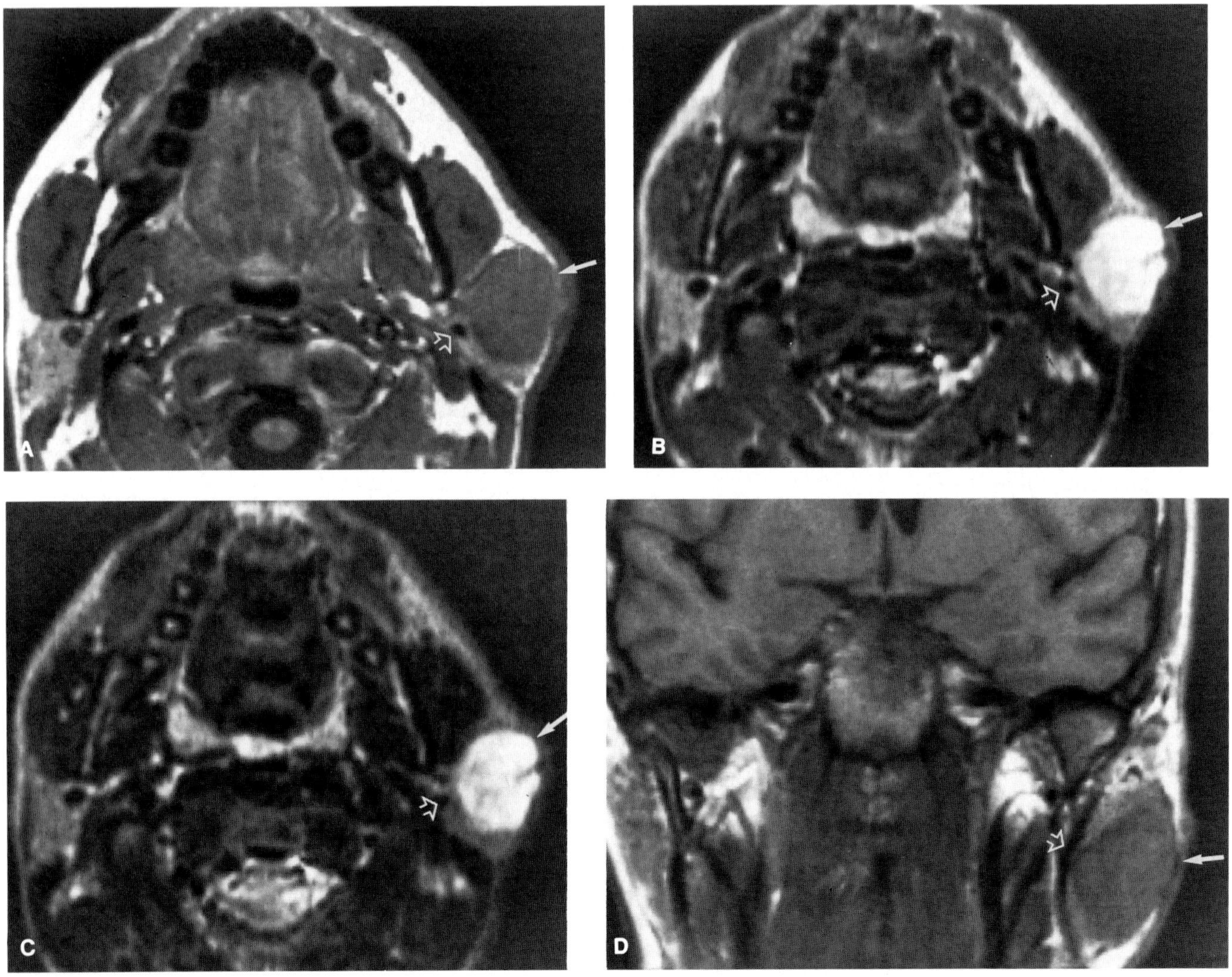

FIGURE 8–21. Superficial parotid gland pleomorphic adenoma. **(A)** T1-weighted, **(B)** proton density, **(C)** T2-weighted axial, and **(D)** T1-weighted coronal images through the parotid glands. The lesion (arrow) in the left parotid gland is superficial to the retromandibular vein (open arrow) and facial nerve. It is isointense with muscle on the T1-weighted images and markedly hyperintense on the T2-weighted images. It has well-defined margins throughout.

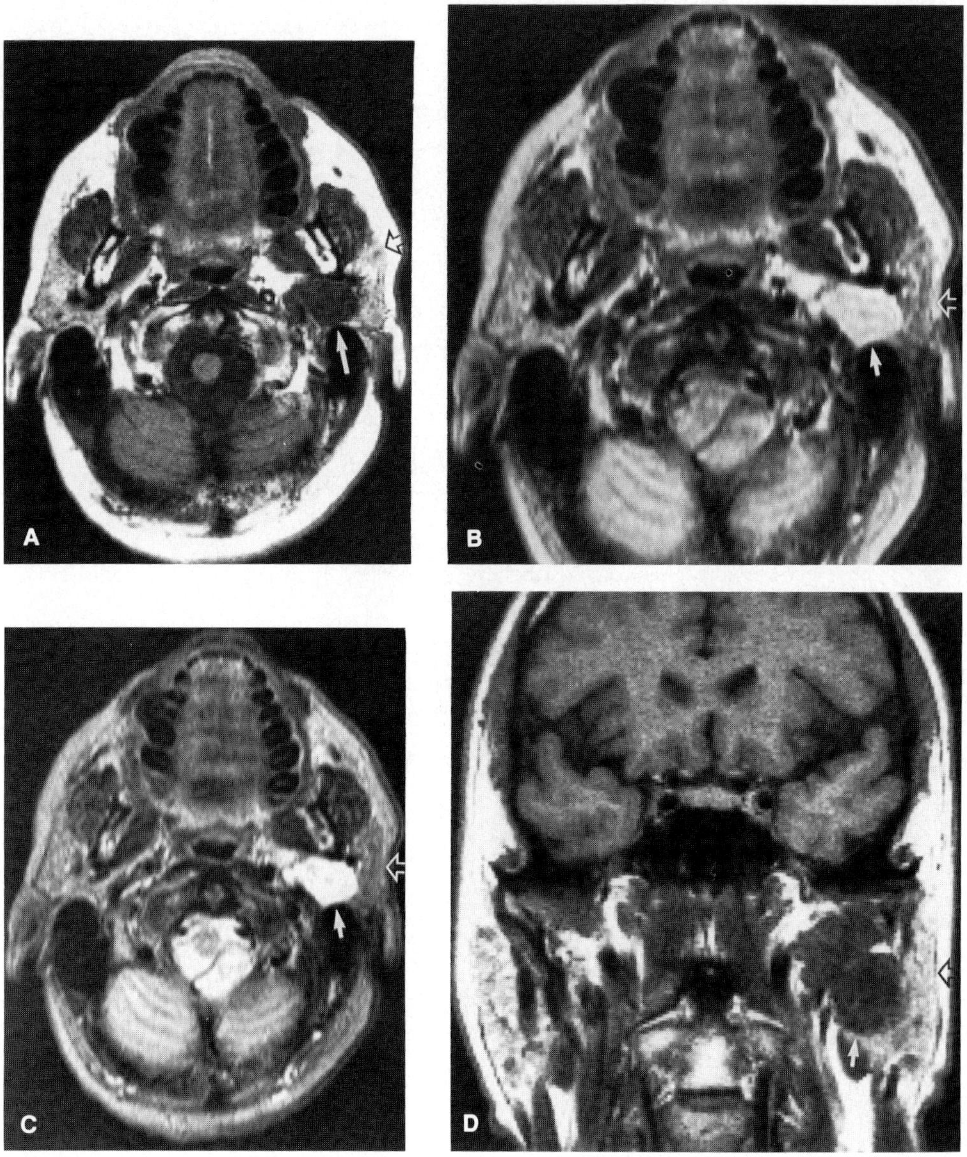

FIGURE 8–22. Pleomorphic adenoma of the deep portion of the left parotid gland. **(A)** T1-weighted, **(B)** proton density, **(C)** T2-weighted axial, and **(D)** T1-weighted coronal images through the parotid glands. The tumor (arrow) is not separated from the parotid gland (open arrow) by a fat plane, indicating a parotid gland origin, rather than parapharyngeal space.

Salivary tumors may arise in either the parotid or submandibular glands, although the most common site is the parotid. Three-quarters of parotid tumors are benign, but submandibular tumors have an approximately 50% chance of malignancy.[19] The majority of the benign tumors of the parotid, and virtually all in the submandibular gland, are pleomorphic adenomas (Figs. 8–21 and 8–22). The other significant benign tumor of the parotid is adenolymphoma or Warthin's tumor. Multiplicity of masses favors Warthin's tumor. The unusual, benign mesenchymal masses, lipomas (Fig. 8–23) and hemangiomas, exhibit characteristic MRI features, as in other areas of the body. Lipomas show very high signal intensities on T1-weighted images and decreased signal on heavily T2-weighted images. Hemangiomas exhibit very high signal on T2-weighted images, often with a characteristic multiseptated appearance.[20]

The malignant masses include mucoepidermoid carcinoma, adenoid cystic carcinoma, adenocarcinoma, acinic cell tumors, squamous cell carcinoma, and the malignant variant of pleomorphic adenoma,

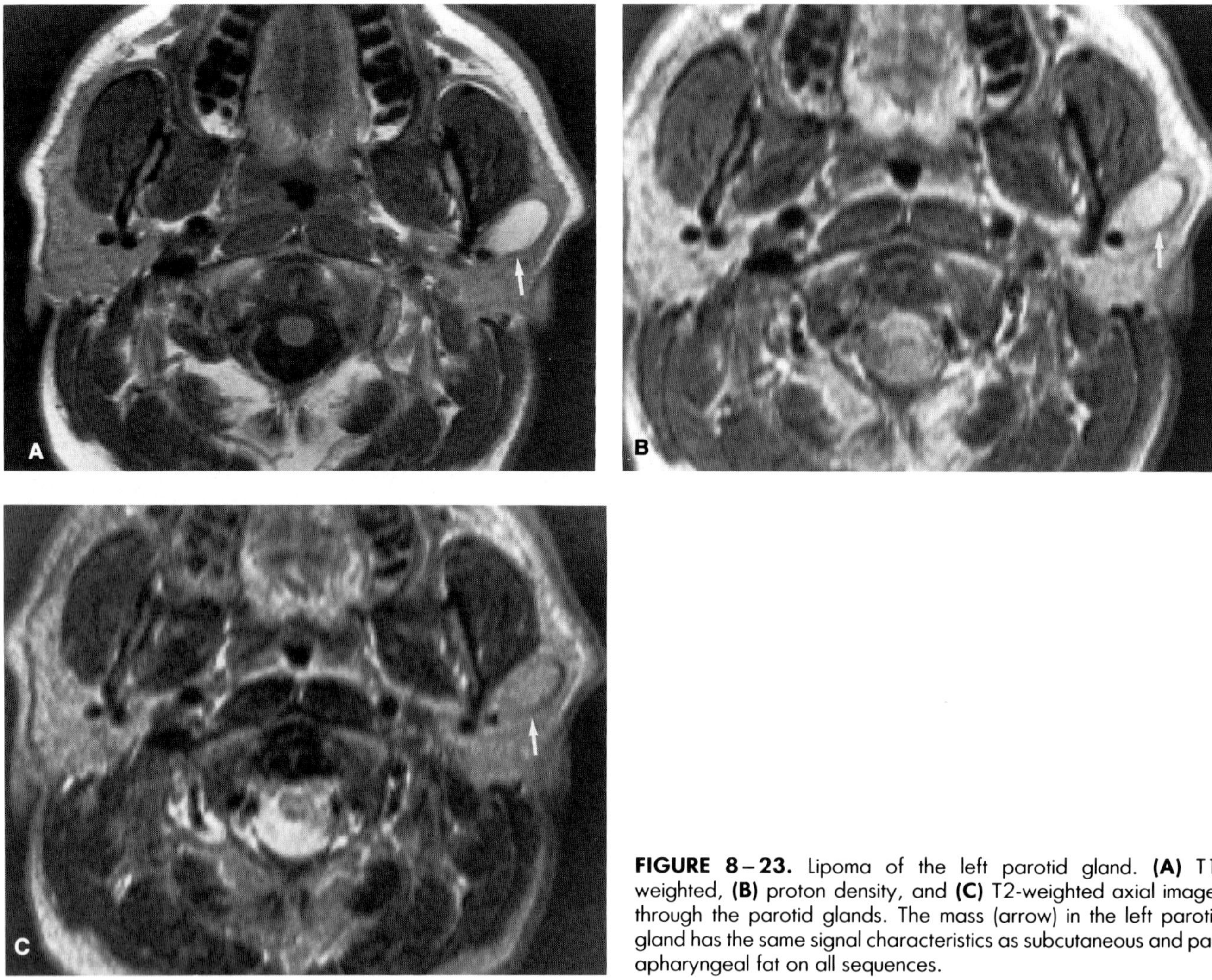

FIGURE 8–23. Lipoma of the left parotid gland. **(A)** T1-weighted, **(B)** proton density, and **(C)** T2-weighted axial images through the parotid glands. The mass (arrow) in the left parotid gland has the same signal characteristics as subcutaneous and parapharyngeal fat on all sequences.

malignant mixed tumors (Figs. 8–24 and 8–25). These tumors are essentially indistinguishable by their MRI characteristics—intermediate intensity on T1-weighted images and high intensity on T2-weighted images—although pleomorphic adenomas are often quite low in signal intensity on T1-weighted sequences in our experience. The contrast of these lesions with the surrounding gland varies with its histologic composition. The relatively greater fat content of the parotid gland gives it higher signal on T1-weighted images, often making parotid lesions easy to visualize on T1-weighted images as lower-signal-intensity masses (similar to muscle) relative to the surrounding gland parenchyma. Early experience has revealed enhancement with Gd DTPA in several primary salivary gland neoplasms (Fig. 8–26 and 8–27).

Marked marginal irregularity and local infiltration favor malignancy, but smooth, regular margins do not ensure benignity. Facial nerve paralysis and pain are ominous signs for malignancy. Metastases, including lymphoma, not uncommonly affect the parotid gland, probably because of numerous intraparotid and periparotid lymph nodes (Figs. 8–28 and 8–29). These nodes drain the face and scalp and are commonly affected by squamous cell carcinomas or melanomas arising in these areas. The MRI appearance will be nonspecific, although multiplicity of lesions is characteristic. Warthin's tumor may also be multifocal and bilateral.

In the evaluation of parotid masses, it is crucial to assess whether the lesion involves the superficial or deep portions of the gland and the relationship of the facial nerve to the tumor, because these features dic-

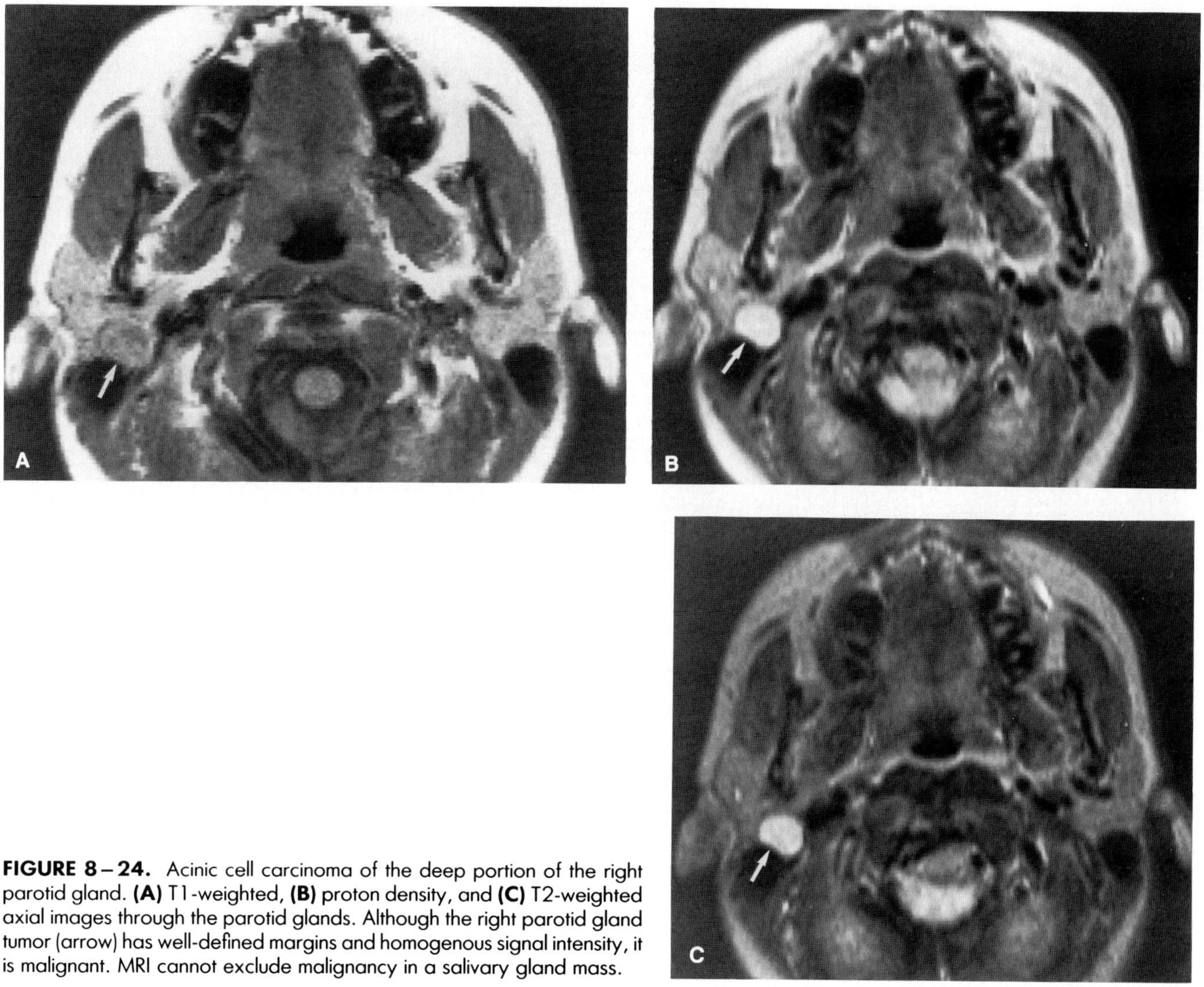

FIGURE 8–24. Acinic cell carcinoma of the deep portion of the right parotid gland. **(A)** T1-weighted, **(B)** proton density, and **(C)** T2-weighted axial images through the parotid glands. Although the right parotid gland tumor (arrow) has well-defined margins and homogenous signal intensity, it is malignant. MRI cannot exclude malignancy in a salivary gland mass.

tate the surgical approach. The superficial and deep portions of the gland are separated by the intraparotid facial nerve, which courses anteriorly from the stylomastoid foramen and laterally to the retromandibular vein. Portions of the nerve may be more commonly seen with MRI than with CT, but even if the nerve is not visualized, its relationship to a mass may be deduced from its expected course. It has been reported that thin (4 mm) cuts angled 30 to 40° caudal to the orbitomeatal line demonstrate the nerve with the greatest reliability.[21]

Tumors that extend from the superficial to the deep portions of the gland characteristically exhibit a waist-like narrowing as they pass between the styloid process and the mandibular condyle. It is important to assess whether deep masses originate in the parotid gland itself or in the parapharyngeal space. This distinction can usually be easily made on MRI by assessing the direction of displacement of the parapharyngeal fat plane: laterally in the case of parapharyngeal masses and medially in the case of deep parotid lesions. If the fat plane is obliterated, an exact determination cannot be made, but statistically, a parotid origin is likely. The coronal plane often helps in evaluating this fat plane.

Although not a common primary indication for MRI of the salivary glands, inflammatory processes in the glands are important because they share the signal characteristics of tumors. They are usually more diffuse than tumors, but focal areas of inflammation or frank abscesses with irregular margins may mimic malignancy. Ductal ectasia may be seen secondary to ductal stenosis and calculi. Salivary duct calculi have

(text continues on page 316)

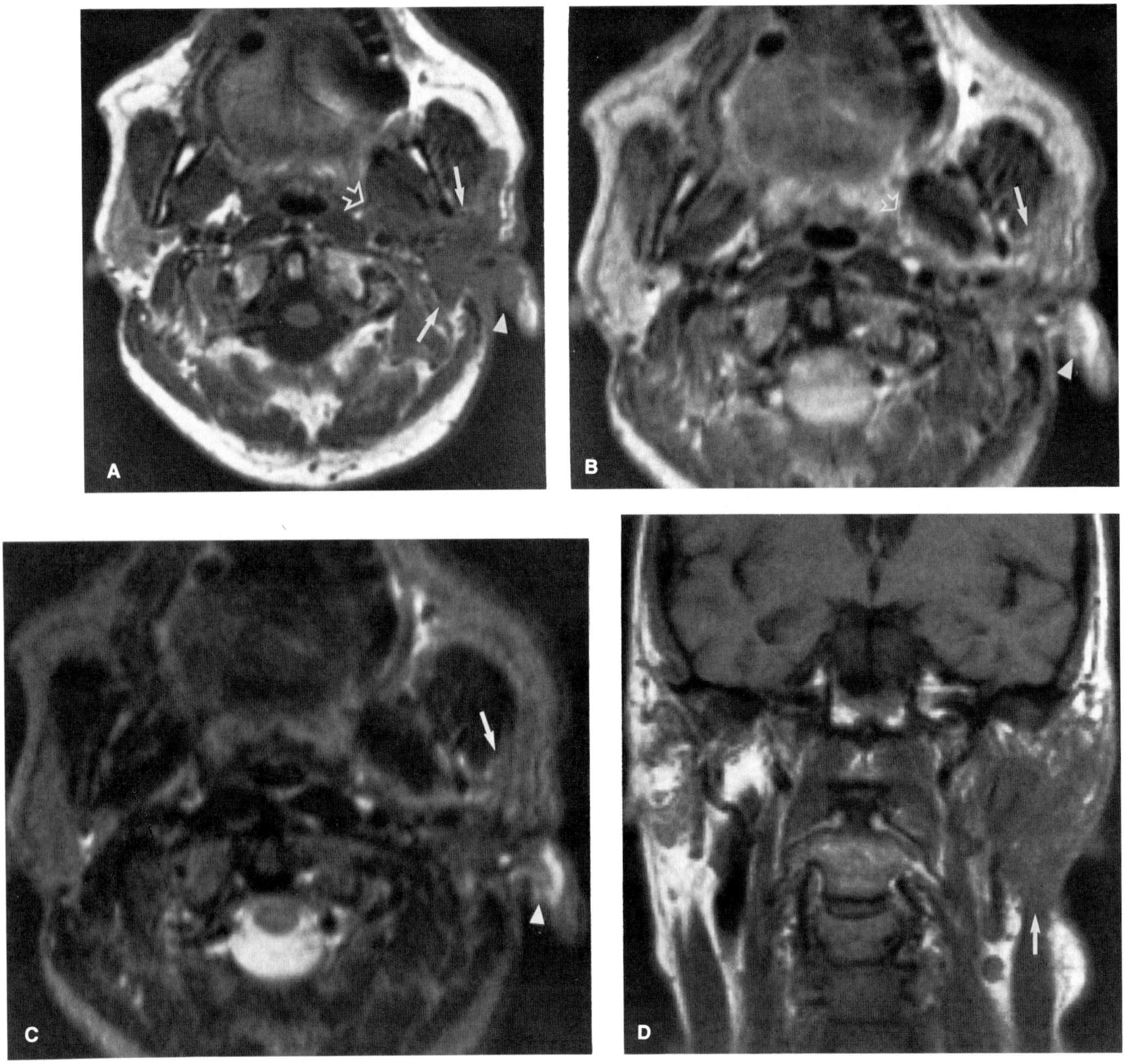

FIGURE 8–25. Recurrent adenosquamous carcinoma of the left parotid gland. **(A)** T1-weighted, **(B)** proton density, **(C)** T2-weighted axial, and **(D)** T1-weighted coronal images through the parotid glands. The left parotid gland is infiltrated by low-signal-intensity tumor (arrow) on the T1-weighted images. The tumor has ill-defined margins and invades the pterygoid muscle and parapharyngeal space medially (open arrow) and pinna laterally (arrowhead). In a case like this, MRI can indicate the malignant nature of a mass. The tumor has an unusually low signal intensity on the T2-weighted image.

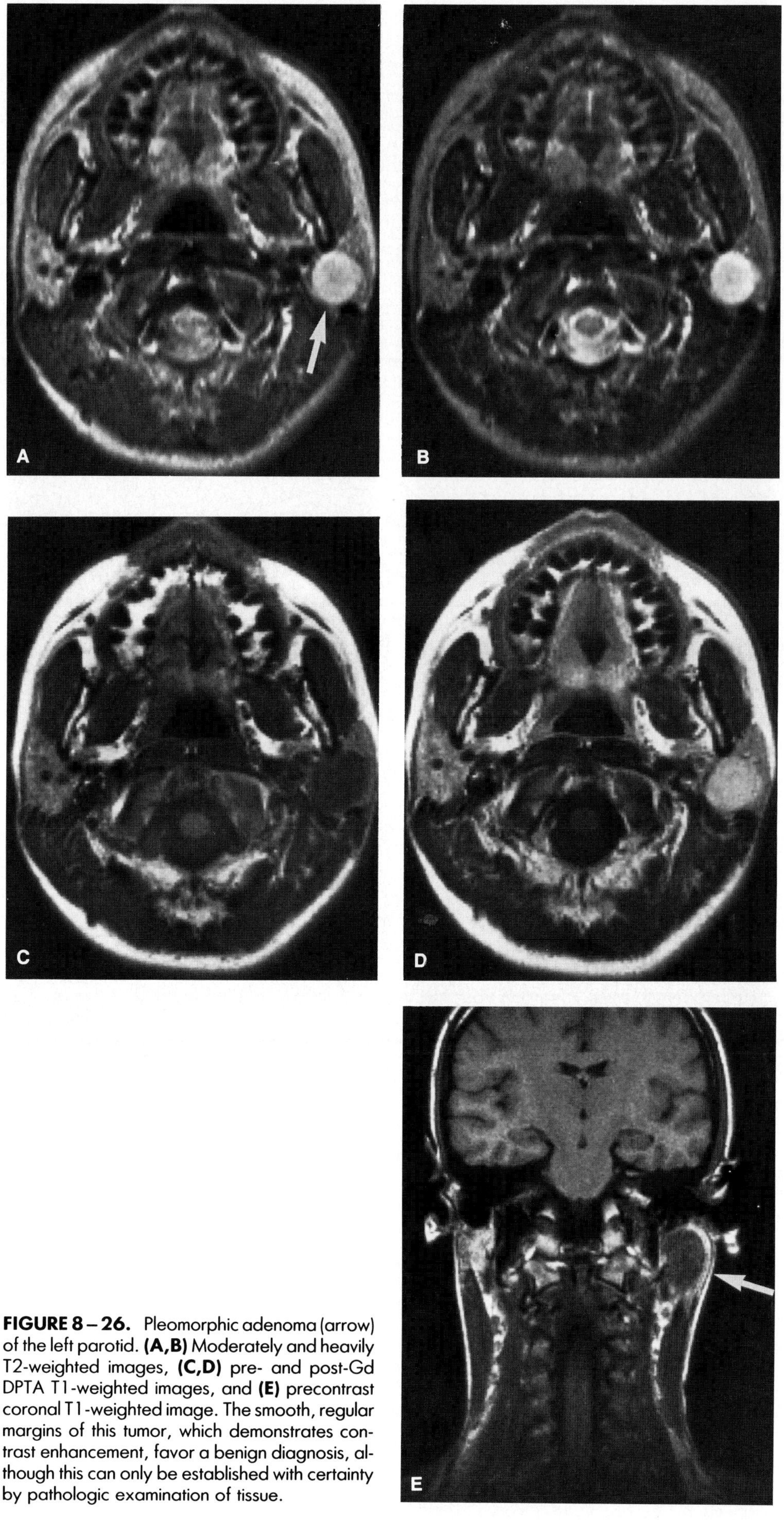

FIGURE 8–26. Pleomorphic adenoma (arrow) of the left parotid. **(A,B)** Moderately and heavily T2-weighted images, **(C,D)** pre- and post-Gd DPTA T1-weighted images, and **(E)** precontrast coronal T1-weighted image. The smooth, regular margins of this tumor, which demonstrates contrast enhancement, favor a benign diagnosis, although this can only be established with certainty by pathologic examination of tissue.

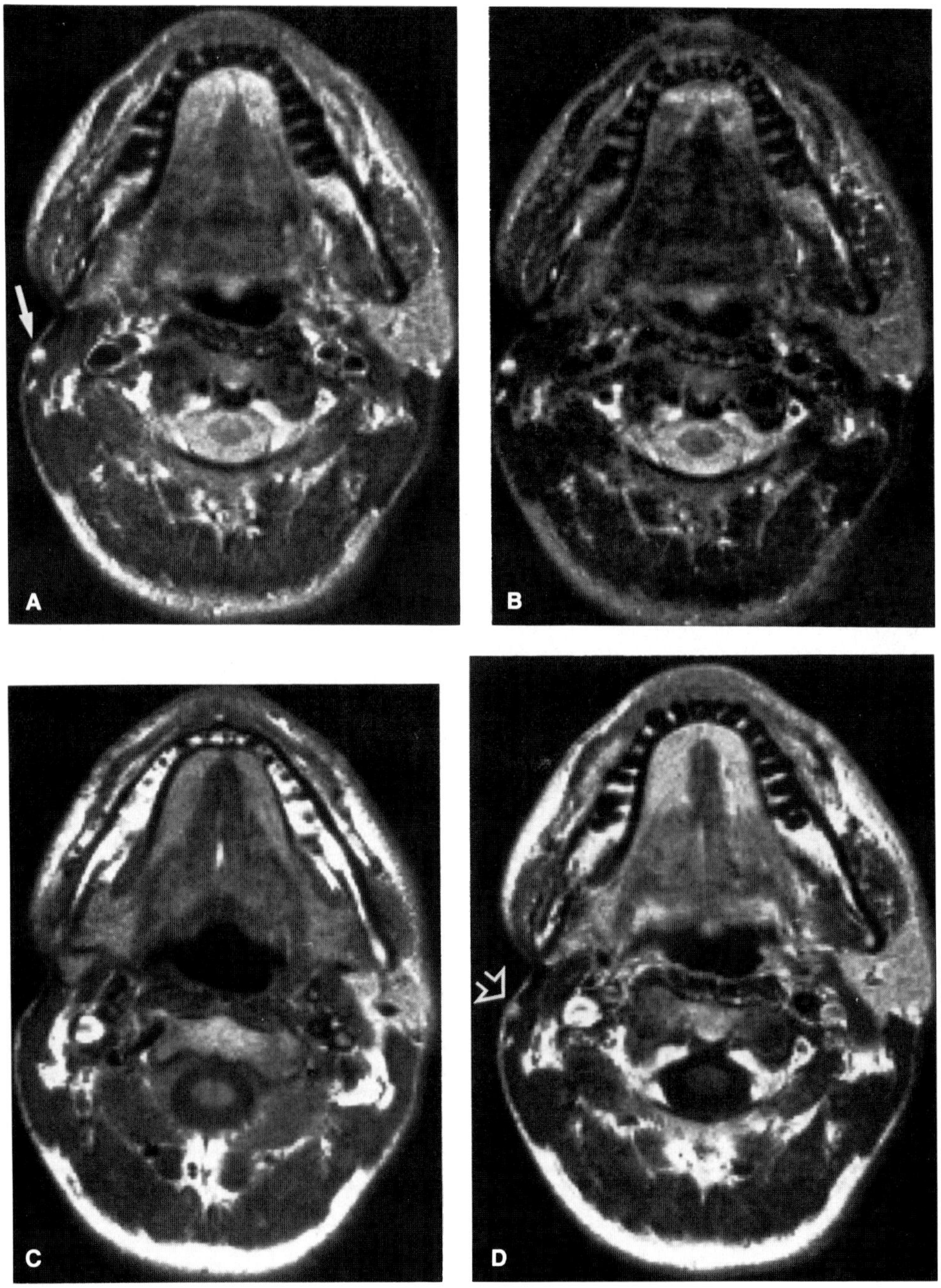

FIGURE 8–27. Recurrent pleomorphic adenoma in a patient after a right parotidectomy with multiple subsequent resections of recurrent tumor. **(A,B)** Moderately and heavily T2-weighted images and **(C,D)** pre- and post-Gd DPTA T1-weighted images. A high-signal-intensity nodule is seen on the T2-weighted images (closed arrow) in the right parotid fossa. Although the area of abnormality is identified on the T2-weighted images, the signal intensity characteristics are nonspecific. Enhancement of this lesion (open arrow) is consistent with recurrent tumor.

FIGURE 8–28. Metastatic squamous cell carcinoma. **(A)** T1-weighted, **(B)** proton density, and **(C)** T2-weighted images through the parotid glands. **(D)** T1-weighted, **(E)** proton density, and **(F)** T2-weighted slices through the masseter muscles. There is a poorly marginated right parotid mass (arrow) and a mass (open arrow) replacing the masseter muscle and invading the zygomatic arch on the right. These masses exhibit heterogeneous signal intensities and were surgically proven to be metastatic squamous cell carcinoma. The more sharply defined mass in the left parotid (curved arrow) was not biopsied, but its appearance is consistent with a pleomorphic adenoma. ▶

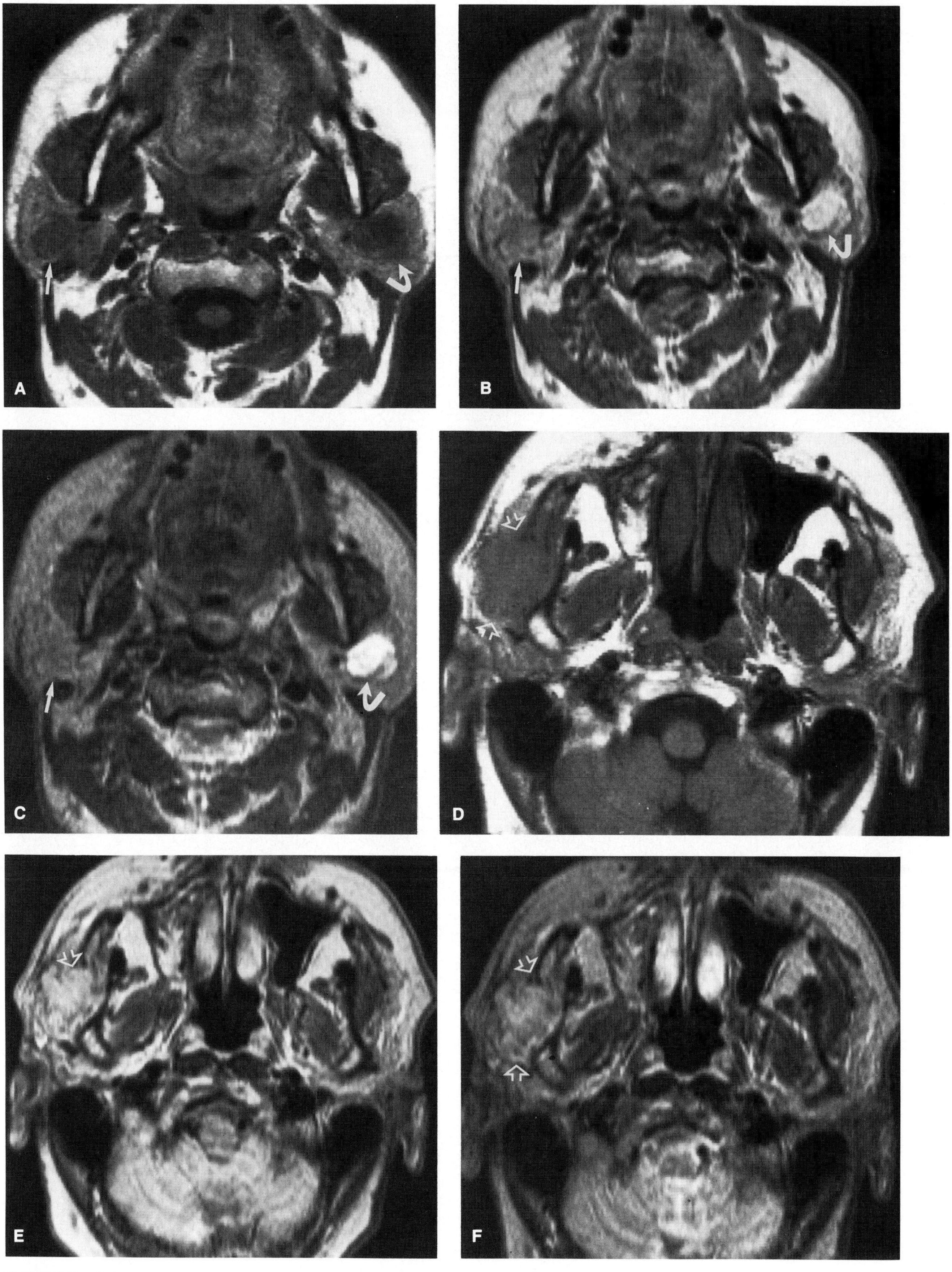

FIGURE 8–28.

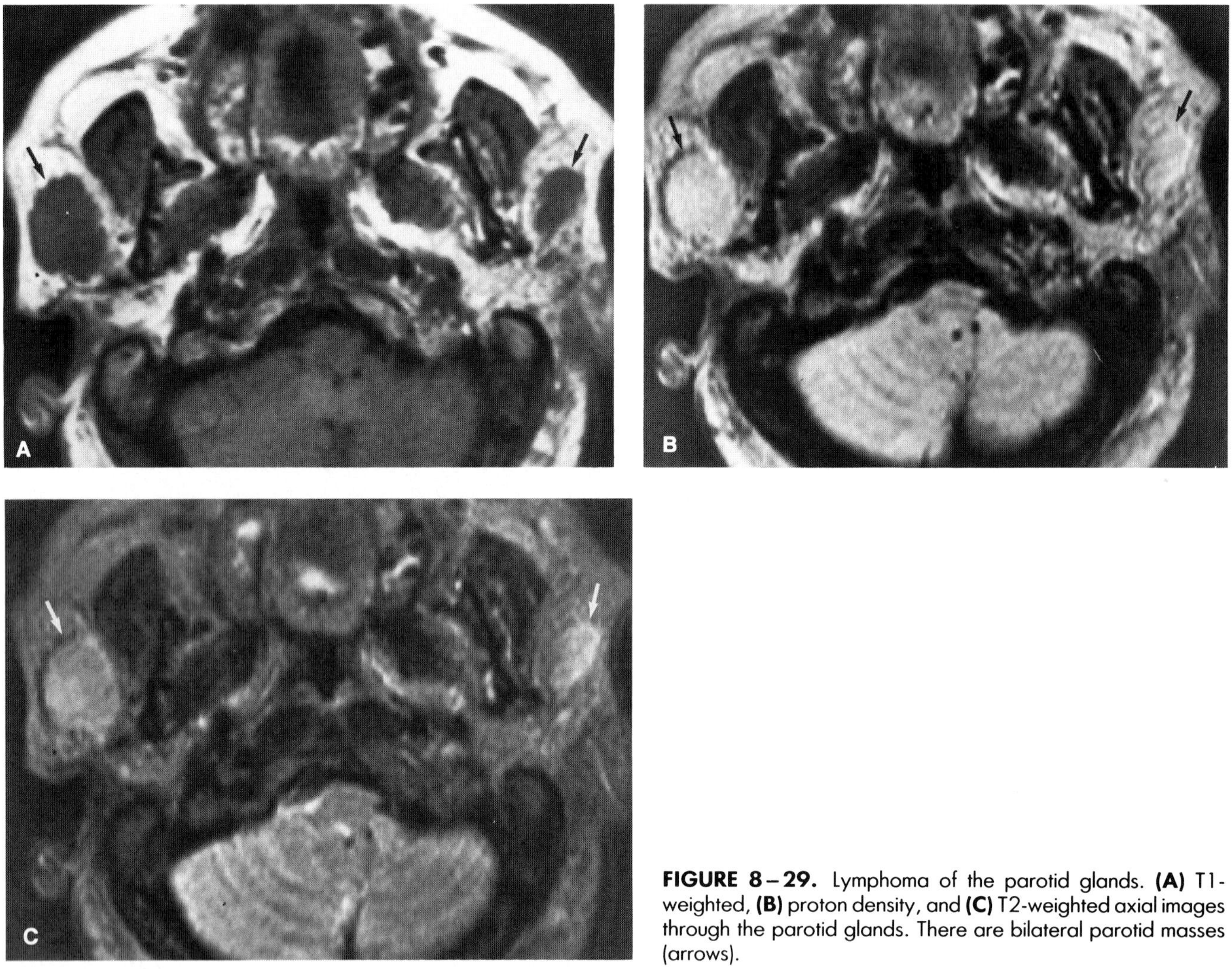

FIGURE 8–29. Lymphoma of the parotid glands. **(A)** T1-weighted, **(B)** proton density, and **(C)** T2-weighted axial images through the parotid glands. There are bilateral parotid masses (arrows).

been reported as foci of signal void on MRI, but are much more reliably imaged with plain films, CT, or sialography (Fig. 8–30).[16] The parotid gland contains numerous lymph nodes. Normal, small nodes and enlarged, inflammatory nodes are commonly imaged during routine scans of the head and face and should not be mistaken for primary or metastatic tumors. The signal characteristics do not help this distinction, so caution must be exercised when small, nonpalpable masses are seen in or adjacent to the parotid gland (Fig. 8–31). Occasionally, unilaterally or bilaterally hypertrophied masseter muscles are mistaken for parotid masses. This distinction is easily made with MRI (Fig. 8–32).

PARANASAL SINUSES

Benign Lesions

The high prevalence of incidentally discovered mucosal thickening in the sinuses is immediately evident to anyone beginning to interpret MRI scans of the head and face.[22] This mucosal thickening exhibits very high signal intensity on T2-weighted images (Fig. 8–33). It may be localized to a portion of one sinus or involve all of the sinuses and tends to be more extensive in pediatric patients. The clinical relevance of this finding is often obscure, and in most of these patients the finding is of no pathologic significance.

Another lesion that is often seen as an incidental finding is the sinus retention cyst. These cysts are usually located in the inferior aspect of the maxillary antrum, exhibit smooth, rounded borders, and have low intensity signals on T1-weighted images and characteristically very high intensity signals on T2-weighted images, identical to fluid. Because retention cysts tend to occupy the most inferior portion of the maxillary antrum, the lowest axial slices through the antrum may simulate sinus fluid. However, on higher axial slices, sinus fluid will exhibit an air-fluid level, and retention cysts have a rounded upper margin. In questionable cases, sagittal views should resolve the issue. Sinus polyps are a much less common lesion and may be indistinguishable from retention cysts,

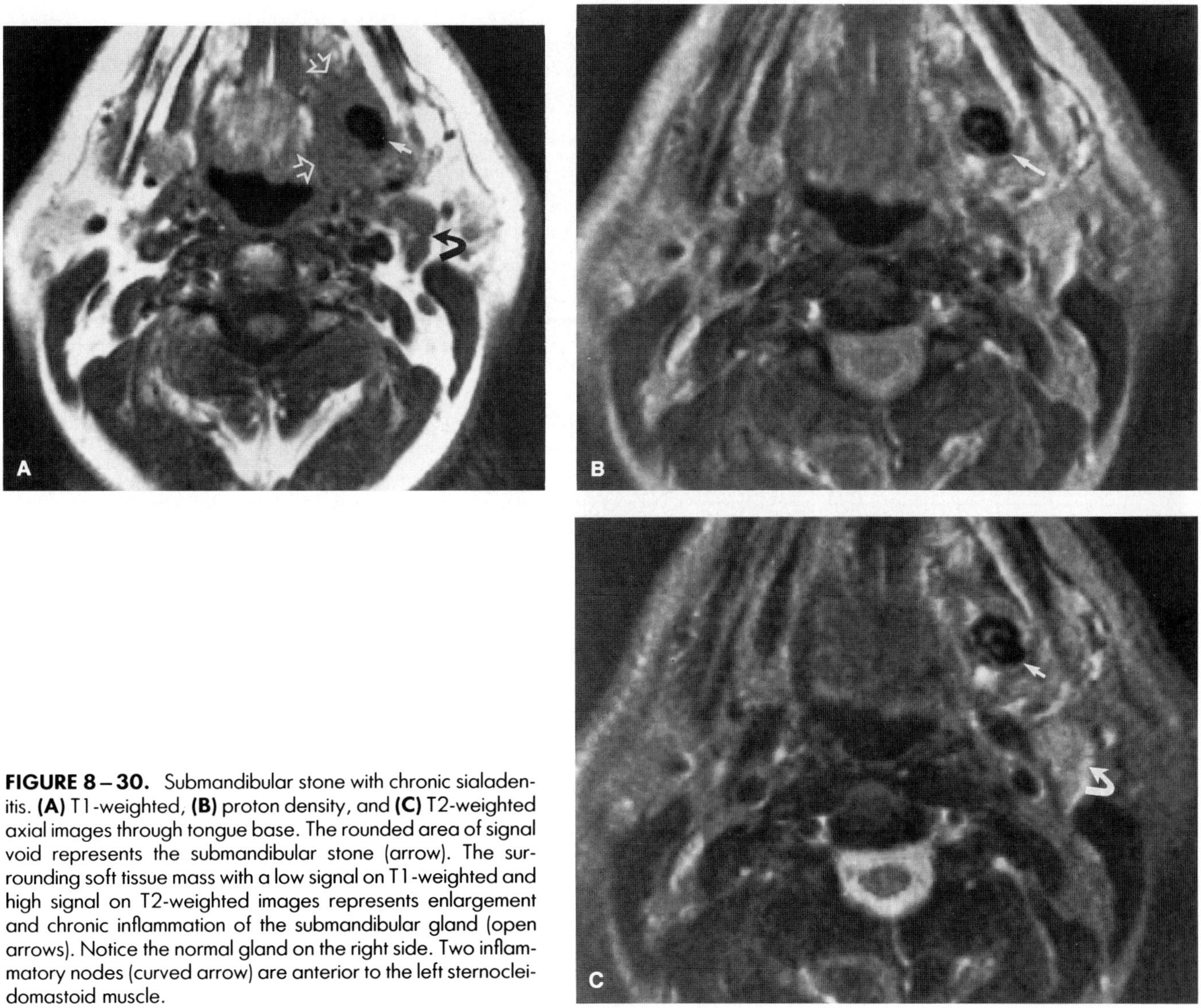

FIGURE 8–30. Submandibular stone with chronic sialadenitis. **(A)** T1-weighted, **(B)** proton density, and **(C)** T2-weighted axial images through tongue base. The rounded area of signal void represents the submandibular stone (arrow). The surrounding soft tissue mass with a low signal on T1-weighted and high signal on T2-weighted images represents enlargement and chronic inflammation of the submandibular gland (open arrows). Notice the normal gland on the right side. Two inflammatory nodes (curved arrow) are anterior to the left sternocleidomastoid muscle.

presenting as smooth, well-defined lesions exhibiting high intensity signals on T2-weighted images.

In acute sinusitis, air-fluid levels are easily diagnosed by MRI, especially on T2-weighted images, on which the high-signal-intensity fluid exhibits the greatest contrast with air. An exception is sinus hemorrhage. Depending on its age, blood may exhibit the highest signal on T1-weighted images. This has been reported following trauma and in patients with a blood coagulopathy.[23,24] The granulomatous diseases that may affect the sinuses, including Wegener's granulomatosis, midline granuloma, sarcoidosis, and tuberculosis, exhibit nonspecific soft tissue signal intensities within the sinuses and may show variable amounts of bone destruction. The degree of bone destruction, however, is more easily appreciated on CT.

Mucoceles and pyoceles exhibit the expected findings of low intensity signals on T1-weighted images and uniform high intensity signals on T2-weighted images, due to their fluid content, with expansion of the sinus and thinning of the sinus wall. Recurrent mucoceles exhibit higher signal intensities on T1-weighted and variable intensity on T2-weighted images due to peri-operative hemorrhage (Fig. 8–34).[7]

The fibro-osseous lesions of the sinuses exhibit decreased signal on both T1-weighted and T2-weighted images. They may have foci of signal void due to areas of dense calcification, although this will usually be easier to appreciate on CT. The aggressive benign lesions of the nose and nasopharynx (i.e., inverted papilloma and juvenile angiofibroma) commonly involve the sinuses, especially the maxillary antrum.

(text continues on page 323)

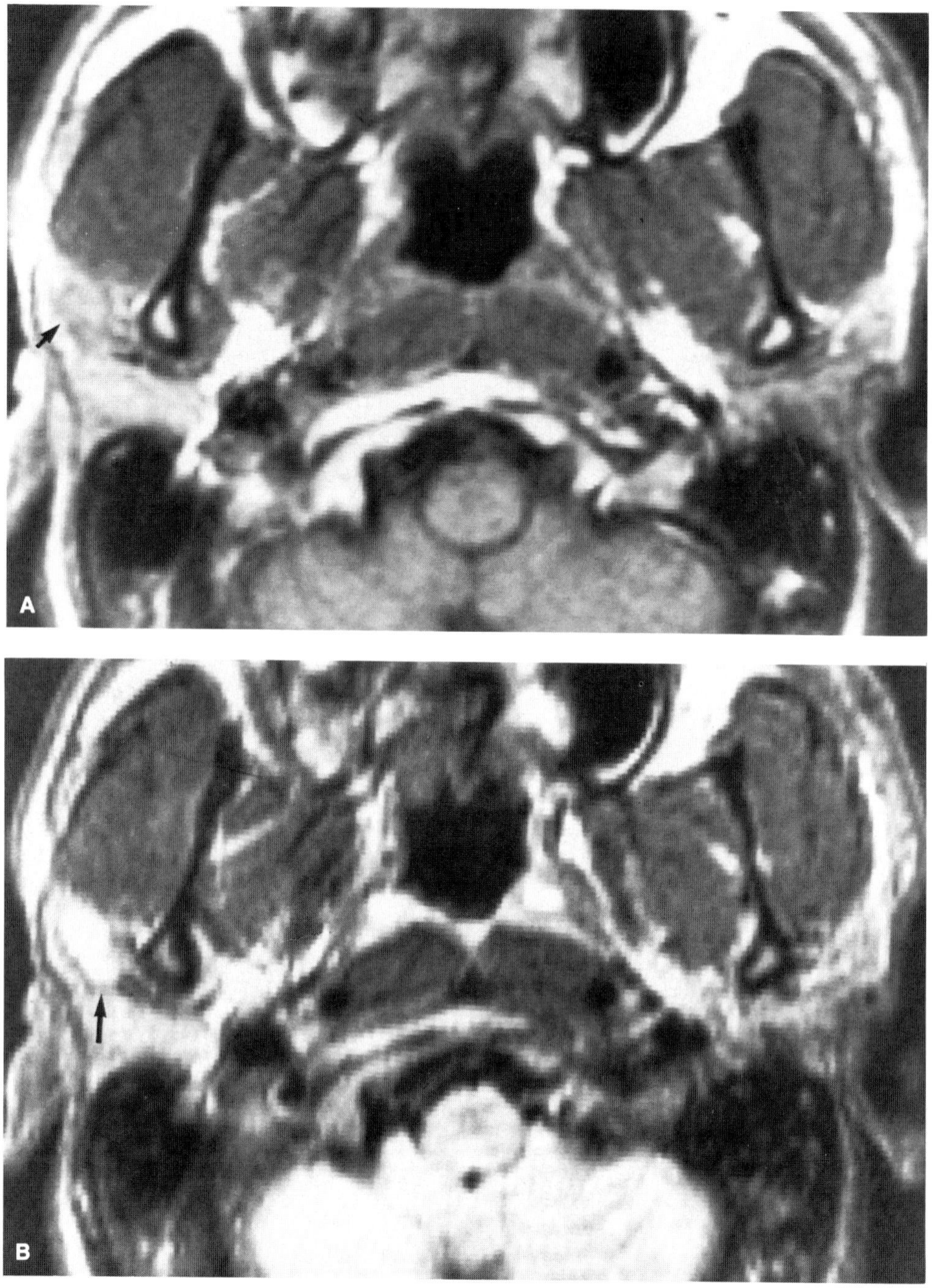

FIGURE 8–31. Benign intraparotid lymph node. **(A)** T1-weighted, **(B)** proton density, **(C)** T2-weighted axial, and **(D)** T1-weighted coronal images demonstrate a small mass (arrow) in the superior aspect of the superficial right parotid gland. This was an incidental finding, and biopsy confirmed normal lymph node tissue.

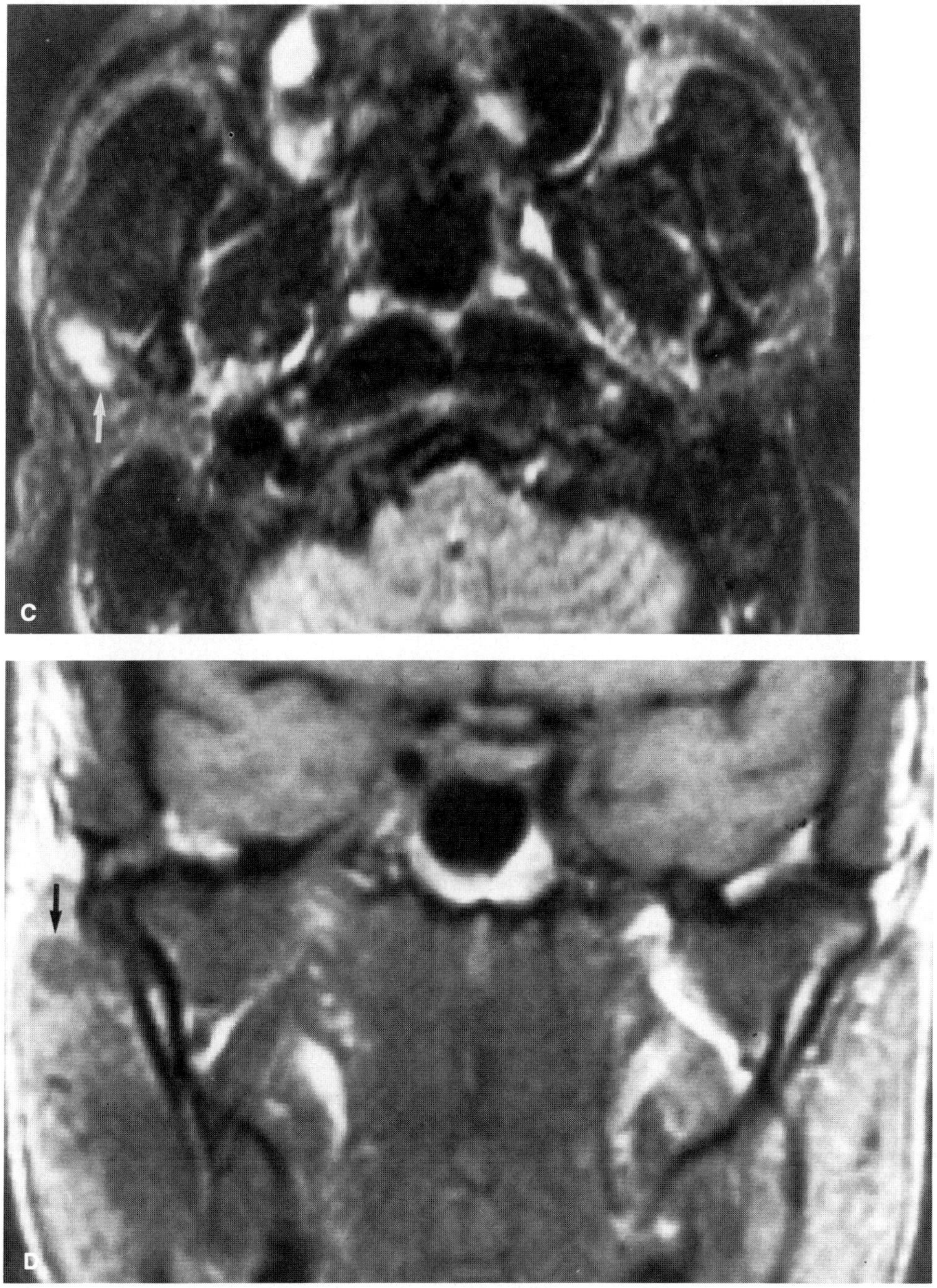

FIGURE 8–31. (Continued)

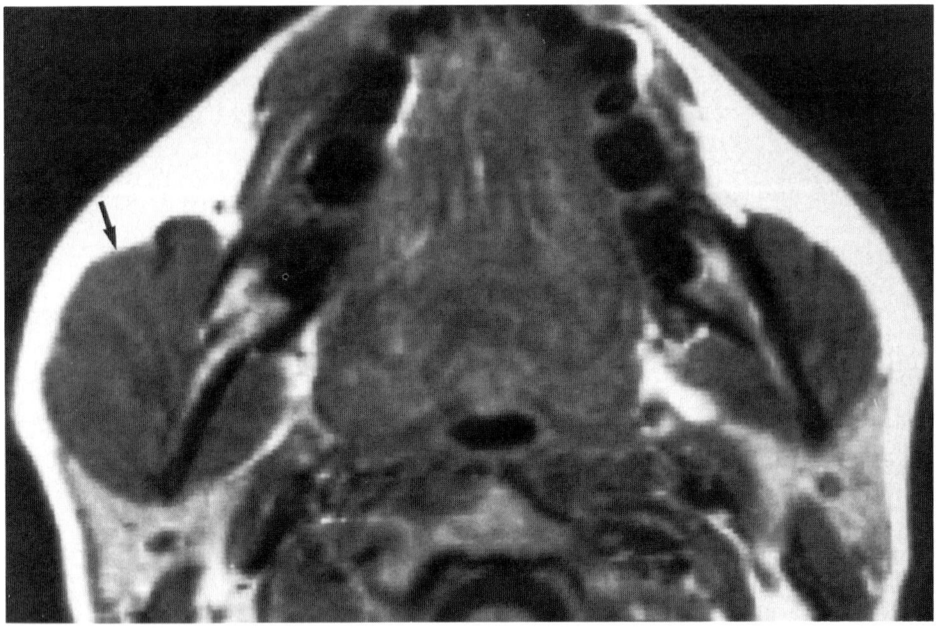

FIGURE 8–32. Unilateral masseter hypertrophy. A T1-weighted axial image clearly demonstrates that the palpable abnormality corresponds to an asymmetrically enlarged right masseter muscle (arrow). The parotid glands were entirely normal.

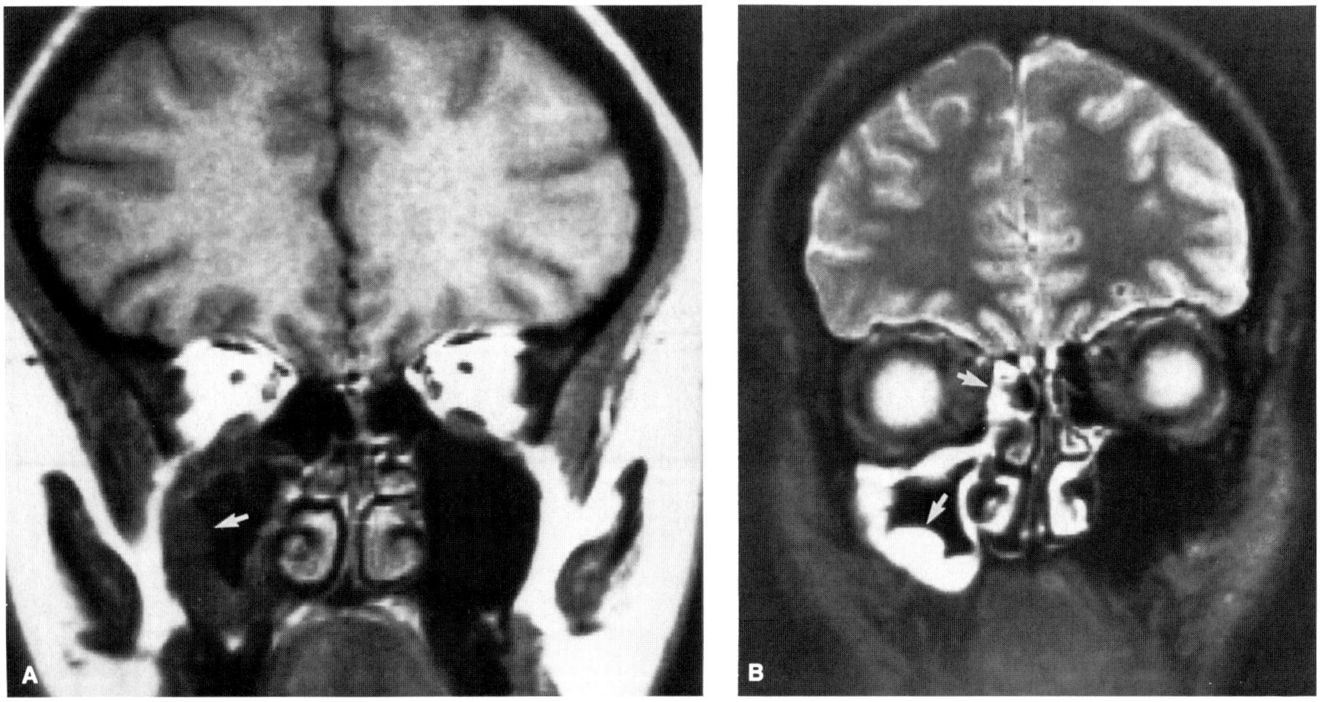

FIGURE 8–33. Sinus mucosal thickening. **(A)** T1-weighted and **(B)** T2-weighted coronal images show marked thickening of the mucosa (arrow) in the right maxillary and ethmoid sinuses in a patient with sinusitis.

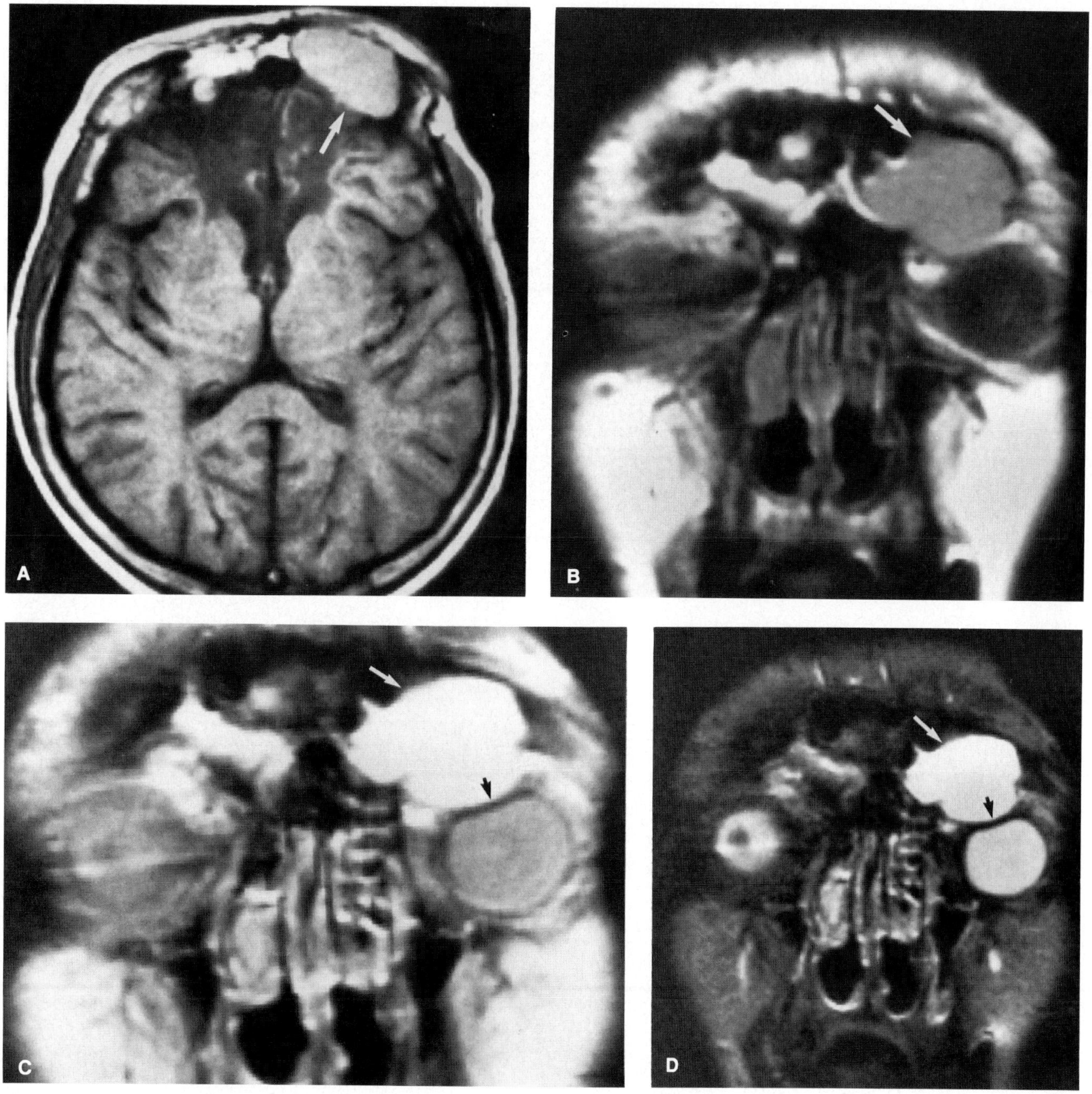

FIGURE 8–34. Recurrent left frontal sinus mucocele. **(A)** T1-weighted axial, **(B)** T1-weighted, **(C)** proton density, and **(D)** T2-weighted coronal images through the frontal sinuses. Fluid fills and expands the left frontal sinus (white arrow). It exhibits high signal intensity on T1-weighted images due to increased protein content or methemoglobin from prior operative hemorrhage. The mucocele is encroaching on the left globe (black arrow).

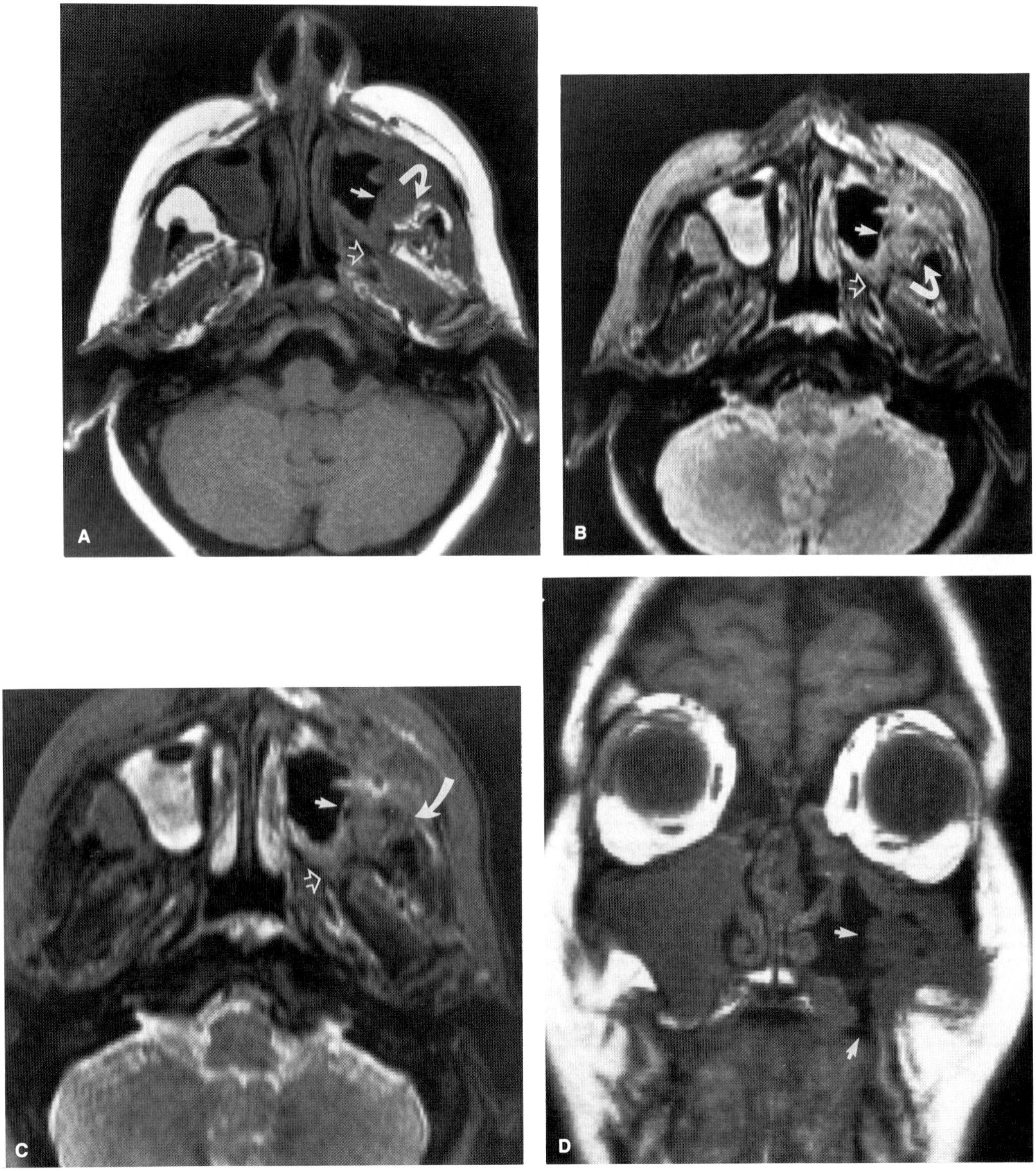

FIGURE 8–35. Squamous cell carcinoma of the left maxillary sinus. **(A)** T1-weighted, **(B)** proton density, **(C)** T2-weighted axial, and **(D)** T1-weighted coronal images through the maxillary sinuses. A soft tissue mass (arrow) in the left maxillary sinus extends back to the pterygopalatine fossa (open arrow) and infratemporal fossa (curved arrow). Bone destruction involving the inferior and lateral walls of the sinus can be appreciated best on the T1-weighted images. Fluid and mucosal thickening is present in the right maxillary sinus. (Carter BL. Tumors of the paranasal sinuses and nasal cavity. In: Valvassori GE, Buckingham RA, Carter BL, et al. Head and neck imaging. New York: Thieme, 1988)

Malignant Lesions

The most common malignant lesion of the paranasal sinuses is squamous cell carcinoma. The hallmark of this lesion on all imaging studies is opacification of a sinus, usually the maxillary antrum, by soft tissue with associated bone destruction. The theoretical advantage of CT in delineating bony detail has not proved to be a significant drawback to MRI for sinus carcinoma. With careful evaluation of the signal voids from cortical bone surrounding the sinuses, bone erosion can almost always be evaluated adequately (Fig. 8-35).

MRI has several advantages over CT. It more easily distinguishes tumor from retained secretions within an obstructed sinus. On T2-weighted images, retained secretions exhibit a uniform very high signal intensity, which contrasts with the inhomogenous, relatively lower signal intensity of the tumor.[6] Extension into surrounding spaces, such as the pterygopalatine fossa, infratemporal fossa, parapharyngeal space, and anterior and middle cranial fossae, is more easily evaluated by MRI. Coronal and sagittal T2-weighted images are especially helpful in evaluating intracranial extension. T1-weighted images are the most helpful in evaluating extension into fat-containing spaces, such as the pterygopalatine and infratemporal fossae and the parapharyngeal space. Axial images usually suffice in evaluating extension into these regions, but the coronal plane may be useful in assessing parapharyngeal space involvement.

Other rare malignancies of the paranasal sinuses include minor salivary gland tumors, rhabdomyosarcoma, plasmacytoma, and lymphoma (Fig. 8-36). These tumors exhibit nonspecific findings on MRI and the differential diagnosis depends on the patient's age, presentation, and biopsy. Metastases may also involve the paranasal sinuses. The most common primary carcinoma to do so is renal cell carcinoma, followed by lung and breast carcinoma. In general, the appearance of these lesions is nonspecific, but highly vascular metastases like renal cell carcinoma may exhibit areas of flow-related signal void.[11]

FACIAL SKELETON

The discussion in this section is limited to the osseous abnormalities of the facial skeleton, with special attention to the mandible and maxilla. Abnormalities of the paranasal sinuses and temporomandibular joints have been discussed in the appropriate sections. MRI is beginning to make a significant contribution to the study of abnormalities of the facial skeleton. Despite the ability of CT to define cortical bone precisely, many pathologic processes of bone predominantly affect the medullary cavity, with later destruction or thinning of the cortex. Most of the work on skeletal MRI has been done on the spine and extremities, and this experience has shown MRI to be much more sensitive to medullary abnormalities than CT, as well as better demonstrating extraosseous soft tissue extension. These principles can be extended to the examination of the facial skeleton.

The multiplanar capabilities of MRI are very useful in evaluating the complex spatial anatomy of the facial skeleton without requiring the patient to assume difficult or uncomfortable positions in the scanner. In addition to a routine initial sagittal scan to serve as a localizer, axial and coronal images are typically obtained. Although the axial images are usually best suited for evaluating the mandible, pathologic processes affecting the maxilla or zygoma may be better appreciated in the coronal plane. This is especially true of the palate, which may be quite difficult to evaluate in the axial plane due to partial volume effects. Four- to five-millimeter slices are adequate for evaluating most bony abnormalities.

As in other areas of the body, both heavily T1-weighted and T2-weighted sequences are essential for evaluating the facial skeleton. Osseous abnormalities are often appreciated as areas of relatively lower signal intensity against the high-signal background of fatty bone marrow on T1-weighted images. There is typically a reversal of the relative signal intensities of bone marrow and abnormality on T2-weighted images due to the relatively high signal of most pathologic processes. This effect is especially important in children, who typically have a more erythropoietic marrow and in whom the bone marrow may be lower in signal intensity on T1-weighted images, producing less contrast with bony abnormalities. Extraosseous involvement of adjacent facial musculature is also better appreciated on T2-weighted images, although the status of the surrounding fat planes is more easily seen on T1-weighted images.

The main pathologic categories of the facial skeleton that can be suitably evaluated with MRI include cystic, neoplastic, and inflammatory lesions. Trauma and congenital abnormalities of the facial skeleton remain the province of radiography and CT, with the exception of frontoethmoidal encephalocele, which is easily evaluated by MRI.

Cystic Lesions

Cystic lesions are especially common in the maxilla and mandible. Those of radiologic interest are of two main types: fissural and odontogenic. Radicular cysts secondary to dental caries rarely require sectional imaging techniques. The fissural cysts, such as the

(text continues on page 327)

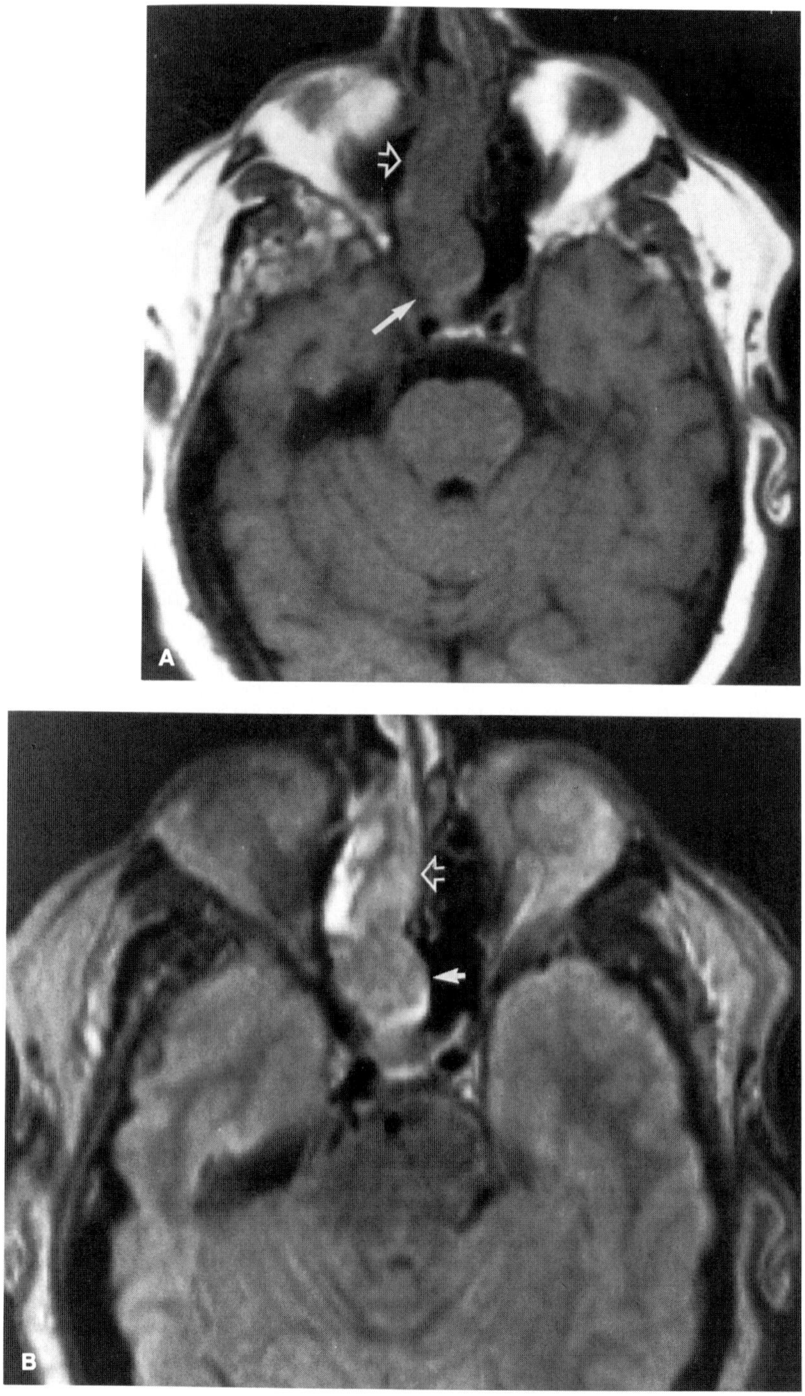

FIGURE 8–36. Adenocarcinoma of the sphenoid sinus. **(A)** T1-weighted, **(B)** proton density, **(C)** T2-weighted axial, and **(D)** T1-weighted sagittal images. There is an intermediate-signal-intensity mass in the sphenoid sinus (arrow), which extends into the ethmoid sinuses (open arrow) and invades the clivus (curved arrow). Destruction of the walls of the sinus can be seen.

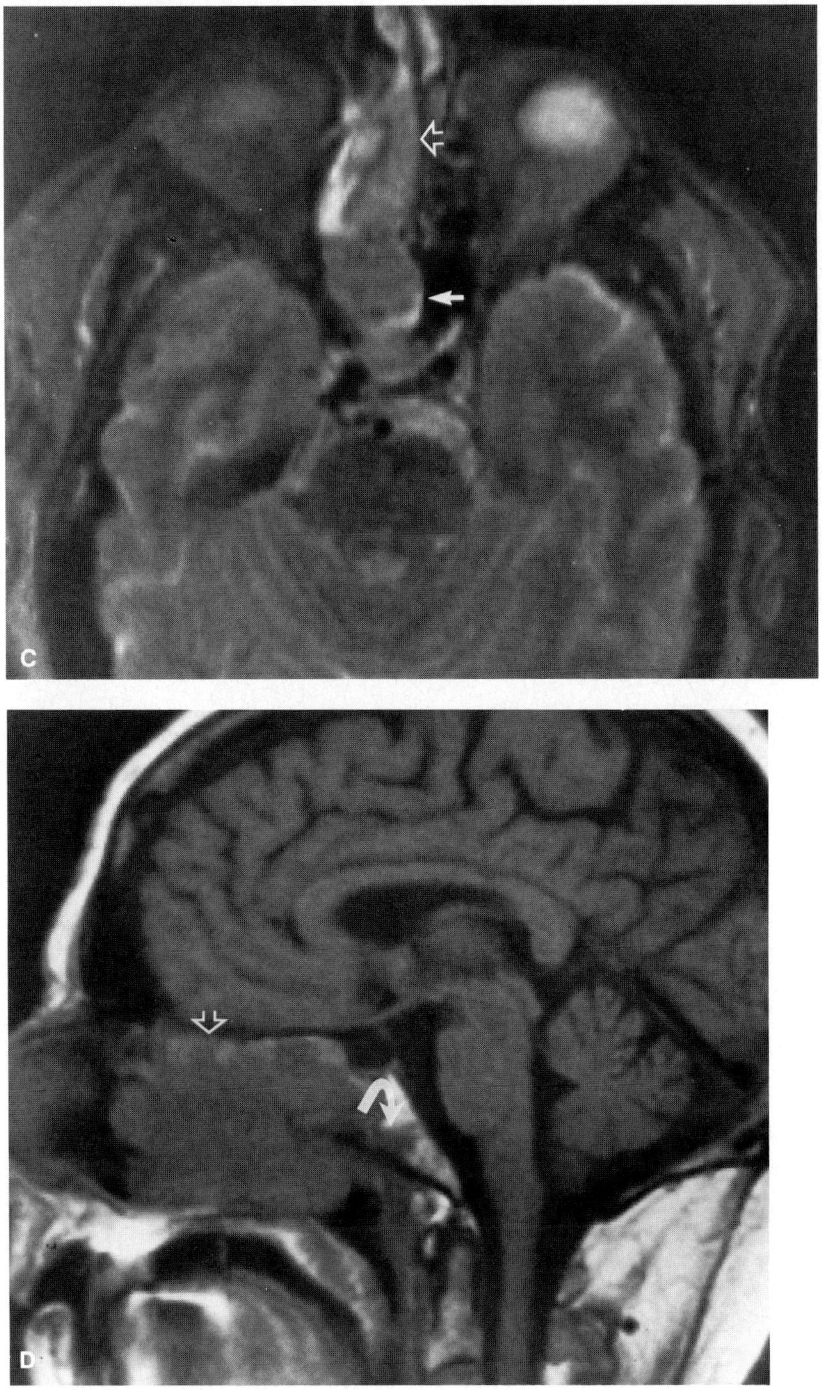

FIGURE 8–36. (Continued)

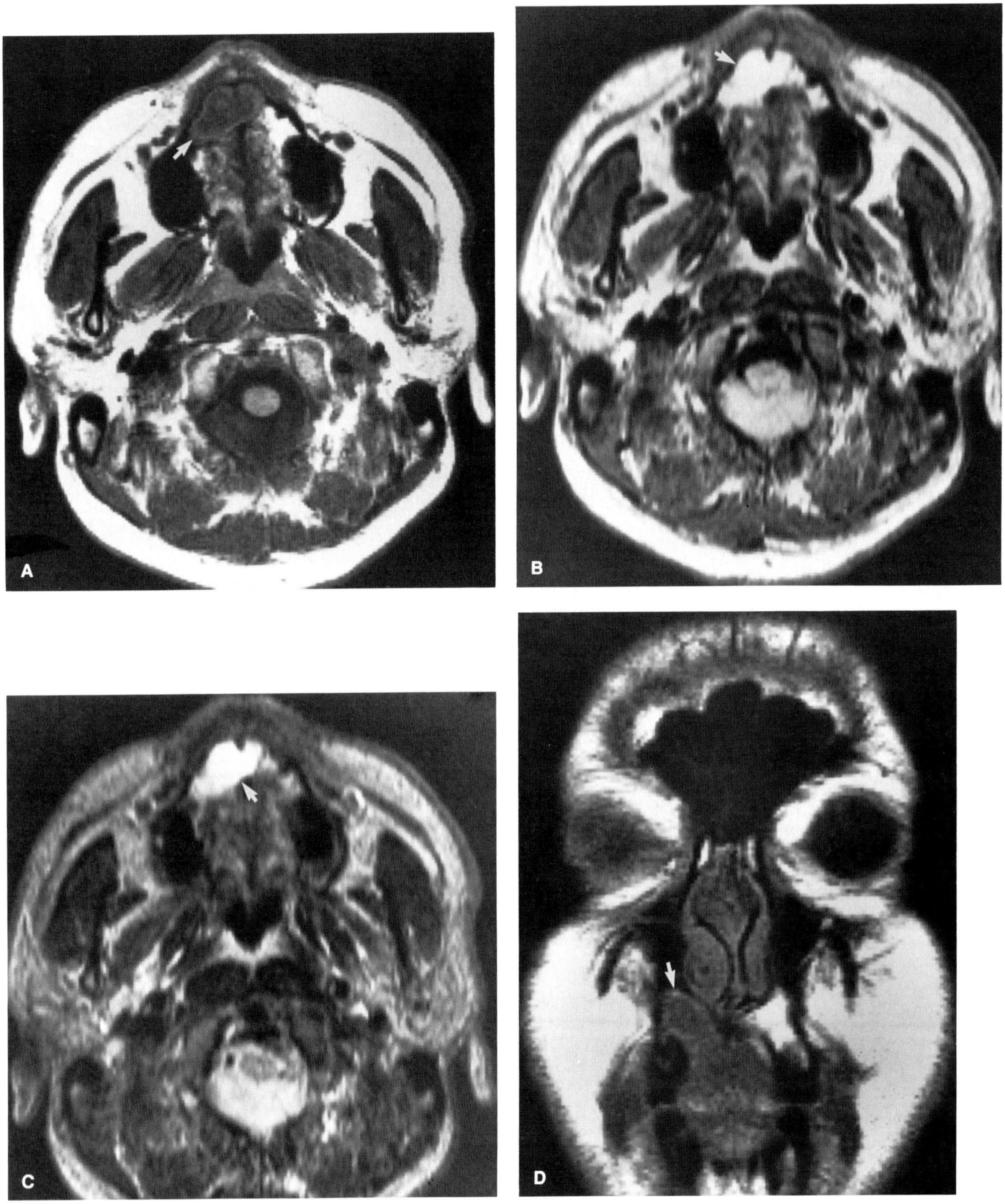

FIGURE 8–37. Nasoalveolar cyst of the maxilla. **(A)** T1-weighted, **(B)** proton density, **(C)** T2-weighted axial, and **(D)** T1-weighted coronal images through the maxilla. The oval-shaped cyst (arrow) in the maxilla exhibits the typical signal characteristics of fluid.

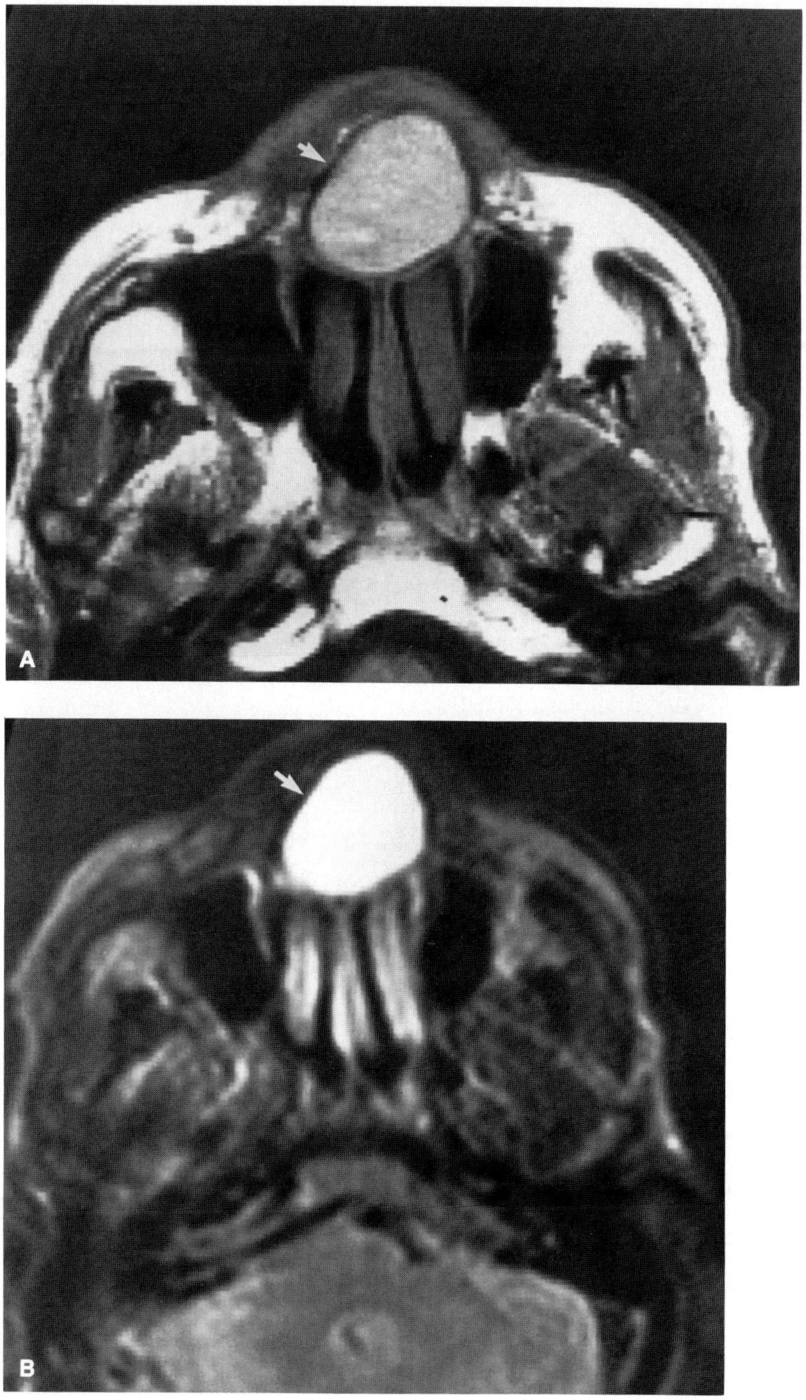

FIGURE 8–38. Incisive cyst of the maxilla. **(A)** T1-weighted and **(B)** T2-weighted axial images through the maxilla. This cyst (arrow) in the region of the incisor canal exhibits high signal intensity on the T1-weighted image most likely due to increased protein content. (Carter BL. Tumors of the paranasal sinuses and nasal cavity. In: Valvassori GE, Buckingham RA, Carter BL, et al. Head and neck imaging. New York: Thieme, 1988)

nasoalveolar cyst, globulomaxillary cyst, and incisive canal cyst, arise in regions of embryonic sutures in the maxilla and mandible (Fig. 8–37). Odontogenic or follicular cysts arise from primordial tooth follicles and may or may not contain a tooth remnant (dentigerous cysts). Occasionally odontogenic cysts develop a keratinizing epithelial lining, in which case they are referred to as odontogenic keratocysts.

The appearances of these lesions are indistinguishable by MRI. They typically exhibit low or intermediate signal intensity on T1-weighted images and very high signal intensity on T2-weighted images.[25] Rarely, these lesions may exhibit high signal intensity on T1-weighted images as well, possibly caused by high protein content or hemorrhage within the cyst (Fig. 8–38). MRI possesses no definite advantages over CT in evaluating cystic lesions of the maxilla and mandible. In fact, the superior delineation of cortical bone on CT may make it easier to define a continuous, expanded cortical rim, allowing the diagnosis of a nonaggressive lesion.

Neoplastic Lesions

The facial bones are subject to the same osseous neoplasms as bones elsewhere in the body, such as fibrosarcoma, osteosarcoma, chondrosarcoma, lymphoma, myeloma, Ewing's sarcoma, metastatic tumors, eosinophilic granuloma, and giant cell tumor. In addition, the maxilla and mandible are subject to the unique amelioblastoma, a locally invasive tumor. These lesions exhibit the typical signal characteristics of tumors anywhere in the body: intermediate signal on T1-weighted and increased signal on T2-weighted images. These tumors may exhibit the greatest contast with normal bone marrow on T1-weighted images. The margins of these lesions vary from well-defined with indolent tumors to irregular and infiltrating with aggressive, malignant lesions (Figs. 8–39 through 8–42). The patterns of ossification and calcification within an osseous neoplasm are better appreciated on CT and radiography due to the decreased sensitivity of MRI to calcium. Densely calcified and fibrotic areas may be seen as foci of decreased signal on both T1-weighted and T2-weighted images (Fig. 8–43).

Inflammatory Lesions

Osteomyelitis, which usually arises from infected teeth, most commonly affects the mandible. It can also be seen in the bony margins of the sinuses, complicating sinusitis. The MRI appearances are nonspecific, with infiltrating, ill-defined low signal on T1-weighted and high signal on T2-weighted images. Disruption of cortical bone may be seen, although CT is probably more sensitive in this regard, but edema of the surrounding soft tissues is better appreciated on T2-weighted MR images (Fig. 8–44).

NECK

Several recent developments, including motion-artifact-suppression techniques, such as gradient refocusing and presaturation, and improved coil designs, such as Helmholtz and specialized surface coils that allow improved SNR with decreased imaging time, promise to significantly widen the applicability of MRI for the neck.[26,27]

The basic imaging protocol for the neck typically includes a sagittal short TR/short TE sequence, which functions as a "scout" image, although in the case of midline lesions, it may also supply useful additional information. Axial short TR/short TE and long TR multiecho sequences are then obtained through the area of interest. The slice thickness on the axial sequences may vary from 5 to 8 mm, depending on the area to be covered, although 5 mm is usually preferable. More slices can be obtained from the long TR than the short TR sequence. For this reason, as well as to provide an additional anatomic perspective, a coronal short TR/short TE sequence may be added.

Lymph Nodes

The lymph nodes of the neck may be categorized by location: submental, submandibular, anterior jugular (i.e., associated with the anterior jugular vein, superficial to the strap muscles); juxtavisceral (i.e., associated with the thyroid gland and tracheo-esophageal groove); internal jugular, which may be further subdivided into high, middle, and low regions using the levels of the carotid bifurcation and cricoid cartilage as dividing lines; and the spinal accessory or posterior triangle chains.[5] Lymph nodes may be involved by metastatic disease from carcinoma of the head and neck or from distant sites, by lymphoma, or by inflammatory disease.

Current MRI technology is probably as accurate as CT in assessing cervical lymph nodes. Axial T1-weighted images are most useful in evaluating the cervical nodes because they provide the highest resolution and clear demarcation between nodes and surrounding fat. Occasionally, coronal scans may provide additional anatomic information. T2-weighted images may help in separating nodes from adjacent muscles, because nodes typically exhibit higher signal intensity than muscle on these sequences.

As with CT, the most reliable criterion for diagnosing pathologic lymph nodes is that of enlargement, a criterion that, unfortunately, has limitations in both sensitivity and specificity. A lymph node diameter of 1.0 cm or greater should be considered pathologic, with the possible exception of the submandibular and jugulodigastric regions, in which isolated nodes up to 1.5 cm in diameter may be normal. The jugulodigastric nodes are located at the point where the posterior belly of the digastric muscle crosses the jugular vein, approximately at the junction of the high and middle internal jugular chains. Necrosis of any node, as indicated by fluid density on CT or fluid signal characteristics on MRI, should be considered pathologic. However, whether a particular pathologic node is involved by neoplastic or inflammatory disease cannot be assessed on the basis of imaging characteristics alone. Conversely, microscopic nodal metastases remain beyond the reach of imaging diagnosis.

Primary head and neck tumors tend to metastasize

(text continues on page 334)

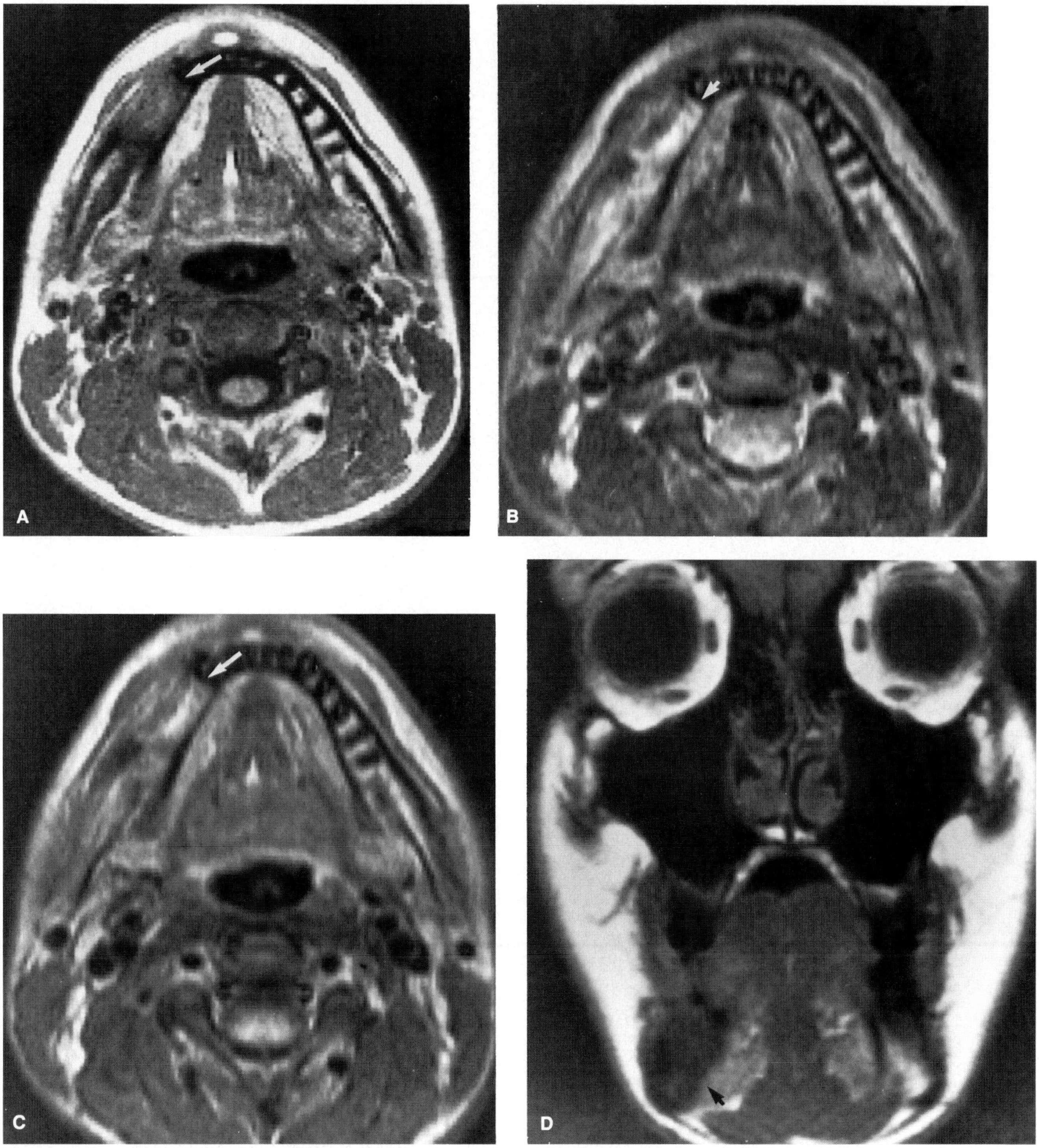

FIGURE 8–39. Eosinophilic granuloma of the mandible. **(A)** T1-weighted, **(B)** proton density, **(C)** T2-weighted axial, and **(D)** T1-weighted coronal images. This rounded lesion (arrow) of intermediate signal intensity replaces the marrow fat, expands the mandible, and thins the cortex laterally.

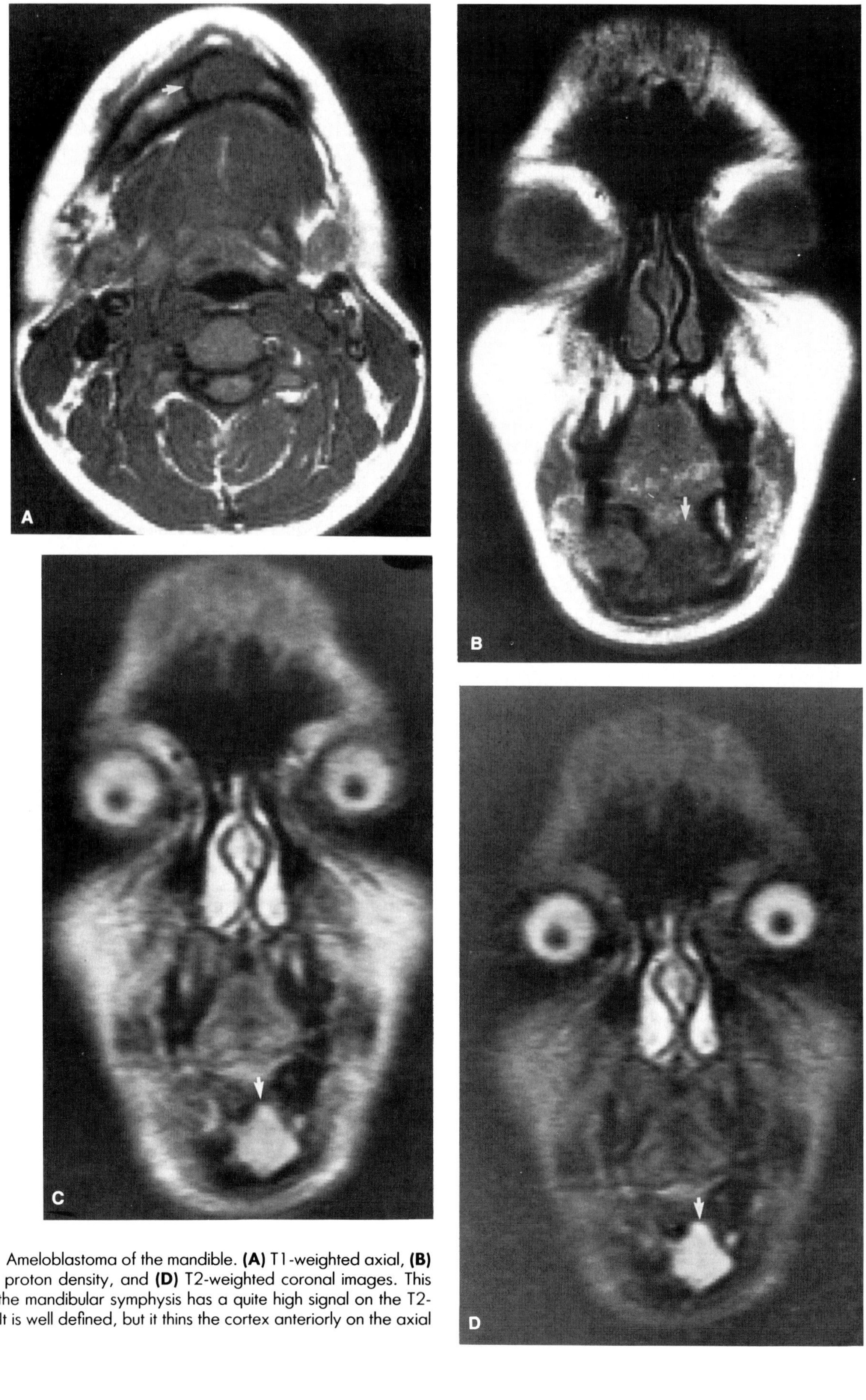

FIGURE 8–40. Ameloblastoma of the mandible. **(A)** T1-weighted axial, **(B)** T1-weighted, **(C)** proton density, and **(D)** T2-weighted coronal images. This lesion (arrow) of the mandibular symphysis has a quite high signal on the T2-weighted image. It is well defined, but it thins the cortex anteriorly on the axial image.

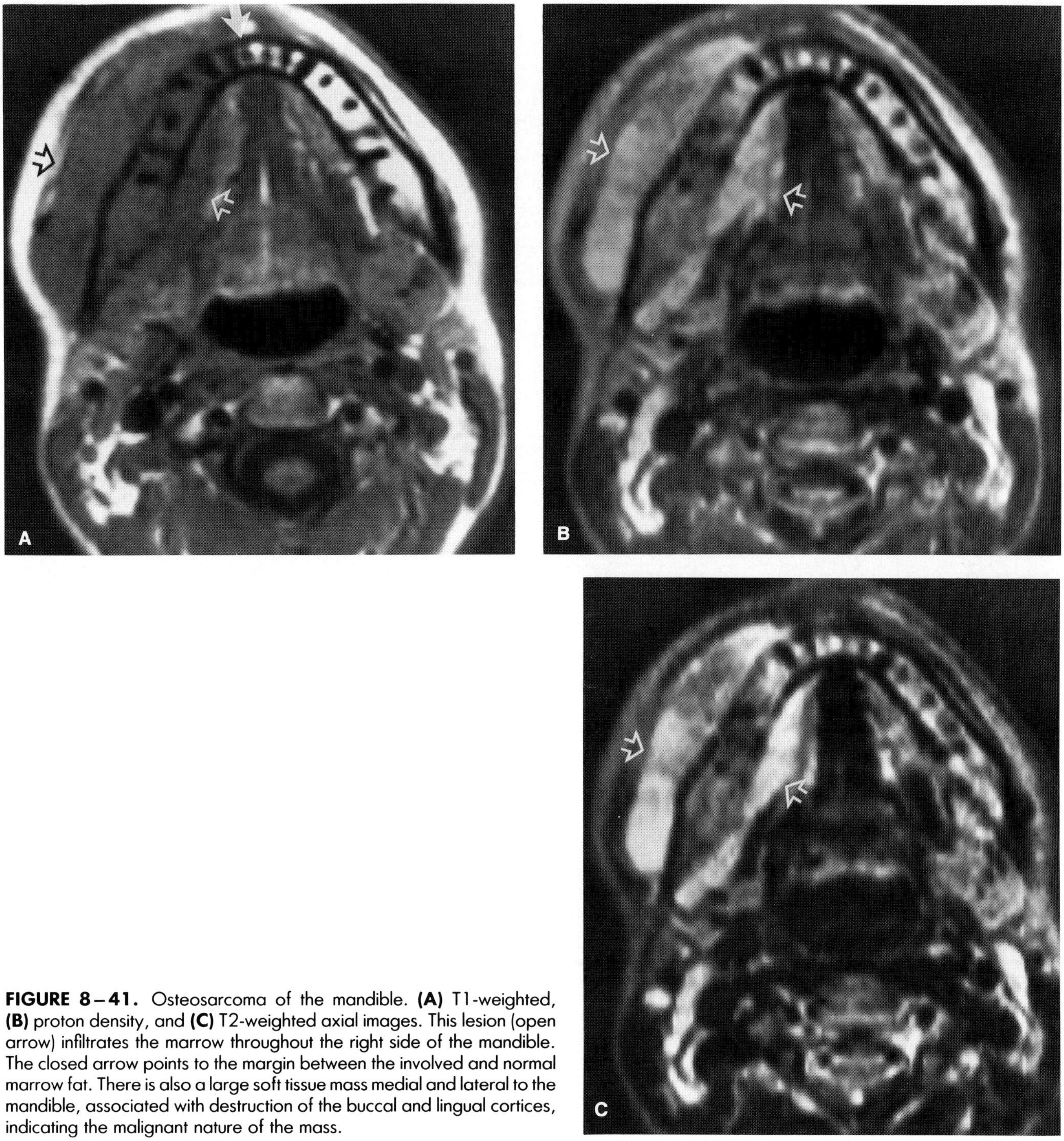

FIGURE 8–41. Osteosarcoma of the mandible. **(A)** T1-weighted, **(B)** proton density, and **(C)** T2-weighted axial images. This lesion (open arrow) infiltrates the marrow throughout the right side of the mandible. The closed arrow points to the margin between the involved and normal marrow fat. There is also a large soft tissue mass medial and lateral to the mandible, associated with destruction of the buccal and lingual cortices, indicating the malignant nature of the mass.

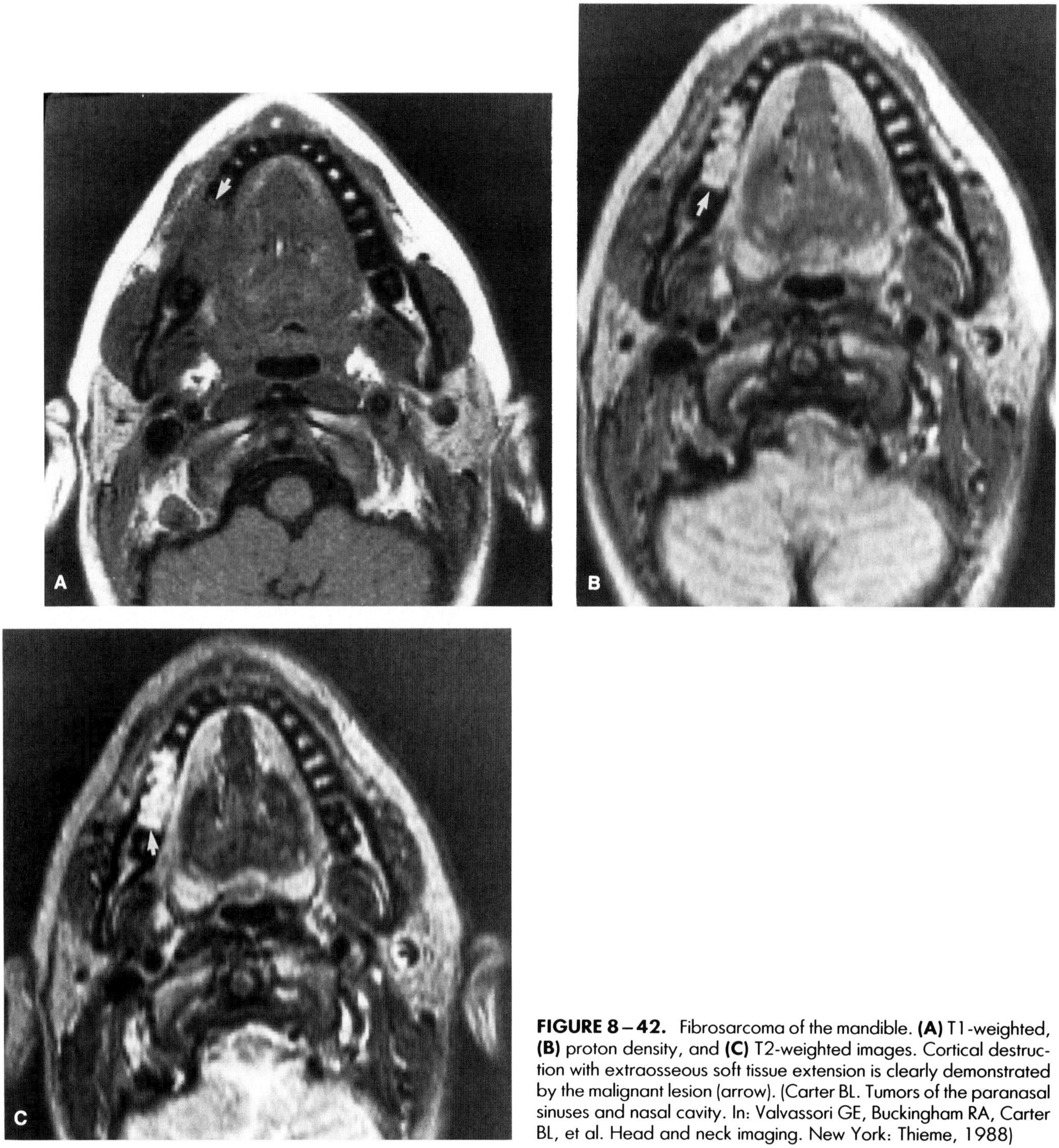

FIGURE 8–42. Fibrosarcoma of the mandible. **(A)** T1-weighted, **(B)** proton density, and **(C)** T2-weighted images. Cortical destruction with extraosseous soft tissue extension is clearly demonstrated by the malignant lesion (arrow). (Carter BL. Tumors of the paranasal sinuses and nasal cavity. In: Valvassori GE, Buckingham RA, Carter BL, et al. Head and neck imaging. New York: Thieme, 1988)

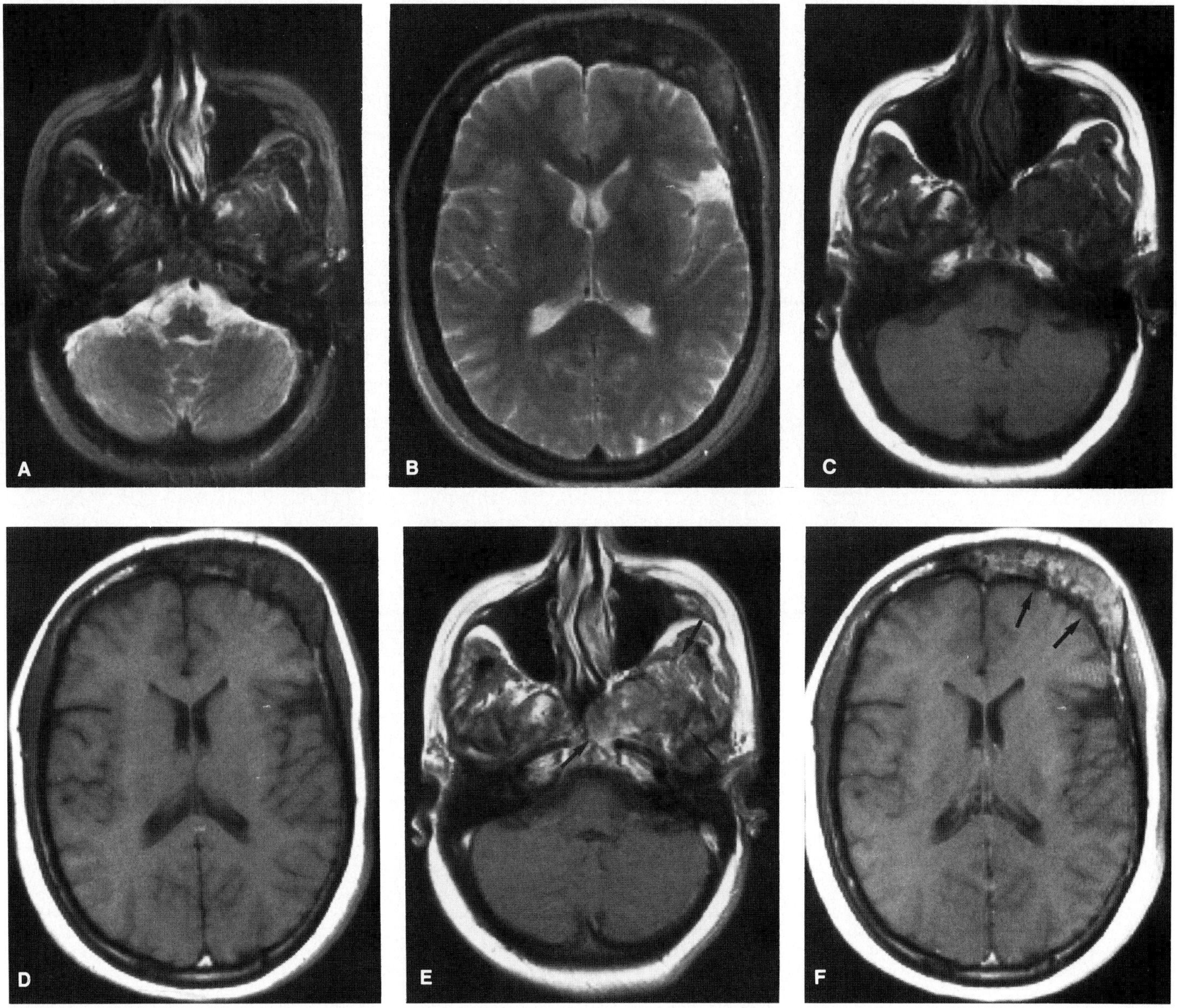

FIGURE 8–43. Polyostotic fibrous dysplasia (Albright's disease). **(A,B)** T2-weighted, **(C,D)** T1-weighted, and **(E,F)** postcontrast T1-weighted images. Involvement of the left frontal bone and sphenoid bone is illustrated. The abnormality demonstrates primarily a low signal intensity on unenhanced T1- and T2-weighted scans, consistent with fibrous tissue. Enhancement is seen (arrows) after Gd DTPA administration.

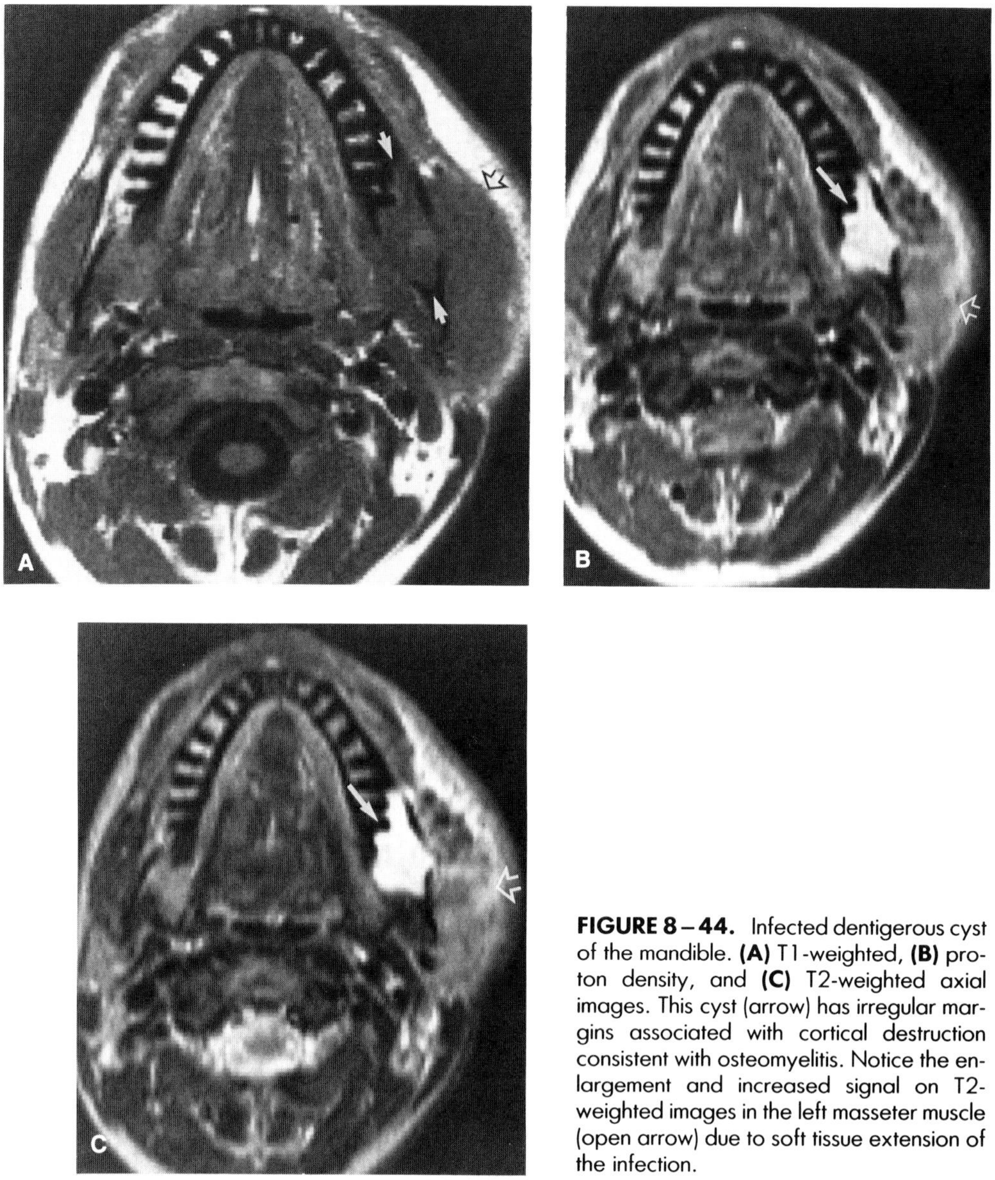

FIGURE 8–44. Infected dentigerous cyst of the mandible. **(A)** T1-weighted, **(B)** proton density, and **(C)** T2-weighted axial images. This cyst (arrow) has irregular margins associated with cortical destruction consistent with osteomyelitis. Notice the enlargement and increased signal on T2-weighted images in the left masseter muscle (open arrow) due to soft tissue extension of the infection.

to the submandibular, internal jugular, and posterior triangle chains. The most commonly involved sites are the jugulodigastric nodes. In general, lesions of the oral cavity tend to spread to the submandibular, submental, and high to middle internal jugular chains, but lesions of the nasopharynx, hypopharynx, and supraglottic larynx may involve nodes at any level along the internal jugular chain and the posterior triangle nodes. Lesions of the tongue base and tonsillar fossa exhibit characteristics more like hypopharyngeal lesions than like other lesions of the oral cavity. Nasopharyngeal carcinoma is noteworthy in having an especially high rate of bilateral nodal metastasis (>30%) and of metastatic disease at presentation (up to 90%), and imaging may play an important role in diagnosing the frequently occult primary lesion in the setting of cervical adenopathy.

Larynx and Hypopharynx

Examination of this anatomic region with MRI has been limited by vascular and respiratory motion artifacts and by limited SNR with previously available imaging technology. Recently developed surface coils and motion-compensating techniques promise improved imaging of this area in the near future.[3,27,28] The submucosal fat planes throughout the hypopharynx and larynx are better imaged on T1-weighted sequences. The various anatomic structures, such as the epiglottis, laryngeal ventricle, true and false cords, and laryngeal skeleton, can be imaged successfully. Additional imaging planes, such as the sagittal for evaluating the epiglottis and coronal for the glottis, can be very helpful.

The true cords may be differentiated from the false cords on axial images using the same criteria as CT: unlike the false cords, the true cords do not have a submucosal fat plane on T1-weighted images, because they consist entirely of fibrous tissue and the vocalis muscles. The vocal process of the arytenoid cartilages is a reliable marker of the true cords. The normal anterior commissure is less than 2 mm thick.

The laryngeal skeleton has a variable appearance on MRI images, depending on the state of ossification of the cartilages.[29] In young patients before significant ossification develops, the laryngeal cartilage exhibits intermediate signal intensity on both T1-weighted and T2-weighted images. As calcification develops, foci of signal void can be seen, and once ossification is complete, a well-defined cortex with fatty marrow can be appreciated. Calcification and ossification of the cartilages take place in an irregular, although more or less symmetrical, pattern, which can make assessment of cartilage destruction problematic.

MRI has shown promise in evaluating squamous cell carcinoma and other lesions of the larynx (Figs. 8-45 and 8-46). As with CT, the primary role of MRI in this disease is assessing submucosal extension before surgery or radiation. T1-weighted images are usually helpful because they have a higher contrast between the intermediate signal tumor and high signal submucosal fat. In addition, T1-weighted images tend to be less degraded by motion artifacts and to have higher SNR characteristics. Also, T1-weighted images are more sensitive for detecting enlarged cervical lymph nodes. T2-weighted images should be obtained as an adjunct because they may help delineate relatively high-signal tumor against surrounding muscles. Both T1-weighted and T2-weighted images need to be carefully examined to assess involvement of the laryngeal skeleton. Even so, definitive assessment may be impossible in the presence of irregularly calcified or ossified cartilages.

Preliminary evidence suggests that MRI may help in evaluating the postoperative or postradiation patient. On T2-weighted images, posttreatment fibrosis tends to be very low in signal intensity, and recurrent tumor should be intermediate or high in signal intensity.[13] Areas of recurrent tumor may exhibit enhancement after administration of Gd DTPA (Fig. 8-47).

Thyroid and Parathyroid

The role of MRI in evaluating parathyroid lesions has been investigated in several reports.[30,31] Parathyroid adenomas characteristically exhibit high signal intensity on T2-weighted images. This and their typical location posterior to the lobes of the thyroid gland (or ectopically in the superior, anterior mediastinum) allow recognition. They exhibit intermediate signal intensity on T1-weighted images, allowing differentiation from cystic lesions. Although high-resolution ultrasound can detect adenomas, it is quite limited for evaluating postoperative patients and those with ectopic parathyroid glands; MRI may have a significant contribution to make in evaluating hyperparathyroidism. However, high-resolution MRI technology with excellent SNR is required for the evaluation of these small lesions on T2-weighted images.

Imaging of the thyroid gland currently is performed with high-resolution ultrasound and nuclear medicine techniques. These are usually sufficient for the routine evaluation of benign thyroid disease. Nevertheless, benign thyroid lesions are quite common and are often seen on neck images obtained for other indications. The normal thyroid gland is of intermediate signal intensity on T1-weighted images and mildly hyperintense on T2-weighted sequences. Thyroid adenomas may exhibit slightly decreased intensity on T1-weighted sequences and markedly increased intensity on T2-weighted images. Cystic areas show marked hypointensity on T1-weighted images and even greater hyperintensity on T2-weighted images. If hemorrhage is present in the lesion, it may be hyperintense on T1-weighted sequences. A multinodular goiter is visualized as an enlarged thyroid with lobulated contours and heterogeneous signal intensity on all imaging sequences, depending on the ratio of normal to adenomatous and cystic areas.

Thyroid carcinoma is indistinguishable from benign disease based on signal characteristics alone. Local invasion, nodal metastates, and vascular involvement can be detected. MRI may have a role in evaluating postoperative recurrence, because there is evidence that postoperative fibrosis may be detectable based on its low signal intensity on T2-weighted images, contrasted with the high signal intensity of recurrent tumor.[13]

Miscellaneous Lesions

The role of MRI in disorders of the neck other than carcinoma and lymphadenopathy has not been widely evaluated. Cystic lesions should exhibit typical fluid characteristics—homogeneous, low signal on T1-weighted and very high signal on T2-weighted images—allowing easy recognition. Complex cysts,

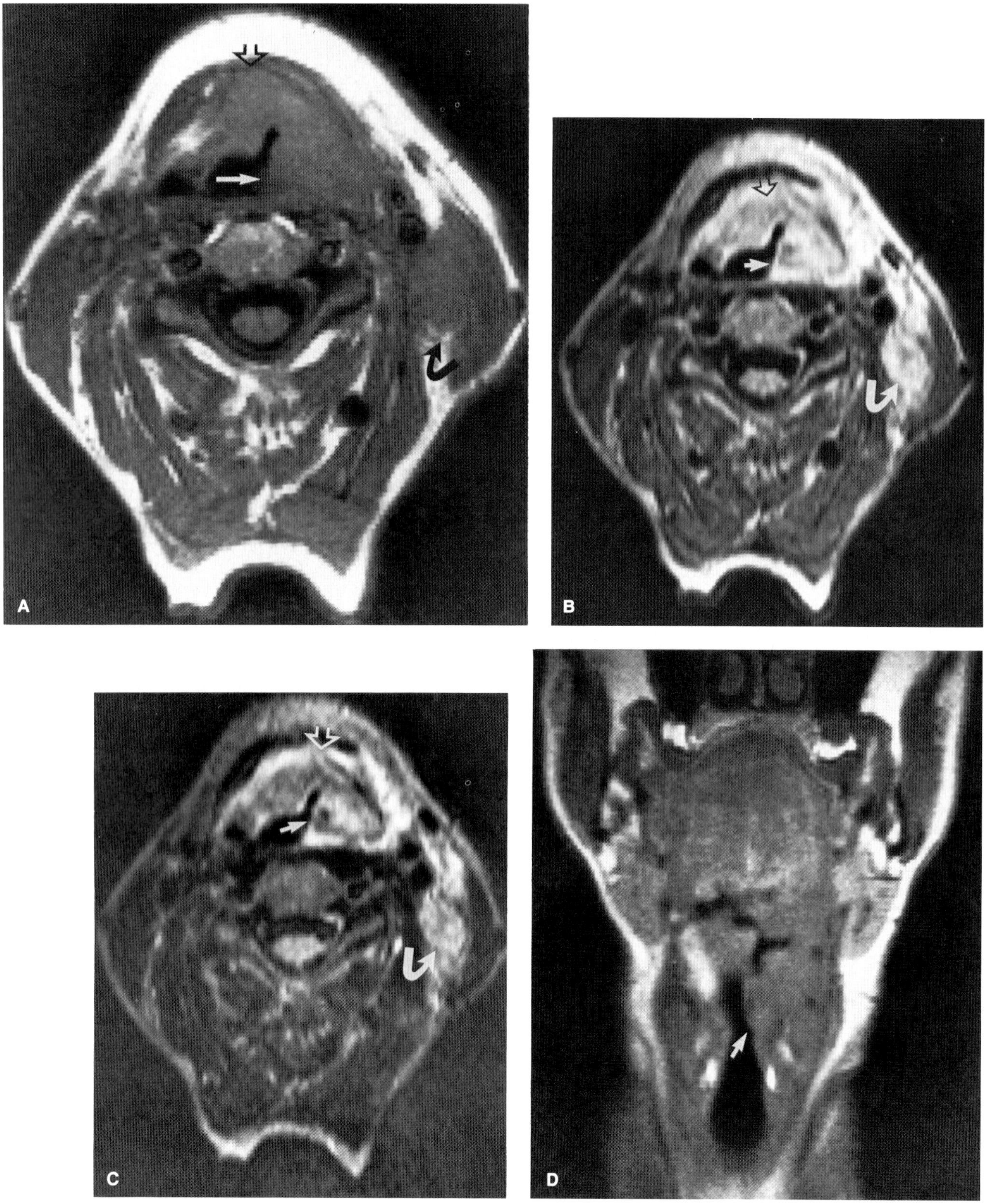

FIGURE 8–45. Supraglottic carcinoma. **(A)** T1-weighted, **(B)** proton density, **(C)** T2-weighted axial, and **(D)** T1-weighted coronal images. A soft tissue mass (arrow) obliterates the left piriform sinus and extends anteriorly across the midline in the pre-epiglottic space (open arrow). Metastatic adenopathy is medial to the sternocleidomastoid muscle (curved arrow).

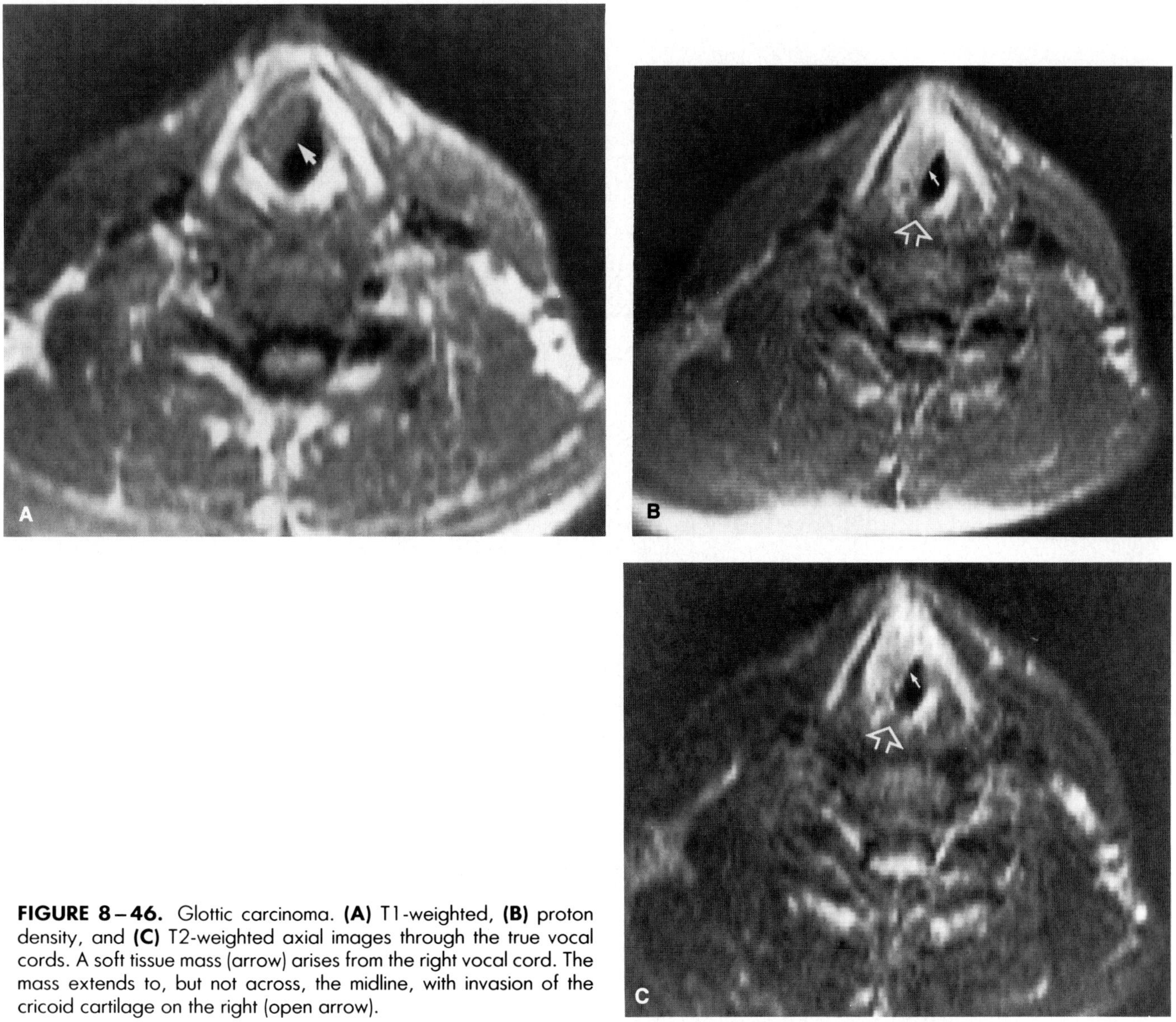

FIGURE 8–46. Glottic carcinoma. **(A)** T1-weighted, **(B)** proton density, and **(C)** T2-weighted axial images through the true vocal cords. A soft tissue mass (arrow) arises from the right vocal cord. The mass extends to, but not across, the midline, with invasion of the cricoid cartilage on the right (open arrow).

such as those containing hemorrhagic, proteinaceous, or infected fluid, may have unusual signal characteristics, most commonly intermediate or high signal on T1-weighted images (Fig. 8–48). Branchial cleft cysts, thyroglossal duct cysts, and cystic hygromas may be differentiated by their characteristic locations in the anterior triangle, midline, and posterior triangle, respectively. Cystic hygromas also typically exhibit a more infiltrative growth pattern with multiple septations. Hemangiomas and other mesenchymal tumors should show the same MRI appearances as in other areas of the body.[20,32] Infection demonstrates infiltration of fat and muscle planes with foci of fluid signal intensity corresponding to liquefaction and abscess formation.

The carotid artery and jugular vein are consistently well visualized on axial images. Partial volume effects may limit depiction on coronal and sagittal images. The presence of flow void within these vessels on spin echo images is diagnostic of patency, but various flow-related artifacts, such as inflow enhancement and even echo rephasing, may make the interpretation of intraluminal signal problematic. Single-slice gradient-echo techniques, which produce a bright signal from flowing blood, frequently help in this situa-

(text continues on page 340)

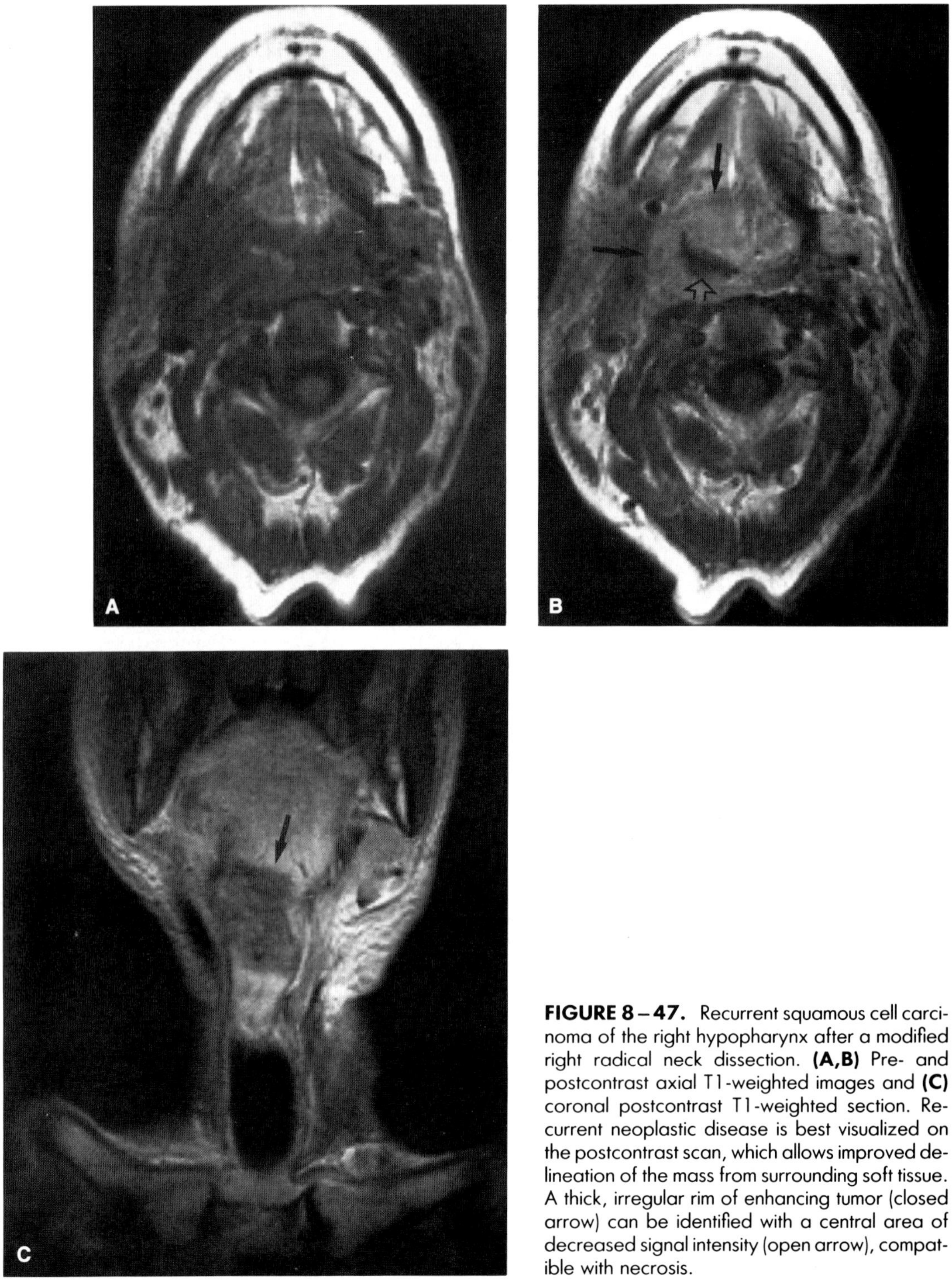

FIGURE 8–47. Recurrent squamous cell carcinoma of the right hypopharynx after a modified right radical neck dissection. **(A,B)** Pre- and postcontrast axial T1-weighted images and **(C)** coronal postcontrast T1-weighted section. Recurrent neoplastic disease is best visualized on the postcontrast scan, which allows improved delineation of the mass from surrounding soft tissue. A thick, irregular rim of enhancing tumor (closed arrow) can be identified with a central area of decreased signal intensity (open arrow), compatible with necrosis.

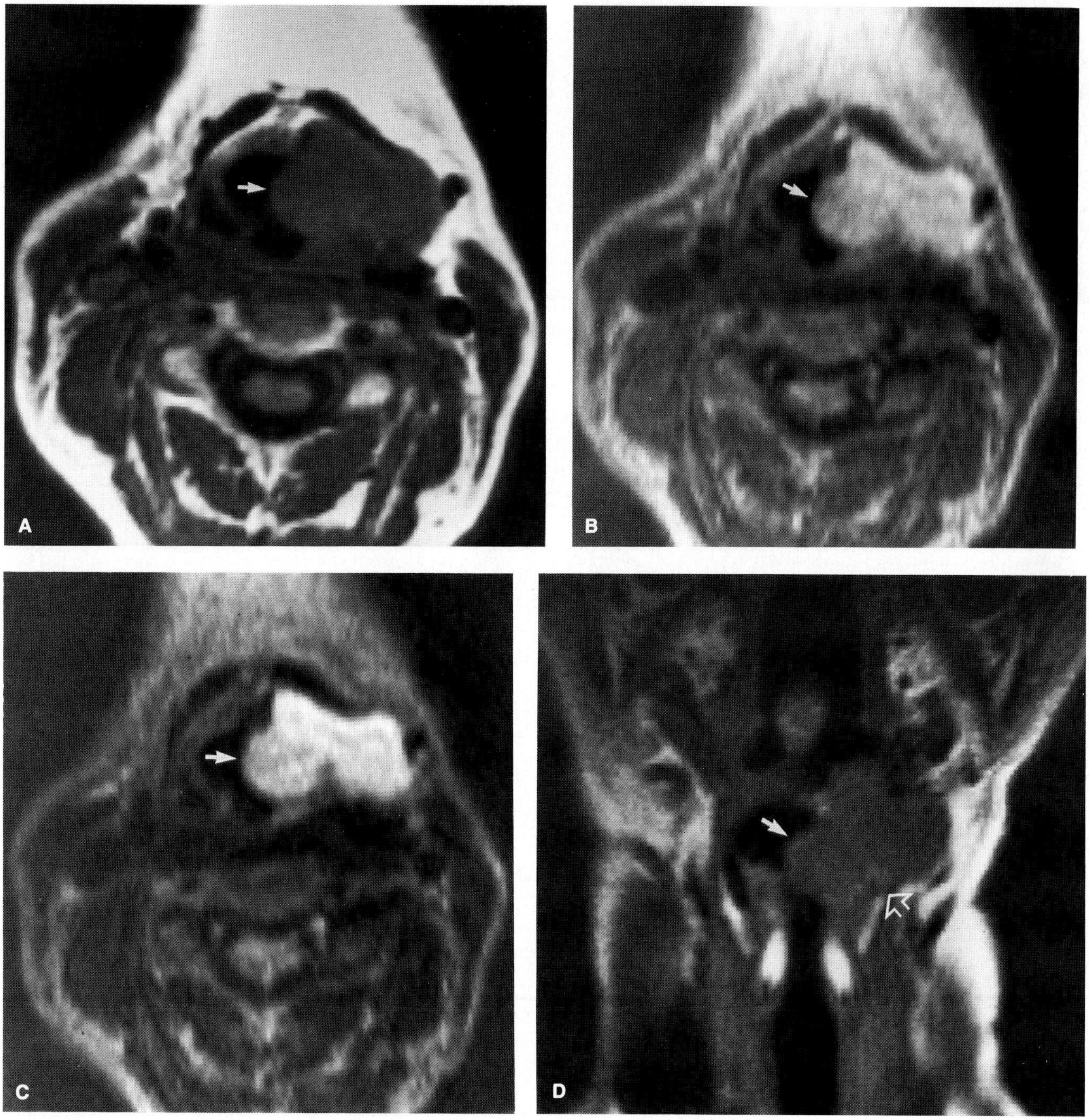

FIGURE 8–48. Obstructed external laryngocele. **(A)** T1-weighted, **(B)** proton density, **(C)** T2-weighted axial, and **(D)** T1-weighted coronal images. There is a cystic mass extending from the laryngeal ventricle superiorly and laterally into the cervical soft tissues. It projects laterally to the thyrohyoid membrane above the thyroid cartilage (open arrow).

tion. Arteriovenous malformations can be identified as complexes of vessels with predominant signal voids on spin echo images but with varying degrees of intraluminal signal due to foci of thrombosis and flow-related artifact. Gradient-echo images usually demonstrate the patent vessels unequivocally.

CONTRAST ENHANCEMENT

There has been limited experience with intravenously enhanced MRI of the head and neck.[14] The mechanisms of enhancement with Gd DTPA are comparable to those with iodinated contrast agents in CT. At the dose of Gd DTPA used in current clinical practice, enhancement is most easily appreciated on T1-weighted images. Normal structures with pronounced vascularity, such as the mucosa of the upper aerodigestive tract, exhibit significant enhancement with Gd DTPA. This is most obvious in the markedly enhancing nasal turbinates. Inflamed and thickened mucosa can be easily demonstrated and differentiated from nonenhancing retained secretions (e.g., in sinusitis), retention cysts, and mucoceles. However, this can also be done on routine T2-weighted images, and the advantages of Gd DTPA for this purpose are limited.

As with CT, vascular tumors such as paraganglioma, neural tumors, angiofibroma, chordoma, and carcinoma, exhibit significant enhancement, which is most easily appreciated on T1-weighted images. Gd-DTPA-enhanced images are most useful in assessing the extension of head and neck tumors into otherwise difficult to evaluate areas, such as intracranially, into muscles, and into small fossae and fissures (e.g., the pterygopalatine fossa). Small mucosal and mesenchymal tumors may also be easier to identify after Gd DTPA administration, but this needs to be more fully evaluated. Gd DTPA enhancement may play a role in the difficult area of differentiating postsurgical and postradiation fibrosis from recurrent tumor, due to significant enhancement of tumor relative to fibrous tissue.

REFERENCES

1. Dillon WP, Mills CM, Kjos B, et al. Magnetic resonance imaging of the nasopharynx. Radiology 1984;152:731.
2. Teresi LM, Lufkin RB, Vinuela F, et al. MR imaging of the nasopharynx and floor of the middle cranial fossa. Part I. Normal anatomy. Radiology 1987;164:811.
3. Valvassori GE, Buckingham RA, Carter BL, et al. Head and neck imaging. New York: Thieme, 1988.
4. Teresi LM, Lufkin RB, Vinuela F, et al. MR imaging of the nasopharynx and floor of the middle cranial fossa. Part II. Malignant tumors. Radiology 1987;164:817.
5. Som PM. Lymph nodes of the neck. Radiology 1987;165:593.
6. Som PM, Shapiro MD, Biller HF, et al. Sinonasal tumors and inflammatory tissues: differentiation with MR imaging. Radiology 1988;167:803.
7. Lloyd GAS, Lund VJ, Phelps PD, Howard DJ. Magnetic resonance imaging in the evaluation of nose and paranasal sinus disease. Br J Radiol 1987;60:957.
8. Som PM, Biller HF, Lawson W, et al. Parapharyngeal space masses: an updated protocol based upon 104 cases. Radiology 1984;153:149.
9. Som PM, Sacher M, Stollman AL, et al. Common tumors of the parapharyngeal space: refined imaging diagnosis. Radiology 1988;169:81.
10. Olsen WL, Dillon WP, Kelley WM, et al. MR imaging of paragangliomas. AJR 1987;148:201.
11. Som PM, Braun IF, Shapiro MD, et al. Tumors of the parapharyngeal space and upper neck: MR imaging characteristics. Radiology 1987;164:823.
12. Schaefer SD, Maravilla KR, Suss RA, et al. Close LG: magnetic resonance imaging vs. computed tomography. Comparison in imaging oral cavity and pharyngeal carcinomas. Arch Otolaryngol 1985;111:730.
13. Glazer HS, Niemeyer JH, Balfe DM, et al. Neck neoplasms: MR imaging. Part II. Posttreatment evaluation. Radiology 1986;160:349.
14. Schiller V, Teresi L, Lufkin R, Hanafee W. Contrast enhanced MRI of the head and neck. In: Runge V, ed. Enhanced magnetic resonance imaging. St. Louis: CV Mosby, 1989.
15. Eneroth CM. Salivary gland tumors in the parotid gland, submandibular gland and the palate region. Cancer 1971;17:1415.
16. Casselman JW, Mancuso AA. Major salivary gland masses: comparison of MR imaging and CT. Radiology 1987;165:183.
17. Mandlebaum SM, Braun IF, Davis PC, et al. Parotid masses: MR imaging. Radiology 1987;163:411.
18. Teresi LM, Lufkin RB, Wortham DG, et al. Parotid masses: MR imaging. Radiology 1987;163:405.
19. Skolnick EM, Friedman M, Becker S, et al. Tumors of the major salivary glands. Laryngoscope 1977;87:843.
20. Levine E, Wetzel LH, Neff JR. MR imaging and CT of extrahepatic cavernous hemangiomas. AJR 1986;147:1299.
21. Teresi LM, Kolin E, Lufkin RB, Hanafee WN. MR imaging of the intraparotid facial nerve. AJR 1987;148:995.
22. Moore J, Potchen M, Waldenmaier N, et al. High-field magnetic resonance imaging of paranasal sinus inflammatory disease. Laryngoscope 1986;96:267.
23. Som PM, Shugar JMA, Troy KM, et al. The use of magnetic resonance and computed tomography in the management of a patient with intrasinus hemorrhage. Arch Otolaryngol 1988;114:200.
24. Zimmerman RA, Bilaniuk LT, Hackney DB, et al. Paranasal sinus hemorrhage: evaluation with MR imaging. Radiology 1987;162:499.
25. Belkin BA, Papageorge MB, Fakitsas J, Bankoff MS. A comparative study of MRI vs. CT for the evaluation of maxillary and mandibular tumors. J Oral Maxillofac Surg 1988;46:1039.
26. Glazer HS, Niemeyer JH, Balfe DM, et al. Neck neoplasms: MR imaging. Part I. Initial evaluation. Radiology 1986;160:343.
27. Lufkin RB, Hanafee WN, Wortham D, Hoover L. Larynx and hypopharynx: MR imaging with surface coils. Radiology 1985;158:747.
28. McArdle CB, Bailey BJ, Amaparo EG. Surface coil magnetic resonance imaging of the normal larynx. Arch Otolaryngol 1986;112:616.
29. Castelijns JA, Gerritsen GJ, Kaiser MC, et al. Invasion of cartilage by cancer: comparison of CT and MR imaging. Radiology 1987;166:199.
30. Hamilton R, Greenberg BM, Gefter W, et al. Successful localization of parathyroid adenomas by magnetic resonance imaging. Am J Surg 1988;155:370.
31. Kier R, Blinder RA, Herfkens RJ, et al. MR imaging with surface coils in primary hyperparathyroidism. J Comput Assist Tomogr 1987;11:863.
32. Itoh K, Hishimura K, Togashi K, et al. MR imaging of cavernous hemangioma of the face and neck. J Comput Assist Tomogr 1985;10:831.

9

Thorax and Heart

Madeleine R. Fisher

Magnetic resonance imaging (MRI) has become an important tool for a variety of conditions presenting within the thorax and cardiovascular system. MRI offers many advantages for imaging of the thorax, including precise delineation of the blood vessels and tracheobronchial tree without the need for contrast media and better soft tissue contrast resolution than computerized tomography (CT). Occasionally difficulty arises when performing CT at the level of the thoracic inlet because artifacts caused by bony structures may obscure lesions. MRI is well-suited evaluating this region because of the multiplanar imaging capability and superb delineation of vascularity. In the cardiovascular system, MRI is beneficial because of the inherent contrast provided between the blood pool and cardiac chambers.

This chapter discusses the MR techniques for imaging of the thorax and heart and reviews several current indications for MR imaging of the thoracic inlet, mediastinum, hila, lung parenchyma, pulmonary vascularity, tracheobronchial tree, and heart.

TECHNIQUE

To obtain adequate images of the structures within the thorax and heart, ECG gating is necessary.[1,2] Several techniques are available, and all typically allow a multislice acquisition. In the routine spin echo gated MR sequence, multiple levels are acquired from the thoracic inlet to diaphragm for thoracic evaluation or only of the heart and great vessels for cardiac evaluation.

Images of the heart are obtained at different phases in the cardiac cycle with this technique. To visualize one anatomic level of the heart from end-diastole to end-systole, two different sequences may be used, either a standard spin echo sequence, often called the rotating gated technique (Fig. 9-1), or a gradient-echo technique (Fig. 9-2).[3,4] To acquire the rotating gated sequence, the order of acquisition of a particular slice level is rotated in time such that it is sampled at different phases in the cardiac cycle.[1,3] The software program formats these images to display one anatomic level throughout the cardiac cycle. Multiple phases in the cardiac cycle at one anatomic level can also be acquired with gradient-echo sequences. Cine images of the heart, aorta, and pulmonary arteries may be obtained with standard spin echo or gradient-echo techniques. Each of these techniques acquires anatomic and functional data.

NORMAL ANATOMY

Comparison of MR imaging with CT shows there is a different gray scale appearance for the structures within the thorax. The lungs are seen as regions of black signal on both MRI and CT. However, the soft tissues have several distinct differences. The subcutaneous fat on MRI has bright signal intensity, as does the fat within the mediastinum. On CT, fat is seen as low attenuation. The muscles on MRI are seen as regions of intermediate signal intensity that change in signal intensity, depending on the pulse sequence employed. On CT, muscles have a homogeneous, intermediate gray attenuation. On MRI, the vascular structures, including the aorta, the main, left, and right pulmonary arteries, and cardiac chambers are seen as regions of signal void (i.e., black) and stand out quite distinctly from the surrounding mediastinal fat and chamber walls.

On noncontrast-CT studies, the aorta and pulmonary arteries are seen as gray attenuation and have a

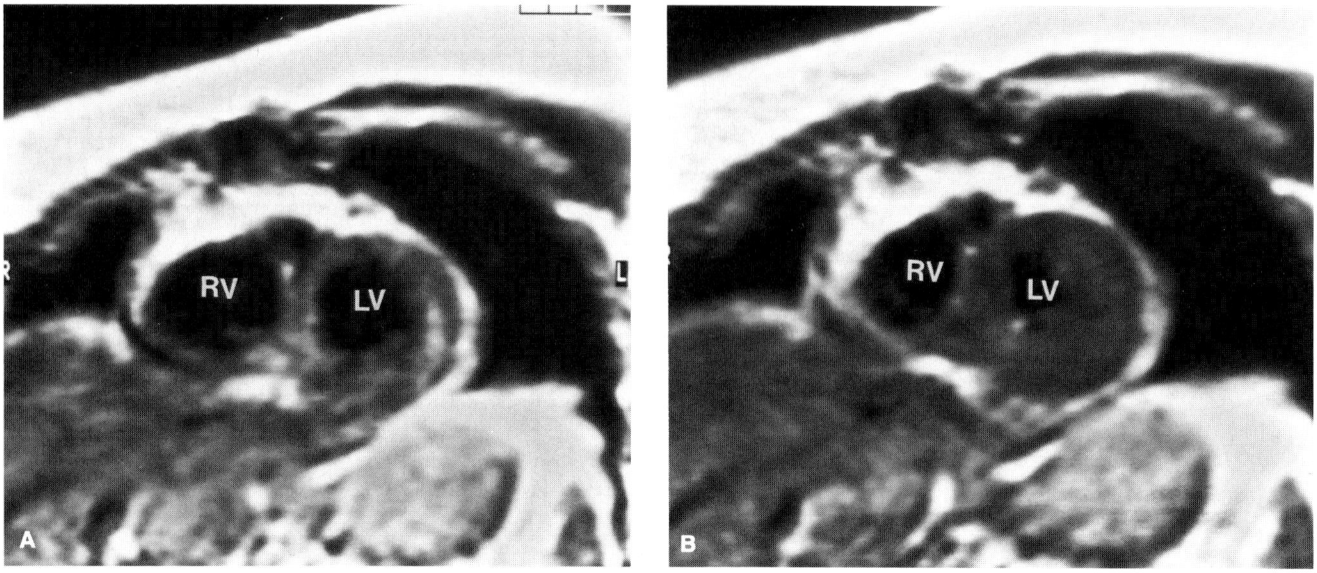

FIGURE 9–1. Rotated gated acquisition. Spin echo gated MR images obtained in a short-axis view demonstrate the left ventricle *(LV)* and right ventricle *(RV)* at end-diastole **(A)** and end-systole **(B).** In this technique, five to six phases in the cardiac cycle are usually obtained, and the blood is seen as regions of signal void within the ventricles.

different appearance from fat. On MRI, the blood vessels are seen as low signal intensity, and masses within the mediastinum typically have an intermediate signal intensity. On a noncontrast-CT study, the vessels and masses have similar attenuations. In order to provide precise differentiation between masses and blood vessels with CT, it is important to provide an adequate bolus of intravenous iodinated contrast media to highlight the blood vessels separately from the surrounding masses.

The bony structures on MRI are seen as bright signal intensity due to the fat within the marrow or as low intensity for cortical bone. On CT, the bony structures have a high attenuation (i.e., white appearance).

On MRI and CT, the tracheobronchial tree is seen as low signal or dark attenuation, similar to the appearance of the lungs, because it is an air-containing structure. On standard gated MR studies of the thorax, it is possible to demonstrate the normal blood vessels, bronchi, mediastinal fat, and cardiovascular structures (Fig. 9–3).[5,6]

Several of the differences between MR and CT images are related to the type of image acquisition for each. MR images are obtained during a period while the patient is breathing. Because MR images are ECG gated, there is good delineation of the blood vessels and cardiovascular structures. However, as a consequence of the breathing, small lesions within the lung parenchyma may move in and out of the imaging plane. CT images are obtained during suspended respiration, and less difficulty arises with partial volume averaging of lesions within the lung parenchyma. Adequate delineation of the blood vessels on CT depends on the timing of intravenous contrast administration. CT has the advantage of obtaining both lung and soft tissue windows. The CT soft tissue windows are very similar to the gated MR studies for anatomic depiction. The lung windows are particularly important in CT for defining small pulmonary nodules that are more difficult to define on the MR study.

Several disadvantages of MRI for imaging of the chest include a prolonged time for data acquisition, partial volume averaging, and limited ability to visualize calcium.[7] Pleural effusions may not be easily visualized with MRI because visualization depends on the type of pulse sequence chosen.[7] By prolonging the repetition time (TR) of the pulse sequence, one may increase the ability to demonstrate pleural effusions. The total imaging time for an MR study of the chest is approximately 1 hour, compared with 30 minutes for a CT examination.

Because of these disadvantages, MRI is usually a complementary procedure to CT. It is a technique employed if CT is equivocal, and it is often used as the first-line modality for patients who have allergies to iodinated contrast media. Additionally, MRI has been used to differentiate tumor recurrence from fibrosis in selected patients.

Since MRI allows multiplanar imaging, it is important to understand the complementary uses of coronal and sagittal planes for evaluating patients with chest disease. This permits optimal acquisition of diagnostic information not available on transverse MR or CT images. The coronal plane of imaging is superior to the

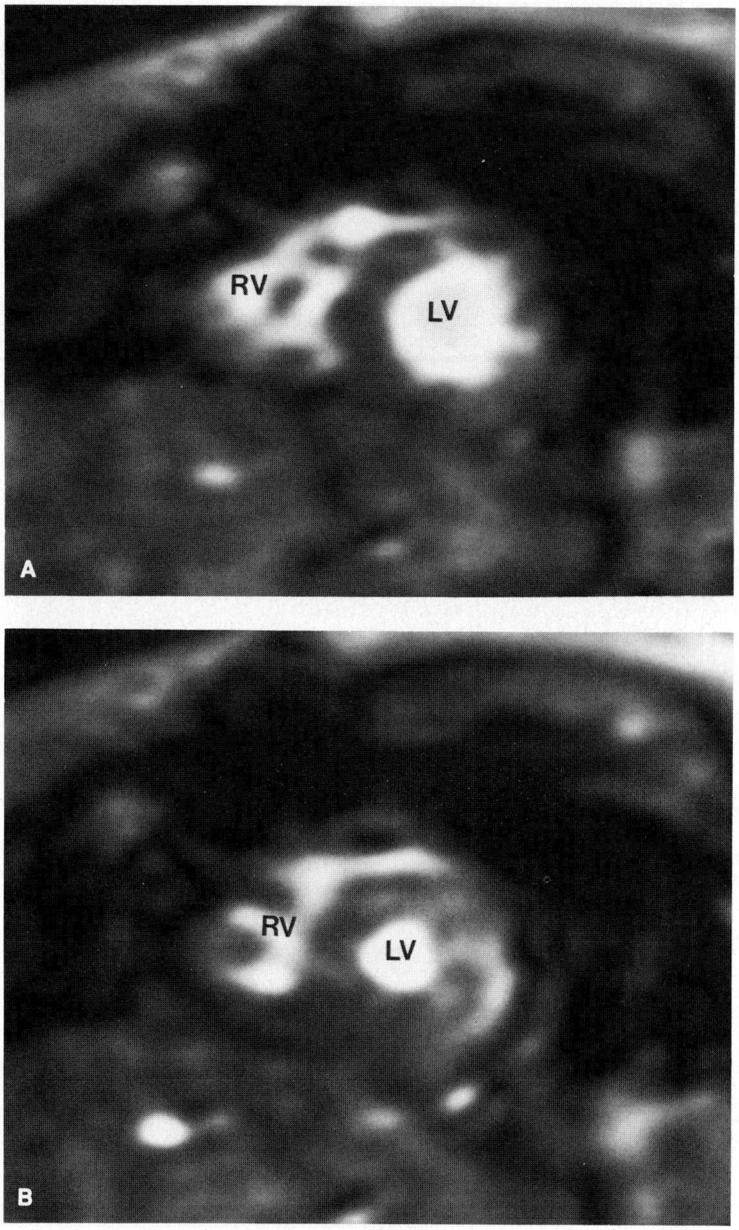

FIGURE 9–2. Gradient echo acquisition. Gradient echo gated MR images obtained in a short axis view demonstrate the left *(LV)* and right ventricle *(RV)* at end-diastole **(A)** and end-systole **(B).** In this technique, 16 or more phases in the cardiac cycle are usually obtained, and the blood is displayed as a high signal intensity within the ventricles.

transaxial plane for evaluating the aortopulmonary window (Fig. 9–4) and for masses within the lung apex or base.[8,9] The transaxial plane is superior for evaluating the pretracheal space, subcarinal space, and hili. At the level of the pulmonary hili, lateral hilar masses are better seen on coronal images than are anterior or posterior hilar masses. The coronal plane, using a short TR sequence, allows evaluation of most node-bearing mediastinal compartments and provides adequate node-to-fat contrast. The sagittal plane is useful for delineating lesions within the lung apices and bases and providing another view of the mediastinal vasculature, which improves evaluation of the effect surrounding masses have on these vessels. Sagittal images are useful for studying the thoracic aorta and for evaluating the relationships of subcarinal masses to the trachea, left atrium, and pulmonary artery.[8,9]

EVALUATION OF THORACIC ABNORMALITIES

Thoracic Inlet

MRI is useful for studying lesions that arise or extend into the thoracic inlet. It is hard to evaluate this area with CT because of artifacts caused by the surrounding bony structures. Additionally, unless an adequate bolus of contrast media is given, the effect of the mass

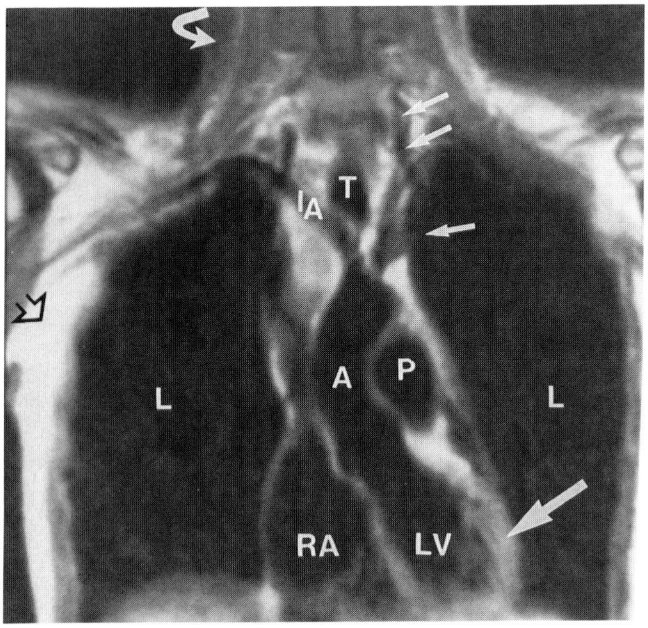

FIGURE 9–3. Normal cardiothoracic anatomy. Gated coronal image (TR/TE = 650/30) through the thorax demonstrates signal void within the cardiac chambers (*LV*, left ventricle; *RA*, right atrium) and great vessels (*A*, aorta; *P*, pulmonary artery) due to the appearance of rapidly flowing blood on MR. The trachea (*T*) and lungs (*L*) are seen as low intensity (black), the appearance of air on MR. The myocardium (white arrow) has an intermediate signal intensity. Notice that fat (open arrow) has a high-intensity (white) and muscle (curved arrow) has an intermediate-intensity signal. The innominate artery (*IA*) and left carotid (small arrows) can also be seen.

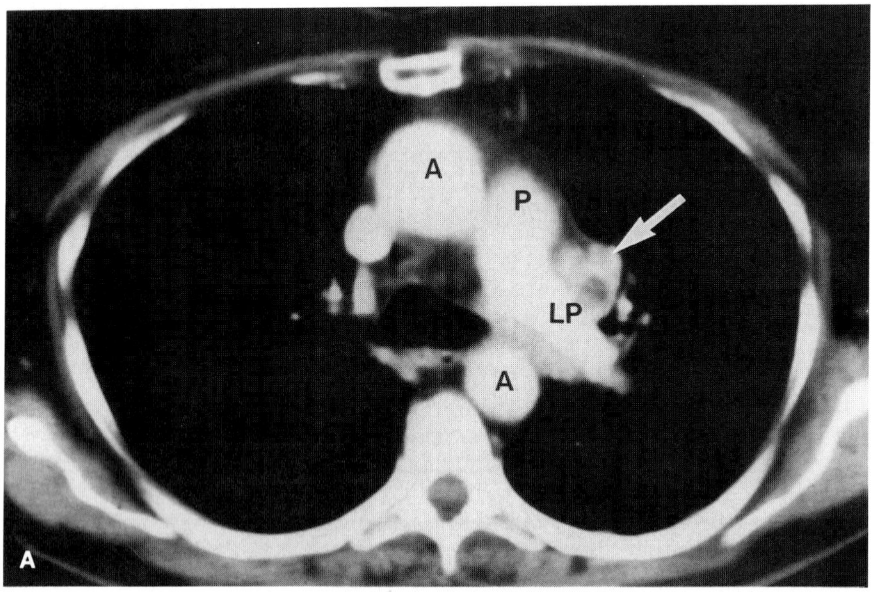

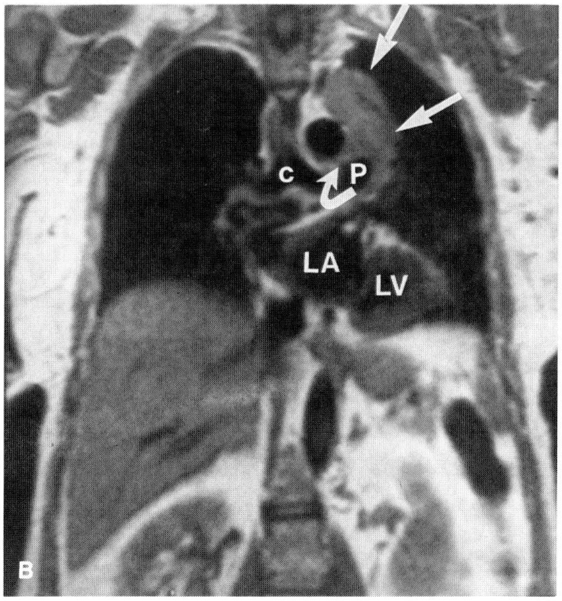

FIGURE 9–4. Coronal MR images of the aortopulmonary window. **(A)** Transverse CT image was obtained immediately after a bolus of contrast media to evaluate the relationship of the bronchogenic carcinoma (white arrows) to the main (*P*) and left (*LP*) pulmonary arteries and to the aorticopulmonary (*AP*) window. The CT sections were inconclusive for evaluation of the AP window (*A*, aorta). **(B)** Coronal gated MR image (TR/TE = 750/30) delineates the tumor (white arrows), which extends into the AP window (curved arrow). Notice the superb depiction of the tumor in relation to the main pulmonary artery (*LA*, left atrium; *LV*, left ventricle; C, carina).

on the blood vessels within the thoracic inlet may not be delineated by CT. Ultrasound may be used for lesions arising within the neck, such as in the thyroid and parathyroid glands, but limitations due to the lung apices and surrounding bony structures prohibit adequate penetration of sound waves.

The direct coronal and sagittal images available with MRI allow a large field of view, greater than that provided by sonography, which improves detection of substernal extension and the retrotracheal components of thyroid masses (Fig. 9–5). Additionally, the directly acquired sagittal and coronal MR images are not possible with CT, and as a result, CT sagittal and coronal images are not optimal image quality. These other planes allow demonstration of the neck, especially the cervical thoracic junction and superior mediastinum. The sagittal and coronal planes provide composite visualization for a greater demonstration of the full extent of lesions within the neck, such as large thyroid malignancies and substernal goiters (Fig. 9–5).

The increased soft tissue contrast provided between neoplasms and normal muscle on MRI helps to assess muscle invasion. Abnormalities involving muscle cause an alteration in the signal intensity. Thyroid neoplasms and goiters have variable signal intensities. MRI does not differentiate between these entities. As demonstrated in Figure 9–5, there is a large mass arising from the thyroid bed and extending into the superior mediastinum. This mass has inhomogeneous signal intensity. The region of bright signal intensity seen posteriorly within the thyroid gland represents an area of colloid degeneration, which was confirmed histopathologically.

Pulmonary Parenchyma

The lungs are seen as regions of low (black) signal intensity on MRI. An abnormality within the lung parenchyma causes an increased signal intensity. A study in 1985 evaluated the capabilities of MRI and CT for detecting pulmonary nodules.[10] Pulmonary nodules less than 1.3 cm were not demonstrated on either CT or MRI. CT better delineated nodules near the diaphragm, the pleura, or each other. MRI better detected nodules adjacent to the blood vessels. In general, most pulmonary nodules were seen using either CT or MR. However, CT usually detected a larger number of small nodules than MRI, but small nodules adjacent to the blood vessels were better displayed on MR images.

One of the reasons small lesions within the lung parenchyma are not as readily identified on MRI as CT is the form of acquisition. MR imaging time is longer and the patients breathe quietly throughout the acquisition of multiple images. Therefore, small lesions can suffer from partial volume averaging during an MR study because they move in and out of the imaging plane. In contrast, CT images are obtained during suspended respiration, which decreases the effect of partial volume averaging of small nodules. Additionally, CT examinations using both soft tissue and lung windows improve identification of small pulmonary nodules.

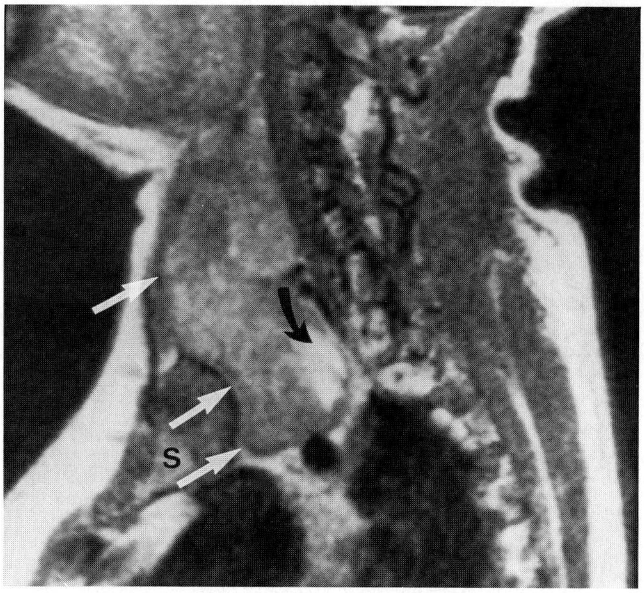

FIGURE 9–5. Thyroid goiter with substernal extension. Sagittal MR image (TR/TE = 1500/30) demonstrates marked enlargement of the thyroid (small arrows), which extends retrosternally (*S*, sternum). The thyroid has mixed signal intensity, and there is a region of colloid degeneration (curved arrow).

The role of MRI in relation to conventional x-ray and CT studies for evaluating bronchogenic carcinoma is controversial. Many studies have reported on the capabilities of the MR technique.[11–14] In one series, both MRI and CT were found to be accurate in assessing hilar and mediastinal adenopathy, with a sensitivity rate of 87%.[11] However, neither method correlated well with mediastinal invasion. Where there was mediastinal invasion, the sensitivity rate was 55% for CT and 64% for MRI.[11]

Another group evaluating MRI, CT, and mediastinoscopy for preoperative assessment of mediastinal nodes in bronchogenic carcinoma found that CT had a sensitivity of 71%, specificity of 87.7%, and overall accuracy of 82.1%.[12] In this review MRI did not provide any benefit over CT for the assessment of mediastinal nodes. Mediastinoscopy had a sensitivity of 87.1%, specificity of 100%, and an accuracy of 95.2%. Mediastinoscopy in this study exceeded the other modalities as the most accurate staging method for bronchogenic carcinoma.[12]

A study evaluating staging of primary lung carcinoma compared MRI and CT and found no statistically significant differences between the two imaging methods for evaluation of tumor extent or node involvement.[13] The multiplanar capabilities of MRI were advantageous for assessing chest wall invasion. The analysis of concordances and discordances did not indicate whether one modality could be substituted for the other or which diagnostic strategy might be more useful.[13] Many times MRI has significantly improved the evaluation of bronchogenic carcinoma particularly for those centrally located (Fig. 9-6) and for extension into the mediastinum, especially the aortopulmonary window (Fig. 9-4).

The literature provides divergent reports about the utility of MR. Many times, as a consequence of the differences between the various MR imaging systems made by different manufacturers and the differences between the MR techniques used in the reported studies, the images used in different studies are not comparable. Perhaps this accounts for the wide variation in the data for evaluating bronchogenic carcinoma. Whether the techniques employed and the images obtained of the chest and heart were of optimal quality must be analyzed in evaluating these studies.

MRI may play an important role in differentiation of radiation fibrosis from recurrent pulmonary neoplasm. It has been used to differentiate mediastinal fibrosis from recurrent tumor within the mediastinum in patients with lymphoma.[15] On the long TR sequence (i.e., T2-weighted sequence), fibrosis has decreased signal intensity, but tumor has increased signal intensity.[16] Usually tumors have an intermediate signal intensity on a T1-weighted sequence and an increased signal intensity on a T2-weighted sequence. If a parenchymal lesion extends into the mediastinum, the tumor may blend with mediastinal fat on the T2-weighted sequence.

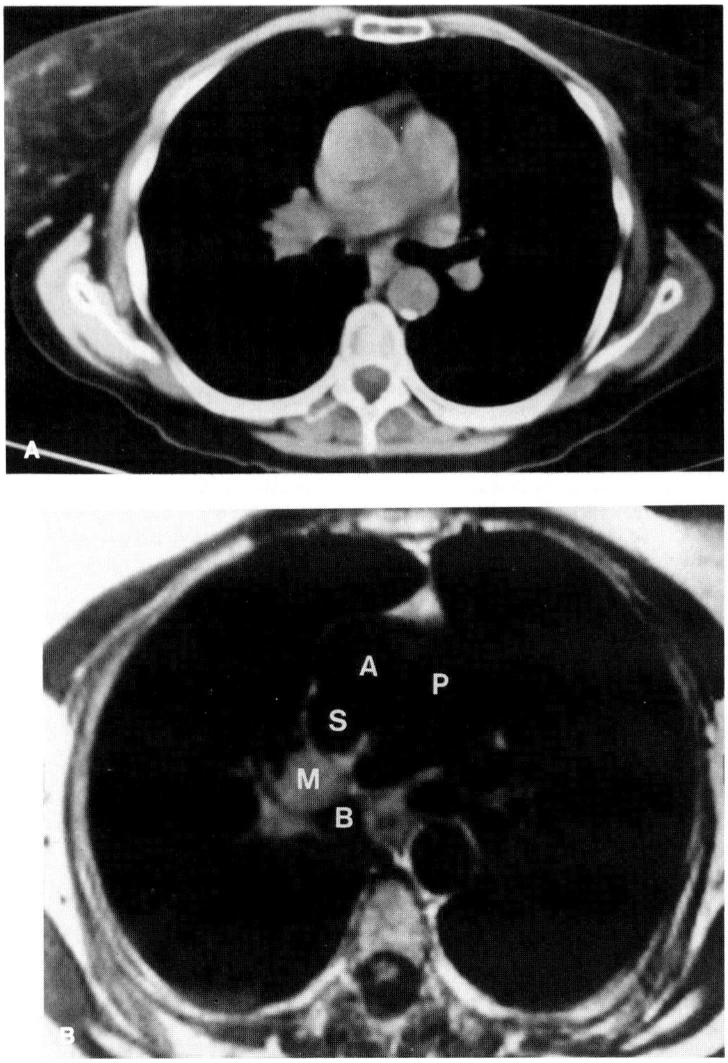

FIGURE 9-6. Masses in the region of the hila. **(A)** Transverse CT image was obtained after a chest x-ray film. The CT was read as equivocal because a definite mass was not identified. **(B)** Transverse MR image (TR/TE = 900/30) delineates a right hilar mass *(M)* posterior to the superior vena cava *(SV)*. Subsequent biopsy results revealed this was a primary bronchogenic carcinoma *(P*, pulmonary artery; *A*, aorta; *B*, bronchi).

The time course of radiation-induced changes within the lungs is important in evaluating patients after radiation therapy. During the early stages, between 6 to 12 weeks after radiation, there is an acute reaction called radiation pneumonitis. During the late or chronic phase of radiation change, normal lung parenchyma is replaced by fibrosis. These changes usually have stabilized by 12 months after radiation therapy has been completed.

Another potential role for MRI is in determining the site for transthoracic biopsy in the patient presenting with a recurrent mass. The areas of increased signal intensity within the mass on a T2-weighted sequence have been correlated with recurrent tumor, and other areas with low signal intensity have been found to represent fibrosis. On the CT study of these masses, there is no differentiation between recurrent tumor and fibrosis.

Pulmonary air space disease has many causes, and it is often difficult to determine the precise pathologic process on clinical examination or with imaging. The consolidation may be secondary to blood, pus, edema, or proteinaceous material. An MR study showed it was not possible to differentiate between the various causes of pulmonary consolidation based on the relaxation times known as T1 and T2.[17] All types of pulmonary consolidation have intermediate intensity on a T1-weighted sequence and increased intensity on a T2-weighted sequence.

MRI has been used to differentiate between a proximal bronchogenic carcinoma and postobstructive lobar collapse. In one study, MRI and CT were equal in the identification of a contour abnormality. However, CT (80%) was more successful than MRI (44%) for differentiating tumor mass from collapsed lung.[18] Other studies have postulated that by increasing the T2 weighting, MR may become more sensitive, because the tumor has a relatively lower signal intensity than the increased signal intensity of fluid within the collapsed lung.[15]

Mediastinum and Hilum

MRI excels in assessment of the mediastinum and hilum. The blood vessels and tracheobronchial tree are both visualized as regions of signal void highlighted by the surrounding fat. Masses in these regions have sufficiently different imaging characteristics to allow their separation from the normal structures and fat (Fig. 9–7). Compared with CT, in which contrast media is often needed to identify a mass and to avoid mistaking a blood vessel for a pathologic region, particularly in the pulmonary hilum (Fig. 9–6), MR imaging provides excellent cross-sectional images of the mediastinum, allowing assessment of mediastinal anatomy that is comparable to CT in quality and clarity.[19] MRI provided greater detail for evaluating disease than CT (Fig. 9–8).[20] MRI was especially valuable for detecting unsuspected metastases in the hilum (Fig. 9–9) and superior mediastinum. Several of the cases in this study had unsuspected hilar metastases and superior mediastinal metastases not delineated by CT but found with MRI.

The optimal sequence for delineating masses within the mediastinum is a gated sequence using a short TR. This allows sharp contrast between the high signal intensity of the fat and the intermediate signal intensity of most masses. The long TR sequence is necessary to optimally characterize mediastinal and hilar masses. It also improves the discrimination between masses and surrounding muscles. A study of mediastinal lesions in children showed that MRI provided similar information to CT about the presence and size of mediastinal masses.[21] MRI allowed better differentiation of mediastinal masses and enlarged nodes from vascular structures. It was also more sensitive than CT in detecting intraspinal extension in patients with posterior mediastinal masses. However, CT was better for demonstrating calcification and bronchial abnormalities that were not easily seen on the MR studies. The study concluded that MRI was

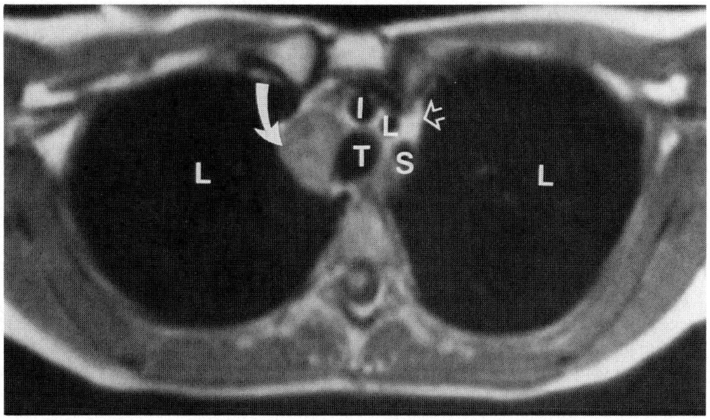

FIGURE 9–7. Lymphomatous lymph nodes. Transverse MR image (TR/TE = 650/30) shows enlarged paratracheal lymph nodes (curved arrow), seen in relation to the high-intensity signal of the fat (open arrow) and the low-intensity signal of the trachea *(T)*, lungs *(L)*, and blood vessels *(I*, innominate artery; *L*, left carotid artery; *S*, left subclavian).

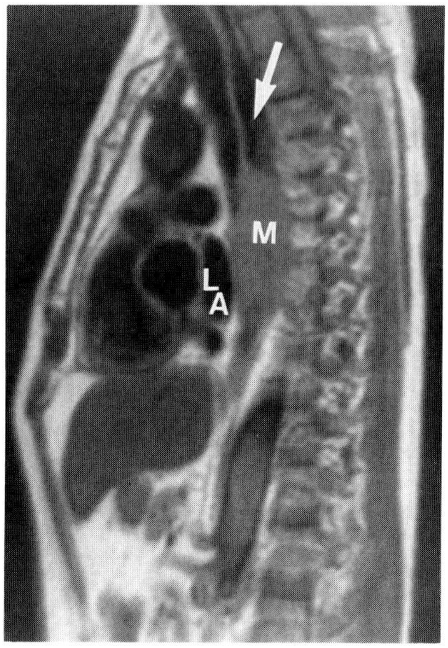

FIGURE 9–8. Posterior mediastinal mass. Sagittal MR image (TR/TE = 900/30) delineates a mass *(M)* compressing the left atrium *(LA)*. This was a large esophageal carcinoma, associated with dilatation of the proximal esophagus (white arrow).

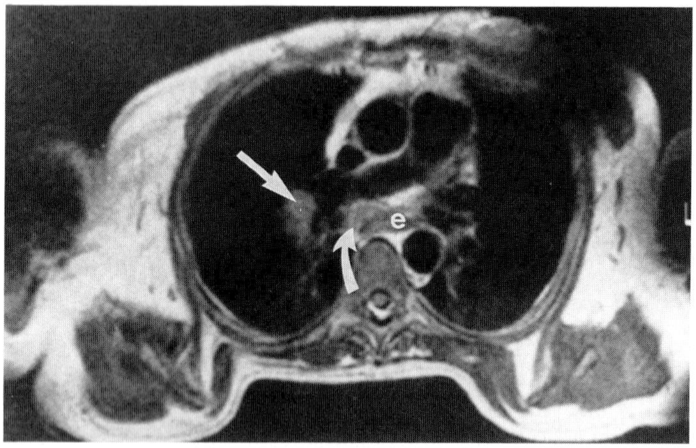

FIGURE 9–9. Hilar and mediastinal masses. Transverse MR image (TR/TE = 530/30) shows metastatic involvement of lymph nodes (white arrow) in the right hila and lymph nodes in the azygo-esophageal recess (curved arrow). The esophagus *(E)* should not be confused with a mass. On the second echo image, the esophagus is often seen with a higher-intensity center and lower-intensity peripheral wall, which can distinguish it from lymph nodes.

more helpful than CT for evaluating posterior mediastinal tumors, but CT remained the primary method for children with suspected mediastinal neoplasms.

Currently, MR is used either as a complimentary procedure for assessing the mediastinum and hilum, or it is used on those patients who have a contraindication for the use of iodinated contrast media or in whom the CT is equivocal, particularly for lesions in the hilum.

Pulmonary Vascularity

Since its introduction, there has been some interest in the use of MRI for evaluating the pulmonary arteries for pulmonary embolism or thrombus. Studies have been performed in animals and humans with pulmonary embolus and/or thrombus.[22-26] Experimental work in dogs showed MRI detected all blood clots greater than 3 mm and only 3 of 20 blood clots less than 3 mm.[22] Other studies in animals showed MRI was also capable of demonstrating the larger pulmonary emboli, especially those centrally located.[23] However, in certain instances central emboli in this series were mistaken for hilar fat.

The studies performed in patients showed MRI detects thrombus as an intraluminal signal within the pulmonary arteries followed by resolution of this signal on repeat examinations after clot lysis.[25,26] Currently, MRI is not the modality of choice for detecting pulmonary emboli. However, in a patient for whom there is an absolute contraindication to contrast and an equivocal ventilation-perfusion scan, MRI may supplement data by demonstrating emboli. If MRI is considered for pulmonary artery evaluation, it is better suited for detection of central than peripheral emboli.

MRI is quite useful for evaluating mediastinal and

thoracic inlet vessels in those patients presenting with obstruction of these vessels. It can provide detailed information about the precise site and extent of venous obstruction.[27] CT with an intravenous contrast infusion can provide information similar to that available with MRI. However, in studies in which an inadequate bolus of contrast is given, CT may not provide the same degree of information as MRI.

Tracheobronchial Tree

Many methods have been used to evaluate airway obstruction. The most often used is conventional radiography. A study in pediatric patients showed MR images in the sagittal and axial plane clearly demonstrated tracheal compression and narrowing from many causes.[28] Endoscopic examination correlated well with the appearance on MRI. In infants, MRI demonstrates the airway and its relationship to the major mediastinal blood vessels, which may play a part in airway obstruction.[28]

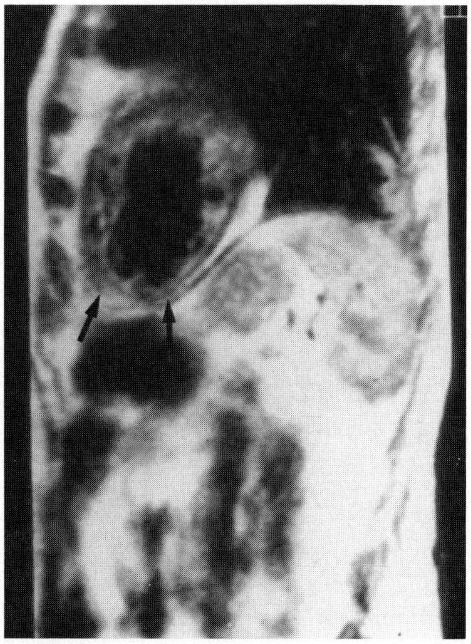

FIGURE 9–10. Left ventricular aneurysm of the inferior wall. Sagittal gated MR image (TR/TE = 700/30) demonstrates abrupt thinning of the inferioapical wall (arrows) at the site of a left ventricle aneurysm. The MR excludes a mural thrombus. Cine images showed dyskinesis at the site of the aneurysm.

CARDIAC IMAGING

An important and frequently used capability of cardiac MRI is in depicting anatomic abnormalities in ischemic heart disease, infection, valvular disease, cardiomyopathies, cardiac tumors, pericardial abnormalities, and congenital heart disease.

MRI is primarily a research tool for evaluating acute ischemic heart disease. It allows direct visualization of the myocardium and can precisely delineate the region of acute infarction.[29,30] Besides demonstrating a discrete abnormality in the myocardium, abnormalities in wall thickness may be seen. Acutely, a discrete region of wall thinning may be seen during systole, and chronically, a permanent region of wall thinning is demonstrable.[31] MRI more often is used to assess complications after acute myocardial infarction, such as left ventricular thrombus and left ventricular aneurysm (Fig. 9–10).

At this time, the standard MR spin echo technique is not optimal for detecting infectious endocarditis. It is not as accurate as echocardiography in demonstrating valvular vegetations. If there is incompetency of the valve secondary to infection, the gradient-echo technique can delineate abnormalities in valve function. However, the standard spin echo images do allow important information about anatomic changes associated with infection, such as fibrin strands within the ventricles or myocardial abscesses.

The efficacy of MRI for valvular disease is currently being studied. The optimal MR method for assessment of valve dysfunction is the gradient-echo technique. On the standard spin echo technique in the cine mode, the valves may be demonstrated (Fig. 9–11), but assessment of stenosis or regurgitation cannot be optimally evaluated. The gradient-echo technique does allow this evaluation (Fig. 9–12).[32–34] With valvular regurgitation, a high-pressure gradient through a narrow orifice causes turbulent flow within the regurgitant chamber. The gradient-echo images demonstrate the turbulence in the regurgitant flow as regions of low signal intensity.

Although standard spin echo techniques do not allow functional analysis of valves, they can demonstrate anatomic abnormalities that affect the valve plane and surrounding region. For example, in a Marfan's syndrome patient, marked dilatation of the sinuses of Valsalva is demonstrable (Fig. 9–13). Other complications, such as aortic dissection, can also be shown. Studies have been done on prosthetic valves to demonstrate the safety of imaging these patients by determining deflection and temperature variations in low-field and high-field MR systems (see Chapter 14).[35]

It is possible to accurately define different types of cardiomyopathies because MRI allows delineation of the endocardial and epicardial surfaces of the myocardium. In ischemic and congested cardiomyopathy, left ventricular dilatation can be quantified. In asymmetric or concentric hypertrophic cardiomyopathies, MRI allows assessment of wall thickness and extent of wall thickening.[36,37] MRI has not provided pathognomonic changes in signal intensity within the myocardium for different types of infiltrative cardiomyopa-

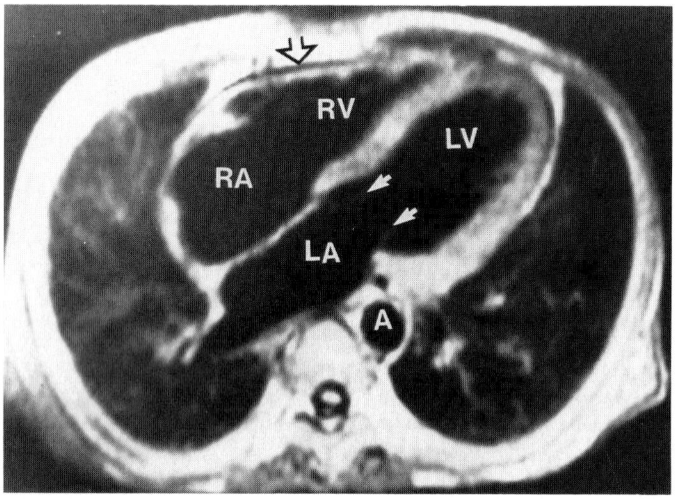

FIGURE 9–11. Spin echo appearance of normal mitral valves and pericardium. Transverse gated MR image (TR/TE = 700/30) in a four-chamber view shows the anterior and posterior mitral valve leaflets (white arrows) during opening. The normal, low-intensity pericardium (open black arrow), approximately 2 mm thick, is highlighted by the epipericardial fat, which has high signal intensity (*LV*, left ventricle; *RV*, right ventricle; *RA*, right atrium; *LA*, left atrium; *A*, aorta).

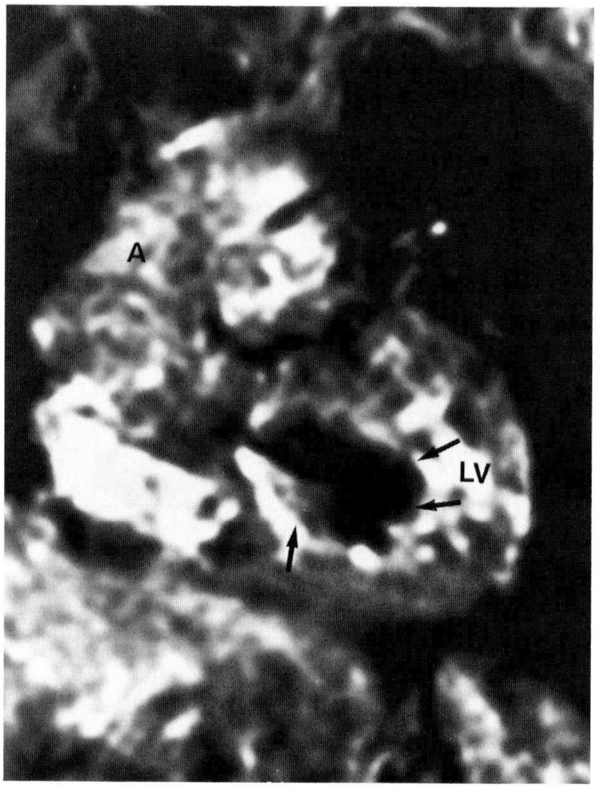

FIGURE 9–12. Aortic regurgitation evaluated with gradient echo MR. Coronal gated gradient echo MR image demonstrates during mid-diastole a region of low signal intensity (small arrows) extending from the aortic valve back into the left ventricle. This is the typical MR appearance for regurgitant blood from a diseased valve (*A*, aorta; *LV*, left ventricle).

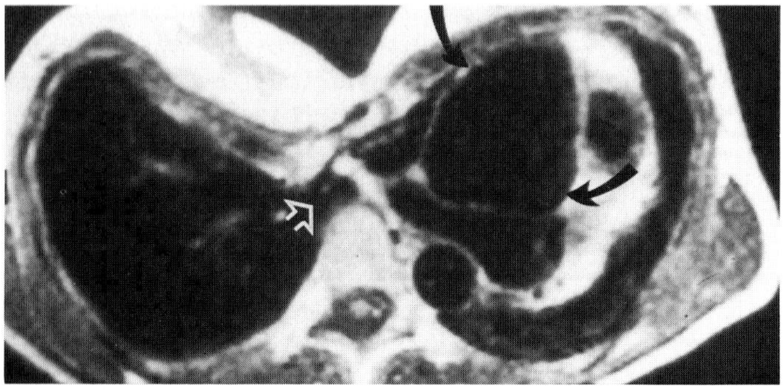

FIGURE 9–13. Patient with Marfan's syndrome with dilated sinuses of Valsalva. Transverse gated MR image (TR/TE = 560/30) demonstrates severe pectus deformity with the sternum almost touching the anterior verterbral body (open arrow). The cardiac structures are shifted into the left hemithorax. Notice the marked dilatation of the sinus of Valsalva (curved arrows) in this patient who also had severe aortic regurgitation.

thies, with the exception of lipomatous hypertrophy of the atrial septum.[38]

An important cardiac application of MRI is in the assessment of cardiac tumors. It is often the technique used after an echocardiographic study. A mass is often seen on the echocardiographic study, and the patient is subsequently evaluated with MRI, in which a mass is shown not to be present.[39,40] Occasionally, difficulties arise in the echocardiographic evaluation of patients (e.g., those with an unusual body habitus or patients with COPD). MRI is useful for confirming the presence of a mass seen by echocardiography by providing a larger field of view in the overall assessment of a mass and allowing better delineation of the mass extent (Fig. 9–14).[41–43]

MR has demonstrated primary tumors (e.g., myx-

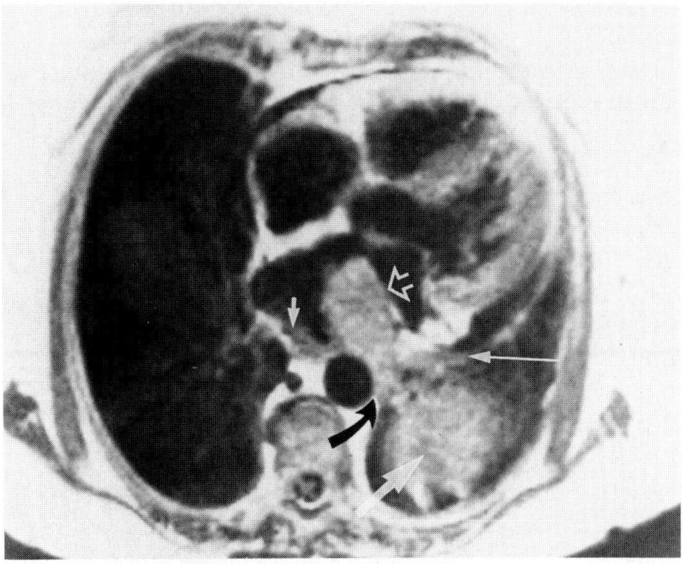

FIGURE 9–14. Intracardiac metastatic sarcoma. Transverse gated MR image (TR/TE = 600/30) shows a mass (open arrow) within the left atrium invading the posterior wall of the left atrium (small white arrow), the fat (arrowhead) anterior to the aorta, and along the fat (curved arrow) in the epipericardial region. There is a posterior pericardial effusion (thin white arrow) and another metastasis in the left lung (large white arrow).

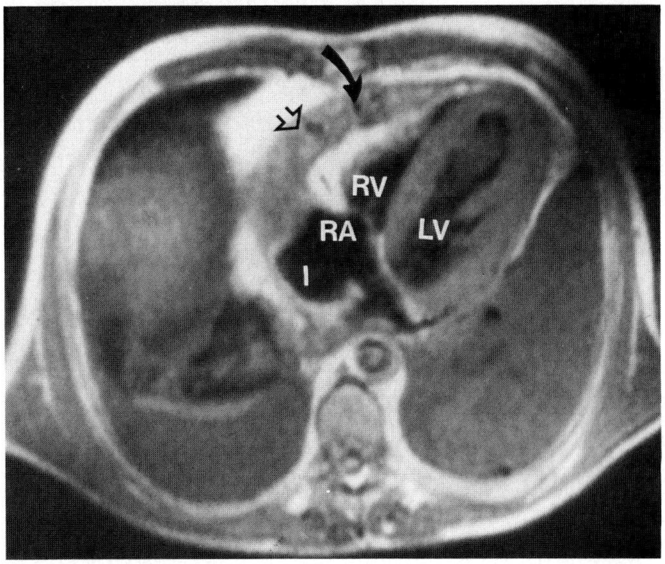

FIGURE 9–15. Staphylococcal pericardial effusion resulting in constrictive pericarditis. Transverse gated MR image (TR/TE = 440/30) demonstrates an intermediate-intensity fluid collection (open arrow) along the right anterior aspect of the right ventricle (*RV*). The collection causes marked compression of the right ventricle, a typical pattern seen with constrictive pericarditis. Notice black intensity foci (curved arrow) within the collection, suggesting air and raising the suspicion of an infection (*RA*, right atrium; *I*, inferior vena cava; *LV*, left ventricle).

omas and benign papillary fibroelastomas) and metastatic disease (e.g., malignant fibrous histiocytoma, breast carcinoma, and melanoma). MRI can show intramyocardial disease, such as multiple masses from cardiac sarcoidosis.[44] MR allows precise evaluation of the relationship of cardiac masses to cardiovascular and mediastinal structures. It is particularly suited for assessing benign masses (e.g., lipomatous hypertrophy of the atrial septum) and is helpful for the echocardiographic analysis.[38] On echocardiography a malignant mass may be suspected and MR allows its benign nature to be demonstrated.

Another important use of MRI is evaluation of the pericardium. The normal pericardium is a thin, low-intensity line around the heart, most often seen along the anterior aspect of the heart on the transverse view (Fig. 9–11).[45] The pericardium probably has a low signal intensity because of its composition, primarily of fibrous tissue and a small amount of pericardial fluid. The normal pericardial thickness is approximately 2 mm.

MRI is used in differentiating patients clinically suspected of having constrictive pericarditis or restrictive cardiomyopathy.[46,47] MRI allows accurate diagnosis of constrictive pericarditis. The pericardium is seen as thickened and may have a variety of signal intensities. It may be entirely of low signal intensity or have a medium or high signal intensity, depending on the cause of the pericarditis. Often the cause of the constriction, better seen on MR, is a loculated pericardial effusion, infected pericardial effusion (Fig. 9–15), or hematoma. MRI allows differentiation between different types of intrapericardial fluid collections better than echocardiography because a subacute hematoma looks quite different from a noncomplex pericardial effusion on MRI.

MRI is useful for assessing congenital heart disease. Cardiac catheterization remains the mainstay of diagnosis for many complex lesions, but MRI and echocardiography are useful for follow-up studies or assessing less-complex lesions. MRI provides an important noninvasive means of assessing the great vessels for defects like coarctation (Fig. 9–16) and pulmonary atresia.[48] It is quite capable of demonstrating ventricular or atrial septal defects, the type of ventricular loop, and visceroatrial situs abnormalities, as well as complex congenital heart lesions, such as single ventricle.[49,50]

The precise role of MRI must be determined. It provides supplementary information in many cases, and it often gives essential preoperative information, such as the size of the pulmonary arteries in patients with severe pulmonary stenosis or atresia, that is not possible to assess with echocardiography or cardiac catheterization.

Functional Capabilities

Both the standard spin echo and gradient-echo techniques may be used for evaluating cardiac function. Images are obtained from the cardiac base to apex to perform calculations of end-diastolic and end-systolic volumes and ejection fraction (Fig. 9–17).[51,52] Additionally, MRI allows assessment of myocardial wall

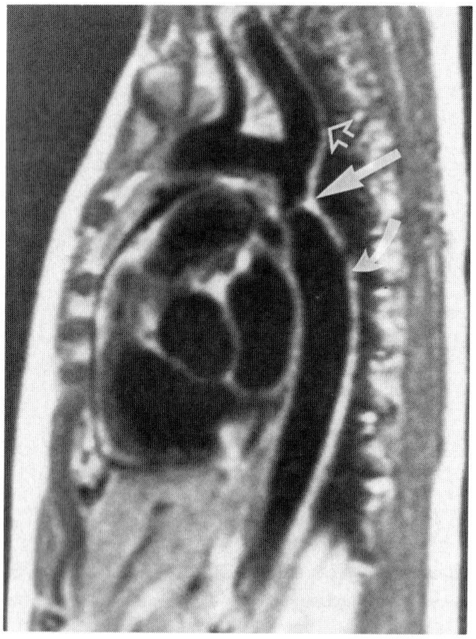

FIGURE 9–16. Juxtaductal coarctation. Sagittal gated MR image (TR/TE = 900/30) shows a region of abrupt narrowing (white arrow) at the juxtaductal portion of the aorta that is typical for a juxtaductal coarctation. Common associated findings are post-stenotic dilatation (curved arrow) of the proximal descending thoracic aorta *(A)* and dilatation of the left subclavian artery (open arrow).

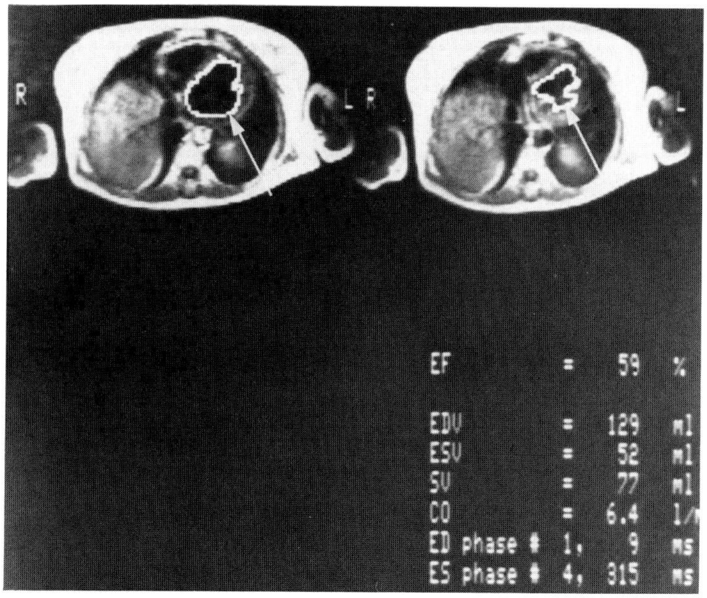

FIGURE 9–17. Functional cardiac MRI. Using a software module on the Philips Gyroscan MR system, it is possible to obtain rapid assessment of ventricular volumes and ejection fractions. This short-axis view of the heart (TR/TE = 610/30) obtained by double angulation technique is optimal for calculating a volume ejection fraction. An irregular region of interest (thin white arrow) is drawn at the endocardial-blood interface for sections from the cardiac base to apex at six different phases in the cardiac cycle. The software program calculates ejection fraction *(EF)*, end-diastolic volume *(EDV)*, end-systolic volume *(ESV)*, stroke volume *(SV)*, and cardiac output *(CO)*.

thickness by obtaining images at end-diastole and end-systole at different cardiac levels. The degree of wall thickening and extent of wall thickening may be determined for the left ventricular walls.[37] With the advent of gradient-echo imaging, cine images of the heart have been obtained in a more efficient manner than was possible with the standard spin echo technique, thereby increasing the utility of MRI because of decreased imaging time. The gradient-echo sequence can be acquired in approximately 2 to 5 minutes, and subsequently cine images are displayed for assessment of cardiac wall motion abnormalities.[53]

MR Tissue Characterization and Spectroscopy

Research continues on myocardial tissue characterization and myocardial spectroscopy. Myocardial tissue characterization has been studied for ischemic myocardial injury, cardiac transplant rejection, and cardiomyopathies due to chemotherapy.[29,30,54,55] Spectroscopic studies are continuing and may provide on a routine basis assessment of myocardial metabolism that will allow early detection of changes within the myocardium caused by diseases.[56,57] Most of the work has evaluated metabolism of phosphorous-31, which provides a potential mechanism for studying high-energy phosphate metabolism clinically.[58]

CONCLUSION

There is continued evolution in the uses of MR for evaluation of thoracic abnormalities. Early studies showed the potential of this technique for imaging the mediastinal and hilar structures and for demonstrating the normal anatomy of the thorax on sagittal, coronal, and transverse MR images. As more data has been compiled, most investigators have compared MRI to CT for its ability to assess mediastinal and hilar adenopathy and masses, bronchogenic carcinoma, and other pulmonary parenchyma lesions, and for assessment of the pulmonary vascularity. In these situations, MRI has generally provided equivalent information to that provided by CT. MRI is still in its infancy, and there still are wide variations in image quality and MR systems. As a result, there is significant variability of the data in the literature. Although the recommended use of MRI may change rapidly, the current opinion is that MRI of the thorax is a complementary procedure to CT, particularly good for those patients with allergies to iodinated contrast material and for defining equivocal lesions seen on CT, such as small central hilar bronchogenic carcinomas.

Cardiac MRI has been proven to be a useful tool for morphologic and functional analysis of the cardiovascular system.

REFERENCES

1. Crooks LE, Barker B, Chang H, et al. Magnetic resonance imaging strategies for heart studies. Radiology 1984;153:459.
2. VanDiijk P. ECG-triggered NMR imaging of the heart. Diagn Imag Clin Med 1984;53:29.
3. Fisher MR, Von Schultness GK, Higgins CB. Multiphasic cardiac magnetic resonance imaging: Normal regional left ventricular thickening. AJR 1985;145:27.
4. Cuppen JJM, Groen JP, Konijh J. Magnetic resonance fast fourier imaging. Medical Physics 1986;13:248.
5. Gamsu G, Webb WR, Sheldon P, et al. Nuclear magnetic resonance imaging of the thorox. Radiology 1983;147:473.
6. Axel L, Kressel H, Thickman D, et al. NMR imaging of the chest. AJR 1983;141:1157.
7. Ross J, O'Donovan PB, Novoa R, et al. Magnetic resonance of the chest: initial experience with imaging and in vivo T1 and T2 calculations. Radiology 1984;152:95.
8. Webb WR, Jensen BG, Gamsu G, et al. Coronal magnetic resonance imaging of the chest: normal and abnormal. Radiology 1984;153:729.
9. O'Donovan PB, Ross JS, Sivak ED, et al. Magnetic resonance imaging of the thorax: the advantages of coronal and sagittal planes. AJR 1984;143:1183.
10. Muller NL, Gamsu G, Webb WR. Pulmonary nodules: detection using magnetic resonance and computed tomography. Radiology 1985;155:687.
11. Martini N, Heelan R, Westcott J, et al. Comparative merits of conventional, computed tomographic and magnetic resonance imaging in assessing mediastinal involvement in surgically confirmed lung carcinoma. J Thorac Cardiovasc Surg 1985;90:643.
12. Patterson G, Ginsberg R, Poon P, et al. A prospective evaluation of MR, CT, and mediastinoscopy in the preoperative assessment of mediastinal node status in bronchogenic carcinoma. J Thorac Cardiovasc Surg 1987;94:679.
13. Musset D, Grenier P, Carette M, et al. Primary lung cancer staging: prospective comparative study of MR imaging with CT. Radiology 1986;160:607.
14. Levitt RG, Glazer HS, Roper C, et al. Magnetic resonance imaging of mediastinal and hilar masses: comparison with CT. AJR 1985;145:9.
15. Kundel HL, Kressel H, Epstein D. The potential role of NMR imaging in thoracic disease. Radiol Clin North Am 1983;21:801.
16. Glazer HS, Levitt RG, Lee JK, et al. Differentiation of radiation fibrosis from recurrent pulmonary neoplasm by MRI. AJR 1984;143:729.
17. Moore E, Webb WR, Muller N, Sollitto R. MRI of pulmonary air space disease: experimental model and preliminary clinical results. AJR 1986;146:1123.
18. Tobler J, Levitt RG, Glazer HS, et al. Differentiation of proximal bronchogenic carcinoma from postobstructive lobar collapse by magnetic resonance imaging. Comparison with CT. Invest Radiol 1987;22:533.
19. Epstein DM, Kressel H, Gefter W, et al. MR imaging of the mediastinum: a retrospective comparison with computed tomography. JCAT 1984;6:670.
20. Cohen AM, Creviston S, Li Puma JP, et al. Nuclear magnetic resonance imaging of the mediastinum and hili: early impressions of its efficacy. AJR 1983;141:1163.
21. Siegel MJ, Nadel SN, Glazer HS, Sagel SS. Mediastinal lesions in children: comparison of CT & MR. Radiology 1986;160:241.
22. Stein M, Crues J, Bradley W, et al. MR imaging of pulmonary emboli: an experimental study in dogs. AJR 1986;147:1133.
23. Gamsu G, Hirji M, Moore E, et al. Experimental pulmonary emboli detected by magnetic resonance. Radiology 1984;153:467.

24. Thickman D, Kressel H, Axel L. Demonstration of pulmonary embolism by MR. AJR 1984;142:921.
25. Moore E, Gamsu G, Stark D, Moon K. Pulmonary embolus: detection and follow-up using magnetic resonance. Radiology 1984;153:471.
26. Fisher MR, Higgins CB. Identification of central thrombi in pulmonary arterial hypertension using MR. Radiology 1986;158:223.
27. Weinreb J, Mootz A, Cohen JM. MRI evaluation of mediastinal and thoracic inlet venous obstruction. AJR 1986;146:679.
28. Fletcher B, Dearborn D, Mulopulos GP. MR imaging infants with airway obstruction: preliminary observations. Radiology 1986;160:245.
29. Fisher MR, McNamara MT, Higgins CB. Acute myocardial infarction: MR evaluation in 29 patients. AJR 1987;148:247.
30. Tscholakoff D, Higgins CB, McNamara MT, Derugin N. Early-phase myocardial infarction: evaluation by MR imaging. Radiology 1986;159:667.
31. Higgins CB, Lanzer P, Stark D, et al. Imaging by NMR in patients with chronic ischemic disease. Circulation 1984;69:523.
32. Pflugfelder PW, Landzberg JS, Aufferman W, et al. Comprehensive evaluation of aortic regurgitation by cine magnetic resonance imaging comparison with echocardiography. [Abstract] SMRM 1987;1:16.
33. Schiebler M, Axel L, Reicheck N, et al. Correlations of cine NMR imaging with two dimensional pulsed Doppler echocardiography in valvular insufficiency. JACT 1987;11:627.
34. Pflugfelder PW, Sechtem UP, Wyite RD, Higgins CB. Evaluation of mitral valvular regurgitation by analysis of systolic left atrial signal loss in cine magnetic resonance images. [Abstract] SMRM 1987;2:729.
35. Soulen R, Budinger T, Higgins CB. Magnetic resonance imaging of prosthetic heart valves. Radiology 1985;154:705.
36. Higgins CB, Byrd BF, Stark JD. MRI of hypertrophic cardiomyopathy. Am J Cardiol 1985;55:1121.
37. Fisher MR, von Schulthess GK, Higgins CB. Multiphasic cardiac magnetic resonance imaging: Normal regional left ventricular wall thickening. AJR 1985;145:27.
38. Levine RA, Weyman AB, Dinsmore RE, et al. Noninvasive tissue characterization: diagnosis of lipomatous hypertrophy of the atrial septum by nuclear magnetic resonance imaging. JACC 1986;7:688.
39. Winkler M, Higgins CB. Suspected intracardiac masses: Evaluation with MR imaging. Radiology 1987;165:117.
40. Freedberg R, Kronzon I, Rumancik W, Liebeskind DJ. The contribution of magnetic resonance to the evaluation of intracardiac tumors diagnosed by echocardiography. Circulation 1988;77:96.
41. Lee R, Fisher MR. Benefits of MR for pre-op evaluation of intracardiac masses. JCAT 1989;13:126.
42. Go RT, O'Donnell JK, Underwood DA, et al. Comparison of gated cardiac MRI and 2D echocardiography of intracardiac neoplasms. AJR 1985;145:21.
43. Amparo EG, Higgins CB, Farmer D, et al. Gated MRI of cardiac and paracardiac masses: Initial experience. AJR 1984;143:1151.
44. Reidy K, Fisher MR. MR of cardiac sarcoidosis. AJR 1988;151:915.
45. Sechtem U, Tscholakoff D, Higgins CB. MRI of normal pericardium. AJR 1986;147:239.
46. Sechtem U, Tscholakoff D, Higgins CB. MRI of abnormal pericardium. AJR 1986;147:239.
47. Soulen R, Stark D, Higgins CB. MRI of constrictive pericardial disease. Am J Cardiol 1985;55:480.
48. von Schulthess GK, Higashino SM, Higgins S, et al. MRI of coarctation of the aorta. Radiology 1986;158:227.
49. Didier D, Higgins CB, Fisher MR, et al. Gated MR in congenital heart disease: Initial experience in 72 patients. Radiology 1986;158:227.
50. Fisher MR, Higgins CB. Magnetic resonance imaging of congenital heart disease. In: Higgins CB, Morganrath J, Pohost G, et al., eds. New concepts in cardiac imaging. Chicago: Year Book Medical Publishers, 1987:231.
51. Fisher MR, Steinberg F, Rogers LF. Evaluation of cardiac function by MR. Association of University Radiologists. [Abstract] April 1987.
52. Stratemeier EJ, Thompson R, Brady JJ, et al. Ejection fraction determination by MR imaging: comparison with left ventricular angiography.
53. Fisher MR, Steinberg F, Rogers LF. Cine MR evaluation of abnormal wall motion in patient status post acute MI. [Abstract] Radiology 1986;161:82.
54. Tscholakoff D, Aherne T, Yee ES, et al. Cardiac transplantation in dogs: evaluation with MR. Radiology 1985;157:698.
55. Thompson RC, Lojeski EW, Ratner AV, et al. Detection of adriamycin cardiotoxicity using proton NMR techniques. [Abstract] Circulation 1982;68:3.
56. Evanochko WE, Reeves RC, Sakai TT, et al. Proton NMR spectroscopy in myocardial ischemic insult. Magn Reson Med 1987;5:23.
57. Cannon PJ, Mandsley A, Hilal SK, et al. NMR imaging of NA-23 in myocardium following coronary artery occulsion and reperfusion. JACC 1986;7:573.
58. Nunnally RC, Bottomley PA. NMR studies of myocardial ischemia and its response to drug therapies. [Abstract] JCAT 1981;5:296.

10

Abdomen

Mark R. Bankoff
Val M. Runge
David D. Stark

The use of magnetic resonance imaging (MRI) in the diagnosis of intra-abdominal diseases has been limited for several reasons. Artifacts caused by respiratory, cardiac, and peristaltic motion significantly degrade the quality of images (Fig. 10–1). The lack of an adequate contrast material for the gastrointestinal system also remains a significant limitation in the MRI examination of the abdomen. Despite these reservations, there are clinical indications for abdominal MRI examinations. This chapter discusses the liver, adrenal glands, and kidneys. In these organs, MRI has a significant contribution to make in the primary evaluation of certain diseases, and some abnormalities are so common that their appearance should be recognized on MRI even if the examination is performed for other reasons.

As MRI technology advances, the limitations for its use in examining the abdomen will be overcome. We can soon expect an acceptable oral contrast agent, and work at many institutions has already shown the great potential for fast scan (breath-hold) sequences.

IMAGING TECHNIQUES

Concepts fundamental to image acquisition and interpretation, particularly for examining the upper abdomen, are discussed in this chapter. For a more detailed discussion of the physics of MRI relative to imaging of the abdomen, see Chapter 13.

The MR examination of the abdomen must compensate for motion. At the current stage of development, methods exist for both respiratory and cardiac gating. These systems decrease artifacts caused by cardiac and respiratory motion, but they also present certain compromises. For example, to achieve a repetition time (TR) of 500 msec, the heart rate must be 120 beats per minute, with slower rates requiring a longer TR. This restriction limits the ability to achieve heavy T1 weighting.

Respiratory gating is limited by the fact that data acquisition can only be performed during certain parts of the respiratory cycle. Imaging time is markedly prolonged depending upon the proportion of the respiratory cycle that is excluded from the imaging process.[1] Newer motion-compensating techniques, such as ROPE (Respiratory Ordering of Phase Encoding), improve on older respiratory gating techniques by using the entire respiratory cycle for imaging. These techniques do not add to imaging time, but the initial set-up time before the scan is prolonged because a respiratory monitor must be employed.

ROPE is operator-dependent. This term is used for techniques that require intervention by an "operator," for example, the process of monitoring the respiratory cycle and successful use of this data for triggering image acquisition. Operator-dependent techniques are more prone to fail because an additional step is added to the imaging process, the successful execution of which cannot be guaranteed. Another limitation to ROPE is blurring of anatomic structures in the final image. This technique does not eliminate the effects of motion, but rather changes the end result. For both reasons, use of ROPE is limited in clinical practice.

If motion is unavoidable (e.g., the upper abdomen), further improvement in image quality requires gradient moment nulling, originally called MAST (Motion Artifact Suppression Technique).[2] Ghost artifacts are caused in part by the effect of motion on transverse magnetization during the time interval TE. Ghosts arise when the dephasing due to motion is different in subsequent TE intervals. Changes in the velocity of motion during imaging are primarily respon-

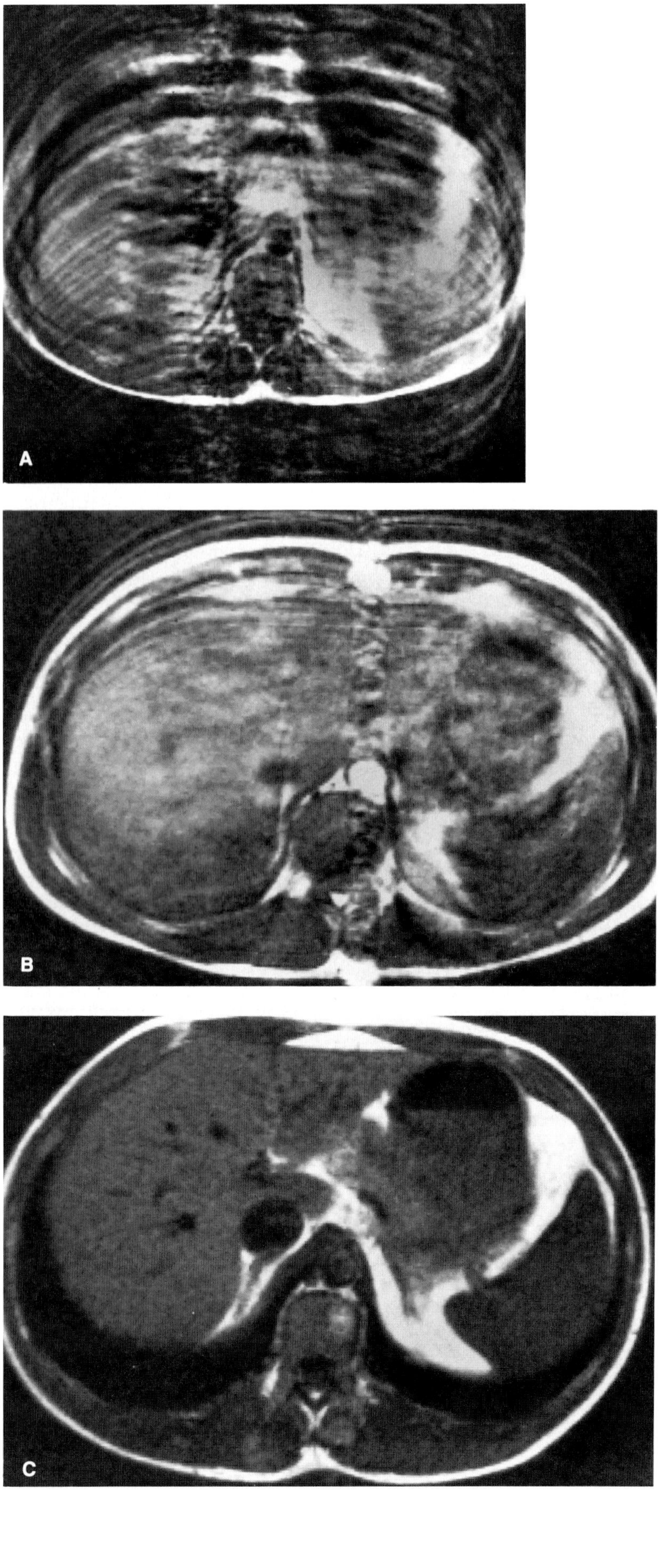

FIGURE 10–1. Breathing produces ghost artifacts and a reduction in the overall signal-to-noise ratio of the primary image on abdominal MRI. The difference between **(A)** heavy breathing, **(B)** normal breathing, and **(C)** breath holding is illustrated in a normal volunteer (TR/TE = 250/17, with one data acquisition). Motion is the major limiting factor in obtaining diagnostic-quality MR images of the upper abdomen.

sible for this effect. Gradient moment nulling directly compensates for changes in the velocity of motion occurring during TE. Higher-order corrections, such as that for acceleration, can also be made (see Chapter 13).

Gradient moment nulling is used routinely in abdominal imaging because it is effective and operator-independent (Fig. 10–2). In this technique, additional gradient pulses are used to cancel the dephasing caused by motion.[3,4] Ghost artifacts can be greatly reduced with no additional patient preparation time, because monitoring is not necessary.

Physical restraints, such as abdominal compression bands, are important in reducing motion artifact. These devices reduce ghosting and should be used in imaging of the abdomen or pelvis. Implementation is limited only by patient tolerance (Fig. 10–3).

Averaging a large number of data acquisitions can reduce artifactual ghosts and improve image quality (Fig. 10–4). If the TR is short, no significant prolongation of imaging time occurs.[5] By this method, respiratory, peristaltic, and cardiac motion artifacts are reduced. Unfortunately, motion causes a loss in signal-to-noise ratio (SNR), which is not avoided by data averaging. Although SNR is improved by the increased number of data acquisitions, the result is inferior to a scan with the same technique during which motion did not occur.

All current motion compensation techniques leave room for improvement. The use of breath-hold images may have a significant impact on abdominal MRI in the near future. Until high-quality breath-hold images can be achieved routinely on all systems, techniques compatible with respiration will continue to play a major role. One additional innovation deserves comment. Saturation pulses (see Chapter 13) can be used to cancel the signal from moving fat (i.e., the abdominal wall), reducing a major source of ghost artifacts. This technique may also be employed to reduce ghosting from through-plane blood flow (e.g., the pulsation artifacts from the aorta and inferior vena cava in axial abdominal images).

LIVER

Focal Masses

Metastatic disease to the liver is a common diagnostic problem. In screening for metastases in the liver, MRI is at least as sensitive as computed tomography (CT) (Fig. 10–5).[6,7] Clearly, lesion detectability is affected by the MR pulse sequences employed. T1-weighted spin echo imaging, used with a short TR and multiple acquisitions, is more sensitive and accurate in detecting metastatic liver lesions than contrast-enhanced CT.[6] At 0.6 T, there was no significant difference between spin echo and inversion recovery T1-weighted images for lesion detection.[6] At high field strengths (1.0–1.5 T), T2-weighted spin echo imaging with gradient moment nulling may be important for detecting liver metastases (Fig. 10–6). The difference between imaging at low and high fields is partially due to the prolongation of spin-lattice relaxation time (T1) with increasing field strength. T2-weighted scans can also be used, regardless of field strength, for improved lesion specificity (Fig. 10–7).

Despite its sensitivity, MRI is still dominated by x-ray CT in screening for liver metastases. The inability to obtain a diagnostic image in some patients, due to breathing artifacts, gross motion, and poor visualization of abnormalities elsewhere in the upper abdomen (i.e., pancreas, para-aortic adenopathy), limit MRI as a primary diagnostic tool.

The ability to identify liver metastases depends on achieving optimal contrast between lesion and liver. Work at 0.6 T revealed better contrast-to-noise ratio (CNR) between metastatic tumor and liver with short TR and TE on T1-weighted spin echo sequences than on the conventional T1-weighted and T2-weighted sequences used in brain imaging.[6,8] On such sequences, the signal intensity of most metastases is lower than that of normal surrounding liver. Because T1 varies with field strength, the relative lesion and liver signal intensities with any specific pulse sequence also change. A good means of assessing pulse sequences to predict their ability to detect metastases is necessary. Because the T1 and T2 relaxation times and the proton density of the spleen are similar to those of the average hepatic metastasis, maximizing the difference in contrast between liver and spleen should produce excellent contrast between a metastasis and liver.[9] At any given field strength, one must choose parameters that produce good CNR between liver and spleen.

To replace x-ray CT in screening for metastatic liver disease, MRI must demonstrate cost-effectiveness, high-image CNR for lesion detection, and high image quality for all patients. Research in pulse techniques has addressed the latter two criteria. Imaging sequences acquired during breath-holding can circumvent the problems associated with patient respiration and improve the consistency of scan quality from patient to patient.[10] To supply adequate CNR, two divergent approaches have been investigated (Fig. 10–8). Gradient-echo techniques, applied with very short TRs and TEs (i.e., $TR \leq 50$ msec, $TE \leq 10$ msec), can produce high CNR images. Acquisition of such an image, with $TR = 40$ msec and 256 phase-encoding steps, can easily be accomplished during breath-holding due to the 10-second scan time. An alternative approach employs spin echo imaging, with the number of phase-encoding steps reduced by appli-

(text continues on page 366)

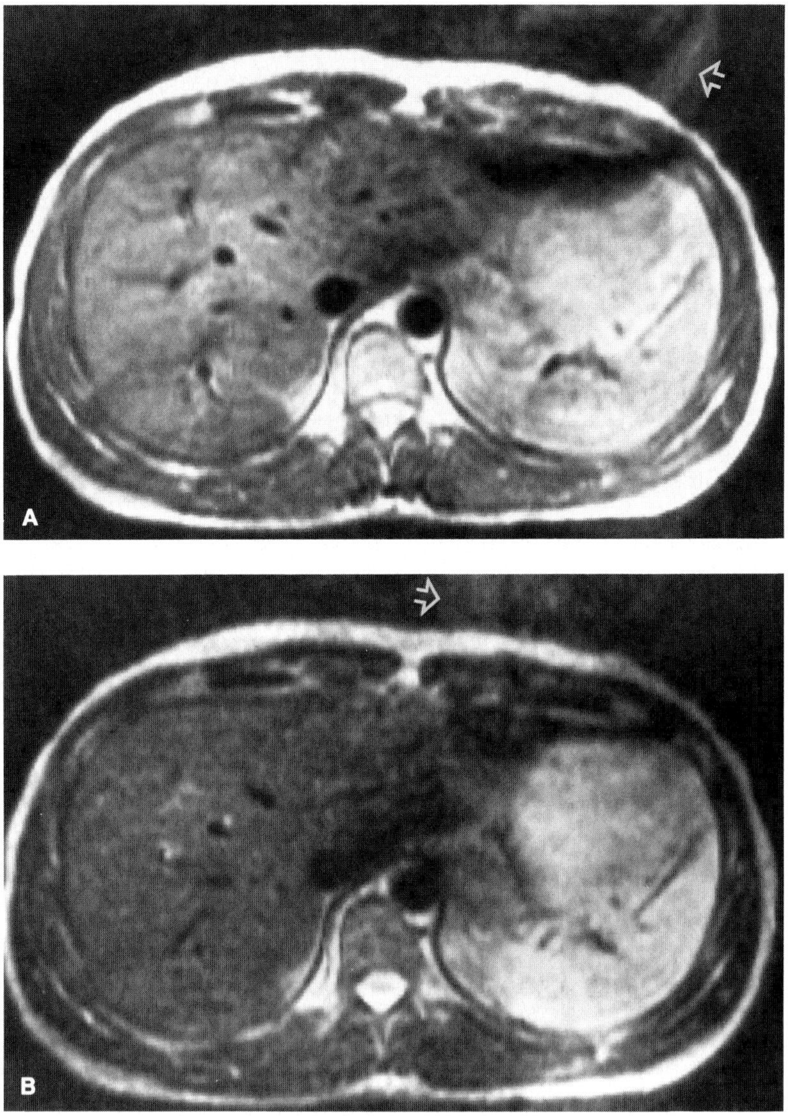

FIGURE 10–2. Reduction of respiratory artifact with gradient moment nulling. With this technique, compensation is made for motion occurring during the time interval TE. First and second echos of a T2-weighted scan (TR/TE = 3000/45,90) are presented **(A,B)** without and **(C,D)** with gradient moment nulling. A first-order correction was employed for the readout and the slice-select gradients. With gradient moment nulling, there is significant reduction of ghost artifact (open arrows). This technique also produces high signal intensity within intrahepatic blood vessels (closed arrows).

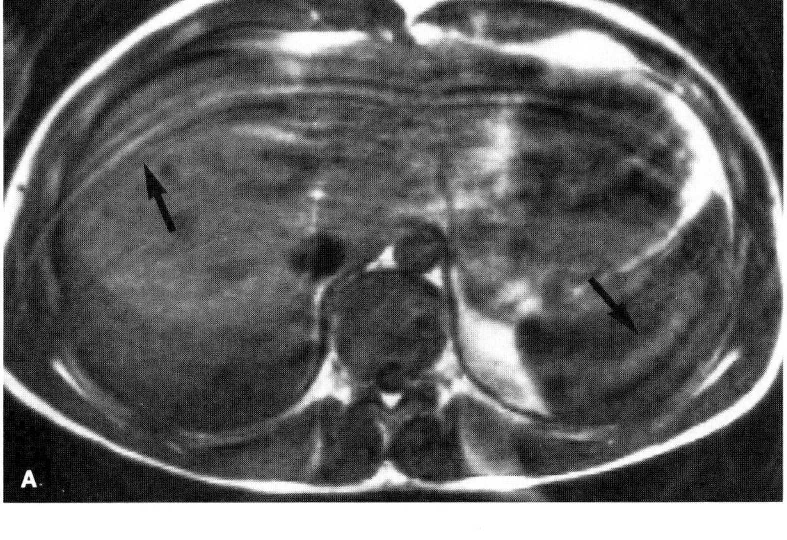

FIGURE 10–3. Reduction of motion artifact by the use of physical restraints. The motion of anterior abdominal fat contributes significantly to image degradation in routine spin echo scans. By restricting displacement of the anterior abdominal fat, artifactual ghosts can be reduced, improving overall image quality. **(A,B)** The only difference between the scans (TR/TE = 400/17, with two data acquisitions) is that a compression band has been used to limit motion of the anterior abdominal wall in the second scan **(B)**. There is a reduction in ghost artifacts (arrows), improving depiction of the liver and spleen. Images presented are from a normal volunteer at 1.0 T.

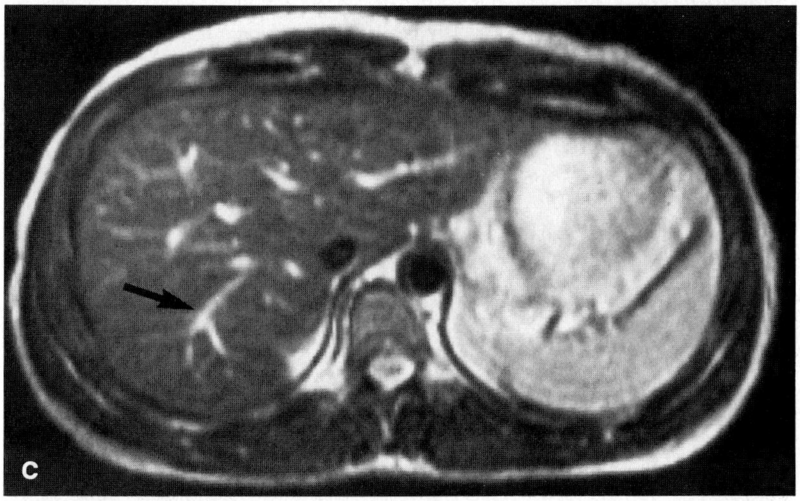

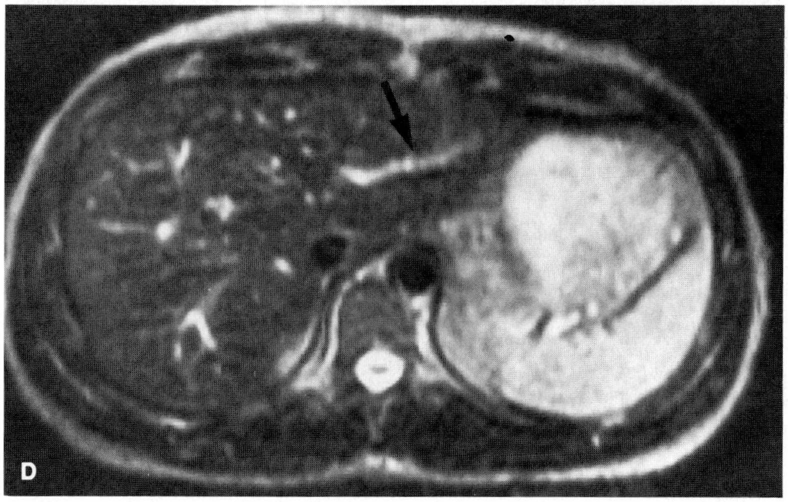

FIGURE 10–2. (Continued)

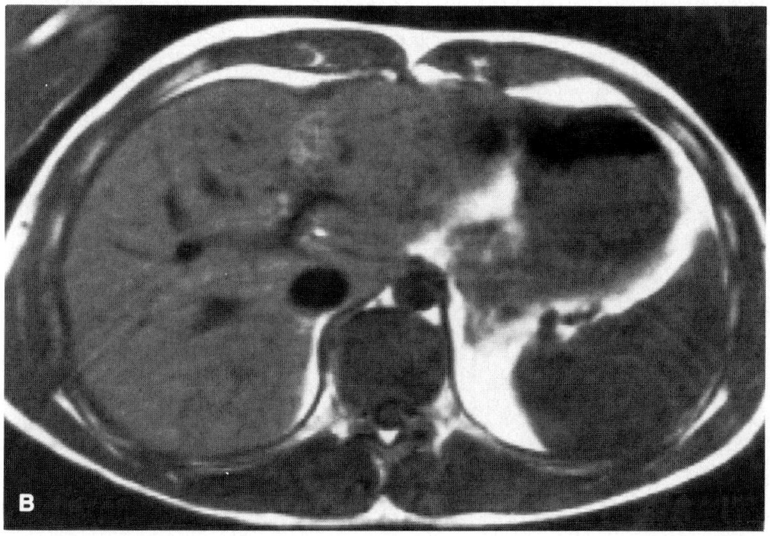

FIGURE 10–3. (Continued)

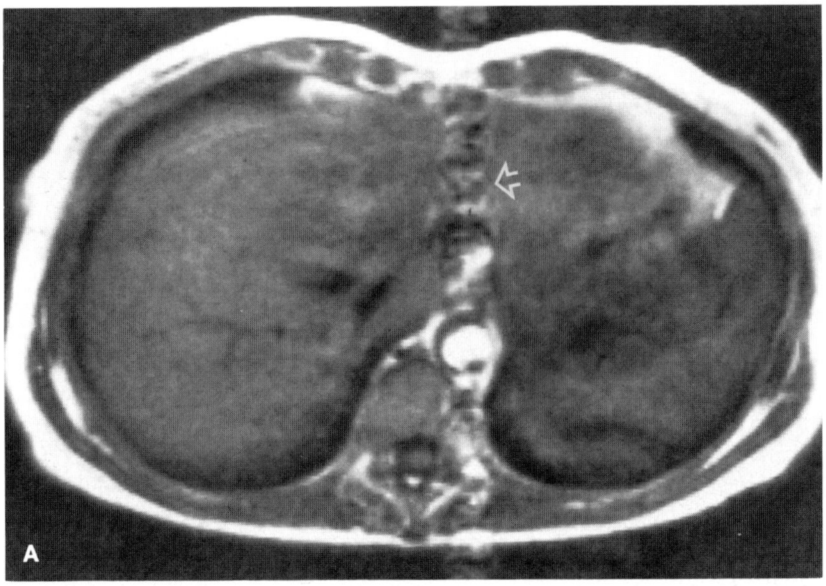

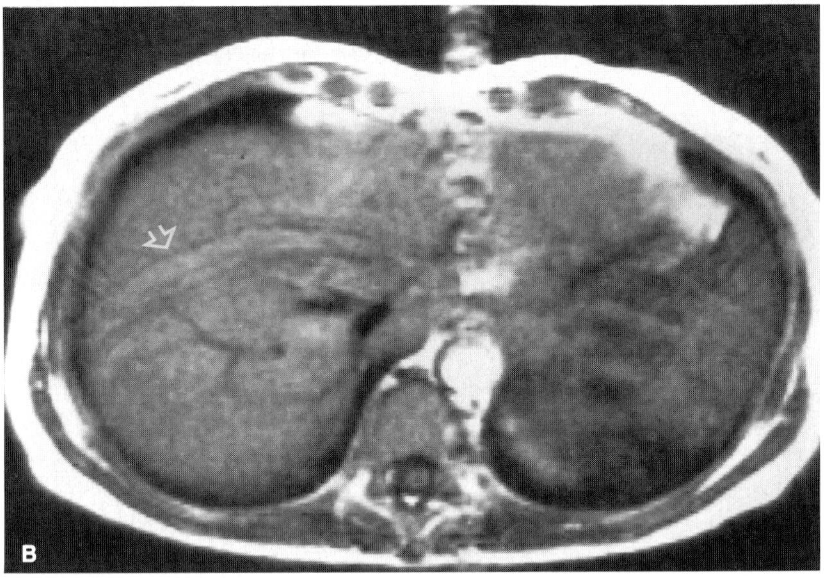

FIGURE 10–4. Data averaging for improved visualization of liver disease. Multiple liver abscesses in a 47-year-old female. Scans with **(A)** one, **(B)** two, **(C)** four, and **(D)** eight acquisitions (TR/TE = 250/17) demonstrate that averaging decreases the prominence of artifactual ghosts (open arrows) caused by respiration and vessel pulsation, improving visualization of an abscess in the right lobe of the liver (closed arrow). The normal hepatic vasculature (curved arrow) is also better depicted.

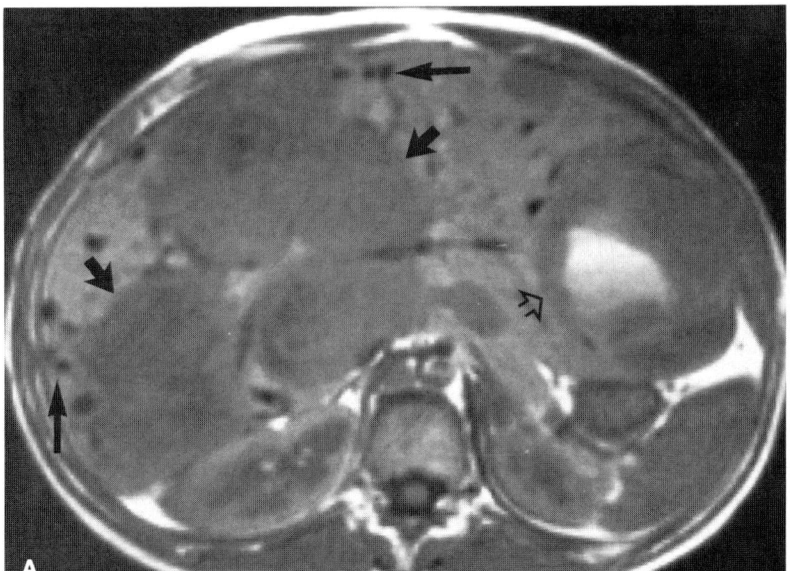

FIGURE 10–5. Metastatic carcinoid in a 17-year-old female. **(A)** T1-weighted (TR/TE = 800/17) and **(B)** T2-weighted (TR/TE = 3000/70) axial sections show marked hepatomegaly. Multiple metastatic lesions (short arrows) are seen with characteristic low signal intensity on T1-weighted and high signal intensity on T2-weighted images. In the left lobe, a single lesion (open arrow) demonstrates high signal intensity on the T1-weighted image, which is consistent with hemorrhage. Multiple dilated intrahepatic ducts (closed arrows) are seen. The inferior vena cava is compressed, but thrombosis can be excluded by the presence of a flow void.

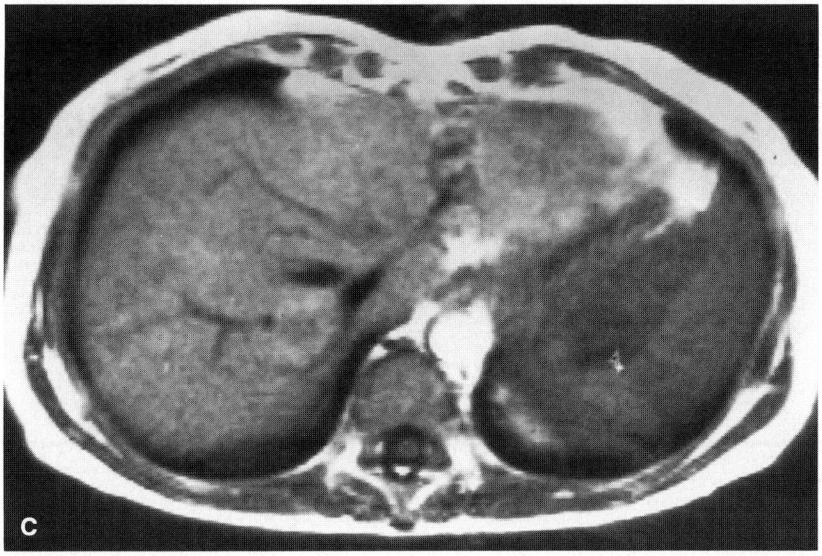

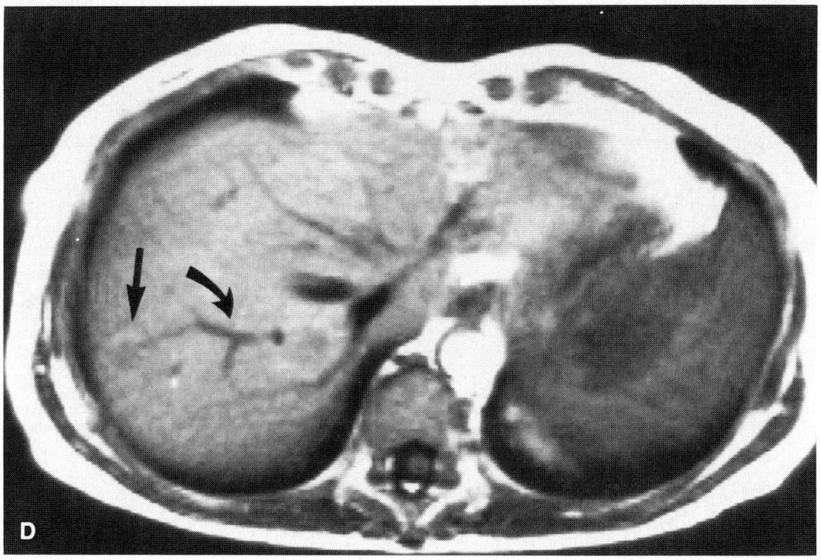

FIGURE 10–4. (Continued)

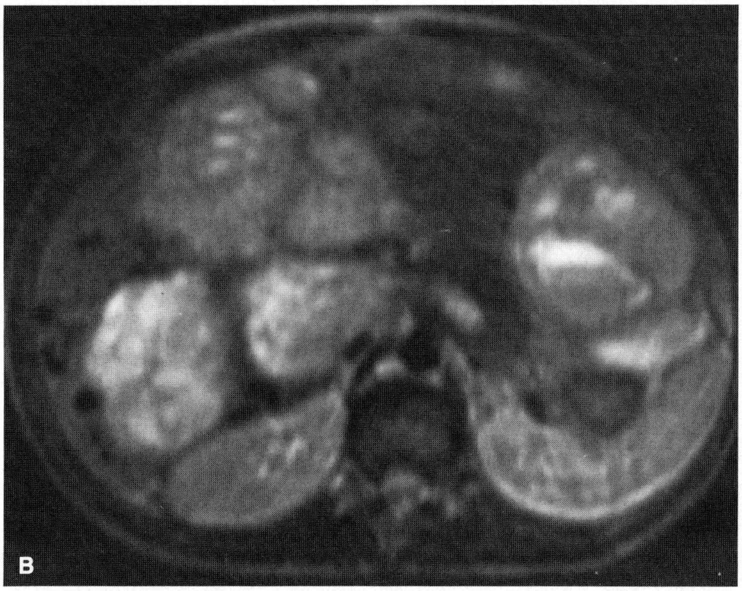

FIGURE 10–5. (Continued)

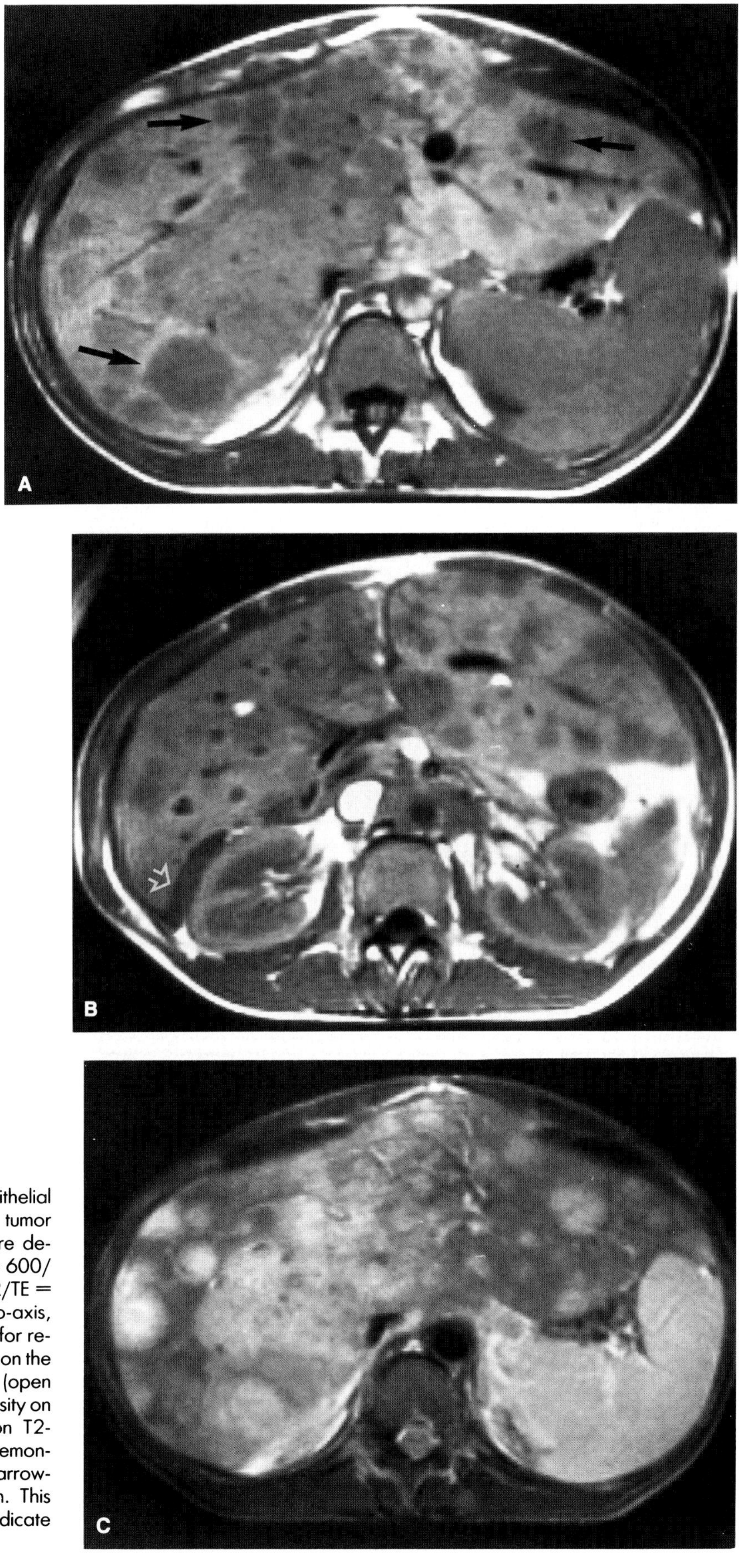

FIGURE 10–6. Metastatic undifferentiated epithelial carcinoma (closed arrows) of an unknown primary tumor in a 27-year-old female. Two anatomic levels are depicted with **(A,B)** T1-weighted sections (TR/TE = 600/17) and T2-weighted sections utilizing **(C,D)** TR/TE = 3000/45 and **(E,F)** TR/TE = 3000/90. Two-axis, first-order gradient moment nulling has been used for reduction of respiratory and vessel pulsation artifacts on the T2-weighted images. A small amount of ascites (open arrow) is demonstrated, with typical low signal intensity on T1-weighted images and high signal intensity on T2-weighted images. Many of the metastatic lesions demonstrate a central area of increased signal intensity (arrowheads) on T2-weighted images, a "target" sign. This finding is not seen in benign liver masses and may indicate central increased water content or necrosis.

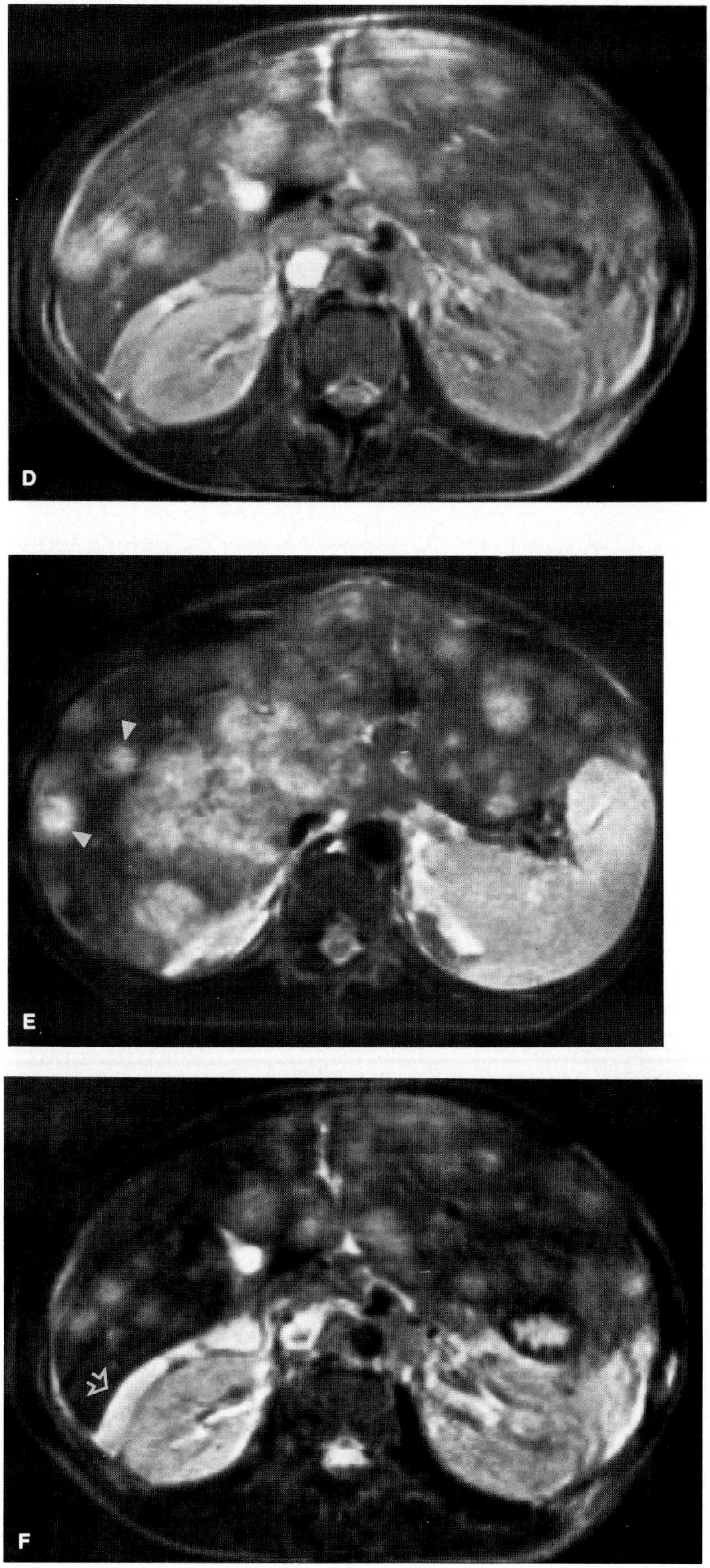

FIGURE 10–6. (Continued)

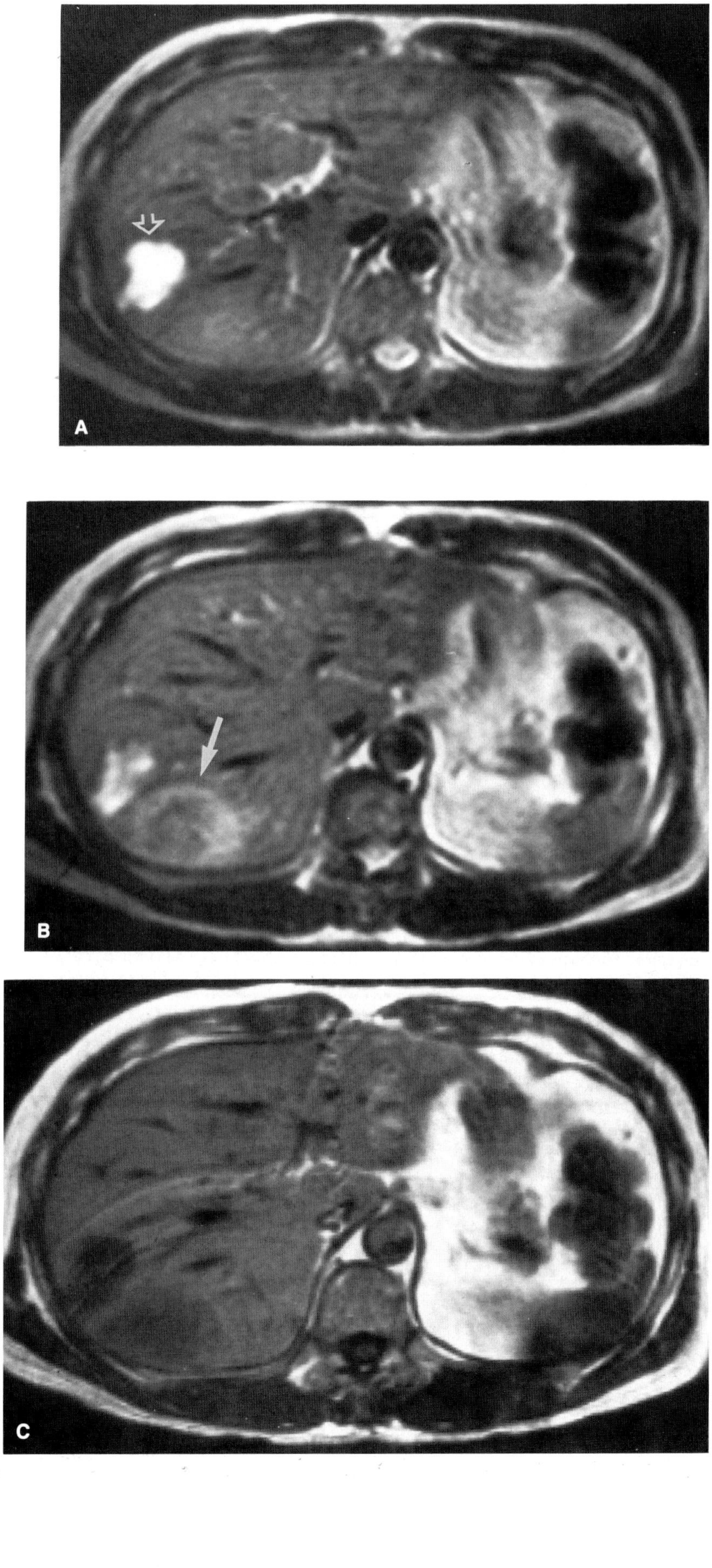

FIGURE 10–7. Metastatic disease to the liver from colon carcinoma in a 65-year-old male. Axial sections at two anatomic levels are illustrated with **(A,B)** T2-weighted images (TR/TE = 2600/70); T1-weighted images (TR/TE = 400/17) using **(C,D)** two data acquisitions and **(E,F)** four data acquisitions; and **(G,H)** breath-hold spin echo scans (TR/TE = 100/17). These sections demonstrate a metastatic lesion (closed arrow) and a cavernous hemangioma (open arrow). Multiple additional metastatic lesions were seen at other levels not displayed. The more posterior lesion demonstrates a bright halo surrounding a lower-signal-intensity central nodule on T2-weighted images, a pattern specific for metastatic disease. The T2 relaxation time of the more anterior lesion is extremely long, characteristic of a cavernous hemangioma. This differentiation can only be made on the T2-weighted image, although the lesions are well depicted on T1-weighted scans. The effect of increasing the number of data acquisitions in reducing ghost artifacts is demonstrated by comparing the two- and four-acquisition T1-weighted image sets. The T1-weighted breath-hold spin echo scans also demonstrate both lesions.

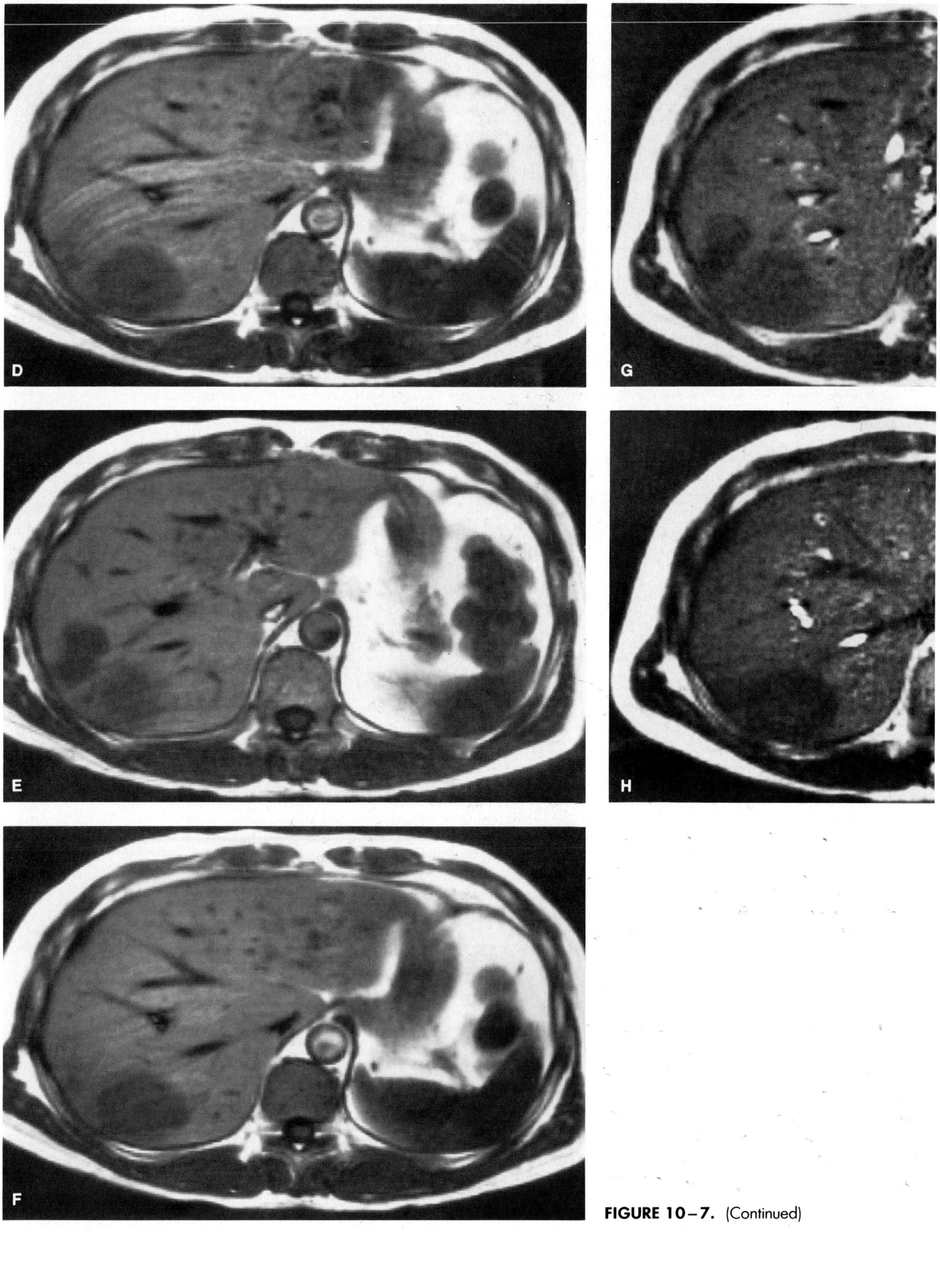

FIGURE 10–7. (Continued)

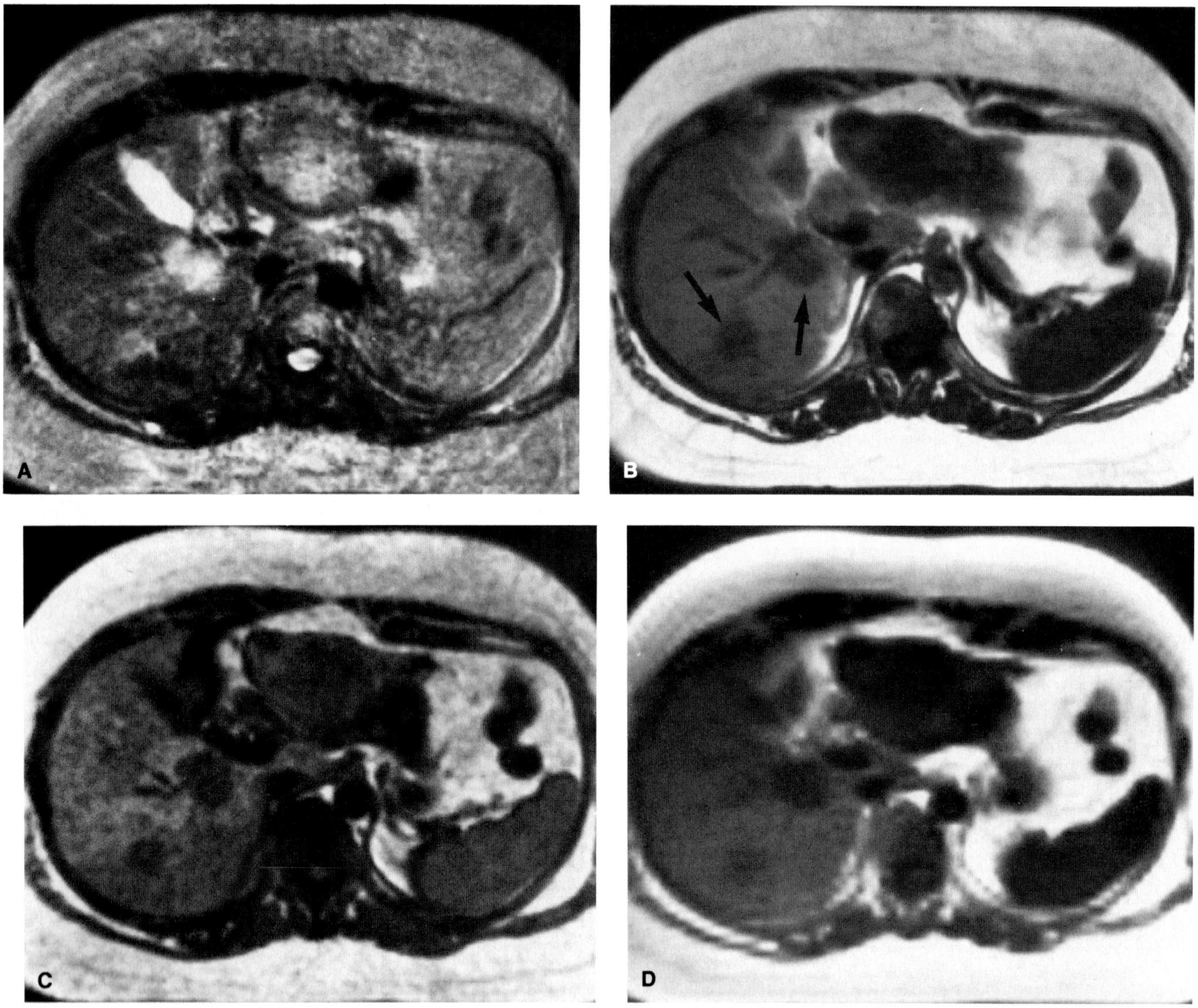

FIGURE 10–8. Metastatic breast carcinoma in a 37-year-old female s/p a left mastectomy. **(A)** T2-weighted scan (TR/TE = 3000/90) with two-axis gradient moment nulling; **(B)** T1-weighted non-breath-hold image (TR/TE = 600/17 with four data acquisitions); **(C,D)** breath-hold gradient echo (TR/TE = 40/10, 50° tip angle) and spin echo (TR/TE = 100/13) images. The two metastatic foci (arrows) are easily identified on the T1-weighted scans **(B–D).** Both the gradient echo and spin echo breath-hold sequences are diagnostic, offering a 60-fold reduction in scan time compared with the data-averaged T1-weighted spin echo scan. The T2-weighted scan suffers from motion degradation despite the use of gradient moment nulling. Sequences acquired during breath holding may emerge in the future as the technique of choice for imaging the upper abdomen.

cation of a rectangular imaging matrix combined with sampling only one polarity of the phase-encoding gradient. The breath-hold spin echo images presented in this chapter were acquired with this approach. The imaging matrix used is 256 × 72 (readout gradient × phase encoding gradient) with a TR of 100 msec, yielding a scan time of 7 seconds. The utility of these two scan techniques is illustrated in a patient with metastatic disease (Fig. 10–8) and other cases. This is investigational work, and further improvements in CNR and resolution are likely.

Simple hepatic cysts usually can be differentiated from other hepatic lesions (Fig. 10–9). The fluid in an uncomplicated cyst is hypointense on T1-weighted images and quite intense on T2-weighted images. In the differentiation of a hepatic cyst from a hemangioma, imaging with a mildly T1-weighted spin echo technique (e.g., TR/TE = 600/30) may be useful. Cysts remain hypointense, but hemangiomas are often isointense compared with normal liver.[11]

Like cysts, hemangiomas have significantly longer T2 relaxation times than liver cancer, and they are

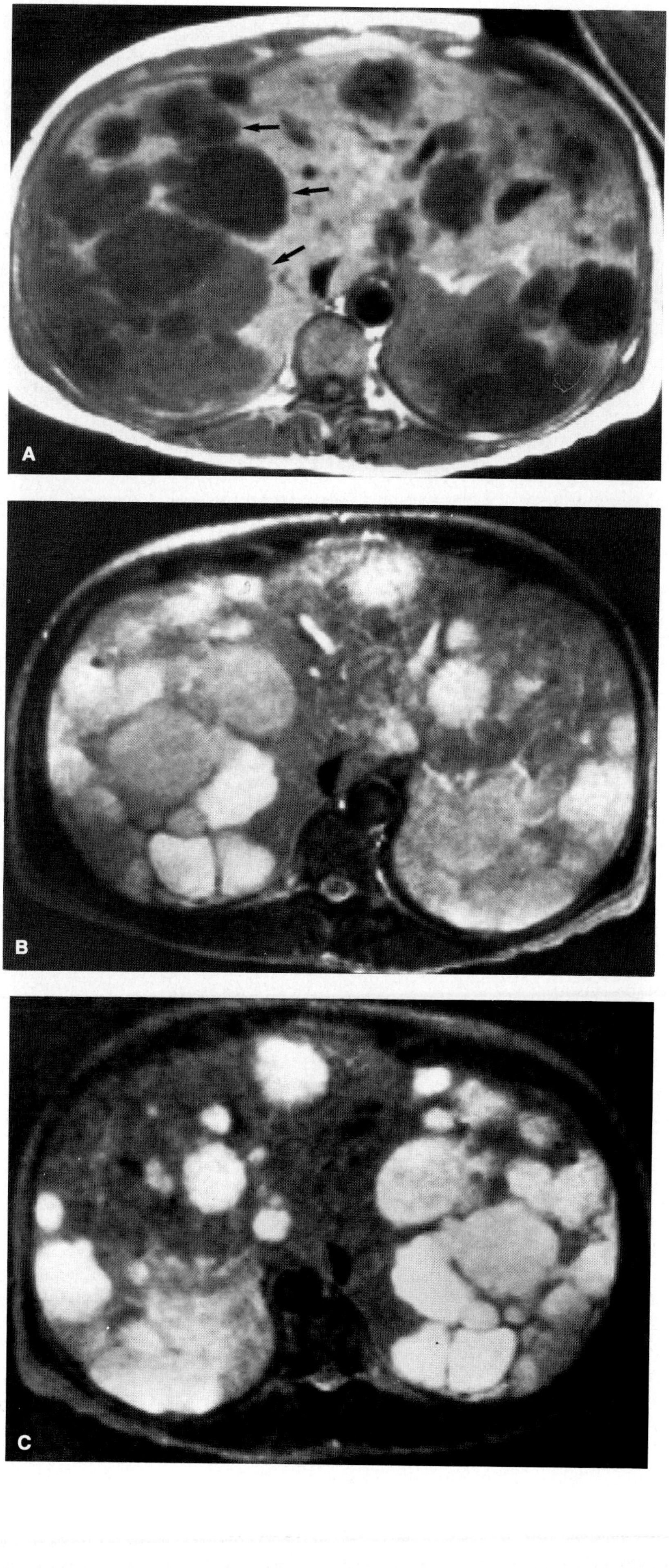

FIGURE 10–9. Polycystic liver disease. **(A)** T1-weighted spin echo scan (TR/TE = 600/17 with four data acquisitions); **(B,C)** T2-weighted spin echo scan (TR/TE = 3000/45,90). Multiple hepatic cysts (arrows) are demonstrated. Complications in this disease include hemorrhage, presumably accounting for the varied signal intensity of the cysts on both T1-weighted and T2-weighted scans.

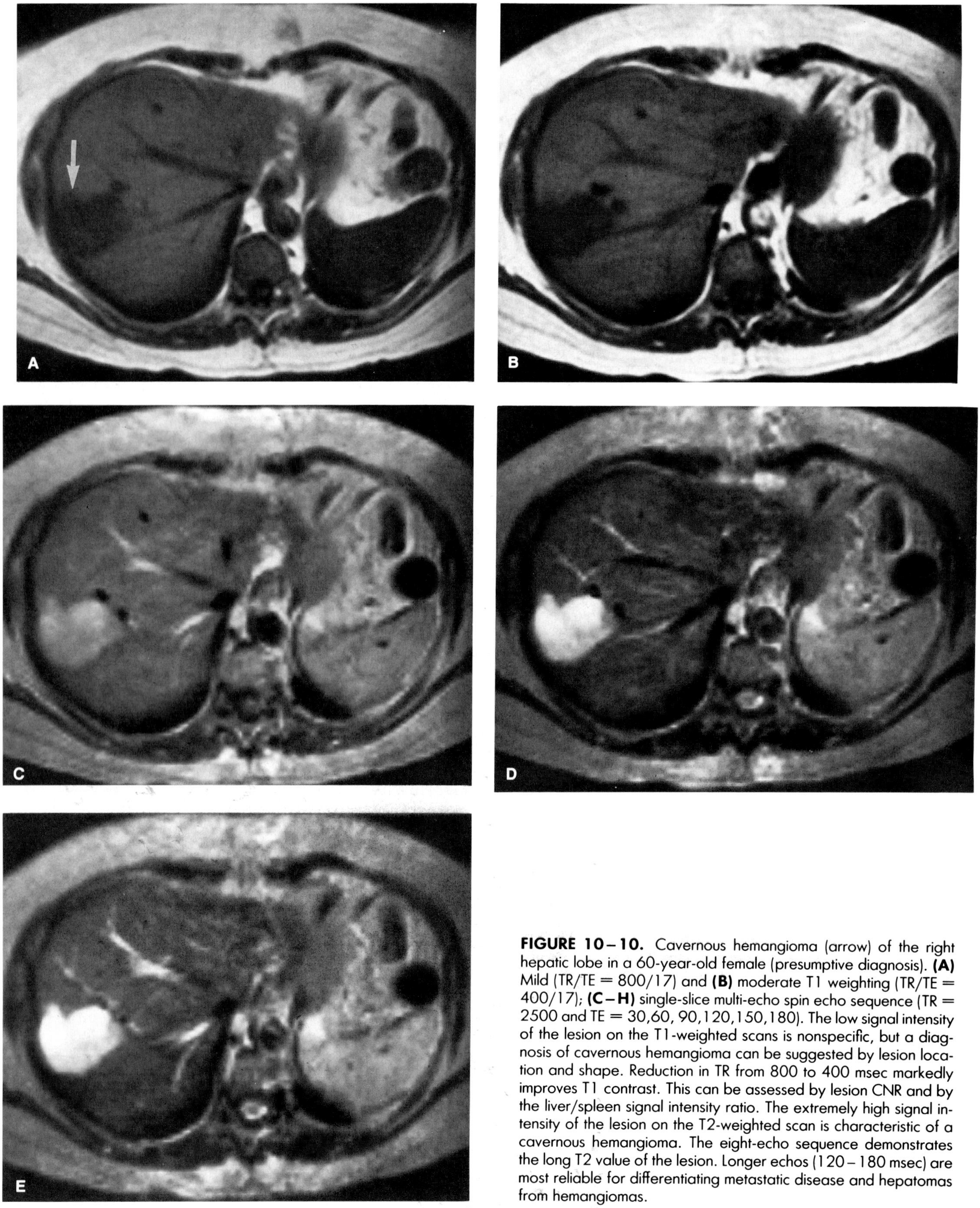

FIGURE 10–10. Cavernous hemangioma (arrow) of the right hepatic lobe in a 60-year-old female (presumptive diagnosis). **(A)** Mild (TR/TE = 800/17) and **(B)** moderate T1 weighting (TR/TE = 400/17); **(C–H)** single-slice multi-echo spin echo sequence (TR = 2500 and TE = 30,60, 90,120,150,180). The low signal intensity of the lesion on the T1-weighted scans is nonspecific, but a diagnosis of cavernous hemangioma can be suggested by lesion location and shape. Reduction in TR from 800 to 400 msec markedly improves T1 contrast. This can be assessed by lesion CNR and by the liver/spleen signal intensity ratio. The extremely high signal intensity of the lesion on the T2-weighted scan is characteristic of a cavernous hemangioma. The eight-echo sequence demonstrates the long T2 value of the lesion. Longer echos (120–180 msec) are most reliable for differentiating metastatic disease and hepatomas from hemangiomas.

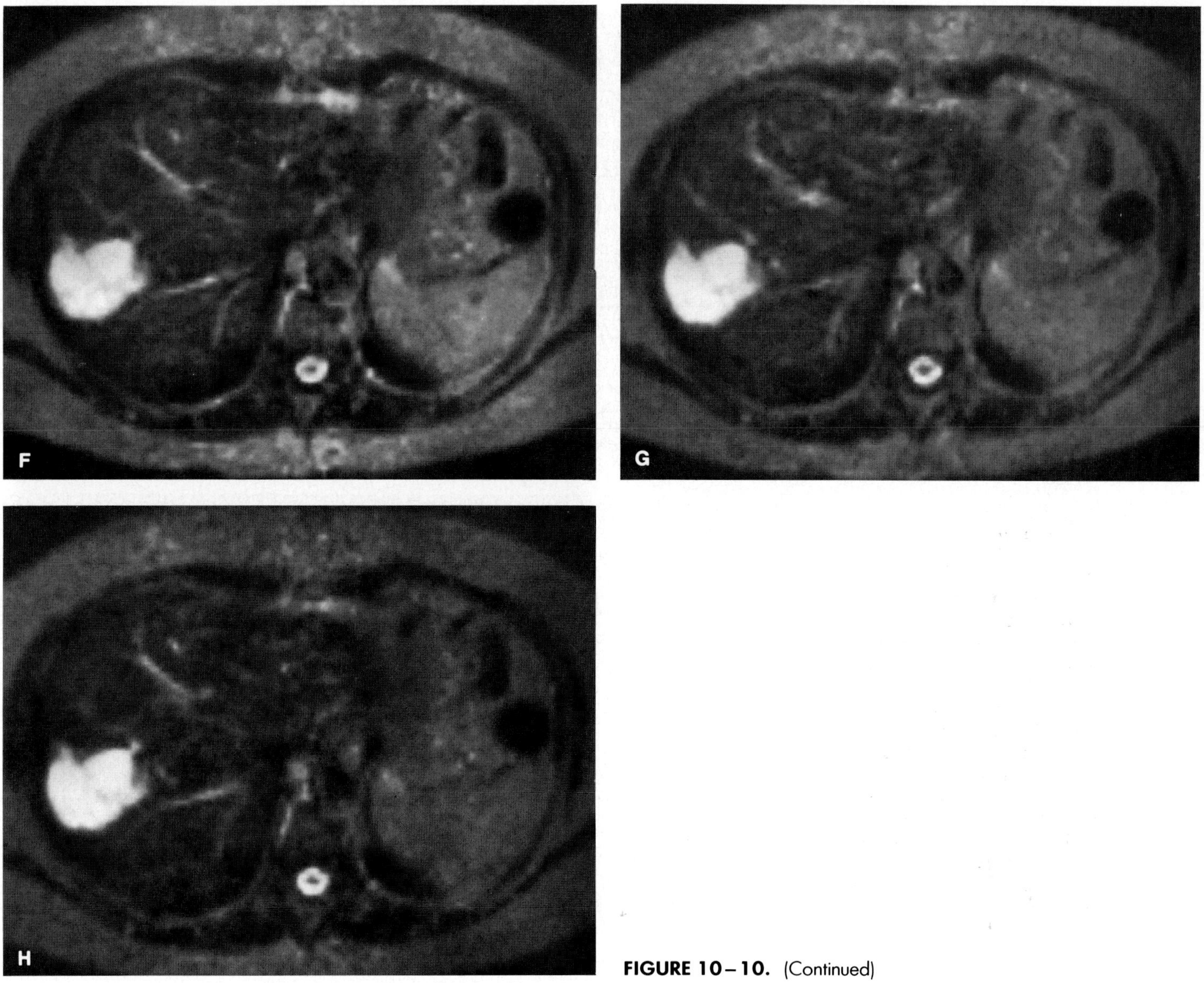

FIGURE 10–10. (Continued)

easily seen as high-signal-intensity lesions on T2-weighted images (Fig. 10–10). Because the T2 relaxation time of hemangiomas is typically much longer (i.e., double) than that of liver cancer, a specific diagnosis of hemangioma can often be made. Characteristic morphologic features of a hemangioma or cancer increase the diagnostic certainty. Most hemangiomas are smoothly marginated and homogeneous in signal intensity (Fig. 10–11). When morphologic features are coupled with intensity criteria, there is a 90% accuracy in differentiating hemangiomas from liver cancer.[12]

Intravenous contrast agents like Gd DTPA may refine imaging of liver hemangiomas (Fig. 10–12). The characteristics of enhancement may improve definitive diagnosis, as in CT, although clinical studies are needed.

Hepatomas can be hyperintense on T1-weighted images (10–15% of cases) because of triglyceride accumulation in tumor cells.[13] Primary hepatocellular carcinoma can also be isointense due to triglyceride content relative to liver on T1-weighted images (Fig. 10–13), necessitating T2-weighted images.[13,14] However, this tumor cannot be differentiated from metastatic disease on the basis of signal intensity.[15] Because hepatocellular carcinomas have fibrous capsules unlike other hepatic neoplasms, the demon-

(text continues on page 372)

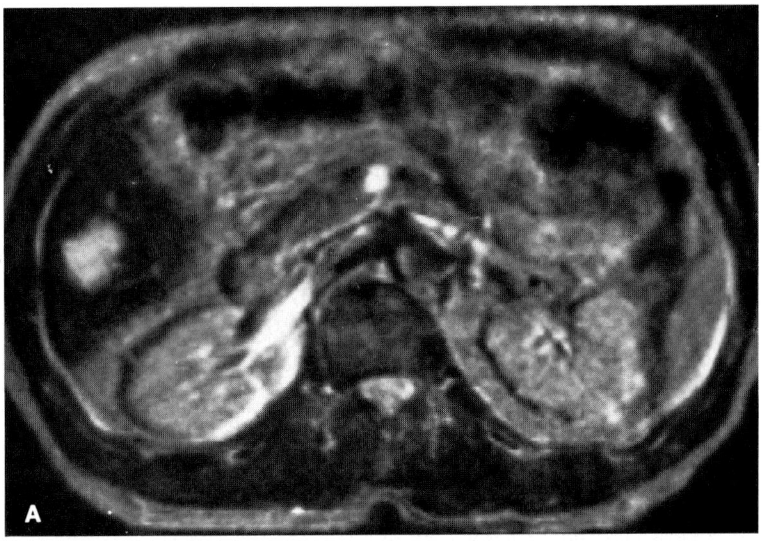

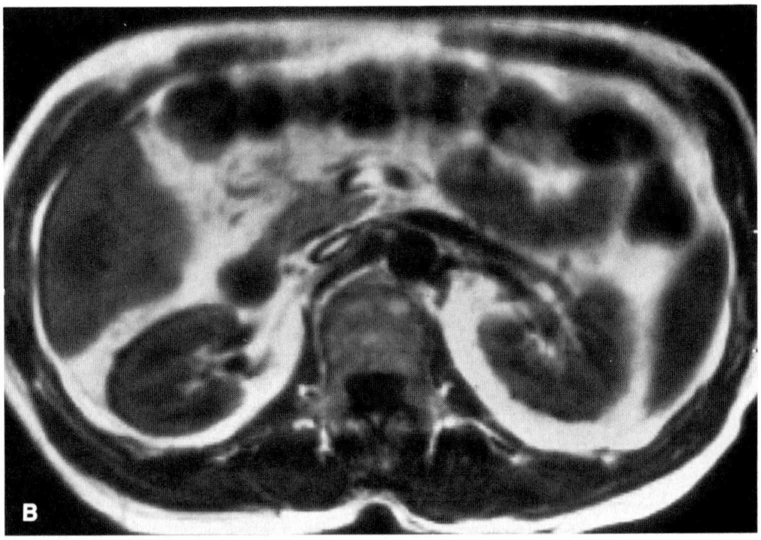

FIGURE 10–11. Cavernous hemangioma (arrow) of the posterior right lobe of the liver in a 64-year-old male (presumptive diagnosis). **(A)** T2-weighted spin echo image (TR/TE = 3000/70); **(B)** T1-weighted spin echo image (TR/TE = 600/17 with four data acquisitions); breath-hold **(C)** gradient echo (TR/TE = 40/10, 50° tip angle) and **(D)** spin echo scans (TR/TE = 100/13, combined half-Fourier and rectangular pixel). This lesion is depicted as a low-signal-intensity mass on all three T1-weighted scans **(B–D).** Morphologic features, such as the homogeneous nature of this lesion and its well-circumscribed appearance, assist in the diagnosis. The T2-weighted image adds specificity for the diagnosis of a cavernous hemangioma due to the very high signal intensity of the lesion. Diagnostic quality breath-hold images can be obtained with present instrumentation, using gradient echo or spin echo techniques. In the future, this approach may replace standard T1-weighted spin echo techniques and, by producing high-contrast, artifact-free images, lead to widespread use of MRI in the upper abdomen.

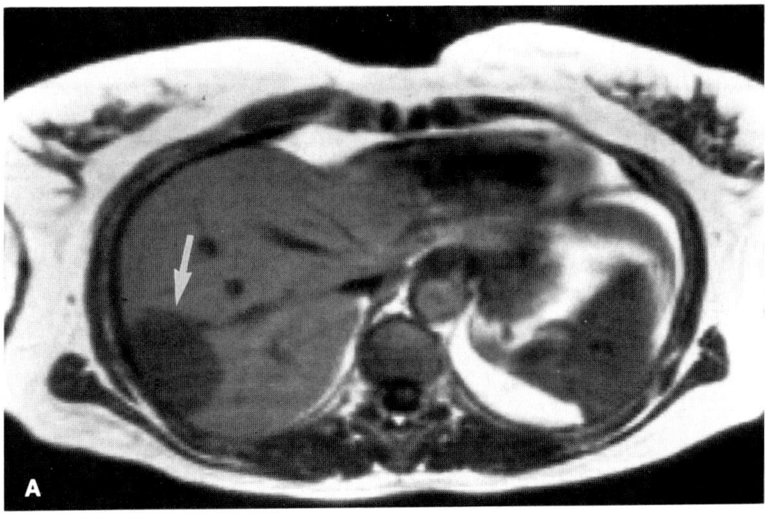

FIGURE 10–12. Cavernous hemangioma (arrow). T1-weighted sections (TR/TE = 500/17) **(A)** before and **(B)** after Gd DTPA enhancement. There is homogeneous enhancement of this peripherally based lesion. (Courtesy of Prof. H. Hundeshagen, Medizinische Hochschule, Hannover, West Germany).

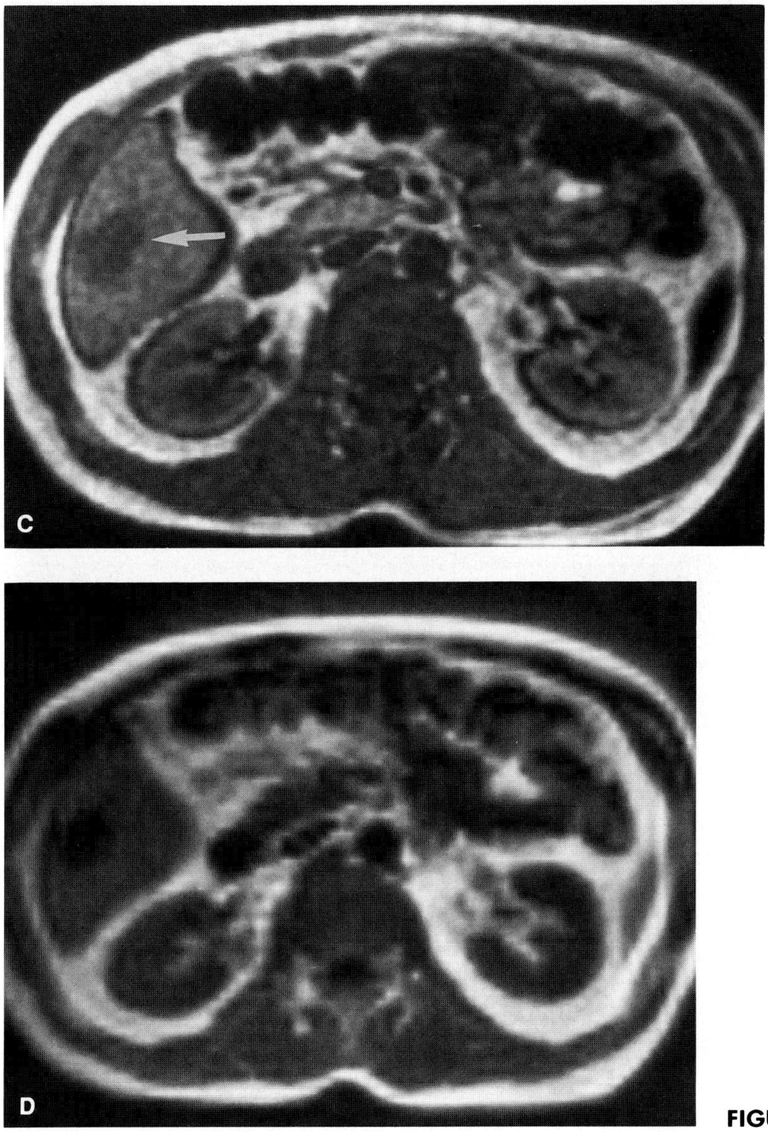

FIGURE 10–11. (Continued)

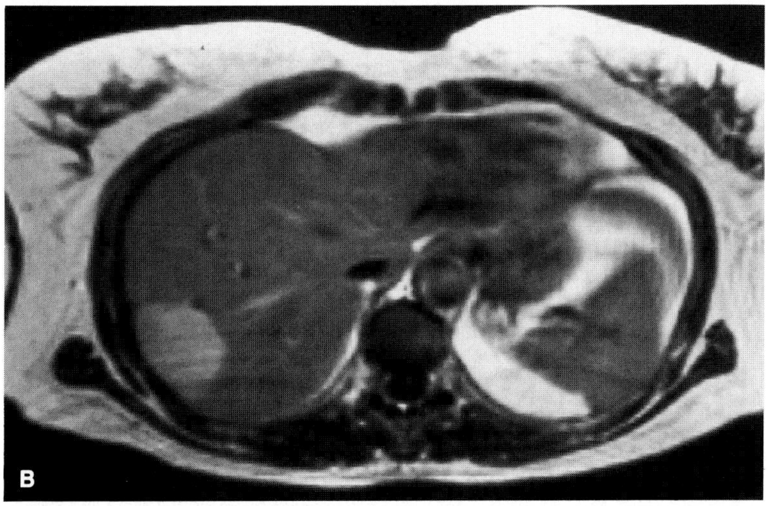

FIGURE 10–12. (Continued)

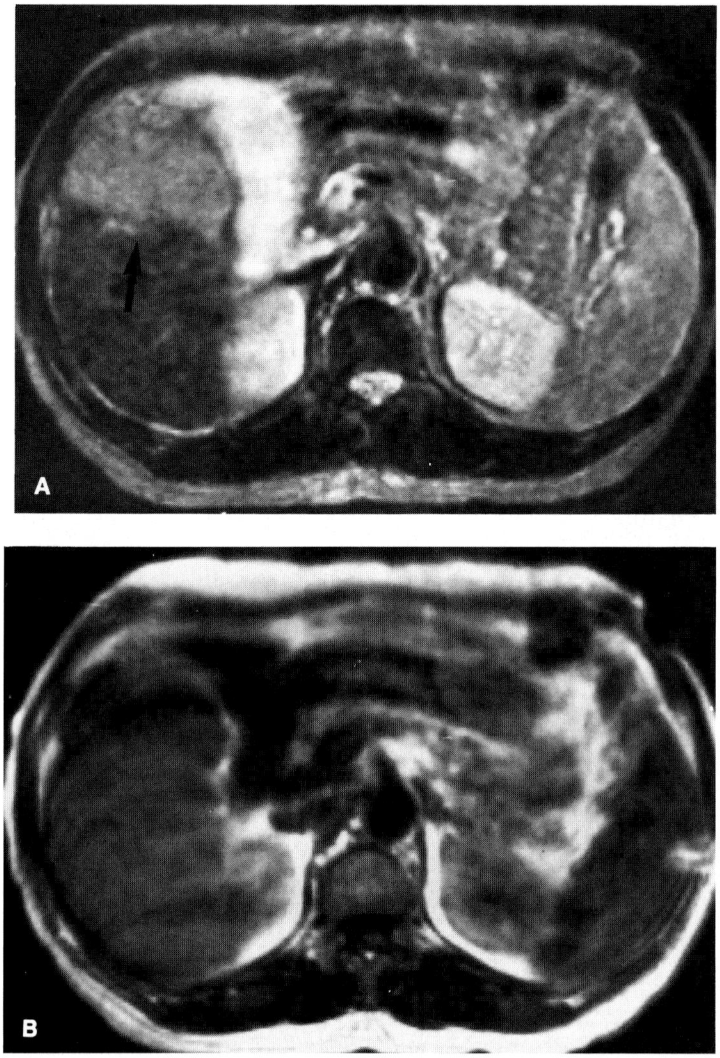

FIGURE 10–13. Hepatocellular carcinoma in a 67-year-old Chinese male with abdominal pain and chronic hepatitis (presumptive diagnosis). **(A)** T2-weighted image (TR/TE = 3000/90); **(B)** T1-weighted spin echo image (TR/TE = 600/17 with four data acquisitions); breath-hold **(C)** gradient echo (TR/TE = 40/10, 50° tip angle); and **(D)** spin echo scans (TR/TE = 100/13). The T2-weighted scan, which incorporates gradient moment nulling, is diagnostic (closed arrow). The 10-minute T1-weighted scan does not depict the lesion due to motion artifact. The lesion is seen on the breath-hold FLASH image **(C)** due to a contour abnormality (arrowheads). The improved contrast of the breath-hold spin echo technique is apparent, revealing the lesion by contour and by its low signal intensity relative to normal liver tissue (open arrow). Two features that often assist in the diagnosis of a hepatoma, a capsule and internal septation, are not seen in this patient.

stration of a capsule supports this diagnosis.[16] The capsule is best seen on T1-weighted spin echo or inversion recovery sequences.[13]

Focal nodular hyperplasia (FNH) and hepatic adenomas are two causes of benign solitary hepatic masses.[17] It is important to differentiate FNH from hepatic adenoma, because the latter has a propensity for hemorrhage and is typically resected. Reports of the appearance of FNH on MRI reveal that the lesion is typically nearly isointense with normal liver on all sequences (slightly hypointense on T1 spin echo images and inversion recovery images and slightly hyperintense on T2 spin echo sequences).[18] FNH shows mass effect with vein displacement. One distinguishing pathologic feature in FNH is a central stellate collagenous scar, which may appear hypointense compared with tumor on T1-weighted images. However, visualization of the scar is variable, and the lesion itself may be isointense.[19] Early results suggest that MRI may be the best imaging method for demonstrating the central scar and differentiating FNH from hepatic adenoma.

Hepatic adenomas have varied MR signal characteristics that make differentiation from hepatic carcinoma difficult. Rarely, they have a low-signal-intensity pseudocapsule on T1-weighted scans, adding further confusion.[15] Secondary signs, such as the lack of vessel invasion and edema, can help differentiate cancer from benign lesions.

Diffuse Disease

Cirrhosis is diagnosed by CT when the characteristic morphologic changes are seen (e.g., enlargement of the caudate lobe, irregular liver contour). MRI can demonstrate these findings, but it cannot make a specific diagnosis of cirrhosis, because without hepatitis the T1 and T2 values are not significantly changed (Fig. 10–14).[20] MRI can identify regenerating nodules within a cirrhotic liver. These nodules are typically

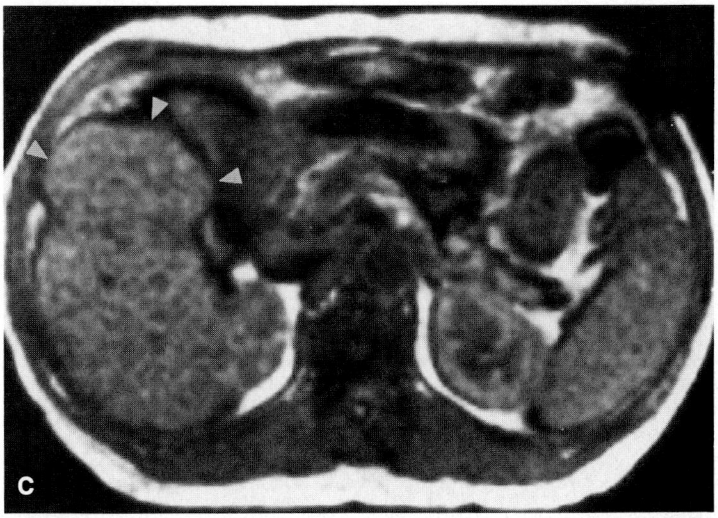

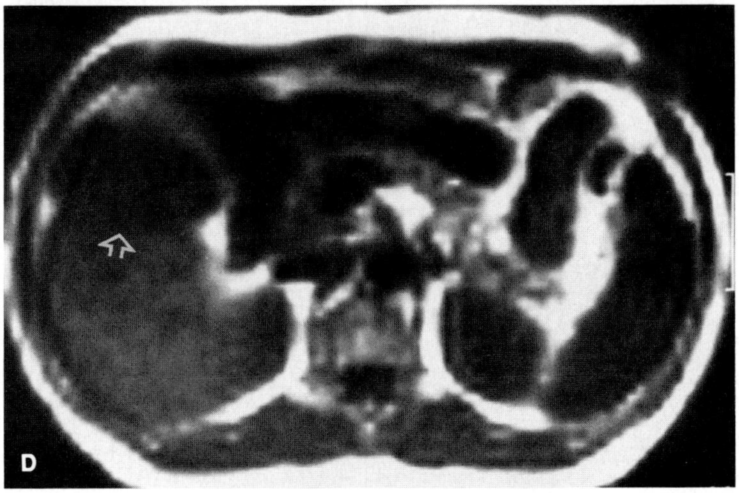

FIGURE 10–13. (Continued)

appreciated on CT only by alterations of liver contour, because they are almost always isodense. Regenerating nodules may be of low signal intensity on T2-weighted images, making them distinguishable from neoplastic disease.[21]

Hemochromatosis can be detected on MRI due to the superparamagnetic properties of ferritin and hemosiderin. For a technique to be clinically useful in this disease, it must be sensitive to small amounts of iron overload and also be able to quantitate iron deposition. Normal liver iron levels are less than 250 $\mu g/g$ (wet weight of liver tissue). Mild overload in chronic liver disease yields levels of 0.5 to 1.5 mg/g. In diseases caused by iron overload, the levels are typically greater than 2 mg/g. At 0.6 T and below, routine spin echo pulse techniques show little change in signal intensity until iron levels are 1 mg/g or greater. However, at 0.6 T, routine sequences can screen for clinically significant overload (> 2 mg/g) and differentiate cirrhosis from hemochromatosis.[22] At higher field strengths, lower levels of iron can be detected (Fig. 10–15). Similarly, MRI can be used to assess therapy, correlating a return to normal signal with good clinical response. It is possible to quantitate elevated iron levels on spin echo sequences by varying the TR and TE and calculating the T1 and T2 relaxation times.[22] T2 relaxation times can be used to determine liver iron stores, forming the basis for therapeutic decisions.

Two contrast agents have been used clinically in the study of liver disease, Gd DTPA and iron oxide.[23,24] This discussion is limited to Gd DTPA, because the particulate agent has yet to receive FDA approval and widespread availability. The effects of intravenous administration of Gd DTPA are time-dependent. On spin echo images requiring greater than 2 minutes for acquisition, Gd DTPA typically increases the signal intensity of a neoplastic lesion. Gd DTPA accumulates preferentially in a liver tumor because it has a greater extracellular space, due to edema and necrosis, than

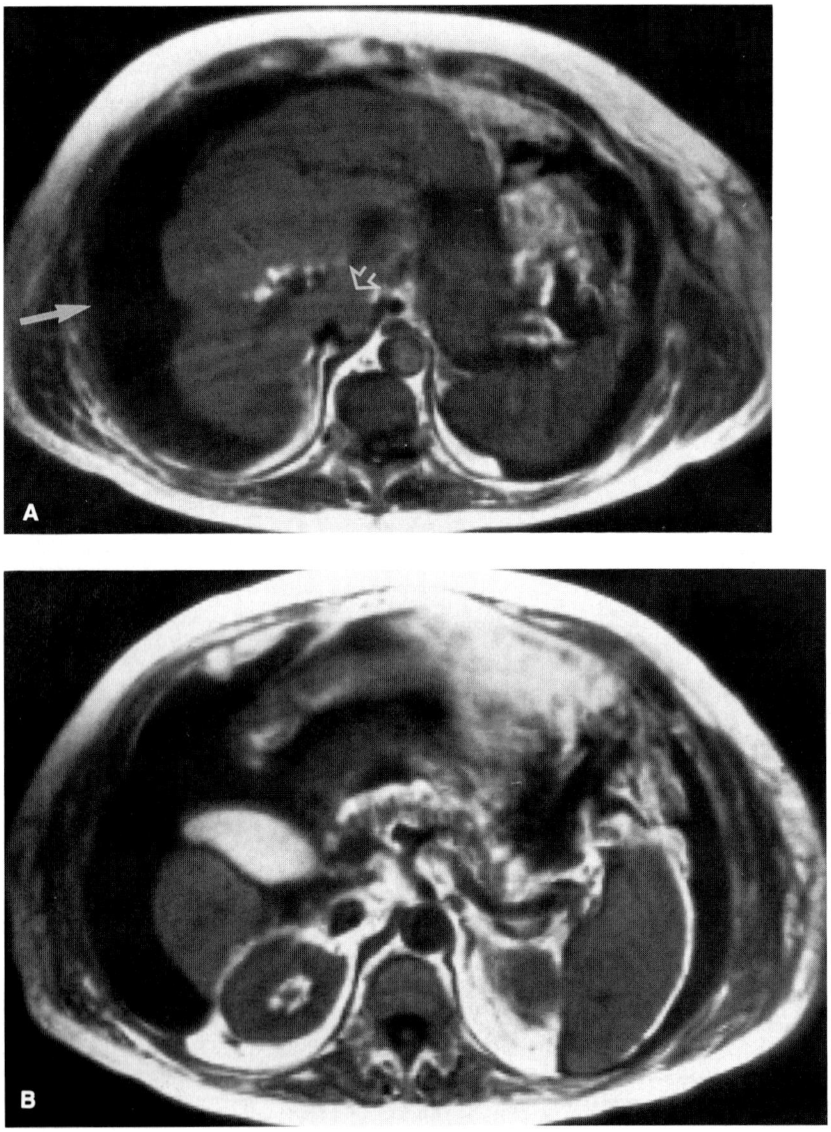

FIGURE 10–14. Liver cirrhosis and abdominal ascites in a 73-year-old male with hepatitis. **(A,B)** T1-weighted sections (TR/TE = 800/17) are illustrated at two anatomic levels. The morphologic changes and associated findings, which have been described on CT, are well depicted by MRI. The nodular appearance of the liver surface and compression of intrahepatic vessels in this patient are caused by nodular regeneration. Caudate lobe hypertrophy (open arrow) has resulted in compression of the intrahepatic inferior vena cava. Secondary extrahepatic findings include ascites (closed arrow), visualized as low-signal-intensity fluid on this T1-weighted exam. Cirrhosis in the absence of hepatitis does not cause a significant change in T1 or T2 relaxation times of liver tissue.

normal liver.[23] This increase in tumor signal intensity can lead to isointensity or decreased intensity differences between tumor and liver.[23] Therefore, optimal lesion detectability is obtained with strongly T1-weighted images without contrast administration.

In the future, fast scanning techniques combined with the use of contrast agents may improve tumor identification. In the first 2 minutes after bolus injection of Gd DTPA, the signal intensity of normal liver is enhanced to a much greater degree than that of neoplastic tissue, presumably on the basis of vascularity. Fast scan techniques can thus demonstrate increased contrast between liver and tumor.[23]

MRI can help in determining the patency of various portal-systemic shunts created for treatment of portal hypertension. Knowledge of the exact anatomy of the various shunt types is necessary for selecting the appropriate scan planes. One report suggests that distal splenorenal shunt patency is best evaluated on axial images.[25] However, depending on shunt location, images in other planes may be more helpful. A flow void demonstrated on spin echo imaging indicates shunt patency. Increased signal intensity caused by bidirectional or impeded flow can be seen in portal venous system branches (e.g., the superior mesenteric vein). Gradient-echo imaging can also be used to demonstrate flow within the shunt.

ADRENAL GLAND

Although CT provides an excellent anatomic depiction of the adrenals with extremely high sensitivity for abnormalities, MRI may increase diagnostic specificity. Commonly encountered lesions in the adrenal include functioning and nonfunctioning adenomas,

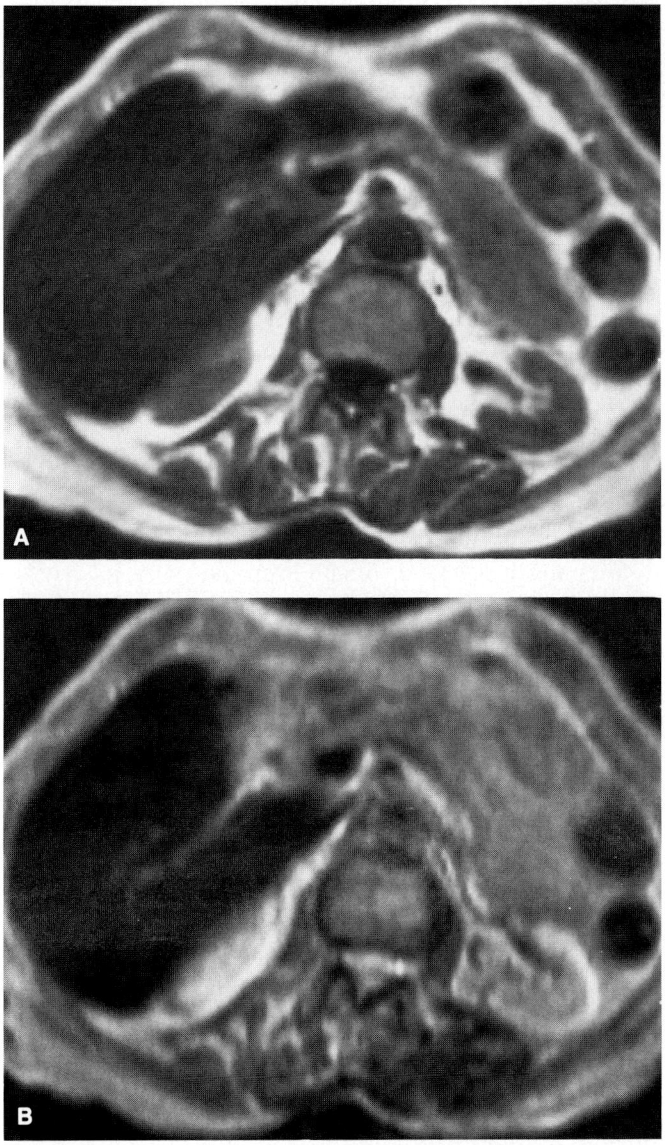

FIGURE 10–15. Hemochromatosis in a 78-year-old female at 1.0 tesla. **(A)** T1-weighted (TR/TE = 600/17) and **(B)** T2-weighted images (TR/TE = 3000/45). At field strengths ≥ 1.0 tesla, conventional spin echo pulse sequences are quite sensitive to abnormal iron deposition in the liver. This produces a reduction in signal intensity of the liver, best visualized on T2-weighted sequences, but also seen on T1-weighted scans. The T2 relaxation enhancement with iron overload is due to the magnetic susceptibility of ferritin and hemosiderin.

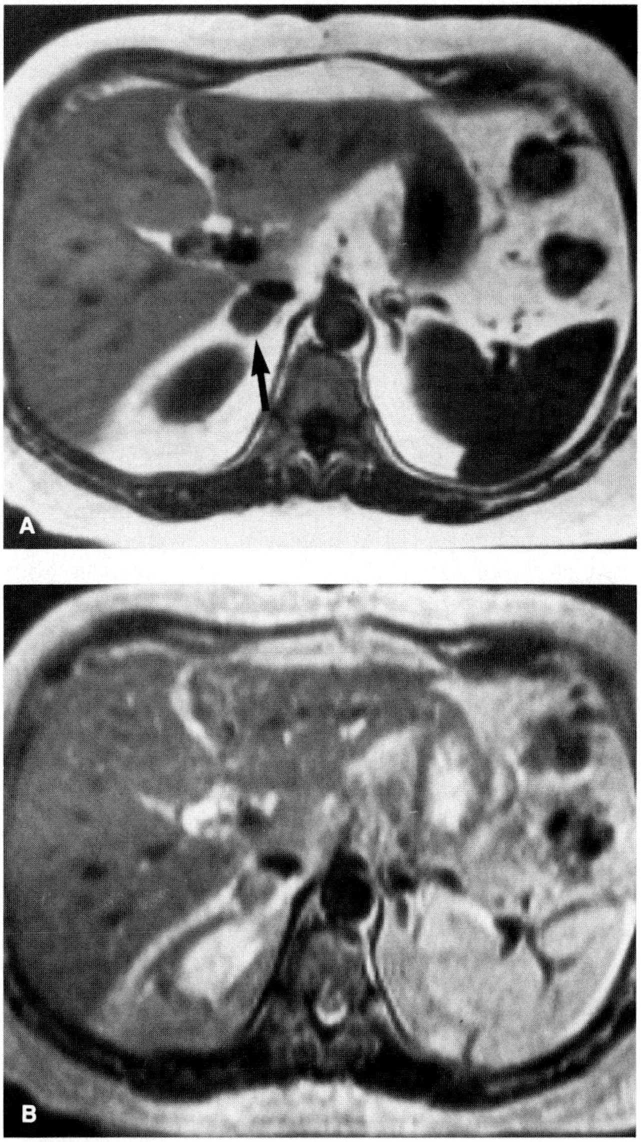

FIGURE 10–16. Adrenal adenoma in a 65-year-old female. **(A)** T1-weighted image (TR/TE = 600/17) and **(B)** T2-weighted image (TR/TE = 3000/70). The right adrenal mass (arrow) is isointense with liver on both sequences, favoring diagnosis of a nonmalignant process.

primary carcinoma, metastasis, and pheochromocytoma.

Given sufficient SNR, imaging of the adrenals should be performed with slice thickness less than or equal to 5 mm. There is significant overlap of signal characteristics of the various adrenal mass lesions. The signal intensity of an adrenal lesion should be measured relative to a normal internal control to aid lesion characterization. For example, using adrenal mass-to-fat ratio, Chang and colleagues were better able to separate adrenal adenomas from malignant neoplasms.[26] Spin echo images were obtained at 0.5 T (TR/TE = 2100/90). All lesions with ratios of ≥0.8 were malignant, and those <0.6 were adenomas. The great variation between systems and imaging sequences limits the practicality of this approach. Even in Chang's study, 31% of lesions could not be categorized.

Functioning and nonfunctioning adenomas cannot be distinguished on MRI (Fig. 10–16). Both are typically isointense compared with liver on T1-weighted spin echo scans and remain isointense on T2-weighted spin echo images (TR/TE = 2500/80 at 0.5 T), with adrenal-to-liver ratios <1.2.[27] Early investigations showed that primary carcinomas and metastases had increased intensities on T2-weighted spin echo images, promoting hope that nonfunctioning and functioning adenomas could be simply and universally distinguished from other lesions. Unfortunately, this has not proven to be the case. One report showed signal-intensity overlaps in 21% of a group with 38 adrenal masses, including adenomas, carcinomas, and metastases. Therefore, biopsy is still necessary.

The typical appearance of an adrenal carcinoma is a mass, usually greater than 5 to 6 cm when diagnosed, having a low signal intensity relative to liver on T1-weighted spin echo images and increased intensity compared with liver on T2-weighted spin echo sequences (Fig. 10–17). Because some carcinomas have intensities on T2-weighted spin echo images that overlap the intensities of benign adenomas, they may be indistinguishable.

The appearance of pheochromocytomas is more specific. At 0.5 T, the pheochromocytomas studied had markedly high signal intensity on T2-weighted spin echo images, giving tumor-to-liver ratios greater than 3.3. The adrenal mass and liver intensities were calculated on spin echo scans (TR/TE = 2500/80). No overlap with other adrenal lesions was seen, but caution is advised, because signal-intensity criteria established on one machine cannot be directly applied to other machines operating at different field strengths.[27] Axial images should be adequate for the study of adrenal masses, but coronal imaging may help in the search for extra-adrenal tumors along the sympathetic chain.

KIDNEY

Compared with intraperitoneal structures, the kidneys are generally more satisfactorily imaged on MRI. Motion artifacts from bowel peristalsis, respiration, and vascular pulsation are significantly reduced in the retroperitoneal region. This location and the surrounding fat, which provides excellent contrast with renal parenchyma, make good-quality MR images possible.

MRI will probably not have a primary role in the diagnosis of simple renal cysts, because they are easily and accurately diagnosed by ultrasound and CT. The typical renal cyst on MRI is round, uniformly thin-walled, and contains simple fluid (Fig. 10–18). Uncomplicated cysts have uniformly low signal intensity on T1-weighted sequences and increasingly high signal intensity with progressive T2 weighting.[28] As expected, complicated cysts may have signal intensities greater than normal renal parenchyma on T1-weighted images, possibly because of increased protein content. Hemorrhagic cysts can demonstrate high signal intensity on both T1-weighted and T2-weighted spin echo images.[29] In polycystic disease, the kidneys are enlarged with multiple cysts. Since there is an increased incidence of hemorrhage into these cysts, compared with isolated, simple cysts, one should expect to find one or more cysts with high signal intensity on both T1-weighted and T2-weighted sequences.

If a renal cyst contains simple fluid, MR characteristics can accurately diagnose a benign cyst. If the signal characteristics of renal masses vary from that of simple fluid, the MR appearance of complicated cysts and solid masses may overlap.[30]

The MR appearance of solid renal masses is varied, and the appearances of different carcinomas and benign adenomas may overlap. Renal cell carcinomas demonstrate variable signal intensities on T1-weighted and T2-weighted images. On T1-weighted images, renal carcinomas typically have heterogeneous signal intensity (Fig. 10–19). Renal cell carcinomas often show some areas of necrosis, which on T1-weighted images produce low signal intensity (Fig. 10–20). If hemorrhage has occurred, the intensity may be high. On T2-weighted images, viable areas of tumor often have high signal intensity. Necrotic or hemorrhagic regions are also typically high in intensity on T2-weighted images.[31] The appearance of renal cell carcinoma on MR has significant overlap with that of metastatic disease (Fig. 10–21).

MRI is limited in its ability to detect renal cell carcinoma because the signal intensity characteristics of normal kidney and tumor are similar. Renal neoplasms often show little contrast with normal renal parenchyma and may be undetectable until they are large enough to cause contour abnormalities. Gd DTPA may improve lesion detection.[32]

Because the initial treatment of renal cell carcinoma is surgical, accurate staging is necessary. MRI in multiple planes can help in defining the local extension of tumor. Although it may be difficult on axial images to assess hepatic or splenic invasion, coronal images may easily provide answers.

Spread of tumor beyond the renal capsule may be inferred, as on CT, from strandy densities in the perinephric fat. Adenopathy may be identified in areas of regional spread, but signal characteristics cannot differentiate hyperplastic from malignant nodes. Local extension into surrounding musculature may also be demonstrated. Venous involvement by tumor may be

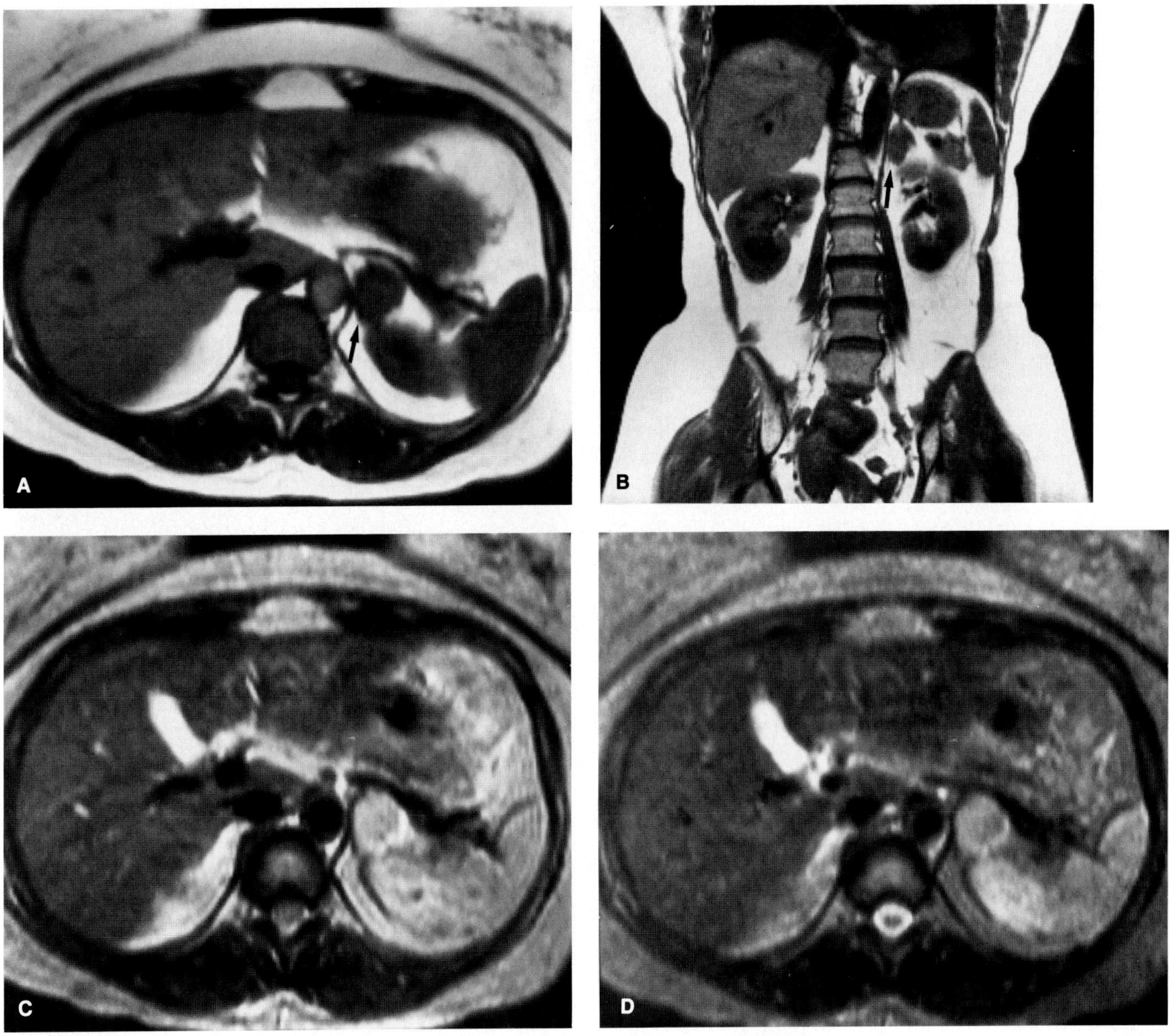

FIGURE 10–17. Left adrenal mass in a 37-year-old female with Cushing's syndrome. **(A,B)** Axial and coronal T1-weighted images (TR/TE = 600/17) and **(C,D)** axial T2-weighted images (TR/TE = 3000/45,90). The left adrenal mass (arrow) is isointense with the spleen on both T1-weighted and T2-weighted scans. Utilization of MRI has focused not only on identifying adrenal lesions but also on whether MRI can offer tissue specific information. Pheochromocytomas characteristically are markedly hyperintense on T2-weighted sequences. One of the most difficult problems in adrenal imaging has been differentiating benign from malignant disease. Most malignancies, like the lesion illustrated, are hyperintense on T2-weighted images compared with liver tissue. Differentiation of malignant from benign lesions, however, cannot be made with certainty on the basis of signal intensity characteristics, as illustrated in this case, which proved, after surgical resection, to be a benign adrenal adenoma.

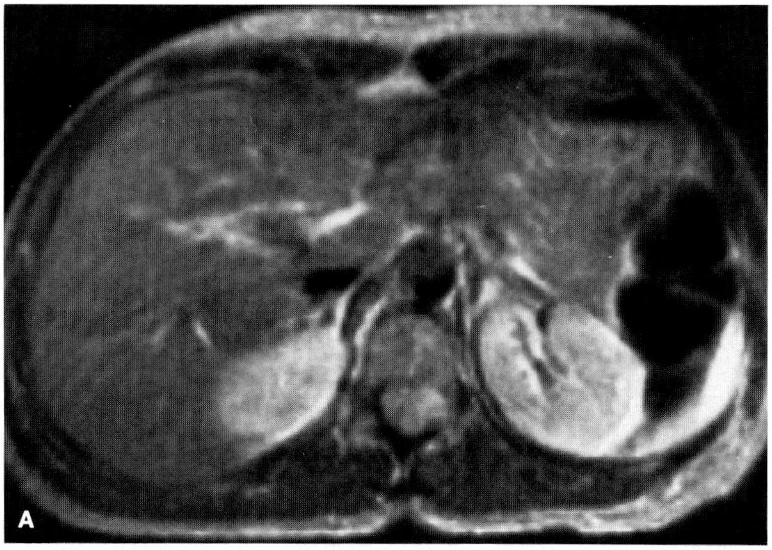

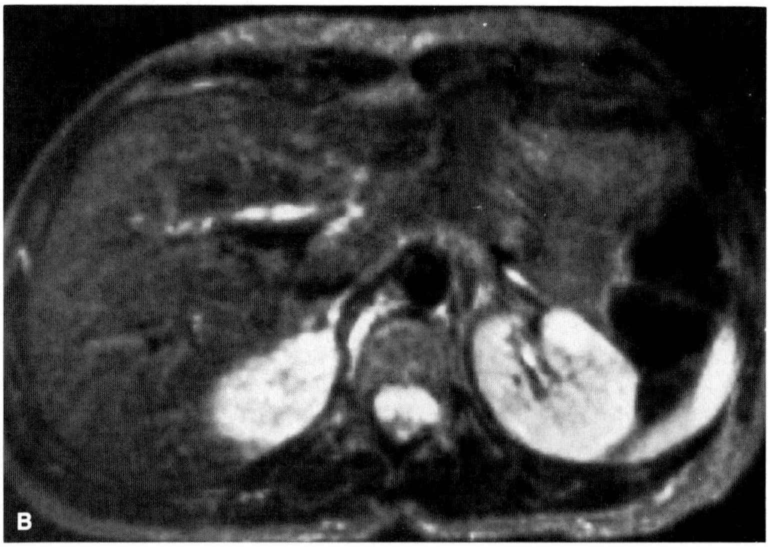

FIGURE 10–18. Simple renal cyst in a 48-year-old female. **(A,B)** Intermediate and heavily T2-weighted spin echo techniques; **(C)** 10-minute data-averaged T1-weighted spin echo technique; **(D)** 10-second breath-hold FLASH acquisition. A small renal cyst is identified in the left kidney (closed arrow). This lesion is isointense with normal renal parenchyma on the intermediate T2-weighted scan. The high signal intensity on heavily T2-weighted scans and low signal intensity on T1-weighted scans are consistent with a simple cyst. The descending colon (arrowheads) appears larger and of lower signal intensity on the gradient echo technique **(D)** due to magnetic susceptibility effects.

demonstrated on MRI by an absence of signal void in the renal vein or the inferior vena cava. It is unknown whether MRI can differentiate intravascular tumor from thrombus.

If small renal neoplasms are isointense on all sequences with normal renal parenchyma, Gd DTPA may help. As demonstrated by Yashiro and colleagues, the enhancement of renal parenchyma after injection of Gd DTPA provides a signal intensity difference from renal neoplasms.[32] This phenomenon is quite similar to enhancement seen with iodinated contrast agents, which increase the contrast between parenchyma and tumor by greater parenchymal enhancement.

If rapid scanning techniques are employed after Gd DTPA injection, tumor enhancement may be seen in relatively hypervascular neoplasms, and an accurate characterization of vascularity can be made. This phenomenon is analogous to the enhancement seen on dynamic CT scanning with iodinated agents.

In renal transplantation, the differentiation of acute tubular necrosis (ATN) from rejection is critical. Basic knowledge of the appearance of a normal kidney is necessary to appreciate the changes in fail-

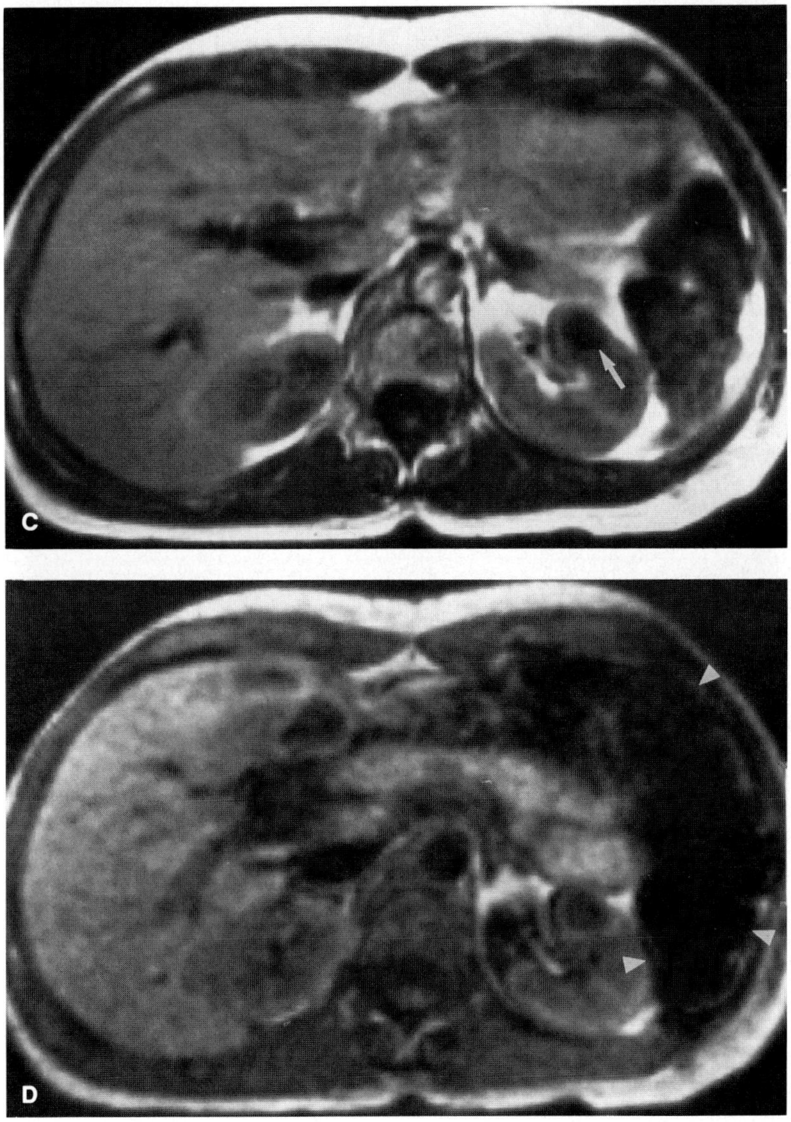

FIGURE 10–18. (Continued)

ing transplants. Healthy transplants should have the same signal characteristics as normal, native kidneys. On T1-weighted spin echo images, the renal cortex should be of intermediate signal intensity, differentiating it from the triangular-shaped areas of lower intensity representing the medullary pyramids. The lower water content of the renal cortex produces the shorter T1 and increased signal intensity relative to the renal medulla. In most normal kidneys, the corticomedullary junction is visible.

The loss of corticomedullary differentiation on T1-weighted images is the most consistent finding in acute or chronic renal transplant rejection, but the loss of corticomedullary differentiation is not specific for rejection.[33–36] Relative or complete loss of corticomedullary differentiation occurs with hydronephrosis, glomerulonephritis, nonspecific renal failure, renal artery stenosis, pyelonephritis, and infiltrative tumor. Various degrees of loss of corticomedullary differentiation can also be seen in ATN. Cyclosporin toxicity has not been definitely associated with this finding.

Perinephric fluid collections, such as postoperative urinomas, seromas, and lymphoceles, are typically

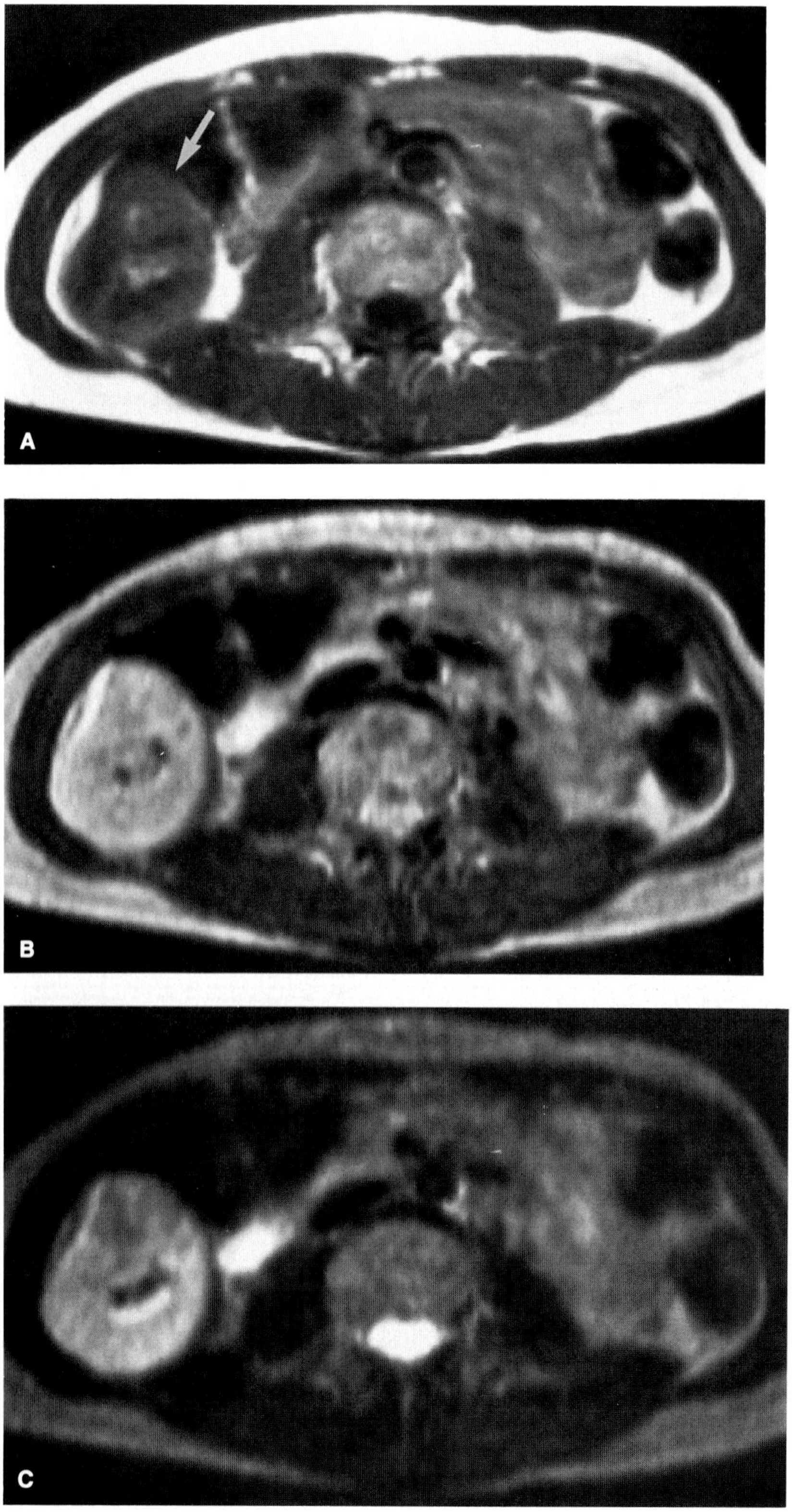

FIGURE 10–19. Renal cell carcinoma in a 35-year-old female. **(A)** T1-weighted (TR/TE = 600/17) and **(B,C)** T2-weighted images (TR/TE = 3000/45,90). A 4-cm-diameter soft tissue mass is identified primarily on the basis of a contour abnormality in the anterior inferior aspect of the right kidney (arrow). This mass is isointense with normal renal cortex on both T1-weighted and T2-weighted scans. Renal cell carcinomas often have signal intensity characteristics similar to those of normal renal tissue. The patient subsequently underwent right nephrectomy.

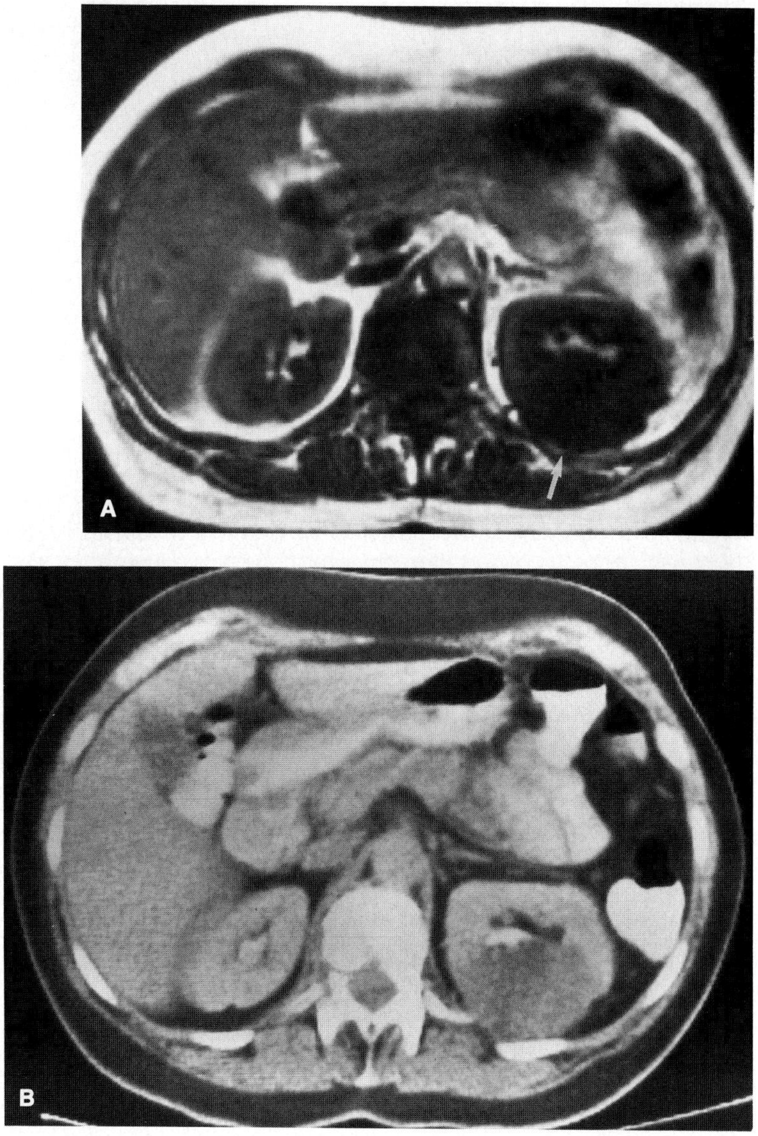

FIGURE 10–20. Renal cell carcinoma in a 50-year-old female, who presented with widespread, bony metastatic disease. The diagnosis was confirmed by CT-directed needle biopsy. **(A)** T1-weighted spin echo scan (TR/TE = 600/17 with four data acquisitions), **(B)** enhanced CT. A large, low-signal-intensity mass (arrow) involves the superior pole of the left kidney on MRI. The lesion is equally well depicted on CT. Although this lesion can be identified on MRI due to its long T1, renal cell carcinomas are often isointense with renal parenchyma.

seen as low intensity on T1-weighted spin echo sequences and intermediate or high intensity on T2-weighted spin echo images, depending upon the TE and TR used. This appearance is similar to other simple fluids.[33] A perinephric abscess is typically heterogeneous and higher in intensity than other fluid collections on intermediate T2-weighted images. Secondary changes in the adjacent kidney may also be seen.[33]

Hematomas vary with age in their MR characteristics. Chronic hematomas have low signal intensities on T1-weighted spin echo sequences and intermediate intensities on T2-weighted spin echo sequences, similar to seromas, urinomas, and lymphoceles. Acute hematomas can be homogeneous in appearance and of intermediate intensity on T1-weighted spin echo images and lower signal intensity on T2-weighted spin echo images. Subacute hematomas (> 1 week) can demonstrate two components, with a central, low-intensity thrombus surrounded by high-intensity serum on T1-weighted images. Thus, in the early postoperative period, MRI should be able to differentiate hematomas from other fluid collections.

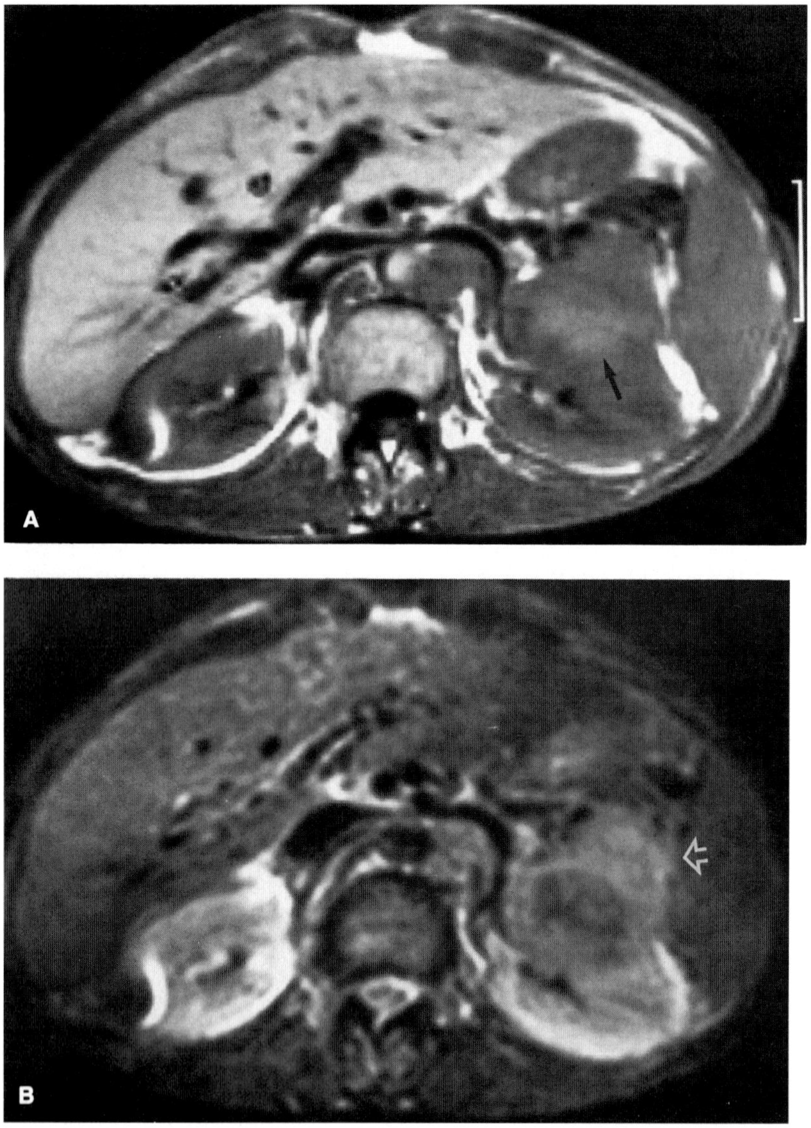

FIGURE 10–21. Left renal metastasis in a 48-year-old male. **(A)** T1-weighted image (TR/TE = 800/17) and **(B)** T2-weighted image (TR/TE = 2400/70). A large tumor mass (open arrow) can be identified in the upper pole of the left kidney. The signal intensity characteristics in the central portion of the lesion (i.e., slightly hyperintense on T1-weighted scan and hypointense on T2-weighted scan) are consistent with hemorrhage (closed arrow). The high signal intensity of the liver on the T1-weighted scan is consistent with fatty infiltration. Conventional spin echo pulse sequences have proved insensitive in most cases for detecting fatty infiltration.

REFERENCES

1. Ehman RL, McNamara MT, Pallack M, et al. Magnetic resonance imaging with respiratory gating: techniques and advantages. AJR 1984;143:1175.
2. Wood ML, Runge VM. Combination of suppression techniques helps reduce MRI motion artifacts. Diagn Imag 1988;6:139.
3. Pattany PM, Phillips JJ, Chiu LC, et al. Motion artifact suppression technique (MAST) for MR imaging. J Comput Assist Tomogr 1987;11:369.
4. Haacke EM, Lenz GW. Improving MR image quality in the presence of motion by using rephasing gradients. AJR 1987;148:1251.
5. Stark DD, Ferrucci JT Jr. Technical and clinical progress in MRI of the abdomen. Diagn Imag 1985;11:118.
6. Stark DD, Wittenberg J, Butch RJ, et al. Hepatic metastases: randomized, controlled comparison of detection with MR imaging and CT. Radiology 1987;165:399.
7. Reinig JW, Dwyer AJ, Miller DL, et al. Liver metastasis detection: comparative sensitivities of MR imaging and CT scanning. Radiology 1987;162:32.
8. Stark DD, Wittenberg J, Edelman RR, et al. Detection of hepatic metastases: analysis of pulse sequence performance in MR imaging. Radiology 1986;159:365.
9. Ferruci JT, Freeny PC, Stark DD, et al. Advances in hepatobiliary radiology. Radiology 1988;168:319.
10. Wolf CR, Runge VM, Wood MR, Carollo BR. Optimizing MR pulse sequences for liver imaging. Magn Reson Imaging 1989;7:177.
11. Kressel HY. Strategies for magnetic resonance imaging of focal liver disease. Radiol Clin North Am 1988;26:607.
12. Stark DD, Felder RC, Wittenberg J, et al. Magnetic resonance imaging of cavernous hemangioma of the liver: tissue-specific characterization. AJR 1985;145:213.
13. Ebara M, Ohto M, Watanabe Y, et al. Diagnosis of small hepatocellular carcinoma: correlation of MR imaging and tumor histologic studies. Radiology 1986;159:371.
14. Rummeny E, Weissleder R, Stark DD, et al. Primary liver tumors: diagnosis by MR imaging. AJR 1989;152:63.
15. Itai Y, Ohtomo K, Furui S, et al. MR imaging of hepatocellular carcinoma. J Comput Assist Tomogr 1986;10:963.
16. Okuda K, Musha H, Nakajima Y, et al. Clinicopathologic fea-

tures of encapsulated hepatocellular carcinoma. A study of 26 cases. Cancer 1977;40:1240.
17. Butch RJ, Stark DD, Malt RA. MR imaging of hepatic focal nodular hyperplasia. J Comput Assist Tomogr 1986;10:874.
18. Mattison GR, Glazer GM, Quint LE, et al. MR imaging of hepatic focal nodular hyperplasia: characterization and distinction from primary malignant hepatic tumors. AJR 1987;148:711.
19. Rummeny E, Stark DD, Weissleder R, et al. Central scar: a nonspecific MR imaging feature of primary liver tumors. Radiology 1988;169:64.
20. Goldberg HI, Moss AA, Stark DD, et al. Hepatic cirrhosis: magnetic resonance imaging. Radiology 1984;153:737.
21. Itai Y, Ohnishi Y, Ohtomo K, et al. Regenerating nodules of liver cirrhosis: MR imaging. Radiology 1987;165:419.
22. Stark DD. Liver. In: Stark DD, Bradley WG, eds. Magnetic resonance imaging. St. Louis: CV Mosby, 1988.
23. Hamm B, Wolf KJ, Felix R. Conventional and rapid MR imaging of the liver with Gd-DTPA. Radiology 1987;164:313.
24. Stark DD, Weissleder R, Elizondo G, et al. Superparamagnetic iron oxide: clinical application as a contrast agent for MR imaging of the liver. Radiology 1988;168:297.
25. Cohen JM, Weinreb JC, Redman HC. Postoperative assessment of splenorenal shunts with MRI: preliminary investigation. AJR 1986;146:597.
26. Chang A, Glazer HS, Lee JKT, et al. Adrenal gland: MR imaging. Radiology 1987;163:123.
27. Reinig JW, Doppman JL, Dwyer AJ, et al. MRI of indeterminate adrenal masses. AJR 1986;147:493.
28. Choyke PL, Kressel HY, Pollack HM, et al. Focal renal masses: magnetic resonance imaging. Radiology 1984;152:471.
29. Hilpert PL, Friedman AC, Radecki PD, et al. MRI of hemorrhagic renal cysts in polycystic kidney disease. AJR 1986;146:1167.
30. Marotti M, Hricak H, Fritzsche P, et al. Complex and simple renal cysts: comparative evaluation with MR imaging. Radiology 1987;162:679.
31. Demas BE, Stafford SA, Hricak H. Kidneys. In: Stark DD, Bradley WG, eds. Magnetic resonance imaging. St. Louis: CV Mosby, 1988.
32. Yashiro N, Masahiro I. T1 weighted magnetic resonance imaging of kidney and adrenal gland using Gd-DTPA as contrast material: dynamic MR imaging of kidney and adrenal gland. In: Runge VM, ed. Enhanced magnetic resonance imaging. St. Louis: CV Mosby. 1989.
33. Hricak H, Terrier F, Demas BE. Renal allografts: evaluation by MR imaging. Radiology 1986;159:435.
34. Baumgartner BR, Nelson RC, Ball TI, et al. MR imaging of renal transplants. AJR 1986;147:949.
35. Geisinger MA, Risius B, Jordan ML, et al. Magnetic resonance imaging of renal transplants. AJR 1984;143:1229.
36. Rholl KS, Lee JKT, Ling D, et al. Acute renal rejection versus acute tubular necrosis in a canine model: MR evaluation. Radiology 1986;160:113.

11

Pelvis

Madeleine R. Fisher

Pelvic anatomy is ideal for MR assessment because image quality is not usually degraded by respirations, the pelvic organs are highlighted by surrounding extraperitoneal fat, and the internal architecture of the organs is seen as a consequence of the superb soft tissue contrast provided by magnetic resonance imaging (MRI).

TECHNIQUE

Successful MR examination of the pelvis requires careful patient preparation, although MR images of the pelvis, compared with those of the abdomen, are better quality because respiratory and intestinal motion are minimal. A useful protocol consists of requiring the patient to fast or have clear liquids at least 4 hours before the MR examination of the pelvis and administering 1 mg of intramuscular glucagon immediately before imaging.[1,2] This decreases the degree of bowel motion and has minimal side-effects. If rectal or sigmoid disease is suspected, place the patient in a prone position, insert a tube used for an air contrast colon examination into the rectum, and instill air into the rectosigmoid colon.

Many times bowel may account for errors in interpreting images of the pelvis by mistaking an unopacified bowel loop for a mass, lymph node, or abscess. Opacification of the small bowel and colon is not routinely performed with MRI because the examinations are designed to image specific organs, such as the bladder, prostate, uterus, or cervix. However, in certain circumstances if there is a question of ovarian or bowel abnormalities, contrast is given. Geritol and ferrite are bowel contrast agents.[3,4] Geritol is readily available and therefore used most frequently for our pelvic imaging. The patient drinks approximately 32 ounces of dilute geritol 1 hour before the MR examination to achieve a high-intensity bowel contrast.[3]

In the computed tomography (CT) examination of the female patient, a tampon is inserted into the vagina to enhance discrimination between the vagina and the cervical, pericervical, and parametrial regions. This is not usually necessary with MRI. The vagina can be seen in either the transverse or sagittal plane without the use of a tampon.

Intravenous contrast is not required to visualize the bladder. The pulse sequences can be varied, manipulating the intensity of urine in the bladder to appear as a low-intensity signal on a T1-weighted spin echo sequence and high-intensity signal on a T2-weighted spin echo sequence. For imaging of the bladder, moderate bladder distension is beneficial in discerning intraluminal and extraluminal abnormalities.

Scans are usually obtained with 10-mm-thick sections at 10-mm intervals. The scans of the pelvis begin at the level of the iliac crest and proceed to the inferior ischial tuberosities. If the MR study is performed for evaluation of the prostate, seminal vesicles, uterus, cervix, or bladder, 5- or 3-mm sections are beneficial. A circumferential surface coil is optimal for pelvic imaging because it significantly increases the signal-to-noise ratio (SNR) compared with the standard body coil. However, when this type of surface coil is not available, the body coil is used for imaging of the pelvic structures.

Depending on the structure imaged, a combination of transverse, coronal, and sagittal images are acquired. The field of view (FOV) chosen depends on the width of the entire pelvis and what is needed to provide optimal SNR according to the slice thickness and number of signal measurements used.

An important artifact in pelvic imaging is chemical shift misregistration. This is seen as a low-intensity line at the junction of perivesical fat and the urinary bladder. This artifact occurs along the frequency-encoding direction. The frequency changes caused by chemical shift differences between fat and water may be seen as artifactual signal displacements in MR images. The chemical shift separation of fat and water protons is approximately 3.0 to 3.5 parts per million.[5] For example, if the frequency-encoding direction in a particular image is from the patient's left to right, the chemical shift misregistration is seen as a low-intensity band on the left side of the bladder and a symmetrical, high-intensity band on the right side of the bladder (Fig. 11-1).

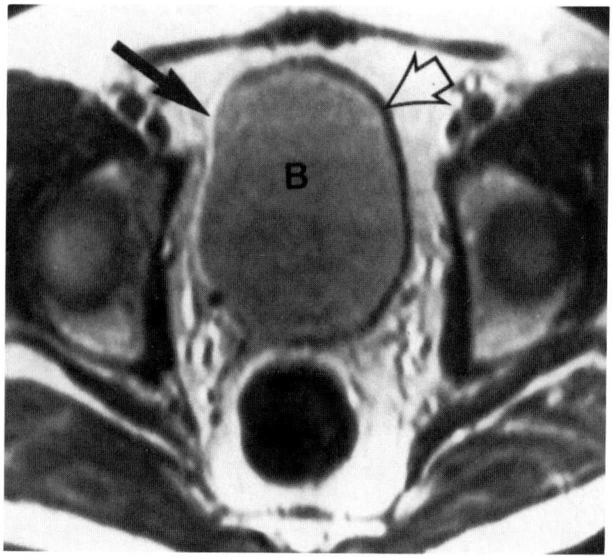

FIGURE 11-1. Transverse image (TR/TE = 2400/60) shows the chemical shift artifact as a band of low intensity (open arrow) on the left side of the bladder **(B)** and a band of high intensity (closed arrow) on the right side of the bladder.

FEMALE PELVIS

Although MRI allows accurate demonstration of female anatomy, sonography remains the screening technique for many uterine and ovarian abnormalities. However, sonography has several limitations, including problems produced by the patient's body habitus, the relative inability to determine tissue characterization, and operator dependence. CT provides a larger FOV and is currently used for staging most pelvic neoplasms. CT also has limitations, including distortion caused by metallic clips from previous surgery, the need for intravenous contrast media, ionizing radiation, and beam hardening artifacts. Therefore, it is important to understand the advantages and limitations of MRI before the technique can be used for evaluation of the female pelvis.

Uterus

The normal uterus on a T1-weighted image is seen as a homogeneous, medium-signal-intensity structure, with relatively indistinct uterine zonal anatomy. On the T2-weighted image, the anatomic uterine division into corpus, isthmus, and cervix is readily delineated. On T2-weighted sequences, the components of the corpus, the myometrium and endometrium, are imaged with different signal intensities, separated by the "junctional zone," a low-signal-intensity line between them (Fig. 11-2).[6-8] The junctional zone represents vascular structures, mainly veins located within the inner third of the myometrium.[8] The low-intensity line is seen on in vivo imaging of the normal menstruating uterus, but is not seen or is indistinct on in vitro imaging.[8]

The uterine appearance on MRI varies with hormonal stimuli.[9-11] Reproductive-age females have changes in uterine appearance during their menstrual cycles.[9-11] The endometrial width changes during the menstrual cycle and is seen at its largest dimension during the midsecretory phase. The volume and signal intensity of the myometrium also varies. During the secretory phase, the myometrium signal intensity is greatest, as seen on the T2-weighted sequence. During the secretory phase, the total uterine volume changes to the greatest extent. Females of reproductive age taking oral contraceptives have a different uterine appearance.[9-11] The separation between the myometrium and endometrium becomes indistinct, and endometrial atrophy is observed with inconsistent demonstration of the junctional zone.

MR images of a premenarchal or postmenarchal uterus differ from the appearance of a reproductive-age uterus. The former uteri are small, and there is absent or atrophic cyclic endometrium (Fig. 11-3). The length of the corpus uteri equals that of the cervix.[7,12] Postmenopausal women on exogenous estrogens have an appearance similar to the uterus of reproductive-age women.

Between 20% and 40% of women over the age of 35 develop leiomyomas, making it the most common benign lesion of the uterus. There is a variable MR appearance of leiomyoma within the uterus that depends on the presence or absence of hyaline, mucinous, myxomatous, cystic, and fatty degeneration and on calcification. MR can provide accurate assessment of the number, size, and precise location of leiomyomas.[8,13-15]

The optimal spin echo imaging technique for the diagnosis of intramural and submucosal leiomyoma is a T2-weighted sequence. However, it is important to obtain both T1-weighted and T2-weighted sequences

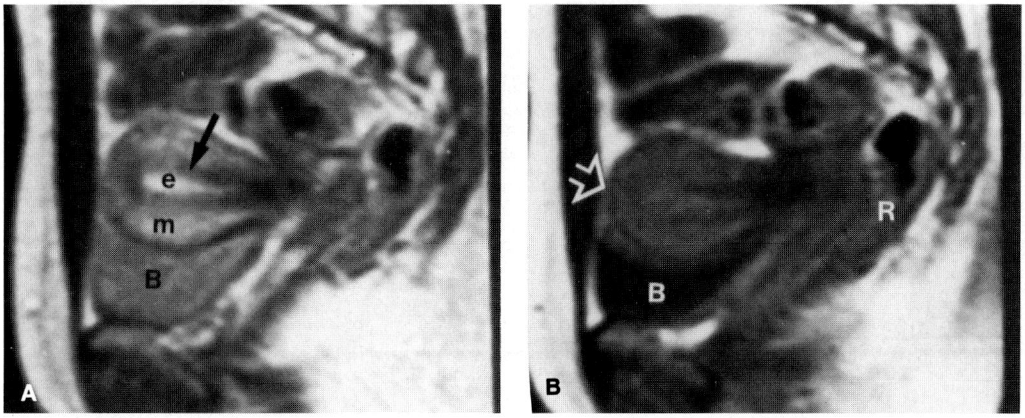

FIGURE 11–2. Normal uterus (open arrow) in a menstruating female. **(A)** Sagittal T2-weighted image (TR/TE = 2000/60) shows an anteverted uterus and the typical uterine zonal anatomy in a patient of this age (*e*, endometrium; *m*, myometrium; *B*, bladder; arrow, junctional zone). **(B)** Sagittal T1-weighted image (TR/TE = 850/30) shows that the uterine zonal anatomy is not as well seen on this sequence (B, bladder; *R*, rectum).

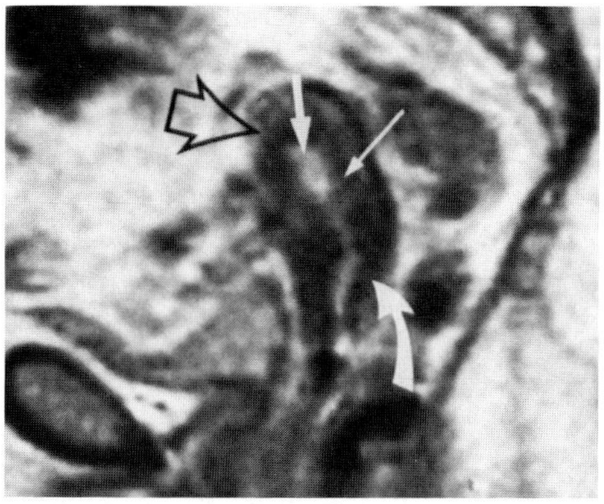

FIGURE 11–3. Postmenarchal uterus. Sagittal image (TR/TE = 2400/60) shows the change in size of the uterus, which is common at this patient's age. The corpus uterus length (open arrow) nearly equals the length of the cervix (curved arrow). The endometrial cavity is wider than normal (white arrow) for this postmenopausal woman, who was diagnosed with Stage I endometrial carcinoma at biopsy. The junctional zone is also seen (thin arrow).

for tissue characterization of myoma or other abnormality within the uterus (Fig. 11–4).

Another benign entity within the uterus that may be demonstrated by MR is adenomyosis. This is a disease typically found in women in their fifth decade. The MR findings in adenomyosis correlate with those of gross pathology.[15] On gross pathologic examination, adenomyosis shows smooth muscle hypertrophy surrounding a focus of basalis endometrium. In diffuse adenomyosis, the uterine body and fundus are diffusely enlarged.[15] On T2-weighted images, diffuse adenomyosis is seen as a wide, low-signal-intensity band that surrounds the normal high-signal-intensity endometrium. The low-signal-intensity band has an uneven distribution or measures thicker than 5 mm. Focal adenomyosis may simulate a leiomyoma, presenting as a focal low signal intensity region within the uterus.[15]

Endometriosis affects approximately 15% of all women during their menstrual life and is usually diagnosed by ultrasound and laproscopy. The MR features of endometriosis usually consist of a high-intensity structure suggestive of blood seen on both the T2-weighted and T1-weighted sequences.[16] The MR diagnosis of this disorder cannot be made without a typical clinical history.

On MRI, endometrial carcinoma is seen as an abnormality within the central endometrial cavity.[12,17–19] This disease most commonly occurs in postmenopausal women. The postmenopausal uterus usually shows a central canal of high signal intensity approximately 3 to 5 mm wide on T2-weighted images. Widening of the endometrial cavity or the presence of endometrial masses are important findings in this postmenopausal group (Fig. 11–5). With endometrial carcinoma, the central high-signal-intensity endometrium is routinely wider.[12] Another important finding is disruption of the low-intensity line, the junctional zone, between the myometrium and endometrium, which may be an important indication of myometrial invasion. Healthy premenopausal women routinely demonstrate the junctional zone on MRI, but it may be absent in normal postmenopausal women. In patients with endometrial carcinoma, visualization of the junctional zone is an indicator that the tumor is confined to the endometrium. However, if the junctional zone is not seen in its entirety, this does not necessarily indicate invasion. Adenomatous hyperplasia and endometrial carcinoma may look similar, and MRI cannot differentiate between them. Supportive pathologic diagnosis is required. However, if endometrial

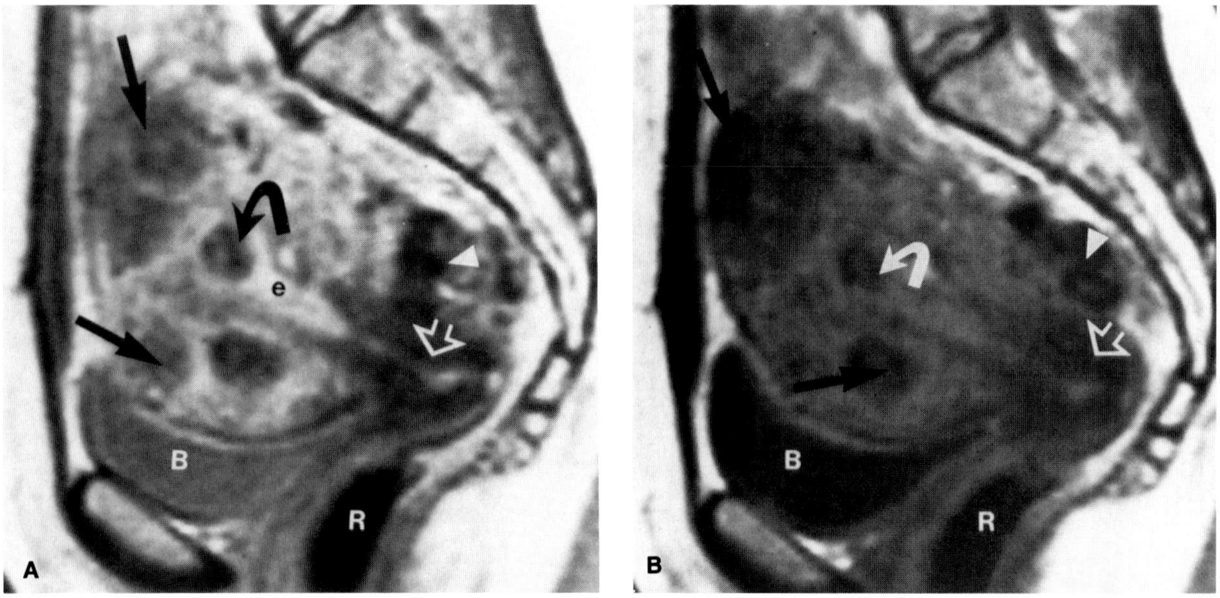

FIGURE 11–4. Leiomyoma. **(A)** Sagittal proton density-weighted image (TR/TE = 2400/30) shows that the uterus is large due to multiple leiomyomas, seen as low signal intensity in submucosal (curved arrows) and intramural (black arrows) locations. Notice that the submucosal leiomyoma is impinging on the endometrial cavity (*e*). (Open arrow, cervix; arrowhead, artifact secondary to bowel peristalsis; *B*, bladder; *R*, rectum). **(B)** Sagittal T1-weighted image (TR/TE = 750/30) shows that the leiomyomas are uniformly low signal intensity, indicating no degeneration.

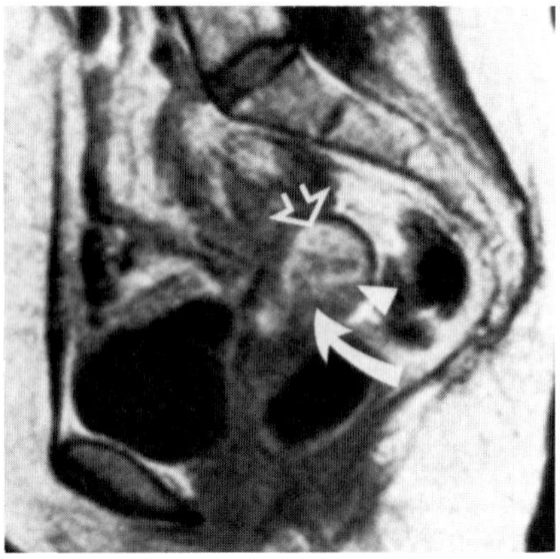

FIGURE 11–5. Endometrial carcinoma. Sagittal T1-weighted image (TR/TE = 750/30) shows widening of the endometrial cavity that is filled with high-intensity (open arrow) and medium-intensity (curved arrow) signals. The tumor is the medium-intensity material. Thinning of the myometrium is seen, and there is invasion into the myometrium (arrowhead). The pathologic specimen confirmed the invasion into the myometrial wall.

carcinoma has been histologically diagnosed by dilatation and curettage, MR may provide excellent local staging.

There is a variable appearance of endometrial carcinoma on MRI. There may be increased size of the high-intensity endometrial cavity without evidence of medium-intensity masses within the cavity on T2-weighted sequences. Another presentation on T2-weighted images shows the tumor as a homogeneous signal intensity lower than the surrounding endometrium. In other patients, there may be high signal intensity or medium signal intensity on a T1-weighted sequence, but on the T2-weighted sequence, the tumor may blend with the surrounding high-intensity endometrium.

Cervix

The cervix is best delineated on the T2-weighted sequence and has at least two separate zones (Fig. 11–6). The central zone is imaged with a high signal intensity and presumably represents the cervical epithelium and mucous.[7] The central canal is surrounded by a discrete region of low signal intensity, presumably representing the fibrous cervical stroma. Occasionally, a third narrow band of medium signal intensity is seen peripheral to the low-intensity band and is very similar to the intensity of the corpus uterus myometrium.[17] The parametrium is seen as low or medium intensity, flanking the cervix on T1-weighted images, and is separate from the low-intensity cervical stroma on both T1-weighted and T2-weighted sequences (Fig. 11–7).[20] On the T2-weighted sequence, there is a relative increase in signal intensity, often blending with fat.[21]

Benign cervical masses occasionally are seen on MRI. The most common lesions demonstrated are small Nabothian cysts. Rare lesions involving the cervix include endometriomas, cervical mucoceles, Gartner duct cysts, cervical pregnancy, and cervical

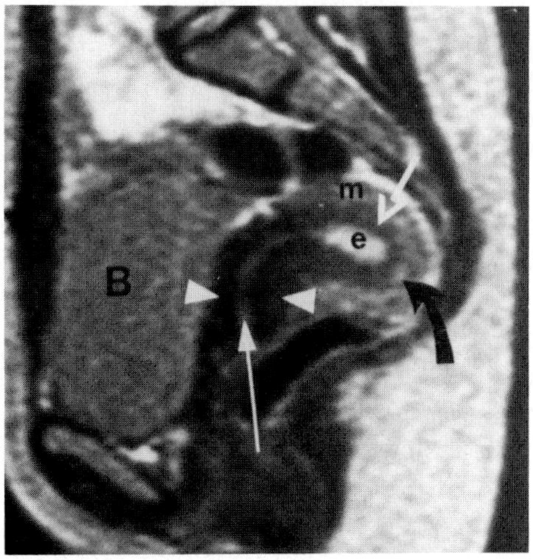

FIGURE 11–6. Normal cervix. Sagittal T2-weighted image (TR/TE = 2400/60) shows two zones of the cervix: the low-intensity mid-portion (arrowheads), representing fibrous cervical stroma, and the high-intensity center (white arrow). The peripheral zone is not seen on this example (curved arrow, uterus; open arrow, junctional zone; *M*, myometrium; *B*, bladder; *e*, endometrium).

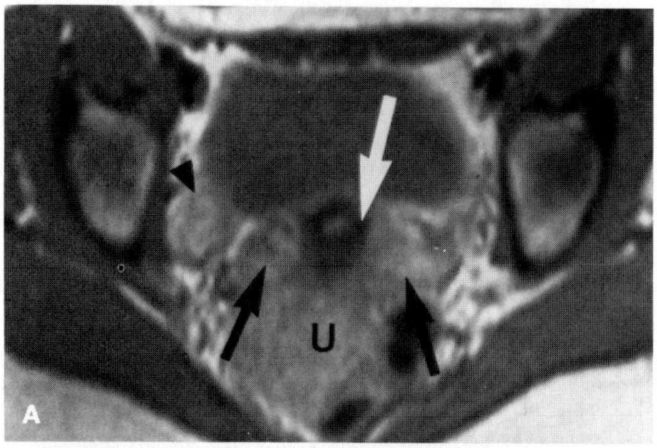

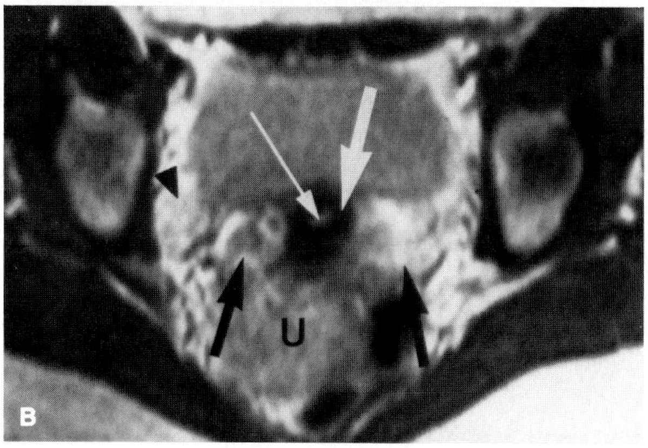

FIGURE 11–7. Normal parametrium. **(A)** Transverse image (TR/TE = 2000/30) shows an intermediate-intensity region (black arrows), on either side of the low-intensity cervical stroma (white arrow), that is the parametrium. The intermediate signal intensity (arrowhead) to the right of the parametrium is the right ovary (*U*, retroverted uterus). **(B)** Transverse T2-weighted image (TR/TE = 2000/60) shows a marked increase in signal intensity of the parametrium (black arrows), this and the right ovary (arrowhead) blend with the surrounding fat on this sequence (white arrow, cervical stroma; thin arrow, endocervical canal; *U*, uterus).

stenosis, which may present as masses and have a variable appearance on MRI depending on the relative composition (e.g. cystic, solid, or hemorrhagic components.)

Because of the increased soft tissue contrast, MRI surpasses CT in the staging of cervical carcinomas (Fig. 11–8).[20,21] The T2-weighted sequence demonstrates the neoplasm as a higher-signal-intensity mass in relation to the normal low signal intensity of the cervical stroma. MRI may be used for assessing tumor extent within the cervical stroma, into the parametrium, and into the vagina. On the T1-weighted sequence, the tumor within the cervical stroma may not be differentiated from the stroma, but tumor extension into the parametrium may be better appreciated due to the tumor's slightly higher signal intensity than that of the parametrium. On the T2-weighted sequence, the parametrium often increases in signal intensity to the same extent as that of tumor. Extension into the lower uterine isthmus or the vagina is optimally seen both on sagittal and coronal planes of imaging, with the transverse images used to complement the findings from the other two sequences (Fig. 11–9). For assessing the primary cervical tumor, sagittal and transverse planes of imaging are optimal; for parametrial extension, an oblique transverse plane angled perpendicular to the long axis of the cervix is helpful.[20,22]

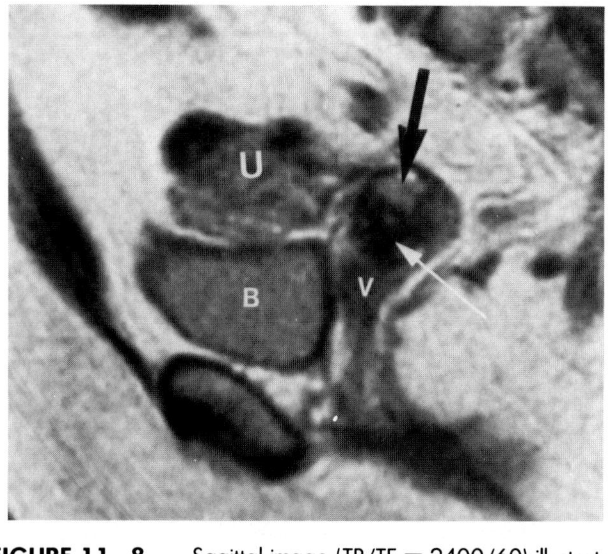

FIGURE 11–8. Sagittal image (TR/TE = 2400/60) illustrates a Stage IB cervical carcinoma arising within the posterior lip (black arrow) of the cervix (white arrow, low-intensity cervical stroma; *U*, uterus; *V*, vagina; *B*, bladder).

Vagina

The vagina is delineated from surrounding structures on T1-weighted and T2-weighted sequences. On T2-weighted sequences, the high-intensity center repre-

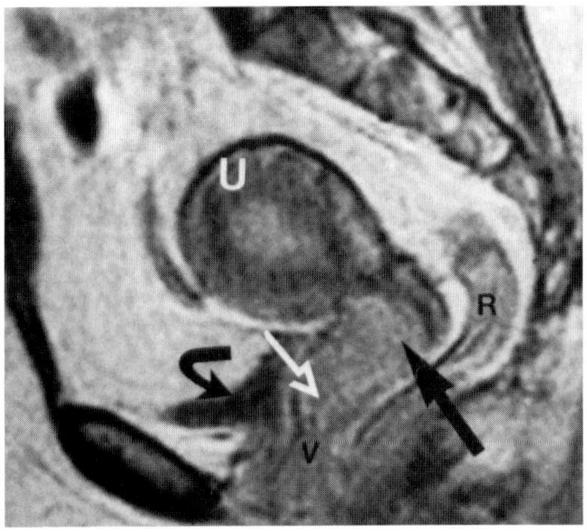

FIGURE 11–9. Sagittal image (TR/TE = 2000/30) illustrates a Stage IIA cervical carcinoma originating from the anterior lip of the cervix (black arrow) with extension into the upper two-thirds of the vagina (open arrow). (Curved arrow, bladder; *U*, uterus; *V*, vagina; *R*, rectum).

sents the vaginal epithelium and mucosa, and the lower signal intensity surrounding the high-signal-intensity center represents the vaginal wall (Fig. 11–10).[7]

Ovary

The normal ovaries are seen as low- or medium-signal-intensity structures on T1-weighted sequences (Fig. 11–11). Occasionally, on T1-weighted sequences, the ovaries may blend with surrounding bowel loops. On T2-weighted sequences, the signal intensity of the ovaries increases and approaches that of fat (Fig. 11–7B). The ideal imaging planes for evaluating the ovaries are the transverse and coronal.[23]

Currently, sonography is the method of choice for evaluation of ovarian masses. MRI often serves as a problem-solving technique after the sonographic study of adnexal abnormalities.[24] Most ovarian masses are benign cysts, such as physiologic follicular cysts, corpus luteum cysts, serous cystadenomas, mucinous cystadenomas, and dermoids. On MRI, simple ovarian cysts are well-circumscribed, homogeneous masses with a smooth interface (Fig. 11–11). If peripherally located, the cyst has a smooth and almost imperceptible wall. On T1-weighted sequences, they are of low signal intensity, often similar to that of urine or slightly greater than urine.[23,24] On a T2-weighted sequence, the signal intensity of the cyst increases and is similar to that of fat on 0.35-T systems and greater than fat on a 1.5-T system.

The dermoid cysts with simple fluid, similar to that contained within simple ovarian cysts, often show localized mural thickening. They have high signal intensity corresponding to that of fat seen on both T1-weighted and T2-weighted sequences.[23]

Ovarian hemorrhagic cysts are well-circumscribed, homogeneous structures with smooth walls of various thickness.[23] The wall is seen as a low-intensity line surrounding the ovarian lesion and corresponds to ovarian tissue or a pseudocapsule. Hemorrhagic cysts have high signal intensity on both T1-weighted and T2-weighted sequences.

Endometriosis has many different appearances on MRI. The most common appearance is similar to that

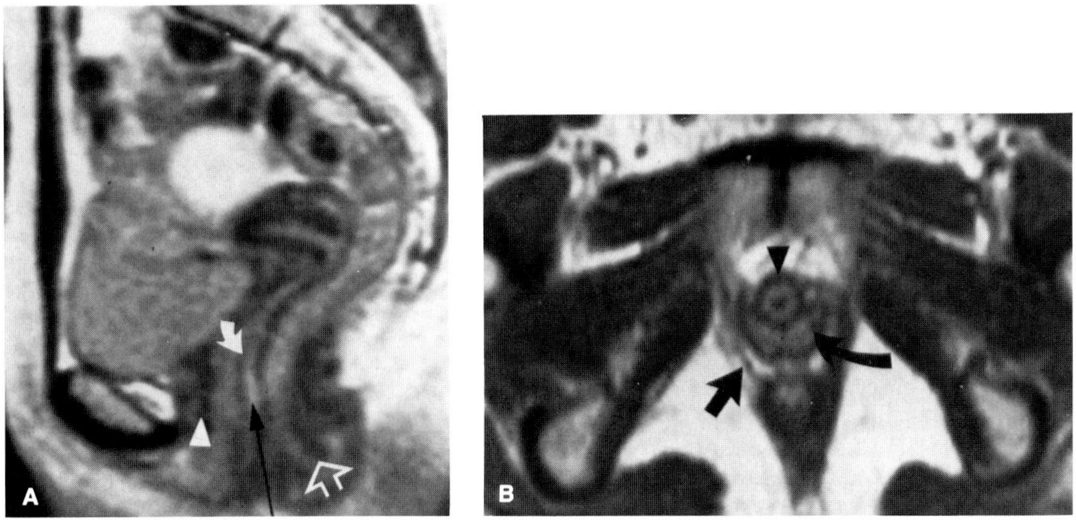

FIGURE 11–10. Normal vagina. **(A)** Sagittal image (TR/TE = 2000/60) shows the vaginal lumen as high intensity (thin black arrow) and the wall as low intensity (curved arrow). Also shown are the urethra (arrowhead) and the anus (open arrow). **(B)** Transverse image (TR/TE = 2000/60) shows the lower third of the vagina (curved arrow) at a level below the bladder base. The urethra (arrowhead) is located anteriorly.

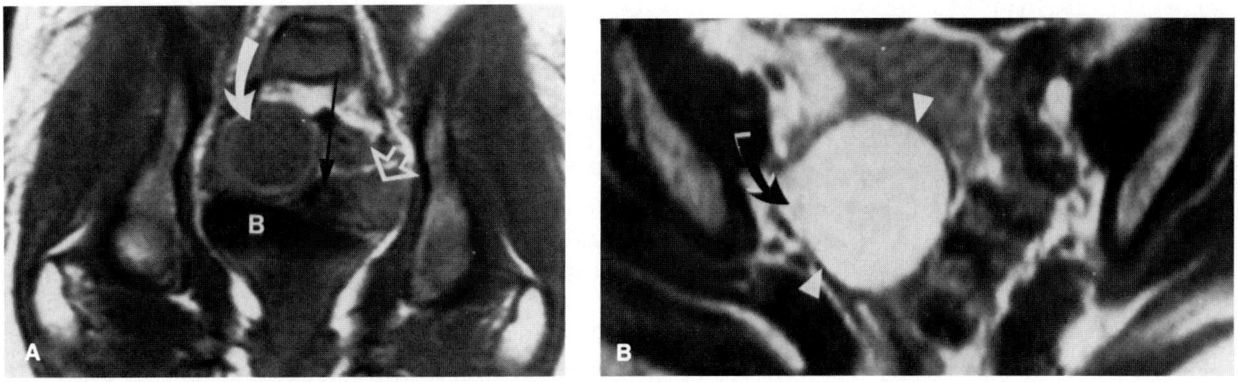

FIGURE 11-11. Ovaries. **(A)** Coronal T1-weighted image (TR/TE = 750/30) shows a benign, simple ovarian cyst arising from the right ovary (curved arrow). This contains fluid with an intensity slighter greater than that of urine. The normal ovarian tissue is compressed by the cyst. The left ovary (open arrow) has normal intensity (thin black arrow, cervix; *B*, bladder). **(B)** Transverse T2-weighted image (TR/TE = 2000/60) shows that the signal of the fluid within the ovarian cyst (curved arrow) increases and is slightly greater than that of fat. The surrounding wall is thin and of low signal intensity (arrowheads).

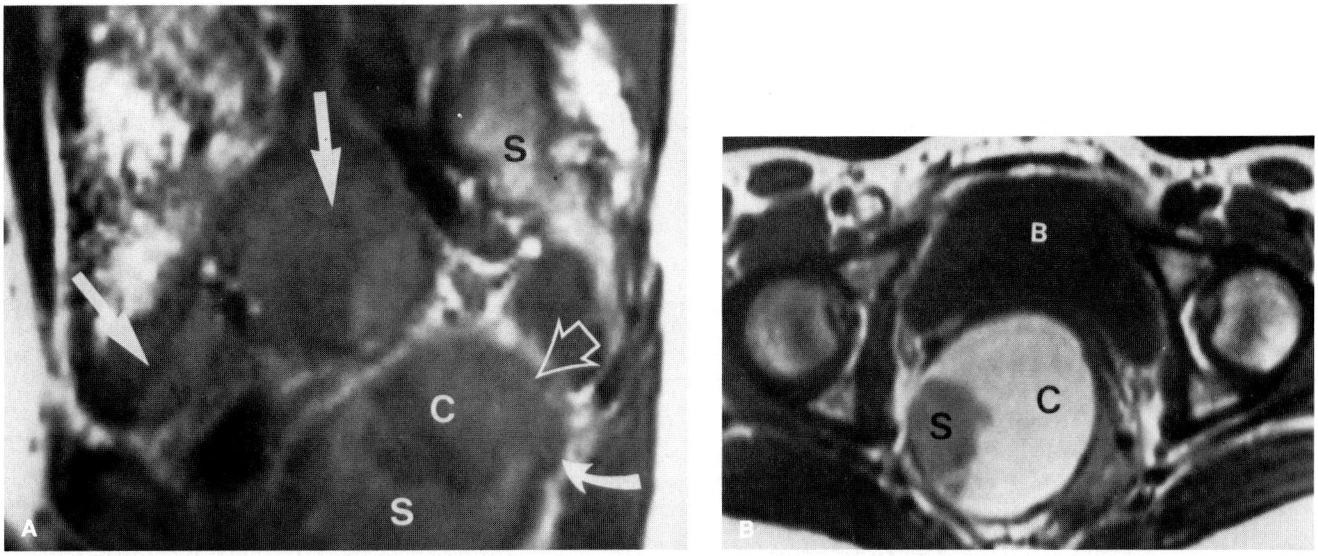

FIGURE 11-12. Ovarian carcinoma. **(A)** Sagittal T1-weighted image (TR/TE = 750/30) shows multiple, complex masses within the pelvis in a patient with ovarian carcinoma. Both solid *(s)* and cystic *(c)* components are seen within the primary lesion (*S*, sacrum). There is extension into the surrounding tissues (curved arrow). Two metastases are seen with the pelvis (arrows). **(B)** Transverse proton density image (TR/TE = 1500/30) shows the lower-intensity solid component *(S)* and the higher-intensity cystic component *(C)* on this sequence within the large ovarian carcinoma (*B*, bladder).

of the hemorrhagic ovarian cyst. Lesions are often heterogenous and are composed of a variety of tissues consisting of a hemorrhagic fluid component, hemorrhagic solid components, and fibrotic tissue.[23-25] Mesenteric endometrial implants are not readily demonstrable.

The precise role of MRI for evaluating patients with ovarian neoplasms has not been defined. Primary ovarian malignancies have a variety of findings and mimic lesions found with pelvic inflammatory disease or cystadenomas.[24] Ovarian carcinoma may present as heterogeneous masses of intermediate signal intensity on T1-weighted sequences with areas of low signal intensity on T2-weighted sequences (Fig. 11-12) or as complex masses best seen on T2-weighted sequences as high signal intensity representing fluid and as solid tissue seen as intermediate signal intensity.[23] Other lesions may have high signal intensity on both T1-weighted and T2-weighted sequences, suggestive of blood.

The primary role of MRI for ovarian imaging is to act as a problem-solving modality after sonography and CT have been performed. MRI is more accurate than ultrasound for tissue characterization in differentiating simple fluid from that of more complex fluids.[23] MRI may supplement the ultrasound examination for defining the nature of an adnexal mass, its extent, and whether there are blood or fat components. However, MRI still may not provide a specific diagnosis of an adnexal mass.

URINARY BLADDER

The optimal spin echo sequence for delineating the normal bladder wall and eccentric or concentric bladder wall hypertrophy is the T2-weighted sequence.[26] The normal bladder wall is easily seen in all planes, but specific regions of the bladder are seen better in certain planes.[27] The region of the base or dome is best visualized in the sagittal plane (Fig. 11-13). In the coronal plane, the bladder dome and lateral walls are easily seen (Fig. 11-14).

Bladder wall hypertrophy is best seen on T2-weighted images (Fig. 11-15). In bladder outlet obstruction, mucosal congestion is occasionally demonstrated within the region of the bladder base. Mucosal congestion is seen with high signal intensity on a T2-weighted image.

Focal wall thickening is the most common presentation of benign disorders involving the bladder. Leiomyoma is the most common benign mesothelial tumor of the bladder. Leiomyomas are seen on MRI as medium-intensity soft tissue tumors on a T1-weighted sequence or the first echo of a T2-weighted sequence. With a longer TE, the urine increases in signal intensity, and the leiomyoma may be seen as a lower signal intensity, or it becomes isointense with urine.[28]

Congenital disorders, such as ureteral bud remnants, may resemble seminal vesicle cysts or Muellerian duct cysts.

If the bladder wall has an unusual configuration, such as a pear-shaped or tear-drop configuration, MRI may readily demonstrate this on coronal sections. MRI may aid in differentiating the cause of the unusual bladder configuration by pelvic hematomas, lymphadenopathy, retroperitoneal fibrosis, lymphocele, inferior vena cava obstruction, iliopsoas muscle hypertrophy, or pelvic lipomatosis (Fig. 11-16).

Morphologic evaluation of malignant bladder tumors include analysis of size, site, and pattern of tumor growth (Fig. 11-17). These are criteria used for MR tumor staging based on the TNM system:

1. TIS (in situ), too small for current resolution.
2. Stage T1 (mucosa and submucosa involvement), tumor confined to bladder wall, with normal outer bladder wall seen as a low-intensity stripe.
3. Stage T2 (superficial muscle invasion), can be considered only when tumor is confined to the bladder wall and normal outer bladder wall is seen as a low-intensity stripe.
4. Stage T3a, gross tumor involvement of the bladder wall seen as a high signal intensity extending through the full thickness of the bladder wall, but not into the perivesical fat.

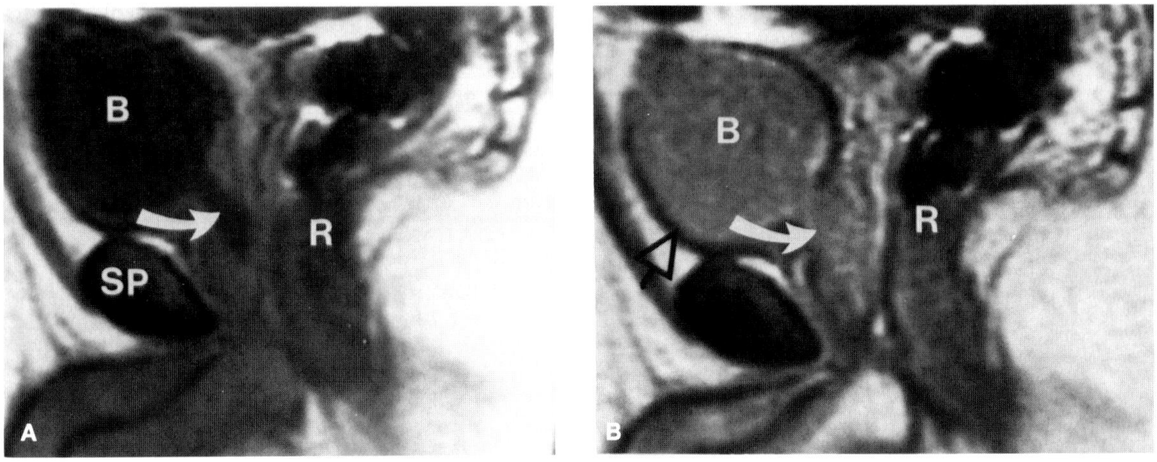

FIGURE 11-13. Bladder. **(A)** Sagittal image (TR/TE = 750/30) demonstrates the low intensity of urine within the bladder and the intermediate intensity of the wall on the T1-weighted image. The base and dome of the bladder are easily seen in the sagittal plane. The prostatic urethra is dilated (curved arrow) in this patient as a result of a transurethral resection of the prostrate (*B*, bladder; *SP*, symphysis pubis; *R*, rectum). **(B)** Sagittal image (TR/TE = 2000/60) shows a relative increase in signal intensity of the urine, providing good contrast with the low-intensity bladder wall (arrow). The wall is best seen on the T2-weighted image. The dilated urethra and prostate tissue blend on this sequence (*B*, bladder; *R*, rectum).

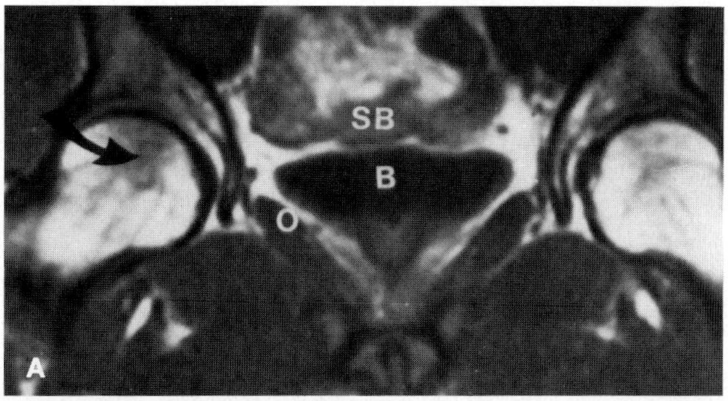

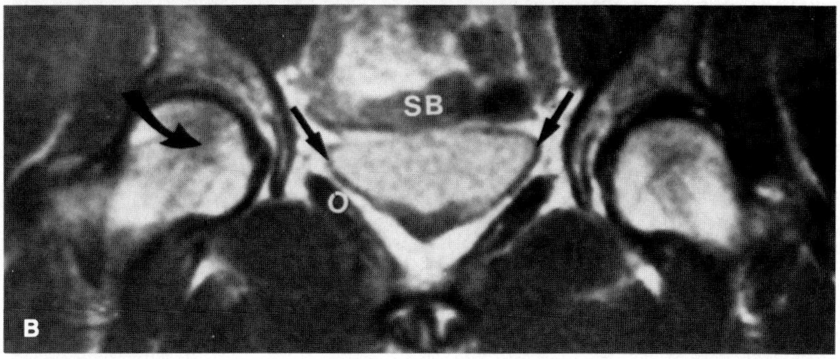

FIGURE 11–14. Bladder. **(A)** Coronal T1-weighted image (TR/TE = 750/30) shows the bladder lumen well as a consequence of the low-intensity urine, but the bladder wall is not easily seen. The coronal plane is useful for delineating the bladder dome, base, and lateral walls (*B*, bladder; *SB*, small bowel; *O*, obturator internis muscle; curved arrow, focal area of avascular necrosis). **(B)** Coronal T2-weighted image (TR/TE = 2400/60) shows a thin, low-intensity line (black arrows), representing the bladder wall, that is easily seen because of the relative increase in signal intensity of the urine.

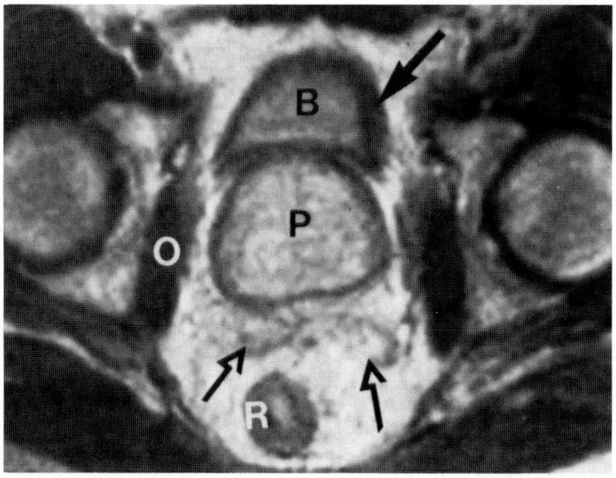

FIGURE 11–15. Bladder wall hypertrophy. Transverse image (TR/TE = 2400/60) shows a thickened bladder wall (black arrow) due to bladder outlet obstruction from prostatic hypertrophy *(P)*. (*B*, bladder; *R*, rectum; *O*, obturator internis muscle; open arrows, seminal vesicles).

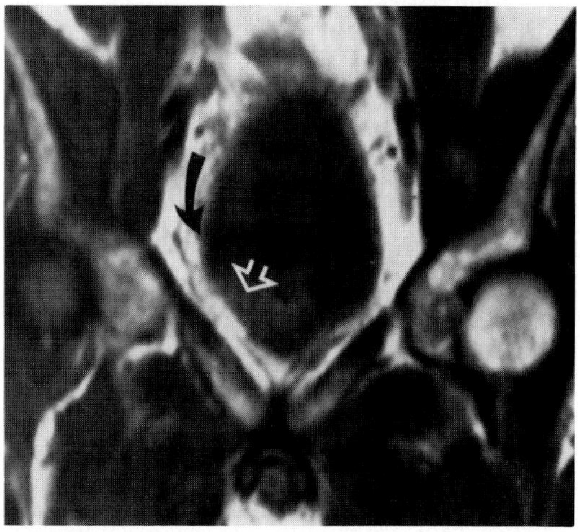

FIGURE 11–16. Pear-shaped bladder. Coronal image (TR/TE = 750/30) shows a pear-shaped configuration of the bladder (curved arrow) caused by pelvic lipomatosis (open arrow, thickened trigone region).

Portions of the bladder wall away from the site of the tumor should be seen as a low-intensity line.

5. Stage T3b, transmural extension of the tumor into the perivesical fat, but not the contiguous structures.
6. Stage T4, invasion of adjacent organs, such as the seminal vesicles, prostate, and rectum or pelvic side wall.[28]

Invasion of the seminal vesicles is demonstrated by an increase in size, diminished signal on a T2-weighted image compared with normal seminal vesicles, and evidence of fat invasion in the angle between the seminal vesicle and posterior bladder wall.[29] Invasion of the prostate and rectum is seen as an abnormal mass and intensity extending into these structures.

The main difficulty in MR staging of bladder carcinoma is differentiation between Stage T1 and T2 and between Stage T2 and a subtle T3a. Disruption of the normal bladder wall should be seen in at least two image planes (Fig. 11–17). If bladder wall disruption is seen in only one plane, it may be a technical artifact.

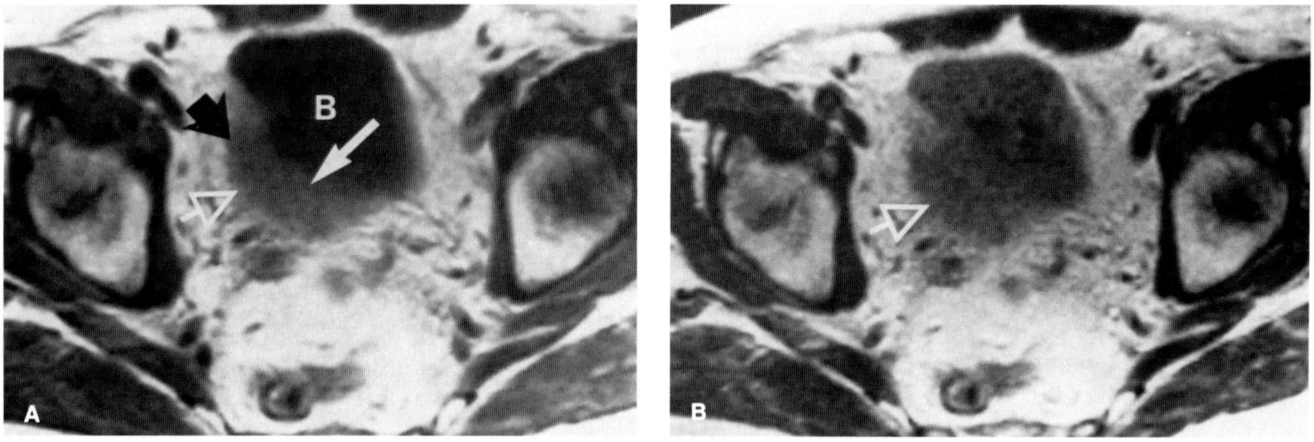

FIGURE 11 – 17. Papillary carcinoma of the bladder. **(A)** Transverse image (TR/TE = 1500/30) reveals a papillary transitional cell carcinoma originating from the right posterolateral aspect of bladder (black arrow). On this proton density image, the luminal component (white arrow) and the extension into the perivesical fat (open arrow) are easily seen (*B*, bladder). **(B)** Transverse image (TR/TE = 1500/60) that is moderately T2 weighted shows the inability to see the papillary component. The extravesical extension (open arrow) is still seen on this sequence, but not as well.

Stage T3a may be difficult to differentiate from a subtle Stage T3b (microscopic extension into perivesical fat).[28-30] On CT, the bladder wall and bladder neoplasms have a similar attenuation value, and bladder wall invasion cannot be adequately assessed.

Understanding chemical shift artifacts and using different imaging planes for interpretation of the MR images allows one to correctly identify artifacts rather than misinterpreting the lack of a low-intensity line as deep muscle invasion. The presence of enlarged lymph nodes should also be assessed when staging bladder neoplasms.

Several studies have shown MR accuracy for extravesical spread of carcinoma to be 77%, compared with 69% with CT.[29] Using the TNM system, MR accuracy has been reported as 64% and 73% by the Jewett-Strong-Marshall system; CT accuracy was 40%.[31]

Several spin echo sequences are necessary for optimal evaluation of bladder carcinoma. The papillary component of carcinoma (Fig. 11 – 17) is best seen on T1-weighted or proton density images. On T2-weighted images, the higher signal intensity of urine may obscure the papillary component of the carcinoma (Fig. 11 – 17). A T2-weighted sequence with a long TE is best for evaluating the infiltrating component of tumor. A short TR sequence is best for evaluating the perivesical extension of the neoplasm into the surrounding adipose tissue. On this sequence, the tumor has an intermediate signal intensity and fat has a high signal intensity.

MALE PELVIS

Prostate

Recently, studies have shown the morphologic appearance of the adult prostate gland to consist of two well-delineated regions within the prostate, rather than lobes.[32-35] The peripheral zone occupies approximately 75% of the gland, and the central zone occupies approximately 20%; the remaining 5% is known as the transitional zone (Fig. 11 – 18). The clinical significance of this distinction is readily seen because the primary site of origin of prostatic carcinoma is usually within the peripheral zone, and the transitional zone is the origin of benign prostatic hyperplasia.

MRI demonstrates the internal architecture of the prostate gland because of increased soft tissue contrast and multiplanar imaging capabilities. Differentiation between the peripheral and central zones is obtained on T2-weighted images.[36-41] On MRI, the prostatic venous plexus is seen both anterior and lateral to the prostate gland. The venous structures are often seen as tubular structures with low signal intensity on a T1-weighted sequence and high signal intensity on a T2-weighted sequence (Fig. 11 – 18).

MRI has been particularly useful for demonstrating prostatic parenchymal abnormalities. Although the technique is very sensitive for depiction of an abnormality, it can not differentiate between the various pathologic types, such as prostatic carcinoma and be-

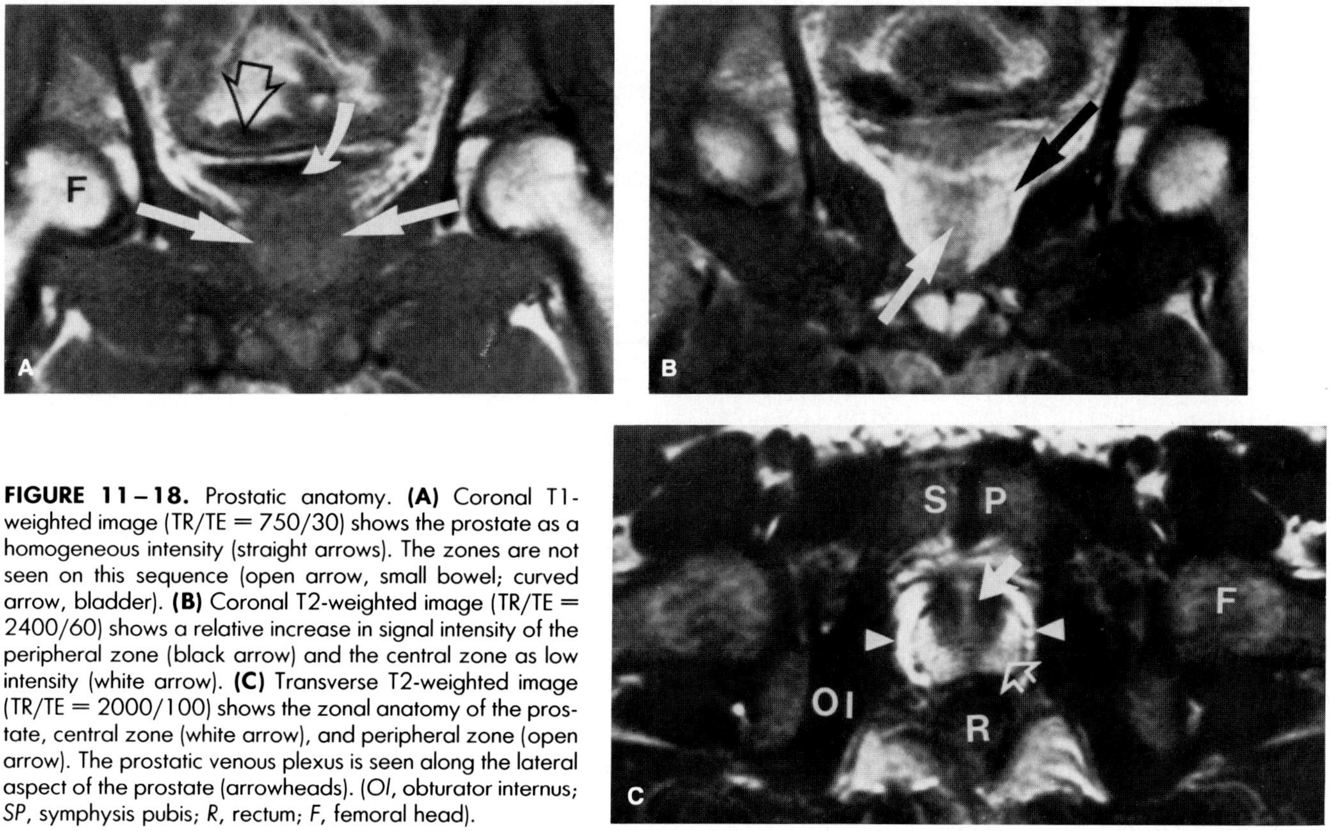

FIGURE 11–18. Prostatic anatomy. **(A)** Coronal T1-weighted image (TR/TE = 750/30) shows the prostate as a homogeneous intensity (straight arrows). The zones are not seen on this sequence (open arrow, small bowel; curved arrow, bladder). **(B)** Coronal T2-weighted image (TR/TE = 2400/60) shows a relative increase in signal intensity of the peripheral zone (black arrow) and the central zone as low intensity (white arrow). **(C)** Transverse T2-weighted image (TR/TE = 2000/100) shows the zonal anatomy of the prostate, central zone (white arrow), and peripheral zone (open arrow). The prostatic venous plexus is seen along the lateral aspect of the prostate (arrowheads). (*OI*, obturator internus; *SP*, symphysis pubis; *R*, rectum; *F*, femoral head).

nign prostatic hyperplasia.[38,39,42,43] Benign prostatic hyperplasia (BPH) has a variable appearance on MRI, a reflection of its heterogeneous composition (Fig. 11–19). Diffuse enlargement caused by BPH may be seen as a homogeneously enlarged gland with a similar signal intensity as that of the normal gland on both T1-weighted and T2-weighted sequences. The intensity of the enlarged gland is moderate on a T1-weighted sequence, increasing in relative signal intensity on a T2-weighted sequence.[43]

Nodular hyperplasia is similar to normal prostatic signal intensity on a T1-weighted sequence. On a T2-weighted sequence, the nodular form may be demonstrated as either a higher or lower signal intensity than that of the surrounding gland.[38,39,42,43]

Limited experience with other benign entities has shown a variable pattern. Most of these benign entities, including acute prostatitis, chronic inflammatory granulomas, and postbiopsy hematomas, are usually seen as a higher signal intensity than that of the surrounding prostatic tissue on T2-weighted sequences.[44]

Prostatic carcinoma is the second leading cause of death due to cancer in American men.[45] Accurate preoperative staging of disease is imperative because the mode of therapy depends on the clinical stage of the condition. Treatment for an intracapsular, Stage B, prostatic carcinoma is usually radical prostatectomy; patients with proven extracapsular extension, Stage C, usually receive external or internal radiation therapy. Clinical examination and current imaging tests have yielded variable degrees of success in defining abnormalities within the prostate gland.

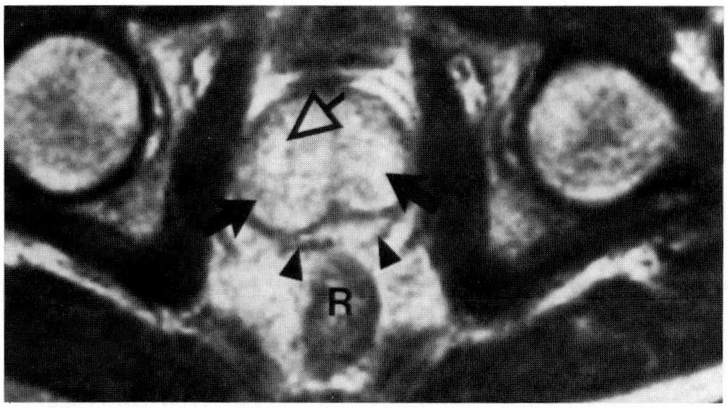

FIGURE 11–19. Benign prostatic hyperplasia. Transverse image (TR/TE = 2400/60) shows diffuse enlargement of the prostate gland secondary to benign prostatic hyperplasia (BPH) (arrows), causing compression of the peripheral zone (arrowheads). A focal nodule of high intensity (open arrow) is seen within the region of BPH (*R*, rectum).

MRI is highly sensitive for detecting an intraprostatic abnormality, although nonspecific in this finding.[38-44,46] Prostatic carcinoma on MRI has been described as a region of hypointensity or hyperintensity on T2-weighted images (Fig. 11-20).[38,42,43,46] On the T1-weighted image, the region of prostatic carcinoma is usually described as hypointense or isointense with the normal prostatic gland.[46-48] Diffuse inhomogeneity of the prostate gland as an indicator of abnormality is perhaps the one description that most researchers can agree on. Currently, it is not possible to distinguish between adenocarcinoma and BPH solely on the basis of signal inhomogeneity.

MRI is important in staging prostatic carcinoma. Determination of whether the carcinoma is confined to the gland or if there is periprostatic extension significantly alters clinical therapy. MR accuracy in differentiating a Stage B from Stage C prostatic carcinoma has been reported as 83% to 89%, compared with 65% CT accuracy.[49,50]

The MR protocol for prostatic carcinoma should include T1-weighted and T2-weighted images in the transverse plane, supplemented by either sagittal or coronal planes with a T2-weighted sequence (Fig. 11-21). It is important that the initial MR study of the prostate be performed before a prostatic biopsy, because focal postsurgical changes may mimic a prostatic abnormality.

Certain features for aiding assessment of extraprostatic extension have been found more useful than others.[50] Of the sites evaluated—periprostatic fat, periprostatic venous plexus, and the seminal vesicles—abnormality of the periprostatic venous plexus is considered the most sensitive indicator of periprostatic involvement.[50]

Seminal Vesicles

The seminal vesicles are demonstrated posterior and superior to the prostate on a sagittal image (Fig. 11-20B,C) and posterior on a transverse image (Fig. 11-22), with a low signal intensity in relation to the fat on a T1-weighted sequence and a higher signal intensity on a T2-weighted sequence (Fig. 11-22).[38,46]

On a T2-weighted sequence there is a relative increase in signal intensity due to the fluid within the seminal vesicles, and the wall is seen as low intensity. Often the signal intensity is greater than that of the surrounding retroperitoneal fat.

Testis and Scrotum

The utility of ultrasound scanning in evaluating scrotal abnormalities has been demonstrated.[51,52] Due to the superb capabilities of ultrasound for displaying the scrotal anatomy and characterization of intratesticular and paratesticular lesions, it is the imaging modality of choice. Recent studies on MR imaging of testicular lesions have shown that MR may demonstrate in great detail the anatomy of the scrotum and inguinal region. MRI is sensitive in demonstrating testicular abnormalities, especially on T2-weighted

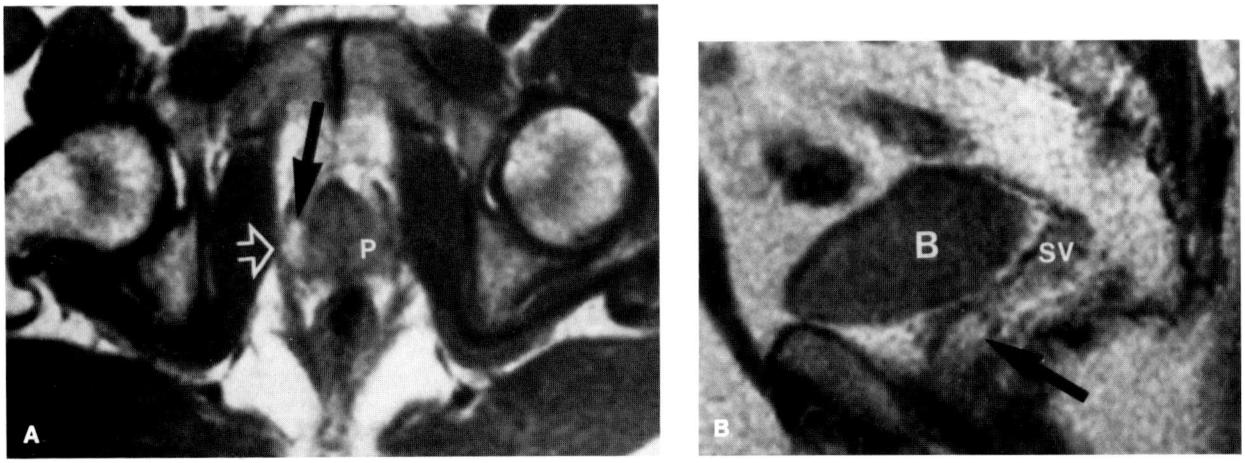

FIGURE 11-20. Prostate carcinoma. **(A)** Transverse image (TR/TE = 1500/30) shows a focal nodule of high intensity (black arrow) within the right peripheral zone (*p*) of the prostate. The levator ani musclae (open arrow) is immediately adjacent to the mass, but there is no evidence of invasion into the muscle. **(B)** Sagittal image (TR/TE = 2400/60) shows the focal nodule with high intensity (black arrow) within the prostate without invasion into the seminal vesicle (*SV*) or bladder.

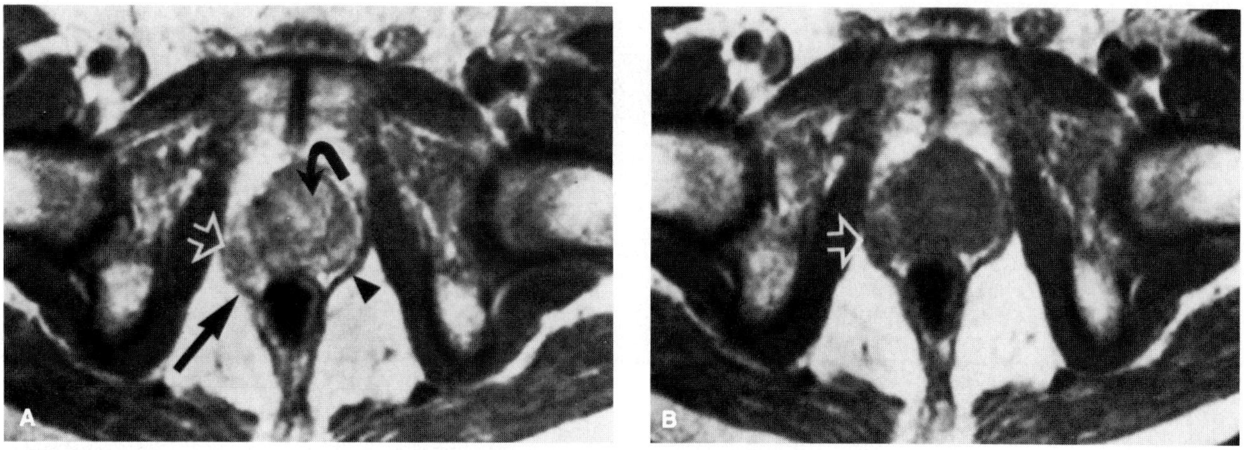

FIGURE 11–21. Prostate carcinoma. **(A)** Transverse image (TR/TE = 2400/30) shows extension of prostate carcinoma (open arrow) into the periprostatic fat, deviating the right levator ani muscle laterally (closed arrow). The entire prostate has inhomogeneous intensity (curved arrow). The left levator ani muscle (arrowhead) is also seen. **(B)** Transverse image (TR/TE = 750/30) better shows periprostatic extension into fat on the T1-weighted sequence. On the T1-weighted image, the prostate is low intensity and homogeneous, without differentiation into zonal anatomy or demonstration of pathology.

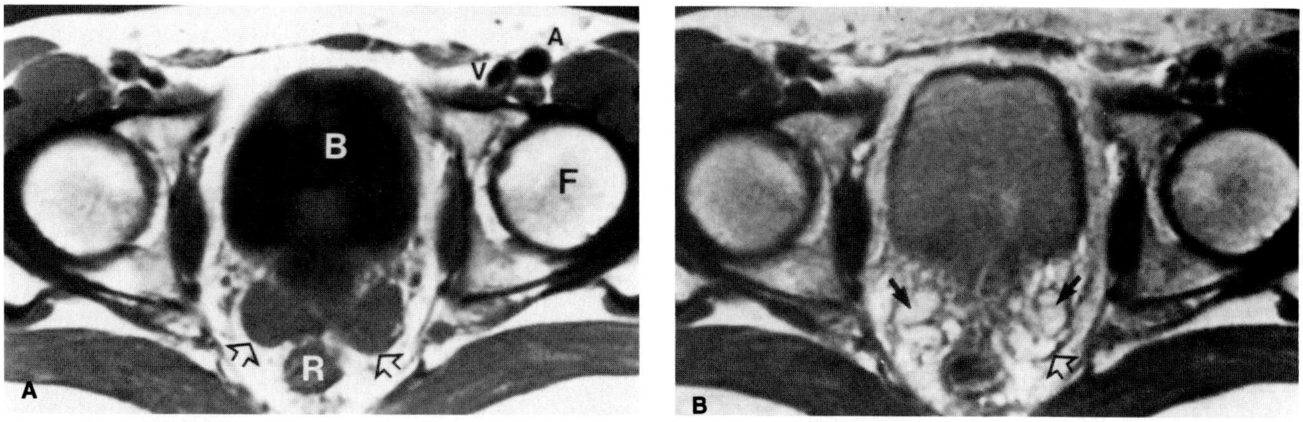

FIGURE 11–22. Seminal vesicles. **(A)** Transverse T1-weighted image (TR/TE = 750/30) shows the seminal vesicles (open arrows) as homogenous intermediate intensity (*B*, bladder; *F*, femoral head; *V*, femoral vein; *A*, femoral artery; *R*, rectum). **(B)** Transverse T2-weighted image (TR/TE = 2400/60) shows a relative increase in signal intensity of the seminal vesicle fluid (small black arrows) and the low intensity of the wall (open arrow). The convoluted pouches of the seminal vesicles are seen best on this sequence.

images.[53,54] MRI currently complements the sonographic studies and is used in cases where further definition is necessary.

The normal testis on MRI is a sharply defined oval structure of homogeneous, intermediate signal intensity on a T1-weighted image and higher signal intensity on a T2-weighted image (Fig. 11–23).[53,55] A low-intensity, 1-mm-thick layer demonstrated around the testis represents the tunica albuginea and the tunica vaginalis. The mediastinum testis, which arises from the tunica, is seen as a region of lower signal intensity than the testis on a T2-weighted sequence and measures approximately 1 to 3 cm long.

Both T1-weighted and T2-weighted sequences are necessary for evaluating the testis and intrascrotal contents. The coronal plane allows visualization of the testis, epididymis, and spermatic cord. This plane allows comparison of the right and left hemiscrotum.

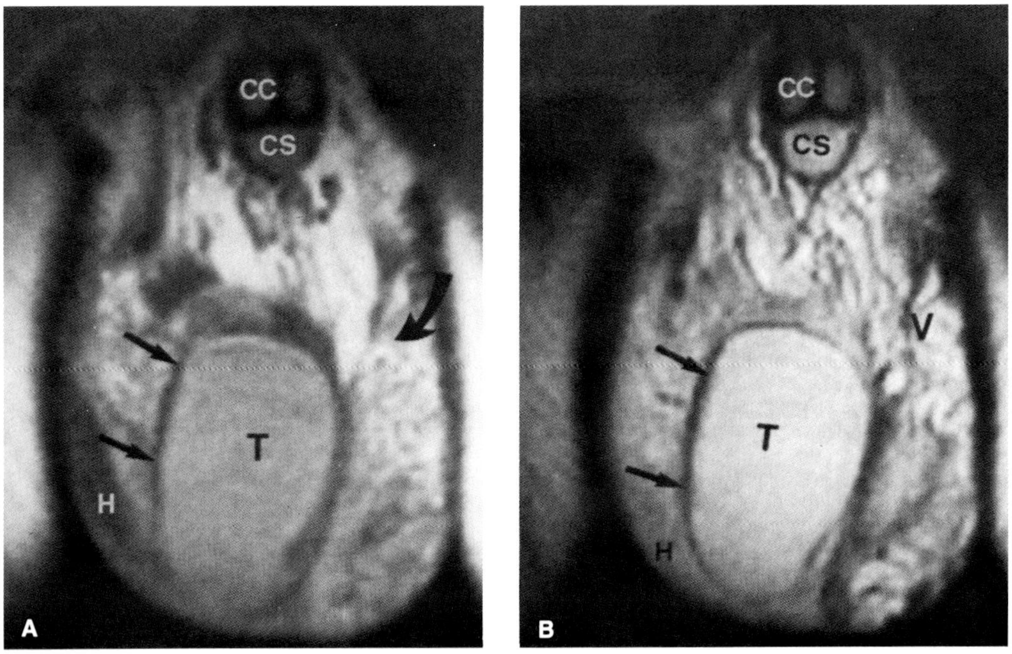

FIGURE 11–23. Normal testis. **(A)** Coronal image (TR/TE = 1000/30) shows an intermediate intensity within the right testis *(T)*, which is lower than the intensity of fat on this intermediate sequence. There is a varicocele (curved arrow) in the left hemiscrotum (*CC*, corpora cavernosa; *CS*, corpus spongiosum; *H*, hydrocele; arrows, the low-intensity line representing the tunica albuginea and tunica vaginalis). **(B)** Coronal T2-weighted image (TR/TE = 2200/60) shows a relative increase in signal intensity of the normal right testis *(T)* that is now similar to fat.

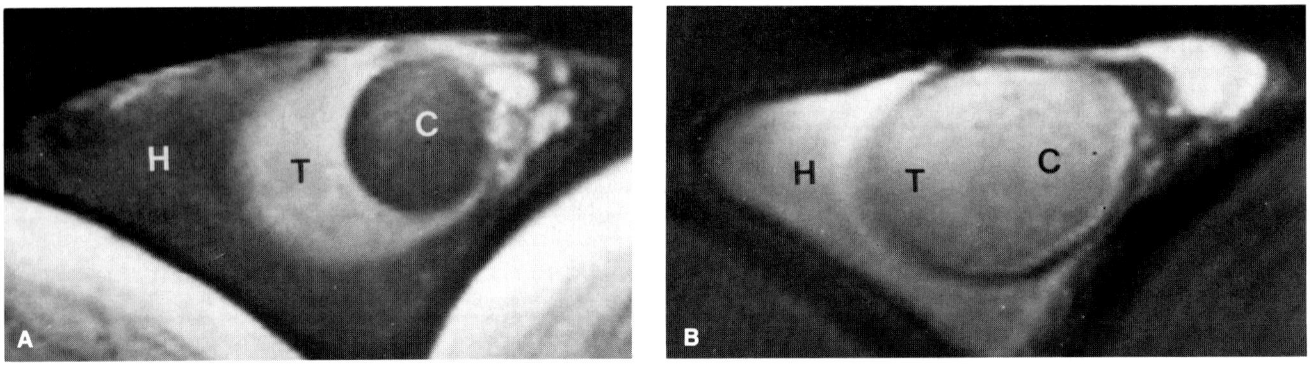

FIGURE 11–24. Testicular cyst. **(A)** Transverse T1-weighted image (TR/TE = 650/30) shows a cyst as a low-intensity, smoothly round structure *(C)* in contrast to the intensity of the surrounding normal testis *(T)*. A hydrocele *(H)* is also detected. **(B)** Transverse T2-weighted image (TR/TE = 2000/100) shows blurring of the cyst *(C)* margins and testicular tissue *(T)* because the cyst is of relatively higher signal intensity on this sequence.

The bare area of the testis and the inguinal canal are best seen in the sagittal plane.[55] The transverse plane allows comparison of the right and left structures and complements the coronal plane.

Testicular cysts are seen as smooth, round lesions on MR images (Fig. 11–24). On the T1-weighted sequence and balanced sequence (e.g., TR/TE = 2000/30), the cyst has low signal intensity compared with the surrounding testicular tissue. On the T2-weighted images, the cyst becomes higher in signal intensity, similar to that of testicular tissue, causing the lesion to appear nearly isointense with the normal testicular parenchyma.

Inflammatory foci within the testis often develop into abscesses. On MRI, inflammatory changes within the testis are seen as a lower signal intensity than the contralateral testis, either focally or diffusely, on T2-weighted images. When an abscess develops, the signal intensity is inhomogeneous, and there is associated poor definition and partial disruption of the tunica albuginea.[54]

MR assessment of patients after trauma has shown that evaluation of the tunica albuginea is important, because the condition of the tunica determines the need for surgical intervention.[56] The traumatized testes are seen as inhomogeneous structures with areas of high and low signal intensity, compared with normal testicular tissue, on both balanced and T2-weighted images.

Testicular tumors are seen as areas of inhomogeneous signal intensity equal to or lower than the intensity of the normal testis on a balanced image (e.g., TR/TE = 2000/30) and markedly lower on a T2-weighted image (e.g., TR/TE = 2000/80) on systems operating at 0.35, 0.5, and 1.5 T.[53,56] The margination and extent of the tumor, as well as the effect on the normal testicular size and shape, are well demonstrated on MR images.[56]

Epididymis

On T1-images, the epididymis is seen as an area of homogeneous, intermediate signal intensity, less than or equal to that of normal testicular tissue. On T2-weighted images it is less intense than that of the testis (Fig. 11–25).[53,55] The head, body, and tail of the epididymis are readily delineated. The epididymis is clearly demarcated from the testis owing to the higher signal intensity of the testis and the low signal intensity of the tunica albuginea.

Hydrocele

Simple hydroceles are seen as lower signal intensity than the testis on T1-weighted images and of similar or slightly lower signal intensity on T2-weighted images (Fig. 11–25).

Penis

The two corpora cavernosa and the corpus spongiosum, which together make up the penis, are readily identified on MRI (Fig. 11–26). The urethra courses through the corpus spongiosum. The corpora cavernosa are seen as medium signal intensity on a T1-weighted sequence and increase in signal intensity on a T2-weighted sequence.[46] The separation between the two corpora cavernosa is delineated by a low-signal-intensity septum. The corpus spongiosum has a similar signal intensity to that of the corpora cavernosa and is distinguishable from the corpora cavernosa by its anatomic location and the surrounding tunica albuginea.[46]

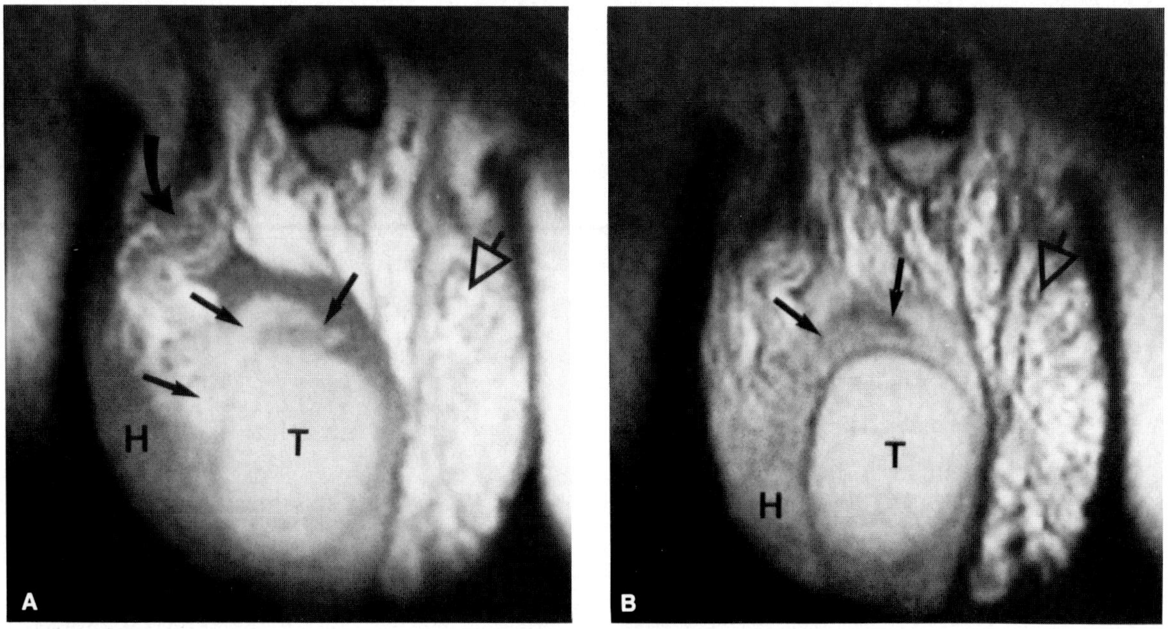

FIGURE 11–25. Epididymis. **(A)** Coronal image (TR/TE = 1000/30) shows the head, body, and tail of the epididymis (small black arrows). The ductus deferens is seen within the spermatic cord (curved arrow) that can be followed to the inguinal canal (open arrow, varicocele; *H*, hydrocele; *T*, testis). **(B)** Coronal T2-weighted image (TR/TE = 2200/60) shows that the epididymis becomes lower in signal intensity (small black arrows) and the testis *(T)* increases in intensity (*H*, hydrocele; open arrow, varicocele).

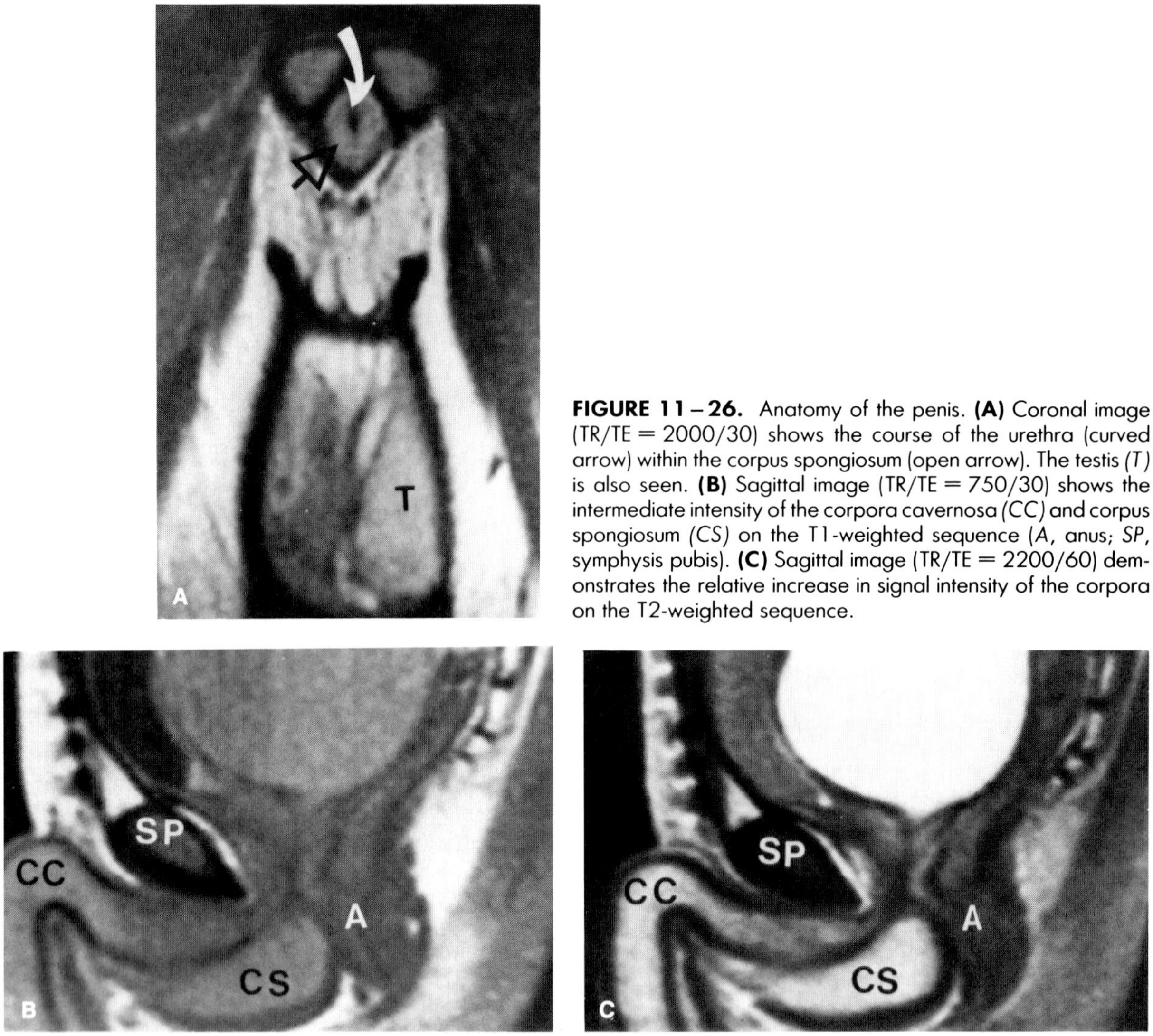

FIGURE 11–26. Anatomy of the penis. **(A)** Coronal image (TR/TE = 2000/30) shows the course of the urethra (curved arrow) within the corpus spongiosum (open arrow). The testis *(T)* is also seen. **(B)** Sagittal image (TR/TE = 750/30) shows the intermediate intensity of the corpora cavernosa *(CC)* and corpus spongiosum *(CS)* on the T1-weighted sequence (*A*, anus; *SP*, symphysis pubis). **(C)** Sagittal image (TR/TE = 2200/60) demonstrates the relative increase in signal intensity of the corpora on the T2-weighted sequence.

REFERENCES

1. Weinreb JC, Maravilla KR, Redman HC. Improved MR imaging of the upper abdomen with glucagon and gas. J Comput Assist Tomogr 1984;8:835.
2. Winkler ML, Hricak H. Pelvis imaging with MR: techniques for improvement. Radiology 1986;158:848.
3. Wesbey GE, Brasch RC, Engelstad BL. Nuclear magnetic resonance enhancement study of the gastrointestinal tract of a human volunteer using nontoxic oral iron solutions. Radiology 1983;149:175.
4. Hahn PF, Stark DD, Saini S, et al. Ferrite particles for bowel contrast in MR imaging: design issues and feasibility studies. Radiology 1987;164:37.
5. Soila KP, Viamonte M, Starewicz PM. Chemical shift misregistration effect in magnetic resonance imaging. Radiology 1984;153:819.
6. Hricak H, Alpers C, Crooks LR, et al. Magnetic resonance imaging of the female pelvis: initial experience. AJR 1983;141:1119.
7. Hricak H. MR of the female pelvis: a review. AJR 1986; 146:1115.
8. Lee JKT, Gersell DJ, Balfe DM, et al. The uterus: In vitro anatomic correlation of normal and abnormal specimens. Radiology 1985;157:175.
9. Demas BE, Hricak H, Jaffe RH, et al. Uterine MR imaging: effects of hormonal stimulation. Radiology 1986;159:123.
10. Haynor DR, Mack LA, Soules MR, et al. Changing appearance of the normal uterus during the menstrual cycle: MR studies. Radiology 1986;161:459.
11. McCarthy S, Tauber C, Gore J. Female pelvic anatomy: MR assessment of variations during the menstrual cycle and with use of oral contraceptives. Radiology 1986;160:119.
12. Hricak H, Stern JL, Fisher MR, et al. Endometrial carcinoma staging by MR imaging. Radiology 1987;162:297.
13. Hricak H, Tscholakoff D, Heinrich L, et al. Uterine leiomyomas: correlation of MR, histopathologic findings, and symptoms. Radiology 1986;158:385.
14. Hamlin DJ, Pettersson H, Fitzsimmons J, et al. MR imaging of uterine leiomyomas and their complications. J Comput Assist Tomogr 1985;9:902.
15. Mark AS, Hricak H, Heinrich LW, et al. Adenomyosis and leiomyoma: differential diagnosis with MR imaging. Radiology 1987;163:527.

16. Hricak H, Schriock E, Lacey C, et al. Gynecologic masses—value of MRI. Am J Obstet Gynecol 1985;153:31.
17. Worthington JL, Balfe DM, Lee JKT, et al. Uterine neoplasms: MR imaging. Radiology 1986;159:725.
18. Butler H, Bryan PJ, Lipuma JP, et al. Magnetic resonance imaging of the abnormal female pelvis. AJR 1984;143:1259.
19. Bies JR, Ellis JH, Kopecky KK, et al. Assessment of primary gynecologic malignancies: comparison of 0.15 T resistive MRI with CT. AJR 1984;143:1249.
20. Davis T, Fisher MR. MR evaluation of cervical cancer. Scientific exhibit of the American Roentgen Ray Society, April 1987, Miami, FL.
21. Balfe DM, Heiken J, McClennan BL. Oncologic imaging for carcinoma of the cervix, ovary and endometrium. In: Bragg DG, Rubin P, Youker JE, eds. Oncologic imaging. New York: Pergamon, 1985;439.
22. Togashi K, Nishimura K, Itoh K, et al. Uterine cervical cancer: assessment with high-field MR imaging. Radiology 1986; 160:431.
23. Dooms GC, Hricak H, Tscholakoff D. Adnexal structures: MR imaging. Radiology 1986;158:639.
24. Mitchell DG, Mintz MC, Spritzer CL, et al. Adnexal masses: MR imaging observations at 1.5 T with US and CT correlation. Radiology 1987;162:319.
25. Nishimura K, Togashi K, Itoh K, et al. Endometrial cysts of the ovary: MR imaging. Radiology 1987;162:315.
26. American Joint Committee on Staging and End-Results. Reporting Manual for Staging of Cancer. Chicago: American Joint Committee, 1978.
27. Fisher MR, Hricak H, Crooks LE. Urinary bladder, MR imaging, part I: normal and benign conditions. Radiology 1985;157:467.
28. Fisher MR, Hricak H. Magnetic resonance imaging of the urinary bladder: neoplasms, part II. Radiology 1985;157:471.
29. Bryan PJ, Butler HE, Lipuma JP, et al. CT and MR imaging in staging bladder neoplasms. J Comput Assist Tomogr 1987;11:96.
30. Rholl KS, Lee JKT, Heiken JP, et al. Primary bladder carcinoma: evaluation with MR. Radiology 1987;167:117.
31. Amendola MA, Glazer GM, Grossman HB, et al. Staging of bladder carcinoma: MR-CT-surgical correlation. AJR 1986; 146:1179.
32. McNeal JE. Regional morphology and pathology of the prostate. Am J Clin Pathol 1968;49:347.
33. McNeal JE. The prostate and prostatic urethra: a morphologic synthesis. J Urol 1972;107:1008.
34. McNeal JE. Normal and pathologic anatomy of the prostate. Urology 1981;17:11.
35. McNeal JE. The zonal anatomy of the prostate. Prostate 1981;2:35.
36. Hricak H, Dooms GC, McNeal JE, et al. Imaging of the prostate gland: normal anatomy. AJR 1987;148:51.
37. Sommer FG, McNeal JE, et al. MR depiction of the zonal anatomy of the prostate at 1.5 T. J Comput Assist Tomogr 1986;10:983.
38. Lee JKT, Rhall KS. MRI of the bladder and prostate. AJR 1986;147:732.
39. Poon PY, McCallum RW, Henkelman MM, et al. Magnetic resonance imaging of the prostate. Radiology 1985;154:143.
40. Fisher MR, Hricak H. MRI of the genitourinary tract. Postgrad Radiol (in press).
41. Fisher MR, Hricak H, Saks BJ. Prostate and urinary bladder. In: Partain L, ed. Magnetic resonance imaging. Philadelphia: WB Saunders, 1988.
42. Ling D, Lee JKT, Heiken JP, et al. Prostatic carcinoma and benign prostatic hyperplasia: inability of MR imaging to distinguish between the two diseases. Radiology 1986;158:103.
43. Carrol CL, Summer FG, McNeal JE, et al. The abnormal prostate: MR imaging 1.5 T with histopathologic correlation. Radiology 1987;163:521.
44. Buonocore E, Hesemann C, Pavlicek W, et al. Clinical and in vitro magnetic resonance imaging of prostate carcinoma. AJR 1984;143:1267.
45. Whitmore WJ Jr. Natural history and staging of prostatic cancer. Urol Clin North Am 1984;11:209.
46. Hricak H, Williams RD, Spring DB, et al. Anatomy of the male pelvis by magnetic resonance imaging. AJR 1983;141:1101.
47. Byran PJ, Butler HE, Lipuma JP, et al. NMR scanning of the pelvis: initial experience with a 0.3 T system. AJR 1983;141:1111.
48. Byran PJ, Butler HE, Nelson AD, et al. Magnetic resonance imaging of the prostate. AJR 1986;146:546.
49. Hricak H, Dooms GC, Jeffrey RB, et al. Prostatic carcinoma: staging by clinical assessment, CT and MR imaging. Radiology 1987;162:331.
50. Biondetti PR, Lee JKT, Ling K, et al. Clinical Stage B prostate carcinoma: staging with MR imaging. Radiology 1987;162:325.
51. Hricak H, Filley RA. Sonography of the scrotum. Invest Radiol 1983;18:112.
52. Leopold GR, Woo VL, Scheible FW, et al. High resolution ultrasonography of scrotal pathology. Radiology 1979;131:719.
53. Rholl KS, Lee JKT, Ling D, et al. MR imaging of the scrotum with high resolution surface. Radiology 1987;163:99.
54. Baker LL, Hajeck PC, Burkhard TK, et al. MR imaging of the scrotum: pathologic conditions. Radiology 1987;163:93.
55. Baker LL, Hajec PC, Burkhard TK, et al. MR imaging of the scrotum: normal anatomy. Radiology 1987;163:89.

12

Musculoskeletal System

Clifford R. Wolf
Val M. Runge

Magnetic resonance imaging (MRI) has emerged as an increasingly effective modality for evaluating the musculoskeletal system. Initially, it was thought that MRI would have limited application in the musculoskeletal system due to its relative inability to detect calcification. It was soon recognized that, despite the lack of visualization of calcium or cortical bone, MRI had better soft tissue contrast than other imaging modalities. Because the musculoskeletal system is comparatively easy to immobilize, motion artifacts are relatively inconsequential. However, MRI had limited utility until the advent of dedicated surface coils, which allowed adequate signal-to-noise ratio (SNR) and improved resolution. The noninvasiveness, lack of ionizing radiation, and multiplanar imaging capabilities are desirable features of MRI.

In the past few years, the indications for MRI in evaluating the musculoskeletal system have increased markedly. MRI is the primary imaging modality for evaluating internal derangements of the knee, meniscal abnormalities in the temporomandibular joint (TMJ), and avascular necrosis, and it is superior for depicting the extent of soft tissue masses and bone marrow abnormalities. MRI is certain to become increasingly important for evaluating the shoulder.

This chapter reviews the current knowledge about MR imaging of the musculoskeletal system, with an emphasis on pathologic conditions and technical parameters for imaging the major joints, including the knee, hip, TMJ, shoulder, wrist, and ankle. The MRI appearances of soft tissue lesions, bone tumors, marrow disease, and infection are also examined.

The author gratefully acknowledges Donald G. Mitchell, MD, from Thomas Jefferson University Hospital for his review of the chapter.

MRI OF THE KNEE

MRI has several advantages compared with other modalities in evaluating the internal architecture of the knee. MRI is noninvasive, painless, and provides excellent soft tissue contrast. The first MRI of the knee was reported in 1985, but initial results were compromised by poor SNR and resolution.[1] The implementation of local coils for extremity imaging and higher-field-strength magnets (1.0–1.5 T) helped to overcome these limitations.[2] MRI plays a dominant role in evaluation of knee abnormalities.

Technique

A complete examination of the knee must evaluate the menisci, ligaments, articular cartilage, and bone marrow. A suggested technique for scanning the knee consists of sagittal T1-weighted (TR/TE = 500–800/15–25) and T2-weighted (TR/TE = 2000–3000/20–90) images and coronal T1-weighted images employing spin echo pulse sequences.[2] Sagittal images with the knee externally rotated 10 to 15° allow optimal depiction of the anterior cruciate ligament. The knee should be repositioned to a neutral position for the coronal scan; this can be done manually or by using oblique scan planes. All scans must be obtained using an extremity coil. Ideal resolution requires a small (e.g., 15 cm) field of view (FOV) to best demonstrate the menisci and ligaments. We obtain our images with two acquisitions, a 256 × 256 matrix, and 4-mm slice thickness. A second set of images filmed with high contrast, a narrow window, and large magnification enhances visualization of the menisci (Fig. 12–1).

Recent studies have shown 3D gradient-echo imaging, specifically FISP and GRASS pulse sequences,

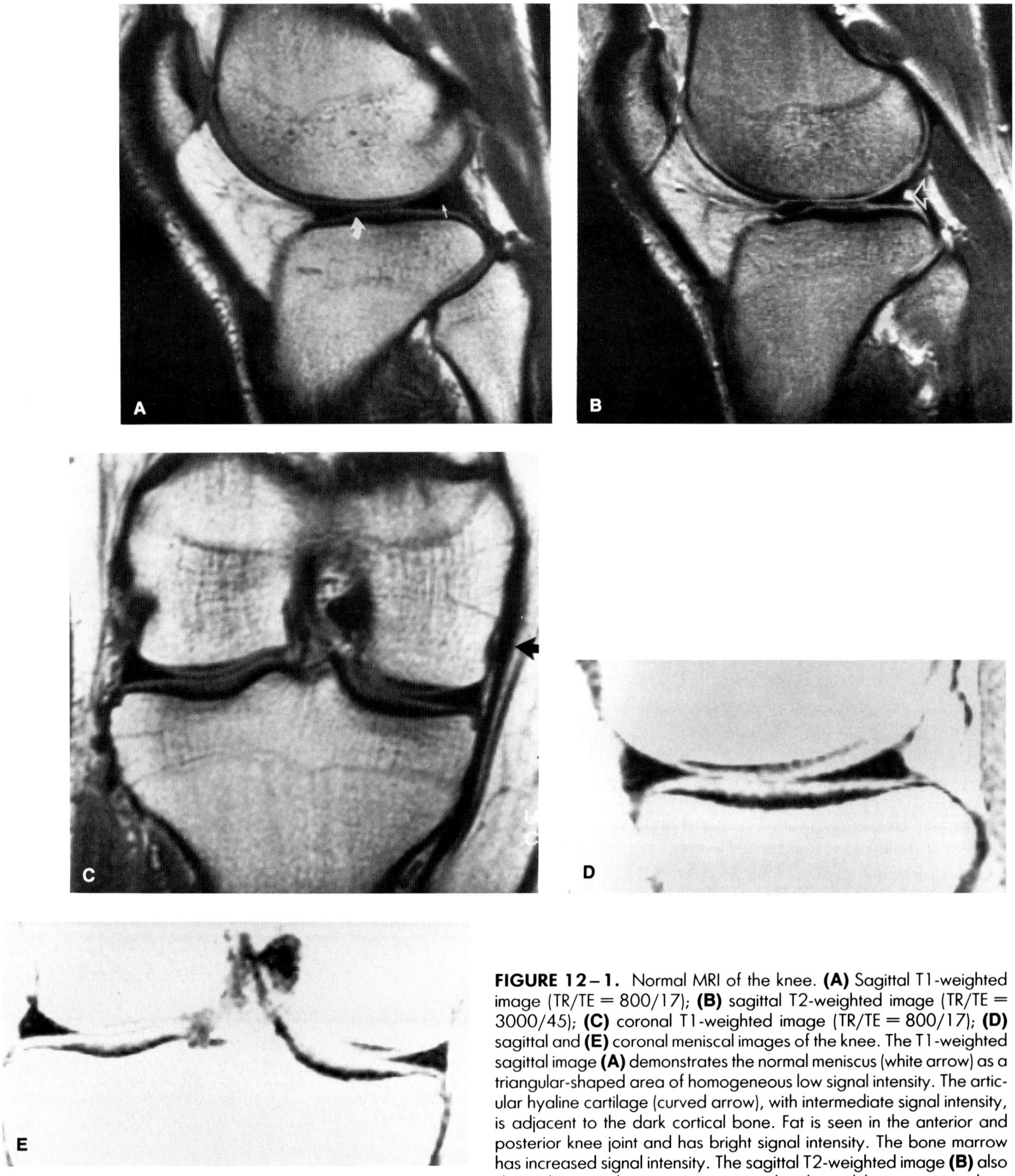

FIGURE 12–1. Normal MRI of the knee. **(A)** Sagittal T1-weighted image (TR/TE = 800/17); **(B)** sagittal T2-weighted image (TR/TE = 3000/45); **(C)** coronal T1-weighted image (TR/TE = 800/17); **(D)** sagittal and **(E)** coronal meniscal images of the knee. The T1-weighted sagittal image **(A)** demonstrates the normal meniscus (white arrow) as a triangular-shaped area of homogeneous low signal intensity. The articular hyaline cartilage (curved arrow), with intermediate signal intensity, is adjacent to the dark cortical bone. Fat is seen in the anterior and posterior knee joint and has bright signal intensity. The bone marrow has increased signal intensity. The sagittal T2-weighted image **(B)** also shows the normal meniscus as a triangular-shaped, homogeneous, low-signal-intensity structure. A small amount of fluid is seen in the posterior knee joint (open arrow). The coronal image **(C)** demonstrates the normal menisci as symmetric, triangular, low-signal-intensity structures. The medial collateral ligament is seen as a continuous linear area of low signal intensity (black arrow). Meniscal windows **(D,E)** optimally demonstrate the menisci and are routinely obtained on all of our knee MRI scans. The normal menisci are seen as triangular-shaped, homogeneous, low-signal-intensity structures.

promising for evaluating the knee.[3-5] These techniques, still under investigation, are reserved for demonstrating the articular cartilage or for obtaining thinner contiguous sections. If the patellofemoral joint space needs to be imaged, axial scans are required. Unfortunately, patient through-put must be considered, and the incorporation of all of the above pulse sequences requires excessive scan time. The 3D FISP/GRASS images and axial scans should be reserved for situations in which the cartilage or patellofemoral joint, respectively, are of specific clinical concern.

Meniscus

The assessment of the meniscus is usually the primary clinical concern in MRI of the knee. The meniscus consists of type I collagen, which contains few excitable protons and should remain dark (low signal intensity) on all pulse sequences.[6] Meniscal tears and degeneration are manifested as increased signal intensity on T1-weighted and T2-weighted sequences within the substance of the meniscus, primarily due to the influx of fluid.[1]

The posterior horn of the medial meniscus is the most common site of injury. Isolated tears of the anterior horn of the meniscus are uncommon.[7] A recent study reported a sensitivity of 95%, specificity of 91%, and accuracy of 93% for MR detection of meniscal tears.[8] This compared favorably with arthroscopy, which had an accuracy of 87 to 95%. The free edge of the meniscus is the most difficult area for MRI to evaluate, and 44% of the diagnostic errors occurred in this portion of the meniscus. The posterior horn of the lateral meniscus is a difficult spot for the arthroscopist to see and therefore is the most common site of diagnostic error in arthroscopy.[7] Because the false-negative rate for MRI of the knee was reported to be almost zero, a normal MRI of the knee should obviate a surgical procedure.[4]

Meniscal abnormalities have been classified by a grading system that has diagnostic and therapeutic implications.[4,9] The grading system is as follows (Fig. 12–2):

Normal—no intrameniscal signal
Grade 1—single round or punctate high signal focus within the meniscal substance (Fig. 12–3)
Grade 2—linear high signal focus within the meniscal substance that does not abut the articular surface (Fig. 12–4)
Grade 3—full- or partial-thickness tears of the meniscus communicating with an articular surface (Fig. 12–5).
Grade 4—meniscal fragmentation or peripheral rim tears (i.e., meniscal capsular separation) (Fig. 12–6)

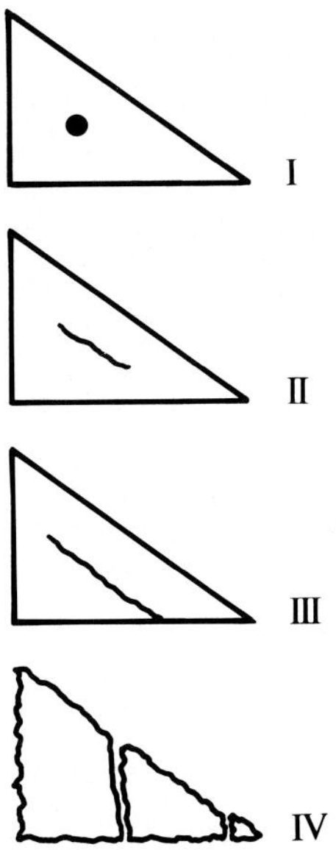

FIGURE 12–2. Grading system for meniscal injury. Grade I is a globular focus of increased signal intensity confined to the substance of the meniscus. Grade II is a linear area of increased signal intensity in the meniscus that does not reach the articular surface. Grade III is a linear area of increased signal intensity in the meniscus, which communicates with the articular surface, indicating a meniscal tear. Grade IV includes meniscal fragmentation and complicated meniscal tears.

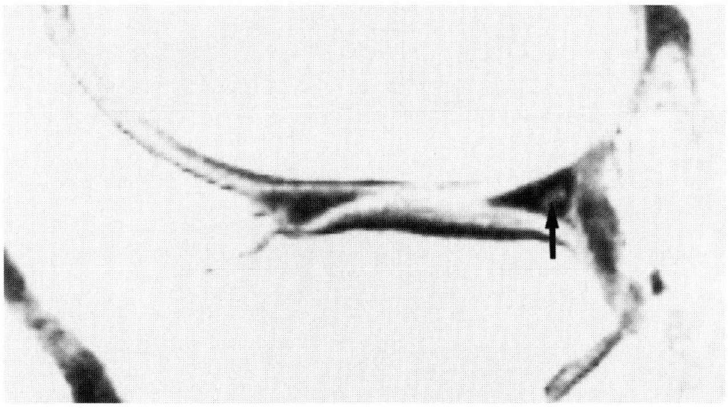

FIGURE 12–3. Grade I meniscal degeneration. Sagittal T1-weighted image (TR/TE = 800/17) filmed with meniscal windows identifies a small globular focus of increased signal intensity (arrow) in the posterior horn of the lateral meniscus. The increased signal intensity does not reach the articular surface.

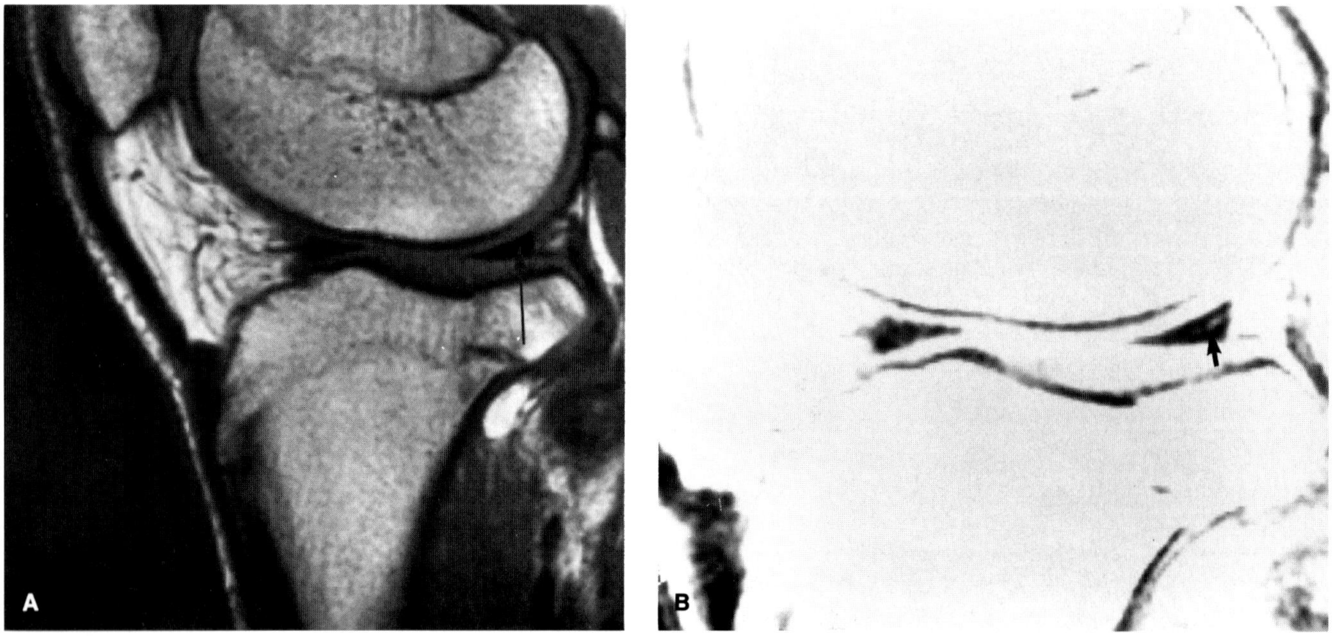

FIGURE 12–4. Grade II meniscal degeneration. **(A)** T1-weighted sagittal image (TR/TE = 800/17) and **(B)** meniscal window image demonstrate a thin, linear area of increased signal intensity (black arrow) in the posterior horn of the medial meniscus due to Grade II degenerative changes. The increased signal intensity within the meniscus does not reach the articular surface.

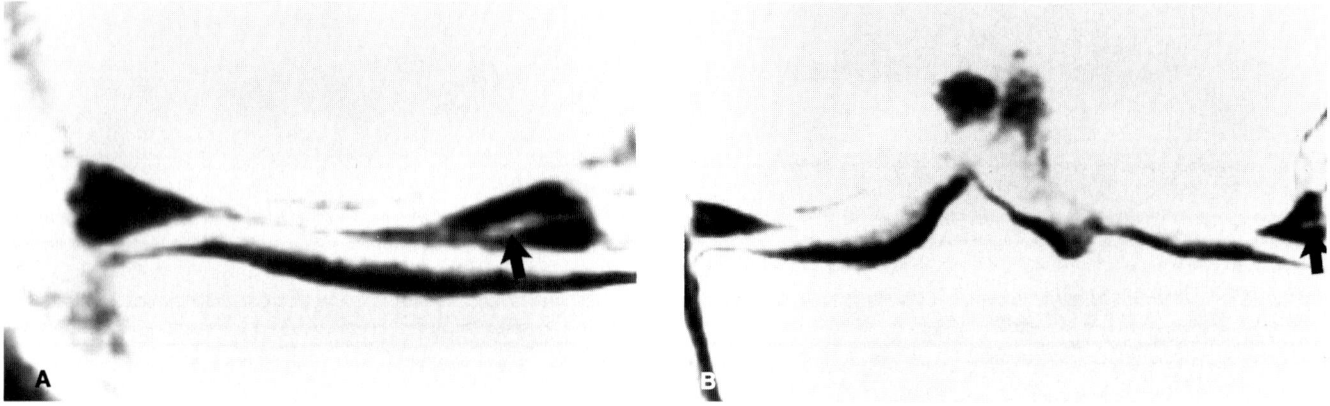

FIGURE 12–5. Grade III meniscal tear on **(A)** sagittal and **(B)** coronal T1-weighted images (TR/TE = 800/17). A linear area of increased signal intensity (arrow), extending to the articular surface, is demonstrated within the meniscus. Arthroscopy confirmed a meniscal tear.

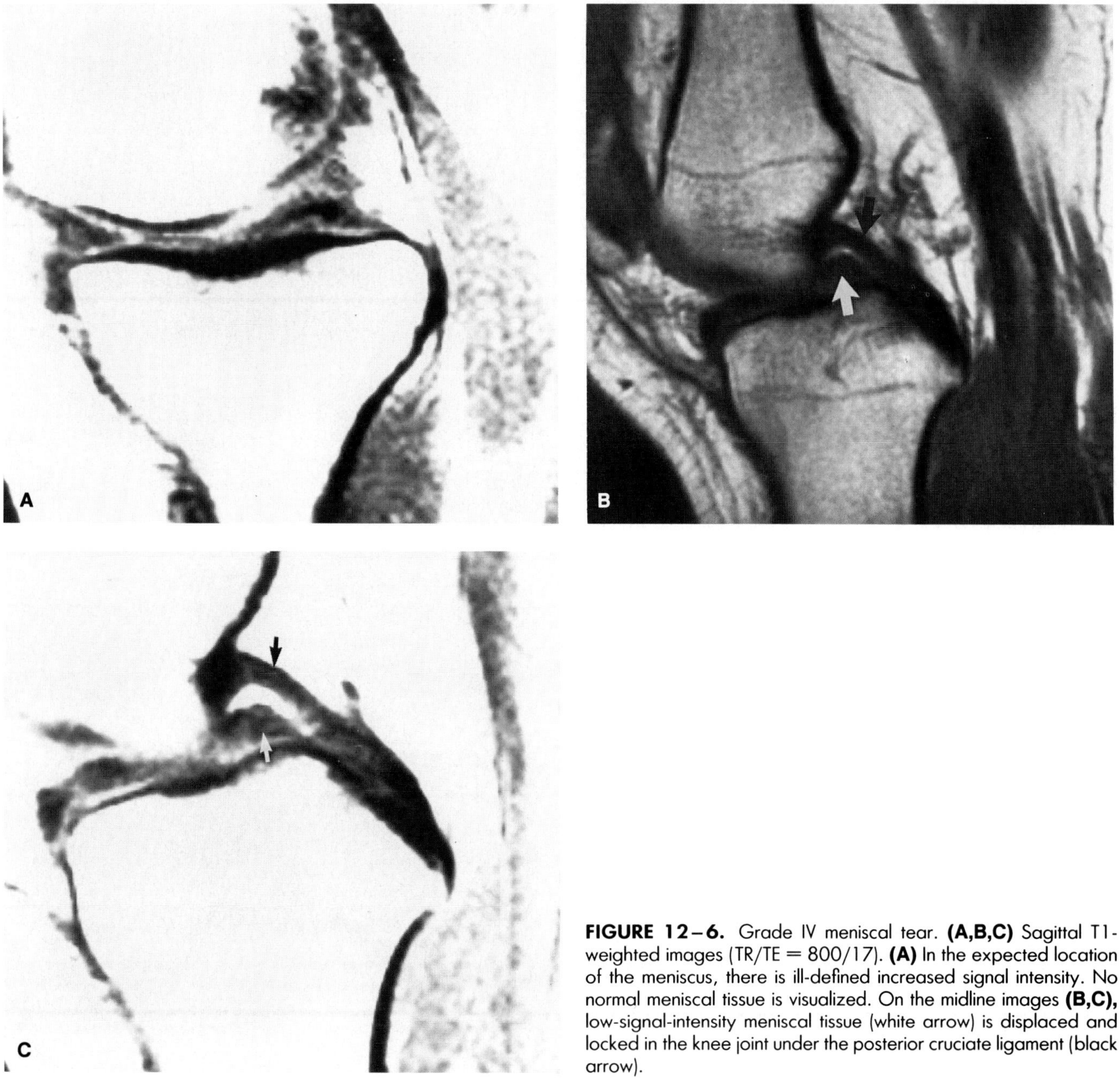

FIGURE 12–6. Grade IV meniscal tear. **(A,B,C)** Sagittal T1-weighted images (TR/TE = 800/17). **(A)** In the expected location of the meniscus, there is ill-defined increased signal intensity. No normal meniscal tissue is visualized. On the midline images **(B,C),** low-signal-intensity meniscal tissue (white arrow) is displaced and locked in the knee joint under the posterior cruciate ligament (black arrow).

A recent study correlated the bright intrameniscal signal (Grade 1 and 2) with meniscal degeneration, which is manifested as a yellow discoloration in arthroscopic and macroscopic inspection. The degeneration, called mucoid or myxoid degeneration, is believed to occur in as many as 60% of patients and increases with age. Initially, collagen bundles enlarge because increased glycan accumulation separates fibrils and induces microcyst formation. Later histologic changes consist of further degeneration of meniscal matrix and collagenization, fragmenting the collagen bundles. The final stage leads to horizontal or oblique meniscal tears along the direction of the collagen fibers.

Other causes of the bright intrameniscal signal do not appear to apply to adult menisci. One group of authors found that the bright signal can be due to perforating vessels in young individuals.[11] Perforating vessels reach the center of the meniscus in children, but not in adults. Stoller and colleagues reported that the increased signal represents a continuum from mucinous degeneration to tear, in which absorbed synovial fluid appears as high signal intensity.[12]

Meniscal tears should be diagnosed only if the high intrameniscal signal intensity reaches an articular surface, as in Grade 3 (Fig. 12–7) and Grade 4 (Fig. 12–8). High signal intensity confined to the meniscus, as in Grades 1 and 2, appears to represent degenera-

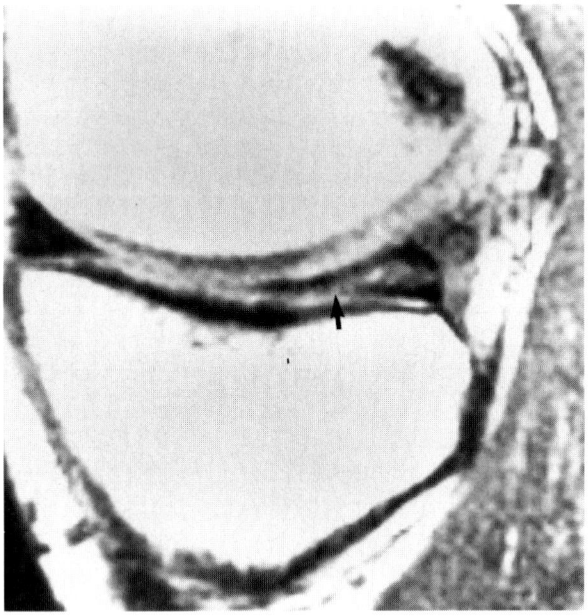

FIGURE 12–7. Grade III meniscal tear. Sagittal T1-weighted image (TR/TE = 800/17) with meniscal windows shows an area of increased signal intensity in the posterior medial meniscus extending to the articular surface (black arrow).

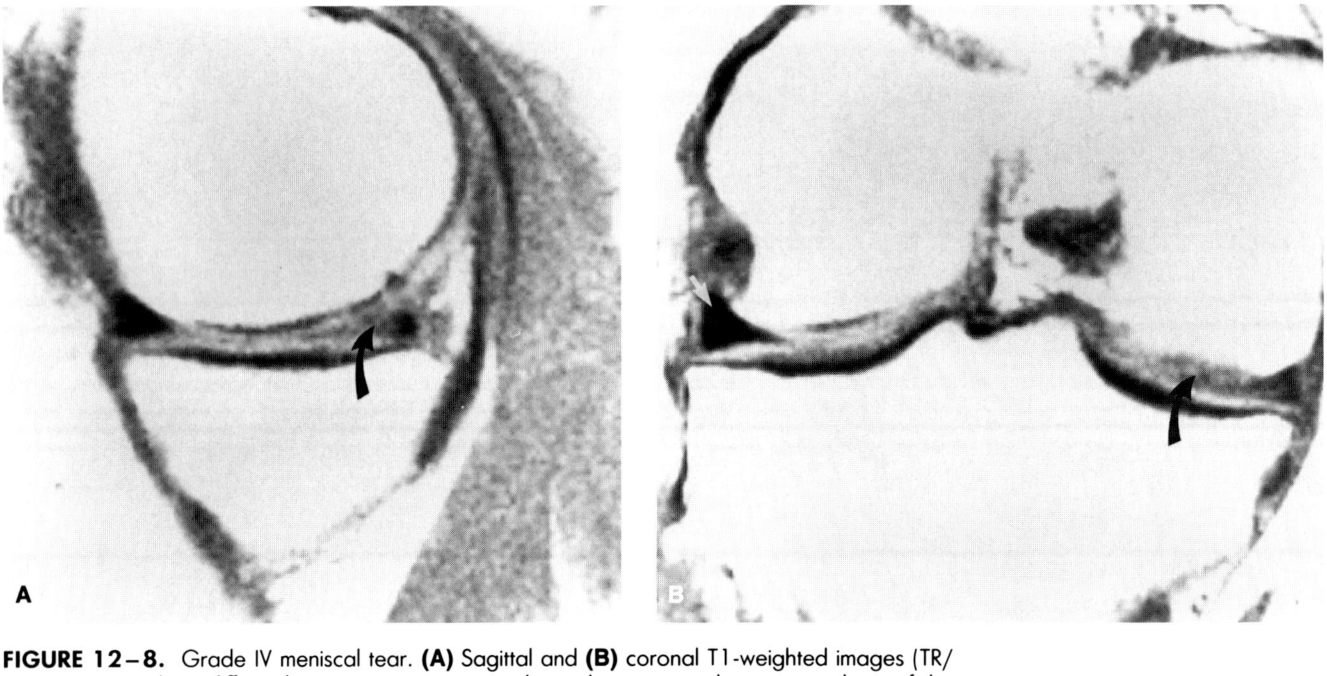

FIGURE 12–8. Grade IV meniscal tear. **(A)** Sagittal and **(B)** coronal T1-weighted images (TR/TE = 750/17) show diffuse, heterogeneous increased signal intensity in the posterior horn of the lateral meniscus (black arrow). There was no prior history of surgery. At arthroscopy, the lateral meniscus was disorganized and revealed multiple tears consistent with a Grade IV meniscal tear. Notice the normal medial meniscus on the coronal image, which has no intrameniscal signal (white arrow).

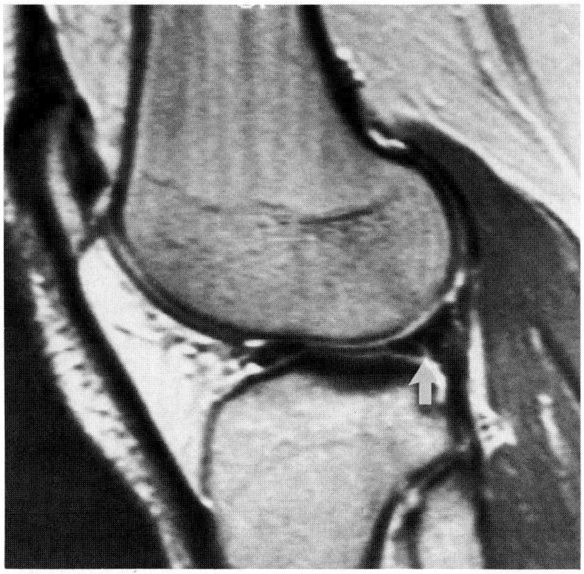

FIGURE 12–9. Bucket-handle tear. Sagittal T2-weighted image (TR/TE = 3000/45) shows a Y-shaped area of increased signal intensity in the posterior horn of the lateral meniscus (arrow). Subtle increased signal intensity extends into the anterior horn of the meniscus. Arthroscopy demonstrated a bucket-handle meniscal tear.

tive changes. Abnormalities confined to the meniscus that do not reach an articular surface may not be seen at arthroscopy. The clinical significance of intrameniscal signal is uncertain, and it is possible that MRI is more sensitive than arthroscopy and may become the gold standard in diagnosing abnormalities of the knee. The decision to perform meniscectomy currently is based exclusively on a surface tear.

Meniscal tears can be categorized by their configuration.[13] A bucket handle tear (Fig. 12–9) usually occurs as a result of an acute injury, most often involving the medial meniscus, beginning posteriorly and extending anteriorly. These tears are often seen as vertical high signal intensities on coronal images. Fragmentation (Grade 4) can produce the appearance of a small meniscus. However, it should be remembered that the posterior horn of the medial meniscus is normally 30% larger than the anterior horn. Horizontal tears (Fig. 12–10) are the most common symptomatic abnormality of the menisci and are usually produced by the late stages of degenerative changes. The parrot beak tear (Fig. 12–11) is a small tear located at the free edge of the body of the lateral meniscus. This is seen as blunting of the free edge of the meniscus, which normally is sharply defined. The discoid meniscus is an anatomic variant in which the body of the meniscus is seen on several (>3) images and often completely covers the tibial plateau.

Overreading of meniscal tears must be avoided so that unnecessary surgical procedures are minimized. Pitfalls in the diagnosis of meniscal tears can be caused by normal low-signal-intensity structures abutting the meniscus.[6] These structures include the

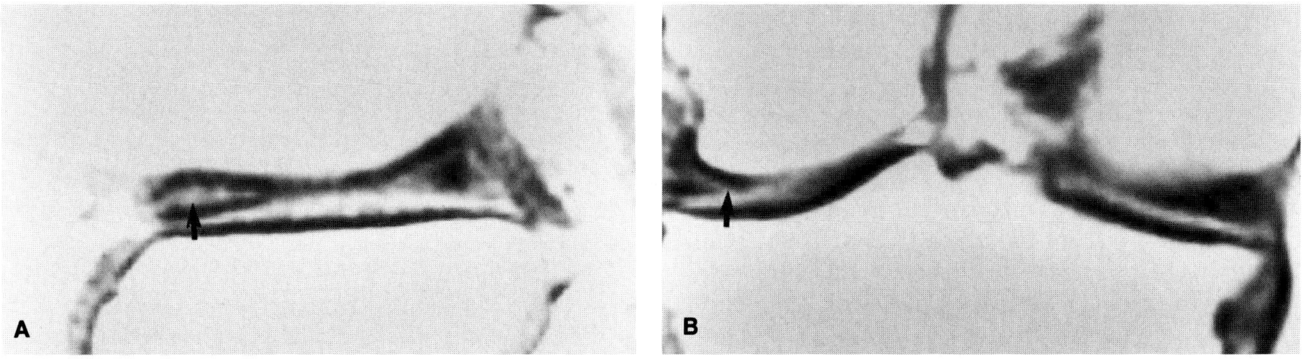

FIGURE 12–10. Horizontal meniscal tear. **(A)** Sagittal and **(B)** coronal T1-weighted images (TR/TE = 800/17). There is a linear area of increased signal intensity within the substance of the anterior lateral meniscus (black arrow) extending to the periphery of the meniscus on the sagittal image. The horizontal meniscal tear extends to the articular surface (black arrow) on the coronal image.

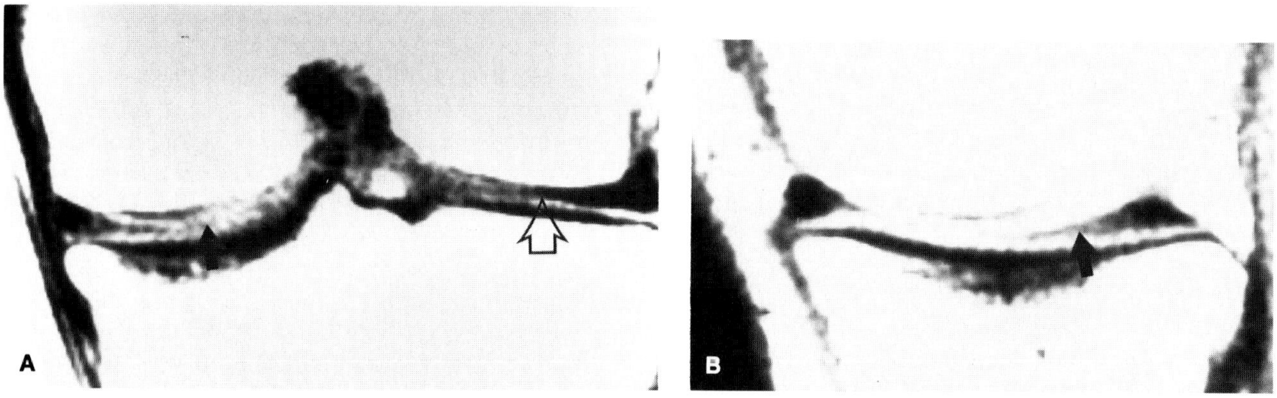

FIGURE 12–11. Parrot-beak meniscal tear. **(A)** Coronal and **(B)** sagittal T1-weighted images (TR/TE = 800/17) show blunting of the posterior medial meniscus (black arrow). There is ill-defined increased signal intensity at the free edge of the meniscus. The normally sharp demarcation of the free edge of the meniscus is not visualized. Compare this with the normal, sharply delineated free edge of the lateral meniscus (open arrow) on the coronal image. These findings represent a parrot-beak meniscal tear, which is the most commonly overlooked meniscal abnormality on MRI scans of the knee.

lateral inferior genicular artery, the transverse ligament, and the popliteus tendon. Pitfalls also arise from volume averaging artifacts.

The lateral inferior genicular artery arises from the popliteal artery at the level of the tibiofemoral joint and courses laterally to the anterior aspect of the knee, where it lies in a fat pad between the meniscus and the lateral collateral ligament. When it lies adjacent to the anterior horn of the lateral meniscus, the space between it and the meniscus may simulate a tear (Fig. 12–12). Usually the artery can be traced on adjacent sagittal images, which help differentiate it from a tear. The coronal images often show the artery as a separate structure from the meniscus.

The transverse ligament, popliteus tendon, and the meniscus are composed of type 1 collagen, and therefore they render no signal on T1-weighted and T2-weighted sequences. The transverse ligament arises from the anterior aspect of the medial meniscus and attaches to the anterior aspect of the lateral meniscus. A space between it and the anterior aspect of the medial meniscus can appear like a tear (Fig. 12–13). The coronal view will help differentiate this from a true tear. The popliteus tendon separates the lateral meniscus from the joint capsule and the lateral collateral ligament. A space between the posterior lateral meniscus and the popliteus tendon can mimic a tear on sagittal images (Fig. 12–14). Coronal views can better delineate the true anatomy.

Volume averaging can also simulate meniscal disease. Sagittal images through the periphery of the meniscus may demonstrate an artifactual, linear high signal intensity in the meniscus due to averaging of fat at the concavity of the periphery of the meniscus. This

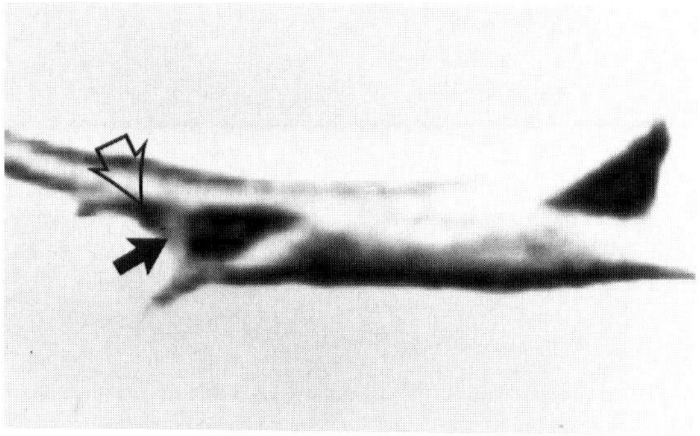

FIGURE 12–12. Lateral inferior genicular artery pitfall simulating a meniscal tear. Sagittal T1-weighted image (TR/TE = 800/17) of the knee shows a linear area of increased signal intensity (black arrow) between the anterior horn of the lateral meniscus and the lateral inferior genicular artery (open arrow), simulating a meniscal tear.

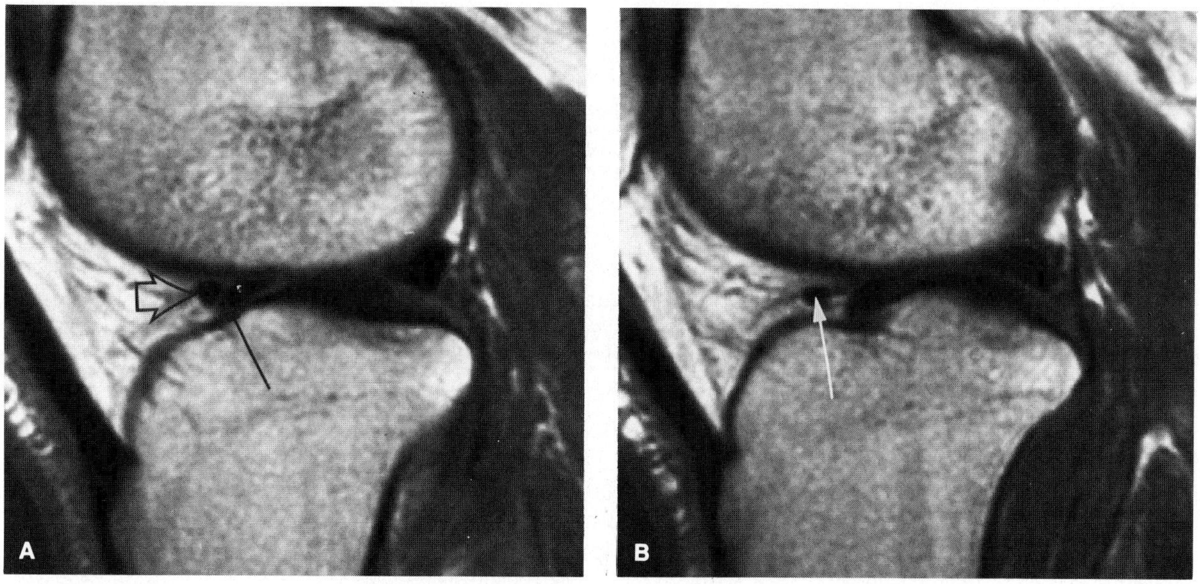

FIGURE 12–13. Transverse ligament pitfall. Sagittal T1-weighted images (TR/TE = 800/17) reveal **(A)** a linear area of increased signal intensity (black arrow) between the anterior medial meniscus and the transverse ligament (open arrow), which simulates a meniscal tear. An adjacent image **(B)** demonstrates the transverse ligament (white arrow) as it moves farther anteriorly from the adjacent medial meniscus.

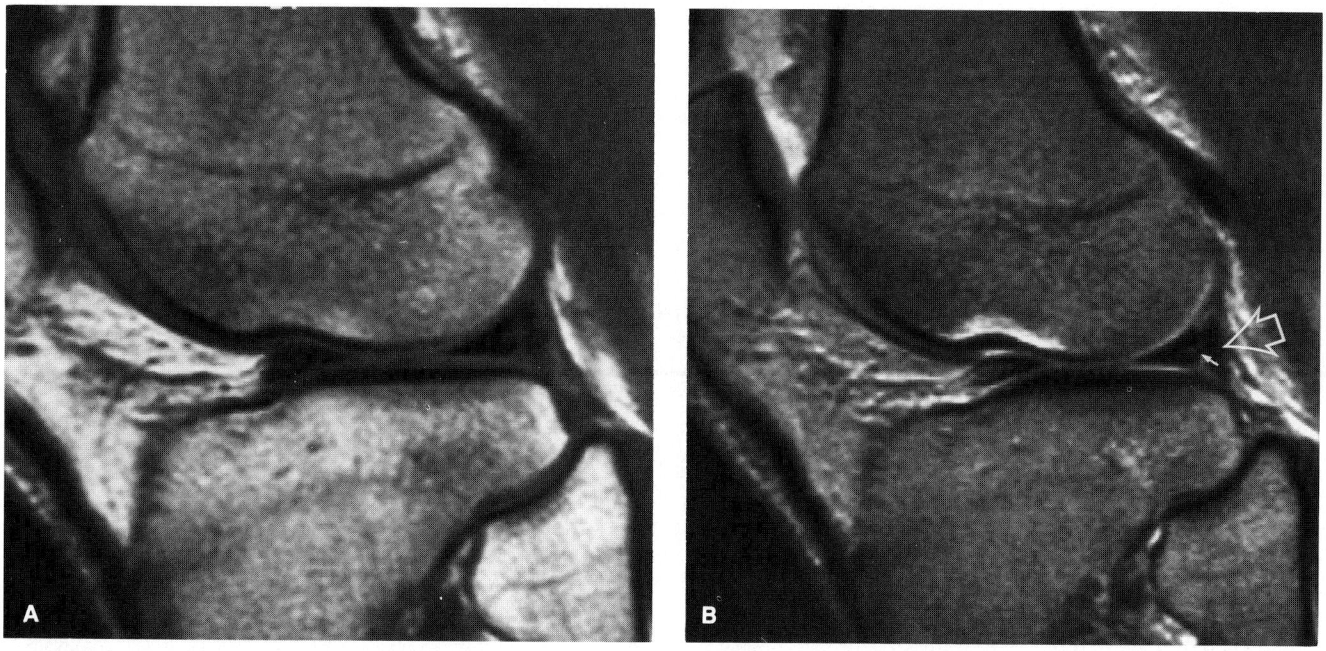

FIGURE 12–14. Popliteus tendon pitfall. **(A)** Sagittal T1-weighted image (TR/TE = 800/17) and **(B)** sagittal T2-weighted image (TR/TE = 3000/45). A linear area of increased signal intensity is demonstrated (arrow) between the posterior lateral meniscus and the popliteus tendon (open arrow), simulating a meniscal tear. Notice the increased signal intensity in the bone marrow of the femoral condyle on the T2-weighted image that is presumably due to previous trauma.

pitfall can be avoided by correlating with coronal images or by using thinner slices (4–5 mm).

Bucket handle tears can be missed on sagittal images because the tear is oriented in the plane of section. This is identified on the coronal images as a vertical high-signal-intensity tear.

The postoperative meniscus presents a difficult challenge for MRI. Comparison with the normal, opposite meniscus and correlation with clinical history are helpful for arriving at the correct diagnosis. After a partial meniscectomy, the residual meniscal tissue appears smaller than the opposite, normal meniscus. After a complete meniscectomy, no residual meniscus is demonstrated (Fig. 12–15). A recent study suggests that the MR characteristics for meniscal tears in the virgin meniscus do not hold well in the postoperative meniscus.[14] In particular, a linear area of increased signal intensity in the meniscus extending to the articular surface suggests retear, but caution must be used because 5 of 17 cases with this finding were false positives. Another common finding is diffuse increased signal intensity in the meniscal remnant, which should be considered to be a stable finding, not indicating a retear. Further work is needed to accurately establish the criteria for retear.

Ligaments

Injuries of the ligaments are common in acute knee trauma. The clinical examination plays a crucial role in evaluating ligamentous injuries, but it can be inaccurate. MR examination of the knee can accurately evaluate the ligaments, including the anterior cruciate ligament (ACL), posterior cruciate ligament (PCL), and the medial and lateral collateral ligaments.

The cruciate ligaments provide stability to the knee. The ACL prevents hyperextension of the knee and acts as a rotational guide for the femoral condyles. The PCL acts as a check against extreme hyperextension and maintains stability of the knee when the joint is flexed.[15] Clinically, a tear of the ACL or PCL is diagnosed by an abnormal anterior drawer sign or posterior drawer sign, respectively. Recent studies show the sensitivity of MRI for ACL tear to be 94% with a specificity of 100%, compared with clinical sensitivity by anterior drawer sign of 78%.[8,16] These studies also demonstrated a 95% accuracy for diagnosing ACL tears by MRI, compared with arthroscopic accuracy ranging from 60 to 95%.[8]

The ACL originates at the posterior inner surface of the lateral femoral condyle and attaches to the tibia anterior and lateral to the anterior tibial spine. The PCL extends from the lateral surface of the medial femoral condyle to a depression behind the interarticular upper surface of the tibia (Fig. 12–16).[15] The cruciate ligaments are best demonstrated on sagittal images, and the ACL is seen best with the knee externally rotated 15°. The collateral ligaments extend from the femur to the tibia, lateral and medial to the joint, and are optimally visualized on neutrally positioned coronal images. Normally, the ligaments are smooth, continuous, low-signal-intensity fibers on

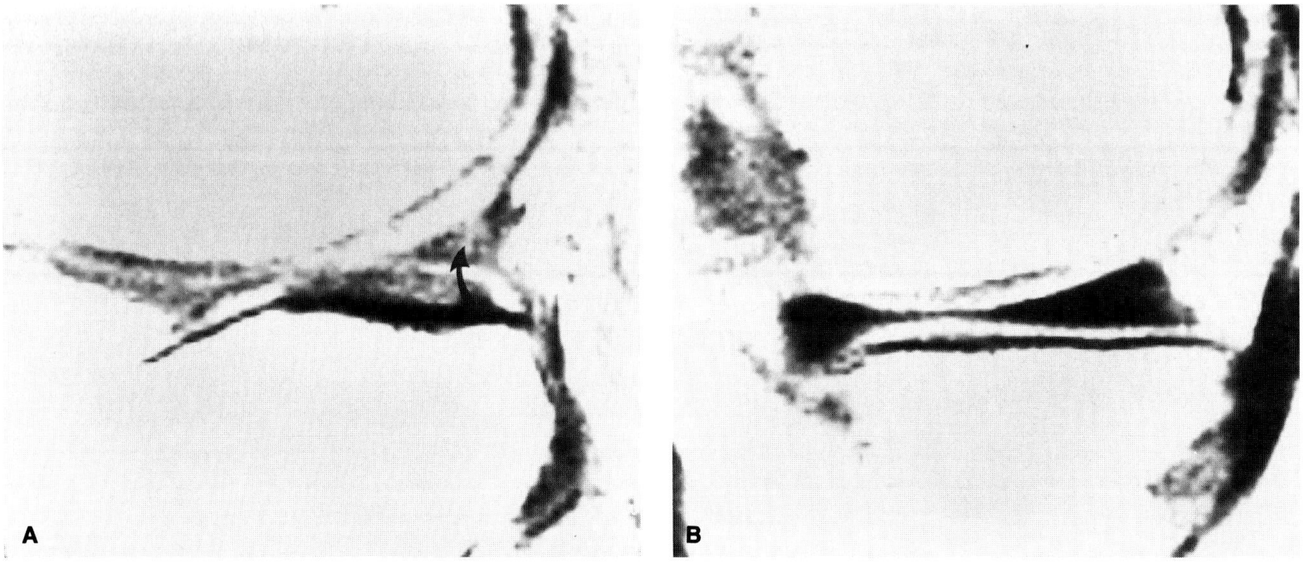

FIGURE 12–15. Lateral meniscectomy. **(A,B)** Sagittal T1-weighted images (TR/TE = 800/17). Image of the lateral meniscus **(A)** shows heterogeneous increased signal intensity in the expected location of the meniscus after a lateral meniscectomy (arrow). No normal meniscal tissue is seen. Compare this with the normal, homogeneous, low-signal-intensity medial meniscus demonstrated on a sagittal T1-weighted image **(B)**.

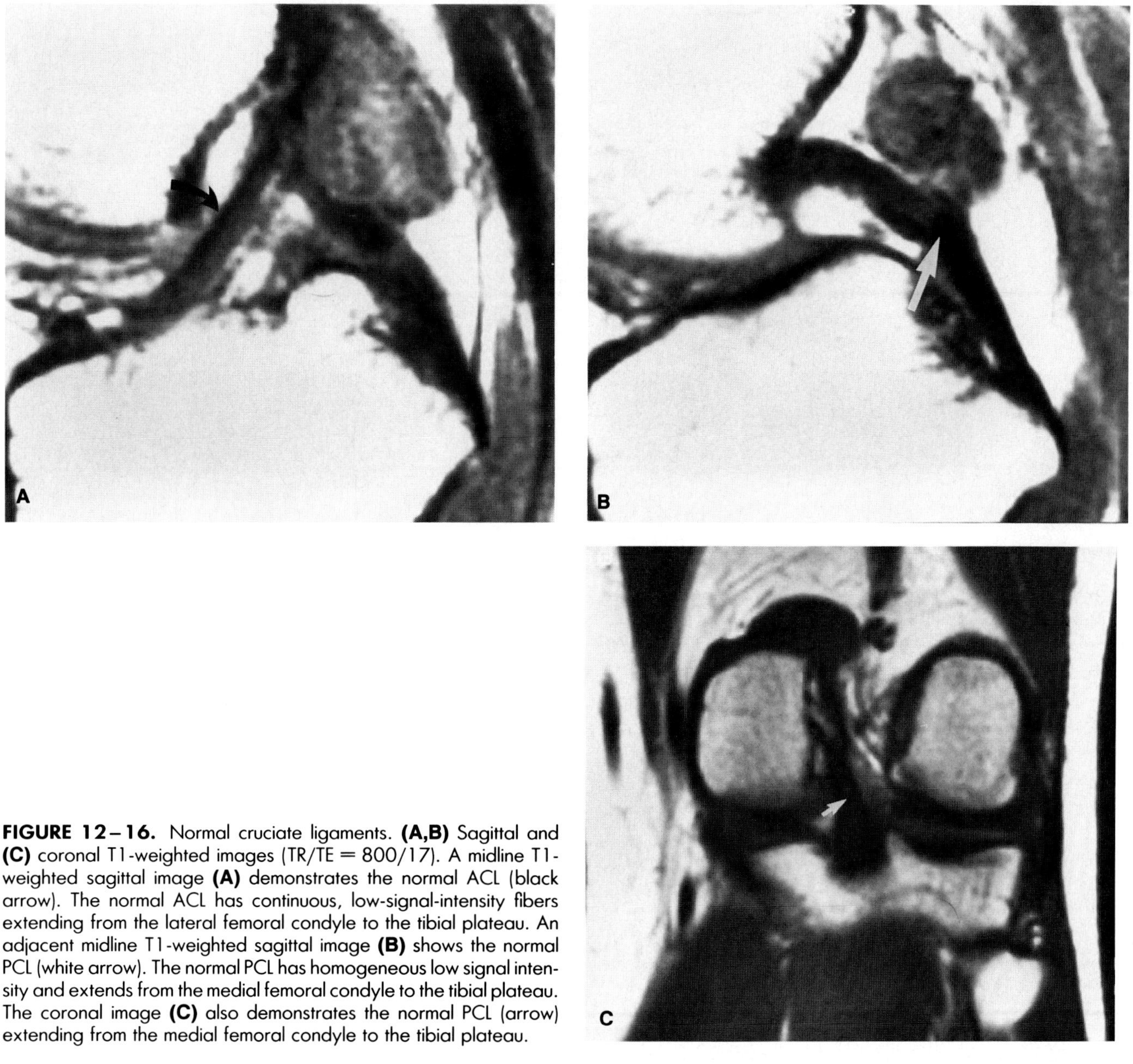

FIGURE 12–16. Normal cruciate ligaments. **(A,B)** Sagittal and **(C)** coronal T1-weighted images (TR/TE = 800/17). A midline T1-weighted sagittal image **(A)** demonstrates the normal ACL (black arrow). The normal ACL has continuous, low-signal-intensity fibers extending from the lateral femoral condyle to the tibial plateau. An adjacent midline T1-weighted sagittal image **(B)** shows the normal PCL (white arrow). The normal PCL has homogeneous low signal intensity and extends from the medial femoral condyle to the tibial plateau. The coronal image **(C)** also demonstrates the normal PCL (arrow) extending from the medial femoral condyle to the tibial plateau.

T1-weighted and T2-weighted images. The normal ACL has a slightly higher signal intensity than the PCL.

Tears of the ACL typically occur in the middle portion of the ligament.[16] Tears usually are caused by external rotational injuries, occurring in abduction and 90° flexion. There are often associated tears of the collateral ligaments or meniscus. The diagnosis of an ACL tear is made on MRI by identifying disruption of the ligament along its normal course (Fig. 12–17).

A finding suggesting a partial tear of the ligament is foci of increased signal intensity within the substance of the ligament, often seen best on T2-weighted images (Fig. 12–18).[8] T2-weighted images create an arthrographic effect, normally showing the straight smooth synovial reflection along the anterior margin of the ACL. Irregularity or waviness of this reflection should suggest a partial tear of the ACL.[16]

Acute angulation of the proximal portion of the PCL is overwhelming evidence for a tear of the ACL. The tear in the ACL causes anterior subluxation of the tibia, which pulls the PCL with it, creating a buckle in the proximal portion of the PCL.[8]

Tears of the PCL are diagnosed by disruption along the course of the ligament or by areas of increased signal intensity within the substance of the ligament (Fig. 12–19). Tears in the collateral ligaments manifest as disruptions of the ligament or as abnormal high

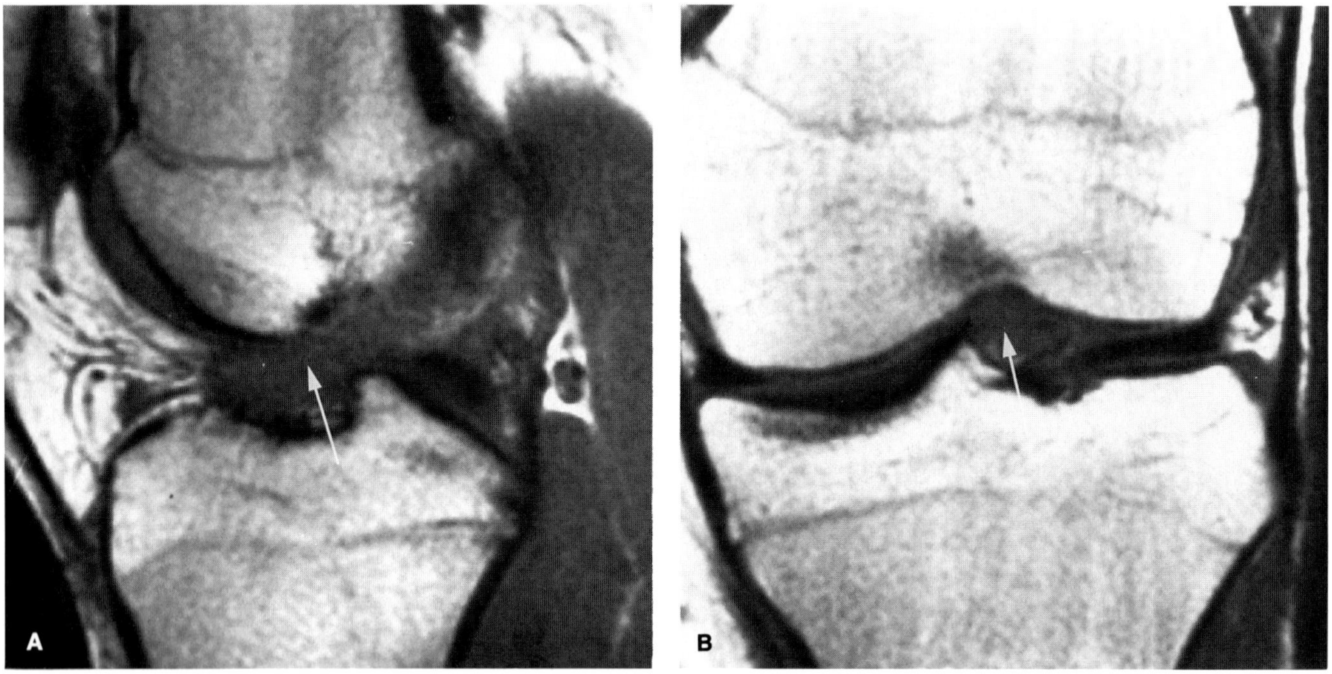

FIGURE 12–17. Complete ACL tear. **(A)** Sagittal and **(B)** coronal T1-weighted images (TR/TE = 800/17) demonstrate abnormal, intermediate-signal-intensity soft tissue in the expected location of the ACL. No normal ACL fibers are identified. These findings indicate a complete ACL tear (arrow).

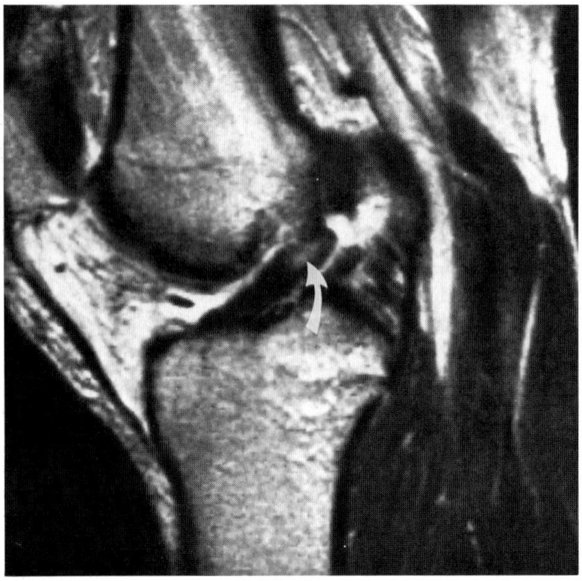

FIGURE 12–18. Partial ACL tear. Sagittal T2-weighted image (TR/TE = 3000/90) identifies a focus of increased signal intensity in the substance of the proximal ACL (arrow).

signal intensity in the adjacent soft tissues that often displaces the ligament, indicating bleeding or edema (Fig. 12–20).[17]

Cartilage

Before MRI, noninvasive techniques capable of imaging the articular cartilage did not exist. Despite all the attention paid to meniscal and ligament damage, injury to hyaline cartilage potentially causes the most serious long-term effects. Damage to the cartilage can predispose patients to premature degenerative arthritis. Injured hyaline cartilage has a limited ability to repair due to its poor vascular supply. Therefore, a noninvasive modality that can assess cartilaginous defects and follow treatment is very useful. On spin echo techniques, hyaline cartilage appears as a gray area overlying the dark subchondral bone.[18] Other authors have reported that gradient-echo techniques, such as FISP or GRASS, may better demonstrate hya-

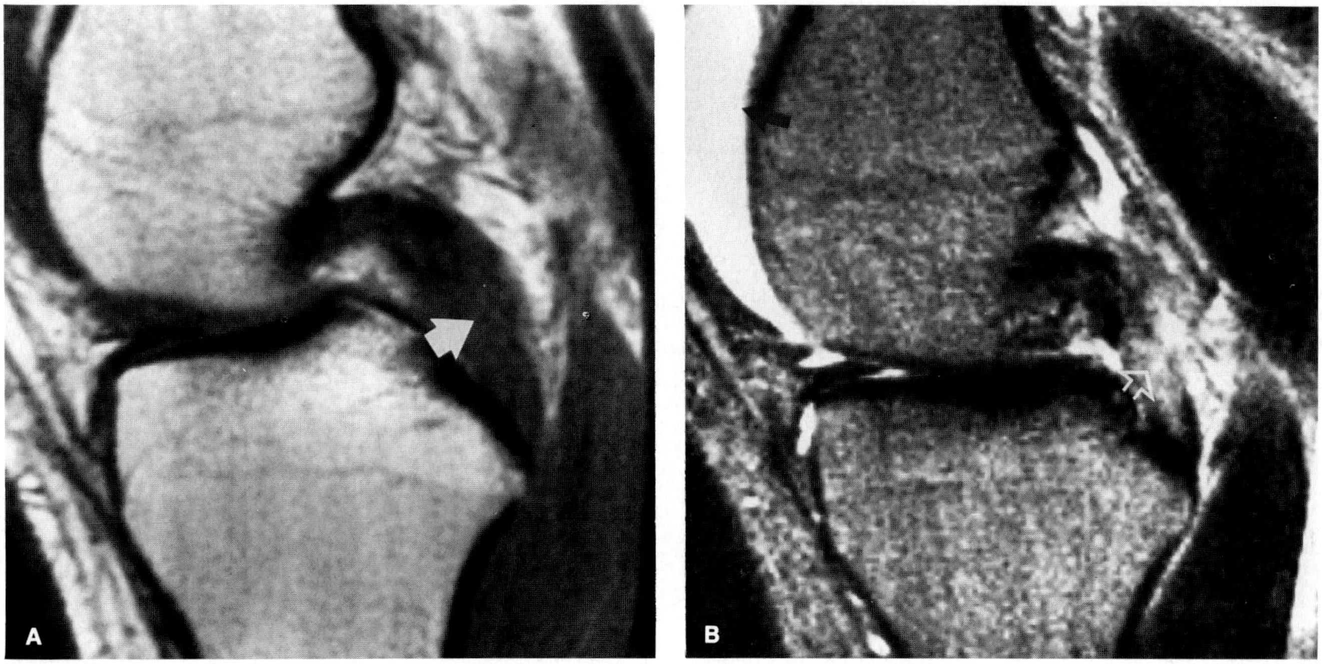

FIGURE 12–19. PCL tear. **(A)** Sagittal T1-weighted image (TR/TE = 800/17) reveals widening of the PCL and intermediate signal intensity within the substance of the PCL consistent with a tear (arrow). **(B)** The T2-weighted sagittal image (TR/TE = 3000/90) shows increased signal intensity within the substance of the PCL, indicating the site of ligament tear (open arrow). Notice also a large joint effusion (black arrow).

line cartilage.[3,5] With these techniques, the cartilage appears as high signal intensity adjacent to the dark cortical bone.

Injuries of the cartilage appear as irregularities or low signal defects. A grading system of cartilage injuries has been proposed:[18]

Grade 0—normal cartilage
Grade 1—surface and texture changes, but no cartilage substance loss
Grade 2—partial-thickness cartilage loss, but no exposed bone
Grade 3—exposed bone

The majority of cartilage defects occur along the femoral condylar surface. A search for cartilaginous injuries is essential to the complete evaluation of the knee.

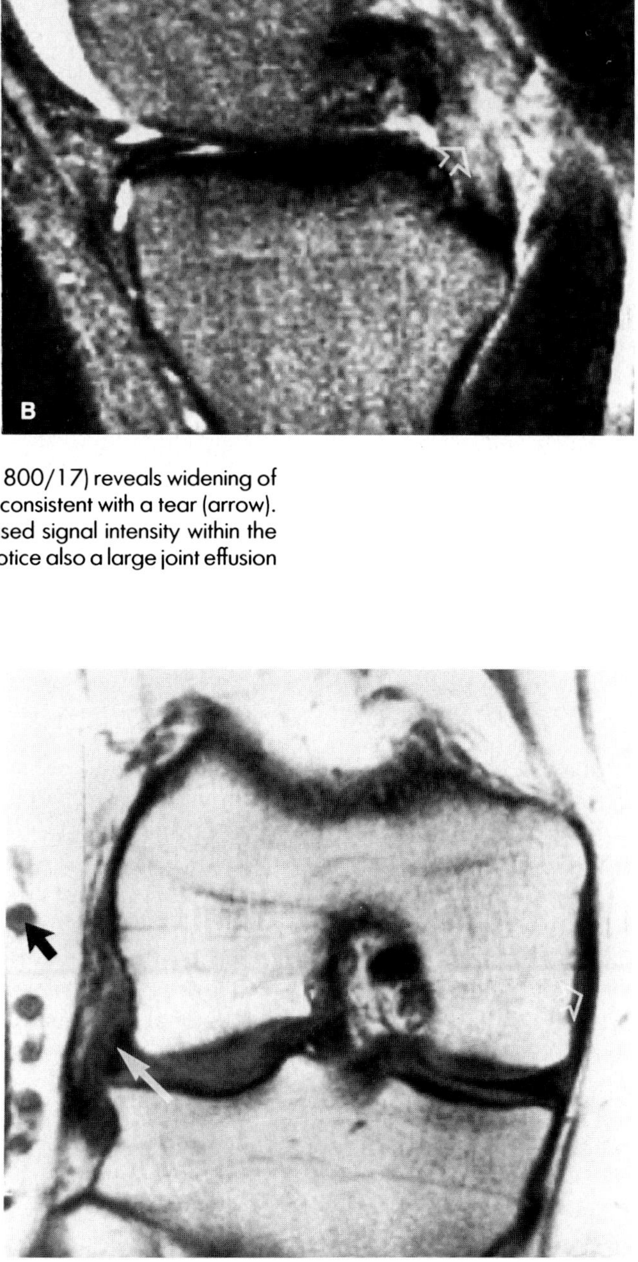

FIGURE 12–20. Lateral collateral ligament tear. Coronal T1-weighted image (TR/TE = 800/17) only partially visualizes the lateral collateral ligament. More importantly, intermediate-signal-intensity and increased-signal-intensity soft tissue is visualized between the lateral collateral ligament and the lateral femoral condyle, representing edema and hemorrhage at the site of the collateral ligament tear (white arrow). Notice the continuous low-signal-intensity, normal medial collateral ligament (open arrow). Incidentally visualized are rounded areas of intermediate signal intensity in the subcutaneous fat at the lateral aspect of the knee, representing varicose veins (black arrow).

Bone Marrow

Many unsuspected abnormalities have been identified within the bone marrow by MRI while scanning the knee. A common finding is an area of decreased signal intensity on T1-weighted images and a corresponding area of increased signal intensity on T2-weighted scans in the subchondral bone marrow (Fig. 12–21). Recent studies have suggested that these areas represent osteonecrosis or microfractures with

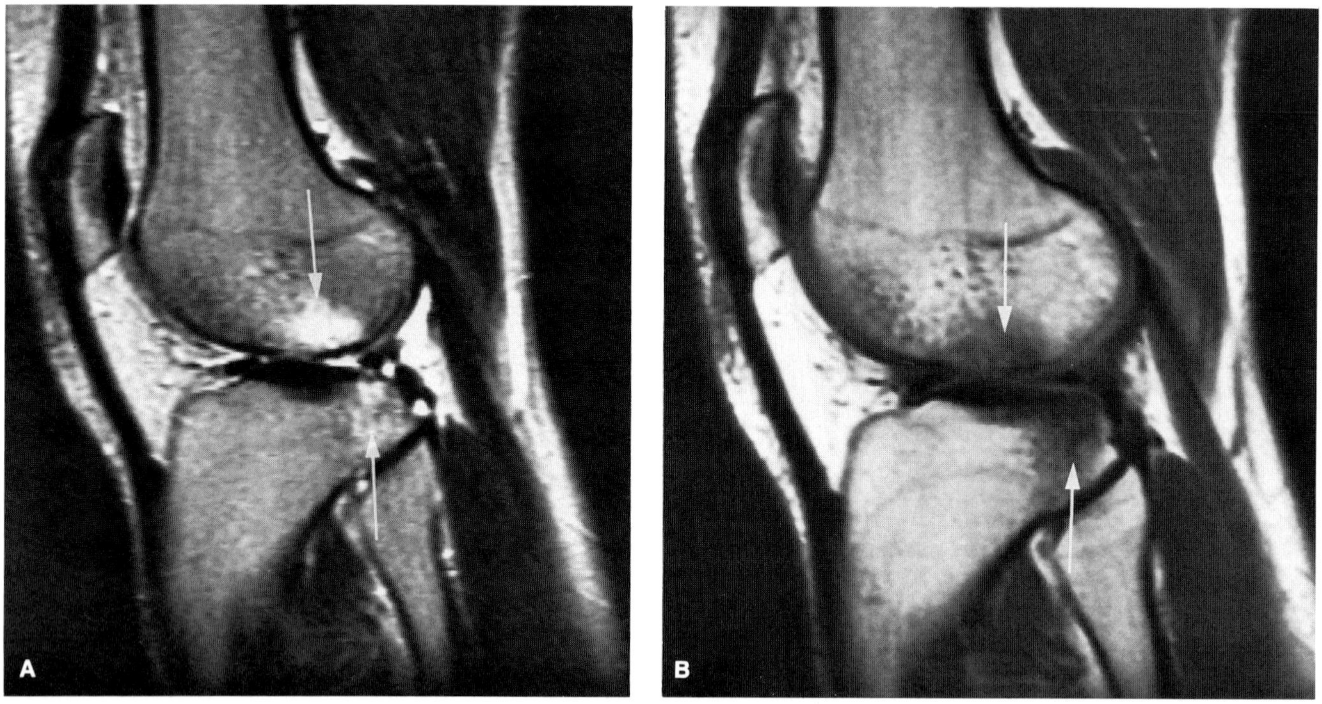

FIGURE 12–21. Bone edema. **(A)** Sagittal T2-weighted image (TR/TE = 3000/90) and **(B)** sagittal T1-weighted image (TR/TE = 800/17). An abnormal area of increased signal intensity is identified in the distal lateral femoral condyle and to a lesser degree in the tibial plateau on the T2-weighted image. This is a common finding, most likely caused by trauma, and presumably represents osteonecrosis or bone edema (arrows). The T1-weighted sagittal image shows low signal intensity in the bone marrow corresponding to the areas of increased signal intensity on the T2-weighted image.

associated edema or hemorrhage.[19,20] Correlative radiographs usually do not show an abnormality. Follow-up MR scans have shown reversibility in some of these lesions.

Another bony abnormality described is medullary infarction, which often presents as a discrete low-signal ring or an area of decreased signal intensity surrounding a high-intensity core on T1-weighted images (Fig. 12–22).[19] Osteochondritis dissecans typically manifests as a fragment of bone with low or moderate signal intensity on T1-weighted images and various degrees of increased signal intensity on T2-weighted images (Fig. 12–23).[21] Separation of the bone fragment, a fluid interface between the fragment and parent bone, or disruption of the articular cartilage represents loosening, which requires surgical treatment.[21] MRI is not very effective in locating small calcified intra-articular loose bodies and computed tomography (CT) or standard radiography is more sensitive.[19]

Joint Fluid

Cystic lesions around the knee are common. By far, the most prevalent of these lesions is the popliteal (Baker's) cyst. This manifests as a rounded focus of intermediate signal intensity on T1-weighted images and increased signal intensity on T2-weighted images (Fig. 12–24). These cysts are usually located posterior to the knee joint, at the region of the gastrocnemius-semimembranosus bursa.[22]

Less common cystic lesions include meniscal and ganglion cysts.[23] These cysts occur in locations atypical for simple popliteal cysts. A meniscal cyst is synovial fluid, forced out through an underlying meniscal tear, which accumulates at the meniscocapsular margin on the medial or lateral surface of the knee joint. Meniscal cysts are always associated with underlying horizontal meniscal tears (Fig. 12–25). Ganglion cysts may occur in atypical locations, attached to tendon sheaths, within muscle bundles, or adjacent to the tibiofibular joint. Ganglion cysts are not associated with meniscal tears. They may or may not have a connection with the joint space. On MRI, meniscal and ganglion cysts have intermediate signal intensity on T1-weighted scans and bright signal intensity on T2-weighted scans.

Effusions can accompany knee injuries or be an isolated finding. Like other fluid, effusions have intermediate signal intensity on T1-weighted scans and increased signal intensity on T2-weighted scans (Fig.

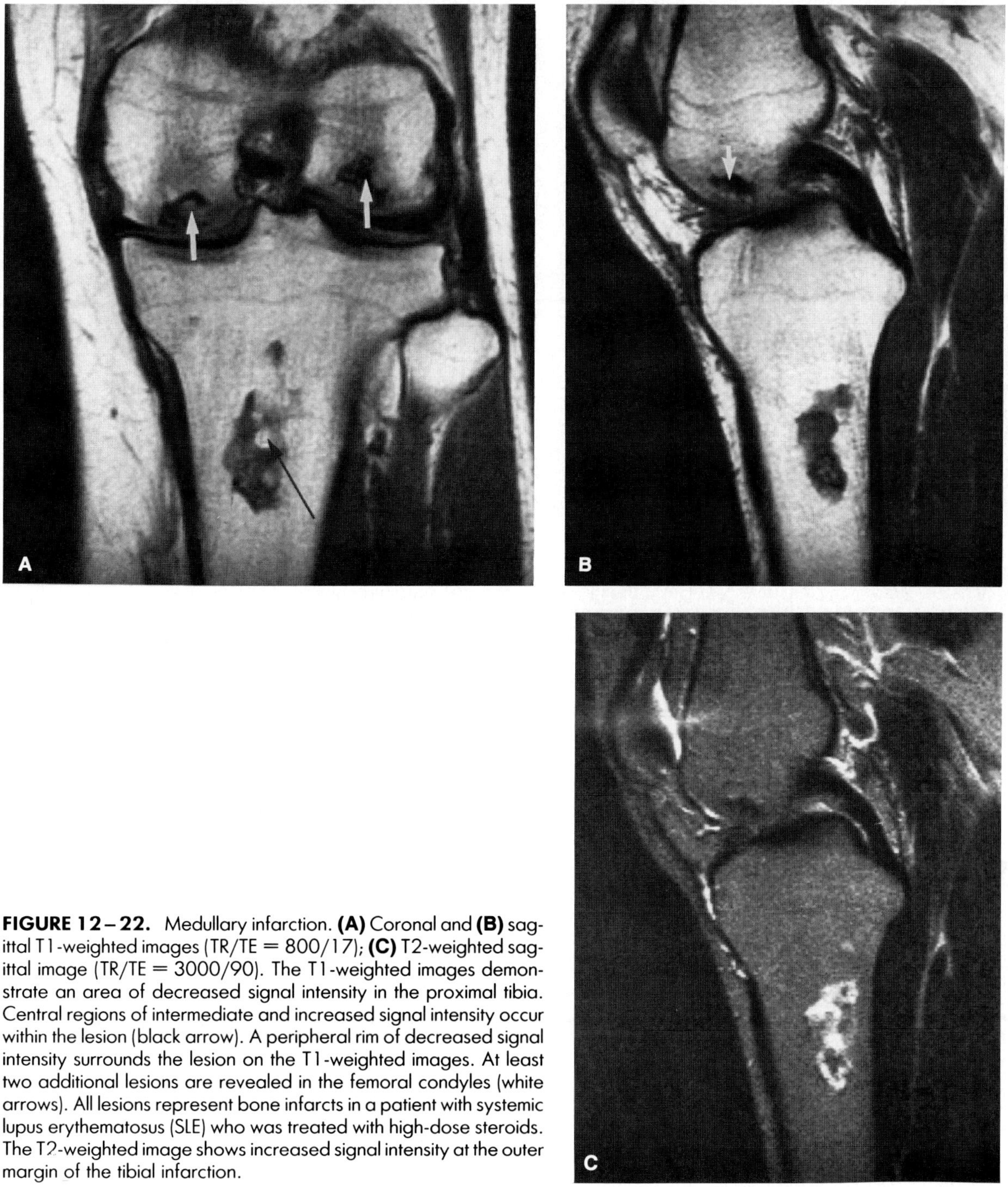

FIGURE 12–22. Medullary infarction. **(A)** Coronal and **(B)** sagittal T1-weighted images (TR/TE = 800/17); **(C)** T2-weighted sagittal image (TR/TE = 3000/90). The T1-weighted images demonstrate an area of decreased signal intensity in the proximal tibia. Central regions of intermediate and increased signal intensity occur within the lesion (black arrow). A peripheral rim of decreased signal intensity surrounds the lesion on the T1-weighted images. At least two additional lesions are revealed in the femoral condyles (white arrows). All lesions represent bone infarcts in a patient with systemic lupus erythematosus (SLE) who was treated with high-dose steroids. The T2-weighted image shows increased signal intensity at the outer margin of the tibial infarction.

12–26). An exception is a bloody effusion, which can, as in hemophilia, have a high signal intensity on T1-weighted images.

Chondromalacia Patella

Chondromalacia patella is a common cause of patellofemoral pain, primarily affecting adolescents and young adults. Most often the cause is repeated minor trauma or an acute traumatic event leading to damage of the posterior patellar hyaline articular cartilage. MRI has been effective in diagnosing chondromalacia patella and correlated with arthroscopic findings in 17 of 19 cases in one study.[24]

The normal patellar hyaline cartilage conforms to the posterior aspect of the patella, completely covers the posterior cortical bone, and has a smooth surface. Various degrees of abnormality can be seen on MRI in

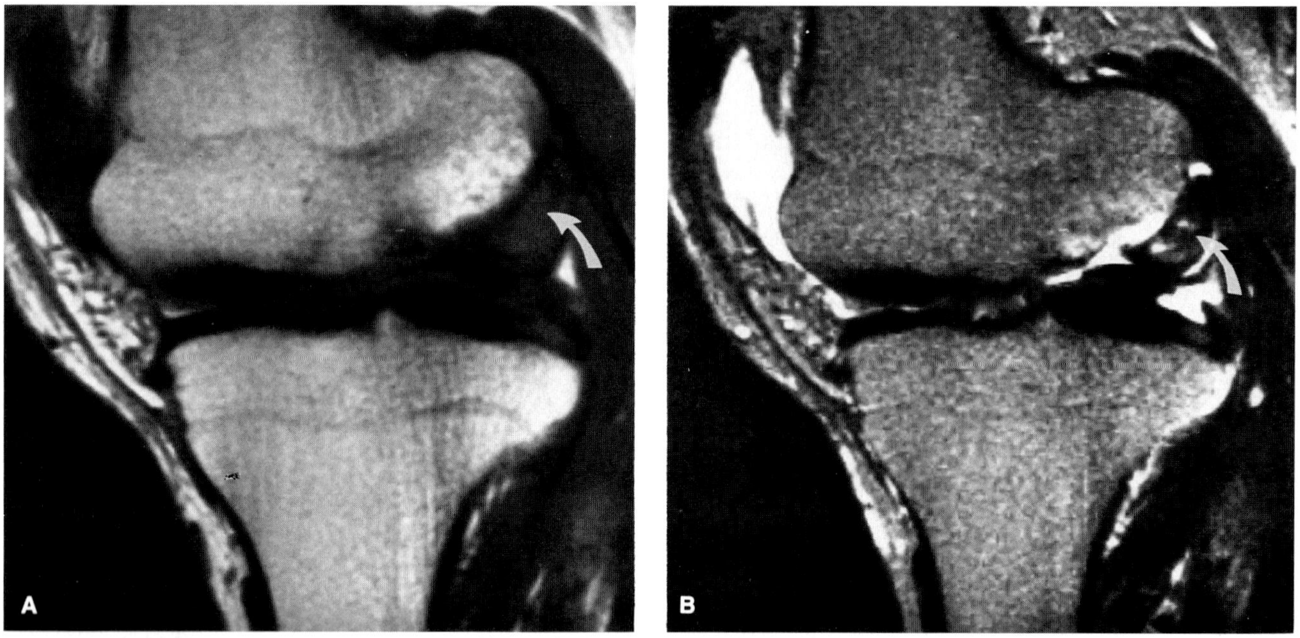

FIGURE 12–23. Osteochondritis dissecans. **(A)** Sagittal T1-weighted image (TR/TE = 800/17) and **(B)** sagittal T2-weighted image (TR/TE = 3000/90). The T1-weighted image shows a large, free bone fragment (arrow), which has decreased signal intensity compared with the normal increased signal intensity in the adjacent parent bone marrow (femur). The T2-weighted image shows heterogeneous signal intensity in the bone fragment (arrow). A bright-signal-intensity rim of fluid surrounds the bone fragment, indicating that the fragment is loose within the joint.

chondromalacia patella.[24] Early findings include focal regions of swelling, with areas of low signal intensity on T1-weighted and T2-weighted images in the patellar cartilage. Later, irregularity of the articular cartilage surface and focal sites of thinning can be seen. In the final stage, absence of the cartilage exposes the subchondral bone. Occasionally, high-signal-intensity synovial fluid can be identified passing through the cartilage defect toward the bone surface on T2-weighted images. To properly evaluate the patellar cartilage, axial and sagittal images must be obtained.

Pigmented Villonodular Synovitis

Pigmented villonodular synovitis (PVNS) is an uncommon disorder of unknown cause. The two best-accepted theories for PVNS are that it represents either a chronic inflammatory response to an unknown, nontraumatic irritant, or a benign neoplasm of synovial or fibrohistiocytic origin.[25] Pathologically, PVNS consists of villous or nodular hyperplasia of the synovium, with hemosiderin and lipid deposition.[25,26] PVNS occurs most commonly in the third to sixth decades of life, with an equal sexual prevalence. Presenting symptoms are progressive pain, swelling, and decreased range of motion of the involved joint. PVNS is usually a monoarticular process, occurring in the knee 80% of the time. Other joints may be involved, particularly the hip, elbow, ankle, and shoulder.[25,27,28]

The radiographic findings in PVNS include soft tissue swelling, which often has increased density in the synovium due to hemosiderin deposition, subchondral cysts, cortical pressure erosions, and late joint-space narrowing.[25] Other conditions that may be confused radiographically with PVNS are uncalcified synovial chondromatosis, tuberculous arthritis, hemophilic arthropathy, and synovial hemangiomas.[25,27]

In diagnosing PVNS, classic MRI signal characteristics have been described.[27,28] On T1-weighted images, the nodules of PVNS have intermediate signal intensity, similar to or slightly higher than muscle. On T2-weighted scans, PVNS has increased signal intensity, representing fluid and congested synovium. Most importantly, on T2-weighted images there are interspersed areas of low signal intensity due to hemosiderin deposition (Figs. 12–27 and 12–28). Combining the clinical history, plain films, and MRI findings enables a specific diagnosis of PVNS to be made most of the time.

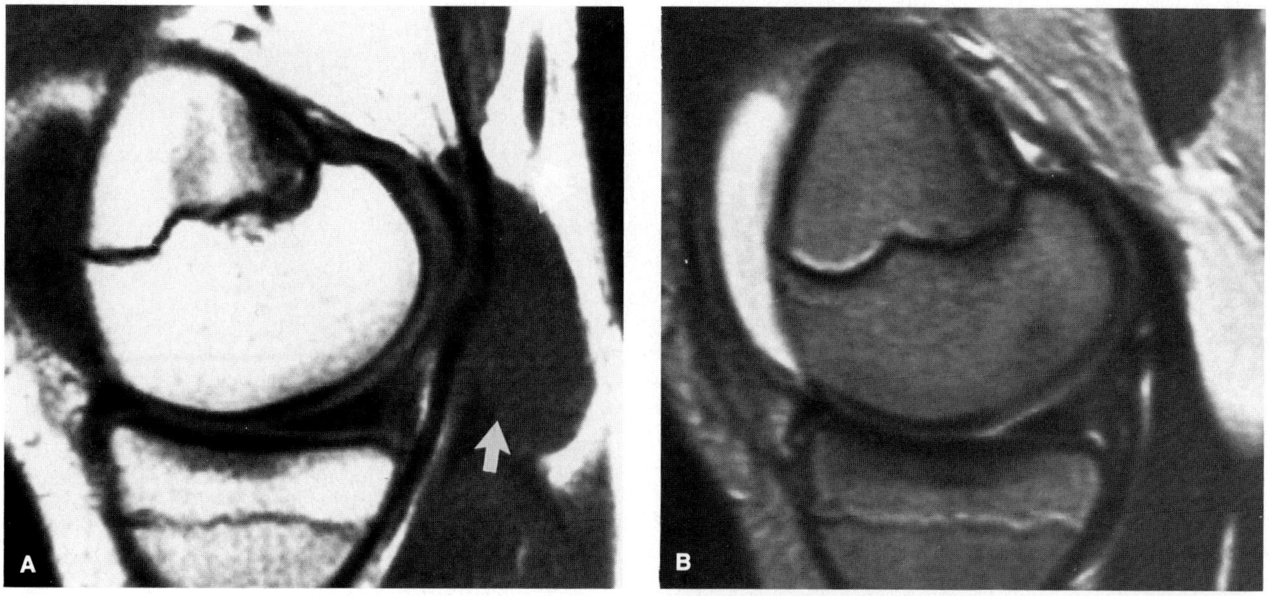

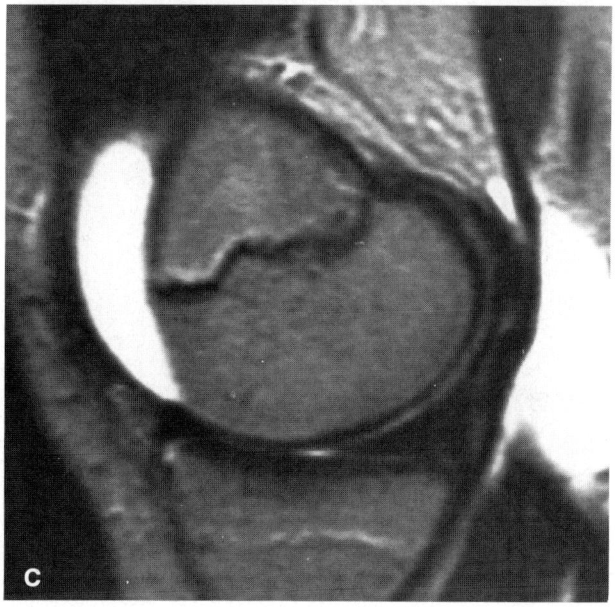

FIGURE 12–24. Popliteal cyst. **(A)** Sagittal T1-weighted image (TR/TE = 800/17) and **(B,C)** T2-weighted images (TR/TE = 3000/45,90). The T1-weighted image shows low signal intensity (arrow) in the gastrocnemius-semimembranosus bursa, representing a popliteal cyst. The T2-weighted images demonstrate marked increased signal intensity in the popliteal cyst. A large anterior knee joint effusion is also present.

MRI OF THE HIP

The primary indication for MRI of the hip is the detection of early avascular necrosis (AVN). The femoral head is the most common site of AVN in the body. Early diagnosis of AVN of the hip allows appropriate treatment, with the goal of arresting or reversing the disease process before collapse of the femoral head.[29,30] MRI is an ideal modality for diagnosing AVN because bone marrow changes can be detected very early in the disease process.[31,32] Many studies have confirmed that MRI is the most sensitive imaging modality for detecting early AVN and is superior to radiography, radionuclide bone scans, and CT.[33–37]

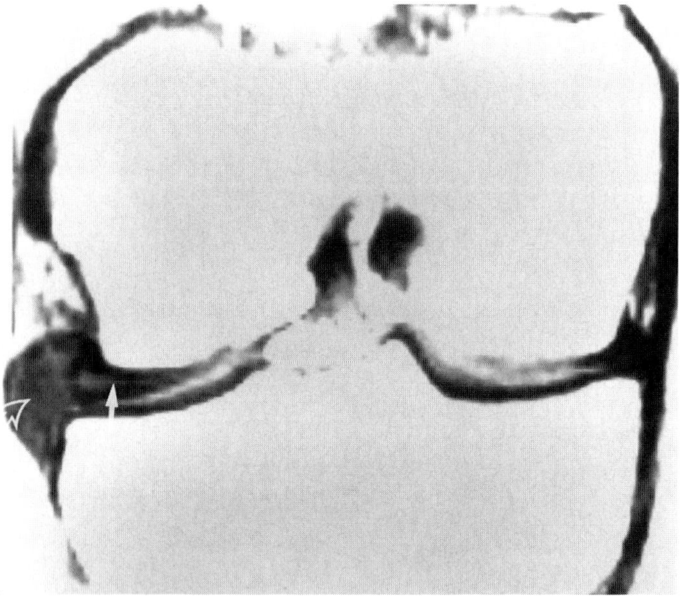

FIGURE 12–25. Meniscal cyst. An intermediate-signal-intensity fluid collection (open arrow) is demonstrated on this coronal T1-weighted image (TR/TE = 800/17) adjacent to the medial meniscus, representing a meniscal cyst. A horizontal area of increased signal intensity due to a horizontal meniscal tear is seen in the medial meniscus (white arrow).

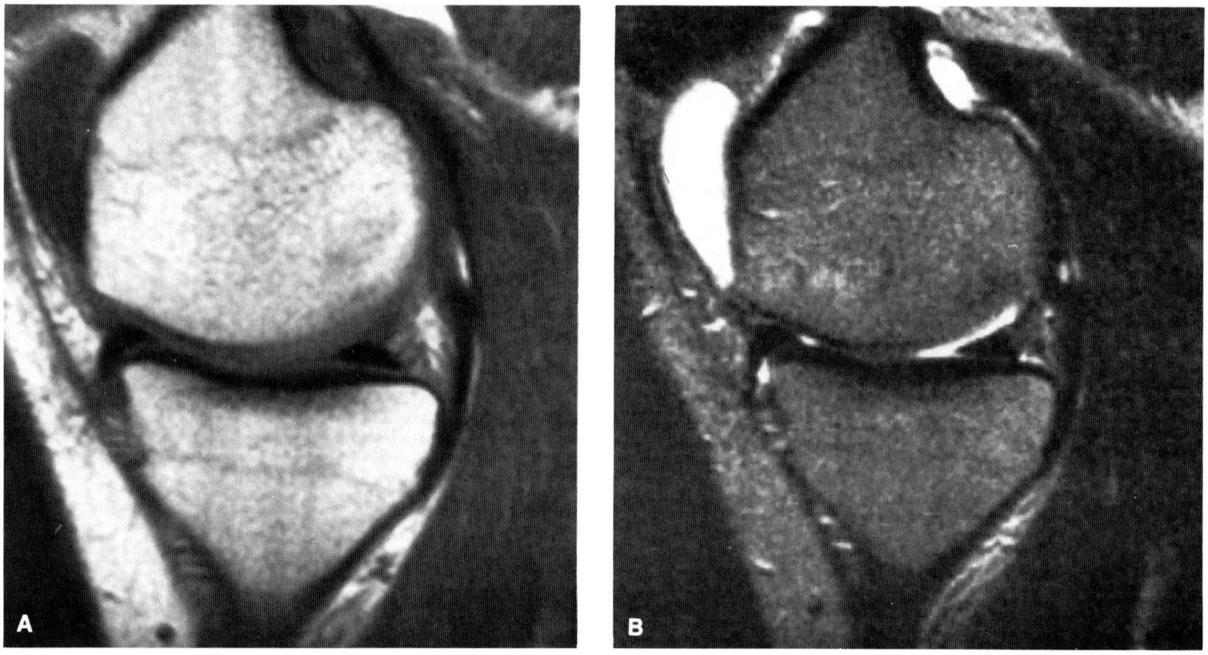

FIGURE 12–26. Joint effusion. **(A)** Sagittal T1-weighted image (TR/TE = 800/17) and **(B)** sagittal T2-weighted image (TR/TE = 3000/90). The T1-weighted image shows low or intermediate signal intensity in the anterior knee joint, representing a large effusion. The T2-weighted image demonstrates corresponding increased signal intensity in the effusion. Smaller areas of increased signal intensity are more easily identified on the T2-weighted image in the posterior joint space and around the posterior horn of the meniscus, also representing joint fluid.

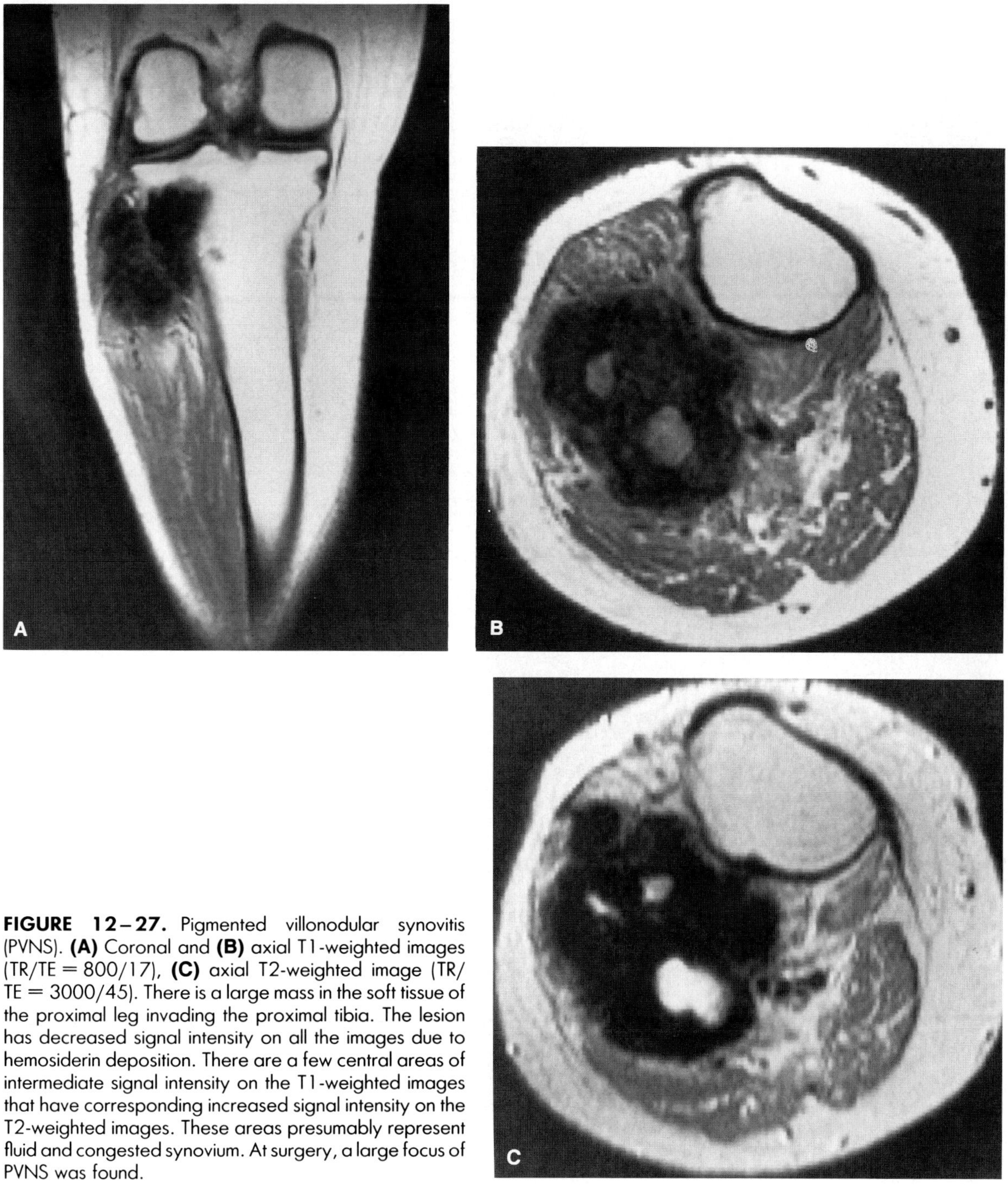

FIGURE 12–27. Pigmented villonodular synovitis (PVNS). **(A)** Coronal and **(B)** axial T1-weighted images (TR/TE = 800/17), **(C)** axial T2-weighted image (TR/TE = 3000/45). There is a large mass in the soft tissue of the proximal leg invading the proximal tibia. The lesion has decreased signal intensity on all the images due to hemosiderin deposition. There are a few central areas of intermediate signal intensity on the T1-weighted images that have corresponding increased signal intensity on the T2-weighted images. These areas presumably represent fluid and congested synovium. At surgery, a large focus of PVNS was found.

Technique

Images of the hip are obtained with the patient supine in the MR scanner, using the body coil as the transmitter and receiver or using dual surface coils. Images are usually acquired in the coronal plane. Routinely, both hips are scanned simultaneously, which permits comparison of the two sides. However, if only one hip is to be scanned, images with superior SNR and resolution can be obtained using a Helmholtz-type coil. T1-weighted (TR/TE = 400–800/15–25) and T2-weighted (TR/TE = 2000–3000/30–90) spin echo pulse sequences are most commonly used. Fatty and hematopoietic bone marrow differentiation is best achieved by using a short TR (400–500 ms). Scans should be obtained with 3- to 5-mm slices, 256 × 128 or 256 scan matrix, and one or two acquisitions (Fig. 12–29). New techniques using chemical shift imaging have been proposed that may better differentiate normal from abnormal bone marrow.[38]

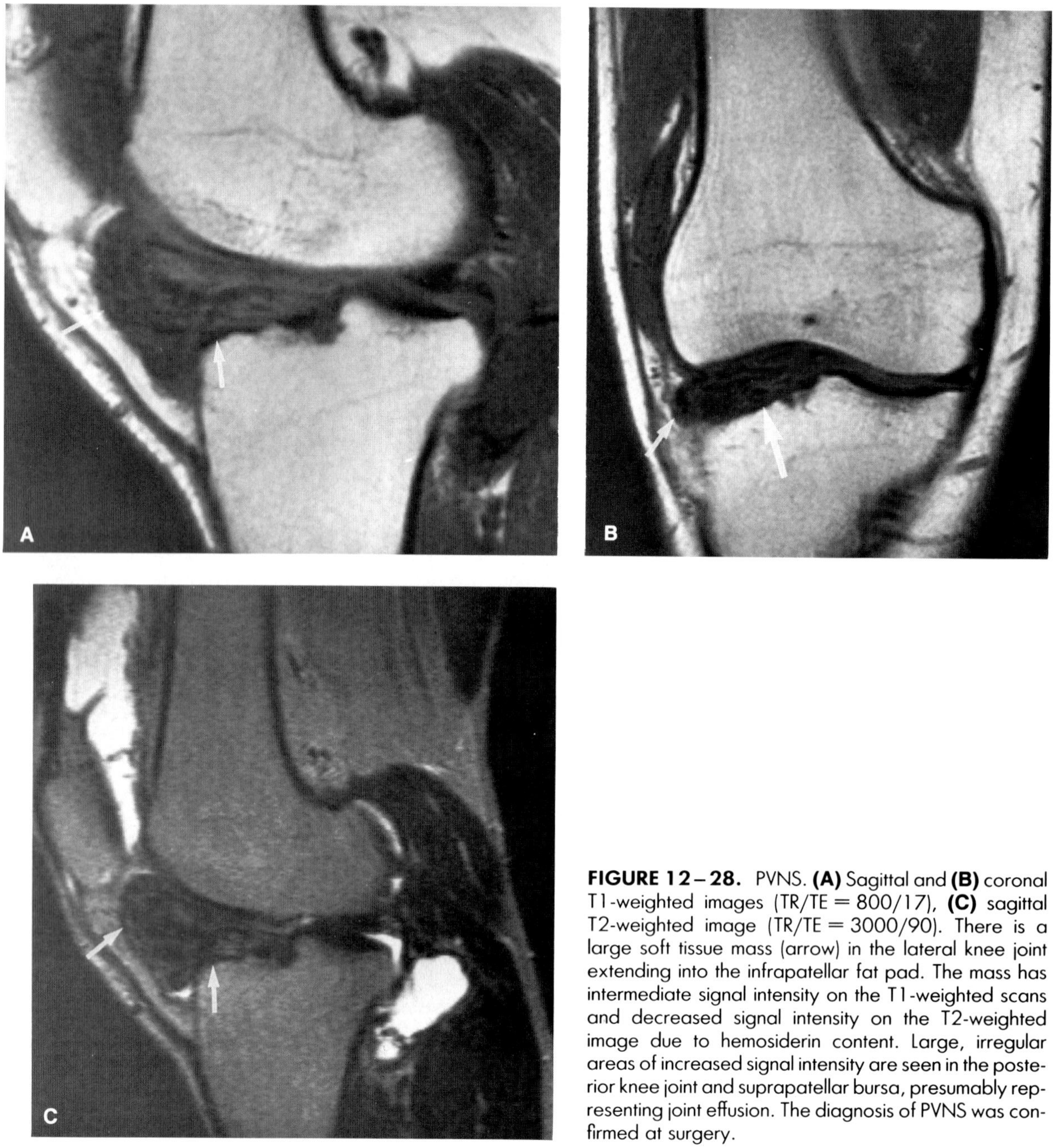

FIGURE 12–28. PVNS. **(A)** Sagittal and **(B)** coronal T1-weighted images (TR/TE = 800/17), **(C)** sagittal T2-weighted image (TR/TE = 3000/90). There is a large soft tissue mass (arrow) in the lateral knee joint extending into the infrapatellar fat pad. The mass has intermediate signal intensity on the T1-weighted scans and decreased signal intensity on the T2-weighted image due to hemosiderin content. Large, irregular areas of increased signal intensity are seen in the posterior knee joint and suprapatellar bursa, presumably representing joint effusion. The diagnosis of PVNS was confirmed at surgery.

Osteonecrosis

Pathogenesis

The cause of AVN can be traumatic or nontraumatic. Traumatic AVN occurs after fractures of the femoral neck, dislocation of the femoral head, or compression fractures of the femoral head, with resultant disruption of the blood supply to the femoral head.[39] Nontraumatic AVN occurs with many conditions, including Gaucher's disease, sickle cell disease, postirradiation necrosis, caisson disease, gout, iron overload, and steroid or alcohol use, or it may be idiopathic. Idiopathic AVN in children is referred to as Legg-Calvé-Perthes disease.[40] The pathogenesis of nontraumatic AVN is unknown, but numerous hypotheses have been proposed, including increased intraosseous pressure that impedes the local blood supply, intraosseous microemboli, and hyperlipidemia.[40,41] Most patients present with symptoms of hip pain that may radiate to the groin, thigh, or knee. Patients often have increased pain with hip motion.

Disease Progression

If left untreated, the natural progression of AVN will be focal bone necrosis and repair, followed by subchondral fractures and collapse of the femoral head,

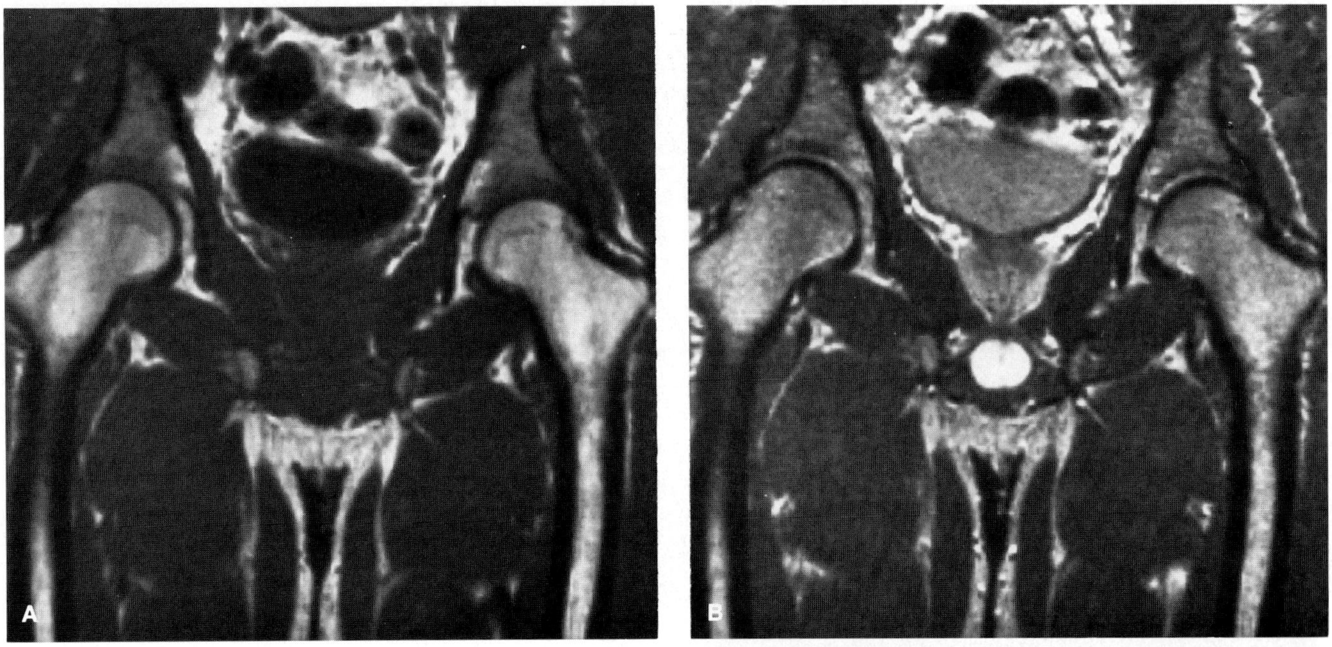

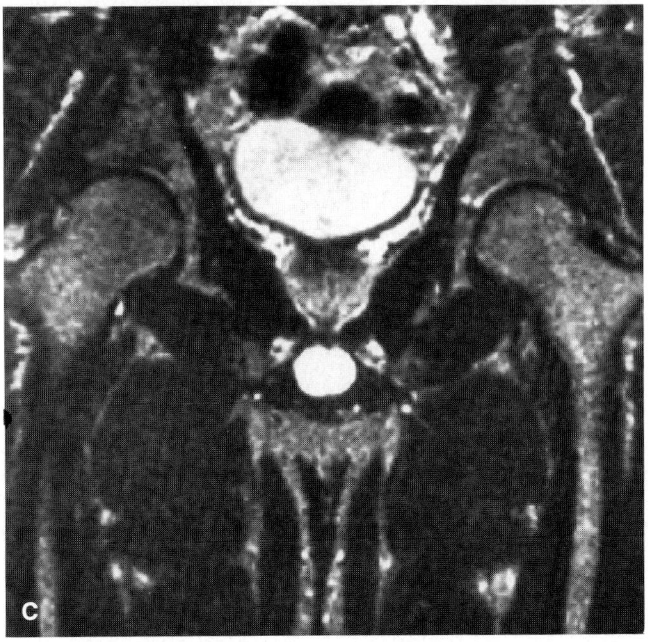

FIGURE 12–29. MRI of the normal adult hip. **(A)** Coronal T1-weighted image (TR/TE = 600/17) and **(B,C)** coronal T2-weighted images (TR/TE = 3000/45,90). The normal bone marrow has increased signal intensity on the T1-weighted image and intermediate signal intensity on the T2-weighted images. A surrounding rim of low-signal-intensity cortical bone is seen on all pulse sequences.

and severe degenerative arthritis of the hip, usually occurring in 3 to 5 years.

The stage of the disease process at the time of diagnosis of AVN determines the treatment. If AVN is diagnosed before collapse or fracture of the femoral head, treatment consists of stress reduction (i.e., crutches and bed rest), core decompression with or without autogenous bone grafts, or an osteotomy. These treatments have arrested or reversed the disease process in some patients, preventing collapse of the femoral head and degenerative arthritis. Core decompression performed before bony fracture can decrease the intramedullary pressure and improve venous drainage and revascularization, with resultant healing.[42] However, treatment of early AVN is still controversial. Once fracture or collapse has occurred, the process is beyond cure and hemiarthroplasty or total hip arthroplasty are the only treatment options.[39–41,43,44]

Pathology

The various MR appearances of AVN are determined by underlying pathologic events.[41–43,45] In early AVN, there is cellular ischemia, with death of osteocytes and marrow cells, leading to bone necrosis and accumulation of necrotic debris in the intertrabecular spaces.

Repair begins with the ingrowth of capillaries and

undifferentiated mesenchymal cells into the necrotic marrow. The necrotic marrow is replaced by proliferating marrow. This marrow differentiates into osteoblasts, which lay down new bone over the dead trabeculae, producing a sclerotic margin. At the same time, osteoclasts are produced to remodel compact bone. During this time, there is a delicate balance between new bone formation and bone resorption. If mechanical forces, such as weight bearing, are excessive, they can overwhelm an area of weak bone and lead to subchondral fractures and subsequent bone collapse.

Radiographic Diagnosis

Before MRI the radiographic diagnosis of AVN relied upon plain film changes and radionuclide bone scans. Radiographic changes are classified as follows:[30]

Stage 0—normal radiographic and radionuclide findings
Stage 1—normal radiographic findings
Stage 2—lucent or sclerotic changes in the femoral head
Stage 3—subchondral lucency and fracture, crescent sign
Stage 4—subchondral collapse with flattening of the femoral head
Stage 5—hip joint narrowing

The diagnosis of AVN is made on bone scans by identifying an area of decreased activity indicating absent or diminished blood supply. Later an area of increased uptake, a hot area, indicates repair and revascularization.[34] MRI has been much more sensitive to early changes of AVN than plain radiographs or bone scans.[34-36] The sensitivity of MRI for AVN has been reported at 88% to 100%, compared with 77% to 81% for bone scans.[34,35] MRI studies revealed a 100% specificity for detection of AVN. One recent study demonstrated that MRI had only a 46% sensitivity for early AVN; radiographs had an 11% sensitivity and bone scans had 18%.[33] Only a small number of patients were studied, a low-field-strength magnet was used, and thick image slices (6-10 mm) were obtained, and the authors stated that small lesions could have been missed.

Another method for diagnosing AVN is bone marrow pressure measurement, an invasive procedure, which was shown to be more sensitive than MRI, but only had a specificity of 57%. Therefore, MRI is the procedure of choice for diagnosing early AVN and is particularly useful in detecting early changes in high-risk patients.

MRI Findings

The normal femoral head (Fig. 12-30) has high signal intensity in the fatty bone marrow on T1-weighted images, surrounded by a thin rim of dark signal intensity representing cortical bone. The most common presentation of AVN is a focal area of decreased signal intensity in the medullary cavity on T1-weighted and T2-weighted images, usually in the superolateral femoral head (Fig. 12-31).[46-48] A classic finding of AVN of the hip is the "double-line sign" (Fig. 12-32). This is a rim of decreased signal intensity on T1-weighted and T2-weighted images, with an inner bright band on T2-weighted scans, surrounding a central lesion of varying signal intensity.[32,42-44,47] The dark peripheral rim was seen in 91% of cases of AVN on T1-weighted and T2-weighted images, and the bright inner band was detected on T2-weighted images in 80% of the cases in one study.[42] The dark peripheral rim is believed to represent the reactive interface between dead and viable bone, where inflammatory and fibroblastic tissue replace marrow fat, and in part may represent an area of sclerosis due to thickened trabecular bone.[31,38,42,43,47] The bright inner band seen on T2-weighted scans is most likely caused by hyperemia in adjacent granulation tissue.[42-44]

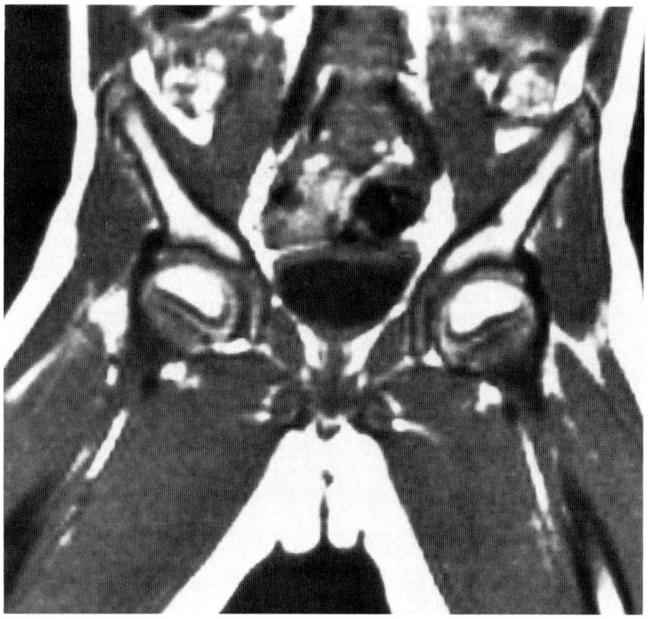

FIGURE 12-30. MRI of a normal hip in a child. Coronal T1-weighted image (TR/TE = 450/17). Normal fatty bone marrow is demonstrated in the epiphyses of the femoral head, which has marked increased signal intensity on this image. The normal alignment of the femoral head with the acetabulum is clearly depicted.

The focus of AVN located within the double line can have a variable signal intensity on T1-weighted and T2-weighted images, depending on the stage of the disease. Mitchell and colleagues correlated the MR signal characteristics of the central lesion with the radiographic stage of disease and histopathologic findings. They devised four MRI classes of AVN.[42] Class A (Fig. 12-33) had a "fat-like" MR appearance, bright on T1-weighted scans and intermediate signal

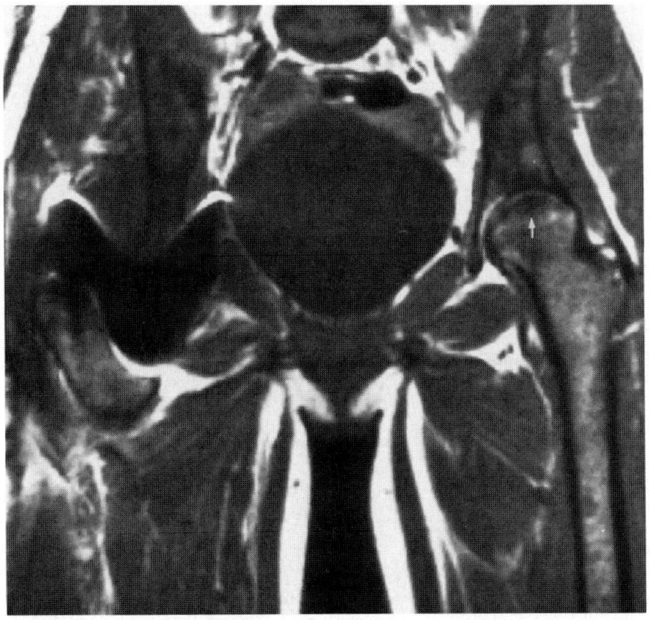

FIGURE 12–31. Avascular necrosis. On the coronal T1-weighted image (TR/TE = 600/17), a focal area of decreased signal intensity is seen in the superolateral aspect of the left femoral head (arrow). This is a common presentation for AVN. Notice the artifact caused by the right hip prosthesis.

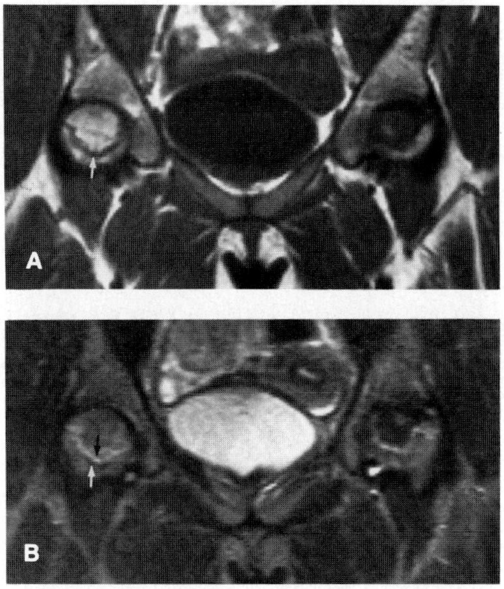

FIGURE 12–32. Double line sign of AVN. **(A)** Coronal T1-weighted image (TR/TE = 600/17) and **(B)** coronal T2-weighted image (TR/TE = 3000/90). The T1-weighted scan shows bilateral AVN. The double line sign is best seen in the right hip. A dark line (white arrow) is seen on both scans, representing sclerosis and fat replacement by fibroblastic tissue. An inner bright-signal-intensity band (black arrow) is seen on the T2-weighted scan, indicating hyperemia and edema in adjacent granulation tissue.

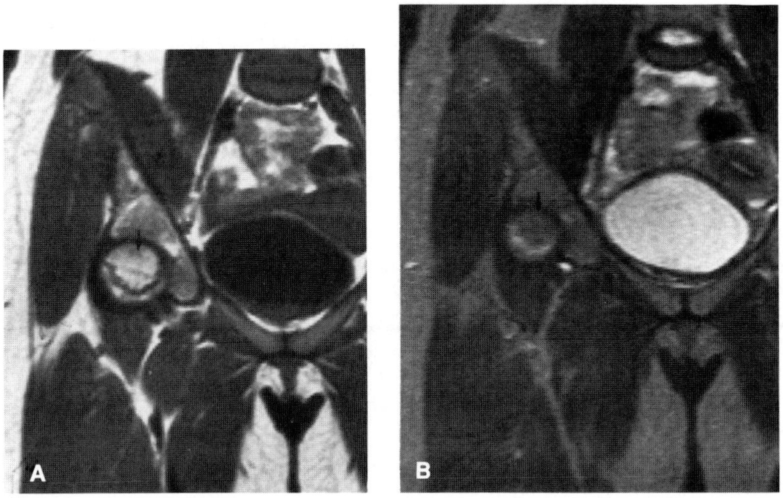

FIGURE 12–33. Class A AVN. **(A)** Coronal T1-weighted image (TR/TE = 600/17) and **(B)** coronal T2-weighted image (TR/TE = 3000/90). On the T1-weighted image, the central focus of AVN (black arrow) has increased signal intensity. A dark-signal-intensity rim surrounds the central lesion. On the T2-weighted image, the central focus of AVN (black arrow) has intermediate signal intensity paralleling that of fat.

intensity on T2-weighted scans. This presumably corresponds to early AVN before revascularization of the central lesion. Class B (Fig. 12–34) had a "blood-like" signal, with bright signal intensity on T1-weighted and T2-weighted images, and was the least common appearance. Class C (Fig. 12–35) is "water-like," with low signal intensity on T1-weighted and high signal intensity on T2-weighted scans. This occurred at early and late stages, presumably indicating inflammation or hyperemia, with decreased lipid content of the femoral head. Class D (Fig. 12–36) is "fibrous-like," with low signal intensity on both T1-weighted and T2-weighted scans, representing advanced AVN, which is complicated by secondary fracture, with predominant fibrosis and sclerosis.

Their classification system correlated well with disease progression and radiographic staging. Early disease before fracture and collapse most often has Class A MR signal characteristics. After fracture or collapse, most cases have Class D MRI findings, with

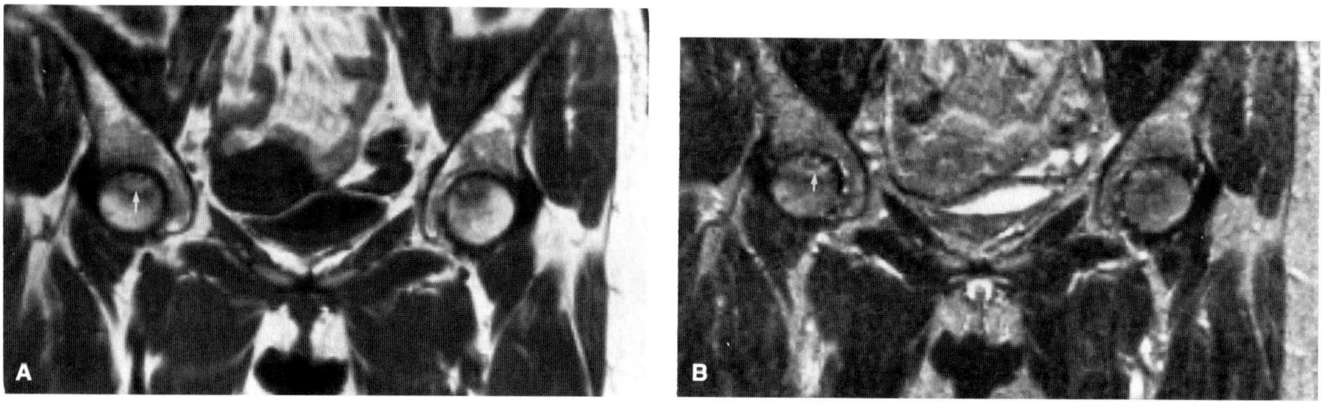

FIGURE 12–34. Class B AVN. **(A)** Coronal T1-weighted image (TR/TE = 500/17) and **(B)** coronal T2-weighted image (TR/TE = 3000/90). The T1-weighted scan shows a focus of AVN (white arrow), which has increased signal intensity. On the T2-weighted scan, the region of AVN also has relatively increased signal intensity (white arrow).

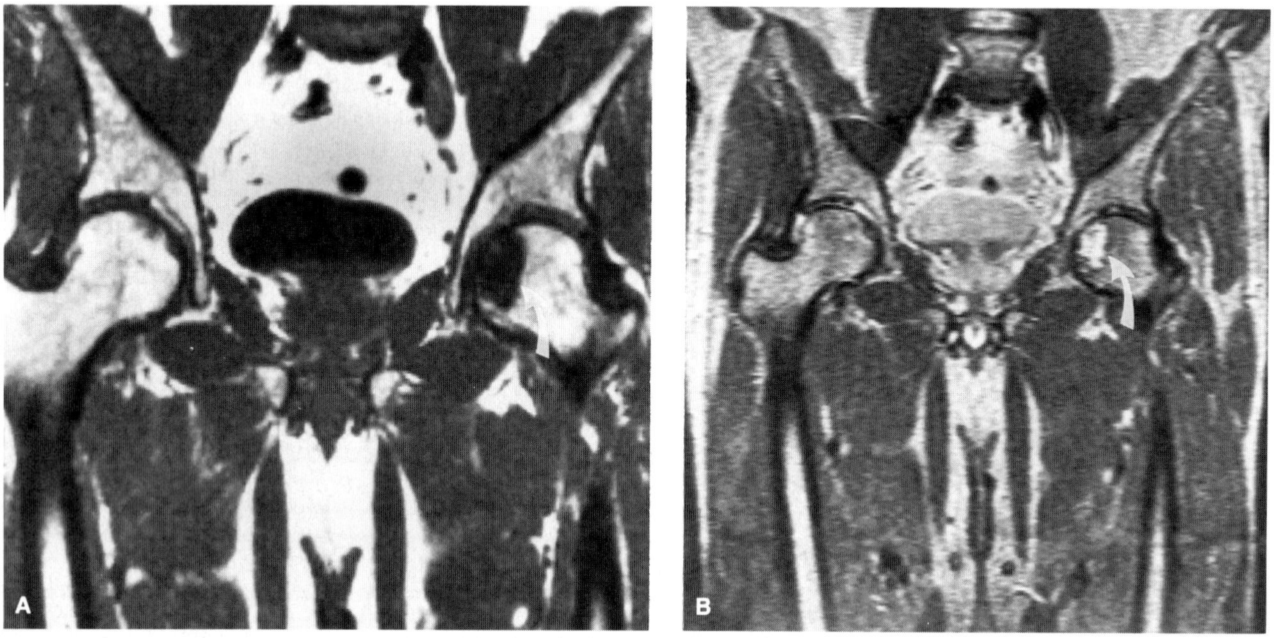

FIGURE 12–35. Class C AVN. **(A)** Coronal T1-weighted image (TR/TE = 600/17) and **(B)** coronal T2-weighted image (TR/TE = 3000/45). There is a focus of AVN involving the medial half of the left femoral head (arrow). The lesion has decreased signal intensity on the T1-weighted scan and increased signal intensity on the T2-weighted scan. The focus of AVN has MR signal characteristics similar to that of fluid.

decreased signal intensity in the central lesion on T1-weighted images. Classes B and C were not as strongly correlated with radiographic stage. The potential impact of MRI on the choice of therapeutic options requires further study.

Additional findings in late AVN include deformity of the femoral head after fracture or collapse (Fig. 12–37). End-stage AVN will show joint space narrowing and osteophyte formation due to severe degenerative arthritis. After a core decompression, a linear area of decreased signal intensity is seen in the femoral head at the site of the core (Fig. 12–38). Because AVN is commonly bilateral, the contralateral hip must be carefully evaluated for early AVN if advanced changes are obvious in the other hip. We have had no difficulties scanning patients with unilateral arthroplasty, other than local distortion of the magnetic field adjacent to the prosthesis (Fig. 12–39).

Excessive joint fluid or early fatty conversion of the bone marrow are common secondary findings in AVN.[49,50] It has been shown that 95% of healthy patients younger than 50 years old have hematopoietic

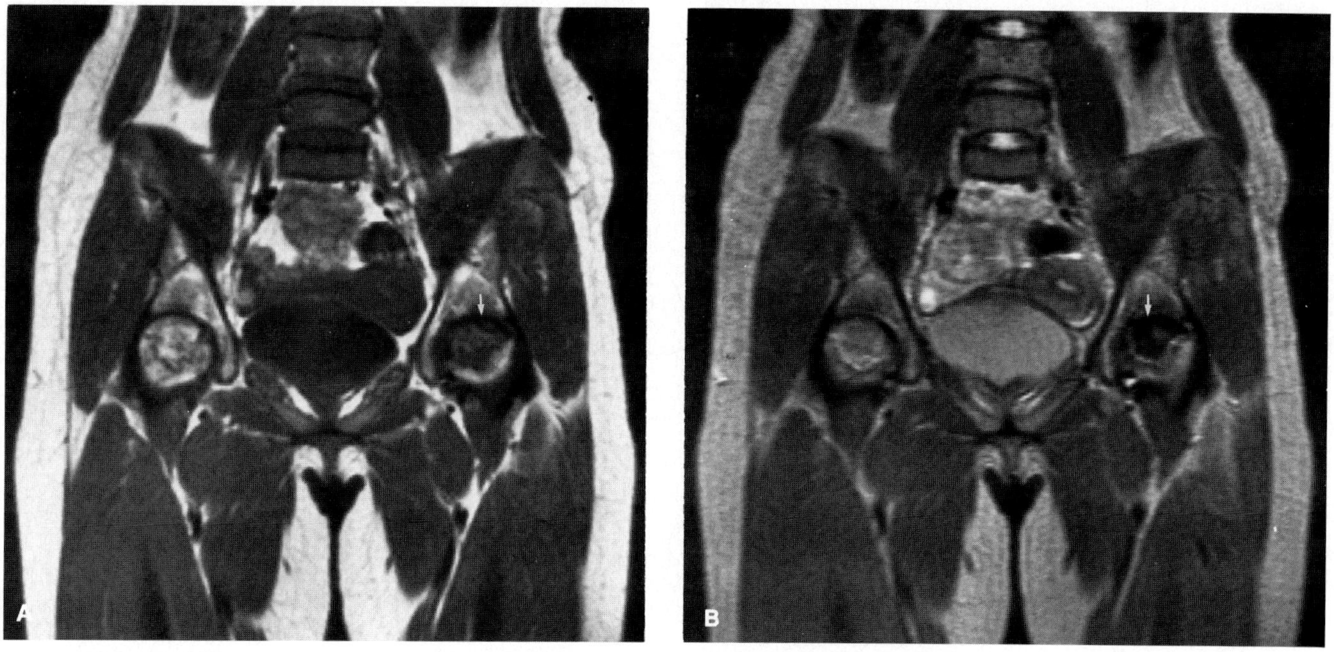

FIGURE 12–36. Class D AVN. **(A)** Coronal T1-weighted image (TR/TE = 600/17) and **(B)** coronal T2-weighted image (TR/TE = 3000/45). Bilateral AVN is identified in the femoral heads. Class D AVN is present in the left femoral head. Decreased signal intensity is visualized in the left femoral head on both scans at the focus of AVN (arrow). This focus of AVN has MR signal characteristics paralleling that of fibrous tissue. Notice also that Class A AVN is seen in the right femoral head.

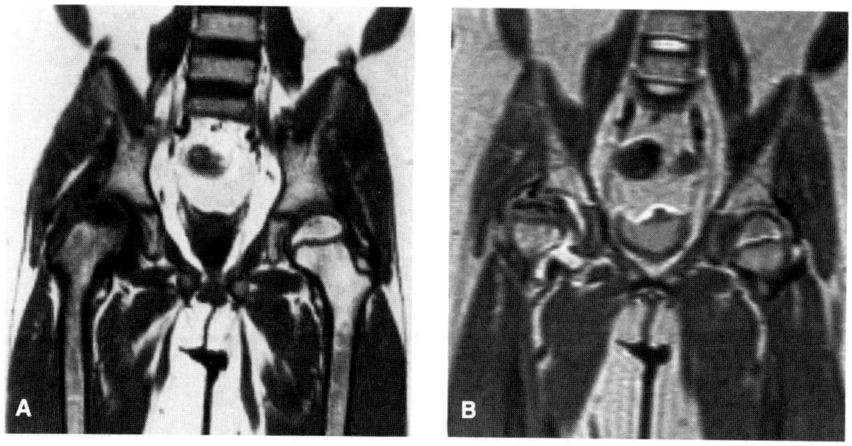

FIGURE 12–37. End-stage AVN with collapse of the right femoral head. **(A)** Coronal T1-weighted image (TR/TE = 600/17) and **(B)** coronal T2-weighted image (TR/TE = 3000/45). Decreased signal intensity is visualized on both scans within the femoral head. There is deformity and collapse of the right femoral head, which is a common occurrence in advanced AVN.

marrow in the intertrochanteric region of the femur, compared with only 33% of patients with AVN (Fig. 12–40).[50] It is postulated that decreased marrow vascularity can hasten the conversion of hematopoietic to fatty marrow, or that premature conversion to fatty marrow predisposes to AVN.

Mitchell et al reported that 84% of normal patients have a small amount of hip joint fluid (Fig. 12–41).[49] However, 58% of patients with AVN and only 5% of normal patients have enough fluid to surround the femoral neck (Fig. 12–42) or distend the joint capsule. In some patients with AVN, symptoms correlate with the presence of an effusion.[44]

Transient Synovitis

Transient synovitis is a common clinical entity in children, of unknown cause, that produces inflammation of the synovium. Symptoms include pain in the hip, limp, decreased range of motion, and associated muscle spasm. Transient synovitis most commonly affects young boys 3 to 10 years old. MRI may be helpful in diagnosing transient synovitis.[51] This may manifest as increased thickness of the synovium, with intermediate signal intensity on T1-weighted images, and increased signal intensity on T2-weighted images in the joint space, like joint effusion (Fig. 12–43).

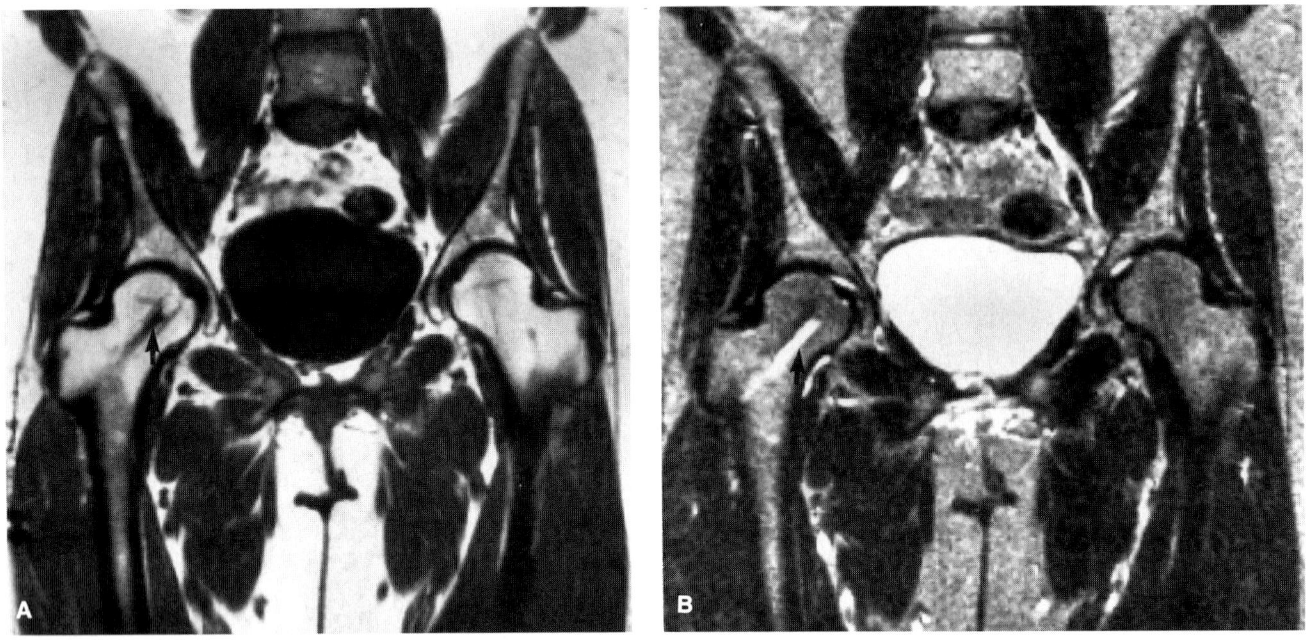

FIGURE 12–38. Core decompression. **(A)** T1-weighted coronal image (TR/TE = 500/17) and **(B)** coronal T2-weighted image (TR/TE = 3000/90). This 31-year-old woman with SLE was treated with high-dose steroids. The patient developed pain in the right hip, and core decompression was performed with the hope of delaying development of AVN. The core decompression (arrow) is visualized as a linear area of decreased signal intensity in the femoral head on the T1-weighted scan and has increased signal intensity on the T2-weighted scan. No evidence of AVN is demonstrated in the femoral heads.

Ultrasound may help confirm that there is only minimal or no joint fluid present.

SHOULDER MRI

The painful shoulder is a common clinical problem with numerous potential causes such as subacromial bursitis, adhesive capsulitis, arthritis, or the various stages of the impingement syndrome, including complete or partial rotator cuff tears and tendinitis. The clinical examination is limited in differentiating these entities. Plain radiographs are helpful for diagnosing calcific tendinitis and arthritis, but they are poor for evaluating the rotator cuff.[52] Arthrography, ultrasound, and CT arthrography have been used to evaluate the rotator cuff with relative success.[53–56] However, arthrography and CT arthrography are invasive procedures and are poor at diagnosing partial rotator cuff tears. Ultrasound is a promising modality, but is exceedingly operator-dependent and can be limited by bone interference. MRI is well-suited for the evaluation of the shoulder because it has excellent soft tissue contrast, multiplanar capability, no bone artifacts, no ionizing radiation, and is noninvasive.[57]

Technique

MRI of the shoulder, first reported in 1986, is gaining acceptance as a primary imaging modality for the shoulder.[56–58] To properly image the shoulder, an extremity coil, such as the Helmholtz design, is essential for obtaining adequate SNR and resolution.[59,60] Oblique nonorthogonal imaging planes are required to optimally visualize the rotator cuff.

Initially, axial 5-mm sections with short TR (500–800) and short TE (15–25) are obtained from the level of the acromion to the inferior aspect of the glenoid. The axial images can be used to position for the oblique scan planes (Fig. 12–44). Two oblique planes are acquired, one parallel to the surface of the glenoid cavity (parasagittal) and another perpendicular to the surface of the glenoid cavity, oriented along the axis of the supraspinatus muscle (paracoronal).[59] Usually, T1-weighted images (TR/TE = 500–800/15–25) are obtained in both oblique planes, along with T2-weighted images in the paracoronal plane (TR/TE = 2000–3000/20–80). Another option is performing double echo T2-weighted scans in both oblique planes, eliminating the T1-weighted scans. Satisfactory images can be achieved with 5-mm sections and a

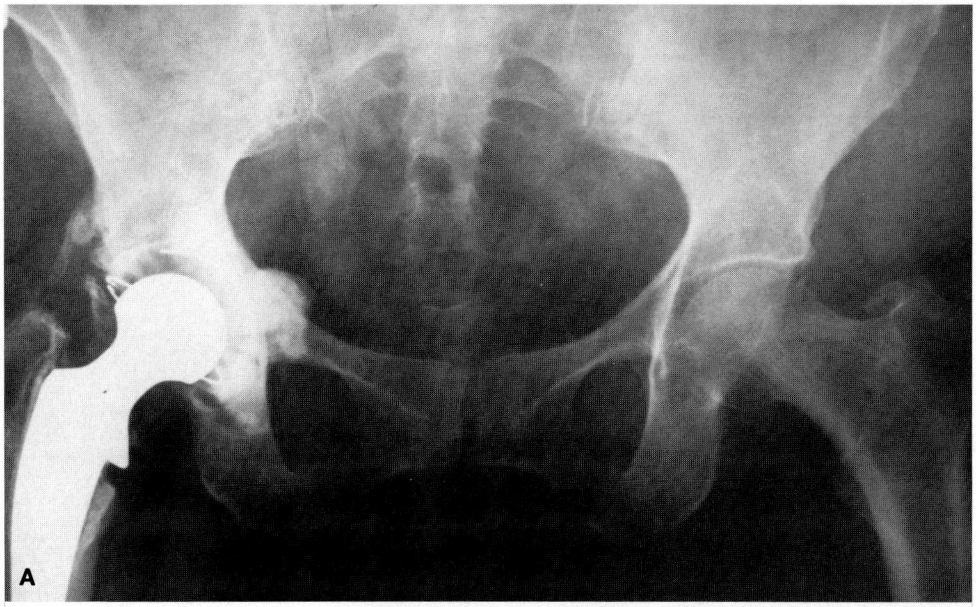

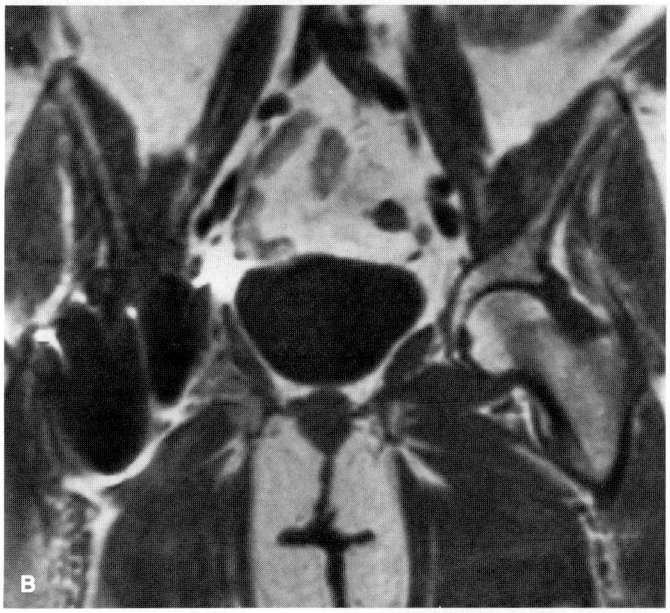

FIGURE 12–39. Right hip arthroplasty. **(A)** Plain film of the pelvis and **(B)** coronal T1-weighted image (TR/TE = 600/17). The plain film reveals a right femoral arthroplasty. The MR image identifies a large artifact, with distortion of the local magnetic environment due to the right hip arthroplasty. Despite the large artifact in the right hip, the normal left hip is clearly visualized.

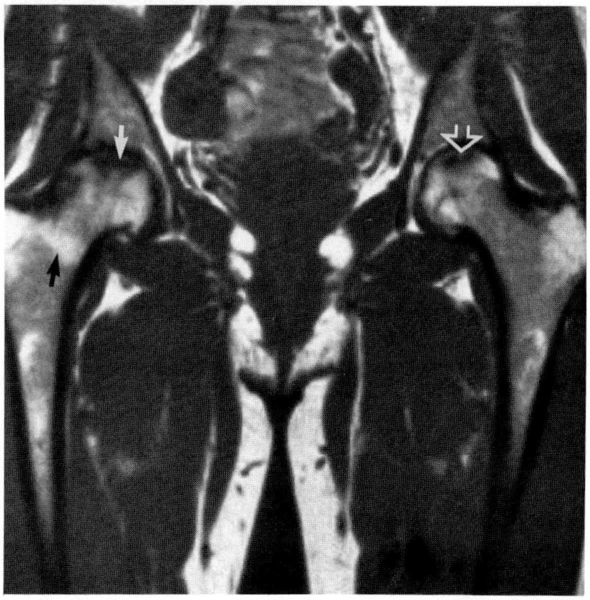

FIGURE 12–40. Early fatty marrow replacement. T1-weighted coronal image (TR/TE = 600/17). This 31-year-old patient was treated with high-dose steroids for ulcerative colitis. An area of decreased signal intensity (white arrow) representing AVN is seen in the superior aspect of the right femoral head. A smaller focus of decreased signal intensity (open arrow) occurring in the left femoral head is also due to AVN. Early fatty marrow replacement is demonstrated as increased signal intensity in the intertrochanteric area of the right femur (black arrow). Early fatty marrow replacement is associated with AVN and is a diagnostically helpful secondary sign. Note that the less involved left femur has normal red marrow distribution in the intertrochanteric area.

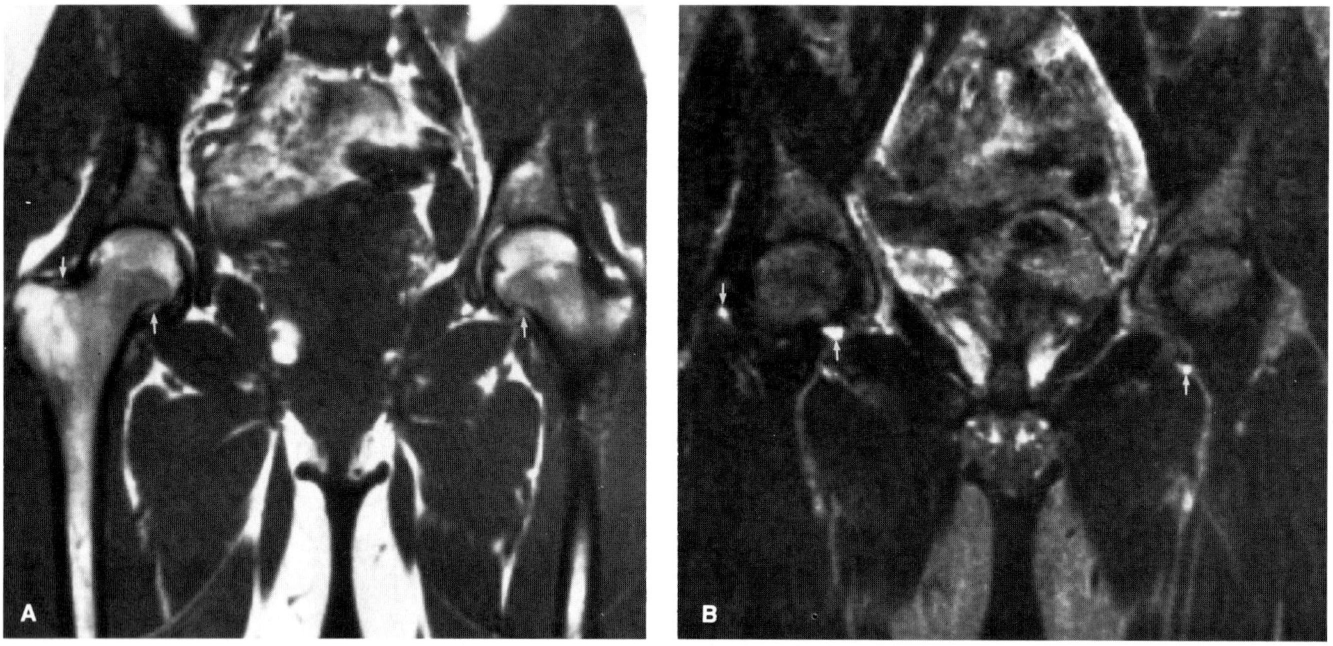

FIGURE 12–41. Normal joint fluid. **(A)** T1-weighted coronal image (TR/TE = 500/17) and **(B)** T2-weighted coronal image (TR/TE = 3000/90). Small foci of intermediate signal intensity (white arrows) are seen adjacent to the femoral heads on the T1-weighted scan. On the T2-weighted scan, these areas have increased signal intensity (white arrows). This degree of joint fluid is within normal limits.

256 × 256 scan matrix with one acquisition for the T2-weighted images and two acquisitions for T1-weighted images or with a 256 × 128 matrix with two acquisitions and a small FOV (16 cm). The patient should be supine, with the arm at the side in a neutral position, thumb up.

Anatomy

The rotator cuff is composed of four muscles. The supraspinatus, infraspinatus, and the teres minor muscles arise from the scapula, and their tendons insert on the greater tuberosity of the humerus.[57,59,60,61] The subscapularis tendon inserts on the lesser tuberosity. Because only 33% of the humeral head is in contact with the surface of the glenoid, joint stability relies heavily upon the integrity of the muscles, tendons, ligaments, and the joint cartilage.

The articular surface of the glenoid cavity and the humeral head are lined by hyaline cartilage, which has intermediate signal intensity on T1-weighted and T2-weighted images. The glenoid labrum and articular surface of the acromioclavicular (AC) joint are composed of fibrocartilage, which has low signal in-

(text continues on page 433)

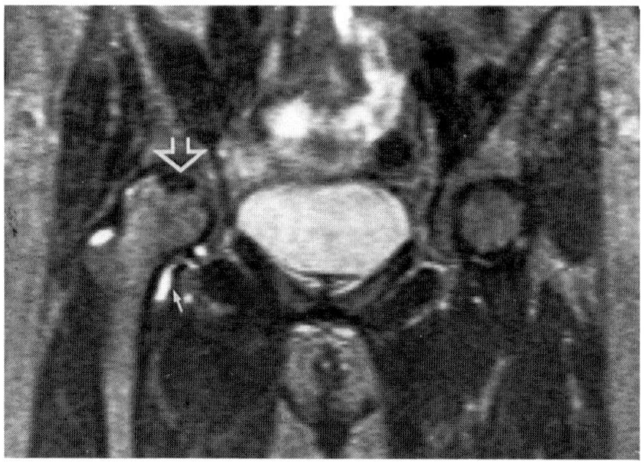

FIGURE 12–42. Joint effusion surrounding the femoral neck. Coronal T2-weighted image (TR/TE = 3000/90). High-signal-intensity fluid (white arrow) surrounds the right femoral neck in a patient with AVN (open arrow). This degree of fluid is abnormal and can be a helpful secondary sign indicating an abnormal hip in patients with AVN.

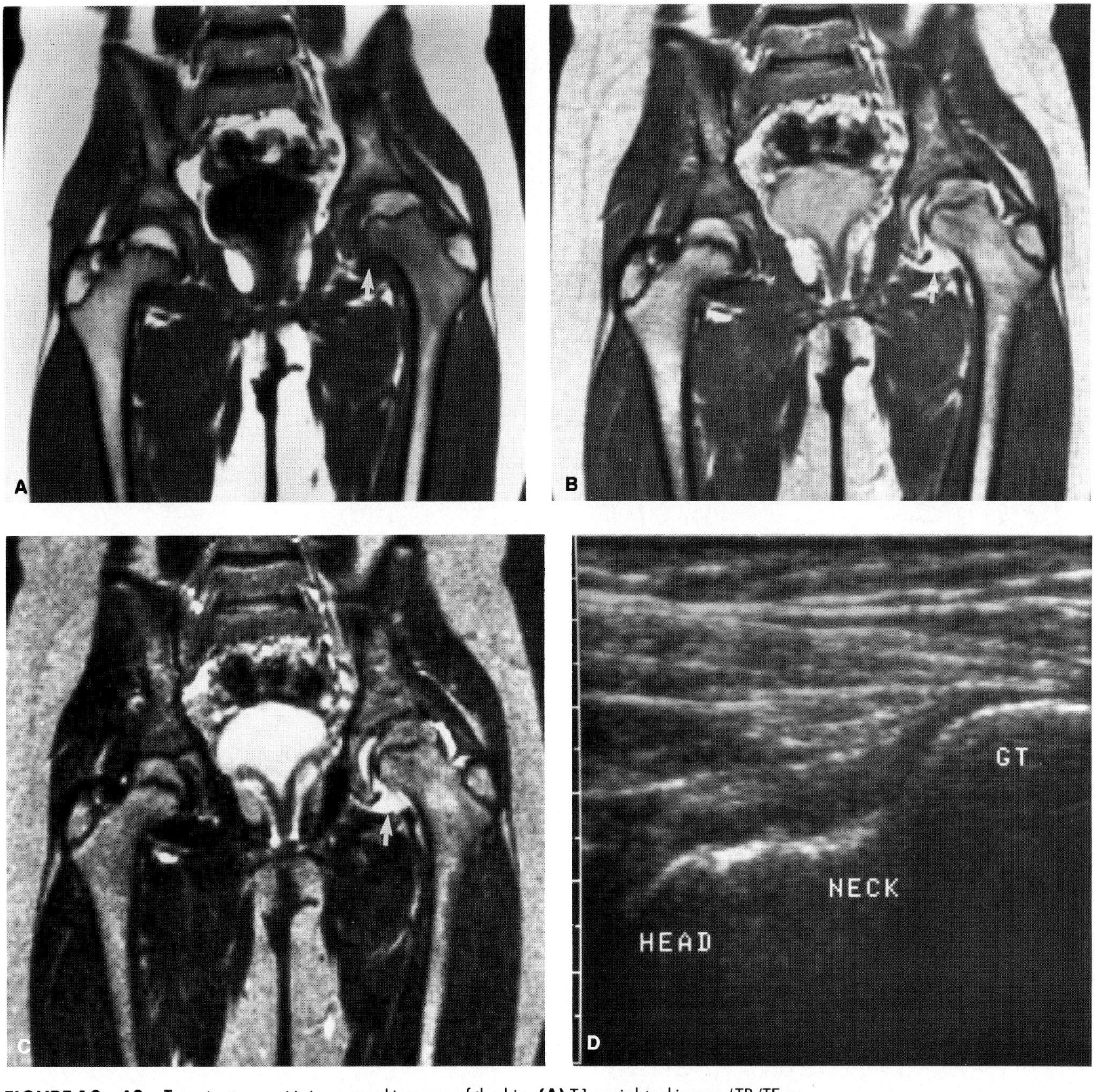

FIGURE 12–43. Transient synovitis in coronal images of the hip. **(A)** T1-weighted image (TR/TE = 500/17); **(B,C)** T2-weighted images (TR/TE = 3000/45,90); **(D)** ultrasound of the left hip. This is a 9-year-old girl with left hip pain. Abnormal intermediate signal intensity (arrow) is seen in the left hip joint on the T1-weighted image, and increased signal intensity (arrow) is visualized in the same location on the T2-weighted images. This represents synovial thickening and inflammation in a patient with proven transient synovitis. The MR signal characteristics of the inflamed synovium are the same as for fluid, and the ultrasound was useful in demonstrating that no joint fluid was present.

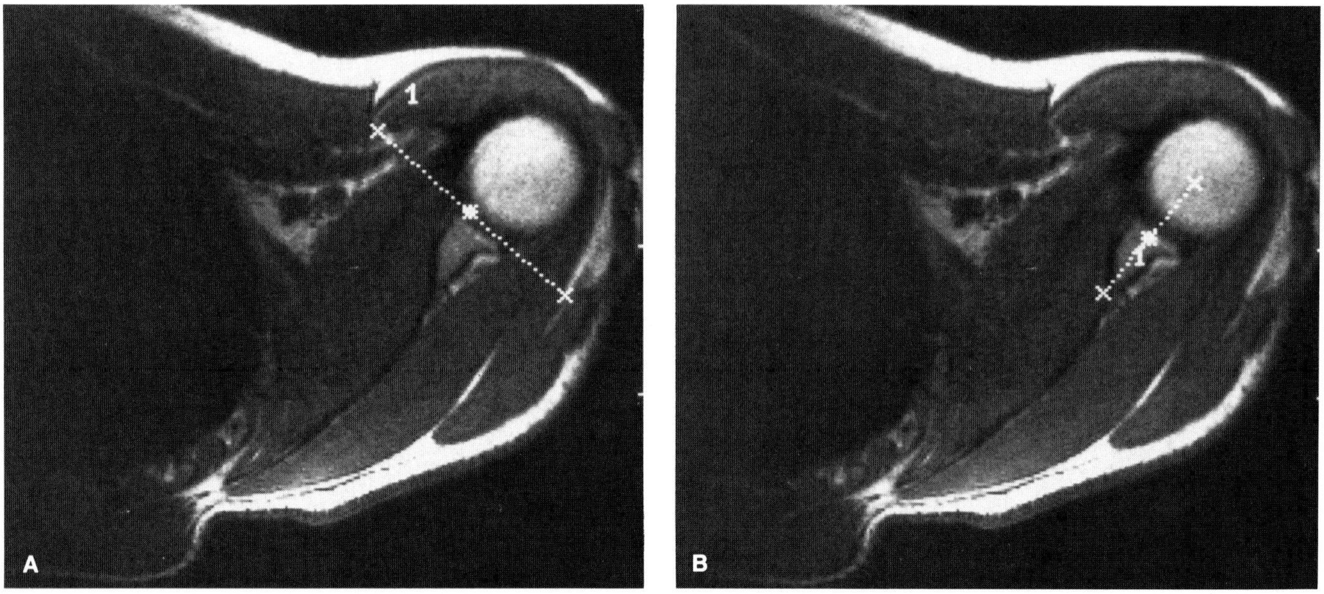

FIGURE 12–44. Positioning for oblique scan planes. **(A,B)** Axial T1-weighted images (TR/TE = 800/25). **(A)** This is the ideal scan plane for obtaining oblique parasagittal scans. The parasagittal images are oriented in a plane parallel to the surface of the glenoid cavity (dotted line). **(B)** This is the scan plane required for acquiring oblique paracoronal images. These images are directed along a line perpendicular to the surface of the glenoid cavity (dotted line).

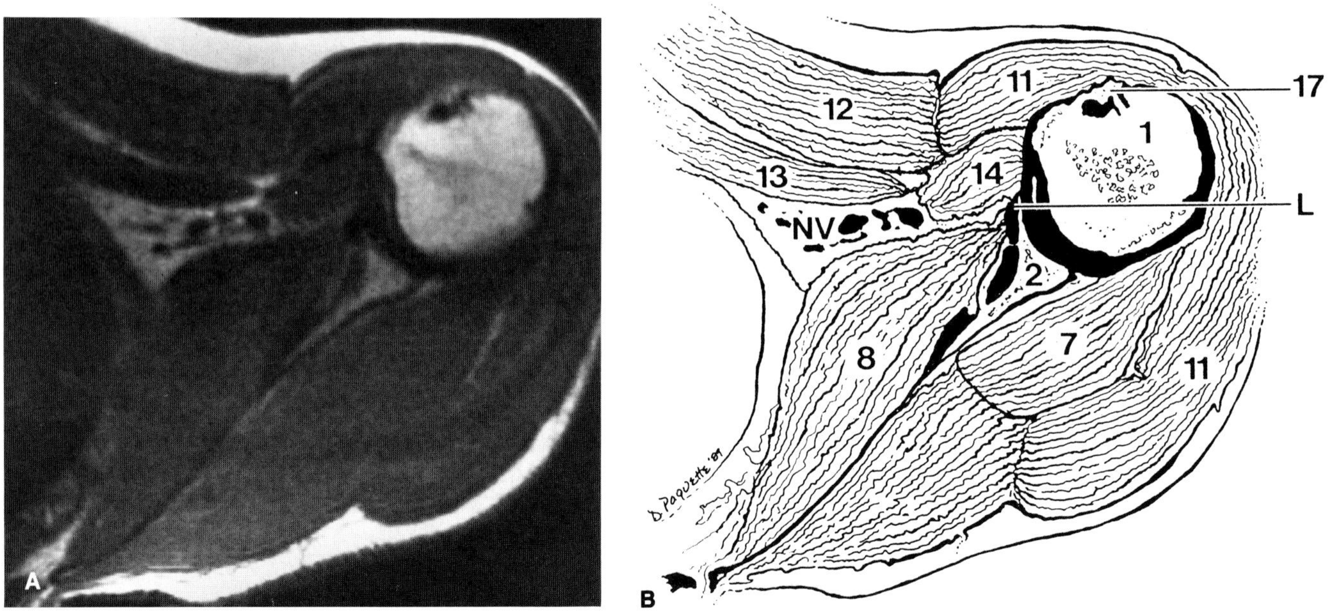

FIGURE 12–45. Normal axial T1-weighted MRI **(A)** and matching anatomic drawing **(B)** of the shoulder. *1*, humerus; *2*, glenoid; *3*, coracoid process; *4*, acromion; *5*, clavicle; *6*, supraspinatus muscle; *6t*, supraspinatus tendon; *7*, infraspinatus muscle; *7t*, infraspinatus tendon; *8*, subscapularis muscle; *8t*, subscapularis tendon; *9*, teres minor muscle; *9t*, teres minor tendon; *10*, teres major muscle; *11*, deltoid muscle; *12*, pectoralis major muscle; *13*, pectoralis minor muscle; *14*, coracobrachialis muscle; *15*, trapezius muscle; *16*, subdeltoid bursa fat pad; *17*, biceps tendon in the bicipital groove; *NV*, neurovascular bundle; *L*, glenoid labrum.

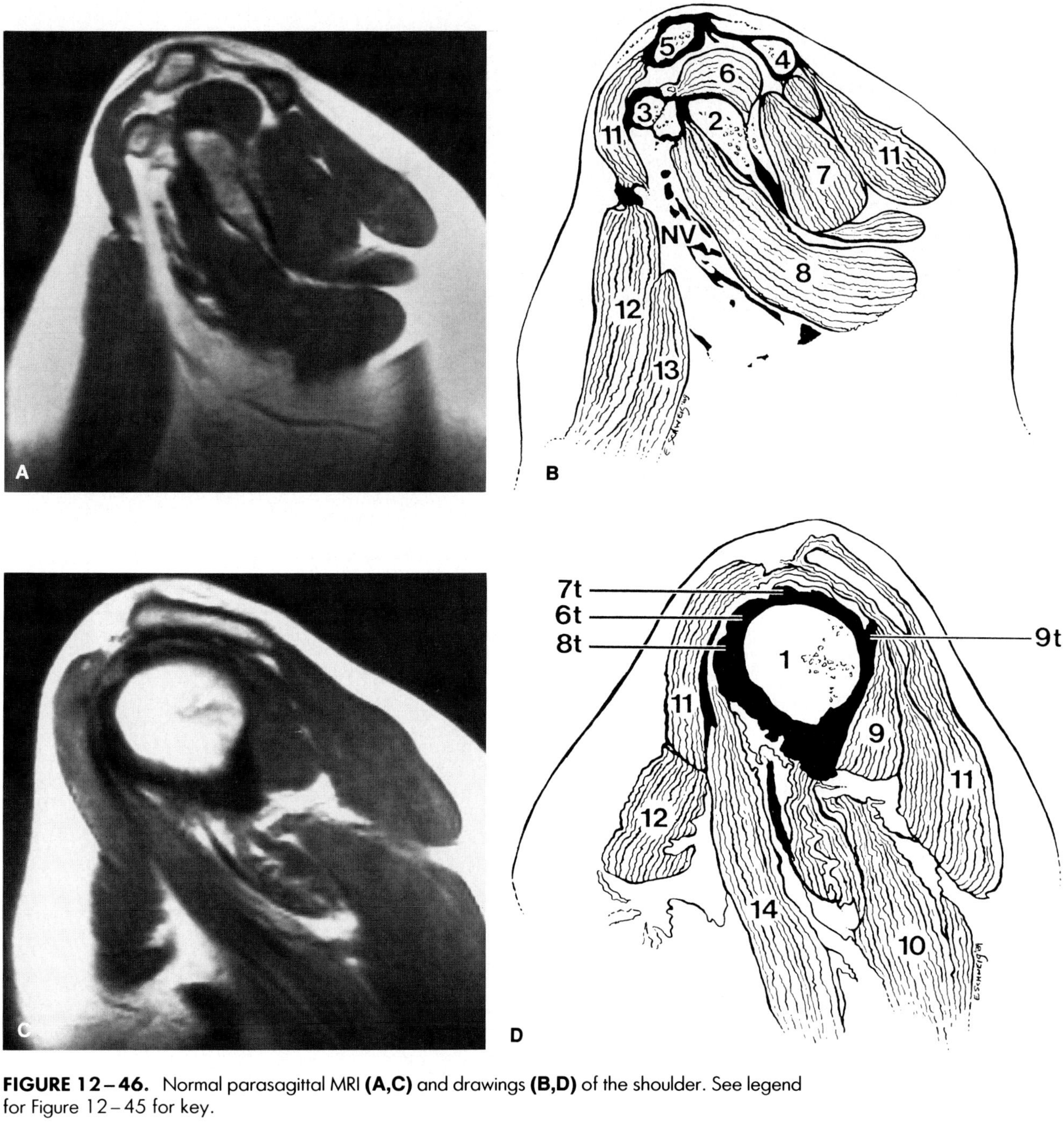

FIGURE 12–46. Normal parasagittal MRI **(A,C)** and drawings **(B,D)** of the shoulder. See legend for Figure 12–45 for key.

tensity on all pulse sequences. The rotator cuff tendons normally have low signal intensity and can be difficult to separate from the adjacent cortical bone of the humeral head.

Axial planes optimally show the relationship between the humeral head and the glenoid cavity (Fig. 12–45). The tendon of the long head of the biceps, the bicipital groove, the glenoid labrum, and the axillary neurovascular bundles are easily seen on the axial images. The oblique plane parallel to the glenoid cavity (i.e., parasagittal) demonstrates the glenoid, coracoid process, and the muscles and tendons of the rotator cuff in cross-section (Fig. 12–46).

The oblique plane perpendicular to the glenoid cavity (i.e., paracoronal) best demonstrates the rotator cuff muscles and tendons (Fig. 12–47). The AC joint, coracoid process, and the subacromial and subdeltoid bursa are also seen. Normally, the subacromial and subdeltoid bursa are potential spaces, and only their fat pads are visualized. These appear as thin straight bands of high signal intensity, located between the rotator cuff tendons and the AC joint and the deltoid

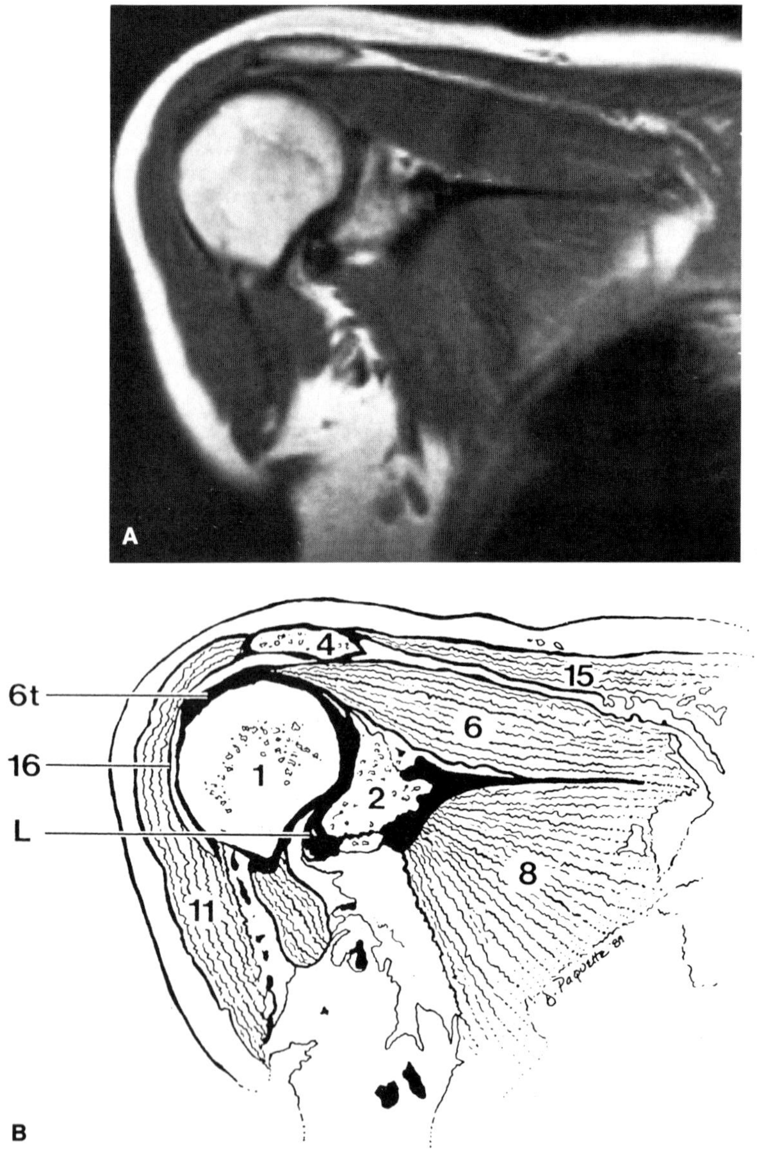

FIGURE 12–47. Normal paracoronal MRI **(A)** and drawing **(B)** of the shoulder. See legend for Figure 12–45 for key.

muscle. The paracoronal plane is optimal for visualizing rotator cuff tears and for other manifestations of the impingement syndrome.

Impingement Syndrome and Rotator Cuff Abnormalities

MRI is well suited for evaluating the shoulder impingement syndrome.[61-63] This is a condition with pain occurring during abduction and external rotation of the arm. The pathophysiology of this syndrome is entrapment of soft tissue, usually the supraspinatus tendon or the long head of the biceps tendon, between the humeral head and the anterior part of the acromion, AC joint, or the coracoacromial ligament. This can cause bursitis, rotator cuff tendinitis, fibrosis, and tearing of the rotator cuff.[64] Neer postulated that 95% of rotator cuff tears are the result of chronic impingement upon the supraspinatus tendon.[64]

Impingement may be caused by repetitive trauma or degenerative disease, which leads to subacromial bone proliferation, spurring or capsular hypertrophy at the inferior AC joint, or degenerative changes with spurring of the humeral head. Rarely, the impingement syndrome is due to a tumor or other mass. Neer believed that rotator cuff injuries represent a continuum of disease that progresses through three stages.[64] Stage I usually occurs in patients younger than 25 years old, who have a history of acute overuse of the shoulder and who develop hemorrhage and edema in the supraspinatus tendon. This stage is reversible, and it is treated conservatively. Stage II typically occurs in patients 25 to 40 years old, who had repeated episodes of minor trauma leading to fibrosis and thickening of the rotator cuff and subacromial bursa. Stage III occurs most often in patients older than 40 years old and manifests as a complete rotator cuff tear. Patients with stage III injuries require surgical correction. The goal of MRI is to diagnose impingement at stages I and II before a complete rotator cuff tear has occurred and to detect and quantify cuff tears to aid surgical planning.

MRI accurately detects rotator cuff tears. A recent study revealed an 89% accuracy for MRI in diagnosing complete rotator cuff tears. The most common site for a rotator cuff tear is a hypovascular zone located approximately 1 cm proximal to the site of insertion of the supraspinatus tendon on the greater tuberosity.[65,66] Before MRI, radiographic evaluation of impingement syndrome and rotator cuff tear had limited success. Plain films are unreliable early, with the classic findings of decreased space (<7 mm) between the acromion and the humeral head and a high position of the humeral head only occurring late in the disease process. Arthrography and CT arthrography cannot detect stage I or II lesions.[63]

A classification scheme of the impingement syndrome has been postulated:[63]

Type 1—Least severe, this represents subacromial bursitis manifested by subacromial bursa thickening, and a normal signal within the supraspinatus muscle and tendon.

Type 2a—There is abnormal high signal intensity in the supraspinatus tendon, but the muscle remains normal. This implies supraspinatus tendinitis (Fig. 12–48).

Type 2b—A very bright signal is seen in the supraspinatus tendon on T2-weighted images, but there is no muscle retraction. This represents disruption of the rotator cuff, with fluid in the cuff substance. The area of increased signal intensity in Type 2b is brighter than that in Type 2a (Fig. 12–49).

Type 3—There is abnormal high signal intensity in the supraspinatus tendon and retraction of the muscle. This implies an extensive rotator cuff tear.

The ability to differentiate tendinitis, partial tears, and small full-thickness tears may not always be possible, because these entities represent a continuum of disease, and their MRI appearances overlap. The necessity of distinguishing these entities depends on the treatment philosophy of the referring orthopedist. Recently, Zlatkin and colleagues[61] reported their MRI findings for 150 patients. Tendinitis (stages I and II) was visualized as high signal intensity on the T1-weighted and proton density scans in the distal supraspinatus tendon, presumably representing edema and inflammation (Fig. 12–50). The rotator cuff tendons remained intact. At this stage, high signal intensity on T2-weighted images representing fluid should not be seen in the subacromial or subdeltoid bursa. The high-signal fat pad of these bursa should be demonstrated on the T1-weighted and proton density images. The diagnosis of small full-thickness tears was made when a small region of increased signal intensity was seen in the supraspinatus tendon, often more focal than with tendinitis. The subdeltoid fat pad was

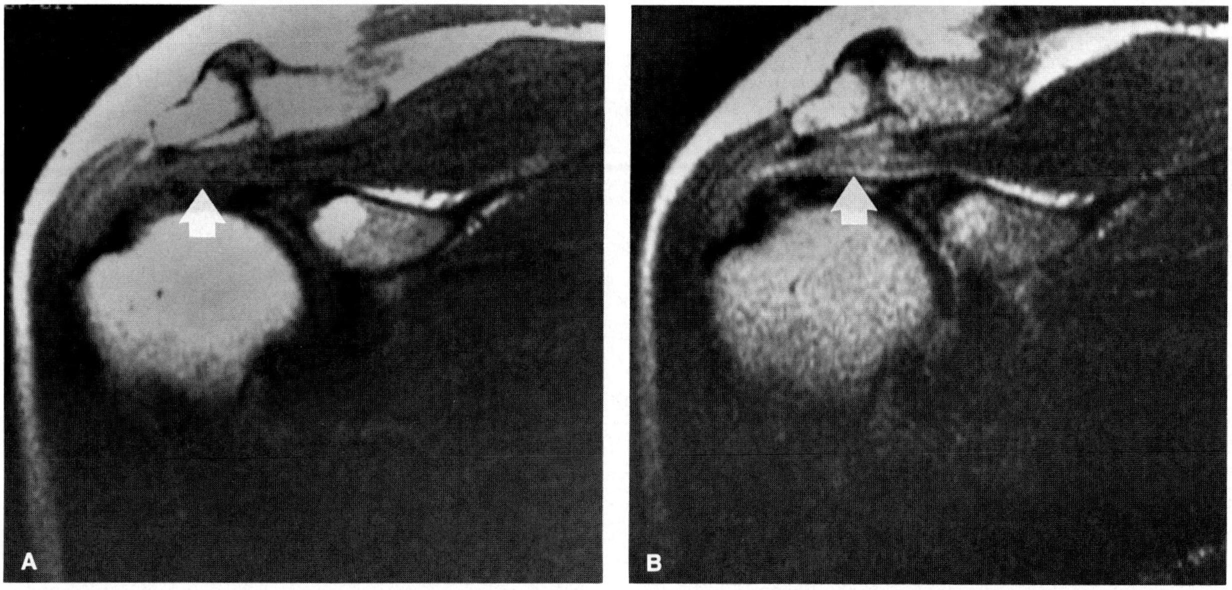

FIGURE 12–48. Tendinitis. **(A)** T1-weighted paracoronal image (TR/TE = 600/25) and **(B)** T2-weighted paracoronal image (TR/TE = 2000/80). A focal area of intermediate signal intensity (arrow) is demonstrated in the supraspinatus tendon on the T1-weighted image. This region has increased signal intensity on the T2-weighted image (arrow). The supraspinatus muscle has a normal position and normal signal intensity. Findings represent tendinitis. (Courtesy of Dr. D. L. Burk, Jr., Thomas Jefferson University Hospital)

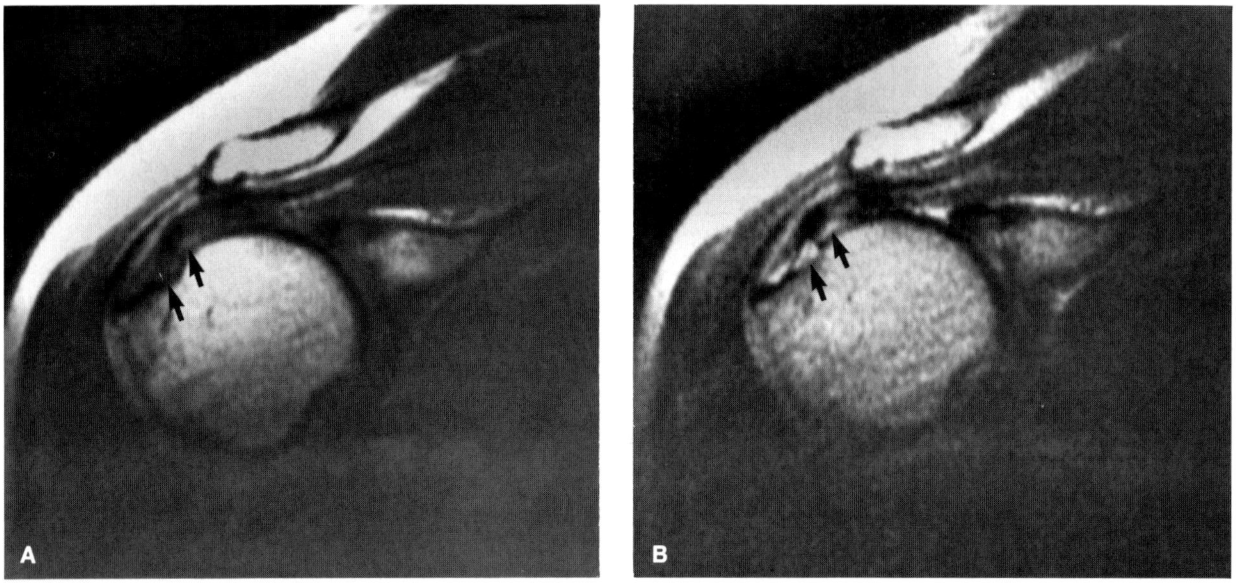

FIGURE 12–49. Partial rotator cuff tear. **(A)** T1-weighted paracoronal image (TR/TE = 600/25) and **(B)** T2-weighted paracoronal image (TR/TE = 2000/80). Abnormal increased signal intensity is seen in the supraspinatus tendon (arrows). The increased signal is brighter on the T2-weighted image, presumably representing fluid within the substance of the rotator cuff. There is no muscle retraction. (Courtesy of Dr. D. L. Burk, Jr., Thomas Jefferson University Hospital)

not well seen on T1-weighted images. On T2-weighted images, the signal intensity in the tendon was further increased and may be associated with increased signal intensity in the subacromial and subdeltoid bursa. Occasionally, discontinuity of the tendons was seen.

The MRI findings of complete rotator cuff tear (stage III impingement) include discontinuity or a gap in the rotator cuff, occasionally with retraction of the muscle-tendon complex in large tears (Fig. 12–51).[61,65–67] Increased signal intensity is commonly seen on T2-weighted images in the supraspinatus tendon in rotator cuff tears. A potential pitfall is that a previous site of steroid or local anesthesia injection can also appear as a bright area on T2-weighted images.[62] With complete rotator cuff tears, increased signal intensity on T2-weighted images may be seen in the subacromial and subdeltoid bursa, presumably representing extension of intraarticular fluid through the cuff tear into the bursa.

Other findings seen on MRI in the impingement syndrome are spurs off the inferior acromion or AC joint, capsular hypertrophy of the AC joint, or inferior displacement of the anterior acromion with respect to the distal clavicle, and pressure effect upon the supraspinatus muscle or tendon. After massive rotator cuff tears, inactivity and instability of the shoulder, along with leaking of synovial fluid, can produce atrophy of the glenohumeral articular cartilage and resorption of subchondral bone, ultimately causing humeral head collapse.[61] Another late finding is atrophy of the rotator cuff, which presents as decreased muscle bulk and increased signal in the muscles on T1-weighted images due to fatty infiltration. Timely acromioplasty can retard the progression of rotator cuff deterioration, and early diagnosis with MRI should facilitate appropriate therapy before the disease progresses to an irreversible stage.[64]

Occasionally, the long head of the biceps tendon is injured in the impingement syndrome as it travels with the supraspinatus tendon under the anterior acromion.[68] The tendon is best evaluated in the axial plane. MRI can help by showing disruption of the tendon and the location of the tendon break.

Instability

The glenohumeral joint is the most mobile joint in the body, and therefore it is also the most unstable joint.[69] The surrounding soft tissues, consisting of the glenoid labrum, synovium, joint capsule, and the rotator cuff muscles and tendons, are vital to joint stability. Instability of the joint most often causes anterior dislocation, pain, weakness, and decreased range of motion. Anterior dislocation can cause tearing of the anterior glenoid labrum and anterior joint capsule.[68,69]

The capsular structures of the joint are best demonstrated on T2-weighted axial images, particularly if there is a joint effusion. The normal anterior glenoid labrum has a triangular shape, and the posterior labrum usually has a rounded configuration. The anterior labrum is normally larger than the posterior labrum. The labrum normally has low signal intensity

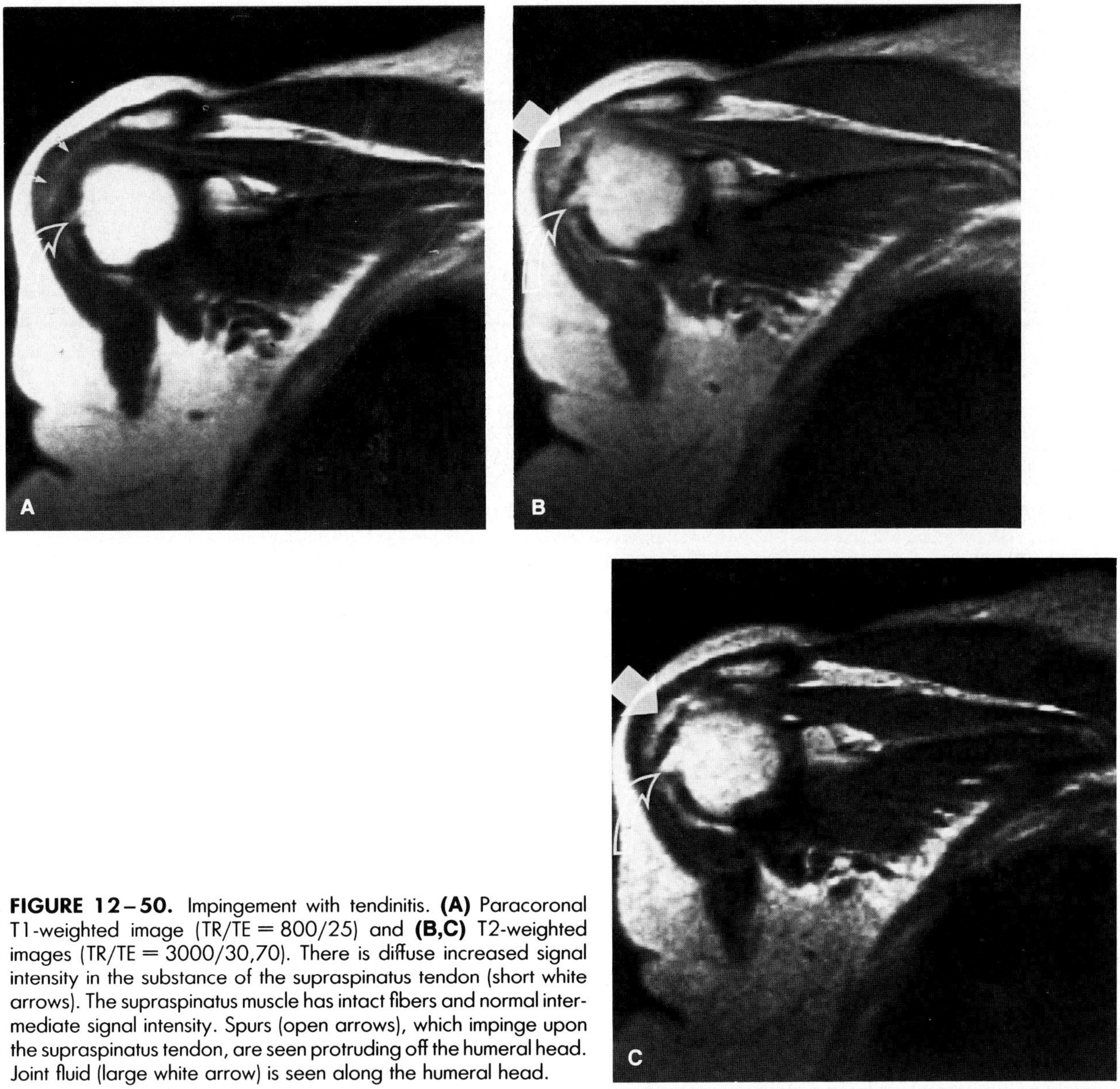

FIGURE 12–50. Impingement with tendinitis. **(A)** Paracoronal T1-weighted image (TR/TE = 800/25) and **(B,C)** T2-weighted images (TR/TE = 3000/30,70). There is diffuse increased signal intensity in the substance of the supraspinatus tendon (short white arrows). The supraspinatus muscle has intact fibers and normal intermediate signal intensity. Spurs (open arrows), which impinge upon the supraspinatus tendon, are seen protruding off the humeral head. Joint fluid (large white arrow) is seen along the humeral head.

on all pulse sequences. The MRI appearance of glenoid labrum tears can manifest as attenuation, irregularity, and indistinct borders of the labrum. Abnormal diffuse or linear areas of increased signal intensity may be seen within the substance of the glenoid labrum on T1-weighted and T2-weighted images.

Recurrent dislocation can produce bony lesions, the Hill-Sachs deformity and the Bankart lesion. Hill-Sachs deformity produces an abnormal contour of the lateral aspect of the humeral head at the level of the coracoid process. The Bankart lesion manifests as high-signal-intensity fluid along the base of the glenoid labrum or along the border of the scapula, indicative of capsular stripping. Fractures of the glenoid rim compatible with Bankart lesions can be identified.[69]

MRI OF THE TEMPOROMANDIBULAR JOINT

The TMJ is a synovial joint that is the articulation between the mandibular condyle, the glenoid fossa, and the articular eminence of the temporal bone. Abnormalities of the TMJ occur in 28% of the adult population.[70] These present as facial pain, joint click, or decreased range of motion of the jaw.

There are several methods for imaging the TMJ. These include plain films, arthrography, and CT arthrography.[71–73] Arthrography and CT arthrography are adequate techniques for evaluating the TMJ, but they are invasive, require specialized technical skill, and deliver a significant radiation dose.[74] MRI

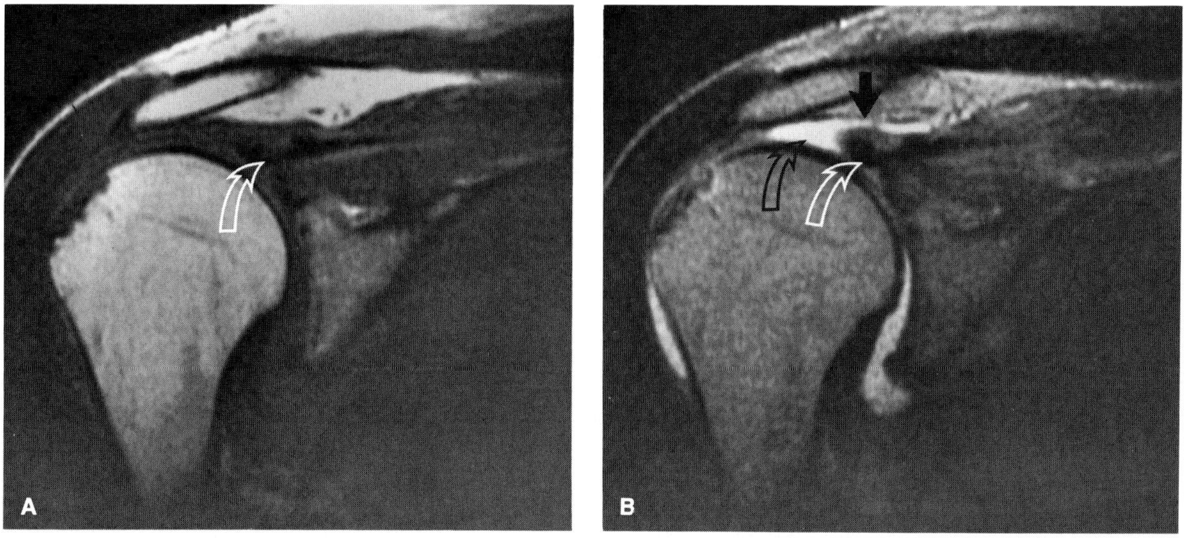

FIGURE 12–51. Complete rotator cuff tear with muscle retraction. **(A)** T1-weighted paracoronal image (TR/TE = 600/25) and **(B)** T2-weighted paracoronal image (TR/TE = 2000/80). Discontinuity and retraction of the rotator cuff musculature are demonstrated on both images (open white arrow). In the expected position of the supraspinatus tendon, at the site of the rotator cuff tear, very bright signal intensity is seen on the T2-weighted scan (open black arrow). Notice the increased signal intensity on the T2-weighted image in the subacromial bursa (black arrow). Presumably the increased signal intensity represents intra-articular fluid, which extends through the rotator cuff tear into the bursa. Also notice the joint effusion surrounding the humeral head. (Courtesy of Dr. D. L. Burk, Jr., Thomas Jefferson University Hospital)

has become the preferred imaging modality for evaluating most abnormalities of the TMJ, especially the position of the meniscus (disc). MRI provides direct visualization of the meniscus, is noninvasive, has excellent soft tissue contrast, is easy to interpret, and does not use ionizing radiation.[75,76]

Technique

To obtain the desired soft tissue resolution and SNR, images must be acquired using a surface coil. Spin echo pulse sequences are currently the imaging technique of choice. Sagittal images are obtained with the mouth closed to determine the position of the meniscus. Open mouth images are then obtained to determine if a dislocated meniscus is reducible and to evaluate the degree of condylar translation. Preferably, images should be acquired with 3-mm slices, 256 × 256 matrix, a small FOV (12–16 cm), two acquisitions, and T1-weighting (TR/TE = 500–1000/20–30). If inflammatory disease, joint fluid, or meniscal degeneration are suspected, T2-weighted images help by demonstrating increased signal intensity in the disc or joint space.[77] T2-weighted images also help to assess the stage of AVN of the mandibular condyle.[78]

Some criticize spin echo MRI's inability to demonstrate functional, dynamic information concerning the joint. These authors suggest obtaining GRASS images at incremental stages of mouth opening (1–3-mm steps). The images are then displayed in a cine mode.[77,79] Other authors suggest adding coronal T1-weighted images to increase accuracy in determining the disc position, specifically medial-lateral displacement.[80,81] New techniques include 3D volume MRI, which can produce thinner contiguous sections and simultaneous bilateral scans.[82] Newer surface coils allow simultaneous bilateral imaging with spin echo technique, which is desired because as many as 50% of these patients have bilateral joint disease. The high incidence of bilateral disease suggests that the mechanical dysfunction of one side may affect the other side.[74]

Anatomy

The mandibular condyle is located anterior to the external auditory meatus (Fig. 12–52). The head of the mandible articulates with the glenoid fossa and articular eminence of the temporal bone. The temporomandibular articulation is divided by the meniscus into upper and lower compartments. The meniscus has a biconcave configuration, with a thick anterior band, a slightly thicker posterior band, and a thin intermediate zone.[83] The normal meniscus has a lower signal intensity than the surrounding soft tissues on both T1-weighted and T2-weighted images.[84] The posterior aspect of the meniscus is attached to the retrodiscal bilaminar zone, which connects the meniscus to

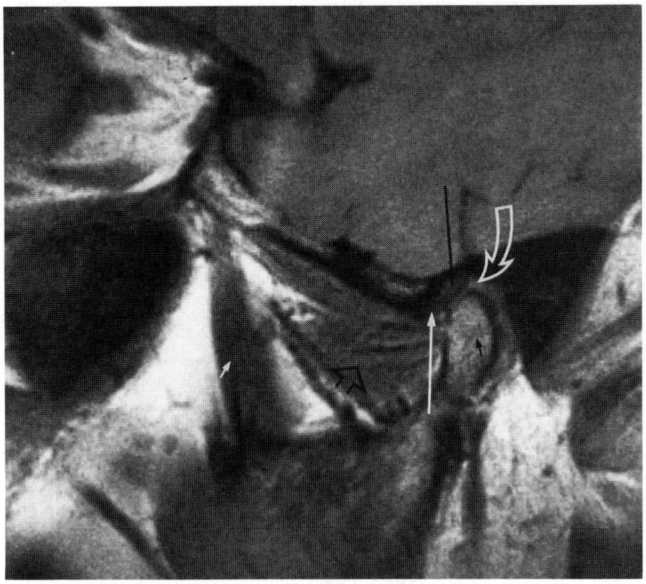

FIGURE 12–52. Normal TMJ. Sagittal T1-weighted image (TR/TE = 800/25) in the closed mouth position. The mandibular condyle (small black arrow) has increased signal intensity with a thin rim of low signal intensity cortical bone surrounding it. The meniscus is a bow-tie-shaped structure that is superior to the mandibular condyle and has low signal intensity. There is a thick anterior band (long white arrow), a thicker posterior band (long black arrow), and a thin intermediate zone. The retrodiscal bilaminar zone (open white arrow) has slightly increased signal intensity and attaches the posterior meniscus to the temporal bone. The temporalis muscle (small white arrow) and the lateral pterygoid muscle (black open arrow) have intermediate signal intensities and are anterior to the mandibular condyle.

the temporal bone behind the condyle.[77] The bilaminar zone contains elastic tissue and fat and has a slightly higher signal intensity than the meniscus.[84]

The lateral pterygoid muscle, located anterior to the meniscus, divides into two heads. The superior belly of the lateral pterygoid muscle inserts into the anteromedial aspect of the meniscus and applies traction on the normal meniscus during forward movement of the condyle. The inferior belly of the lateral pterygoid muscle inserts at the anatomic neck of the mandibular condyle and pulls the condyle forward during contraction.[77]

Normal TMJ Motion

With the mouth closed, the mandibular condyle lies centered in the glenoid fossa, with the disc located between the condyle and the glenoid fossa. Normally, the posterior band of the disc lies at "12 o'clock" relative to the mandibular condyle. Upon opening the mouth, the mandibular condyle translates anteriorly to a position under the articular eminence of the temporal bone (Figs. 12–53 and 12–54). Occasionally, the mandibular condyle will translate anterior to the articular eminence in a normal TMJ. The meniscus also moves anteriorly upon opening the mouth and should remain between the articular eminence and the mandibular condyle.[85]

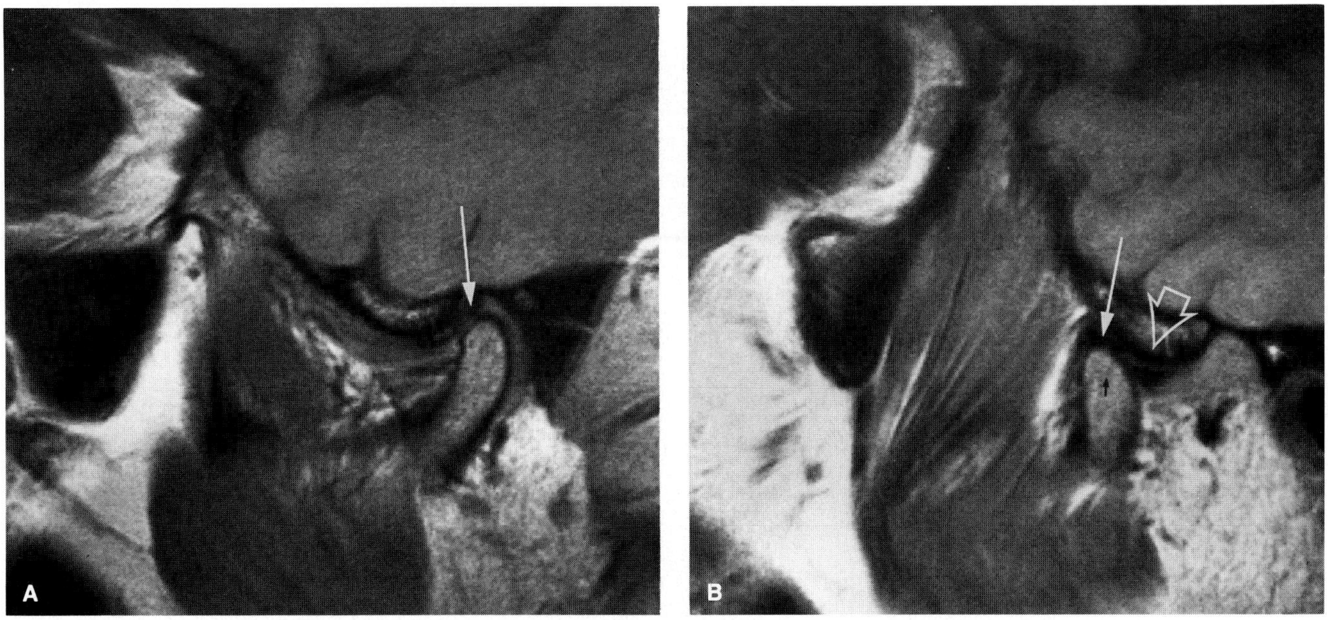

FIGURE 12–53. Normal motion of the TMJ. **(A)** Closed-mouth position and **(B)** open-mouth position sagittal T1-weighted images (TR/TE = 800/25). In the closed-mouth position, the meniscus (white arrow) is located between the mandibular condyle and the glenoid fossa. Normally the posterior band of the meniscus lies at a "12 o'clock" position relative to the mandibular condyle. Upon opening the mouth, the mandibular condyle (small black arrow) translates anteriorly to a position under the articular eminence (open arrow) of the temporal bone. The meniscus (white arrow) moves anteriorly with the condyle and should remain between the articular eminence and the mandibular condyle.

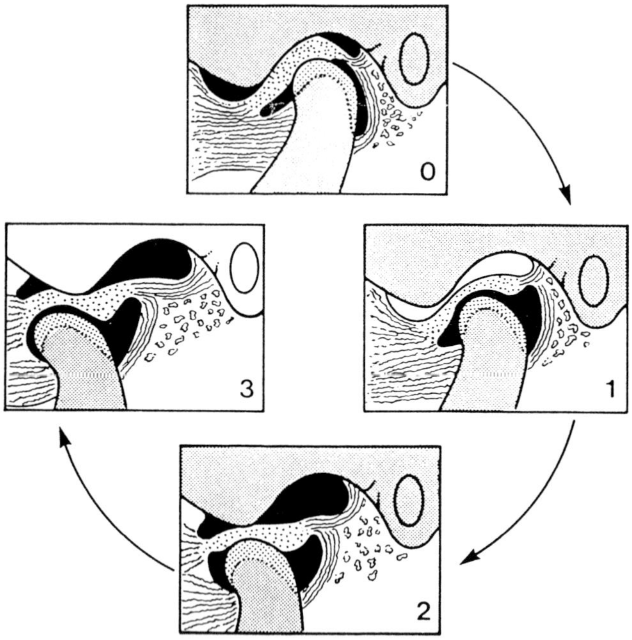

FIGURE 12–54. Diagram of normal motion of the TMJ. In the closed mouth position *(0)*, the normal meniscus is located between the condyle and the glenoid fossa, with the posterior band of the meniscus at "12 o'clock" with respect to the condyle. Upon opening *(1)*, the condyle rotates under the disc, and further opening *(2)*, causes the meniscus and condyle to translate anteriorly to a position under the articular eminence *(3)*. (Adapted from Harms SE, Wilk RM. Magnetic resonance imaging of the temporomandibular joint. Radiographics 1987;7:521)

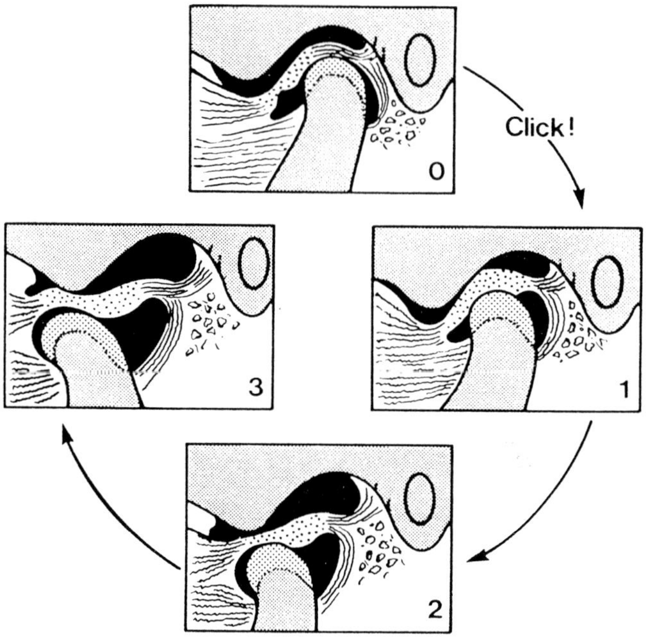

FIGURE 12–55. Diagram of anteriorly displaced meniscus with reduction. In the closed mouth position *(0)*, the meniscus is displaced anterior to the condyle. Upon opening *(1)*, the condyle translates anteriorly under the intermediate zone of the meniscus. A click or pop is often heard. With further opening *(2)*, the disc and condyle translate to a normal position under the articular eminence *(3)*. (Adapted from Harms SE, Wilk RM. Magnetic resonance imaging of the temporomandibular joint. Radiographics 1987;7:521)

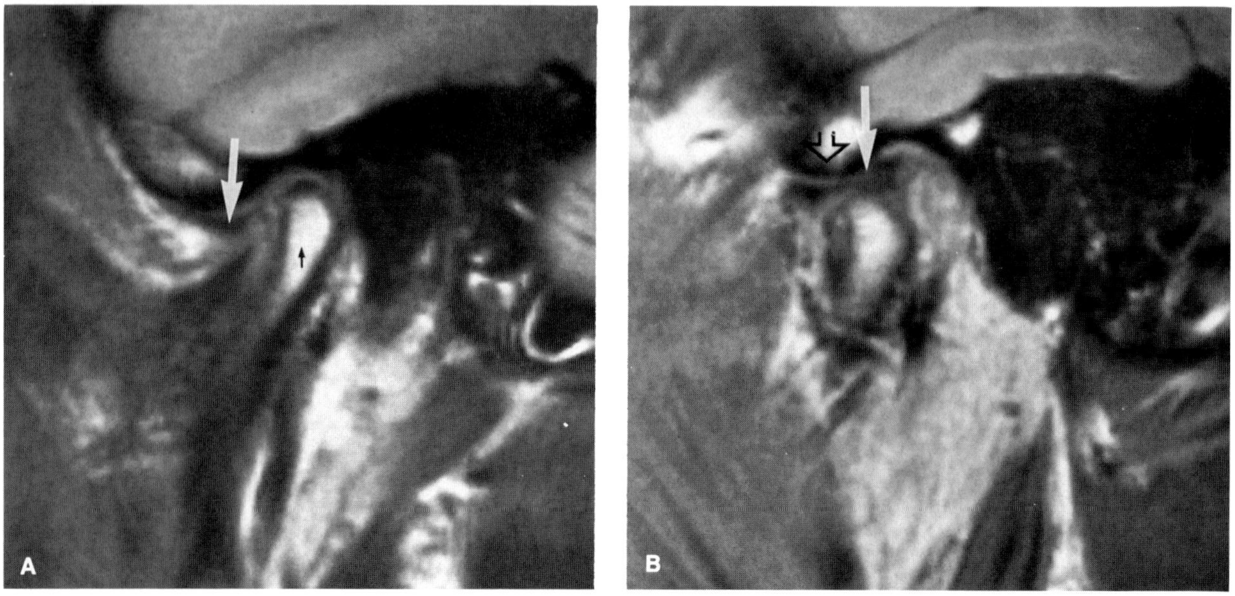

FIGURE 12–56. Anteriorly dislocated meniscus with reduction. **(A)** Closed-mouth position and **(B)** open-mouth position T1-weighted sagittal images (TR/TE = 700/25). In the closed-mouth position, the meniscus (white arrow) is anterior to the mandibular condyle (black arrow). Upon opening the mouth, the meniscus (white arrow) resumes a normal position between the mandibular condyle and the articular eminence of the temporal bone (open arrow). An anterior osteophyte also can be seen along the articular surface of the condyle.

TMJ Dysfunction

The most common symptoms of an abnormal TMJ are facial pain, click, and decreased range of motion of the jaw. Anterior dislocation of the disc is the most common cause.[77] In an anterior reducible dislocation, the meniscus is located anterior to the mandibular condyle, with the condyle resting on the retrodiscal tissue in the closed position (Figs. 12–55 and 12–56). On opening, the condyle translates anteriorly under the posterior band of the meniscus, with a resultant click. The condyle then assumes a normal position, with the mandibular condyle located under the intermediate zone of the meniscus in the open-mouth position.[85]

With a fixed (nonreducible) anterior dislocation, the meniscus is located anterior to the mandibular condyle when the mouth is closed and often has a deformed, bunched-up appearance (Figs. 12–57 and 12–58). In the open-mouth position, the disc remains dislocated anterior to the condyle. Often there is also mechanical obstruction to condylar translation, producing a locked condyle.[85] Sideward displacement of the meniscus, most often medially, commonly accompanies anterior displacement of the meniscus and advanced internal derangements of the TMJ (Fig. 12–59). Coronal images can help in demonstrating medial or lateral displacement, but often sagittal images are sufficient.[77,81]

It is postulated that when the disc is anteriorly dis-

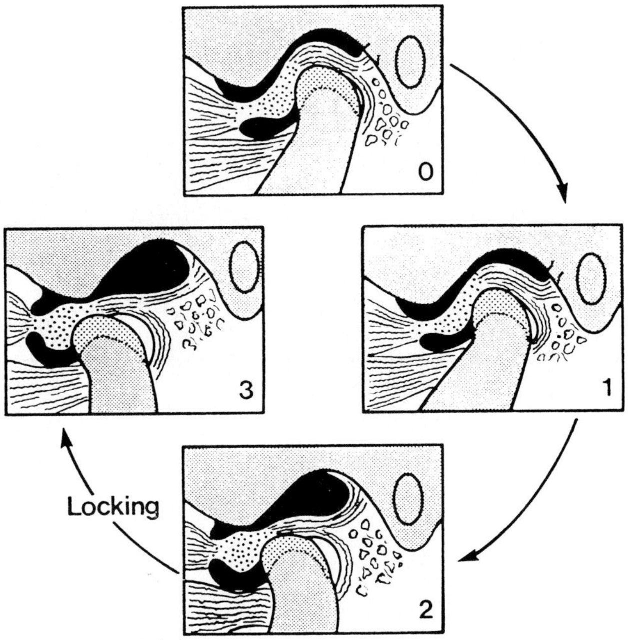

FIGURE 12–57. Diagram of anterior dislocation without reduction. In the closed mouth position *(0)*, the meniscus is displaced anteriorly to the condyle, with the condyle resting on the retrodiscal tissue. Upon opening *(1)*, the disc remains anterior to the condyle. Further opening *(2)* causes compression of the disc by the condyle. The disc acts as a mechanical obstruction, locking the mandible and preventing translocation *(3)*. (Adapted from Harms SE, Wilk RM. Magnetic resonance imaging of the temporomandibular joint. Radiographics 1987;7:521)

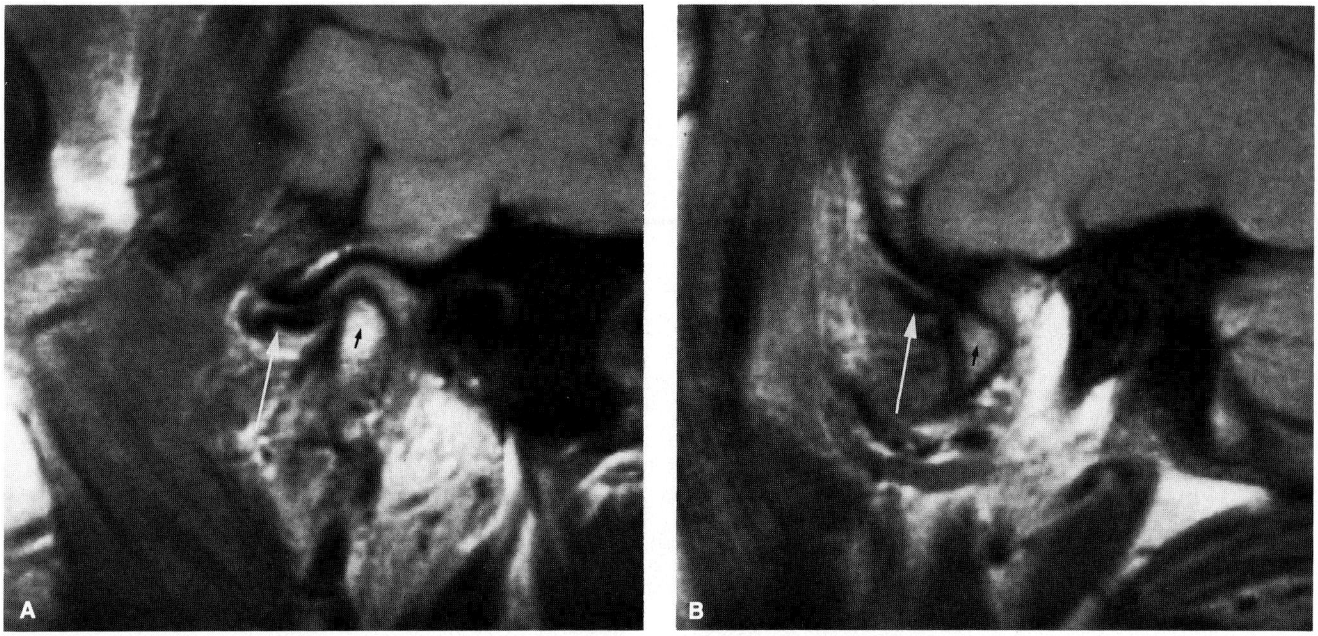

FIGURE 12–58. Anteriorly dislocated meniscus without reduction. **(A)** Closed-mouth position and **(B)** open-mouth position T1-weighted sagittal images (TR/TE = 800/25). In the closed-mouth position, the meniscus (white arrow) is displaced anterior to the mandibular condyle (black arrow) and has a buckled distorted shape. Upon opening the mouth, the meniscus (white arrow) remains dislocated anterior to the mandibular condyle (black arrow).

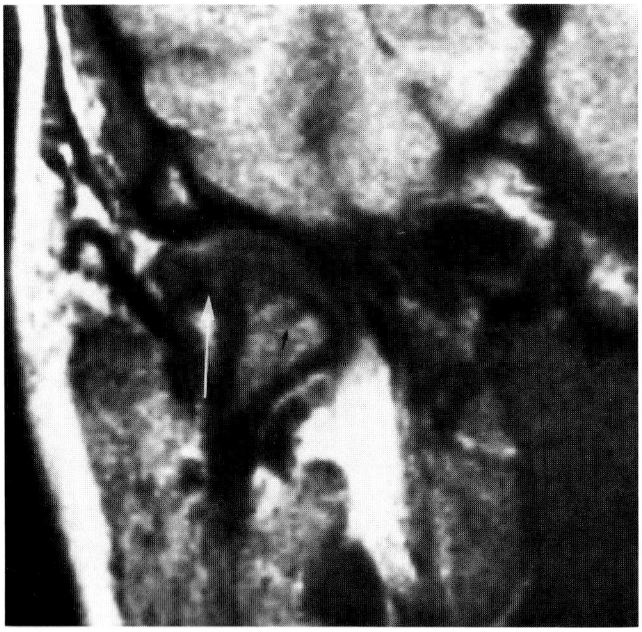

FIGURE 12–59. Laterally dislocated meniscus. T1-weighted coronal image (TR/TE = 800/25) identifies the meniscus (white arrow) laterally displaced with respect to the mandibular condyle (black arrow).

placed, the condyle articulates with the posterior attachment of the disc, rather than with the disc itself. This leads to inflammation and often to perforation of the posterior meniscal attachment. Once perforation has occurred, the direct contact between the articular surfaces of the mandibular condyle and the temporal bone erodes the articular cartilage and causes degenerative arthritis (Fig. 12-60).[75,86]

Perforations of the meniscus are easily diagnosed by arthrography by demonstrating contrast entering the substance of the meniscus or contrast filling the superior joint compartment after injection of the inferior compartment.[75] MRI has only marginal success in demonstrating perforations. At present, only large perforations with separation of the disc fragments can be reliably demonstrated. Many smaller tears that could be seen with arthrography go undetected with MRI.[75,76,87] One study demonstrated several false-positive perforations diagnosed by MRI. This was caused by an attenuated appearance of the stretched bilaminar zone in chronic anterior disc displacement.[77] Because disc perforation is often a relatively late occurrence in the abnormal TMJ, the diagnosis of internal derangement of the TMJ should be based on ear-

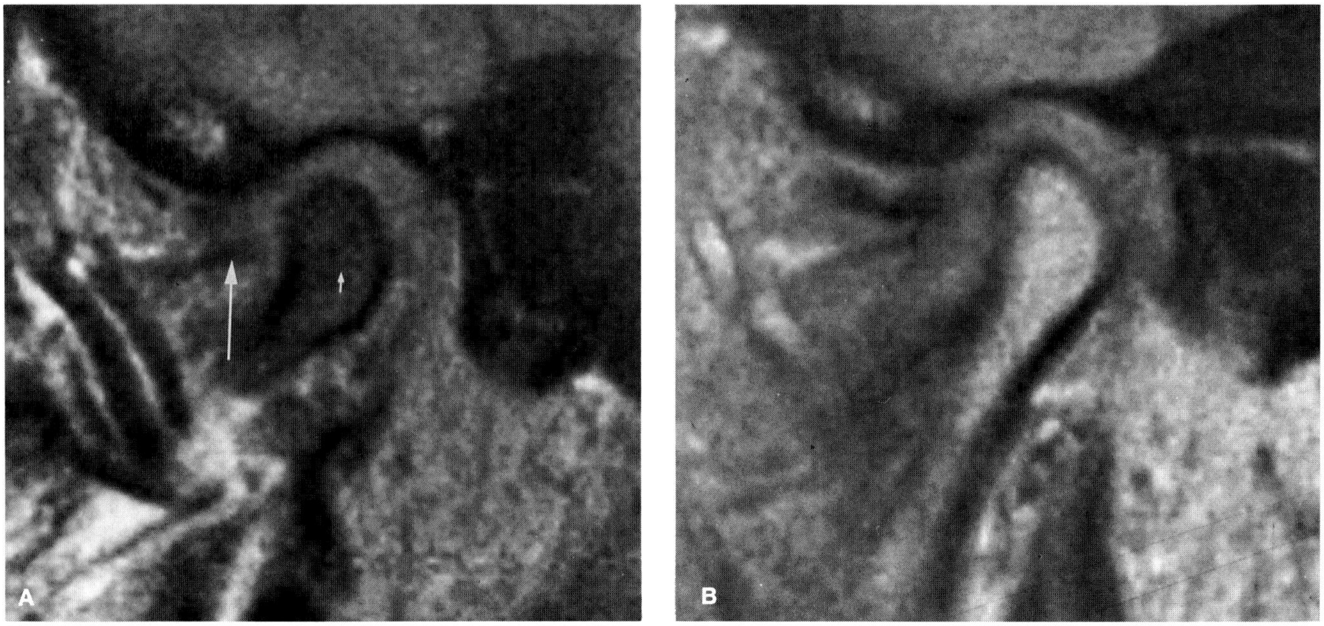

FIGURE 12–60. Degenerative changes in the mandibular condyle. **(A)** Right TMJ and **(B)** left TMJ, T1-weighted sagittal images (TR/TE = 800/25). Sagittal image of the right TMJ demonstrates diffuse decreased signal intensity in the bone marrow of the right mandibular condyle (short white arrow), representing degenerative changes. Notice the meniscus is anteriorly displaced (long white arrow). Compare with the left TMJ, which shows normal high signal intensity in the marrow of the mandibular condyle.

lier findings, such as anterior disc displacement. MRI is very accurate in determining the disc position, and therefore has become the procedure of choice for evaluating TMJ meniscal abnormalities.[88]

Chronic anterior disc displacement can lead to changes in the meniscus, muscles, and the adjacent bony structures. Myxoid degeneration of the meniscus fibrocartilage may cause increased signal intensity in the substance of the abnormal meniscus on T2-weighted images.[77] Fibrosis, atrophy, and contracture of the superior belly of the lateral pterygoid muscle can occur following chronic anterior disc dislocation and present as fatty replacement (increased signal intensity on T1-weighted images) and attenuation of the muscle.[77] Thickening of the fascia in the inferior belly of the lateral pterygoid muscle may indicate chronic anterior disc displacement.[89] Later, osteoarthritic changes can be seen in the mandibular condyle and along the glenoid fossa, which manifest as osteophytes (Fig. 12–61) and bony deformities (Fig. 12–62).[75]

Internal derangement of the TMJ may induce osteochondritis or AVN of the mandibular condyle. MRI findings of AVN include loss of the normal fatty marrow signal intensity, with resultant low signal intensity in the marrow of the mandibular condyle on short TR/TE scans.[78] Early and reparative AVN have an increased signal intensity in the marrow on T2-weighted scans, while late AVN has decreased signal intensity in the marrow. There is often associated contour deformity of the mandibular condyle. Osteochondritis presents as a focal subarticular bone defect, which often has a low signal intensity centrally, surrounded by high signal intensity on both T1-weighted and T2-weighted scans.[78]

Simple meniscectomy is the surgical treatment of choice in patients who have meniscal degeneration and in patients with pain and dysfunction of the TMJ secondary to anterior displacement of the meniscus. This may be accompanied by temporary meniscal implants to prevent adhesions in the early postoperative period.[77,90] The rationale for meniscectomy is to increase the articular-bearing surface between the temporal bone and the mandibular condyle to decrease the focal stress on the articular surface cartilage, thereby decreasing the likelihood that osteoarthritis will develop.[75] Other surgical procedures include meniscus plication, condylectomy, and reduction osteotomy of the articular eminence.[77]

The postoperative TMJ is a challenge to MRI. Typi-

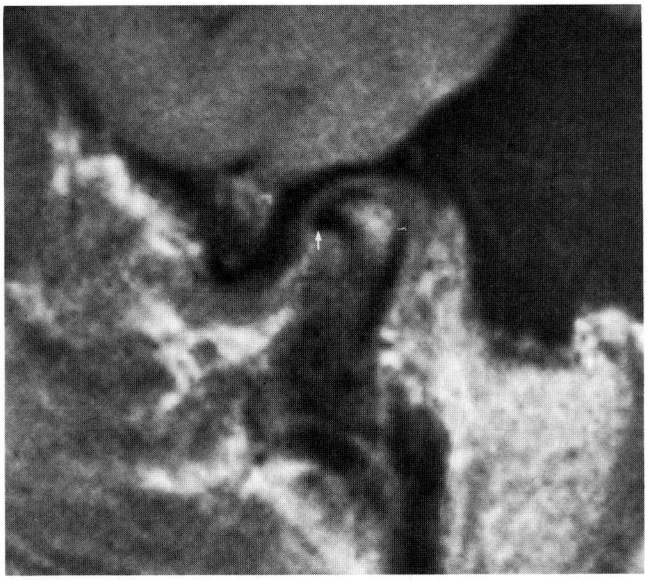

FIGURE 12–61. Mandibular condyle osteophyte. T1-weighted sagittal image (TR/TE = 800/25). This closed-mouth-position image shows decreased signal intensity along the anterior aspect of the head of the mandibular condyle, representing a degenerative osteophyte (white arrow), which is a common secondary finding in chronic anterior disc displacement. Notice that the meniscus is anteriorly dislocated.

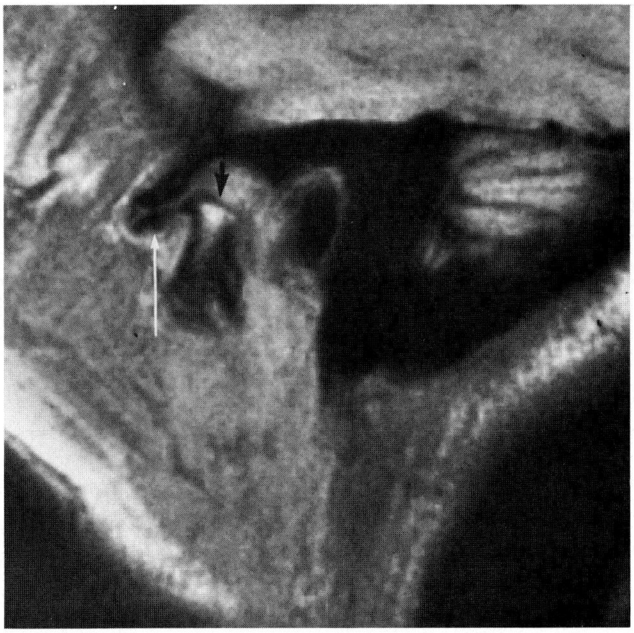

FIGURE 12–62. Advanced osteoarthritic changes in the mandibular condyle. Sagittal T1-weighted image (TR/TE = 800/25) shows chronic anterior dislocation of the meniscus (long white arrow). Osteoarthritic changes, with marked deformity and flattening of the mandibular condyle (black arrow), resulted.

cally, after meniscectomy, the amputated posterior and anterior meniscal attachments are seen at the margins of the articular space. There is often some remodeling of the TMJ, with thickening of the articular cartilage surfaces of the glenoid fossa and mandibular condyle and often slight flattening of these structures.[77] The articular space is maintained by the surface fibrocartilage, although often relatively narrowed, but without functional disturbance.

If a prosthesis is placed, it can be identified as an area of signal void between the mandibular condyle and the temporal bone (Fig. 12-63). Approximately 25% of prostheses will fragment or fracture. Any discontinuity of the prosthesis should be interpreted as a fracture.[90] Other complications of failed Proplast-Teflon implants include erosions, foreign-body reactions, and AVN.[91] Erosions can affect both the mandibular condyle and the temporal bone. Foreign-body granulomatous reactions and AVN of the condyle are not uncommon.[91] Either of these processes can present as decreased signal intensity in the marrow of the condyle. Granulomatous reactions often have accompanying soft tissue masses and cortical erosions. AVN is distinguished by bony deformity and collapse. Other complications after surgery include joint fluid, bony ankylosis, and adhesions, often seen as thick fibrous connective tissue bands that are isointense with soft tissue.[77,90]

Strict attention must be paid to MRI technique so that images with proper SNR and resolution are obtained. Rapid scanning and 3D scanning may soon play a more prominent role and provide functional information about the TMJ.

MRI OF THE WRIST

Despite the proven efficacy of MRI for the musculoskeletal system, only limited experience exists for the wrist. As in most other joints, high-resolution scans of the wrist with adequate SNR require surface coil imaging, preferably performed at high field strength (1.0-1.5 T). Current indications for MRI of the wrist include the evaluation of osseous abnormalities, such as AVN, soft tissue masses, and the carpal tunnel syndrome.

Technique

The most successful position for imaging the wrist requires a prone patient in the gantry with the arm extended overhead. Surface coil imaging is manda-

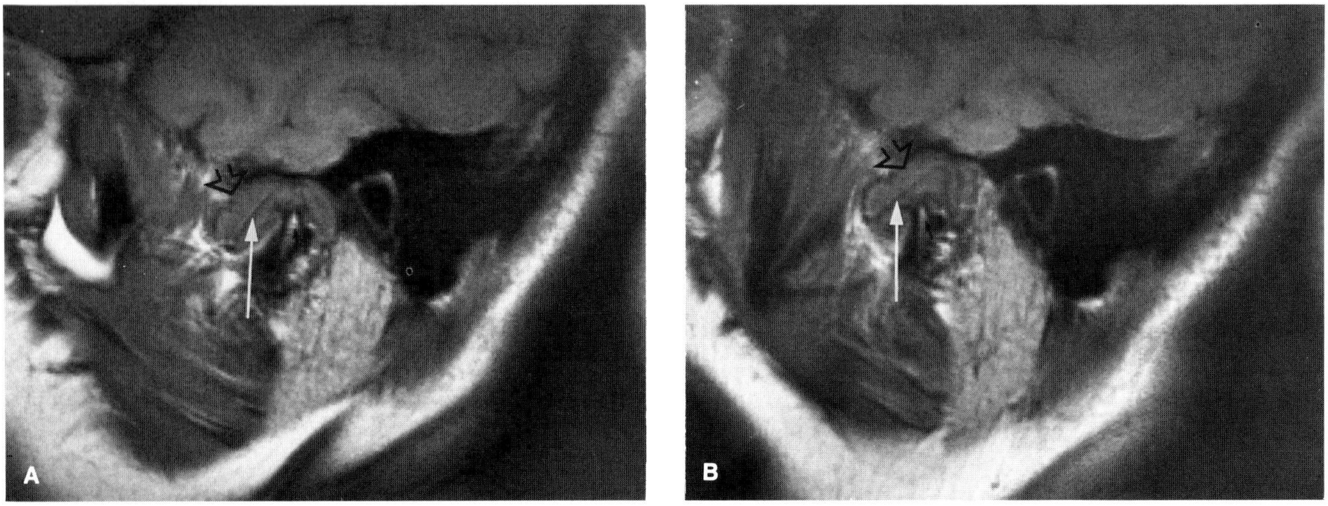

FIGURE 12-63. Meniscal prosthesis. **(A)** Closed-mouth position and **(B)** open-mouth position on T1-weighted sagittal images (TR/TE = 800/17). The closed-mouth scan identifies no normal meniscal tissue. A linear, low-signal-intensity prosthesis (long white arrow) is interposed in the joint space between the deformed mandibular condyle (black arrow) and the articular tubercle of the temporal bone. Upon opening the mouth, there is anterior translation of the mandibular condyle (black arrow), accompanied by the meniscal prosthesis (long white arrow), to a normal position under the articular eminence. On both images, a soft tissue mass representing reactive granulation tissue (open arrow) is seen surrounding the meniscal prosthesis.

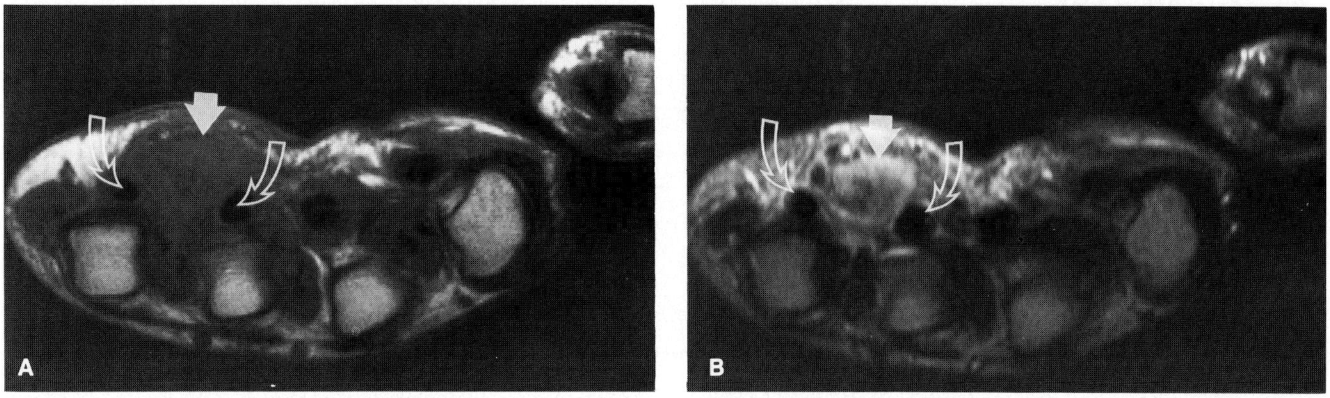

FIGURE 12–64. Soft tissue sarcoma. **(A)** Axial T1-weighted image (TR/TE = 700/25) and **(B)** T2-weighted axial image (TR/TE = 3000/90). A rounded soft tissue mass is visualized on both images. The mass (white arrow) has intermediate signal intensity on the T1-weighted scan and increased signal intensity on the T2-weighted scan. The adjacent, low-signal-intensity tendons (white open arrows) are splayed by the soft tissue mass. At surgery, a soft tissue sarcoma was found.

tory for adequate SNR and resolution. The wrist is placed palm down on a surface coil, circular or planar, and then taped or sand-bagged firmly to minimize motion. Other techniques can be used, such as elevating the wrist on foam pads and placing a surface coil tightly against the dorsal aspect of the wrist. Small circumferential transmit-receive coils are also effective. Most commonly, spin echo pulse sequences are used with T1-weighted (TR/TE = 500–700/20–30) scans obtained in coronal and axial planes. T2-weighted scans (TR/TE = 2500–3000/20–90) should be obtained in the scan plane that will best delineate the abnormality. Generally, coronal planes are best for osseous abnormalities, such as AVN, and axial planes are best for the carpal tunnel and to evaluate the extent of soft tissue masses (Fig. 12–64). A small FOV is essential for attaining good resolution. Recommended scan parameters for wrist imaging are 3- to 4-mm slices, 256 × 256 scan matrix, 8 to 12 cm FOV, and one acquisition for T2-weighted images and two to four acquisitions for T1-weighted scans.

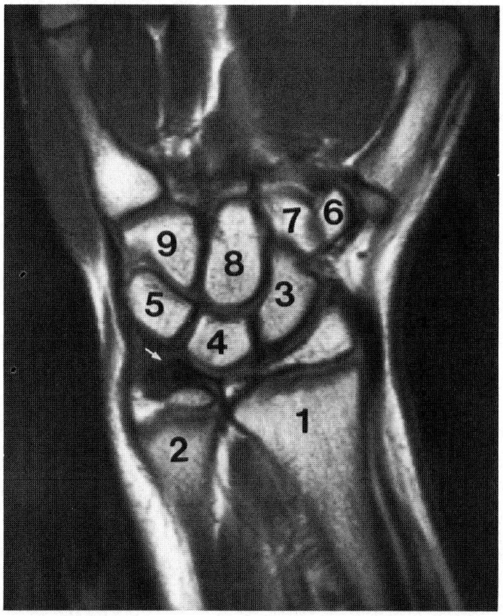

FIGURE 12–65. Normal wrist in a coronal T1-weighted image (TR/TE = 700/25). The coronal scan plane ideally shows the relationship of the carpal bones to the metacarpal bones and the radius and ulna. The triangular fibrocartilage is demonstrated by low signal intensity (white arrow). *1*, radius; *2*, ulna; *3*, scaphoid; *4*, lunate; *5*, triquetrium; *6*, trapezium; *7*, trapezoid; *8*, capitate; *9*, hamate.

Anatomy

The tendons and ligaments of the wrist usually have low signal intensity on all pulse sequences. Bone marrow has high signal intensity on T1-weighted images, due to fat, which is surrounded by low-signal-intensity cortical bone. Muscles and nerves have an intermediate signal intensity on all pulse sequences.[92–95]

Coronal images (Fig. 12–65) best show the relationship of the carpal bones to the metacarpal bones, the ulna, and the radius. The course of nerves, vessels, and tendons is also well visualized. The triangular fibrocartilage is seen on coronal images as a triangular region of low signal intensity on T1-weighted and T2-weighted images.

The axial plane is superior for imaging the carpal tunnel (Fig. 12–66).[96] The carpal tunnel is primarily occupied by the tendons of the flexor muscles of the hand and the median nerve. Carpal bones form the dorsal surface of the carpal tunnel. The palmar surface is formed by a ligamentous band called the flexor retinaculum. The flexor retinaculum extends medially from the hook of the hamate and pisiform bone laterally to the scaphoid and trapezium. The flexor retinaculum appears as a thin band of low signal in-

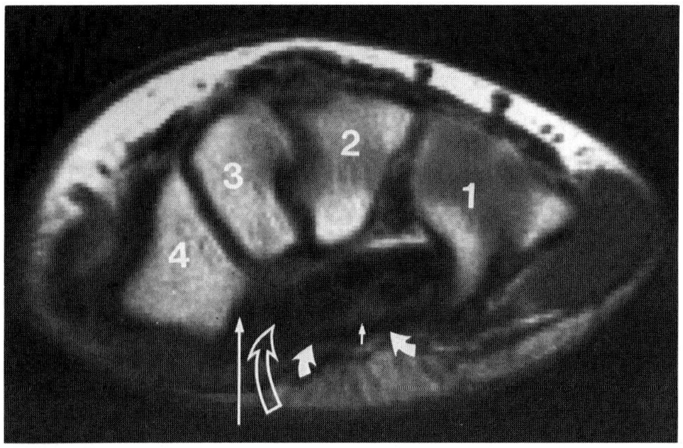

FIGURE 12–66. Axial T1-weighted (TR/TE = 700/25) MRI of the normal wrist. The axial plane best demonstrates the carpal tunnel. The tendons have low signal intensity, and the median nerve has intermediate signal intensity (small white arrow). The flexor retinaculum is a thin, low-signal-intensity band forming the palmar surface of the carpal tunnel (curved white arrows). Adjacent to the median nerve are the flexor digitorum superficialis tendons. The deepest tendons are the flexor digitorum profundus tendons. *1*, hamate; *2*, capitate; *3*, trapezoid; *4*, trapezium, long white arrow, flexor carpi radialis tendon; curved open arrow, flexor pollicus longus tendon.

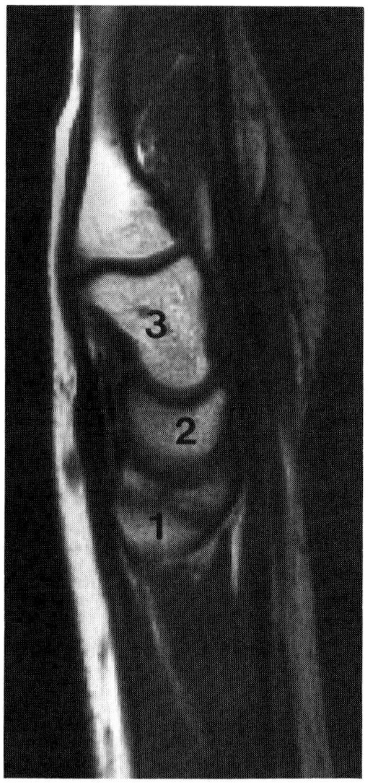

FIGURE 12–67. Sagittal T1-weighted image (TR/TE = 700/25) of the normal wrist. The sagittal plane can demonstrate the alignment of the radius, lunate, capitate, and the 3rd metacarpal bone. *1*, radius; *2*, lunate; *3*, capitate.

tensity on all pulse sequences. Just deep to the flexor retinaculum lie the tendons of the flexor digitorum superficialis muscles, which divide into four tendons as they pass through the carpal tunnel. Lateral and deep to these tendons is the tendon of the flexor pollicis longus muscle. Lateral to the flexor pollicis longus tendon is the flexor carpi radialis tendon, which actually lies outside and adjacent to the carpal tunnel. The deepest tendons in the carpal tunnel are the four tendons of the flexor digitorum profundus muscles, which lie deep to the flexor digitorum superficialis tendons. The tendons in the carpal tunnel have low signal intensity on all pulse sequences and are outlined by higher-signal-intensity sheaths. The median nerve usually is located against the flexor retinaculum near the second flexor digitorum superficialis tendon. The median nerve has intermediate signal intensity on all pulse sequences, paralleling that of muscle, in contrast to the low-signal-intensity tendons.

The sagittal plane is usually the least informative. It can help in evaluating the digits, especially the insertion of tendons upon the phalanges. Sagittal images also offer an additional view of the relationship of the radius and ulna with respect to the carpal bones (Fig. 12–67).

Pathology

Ganglion cysts are the most common tumors of the hand, often presenting with wrist or hand pain.[97] From 10 to 20% occur in close proximity to a major vessel, which must be avoided during aspiration. MRI can demonstrate the relationship of the ganglion to adjacent vessels and nerves. Most ganglion cysts have typical MRI signal characteristics with intermediate signal intensity on T1-weighted images and high signal intensity on T2-weighted images (Fig. 12-68). Often ganglion cysts splay the adjacent tendons.

AVN commonly occurs in the wrist after trauma and presents with local wrist pain. Fractures of the proximal or middle portion of the scaphoid bone often lead to AVN of the proximal pole of the scaphoid (Fig. 12–69). Minor repetitive trauma can cause AVN of the lunate bone, Kienböck's disease (Fig. 12–70), or rarely may involve other carpal bones (Fig. 12–71). MRI is very sensitive for AVN and often shows abnormalities before radiographic changes. MRI is more specific for AVN than radionuclide bone scans. The most common MRI presentation of AVN is decreased signal intensity in the bone marrow on T1-weighted scans. To increase specificity, it has been suggested that AVN should have decreased signal intensity in the marrow on T2-weighted scans, which matches an expected vascular territory.[98]

The carpal tunnel syndrome is caused by numerous pathologic conditions, including thickening and fibrosis of the flexor tendon sheaths, scar tissue, tumor compressing the median nerve, or inflammation producing swelling of the median nerve.[96] The normal size of the median nerve is 4.5 × 2.0 mm at the level of

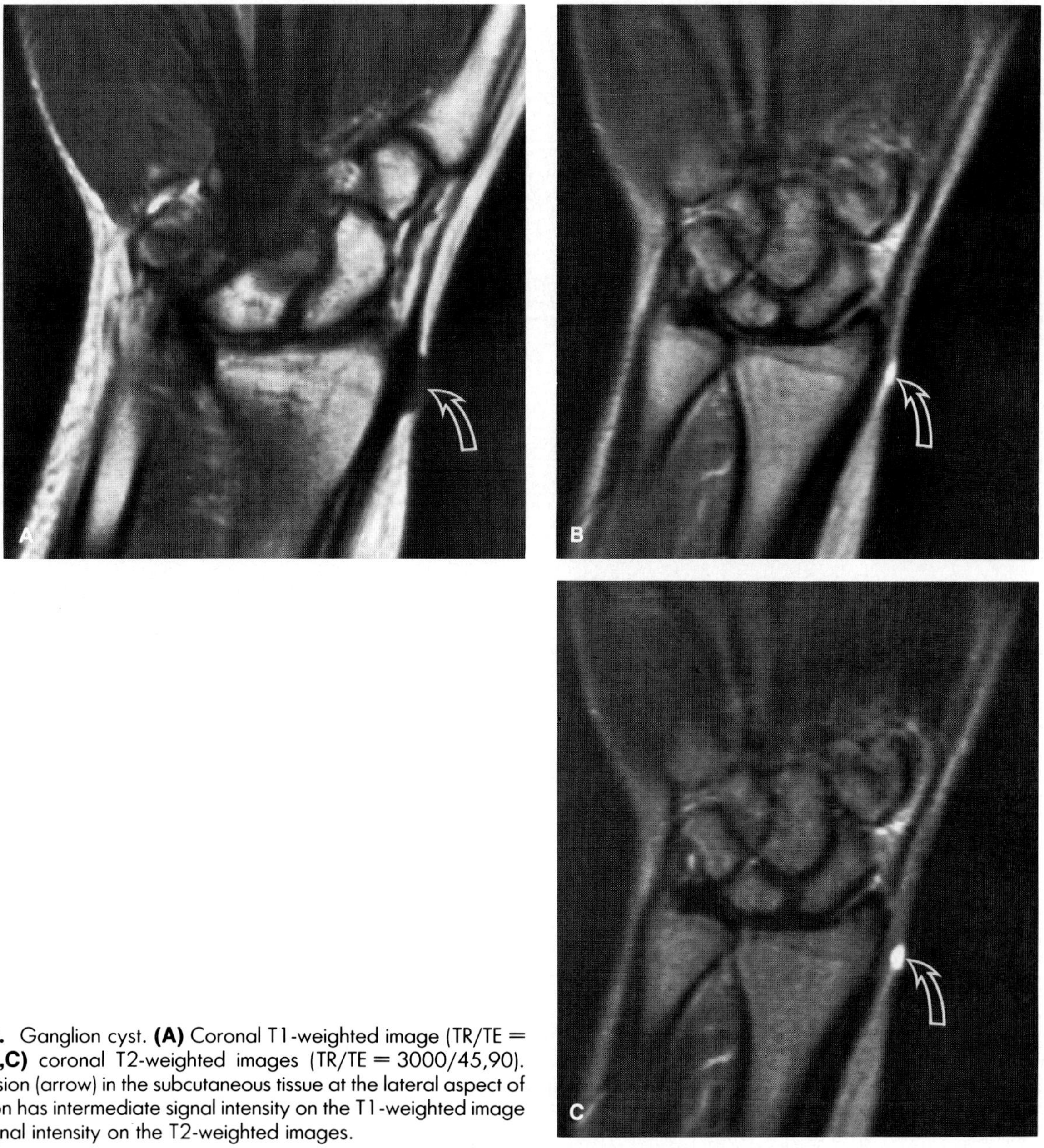

FIGURE 12–68. Ganglion cyst. **(A)** Coronal T1-weighted image (TR/TE = 700/25) and **(B,C)** coronal T2-weighted images (TR/TE = 3000/45,90). There is a small lesion (arrow) in the subcutaneous tissue at the lateral aspect of the wrist. The lesion has intermediate signal intensity on the T1-weighted image and increased signal intensity on the T2-weighted images.

the pisiform bone, and 4.9 × 2.1 mm at the level of the hook of the hamate.[96] Abnormalities of the median nerve, causing the carpal tunnel syndrome, should be suspected when the median nerve measures greater than two standard deviations above the mean. Also, increased signal intensity may be seen within the median nerve on T2-weighted images, indicating swelling or edema. Scar tissue, fibrosis of tendon sheaths, and tumors displacing and distorting the median nerve are easily identified with MRI. Often comparison with the contralateral normal wrist makes the diagnosis easier.

A few cases have been reported in which MRI detected fractures of the hook of the hamate that could not be identified on plain films.[97] MRI reveals pannus formation around carpal and interphalangeal joints in patients with rheumatoid arthritis. Acutely inflamed pannus has decreased signal intensity on T1-weighted images and increased signal intensity on T2-weighted images, and chronic pannus has decreased signal intensity on both T1-weighted and T2-weighted scans.[97]

MRI OF THE ANKLE

The ankle is a commonly injured joint, primarily imaged with plain radiographs or radionuclide bone scans and less commonly delineated by arthrography and CT. MRI plays only a limited role in evaluating

(text continues on page 450)

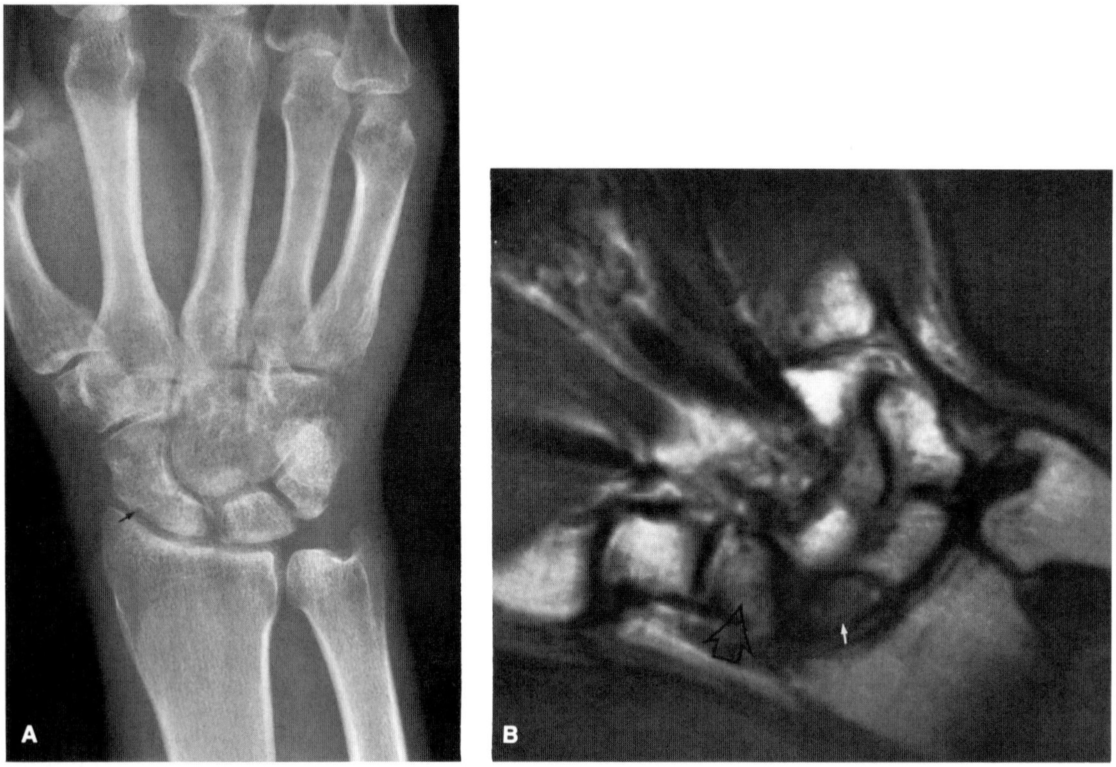

FIGURE 12–69. AVN of the proximal pole of the scaphoid bone after fracture. **(A)** Plain radiograph of the wrist and **(B)** coronal T1-weighted image (TR/TE = 700/25). Plain film reveals a fracture through the waist of the scaphoid bone (black arrow). Notice the mild sclerosis of the proximal pole of the scaphoid, indicating AVN. The MRI scan shows marked decreased signal intensity in the proximal pole of the scaphoid due to AVN (white arrow). There is normal increased signal intensity in the visualized portion of the distal pole of the scaphoid bone (open arrow).

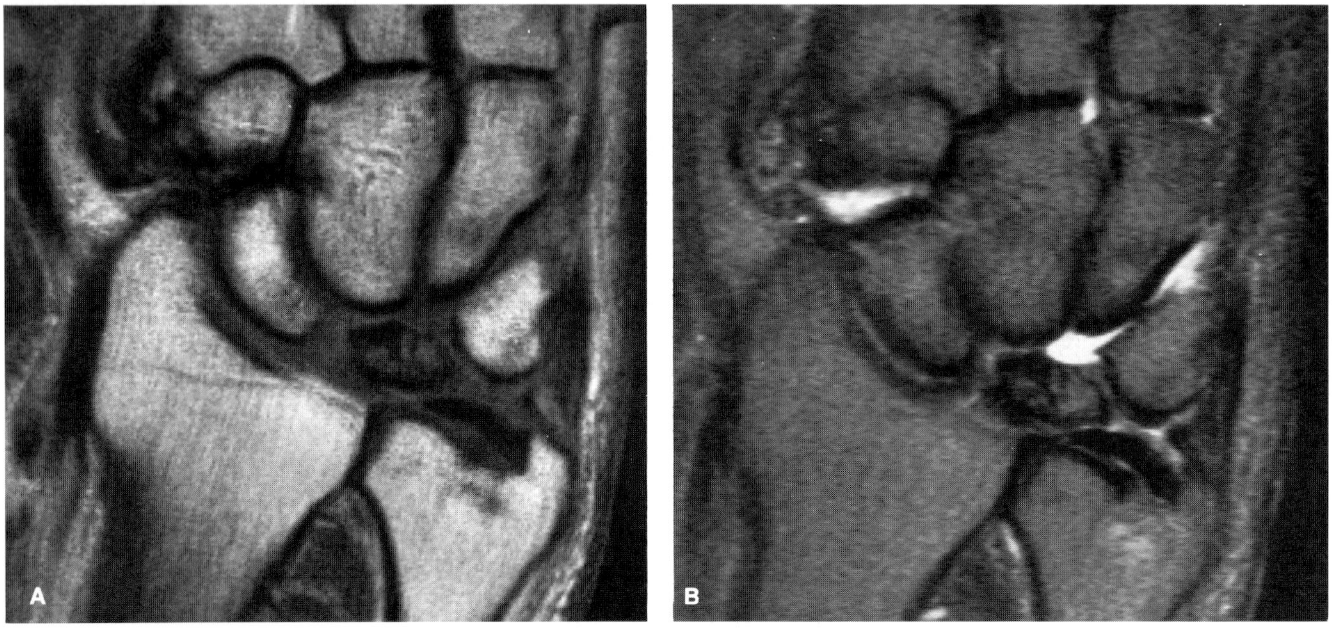

FIGURE 12–70. Kienböck's disease. **(A)** Coronal T1-weighted image (TR/TE = 700/25) and **(B)** coronal T2-weighted image (TR/TE = 3000/90) show decreased signal intensity in the lunate bone. This is the classic MR appearance of AVN in the wrist. Notice the increased-signal-intensity joint fluid on the T2-weighted scan.

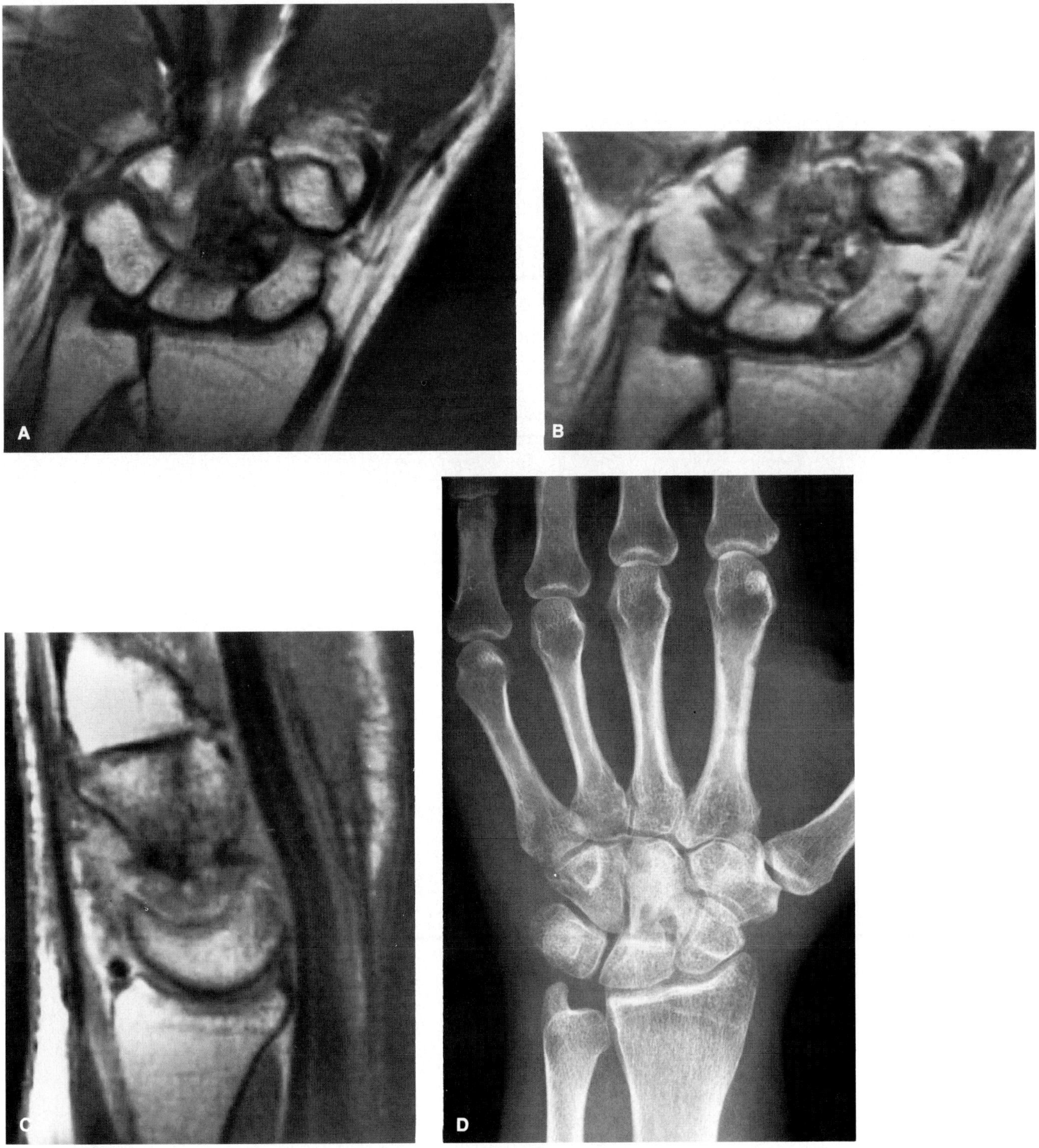

FIGURE 12–71. AVN of the capitate. **(A)** Coronal T1-weighted image (TR/TE = 700/25); **(B)** coronal T2-weighted image (TR/TE = 3000/45); **(C)** sagittal T1-weighted image (TR/TE = 800/25); **(D)** radiograph of the wrist. There is heterogeneous decreased signal intensity in the capitate bone on the T1-weighted and T2-weighted images, representing AVN. A few small areas of intermediate or high signal intensity are seen in the capitate bone on the T2-weighted scan, which are the result of previous bone graft. The plain film demonstrates increased density in the capitate bone due to AVN and postoperative changes.

ankle abnormalities, although MRI is capable of delineating the complex anatomy of the ankle joint.[99-101] As in other joints, MRI is useful for evaluating soft tissue masses, bone marrow abnormalities, ligaments, tendons, and articular cartilage.

Technique

The attainment of adequate SNR and resolution requires the use of local coils. The ankle may be placed within a volume coil, such as the knee or head coil, with the patient lying supine in the gantry. Other possibilities include the patient lying on his side with the ankle on a flat planar surface coil, such as the spine coil. The ankle must be immobilized to minimize motion during the scan. Spin echo T1-weighted (TR/TE = 400–600/20–30) and T2-weighted (TR/TE = 2000–3000/20–90) pulse sequences are most often employed. Suggested image parameters are 3- to 4-mm slices, 256 × 256 scan matrix, 12-cm FOV, and two acquisitions for T1-weighted and one acquisition for T2-weighted scans.

Anatomy

The excellent soft tissue contrast of MRI clearly delineates the complex anatomy of the ankle joint (Fig. 12–72).[99-101] The tendons and ligaments have very

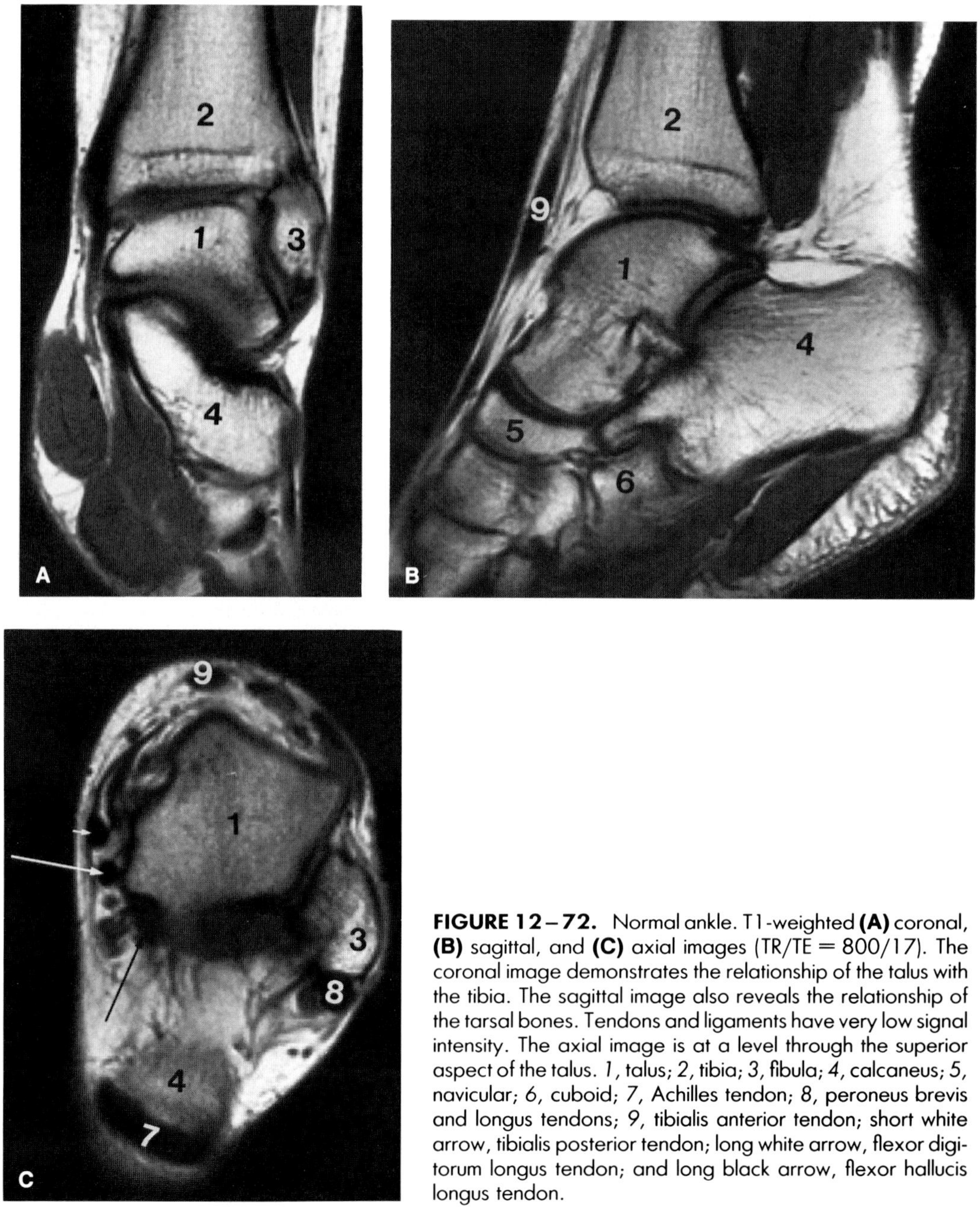

FIGURE 12–72. Normal ankle. T1-weighted **(A)** coronal, **(B)** sagittal, and **(C)** axial images (TR/TE = 800/17). The coronal image demonstrates the relationship of the talus with the tibia. The sagittal image also reveals the relationship of the tarsal bones. Tendons and ligaments have very low signal intensity. The axial image is at a level through the superior aspect of the talus. *1*, talus; *2*, tibia; *3*, fibula; *4*, calcaneus; *5*, navicular; *6*, cuboid; *7*, Achilles tendon; *8*, peroneus brevis and longus tendons; *9*, tibialis anterior tendon; short white arrow, tibialis posterior tendon; long white arrow, flexor digitorum longus tendon; and long black arrow, flexor hallucis longus tendon.

low signal intensity on all pulse sequences and are contrasted by the high signal intensity of adjacent fat. Bone marrow has increased signal intensity on T1-weighted images and is surrounded by the decreased signal of cortical bone. Muscles have an intermediate signal intensity on all pulse sequences. Hyaline cartilage also has intermediate signal intensity and is well visualized against the neighboring black (low intensity) cortical bone.

Coronal images show the relationship of the tibia and fibula to the adjoining tarsal bones, particularly the talus (Fig. 12–72A). The collateral ligaments are also easily visualized on coronal images.

Sagittal images optimally show the course of the tendons (Fig. 12–72B). The tibialis anterior, peroneus tertius, extensor hallucis longus, and extensor digitorum longus tendons reside anteriorly, and the peroneus longus and brevis tendons are seen laterally. Seen medially are the tibialis posterior, flexor hallucis longus, and flexor digitorum longus tendons. The Achilles tendon lies posteriorly. The tendons normally have low signal intensity on all pulse sequences. Sagittal images also demonstrate the articular surfaces of the tibia, fibula, and talus.

Axial images are useful for characterizing soft tissue masses and determining their extent (Fig. 12–72C). The Achilles tendon and the other ankle tendons are seen in cross-section on axial images.

Pathology

Very few pathologic cases have been reported with MRI of the ankle. Despite this, the MRI data for other joints can be extrapolated to the ankle. Soft tissue masses (Fig. 12–73) and bone tumors can plainly be depicted with MRI, along with their extent of involvement. Complex fractures and osteochondral fractures may be demonstrated with MRI while other imaging modalities can fail to recognize the degree of abnormality, such as nonviability of a fracture fragment (Fig. 12–74).[99] AVN of the talus (Fig. 12–75) or other tarsal bones (Fig. 12–76) is not uncommon. AVN manifests as decreased signal intensity on T1-weighted and T2-weighted scans. Cartilaginous defects, thinning of the cartilage, and synovial abnormalities (Fig. 12–77), as well as ligamentous injuries, may be seen by MRI.[99] Further work will determine the exact indications for MRI in the ankle.

One entity unique to the ankle for which MRI has been useful is an abnormality of the Achilles tendon. The normal Achilles tendon has a low, black signal intensity on all pulse sequences, with no intratendinous signal (Fig. 12–78). The Achilles tendon is seen best on sagittal and axial images. In cross section, on axial images, the normal Achilles tendon is flat with a slight concavity anteriorly and slight convexity posteriorly. The lateral and medial margins have a rounded configuration. The incidence of Achilles tendon injuries is increasing and commonly occur in joggers or after blunt trauma. The most common site of injury is 2 to 3 cm proximal to its insertion on the calcaneus.

The hallmark of an Achilles tendon injury is thickening and swelling of the tendon, with or without increased intratendinous signal intensity. Acute complete tendon tears show disruption of the tendon fibers. There are foci of increased signal intensity on T2-weighted images adjacent to the tear, representing edema or hemorrhage. Partial tears of the tendon produce thickening of the tendon, partial discontinuity of the tendon fibers, and abnormal increased signal in-

(text continues on page 455)

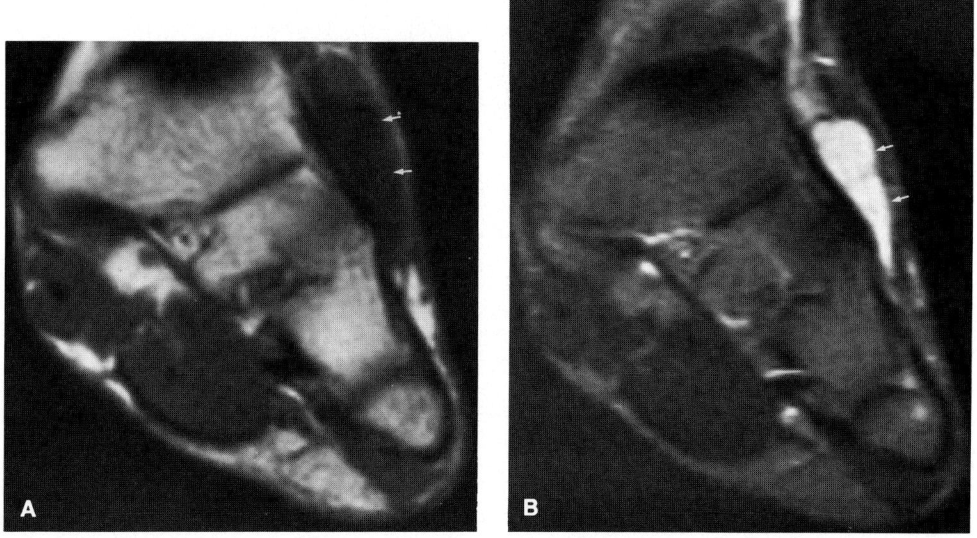

FIGURE 12–73. Ganglion cyst. **(A)** T1-weighted sagittal image (TR/TE = 600/17) and **(B)** T2-weighted sagittal image (TR/TE = 3000/90). There is a multiloculated cystic mass (arrows) in the subcutaneous tissue of the anterior ankle. The mass has intermediate signal intensity on the T1-weighted image and marked increased signal intensity on the T2-weighted image.

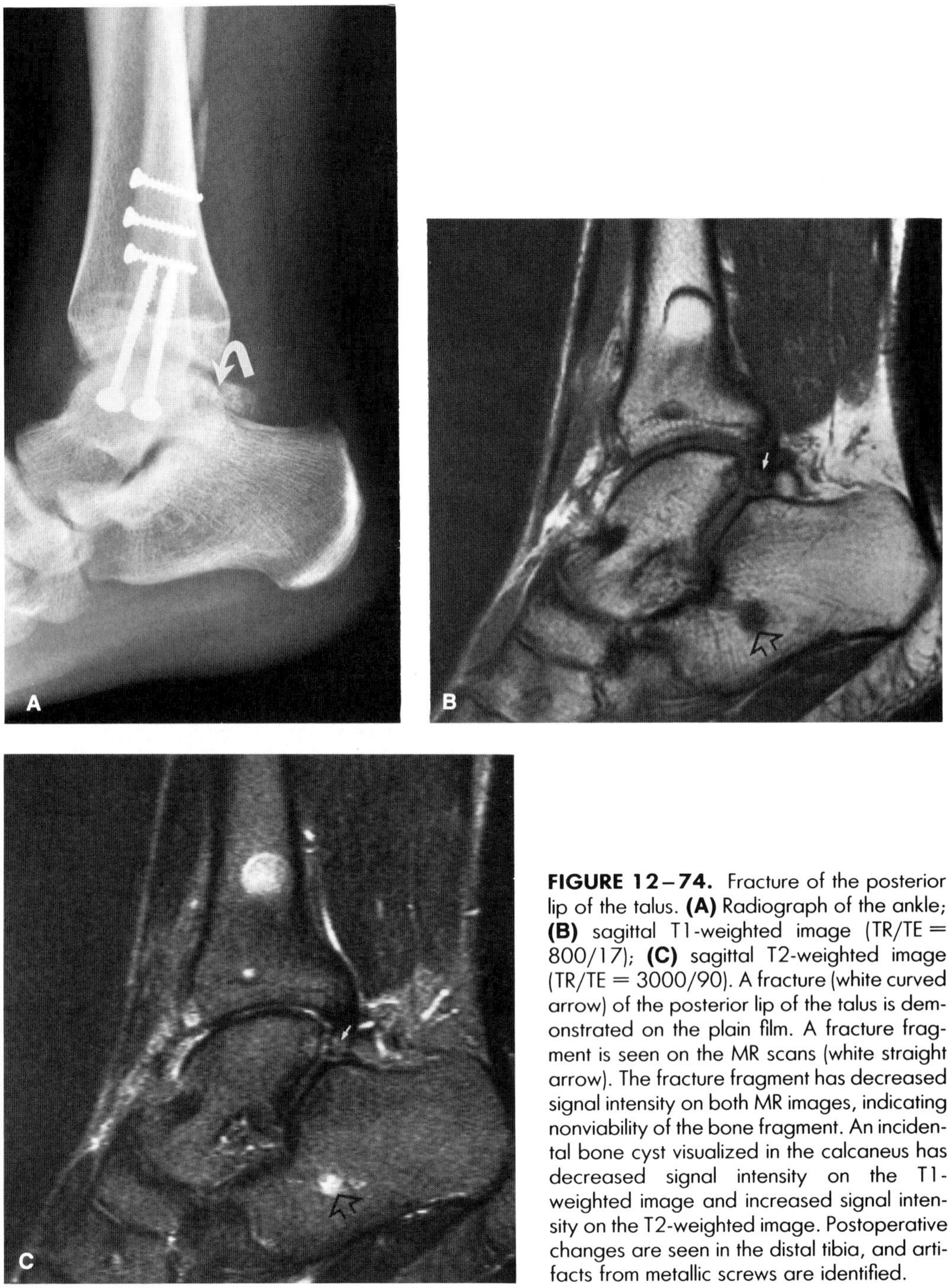

FIGURE 12–74. Fracture of the posterior lip of the talus. **(A)** Radiograph of the ankle; **(B)** sagittal T1-weighted image (TR/TE = 800/17); **(C)** sagittal T2-weighted image (TR/TE = 3000/90). A fracture (white curved arrow) of the posterior lip of the talus is demonstrated on the plain film. A fracture fragment is seen on the MR scans (white straight arrow). The fracture fragment has decreased signal intensity on both MR images, indicating nonviability of the bone fragment. An incidental bone cyst visualized in the calcaneus has decreased signal intensity on the T1-weighted image and increased signal intensity on the T2-weighted image. Postoperative changes are seen in the distal tibia, and artifacts from metallic screws are identified.

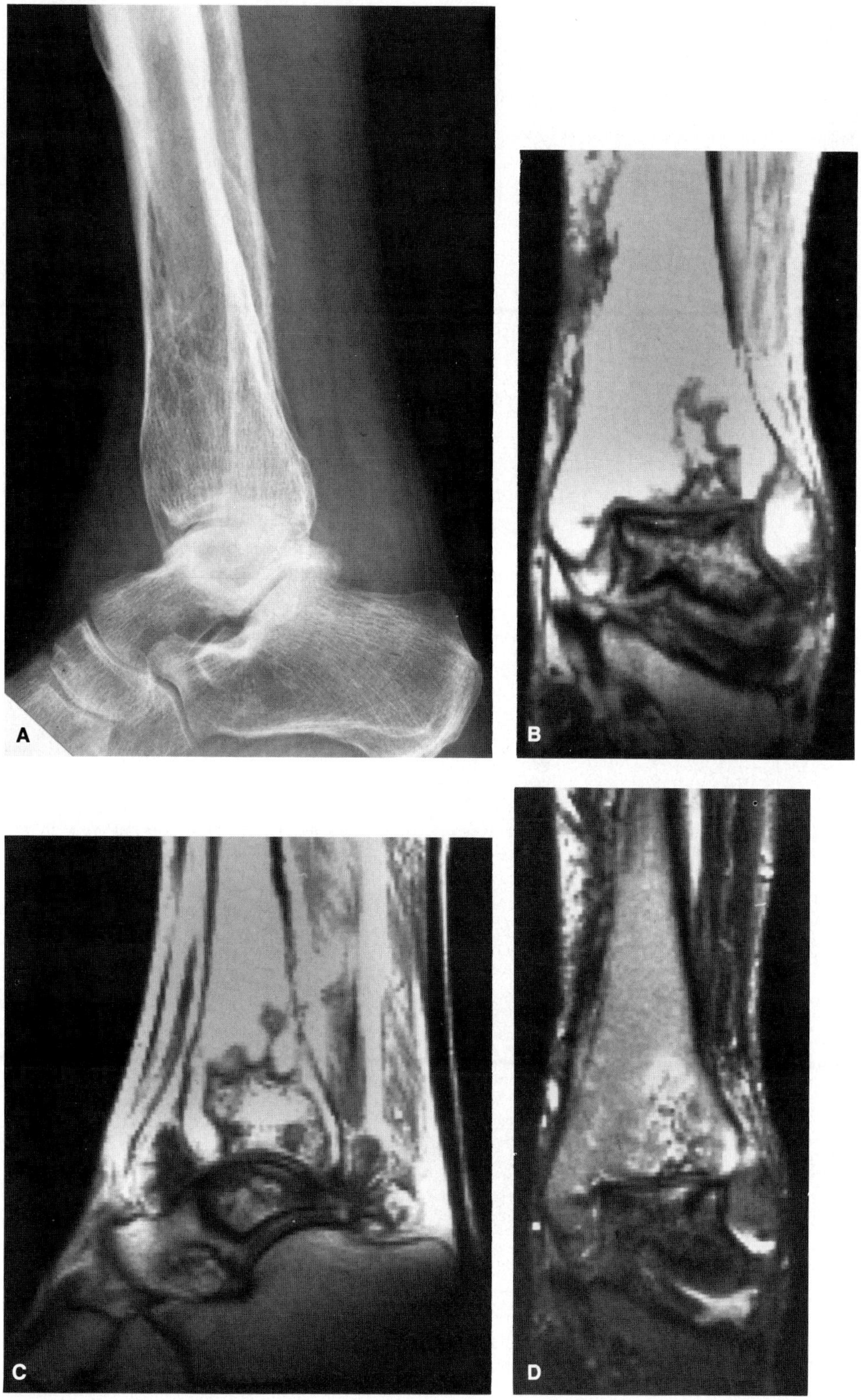

FIGURE 12–75. AVN of the talus. **(A)** Radiograph of the ankle; **(B)** coronal and **(C)** sagittal T1-weighted images (TR/TE = 500/17); **(D)** coronal T2-weighted image (TR/TE = 3000/90). The plain film of the ankle shows sclerosis in the talus due to AVN. Post-traumatic changes are seen in the tibia. The T1-weighted images demonstrate heterogeneous areas of increased and decreased signal intensity in the talus. The T2-weighted image shows decreased signal intensity in the talus. These findings represent AVN. There is a bone infarct in the distal tibia, which has a central region of increased signal intensity on the T1-weighted and T2-weighted images and a surrounding rim of decreased signal intensity on the T1-weighted images.

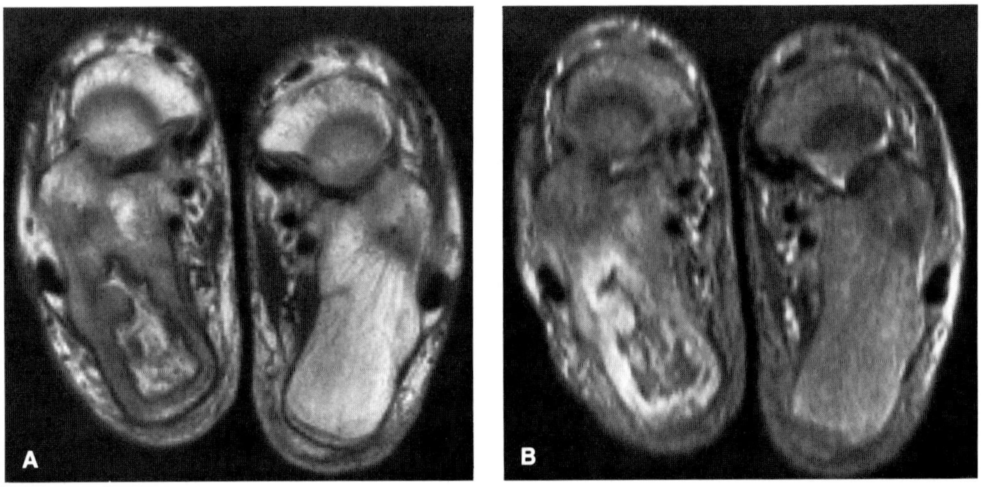

FIGURE 12–76. Calcaneal infarct. **(A)** T1-weighted axial image (TR/TE = 600/17) and **(B)** T2-weighted axial image (TR/TE = 2500/90). The patient has a history of Crohn's disease and long-term treatment with steroids. There is a large infarct in the right calcaneus that has a central region of increased signal intensity, with a surrounding rim of decreased signal intensity on the T1-weighted scan. This lesion has heterogeneous intermediate signal intensity centrally on the T2-weighted image, with an area of increased signal intensity surrounding the lesion.

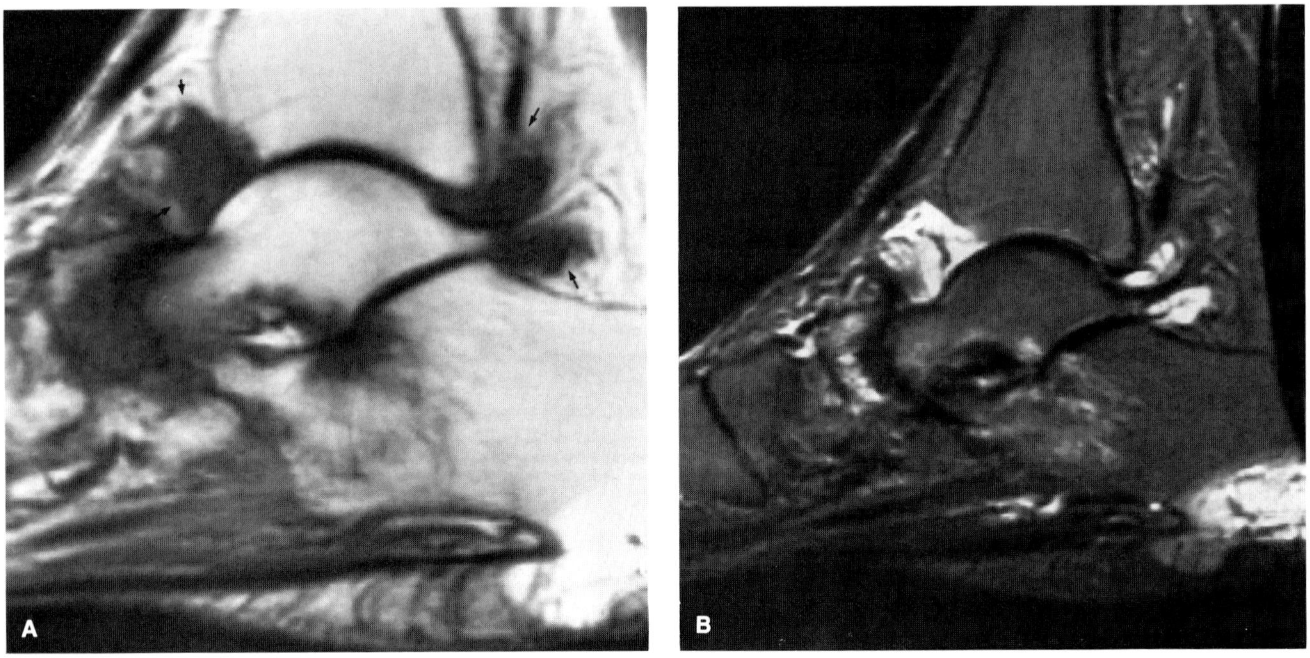

FIGURE 12–77. Synovitis. **(A)** Sagittal T1-weighted image (TR/TE = 600/17) and **(B)** sagittal T2-weighted image (TR/TE = 3000/90). There is a soft tissue lesion (arrows) filling the joint space anterior and posterior to the talus. This represents thickened inflamed synovium, which has intermediate signal intensity on the T1-weighted image and marked increased signal intensity on the T2-weighted image. This has similar MR signal characteristics to that of fluid, but at surgery, inflamed synovium was resected.

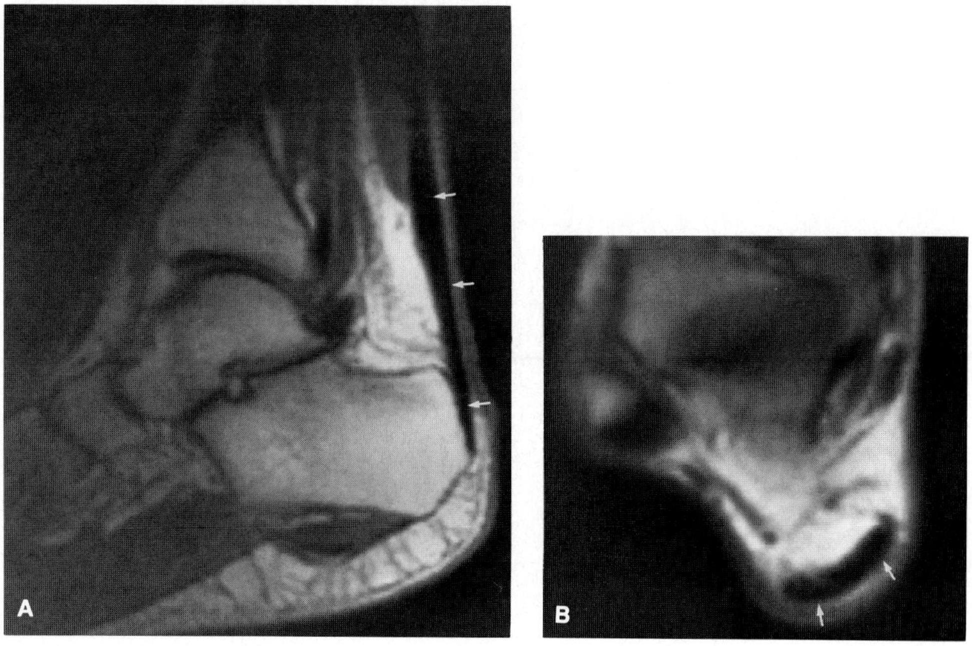

FIGURE 12–78. Normal Achilles tendon. **(A)** Sagittal and **(B)** axial T1-weighted images (TR/TE = 800/17). The normal Achilles tendon (white arrows) has low signal intensity with no intratendinous signal. The tendon is flat, with slight anterior concavity and posterior convexity on the axial scan.

tensity within the tendon on T2-weighted images and intermediate signal intensity on T1-weighted images. Tendinitis manifests as diffuse tendon thickening, with a rounded configuration, with or without an intratendinous signal (Fig. 12–79).[102]

MUSCULOSKELETAL TUMORS, MARROW DISEASE AND INFECTION

MRI is becoming an increasingly useful imaging modality for detecting bone and soft tissue tumors, especially for preoperative planning. The multiplanar capability, excellent contrast resolution between neoplastic and normal tissue, lack of artifacts from dense bone, and absence of ionizing radiation are desirable features. MRI is very sensitive for detecting and defining the extent of soft tissue and bone marrow disease.

Anatomy and Technique

Normal bone marrow contains a large amount of fat and therefore has intermediate or high signal intensity on T1-weighted images, depending on the marrow composition. The surrounding bone cortex has very low, black signal intensity on all pulse sequences. Most pathologic lesions lead to replacement of marrow fat, causing decreased signal intensity on T1-weighted images. Normal soft tissue, such as muscle, has an intermediate or low signal intensity on T2-weighted scans. Most pathologic soft tissue lesions have greater fluid content, which produces an increased signal intensity on T2-weighted images.

Spin echo pulse sequences are ideal for differentiating normal bone marrow and soft tissue from pathologic conditions. Short TR/TE (T1-weighted) sequences emphasize the difference between normal and abnormal marrow fat composition. Long TR/TE (T2-weighted) sequences distinguish normal from abnormal soft tissues.[103–106] T1-weighted and T2-weighted axial images through a tumor best show the characteristics of the mass, specifically the signal intensity of the lesion, soft tissue extension, and cortical involvement. Sagittal or coronal T1-weighted images are ideal for showing the extent of bone marrow involvement and skip lesions.[107,108] Sagittal and coronal T2-weighted images can help in delineating the cephalocaudad extent of soft tissue abnormalities.

Soft Tissue and Bone Tumors: General Characteristics

MRI is the most sensitive imaging modality for detecting soft tissue and bone marrow lesions.[104,105,108–111] Most osteolytic lesions have low signal intensity on T1-weighted images and high signal intensity on T2-

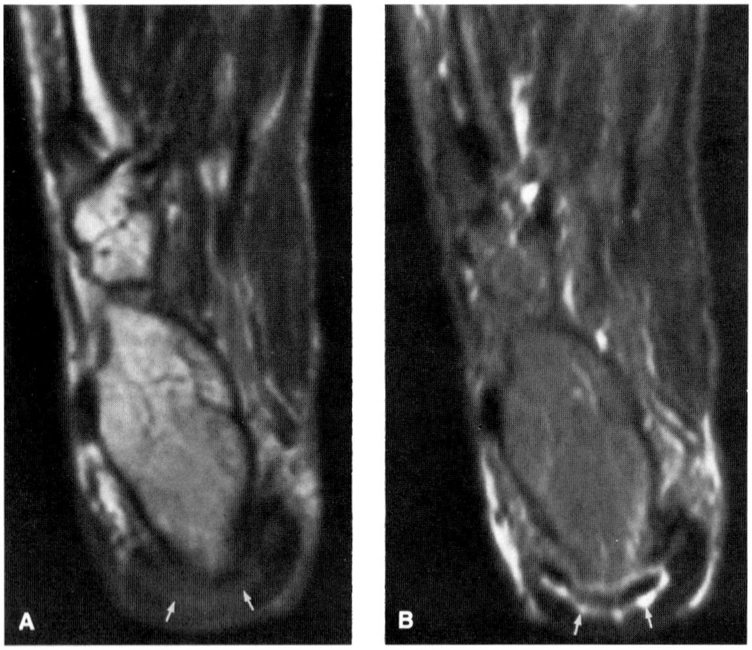

FIGURE 12–79. Achilles tendinitis. **(A)** Axial T1-weighted image (TR/TE = 700/17) and **(B)** T2-weighted axial image (TR/TE = 3000/90). Both images demonstrate diffuse thickening of the Achilles tendon. There is abnormal intermediate signal intensity on the T1-weighted image and marked increased signal intensity on the T2-weighted image in the substance of the Achilles tendon (arrow).

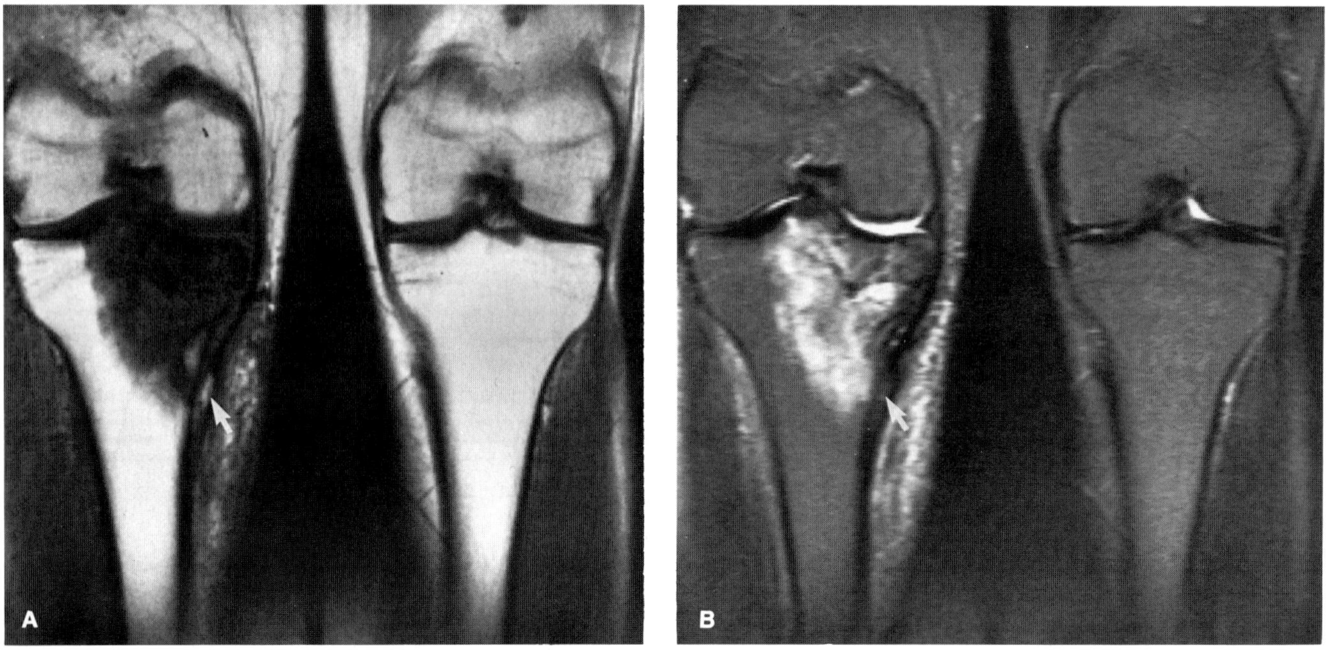

FIGURE 12–80. Lymphoma. Coronal **(A)** T1-weighted image (TR/TE = 600/17) and **(B)** T2-weighted image (TR/TE = 3000/90). There is a mass, which has low signal intensity on the T1-weighted image, involving the proximal right tibia extending into the epiphysis. This lesion has inhomogeneous increased signal intensity on the T2-weighted image. Notice the mildly increased signal intensity on both images in the medial tibial cortex (arrow), indicating cortical break-through of the tumor. The normal signal void of the cortical bone is absent. This lesion has nonspecific MR signal characteristics, like the majority of osteolytic lesions. At surgery, this lesion proved to be lymphoma.

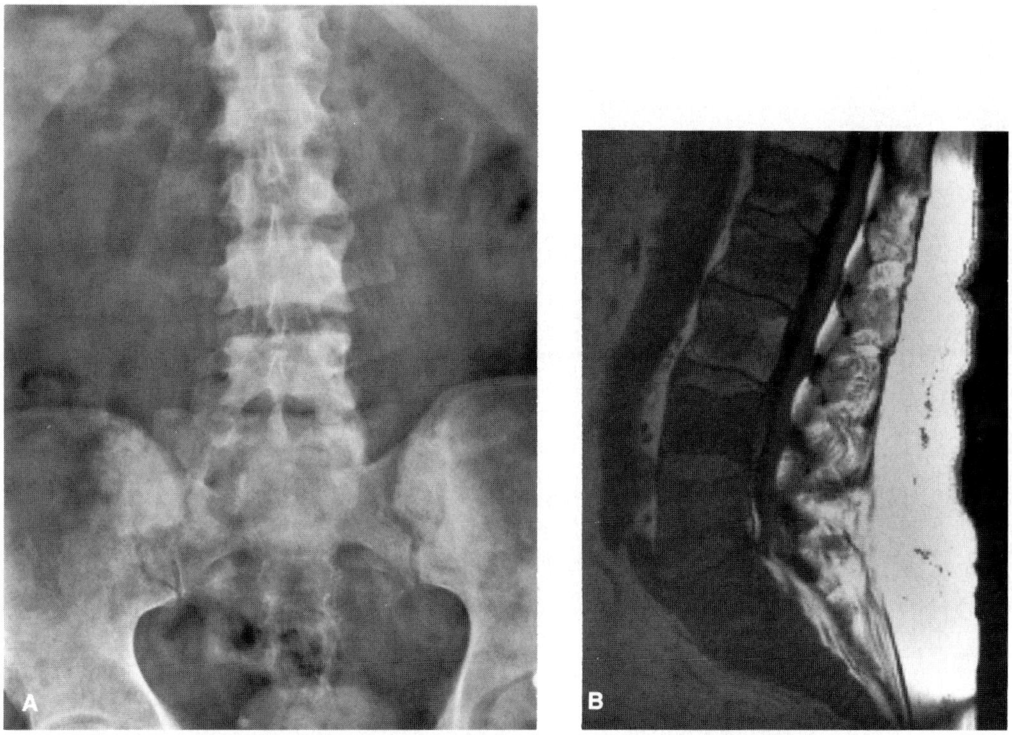

FIGURE 12–81. Blastic metastasis. **(A)** Radiograph of the lumbar spine and **(B)** sagittal T1-weighted image (TR/TE = 600/17). Blastic metastases are visualized throughout the lumbar spine and in the pelvis on the plain film of this patient with known metastatic prostate carcinoma. On the T1-weighted scan, there is decreased signal intensity in the bone marrow of the lumbar vertebral bodies due to metastatic marrow infiltration. Notice that the discs have a higher signal intensity than the adjacent vertebral bodies.

weighted images (Fig. 12–80). Tumors that produce bone or elicit a sclerotic response, such as sclerotic osteosarcoma and blastic metastases (Fig. 12–81), often have low signal intensity on both T1-weighted and T2-weighted images.[110] Low-signal-intensity tumors on T2-weighted images tend to be fibrotic and hypocellular.[112] Most soft tissue lesions have decreased signal intensity on T1-weighted images and increased signal intensity on T2-weighted images. The differentiation between malignant and benign soft tissue masses is limited, but malignant lesions often have a more heterogeneous signal intensity (Fig. 12–82).[107] Despite these advantages, a major criticism of MRI is its lack of lesion specificity.

Soft Tissue Masses

As more experience is gained with MRI, the specificity continues to improve. There are several characteristic findings that may improve diagnostic specificity with soft tissue lesions. Lipomas have an increased signal intensity on T1-weighted images and intermediate signal intensity on T2-weighted images, paralleling body fat.[113] Benign lipomas have a very short T1, producing very high signal intensity on T1-weighted images, and therefore can often be distinguished from liposarcomas, which are usually less intense on T1-weighted scans.

Hematomas have various signal intensities, depending on the stage of hemoglobin degradation, and sequential scans can show progression of clot resorption (Fig. 12–83). Unlike hematomas within the brain parenchyma, chronic soft tissue hematomas have signal characteristics of fluid and usually do not contain a significant amount of hemosiderin. Hemangiomas and lymphangiomas are usually well-circumscribed and have decreased signal intensity on T1-weighted images and very high signal intensity on T2-weighted images (Fig. 12–84).[107]

Neurofibromas may have mildly increased signal intensity on T1-weighted images and markedly in-

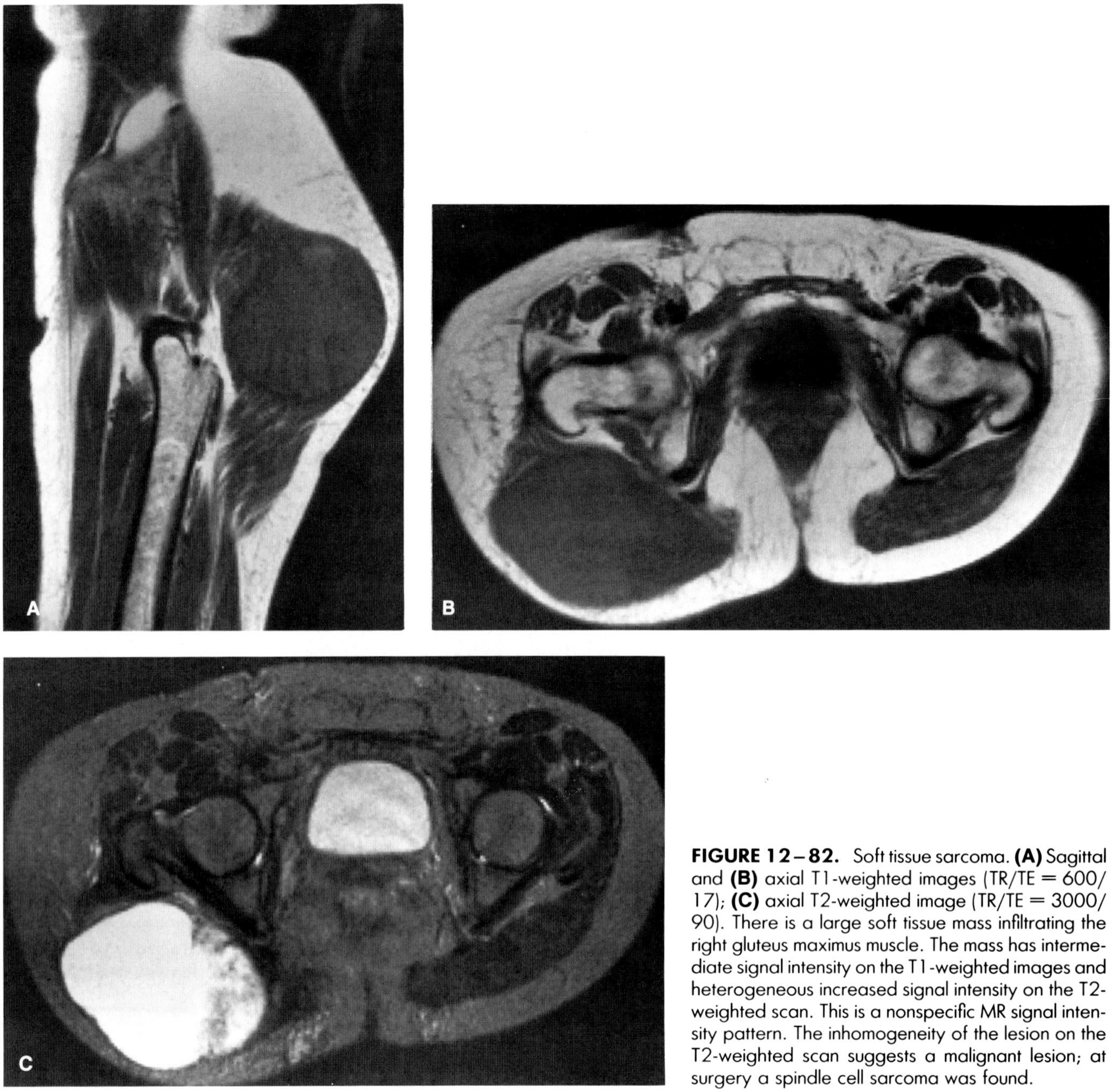

FIGURE 12–82. Soft tissue sarcoma. **(A)** Sagittal and **(B)** axial T1-weighted images (TR/TE = 600/17); **(C)** axial T2-weighted image (TR/TE = 3000/90). There is a large soft tissue mass infiltrating the right gluteus maximus muscle. The mass has intermediate signal intensity on the T1-weighted images and heterogeneous increased signal intensity on the T2-weighted scan. This is a nonspecific MR signal intensity pattern. The inhomogeneity of the lesion on the T2-weighted scan suggests a malignant lesion; at surgery a spindle cell sarcoma was found.

creased signal intensity on T2-weighted images, often with a central area of decreased signal intensity due to dense fibrous tissue condensations (Fig. 12–85).[107] Aggressive fibromatosis is a rare soft tissue lesion that usually has low signal intensity on T1-weighted and T2-weighted images due to dense fibrous tissue (Fig. 12–86).[109] Depending on the degree of cellularity, aggressive fibromatosis may have high signal on T2-weighted images.[112] Benign soft tissue cysts are typically well defined, with homogeneous signal intensity equal to or less than muscle on T1-weighted images and hyperintense on T2-weighted images. Proteinaceous cysts have increased signal intensity on both T1- and T2-weighted scans.[107]

Bone Tumors

The hallmark of a benign bone tumor on MRI is a well-defined peripheral margin of decreased signal intensity on all pulse sequences, separating the lesion from the adjacent normal marrow.[107] Some specific

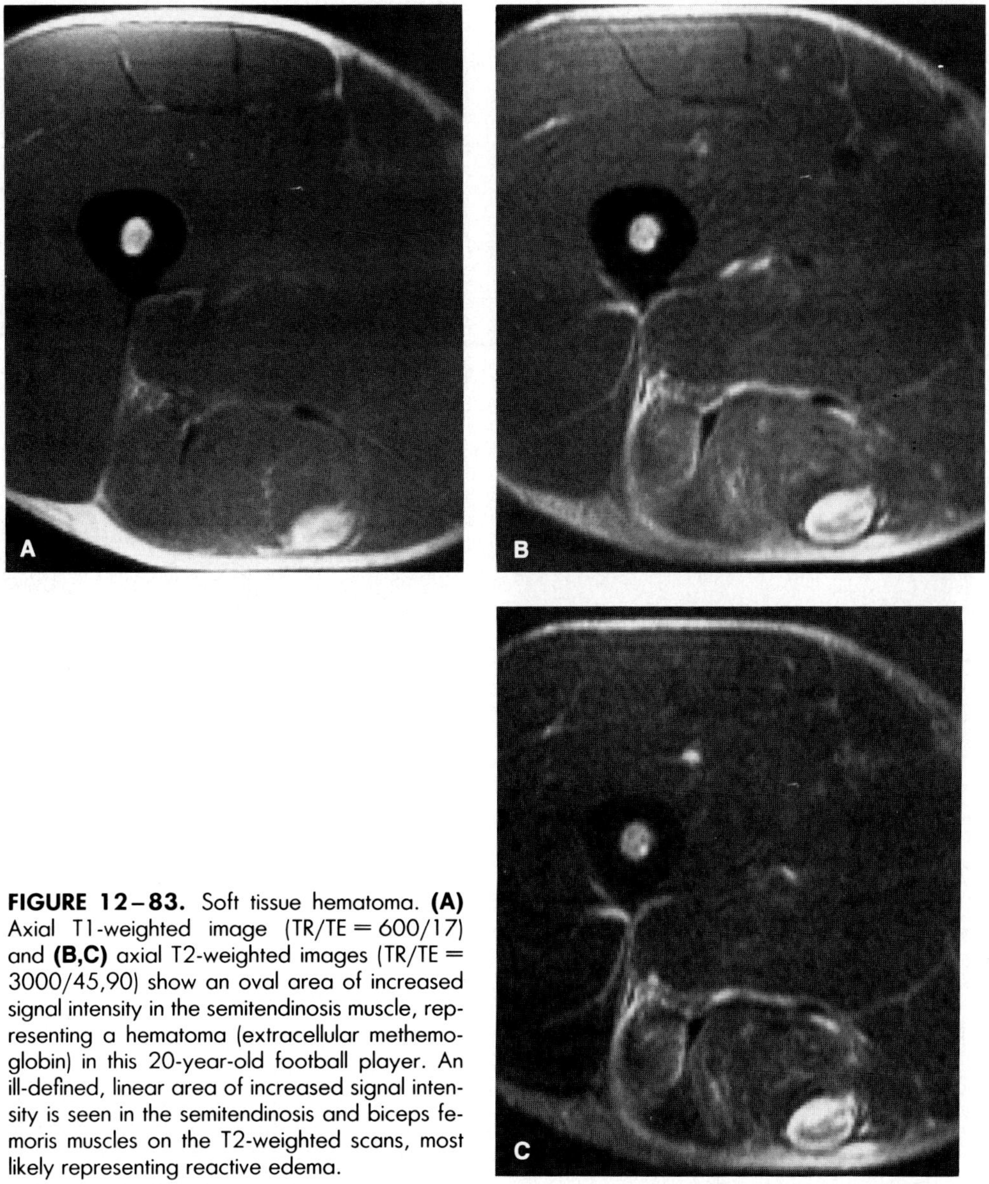

FIGURE 12–83. Soft tissue hematoma. **(A)** Axial T1-weighted image (TR/TE = 600/17) and **(B,C)** axial T2-weighted images (TR/TE = 3000/45,90) show an oval area of increased signal intensity in the semitendinosis muscle, representing a hematoma (extracellular methemoglobin) in this 20-year-old football player. An ill-defined, linear area of increased signal intensity is seen in the semitendinosis and biceps femoris muscles on the T2-weighted scans, most likely representing reactive edema.

findings for bone tumors have been published. Hyaline cartilage matrix lesions including enchondromas (Fig. 12–87), osteochondromas, and most chondrosarcomas (Fig. 12–88) may have a unique appearance on T2-weighted scans.[114] Various sizes of lobules of homogeneous increased signal intensity separated by thin, low-intensity septa are characteristic of these lesions. The septated appearance and homogeneity of the signal intensity allows differentiation of hyaline cartilage lesions from most other masses with increased signal intensity on T2-weighted images.

Fibroxanthomas typically have predominantly decreased signal intensity on T1-weighted and T2-weighted images, due to hemosiderin pigment or increased amounts of collagen.[115] Osteoid osteoma classically has low signal intensity in the nidus of the lesion on T1-weighted and T2-weighted scans, with a surrounding area of increased signal intensity on T2-weighted scans (Fig. 12–89).[116]

Osteochondromas show continuity of the cortex of the lesion with the parent bone and of the parent

(text continues on page 464)

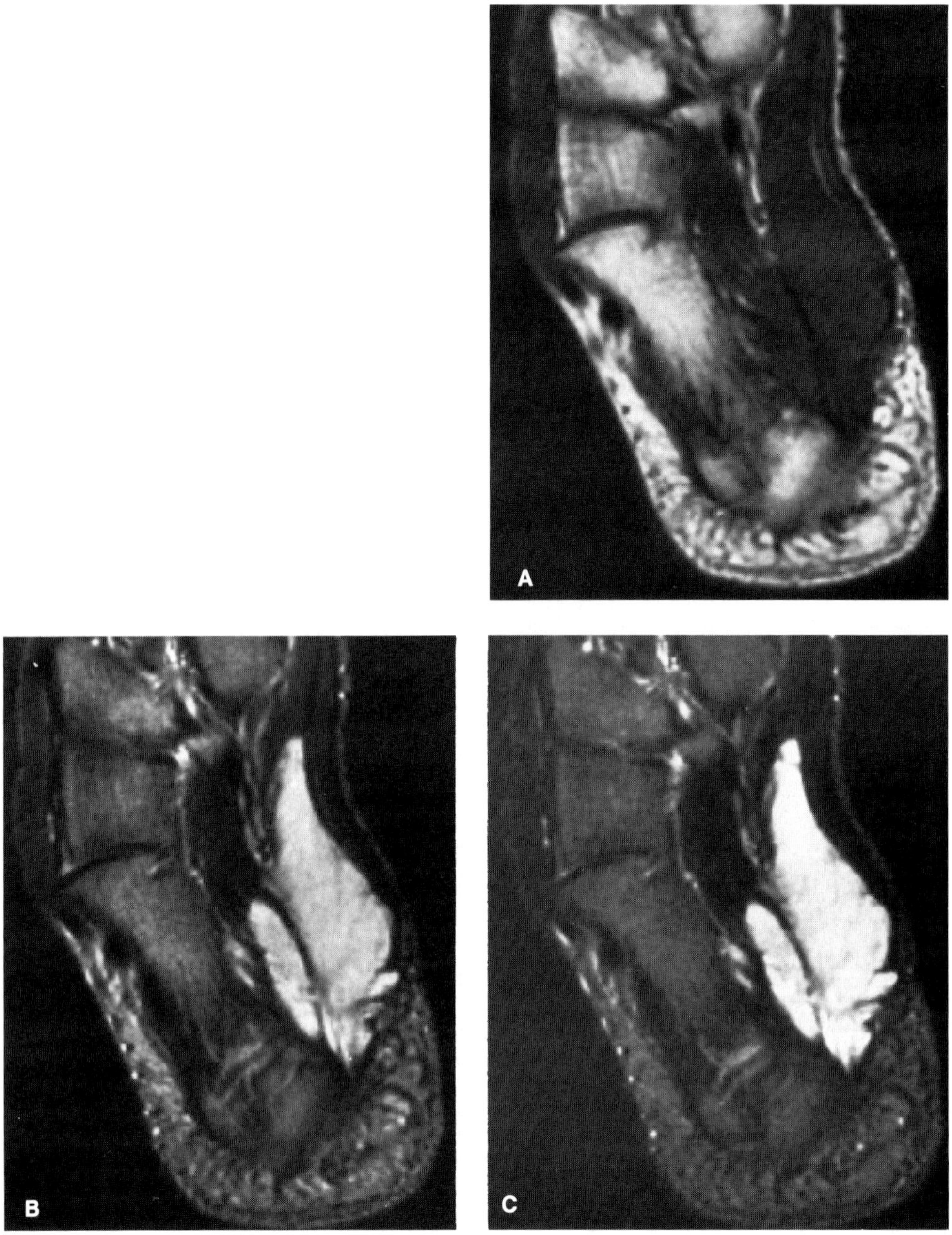

FIGURE 12–84. Soft tissue hemangioma. **(A)** Axial T1-weighted image (TR/TE = 750/17) and **(B,C)** axial T2-weighted images (TR/TE = 3000/45,90). There is a soft tissue mass involving the flexor plantar muscles of the foot that has an isointense signal on the T1-weighted image and markedly hyperintense signal on the T2-weighted images. At surgery, a large hemangioma was resected.

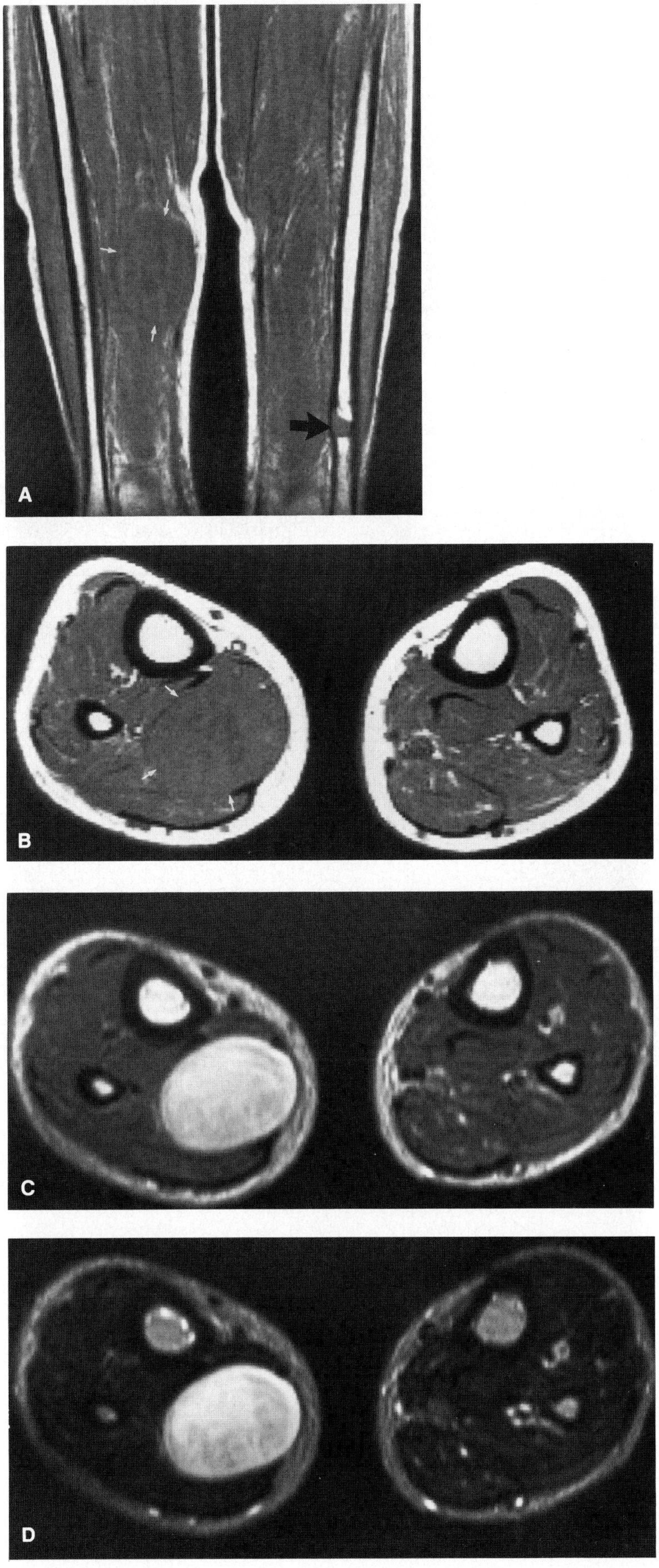

FIGURE 12–85. Neurofibroma. **(A)** Coronal and **(B)** axial T1-weighted images (TR/TE = 600/17); **(C,D)** axial T2-weighted images (TR/TE = 2500/45,90). There is a well-defined soft tissue mass (white arrows) located between the gastrocnemius and soleus muscles. The lesion is isointense with muscle on the T1-weighted images and hyperintense on the T2-weighted images. There is a central area of necrosis in the lesion. A pseudoarthrosis (black arrow) of the distal left fibula is seen on the coronal image. This patient has neurofibromatosis and presented with an enlarging, painful right leg mass.

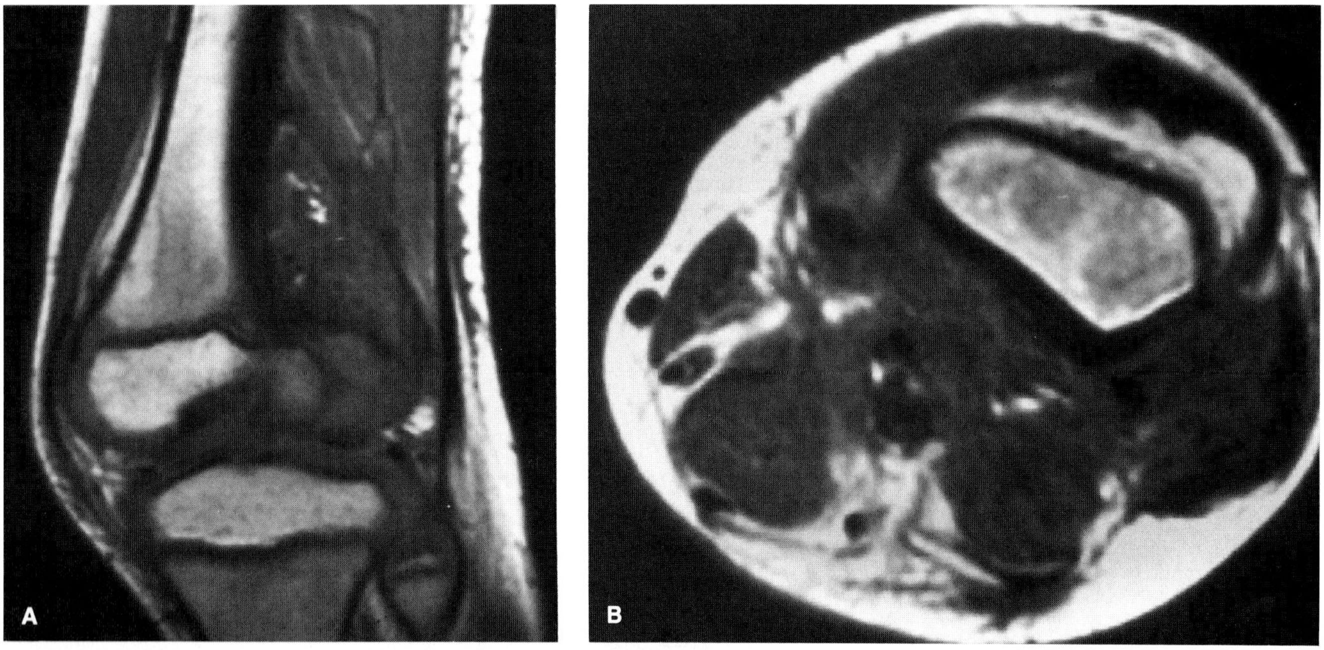

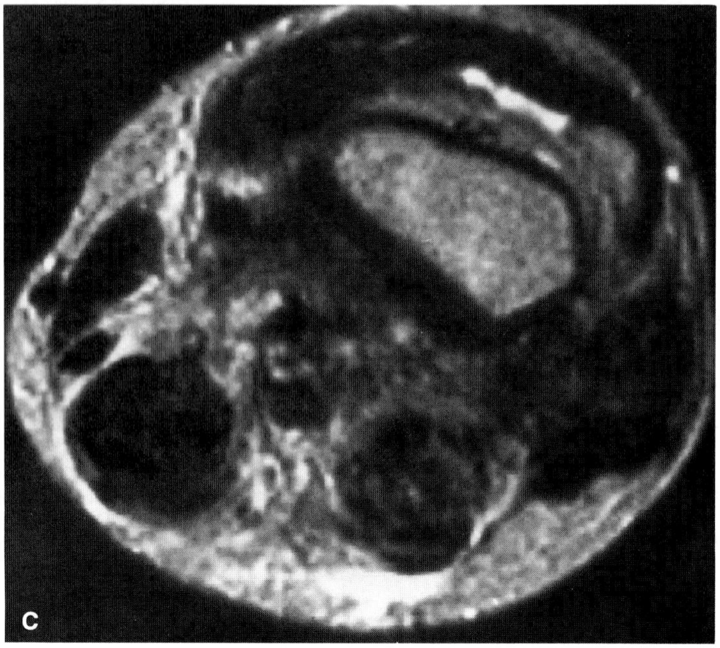

FIGURE 12–86. Aggressive fibromatosis. **(A)** Sagittal and **(B)** axial T1-weighted images (TR/TE = 800/17); **(C)** axial T2-weighted image (TR/TE = 3000/90). An infiltrating soft tissue mass is identified in the lower left thigh adjacent to the femur. The lesion has low signal intensity on all images. The normal muscles and fat planes are not clearly delineated due to tumor infiltration. This is a classic MRI appearance of aggressive fibromatosis.

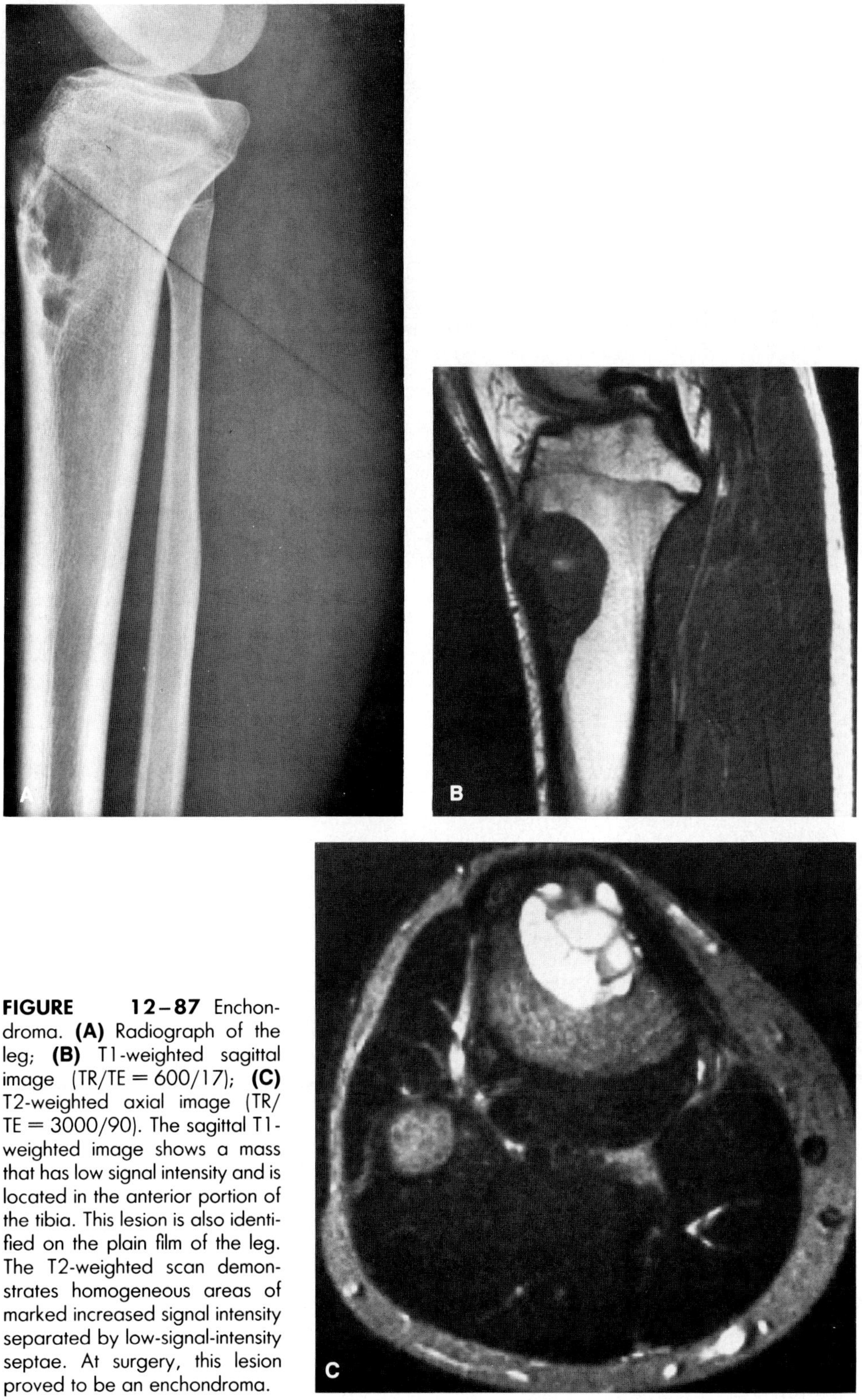

FIGURE 12–87 Enchondroma. **(A)** Radiograph of the leg; **(B)** T1-weighted sagittal image (TR/TE = 600/17); **(C)** T2-weighted axial image (TR/TE = 3000/90). The sagittal T1-weighted image shows a mass that has low signal intensity and is located in the anterior portion of the tibia. This lesion is also identified on the plain film of the leg. The T2-weighted scan demonstrates homogeneous areas of marked increased signal intensity separated by low-signal-intensity septae. At surgery, this lesion proved to be an enchondroma.

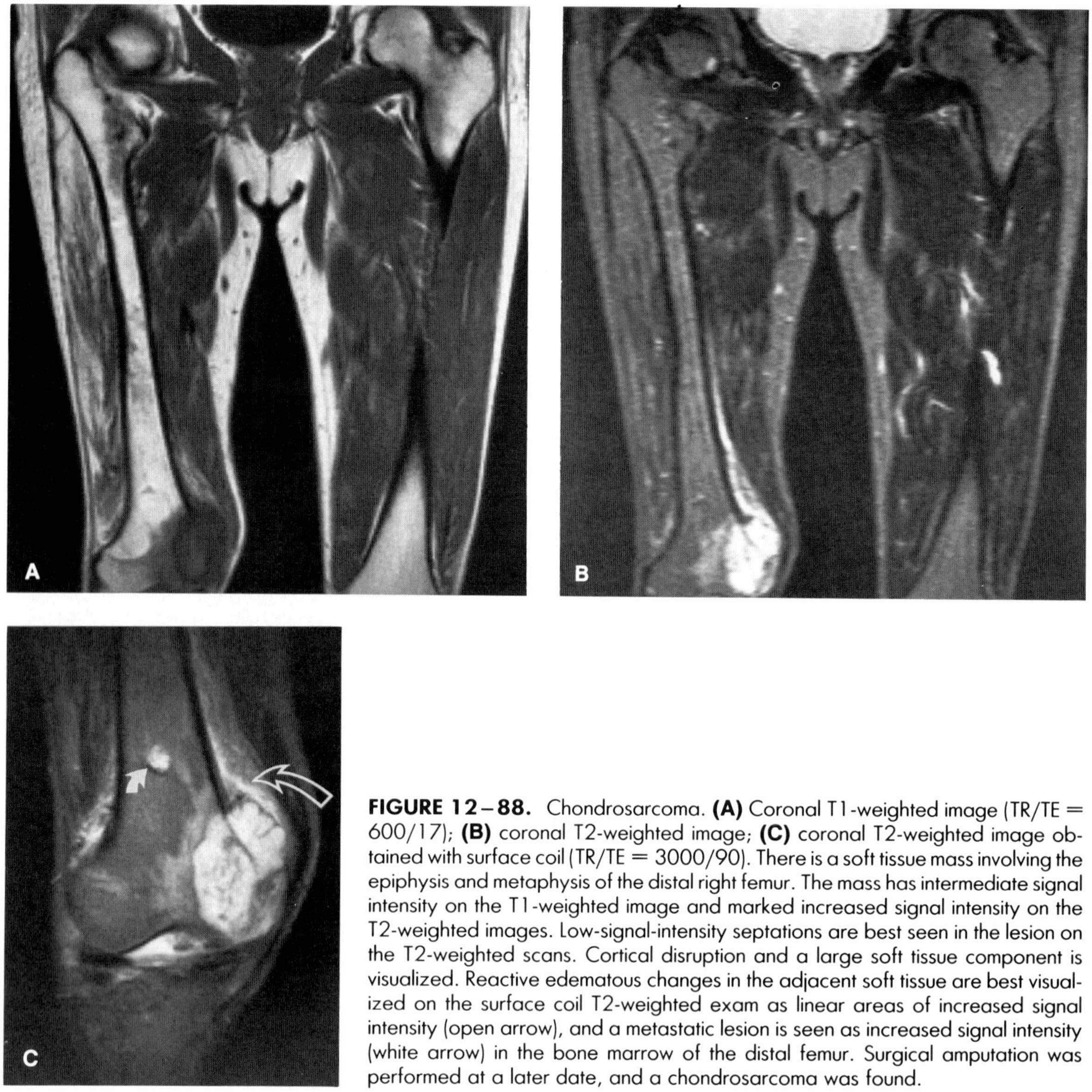

FIGURE 12–88. Chondrosarcoma. **(A)** Coronal T1-weighted image (TR/TE = 600/17); **(B)** coronal T2-weighted image; **(C)** coronal T2-weighted image obtained with surface coil (TR/TE = 3000/90). There is a soft tissue mass involving the epiphysis and metaphysis of the distal right femur. The mass has intermediate signal intensity on the T1-weighted image and marked increased signal intensity on the T2-weighted images. Low-signal-intensity septations are best seen in the lesion on the T2-weighted scans. Cortical disruption and a large soft tissue component is visualized. Reactive edematous changes in the adjacent soft tissue are best visualized on the surface coil T2-weighted exam as linear areas of increased signal intensity (open arrow), and a metastatic lesion is seen as increased signal intensity (white arrow) in the bone marrow of the distal femur. Surgical amputation was performed at a later date, and a chondrosarcoma was found.

medullary cavity with the lesion (Fig. 12–90).[117] A bright signal intensity cartilage cap can be demonstrated on T2-weighted images. As a general rule, the thicker the cartilage cap, the more likely the lesion has undergone malignant change. Most cartilage caps less than 3 mm thick are benign.[117] A dark rimmed perichondrium can be seen around the cartilage cap. It is important to delineate this preoperatively because incomplete removal of the perichondrium can allow tumor regrowth postoperatively.

Aneurysmal bone cysts (Fig. 12–91) and giant cell tumors (Fig. 12–92) frequently have increased signal intensity on T1-weighted images due to central areas of hemorrhage.[118,119] On T2-weighted images, these lesions have increased signal intensity and may contain fluid-fluid levels. Vertebral hemangiomas have a unique MR appearance, with mottled, rounded areas of increased signal intensity on T1-weighted and T2-weighted scans interspersed with areas of decreased signal intensity.[120] The increased signal intensity on T1-weighted images represents fatty components of the lesion. Despite these specific findings, plain films are the mainstay in determining the differential diagnosis of most bone tumors.[106]

The primary use of MRI in bone tumors is for staging. MRI is superior to other imaging modalities in determining intramedullary tumor extent.[106,108,110,111,121–123] MRI also detects the skip lesions that occur with bone sarcomas.[111,124] T1-weighted coronal or sagittal images are often best for showing the

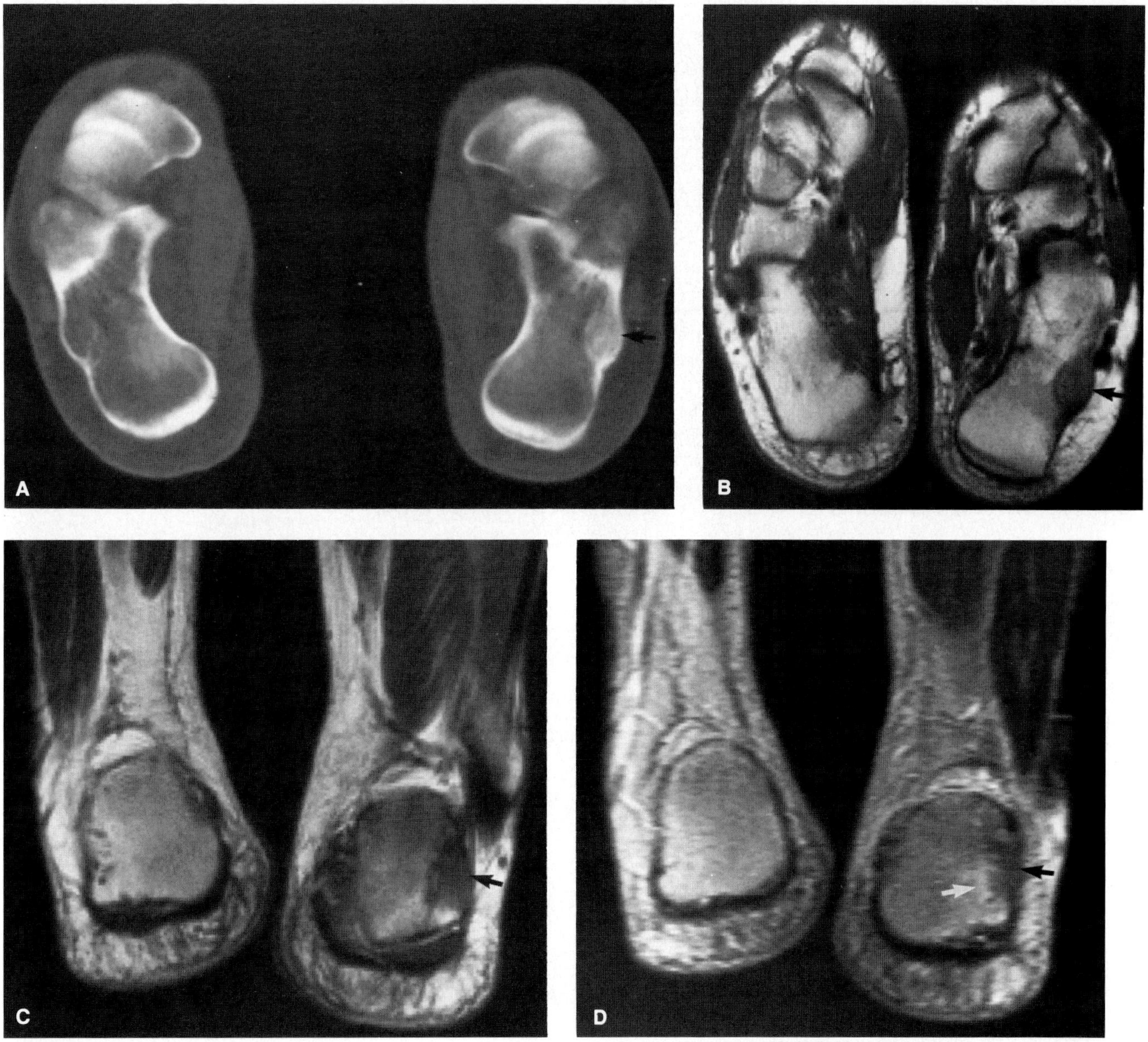

FIGURE 12–89. Osteoid osteoma. **(A)** CT scan of the foot; **(B)** axial and **(C)** coronal T1-weighted images (TR/TE = 600/17); **(D)** coronal T2-weighted image (TR/TE = 2500/17). There is a sclerotic lesion (black arrow) in the lateral aspect of the left calcaneus on the CT scan. The MRI scan shows a corresponding area of intermediate signal intensity in the center of the lesion on T1-weighted and T2-weighted images. There is a rim of surrounding increased signal intensity (white arrow) on the T2-weighted scan.

intramedullary tumor extent (Fig. 12–93). Assessment of invasion or breakthrough of the bony cortex is important preoperatively. Long TR/short TE images usually show cortical invasion best. Bone cortex invasion manifests as slightly increased signal intensity compared with the normal signal void of cortical bone. Gross cortical destruction produces interruption of the normal cortical signal void.[111,122,124]

MRI is superior to other imaging modalities in detecting and demonstrating the extent of soft tissue involvement. The local soft tissue extension of tumor is best seen on T2-weighted axial images.[103,108,110] Gd DTPA enhances viable tumor, further improving tumor conspicuity and visualization of the extent of soft tissue involvement on T1-weighted images (Fig. 12–94).[110] MRI may also differentiate soft tissue tumor extension from reactive edema in the muscles.

(text continues on page 470)

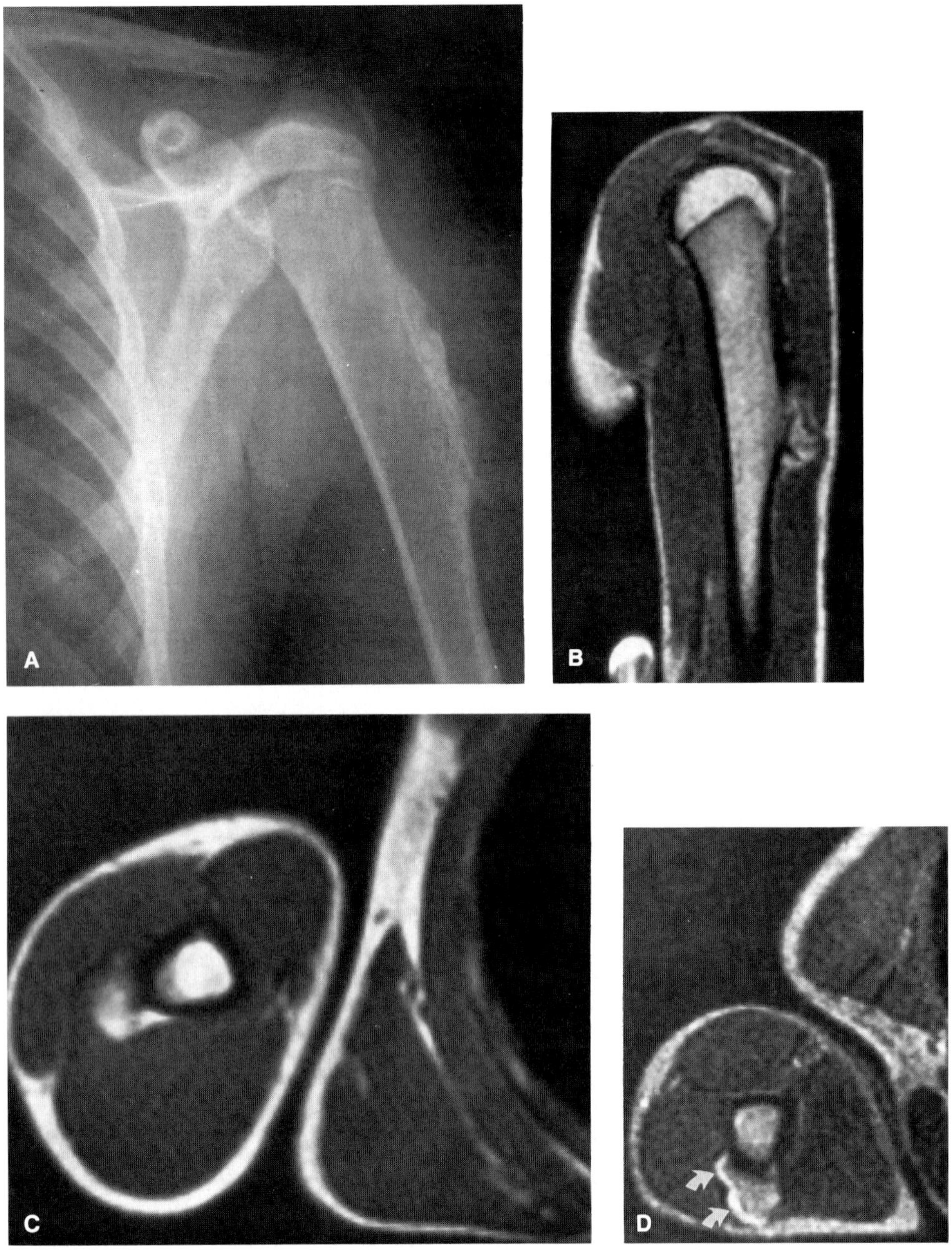

FIGURE 12–90. Osteochondroma. **(A)** Radiograph of the right arm; **(B,C)** T1-weighted images (TR/TE = 650/17); **(D)** axial T2-weighted image (TR/TE = 3000/45). The plain film demonstrates a large osteochondroma in the right humerus. The lesion is also demonstrated on MRI and has a central area of increased signal intensity on the T1-weighted images representing bone marrow. Notice that the lesion has a similar signal intensity to the adjacent normal marrow in the humerus. There is a dark, low-intensity rim surrounding the lesion on the T1-weighted images. The T2-weighted image reveals a rim of hyperintensity at the periphery of the lesion, which represents the cartilaginous cap (arrows).

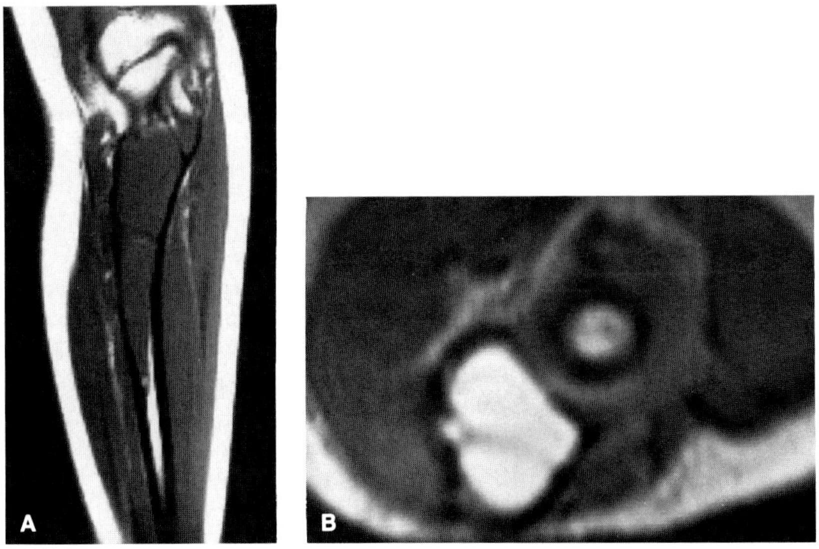

FIGURE 12–91. Aneurysmal bone cyst. **(A)** Sagittal T1-weighted image (TR/TE = 600/17) and **(B)** axial T2-weighted image (TR/TE = 3000/35) of the right elbow. There is an expansile soft tissue mass in the ulna that has intermediate signal intensity on the T1-weighted scan and markedly increased signal intensity on the T2-weighted scan. Septations are identified as low-signal-intensity bands within the mass. At surgery an aneurysmal bone cyst was found.

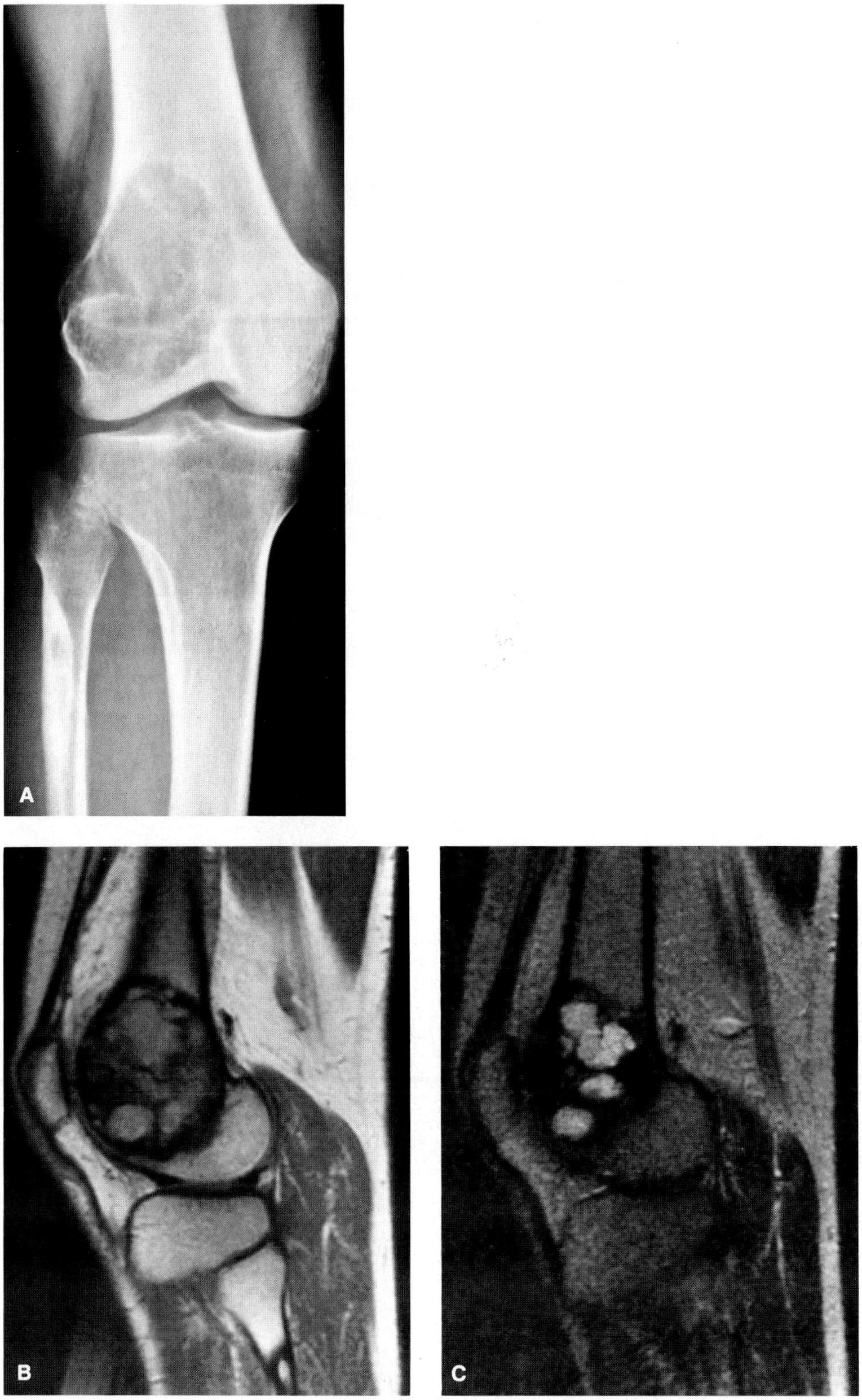

FIGURE 12–92. Giant cell tumor. **(A)** Plain film of the knee; **(B)** sagittal T1-weighted image (TR/TE = 600/25); **(C)** sagittal T2-weighted image (TR/TE = 2000/80). The plain film demonstrates a lytic lesion in the distal femur. The lesion has intermediate signal intensity slightly greater than muscle on the T1-weighted image. The lesion has foci of marked increased signal intensity on the T2-weighted scan. At surgery this proved to be giant cell tumor.

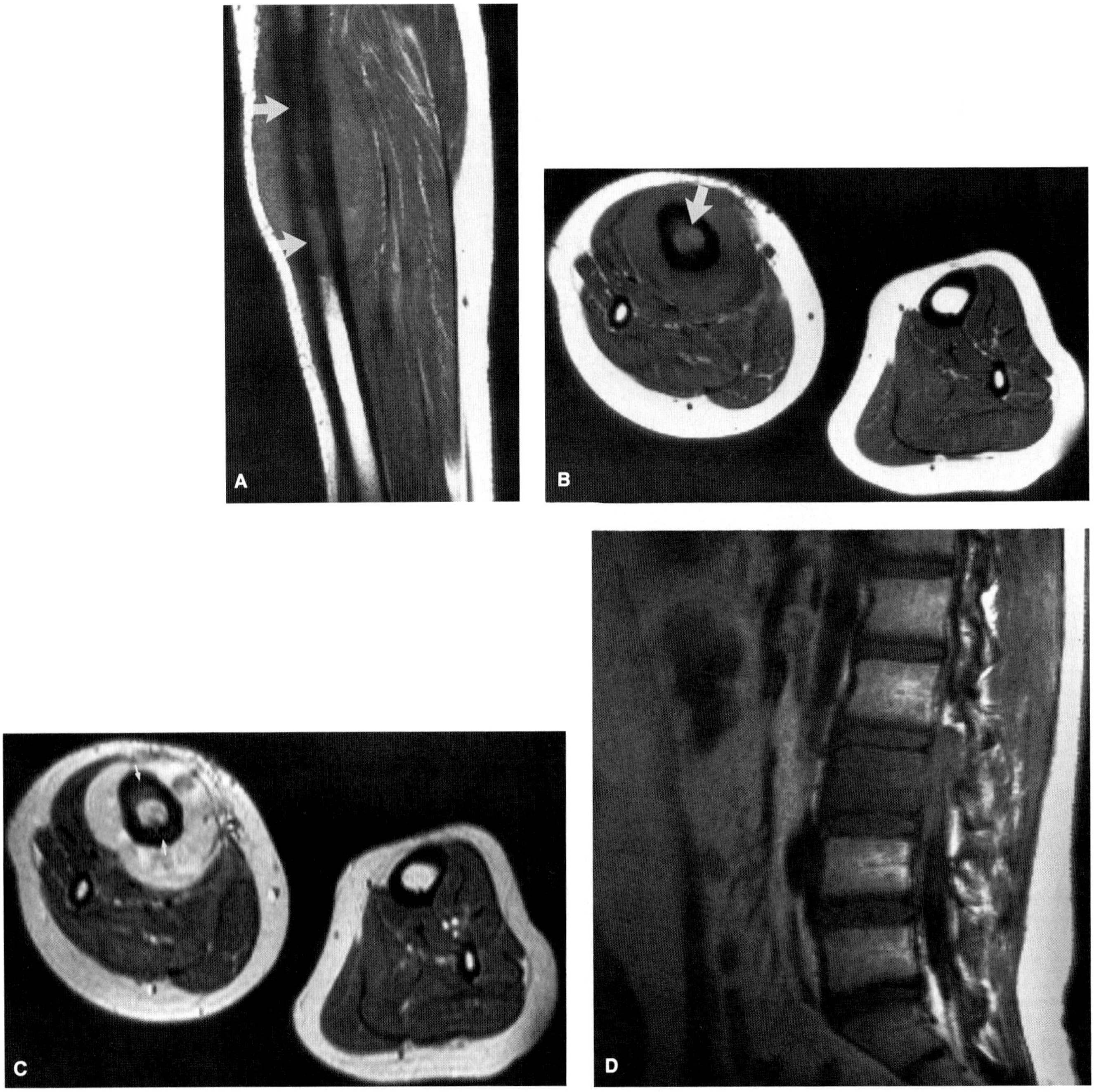

FIGURE 12–93. Ewing's sarcoma. **(A)** Sagittal and **(B)** axial T1-weighted images (TR/TE = 600/17); **(C)** axial T2-weighted image (TR/TE = 3000/45); **(D)** sagittal T1-weighted image of the lumbar spine (TR/TE = 650/20). The T1-weighted images **(A,B)** demonstrate loss of the normal increased signal intensity of the marrow fat in the right tibia, indicating marrow infiltration (arrow). The extent of marrow infiltration is best seen on the sagittal image. Soft tissue extension is ideally visualized on the axial images **(B,C)**, with intermediate signal intensity on the T1-weighted scan and increased signal intensity on the T2-weighted scan. Additionally, cortical invasion is identified on the T2-weighted exam as intermediate signal intensity in the normally signal-void bony cortex (small white arrow). Despite chemotherapeutic treatment, the patient developed back pain. A scan of the lumbar spine **(D)** revealed metastatic disease involving the L3 vertebral body and an associated extradural soft tissue mass, which caused nerve compression at this level. Notice the decreased signal intensity in the L3 vertebral body due to bone marrow infiltration.

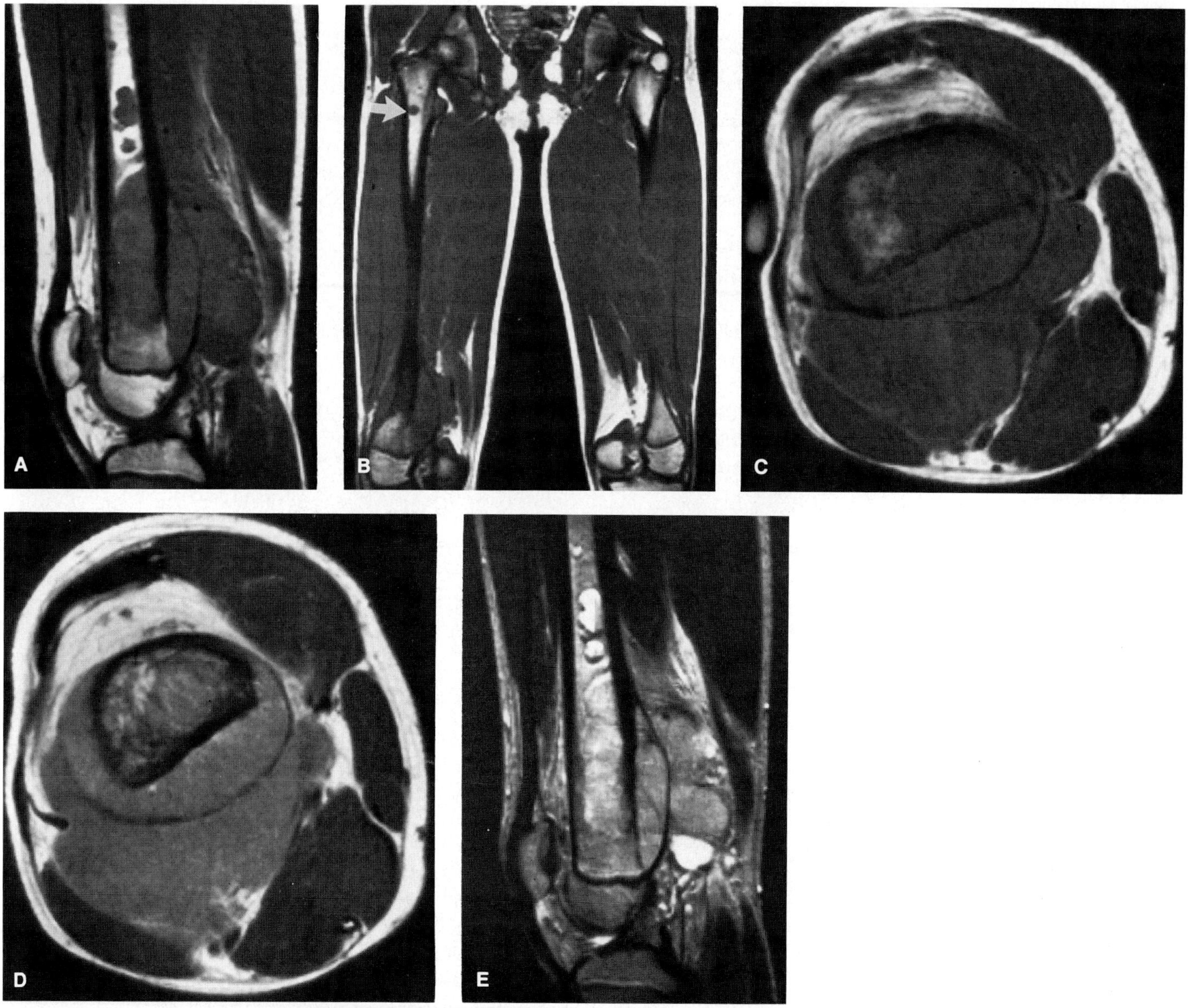

FIGURE 12–94. Ewing's sarcoma. **(A)** Sagittal, **(B)** coronal, **(C)** axial, and **(D)** axial post-Gd-DTPA T1-weighted images (TR/TE = 800/17); **(E)** sagittal T2-weighted image (TR/TE = 3000/45). The T1-weighted scans **(A,C)** show intermediate signal intensity in the bone marrow of the distal right femur due to tumor infiltration. A large soft tissue mass is also demonstrated adjacent to the distal femur. After Gd DTPA administration **(D),** there is homogeneous enhancement of the soft tissue component of the mass, enabling clear depiction of the tumor extent. There is also inhomogeneous enhancement of the infiltrated bone marrow. The T2-weighted image **(E)** also demonstrates the soft tissue extent of the lesion as an area of increased signal intensity. Skip lesions are a common finding with Ewing's sarcoma. The coronal image **(B)** reveals a small focus of decreased signal intensity in the proximal right femur (arrow), remote from the primary tumor site and representing a metastatic lesion.

Both of these conditions present as increased signal intensity in the muscle adjacent to a tumor on T2-weighted scans. If the tumor is well-demarcated from the adjacent increased signal intensity in the muscle, the muscle signal is most likely caused by edema. If the distinction between the muscle and the mass is poor, it most likely represents tumor invasion.[125] Contrast enhancement with Gd DTPA should improve differentiation of tumor from edema.

MRI is superior to other imaging modalities in detecting joint involvement and neurovascular encasement, obstruction, and displacement. MRI can obviate the need for angiography by offering sufficient information about vascular involvement. One downfall of MRI is the poor detection of calcifications and ossification of tumor matrix, which limits the specificity of the technique. Also, thin bony rims and subtle cortical breaks may not be seen with MRI.[109,111]

Postoperative Tumor Detection

MRI may be valuable for assessing the success of bone tumor surgery and for evaluating postoperative masses. One study revealed that, if a mass was demonstrated postoperatively and was found to have a low signal intensity on T2-weighted images, 96% of these lesions were benign. However, if the lesion has increased signal intensity on T2-weighted images, it probably is malignant.[126]

MRI may be useful for evaluating the response of tumors to chemotherapy.[110] A satisfactory chemotherapeutic response is seen as decreased tumor volume; decreased signal intensity on T2-weighted images due to dehydration of the tumor, calcification, or fibrosis; or marked increased signal intensity on T2-weighted images due to necrosis or hemorrhage. An unsatisfactory response manifests as stable signal intensity and tumor volume or as increased tumor volume. A potential application of MR spectroscopy is to monitor treatment of tumors. ^{31}P MR spectroscopy may be able to obtain data concerning tumor metabolism and thereby detect earlier evidence of tumor regression or relapse during chemotherapy.[127]

Bone Marrow Disease

Normal bone marrow is composed of red marrow, which is hematologically active, and yellow (fatty) marrow, which is hematologically inactive. Fatty marrow has increased signal intensity on T1-weighted spin echo images and intermediate signal intensity on T2-weighted images. Red marrow MR signal characteristics are formed by a combination of lipid and water. The T1-weighted signal intensity of red marrow is less than that of yellow marrow.

During growth, there is continual conversion of red to yellow marrow. At birth, almost the entire marrow space contains red marrow. Conversion to yellow marrow begins in the appendicular skeleton. By 25 or 30 years of age, an adult pattern is reached. The normal adult pattern has red marrow in the axial skeleton (skull, vertebrae, ribs, sternum, and pelvis) and in the proximal appendicular skeleton (proximal femur and humerus). Epiphyses and apophyses contain fatty marrow, even in infants. Slow, progressive conversion of red to yellow marrow continues throughout adulthood. This is most noticeable in the vertebral bodies in which focal fatty conversion is a common finding with increasing age.[128]

Several experimental MRI techniques exist for evaluating the marrow.[128] STIR is a specific form of inversion recovery that obliterates the signal from yellow fatty marrow. Pathologic lesions can be readily detected in fatty marrow as bright areas. Limitations of STIR are loss of anatomic definition and poor SNR. Chemical shift imaging is another technique that can enhance the differences among fatty marrow, hematopoietic marrow, and abnormal marrow by forming "fat minus water" images or exclusively fat or water images.[128]

When using spin echo pulse sequences, the differentiation of fatty marrow, hematopoietic marrow, and pathologic marrow depends on detecting the amount of fat content in the marrow. Therefore, highly T1-weighted images, which ideally show fat, are essential. The shorter the TR the better the T1-weighted contrast will be. Therefore images should be acquired with TR < 500.

Pathologic processes involving the bone marrow replace normal marrow fat cells and produce decreased signal intensity on T1-weighted spin echo images. MRI is very sensitive to bone marrow infiltration, but it is nonspecific.[104,105] Lymphoma, leukemia, myelofibrosis (Fig. 12–95), metastatic disease (Fig. 12–81), multiple myeloma, Gaucher's disease, and severe anemias can present similarly as focal or diffuse areas of decreased signal intensity in the bone marrow on T1-weighted images. MRI can distinguish between hypercellular and fibrotic marrow. Marked increased signal intensity in the bone marrow on T1-weighted images, due to fatty replacement, can be seen with aplastic anemia and after radiation therapy (Fig. 12–96).[118]

Osteomyelitis

The diagnosis of osteomyelitis is a clinical dilemma.[129,130] Radionuclide bone scans are the primary imaging modality for diagnosing osteomyelitis, but they have poor spatial resolution and require hours to be completed. MRI is a useful adjunctive imaging modality that is very sensitive to osteomyelitis. Osteomyelitis appears as decreased signal intensity on

T1-weighted and increased signal intensity on T2-weighted scans (Fig. 12–97). The specificity of MRI is poor and does not allow differentiation from other conditions, such as neoplasm or trauma. However, osteomyelitis tends to be less well-defined than tumors. MRI is useful for determining the extent of bone and soft tissue involvement.

Stress Fractures

Stress fractures are most often caused by repeated minor trauma and present with focal pain. They are usually located in the metaphysis or diaphysis of long bones. Radiographs are notoriously poor for diagnosing stress fractures. Radionuclide bone scans are very sensitive for detecting stress fractures, but they are nonspecific. MRI is at least as sensitive as radionuclide bone scans, but much more specific for diagnosing stress fractures.[131]

MRI findings of stress fracture are a thin band of very low signal intensity in the bone marrow, which extends to the cortical surface and is seen on both T1- and T2-weighted images (Fig. 12–98).[131] This represents microfracture or bone sclerosis. A larger surrounding area of relatively decreased signal intensity is also seen in the bone marrow on T1-weighted

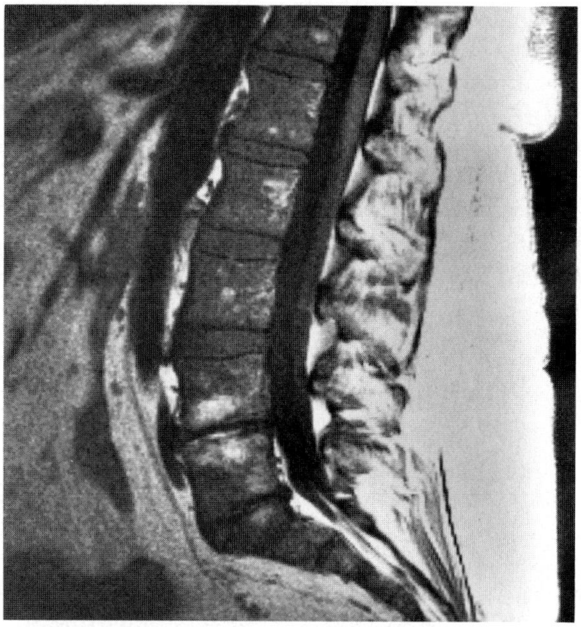

FIGURE 12–95. Bone marrow infiltration: myelofibrosis. T1-weighted sagittal image of the lumbar spine (TR/TE = 450/20) shows marked decreased signal intensity in the vertebral bodies of the lumbar spine. The intervertebral discs are isointense with the adjacent vertebral bodies. This indicates marrow infiltration and can occur in many pathologic conditions.

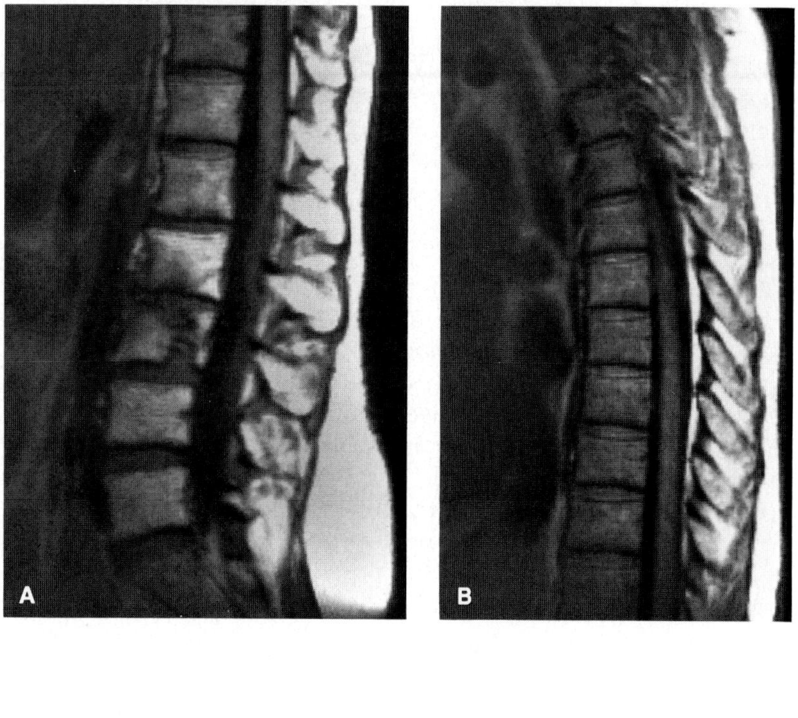

FIGURE 12–96. Marrow changes after radiation therapy. **(A)** T1-weighted sagittal image of the lumbar spine (TR/TE = 650/20) and **(B)** T1-weighted sagittal image of the thoracic spine (TR/TE = 970/20). This is a 49-year-old woman with breast cancer metastatic to L3. The patient received radiation therapy locally in the lumbar spine. A metastatic lesion is demonstrated in the L3 vertebral body as an area of low signal intensity. The adjacent vertebral bodies in the lumbar spine have increased signal intensity, which is a common finding after radiation therapy. For comparison, the nonradiated thoracic spine has intermediate or mildly increased signal intensity in the normal vertebral bodies.

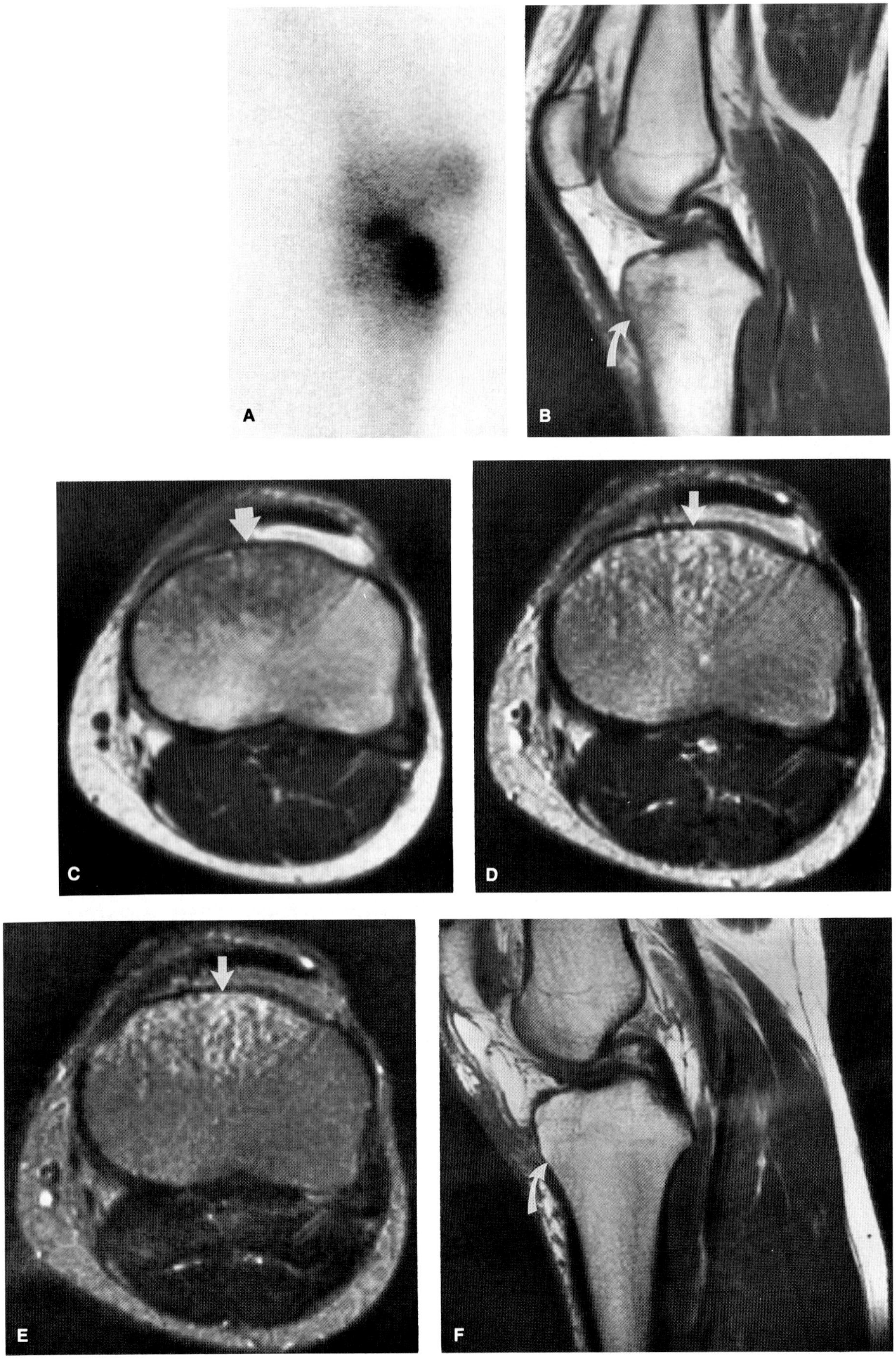
A
B
C
D
E
F

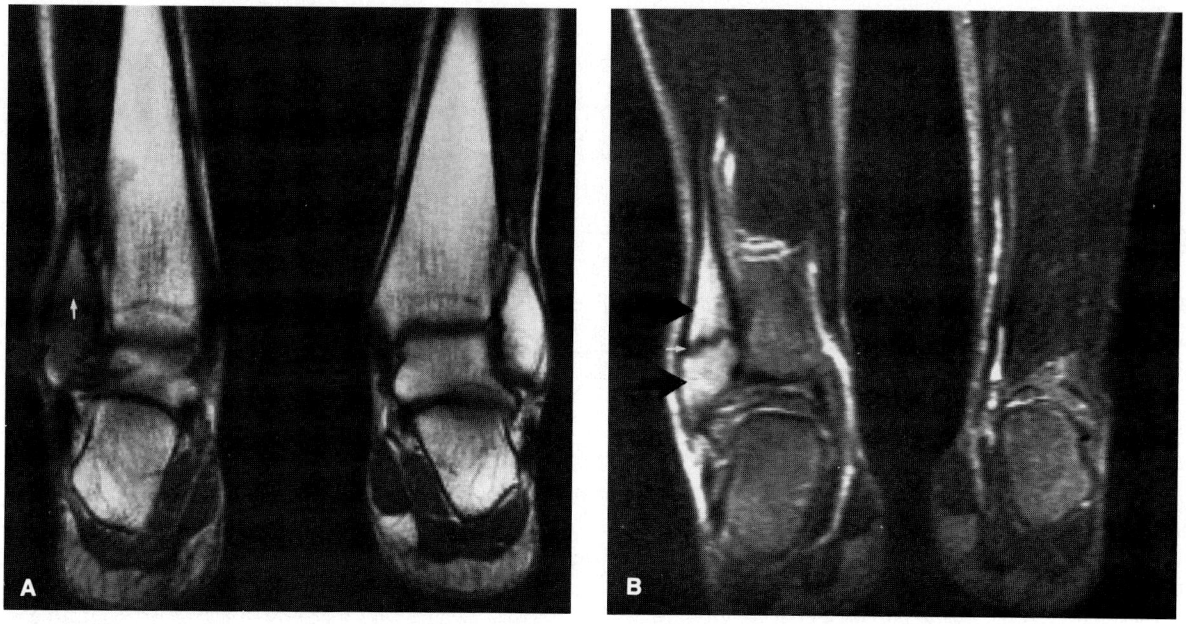

FIGURE 12–98. Stress fracture. **(A)** Coronal T1-weighted image (TR/TE = 600/17) and **(B)** coronal T2-weighted image (TR/TE = 2500/90). There is a linear area of very low signal intensity (small white arrow) on both images in the distal right fibula, which extends to the bony cortex and represents a fracture line. There is a surrounding area of decreased signal intensity on the T1-weighted image and increased signal intensity (black arrows) on the T2-weighted image in the bone marrow of the distal fibula. This presumably represents adjacent bone edema. Notice the normal high signal intensity on the T1-weighted image and intermediate signal intensity on the T2-weighted image in the adjacent normal marrow of the tibia.

◀ **FIGURE 12–97.** Osteomyelitis. **(A)** Bone scan; **(B)** sagittal and **(C)** axial T1-weighted images (TR/TE = 800/17); **(D,E)** axial T2-weighted images (TR/TE = 3000/45,90); **(F)** sagittal T1-weighted image after treatment (TR/TE = 800/17). The bone scan shows increased uptake in the region of the proximal tibia. Ill-defined decreased signal intensity is demonstrated in the anterior proximal tibia on the T1-weighted images **(B,C).** Corresponding areas of heterogeneous increased signal intensity (arrows) are seen in the tibia on the T2-weighted scans **(D,E).** After antibiotic treatment, the patient's symptoms resolved, and a follow-up MRI **(F)** showed resolution of the marrow abnormality, with reappearance of the normal homogeneous high signal intensity marrow at the previous site of osteomyelitis (arrow).

images. On T2-weighted images, there is an area of increased signal intensity in the marrow around the thin band of low signal. This represents hemorrhage or edema.

ACKNOWLEDGMENT

The author thanks Bert Carollo, Nancy Wysocki, Martha Pacetti, and Adam Flanders and his wife Robin, for their support and assistance.

REFERENCES

1. Reicher MA, Bassett LW, Gold RH. High-resolution magnetic resonance imaging of the knee joint: pathologic correlations. AJR 1985;145:903.
2. Burk DL Jr, Kanal E, Brunberg JA, et al. 1.5-T surface coil MRI of the knee. AJR 1986;147:293.
3. Tyrrell RL, Gluckert K, Pathria M, et al. Fast three-dimensional MR imaging of the knee: comparison with arthroscopy. Radiology 1988;166:865.
4. Haggar AM, Froelich JW, Hearshen DO, et al. Meniscal abnormalities of the knee: 3DFT fast-scan GRASS MR imaging. AJR 1988;150:1341.
5. Spritzer CE, Vogler JB, Martinez S, et al. MR imaging of the knee: preliminary results with a 3DFT GRASS pulse sequence. AJR 1988;150:597.
6. Herman LJ, Beltran J. Pitfalls in MR imaging of the knee. Radiology 1988;167:775.
7. Reicher MA, Hartzman S, Duckwiler GR, et al. Meniscal injuries: detection using MR imaging. Radiology 1986;159:753.
8. Mink JH, Levy T, Crues JV III. Tears of the anterior cruciate ligament and menisci of the knee: MR imaging evaluation. Radiology 1988;167:769.
9. Crues JV III, Mink J, Levy TL, et al. Meniscal tears of the knee: accuracy of MR imaging. Radiology 1987;164:445.
10. Hajek PC, Gylys-Morin VM, Baker LL, et al. The high signal intensity meniscus of the knee: magnetic resonance evaluation and in vivo correlation. Invest Radiol 1987;22:883.

11. Quinn SF, Muus C, Sara A, et al. Meniscal tears: pathologic correlation with MR imaging. Radiology 1988;167:580.
12. Stoller DW, Martin C, Crues JV III, et al. Meniscal tears: pathologic correlation with MR imaging. Radiology 1987:163:731.
13. Harms SE, Greenway A. Musculoskeletal system. In: Stark DD, Bradley WG Jr, eds. Magnetic resonance imaging. St. Louis: CV Mosby, 1988:1323.
14. Deutch AL, Mink JH. MR imaging of the postoperative meniscus. Radiology 1988;169(P):20.
15. Girgis FG, Marshall JL, Al Monajem ARS. The cruciate ligaments of the knee joint: anatomical, functional and experimental analysis. Clin Orthop 1975;106:216.
16. Lee JK, Yao L, Phelps CT, et al. Anterior cruciate ligament tears: MR imaging compared with arthroscopy and clinical tests. Radiology 1988;166:861.
17. Turner DA, Prodromos CC, Petasnick JP, et al. Acute injury of the ligaments of the knee: magnetic resonance evaluation. Radiology 1985;154:717.
18. Wojtys E, Wilson M, Buckwalter K, et al. Magnetic resonance imaging of knee hyaline cartilage and intraarticular pathology. Am J Sports Med 1987;15:455.
19. Reicher MA, Hartzman S, Bassett LW, et al. MR imaging of the knee. Part I. Traumatic disorders. Radiology 1987;162:547.
20. Yao L, Lee JK. Occult intraosseous fracture: detection with MR imaging. Radiology 1988;167:749.
21. Mesgarzadeh M, Sapega AA, Bonakdarpour A, et al. Osteochondritis dissecans: analysis of mechanical stability with radiography, scintigraphy, and MR imaging. Radiology 1987;165:775.
22. Hartzman S, Reicher MA, Bassett LW, et al. MR imaging of the knee. Part II. Chronic disorders. Radiology 1987;162:553.
23. Burk DL Jr, Dalinka MK, Kanal E, et al. Meniscal and ganglion cysts of the knee: MR evaluation. AJR 1988;150:331.
24. Yulish BS, Montanez J, Goodfellow DB, et al. Chondromalacia patellae: assessment with MR imaging. Radiology 1987;164:763.
25. Goldman AB, DiCarlo EF. Pigmented villonodular synovitis diagnosis and differential diagnosis. Radiol Clin North Am 1988;126:1327.
26. Jaffe HL, Lichtenstein L, Sutro CJ. Pigmented villonodular synovitis, bursitis, and tenosynovitis. Arch Pathol 1941;31:731.
27. Spritzer CE, Dalinka MK, Kressel HY. Magnetic resonance imaging of pigmented villonodular synovitis: a report of two cases. Skeletal Radiol 1987;16:316.
28. Kottal R, Vogler JB III, Matamoros A, et al. Pigmented villonodular synovitis: a report of MR imaging in two cases. Radiology 1987;163:551.
29. Siegel SC, Haggar AM, Froelich JW, et al. An overview of magnetic resonance imaging of the appendicular musculoskeletal system. Henry Ford Hosp Med J 1987;35:234.
30. Steinberg ME, Brighton CT, Hayken GD, et al. Early results in the treatment of avascular necrosis of the femoral head with electrical stimulation. Orthop Clin North Am 1984;15:163.
31. Takatori Y, Kamogawa M, Kokubo T, et al. Magnetic resonance imaging and histopathology in femoral head necrosis. Acta Orthop Scand 1987;58:499.
32. Mikhael MA, Paige ML, Widen AL. Magnetic resonance imaging and the diagnosis of avascular necrosis of the femoral head. Comput Radiol 1987;11:157.
33. Genez BM, Wilson MR, Houk RW, et al. Early osteonecrosis of the femoral head: detection in high-risk patients with MR imaging. Radiology 1988;168:521.
34. Beltran J, Herman LJ, Burk JM, et al. Femoral head avascular necrosis: MR imaging with clinical-pathologic and radionuclide correlation. Radiology 1988;166:215.
35. Markisz JA, Knowles RJR, Altchek DW, et al. Segmental patterns of avascular necrosis of the femoral heads: early detection with MR imaging. Radiology 1987;162:717.
36. Mitchell MD, Kundel HL, Steinberg ME, et al. Avascular necrosis of the hip: comparison of MR, CT, and scintigraphy. AJR 1986;147:67.
37. Thickman D, Axel L, Kressel HY, et al. Magnetic resonance imaging of avascular necrosis of the femoral head. Skeletal Radiol 1986;15:133.
38. Mitchell DG, Joseph PM, Fallon M, et al. Chemical-shift MR imaging of the femoral head: an in vitro study of normal hips and hips with avascular necrosis. AJR 1987;148:1159.
39. Meyers MH. Osteonecrosis of the femoral head: pathogenesis and long-term results of treatment. Clin Orthop 1988;231:51.
40. Hungerford DS, Lennox DW. The importance of increased intraosseous pressure in the development of osteonecrosis of the femoral head: implications for treatment. Orthop Clin North Am 1985;16:635.
41. Cruess RL. Osteonecrosis of bone: current concepts as to etiology and pathogenesis. Clin Orthop 1986;208:30.
42. Mitchell DG, Rao VM, Dalinka MK, et al. Femoral head avascular necrosis: correlation of MR imaging, radiographic staging, radionuclide imaging, and clinical findings. Radiology 1987;162:709.
43. Lang P, Jergesen HE, Moseley ME, et al. Avascular necrosis of the femoral head: high-field strength MR imaging with histologic correlation. Radiology 1988;169:517.
44. Coleman BG, Kressel HY, Dalinka MK, et al. Radiographically negative avascular necrosis: detection with MR imaging. Radiology 1988;168:525.
45. Sweet DE, Madewell JE. Pathogenesis of osteonecrosis. In: Resnick NK, Niwayama G, eds. Diagnosis of bone and joint disorders. Philadelphia: WB Saunders, 1988:3188.
46. Rush BH, Bramson FT, Ogden JA. Legg-Calve-Perthes disease: detection of cartilaginous and synovial changes with MR imaging. Radiology 1988;167:473.
47. Ehman RL, Berquist TH, McLeod RA. MR imaging of the musculoskeletal system: a 5-year appraisal. Radiology 1988;166:313.
48. Bassett LW, Gold RH, Reicher M, et al. Magnetic resonance imaging in the early diagnosis of ischemic necrosis of the femoral head. Preliminary results. Clin Orthop 1987;214:237.
49. Mitchell DG, Rao V, Dalinka M, et al. MRI of joint fluid in the normal and ischemic hip. AJR 1986;146:1215.
50. Mitchell DG, Rao VM, Dalinka M, et al. Hematopoietic and fatty bone marrow distribution in the normal and ischemic hip: new observations with 1.5 T MR imaging. Radiology 1986;161:199.
51. Toby EB, Koman LA, Bechtold RE. Magnetic resonance imaging of pediatric hip disease. J Pediatr Orthop 1985;5:665.
52. Mitchell MJ, Causey G, Berthoty DP, et al. Peribursal fat plane of the shoulder: anatomic study and clinical experience. Radiology 1988;168:699.
53. Mink JH, Harris E, Rappaport M. Rotator cuff tears: evaluation using double-contrast shoulder arthrography. Radiology 1985;157:621.
54. Mack LA, Matsen FA III, Kilcoyne RF, et al. US evaluation of the rotator cuff. Radiology 1985;157:205.
55. Rafii M, Firooznia H, Golimbu C, et al. CT arthrography of capsular structures of the shoulder. AJR 1986;146:361.
56. Beltran J, Gray LA, Bools JC, et al. Rotator cuff lesions of the shoulder: evaluation by direct sagittal CT arthrography. Radiology 1986;160:161.
57. Huber DJ, Sauter R, Mueller E, et al. MR imaging of the normal shoulder. Radiology 1986;158:405.
58. Kneeland JB, Carrera GF, Middleton WD, et al. Rotator cuff tears: preliminary application of high-resolution MR imaging with counter rotating current loop-gap resonators. Radiology 1986;160:695.
59. Kieft GJ, Bloem JL, Obermann WR, et al. Normal shoulder: MR imaging. Radiology 1986;159:741.
60. Seeger LL, Ruszkowski JT, Bassett LW, et al. MR imaging of the normal shoulder: anatomic correlation. AJR 1987;148:83.
61. Zlatkin MB, Dalinka MK, Kressel HY. Magnetic resonance imaging of the shoulder. Magn Reson Q 1989;5:3.
62. Kieft GJ, Bloem JL, Rozing PM, et al. Rotator cuff impingement syndrome: MR imaging. Radiology 1988;166:211.
63. Seeger LL, Gold RH, Bassett LW, et al. Shoulder impingement syndrome: MR findings in 53 shoulders. AJR 1988;150:343.
64. Neer CS II. Impingement lesions. Clin Orthop 1983;173:70.

65. Evancho AM, Stiles RG, Fajman WA, et al. MR imaging diagnosis of rotator cuff tears. AJR 1988;151:751.
66. Reeder JD, Andelman S. The rotator cuff tear: MR evaluation. Magn Reson Imaging 1987;5:331.
67. Kneeland JB, Middleton WD, Carrera GF, et al. MR imaging of the shoulder: diagnosis of rotator cuff tears. AJR 1987;149:333.
68. Crues JV III. Applying MRI to shoulder poses special problems. Diagn Imag 1988;10:164.
69. Seeger LL, Gold RH, Bassett LW. Shoulder instability: evaluation with MR imaging. Radiology 1988;168:695.
70. Katzberg RW, Dolwick MF, Helms CA, et al. Arthrotomography of the temporomandibular joint. AJR 1980;134:995.
71. Katzberg RW, Dolwick MF, Bales DJ, et al. Arthrotomography of the temporomandibular joint: new technique and preliminary observations. AJR 1979;132:949.
72. Norgaard F. Arthrography of the joint. Acta Radiol 1944;25:679.
73. Mafee MF, Heffez L, Campos M, et al. Temporomandibular joint: role of direct sagittal CT air-contrast arthrogram and MRI. Otolaryngol Clin North Am 1988;21:575.
74. Sanchez-Woodworth RE, Tallents RH, Katzberg RW, et al. Bilateral internal derangements of temporomandibular joint: evaluation by magnetic resonance imaging. Oral Surg Oral Med Oral Pathol 1988;65:281.
75. Schellhas KP, Wilkes CH, Omile MR, et al. The diagnosis of temporomandibular joint disease: two-compartment arthrography and MR. AJR 1988;151:341.
76. Schach RT, Sadowsky PL. Clinical experience with magnetic resonance imaging in internal derangements of the TMJ. Angle Orthod 1988;58:21.
77. Schellhas KP, Wilkes CH, Fritts HM, et al. Temporomandibular joint: MR imaging of internal derangements and post-operative changes. AJR 1988;150:381.
78. Schellhas KP, Wilkes CH, Fritts HM, et al. MR of osteochondritis dissecans and avascular necrosis of the mandibular condyle. AJNR 1989;10:3.
79. Burnett KR, Davis CL, Read J. Dynamic display of the temporomandibular joint meniscus by using "fast-scan" MR imaging. AJR 1987;149:959.
80. Westesson P-L, Katzberg RW, Tallents RH, et al. Temporomandibular joint: comparison of MR images with cryosectional anatomy. Radiology 1987;164:59.
81. Katzberg RW, Westesson P-L, Tallents RH, et al. Temporomandibular joint: MR assessment of rotational and sideways disk displacements. Radiology 1988;169:741.
82. Wilk RM, Harms SE. Temporomandibular joint: multislab, three-dimensional fourier transformation MR imaging. Radiology 1988;167:861.
83. Avrahami E, Schreiber R, Benmair J, et al. Magnetic resonance imaging of the temporo-mandibular joint and meniscus dislocation. Br J Radiol 1986;59:1153.
84. Schellhas KP, Wilkes CH, Heithoff KB, et al. Temporomandibular joint: diagnosis of internal derangements using magnetic resonance imaging. Minn Med 1986;69:516.
85. Harms SE, Wilk RM. Magnetic resonance imaging of the temporomandibular joint. Radiographics 1987;7:521.
86. Hellsing G, L'Estrange P, Holmlund A. Temporomandibular joint disorders: a diagnostic challenge. J Prosthet Dent 1986;56:600.
87. Harms SE, Wilk RM, Wolford LM, et al. The temporomandibular joint: magnetic resonance imaging using surface coils. Radiology 1985;157:133.
88. Donlon WC, Moon KL. Comparison of magnetic resonance imaging, arthrotomography and clinical and surgical findings in temporomandibular joint internal derangements. Oral Surg Oral Med Oral Pathol 1987;64:2.
89. Laurell KA, Tootle R, Cunningham R, et al. Magnetic resonance imaging of the temporomandibular joint. Part II: comparison with laminographic, autopsy, and histologic findings. J Prosthet Dent 1987;58:211.
90. Kneeland JB, Ryan DE, Carrera GF, et al. Failed temporomandibular joint prostheses: MR imaging. Radiology 1987;165:179.
91. Schellhas KP, Wilkes CH, Deeb ME, et al. Permanent proplast temporomandibular joint implants: MR imaging of destructive complications. AJR 1988;151:731.
92. Weiss KL, Beltran J, Shamam OM, et al. High-field MR surface coil imaging of the hand and wrist. Part I. Normal anatomy. Radiology 1986;160:143.
93. Koenig H, Lucas D, Meissner R, et al. The wrist: a preliminary report on high-resolution MR imaging. Radiology 1986;160:463.
94. Baker LL, Hajek PC, Bjorkengren A, et al. High-resolution magnetic resonance imaging of the wrist: normal anatomy. Skeletal Radiol 1987;16:128.
95. Binkovitz LA, Cahill DR, Ehman RL, et al. Magnetic resonance imaging of the wrist: normal cross sectional imaging and skeletal abnormal cases. Radiographics 1988;8:1171.
96. Middleton WD, Kneeland JB, Kellman GM, et al. MR imaging of the carpal tunnel: normal anatomy and preliminary findings in the carpal tunnel syndrome. AJR 1987;148:307.
97. Weiss KL, Beltran J, Lubbers LM. High-field MR surface-coil imaging of the hand and wrist. Part II. Pathologic correlations and clinical relevance. Radiology 1986;160:147.
98. Reinus WR, Conway WF, Totty WG, et al. Carpal avascular necrosis: MR imaging. Radiology 1986;160:689.
99. Beltran J, Noto AM, Mosure JC, et al. Ankle: surface coil MR imaging at 1.5 T. Radiology 1986;161:203.
100. Kneeland B, Macrandar S, Middleton WD, et al. MR imaging of the normal ankle: correlation with anatomic sections. AJR 1988;151:117.
101. Hajek PC, Paker LL, Bjorkengren A, et al. High-resolution magnetic resonance imaging of the ankle: normal anatomy. Skeletal Radiol 1986;15:536.
102. Quinn SF, Murray WT, Clark RA, et al. Achilles tendon: MR imaging at 1.5 T. Radiology 1987;164:767.
103. Rosenthal DI. Tumors of the musculoskeletal system: magnetic resonance imaging and computed tomography. Bull NY Acad Med 1987;63:493.
104. Porter BA, Shields AF, Olson DO. Magnetic resonance imaging of bone marrow disorders. Radiol Clin North Am 1986;24:269.
105. Daffner RH, Lupetin AR, Dash N, et al. MRI in the detection of malignant infiltration of bone marrow. AJR 1986;146:353.
106. Haggar AM, Froelich JW. MR imaging strategies in primary and metastatic malignancy. Radiol Clin North Am 1988;26:689.
107. Kanal E, Burk DL Jr, Brunberg JA, et al. Pediatric musculoskeletal magnetic resonance imaging. Radiol Clin North Am 1988;26:211.
108. Pettersson H, Gillespy T III, Hamlin DJ, et al. Primary musculoskeletal tumors: examination with MR imaging compared with conventional modalities. Radiology 1987;164:237.
109. Aisen AM, Martel W, Braunstein EM, et al. MRI and CT evaluation of primary bone and soft-tissue tumors. AJR 1986;146:749.
110. Bloem JL, Bluemm RG, Taminiav AHM, et al. Magnetic resonance imaging of primary malignant bone tumors. Radiographics 1987;7:425.
111. Wetzel LH, Levine E, Murphy MD. A comparison of MR imaging and CT in the evaluation of musculoskeletal masses. Radiographics 1987;7:851.
112. Sundaram M, McGuire MH, Schajowicz F. Soft-tissue masses: histologic basis for decreased signal (short T2) on T2-weighted MR images. AJR 1987;148:1247.
113. Dooms GC, Hricak H, Sollitto RA, et al. Lipomatous tumors and tumors with fatty component: MR imaging potential and comparison of MR and CT results. Radiology 1985;157:479.
114. Cohen EK, Kressel HY, Frank TS, et al. Hyaline cartilage-origin bone and soft-tissue neoplasms: MR appearance and histologic correlation. Radiology 1988;167:477.
115. Kransdorf MJ, Utz JA, Gilkey FW, et al. MR appearance of fibroxanthoma. J Comput Assist Tomogr 1988;12:612.
116. Yeager BA, Schiebler ML, Wertheim SB, et al. MR imaging of osteoid osteoma of the talus. J Comput Assist Tomogr 1987;11:916.

117. Lee JK, Yao L, Wirth CR. MR imaging of solitary osteochondromas: report of eight cases. AJR 1987;149:557.

118. McKinstry CS, Steiner RE, Young AT, et al. Bone marrow in leukemia and aplastic anemia: MR imaging before, during, and after treatment. Radiology 1987;162:701.

119. Herman SD, Mesgarzadeh M, Bonakdarpour A, et al. The role of magnetic resonance imaging in giant cell tumor of bone. Skeletal Radiol 1987;16:635.

120. Ross JS, Masaryk TJ, Modic MT, et al. Vertebral hemangiomas: MR imaging. Radiology 1987;165:165.

121. Gillespy T III, Manfrini M, Ruggieri P, et al. Staging of intraosseous extent of osteosarcoma: correlation of preoperative CT and MR imaging with pathologic macroslides. Radiology 1988;167:765.

122. Boyko OB, Cory DA, Cohen MD, et al. MR imaging of osteogenic and Ewing's sarcoma. AJR 1987;148:317.

123. Sundaram M, McGuire MH, Herbold DR, et al. Magnetic resonance imaging in planning limb-salvage surgery for primary malignant tumors of bone. J Bone Joint Surg 1986;68A:809.

124. Zimmer WD, Berquist TH, McLeod RA, et al. Magnetic resonance imaging of osteosarcomas: comparison with computer tomography. Clin Orthop 1986;208:289.

125. Beltran J, Simon DC, Katz W, et al. Increased MR signal intensity in skeletal muscle adjacent to malignant tumors: pathologic correlation and clinical relevance. Radiology 1987;162:251.

126. Vanel D, Lacombe M-J, Covanet D, et al. Musculoskeletal tumors: follow-up with MR imaging after treatment with surgery and radiation therapy. Radiology 1987;164:243.

127. Ross B, Helsper JT, Cox IJ, et al. Osteosarcoma and other neoplasms of bone. Magnetic resonance spectroscopy to monitor therapy. Arch Surg 1987;122:1464.

128. Vogler JB III, Murphy WA. Bone marrow imaging. Radiology 1988;168:679.

129. Berquist TH, Brown ML, Fitzgerald RH Jr, et al. Magnetic resonance imaging: application in musculoskeletal infection. Magn Reson Imag 1985;3:219.

130. Modic MT, Pflanze W, Feiglin DHI, et al. Magnetic resonance imaging of musculoskeletal infections. Radiol Clin North Am 1986;24:247.

131. Lee JK, Yao L. Stress fractures: MR imaging. Radiology 1988;169:217.

13

Imaging Technique

Michael L. Wood

A bewildering array of conditions influence the quality of magnetic resonance (MR) images. Not only do numerous imaging techniques exist, but each technique also presents its own options. With superior visualization of lesions as the general goal, desirable imaging techniques strive for the highest contrast between tissues and the least noise. Constraints upon imaging time and spatial resolution make this objective elusive. Almost any imaging technique could produce acceptable images if sufficient time was available, but for practical reasons, it is imperative that imaging techniques demand as little time as possible. Another desirable characteristic of MR images is high spatial resolution. Unfortunately, higher-resolution images take too long to create or are noisier.

This chapter explains basic principles of the most common MRI techniques, which are called spin echo and gradient echo. The material is presented at an introductory level intended for practical use primarily by physicians with minimal experience in MRI.

ACHIEVING CONTRAST BETWEEN TISSUES

Contrast and Contrast-to-Noise Ratio

One of the most basic goals of a medical imaging procedure is to give an abnormality an intensity distinct from other tissues, or in other words, to generate contrast. There are several definitions of contrast, all of which involve the difference in intensity of two structures relative to a reference level. The specification of a reference produces various definitions of contrast.

One possible reference level for the definition of contrast is the average intensity of the two structures under comparison. Contrast, defined as the intensity difference of two structures divided by their average intensity, is called relative contrast and it is used most frequently in screen-film radiography. However, this relative contrast is inappropriate for digital imaging modalities, such as MRI or x-ray computed tomography (CT), because the appearance of digital images can be altered simply through adjustments to the window and center of the display. In particular, higher contrast can be achieved if the display window is reduced, so that a smaller range of intensity values is assigned to the same shades of gray. In practice, noise limits the usefulness of displaying a digital image with arbitrarily high contrast. Therefore, it is pertinent to express contrast in MRI relative to the level of noise.

The intensity difference between two tissues divided by the standard deviation of the noise is called the contrast-to-noise-ratio (CNR). The CNR is regarded as a good indicator of tissue differentiation in MRI.[1] Because this section is not concerned with conditions that alter noise, it will be more convenient to use the term contrast as a simplification of CNR. The term contrast in this chapter refers to the intensity difference between two tissues relative to a fixed level of noise. To compare contrast in images with different noise, the intensity of each image must be multiplied by a number to equalize the level of noise in all images.

Obviously, each imaging modality has a different mechanism for achieving contrast between tissues. For example, x-ray imaging modalities exploit differences in the attenuation of x-rays, which results from interactions between x-ray photons and atomic electrons. Mechanisms of contrast in MRI are less obvious than in x-ray imaging, perhaps because MRI has more variables to consider. Instead of electron density, the contrast between tissues in MRI depends primarily on three other parameters: proton density and the so-called T1 and T2 relaxation time constants.

Nuclear Magnetic Resonance

Proton density and the T1 and T2 relaxation processes are characteristic of nuclear magnetic resonance (NMR), which is the phenomenon responsible for giving tissues their intensity in MRI. More than 40 years have passed since the discovery of NMR in 1946.[2,3] Nuclei with an odd number of protons or neutrons exhibit NMR. Hydrogen nuclei, which are simply protons, produce the strongest NMR signals in the human body, due to the abundance of water and the inherent sensitivity of protons to NMR. Many articles provide details about the physical principles of NMR relevant to MRI.[4–7]

A group of protons in a magnetic field behaves somewhat like a magnetic dipole. A tiny magnetic field is produced by a group of protons, and the field is characterized by a vector called the magnetic moment. (A vector is an entity that has both a magnitude and a direction, and it is denoted by an arrow.) Most of the phenomena encountered in MRI can be explained through analysis of the resultant contribution of groups of protons, which are referred to as magnetization components. The so-called net magnetization is manipulated and observed in NMR.

At equilibrium, tissues in the body acquire a net magnetization, which tends to be aligned parallel to the magnetic field. (Both the net magnetization and the magnetic field are vectors.) The net magnetization can be observed after its equilibrium orientation has been disturbed by a pulse of radio-frequency (RF) energy. For it to be effective, the RF pulse must have a specific frequency, depending on the magnetic field strength (42.6 MHz at 1.0 T and 63.9 MHz at 1.5 T). An RF pulse can tip the net magnetization by an amount determined by the amplitude and duration of the pulse.

Tipping the net magnetization creates a transverse component from the longitudinal magnetization, which is the component parallel to the magnetic field. An RF pulse that tips the magnetization through 90° is called a 90° RF pulse. A 90° RF pulse converts all of the longitudinal magnetization into transverse magnetization (and vice versa, if any transverse magnetization existed before the RF pulse). The transverse magnetization precesses, or rotates, about the direction of the magnetic field at a frequency called the Larmor frequency. The Larmor frequency is 42.6 MHz if the magnetic field strength is 1.0 T.

The changing magnetic field caused by the precession of transverse magnetization can induce an electrical voltage in a receiver coil. The voltage is directly proportional to the amount of transverse magnetization. The voltage oscillates with the same frequency as the frequency of precession, and it also decreases as the transverse magnetization decays. Measurements of this voltage constitute NMR signals. When NMR signals are assigned to a volume element (voxel) or picture element (pixel) in an MR image, voxels or pixels that have greater intensity represent regions that produced stronger NMR signals. Throughout the text, the term NMR signal is used to distinguish the measurements of data from the intensity of pixels in MR images.

Spatial Encoding with Magnetic Field Gradients

The procedure for encoding spatial information into NMR signals, so that they can be assigned to distinct voxels in a digital MR image, involves numerous steps, the details of which are not pertinent here.[8,9] The equipment for MRI includes components called gradient coils, which are activated for periods of several milliseconds (ms). A magnetic field gradient makes the magnetic field increase linearly along one direction. There is a gradient coil for each of the three orthogonal directions. Magnetic field gradients are employed in several subtle ways to encode spatial information into NMR signals. One gradient is activated so that an RF pulse tips the magnetization from only the structures in a slice; this is called selective excitation.

A second gradient, called the frequency-encoding gradient, is applied while NMR signals are being measured, which makes the Larmor frequency vary linearly along one axis. In this way, components situated at different positions along the frequency-encoding direction contribute NMR signals that oscillate at different rates. The individual contributions give the resultant NMR signal a beat pattern, analogous to a combination of musical notes. The shape and position of structures that produced the NMR signals can be derived by subjecting these signals to computer processing.

Frequency encoding provides information about one direction in a plane. The other direction can be resolved through a procedure called phase encoding. Phase encoding uses a third magnetic field gradient, which is turned on only for a few milliseconds and then turned off before any measurements. This affects NMR signals, depending on the strength and duration of the gradient, and of course, the characteristics of the anatomic structures in the slice. Phase encoding requires numerous NMR signals to be produced and measured, the number depending on the desired spatial resolution. For example, resolving 256 pixels along the phase-encoding direction of an MR image takes 256 different NMR signals. Each application of the phase-encoding gradient to produce a different NMR signal is called a phase-encoding step. The phase-encoding gradient is incremented in amplitude each time it prepares another NMR signal. Sometimes phase-encoding steps are repeated so that measurements can be averaged to reduce noise. The number of identical repetitions are often called number of excitations (NEXs), acquisitions, or averages.

Consecutive NMR signals are generated after a delay of TR, which is called the repetition time. As will be seen below, TR ranges from about 10 ms to several seconds. It takes a longer time to acquire data for an MR image if the TR is longer. This measurement time is referred to commonly as the imaging time, even though it excludes the time needed to convert the measurements into an MR image, which can be as long as 5 seconds for each image.

Techniques for MRI

The signals from NMR depend on details of the associated technique, specifically the characteristics, sequence, and timing of the various RF pulses. The most common NMR technique is called saturation recovery spin echo, or simply spin echo, and it is described more fully in a later section. A spin echo is a type of NMR signal, which can be generated through the action of a 180° RF pulse. After a general analysis of the spin echo techniques, a category of simpler techniques, which refocus NMR signals by reversing the polarity of a magnetic field gradient, are introduced. Gradient-echo techniques allow images to be acquired more rapidly. In fact, gradient-echo techniques can produce a two-dimensional (2D) image of a slice in a few seconds instead of minutes, or a three-dimensional (3D) volume image in minutes instead of hours. Shorter imaging times allow abdominal images to be acquired during periods of continuous breath holding. Examples of 3D gradient-echo MR images have already been presented in this book. These images show that 3D techniques can cover extensive regions of anatomy with thin slices.

There are other techniques that also deserve mention. Inversion recovery is distinguished by an additional RF pulse that tips the longitudinal magnetization by 180° before the application of the customary 90° RF pulse that creates a transverse component of magnetization from the longitudinal component.[10] Ordinarily, inversion recovery provides strong T1-weighted contrast, although it is also possible to use inversion recovery to exploit differences in T2. Images can also be formed from NMR signals called stimulated echoes.[11,12] In echo-planar imaging, and its variants, enough measurements to form an image are collected within about 35 msec after a single RF pulse.[13,14] There are also techniques that attempt to establish a steady state for the transverse magnetization, which tends to enhance the signals from fluids.[15] Although these techniques have limited applicability, they should not be ignored, because the inherent flexibility of MRI is one of its strongest attributes. Specialized techniques should enhance the capability of MRI as the technology matures.

Most techniques achieve contrast because of differences in proton density, T1, or T2. However, other conditions can affect NMR signals, including motion and differences in magnetic susceptibility, which is simply a measure of the extent to which a material becomes magnetized in a magnetic field. Flowing blood can have an appearance different from stationary blood, and this property has been employed to assess the patency of arterial vessels. Not surprisingly, some specialized techniques exploit various secondary NMR parameters to derive contrast between tissues.

It has long been known that diffusion affects NMR signals.[16] Techniques have been demonstrated that provide information related to diffusion, which occurs more readily in certain tissues.[17] Techniques intended primarily to assess diffusion have not yet received widespread use. On the other hand, contrast agents, such as Gd DTPA, have more general applicability and are being used routinely to enhance the capabilities of MRI.

Proton Density, T1, and T2

Tissues have at least three characteristics that are pertinent to MRI: proton density and the T1 and T2 relaxation time constants. Proton density is a dimensionless quantity representing the number of protons that are available to contribute to the signals measured in MRI. Most of the NMR signals relevant to MRI arise from the protons of water molecules. Lipids in adipose tissue also produce strong NMR signals, and proteins and other macromolecules contribute to a small part. Because of the abundance of water, proton density in MRI is correlated largely with water content.

It is difficult to measure proton density, but several properties are well-known. There is little difference between the density of protons in liver, spleen, and kidney.[6,18,19] Therefore, proton density is not useful for creating contrast between abdominal tissues. On the other hand, the density of protons in gray matter exceeds that of white matter by approximately 10%, which is sufficient to create contrast between these two tissues in an MR image.[20]

The more protons, the stronger the NMR signal and the greater the image intensity. Proton density would govern the intensity of tissues in MRI if TR were infinitely long and TE were zero, both of which are obviously impossible. In practice, T1 and T2 relaxation processes also influence NMR signals and, consequently, image intensity.

The T1 relaxation process concerns the recovery of longitudinal magnetization to its equilibrium state after having been affected by an RF pulse. This recovery occurs exponentially with a time constant, T1, which means that the recovery slows down as equilibrium is approached. After an interval equal to T1, the longitudinal magnetization recovers about 63% of the difference between its actual state and its equilibrium value. Similar to the familiar story about a race between a tortoise and a hare, it would appear to take forever for the longitudinal magnetization to regain equilibrium. However, the difference between the actual state of the longitudinal magnetization and its equilibrium value becomes negligible as time passes. The time necessary for sufficient T1 relaxation in MRI depends on the tissue of interest.

The conversion of longitudinal magnetization into transverse magnetization requires energy, which is supplied by an RF pulse, and this energy is returned to the surroundings during T1 or spin-lattice relaxation. Spin-lattice relaxation does not occur spontaneously, but is stimulated by the random tumbling of nearby protons. Tumbling changes the direction of the tiny magnetic fields of protons, which is analogous to pulses of radio-frequency energy. The rate of tumbling depends on the size of the molecules to which the protons are linked. Efficient T1 relaxation occurs when the frequency of tumbling is near the Larmor frequency. Therefore, the strength of the magnetic field influences T1 relaxation. For the conditions encountered in MRI, T1 relaxation depends on the number and environment of water molecules, more precisely on the extent to which water is associated with various macromolecules.[21]

Mechanisms for T1 relaxation are reasonably well understood for protons in homogeneous environments. Figure 13–1A presents estimates of T1 for various materials at a magnetic field strength of 1.0 T.[22–24] The most striking observation is that the range of T1 is much greater than the range of proton density. Under the conditions encountered in MRI, both liquids and solids tend to have T1 time constants on the order of seconds. The reason for the long T1s is the mobility of these molecules, specifically the likelihood for tumbling to occur at frequencies close to the Larmor frequency. The atoms of solid materials are generally locked too rigidly into a lattice to tumble rapidly enough. At the other extreme, molecules in the liquid state tumble with such a broad spectrum of frequencies that only a small fraction fall into the desired range near the Larmor frequency. The T1 of adipose tissue is short, because the associated molecules are intermediate in size and tend to tumble at frequencies clustered near the Larmor frequency.

Of more interest are the T1 time constants for other common biologic soft tissues, but models for T1 relaxation become complicated for precisely these inhomogeneous tissues. Whatever the exact mechanism, it is

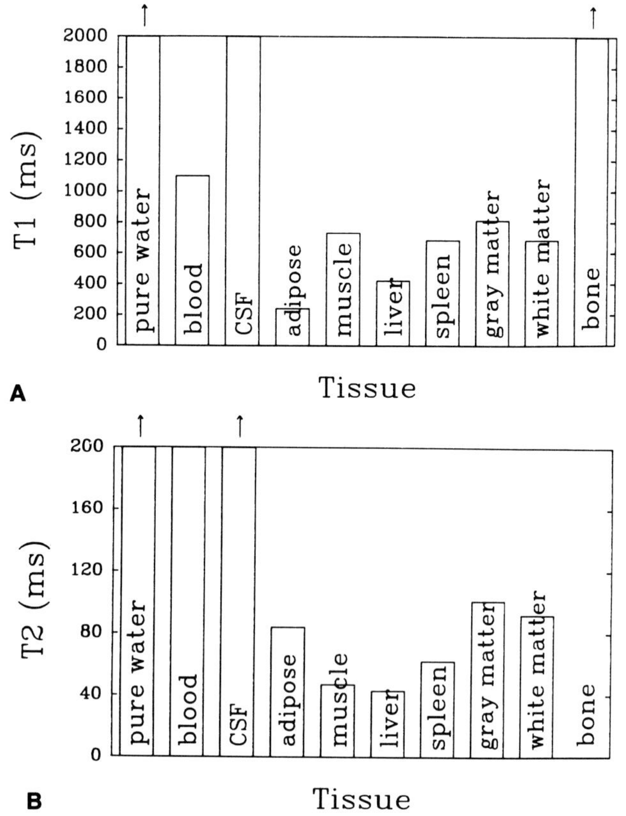

FIGURE 13–1. **(A,B)** Estimates of the NMR time constants T1 and T2, which were compiled from references 18 to 24. The T1 values tabulated **(A)** apply to a magnetic field strength of 1.0 tesla and would generally be longer in a stronger magnetic field.

most opportune that many normal and pathologic tissues have different T1 values. This property can be exploited to distinguish between different tissues in MRI. The longer the T1, the weaker the NMR signals and the image intensity associated with a particular tissue. In this manner, a long T1 time constant handicaps the intensity of a tissue on an MR image.

A distinct process called T2 or spin-spin relaxation describes the decay of NMR signals. T2 relaxation concerns processes that cause the various transverse magnetization components to precess at different rates and thereby lose synchrony. The magnetization components themselves contribute a small and temporally varying magnetic field in addition to the field established by the magnet. Consequently, the rate of precession of a particular magnetization component is influenced by nearby components. The additional magnetic field contributed by magnetization components changes according to their relative motion. The longer that nearby components remain mutually aligned, the shorter the T2. This is the reason for the characteristically microsecond-long T2 time constants of solid materials, such as cortical bone. Estimates of T2 for other biologic tissues are presented in

Figure 13-1B. The long T2s observed for liquids are explained by the relatively free motion of the molecules. The motion of the polar lipids that constitute membranes is severely restricted, and consequently, T2 is so short that membrane lipids are effectively invisible in MRI.[21] The nonpolar lipids found in adipose tissue are more mobile, and their T2 is much longer.

In practice, the decay of NMR signals in MRI is more rapid than described by the time constant T2. The decay is accelerated by magnetic field inhomogeneities, which arise from imperfections in the construction of the magnet. Patients also introduce magnetic field inhomogeneities, because certain tissues have different magnetic susceptibilities. Magnetic susceptibility is a measure of the amount by which a material becomes magnetized in a magnetic field. For example, near the border between an air sinus and a soft tissue, differences in magnetic susceptibility can make the magnetic field inhomogeneous enough to cause NMR signals at the edge of the soft tissue to vanish before measurement. This loss of signal distorts images by enlarging the apparent size of the sinus.

A clever technique called a spin echo can reverse the contributions of magnetic field inhomogeneities to the decay of NMR signals.[16] Spin echo techniques employ a 180° RF pulse in such a manner that more rapidly precessing magnetization components are given a handicap, which allows slower components to regain synchrony and produce an echo. This 180° pulse is applied midway between the 90° pulse and the intended peak of the echo. Most MR images arise from spin echoes. Note, however, that spin echoes are compensated for signal losses caused by static imperfections, but not usually for patient movement or temporal fluctuations of the magnetic field.

Spin Echo Techniques

The contrast between tissues in saturation recovery spin echo MR images, which so far has been the most common imaging technique, depends primarily on differences in proton density, T1, and T2.[20,24-32] Given the knowledge of these three NMR parameters, the contrast between tissues can be predicted with considerable accuracy. Because of uncertainty in the actual values of proton density, T1, and T2, statistical techniques have been developed to optimize contrast.[30,31] Even though the mathematical equations that describe the contrast in spin echo images are simple, it is possible to appreciate the most general features of image contrast without resorting to mathematics.

One of the most obvious observations regarding NMR signals, and by extension, MR image intensity, is that the influence of T1 decreases as TR becomes longer. It is also clear that T2 exerts less influence on contrast when TE is short. These trends are important, but more detailed knowledge of the extent to which TR and TE affect image contrast is necessary for optimizing imaging conditions. Several images of the head and abdomen of volunteers have been produced using a wide range of TR and TE times (Figs. 13-2 through 13-8).

Under the conditions of long TR and short TE, the contrast between tissues depends primarily on differences in the density of protons. It would take an infinitely long TR and a negligibly short TE to eliminate the effects of T1 and T2 entirely and make the image intensity simply proportional to proton density. In spite of practical limitations, strongly proton density weighted images of the head can be seen in Figures 13-2 and 13-3. The TR/TE = 3000/13 ms image in Figure 13-2A is the most heavily proton-density-weighted image. The intensity of gray matter in this image exceeded that of white matter, which in turn, was greater than cerebrospinal fluid (CSF). The density of protons in gray matter is about 10% greater than in white matter, explaining the higher intensity of gray matter.

The images in Figure 13-2 and the other head images were produced using a receiver coil designed originally for examinations of the knee and other extremities. This extremity coil is smaller than most head coils, and it was used because it yields images with less noise. A limitation associated with the use of the extremity coil for head imaging is the nonuniformity of intensity, which can be appreciated from Figure 13-2. There are noticeable "hot spots" on the right and left posterior surface of the head. However, the loss of uniformity was an acceptable sacrifice, because the images were about 40% less noisy than with the standard head coil. With the head coil, twice as many measurements of data must be averaged to achieve a similar reduction of noise, taking twice as long.

Further inspection of the images in Figure 13-2 shows that the intensity of CSF remained low relative to the other tissues. Notice that the curve portraying the intensity of CSF did not become nearly as flat as the other curves as TR increased. There was no apparent plateau for the intensity of CSF while TR remained below 3.0 seconds. Therefore, significantly more T1 relaxation could have occurred had longer values of TR been used. The graph also reveals that all tissues became less intense for shorter values of TR. Obviously, a longer TR allows for more complete recovery of the longitudinal magnetization, which provides for stronger NMR signals.

Although it is desirable for tissues to emit strong NMR signals and thereby have high image intensity, a large difference between the strength of NMR signals from different tissues is more important. For example, consider the task of discriminating between gray

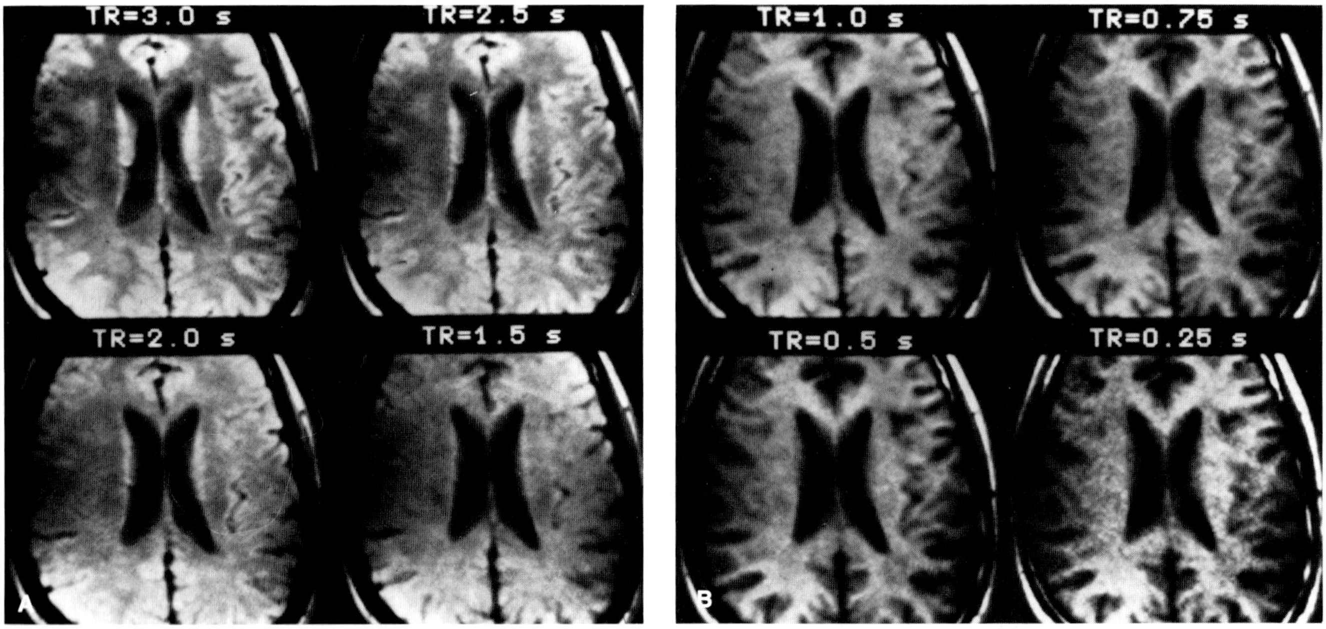

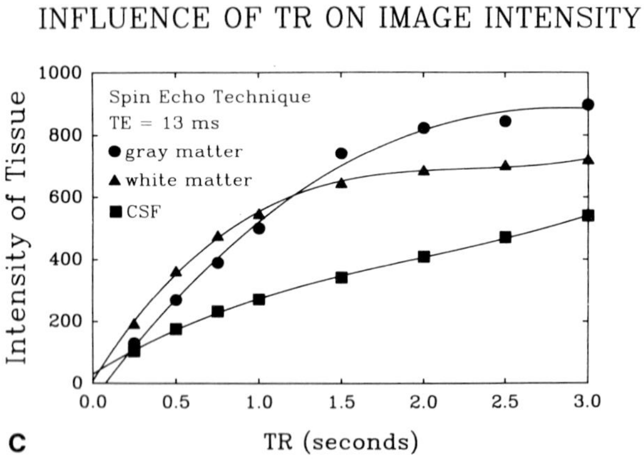

FIGURE 13–2. Influence of the repetition time, TR, on the intensity of various cranial tissues. The axial images **(A,B)** were acquired from a normal volunteer in a 1.0 tesla magnetic field. All of the images were produced under similar conditions, except for the TR, which is indicated directly on each image. There was only one slice, and TE was 13 milliseconds (ms). The field of view was 300 mm, and with 256 pixels in each direction, the spatial resolution was 1.2 mm. There was no averaging of data, and there were only 136 phase-encoding steps (half-Fourier imaging). The intensity of pixels representative of gray matter, white matter, and cerebrospinal fluid measured from the images **(A,B)** is plotted **(C)**. These measurements were used to give white matter a common intensity, thereby facilitating the visual comparison of the images.

matter and white matter. Under the conditions used for Figure 13–2 (TE = 13 ms; 1.0 T), a TR of about 1.0 second would have been the worst choice. The graph in Figure 13–2 shows that white matter was more intense than gray matter for long TR, but less intense than gray matter for short TR. When TR slightly exceeded 1 second, white matter and gray matter were equally intense (isointense). Thus, a reversal of contrast between gray matter and white matter occurred for a value of TR near 1 second.

The image in Figure 13–3A (TR/TE = 3000/28) is also heavily proton density weighted. Under these conditions, CSF was more intense than white matter, although still less than gray matter. In comparison, Figure 13–2 showed CSF to be less intense than white matter at a TE of 13 ms. As expected, the long T2 of CSF had more influence on the image intensity at a TE of 28 ms than at 13 ms. Because CSF was more intense than white matter when TE was 28 ms, and the reverse was true for a 13-ms TE, it follows that CSF and white matter were isointense at a particular intermediate value of TE.

The other images in Figure 13–3 show that CSF grew more intense relative to the other tissues as TE became longer. This feature is demonstrated by the graph. The curve that fits the intensity measurements of each tissue in the eight images depicts the T2 decay. As expected, the curves show that the image intensity or NMR signals decayed approximately exponentially. Moreover, the T2 time constants for this decay were calculated to be 700, 100, and 80 ms for CSF, white matter, and gray matter, respectively. The values for gray matter and white matter are consistent with the nominal values reported in Figure 13–1B. The T2 calculated for CSF was low because of imperfections associated with the imaging technique.

The contrast between gray matter and white matter depends on TE, because the two tissues have different T2 time constants. Both the proton density and T2 of gray matter exceed that of white matter. It

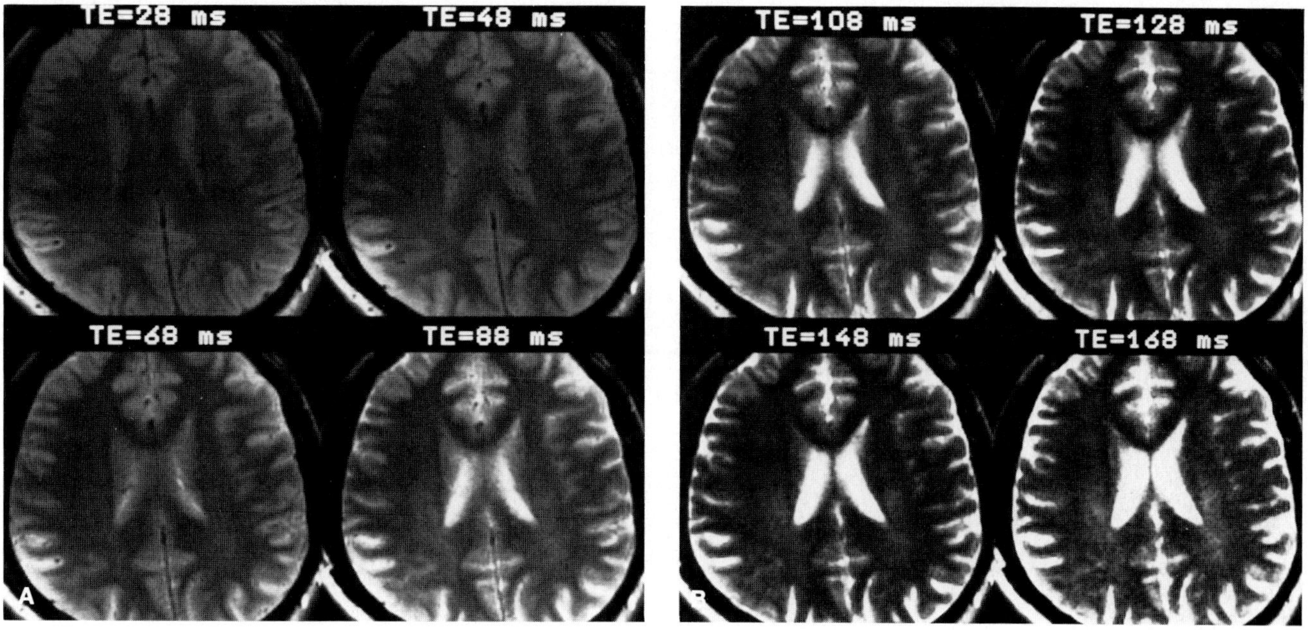

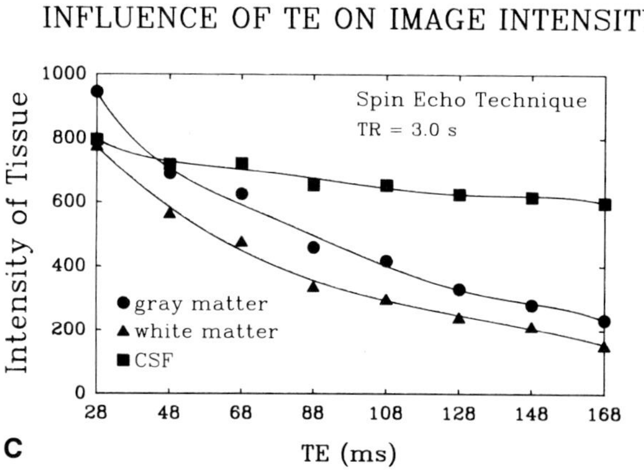

FIGURE 13–3. Influence of echo time, TE, on the intensity of cranial tissues for a long TR of 3.0 seconds. The TE is indicated directly on each image **(A,B)** of a normal volunteer in a field strength of 1.0 tesla. The imaging technique collected eight echoes from one 5-mm-thick slice. These eight echoes correspond to the eight images shown. The field of view was 300 mm, and there were 256 phase-encoding steps, which achieved a 1.2-mm spatial resolution. There was no averaging of data. For display purposes only, the images were scaled to give white matter a similar intensity. Measurements of the intensity of gray matter, white matter, and cerebrospinal fluid are compared **(C)**. The measurements were taken from **(A)** and **(B)** before the images were scaled to give white matter a common intensity.

seems reasonable to expect that the difference in T2 can be exploited through the use of a long TE, but as TE becomes longer, the strength of NMR signals decreases. Not only does the intensity of gray matter and white matter become weaker at longer TE, but the intensity difference between the two tissues shrinks. In Figure 13-3, the greatest difference between the intensity of gray matter and white matter occurs for a TE near 70 ms, although the intensity difference is not substantially less at shorter values of TE. It is generally accepted that TE values near the T2 of both tissues achieve the greatest contrast.[32]

The imaging conditions for Figure 13–3 would have made CSF and white matter isointense for a TE somewhere between 13 and 28 ms. CSF and gray matter became isointense at a TE of about 45 msec. It is common to choose special values of TE that make CSF isointense with either white matter or gray matter, but the exact TE at which two tissues appear isointense depends on the choice of TR. Consider, for example, the images in Figure 13–4, which were created under conditions similar to those in Figure 13–3, except that TR was only half as long. The images were displayed with the same scale, yet corresponding images in Figures 13–3 and 13–4 exhibit significantly different contrast.

The differences between Figures 13–3 and 13–4 are perhaps most striking for the shorter TE images. When TR was only 1.5 seconds, instead of 3.0 seconds, CSF was actually less intense than white matter at a TE of 28 ms. The shorter TR allowed T1 to exert more influence. The graphs show that all three of the measured tissues were less intense when TR was shorter, especially CSF, which decreased in intensity by almost half. CSF was affected most because it has a much longer T1 than white matter or gray matter.

In addition to reducing the intensity of the cranial tissues, the use of a short TR also altered the contrast.

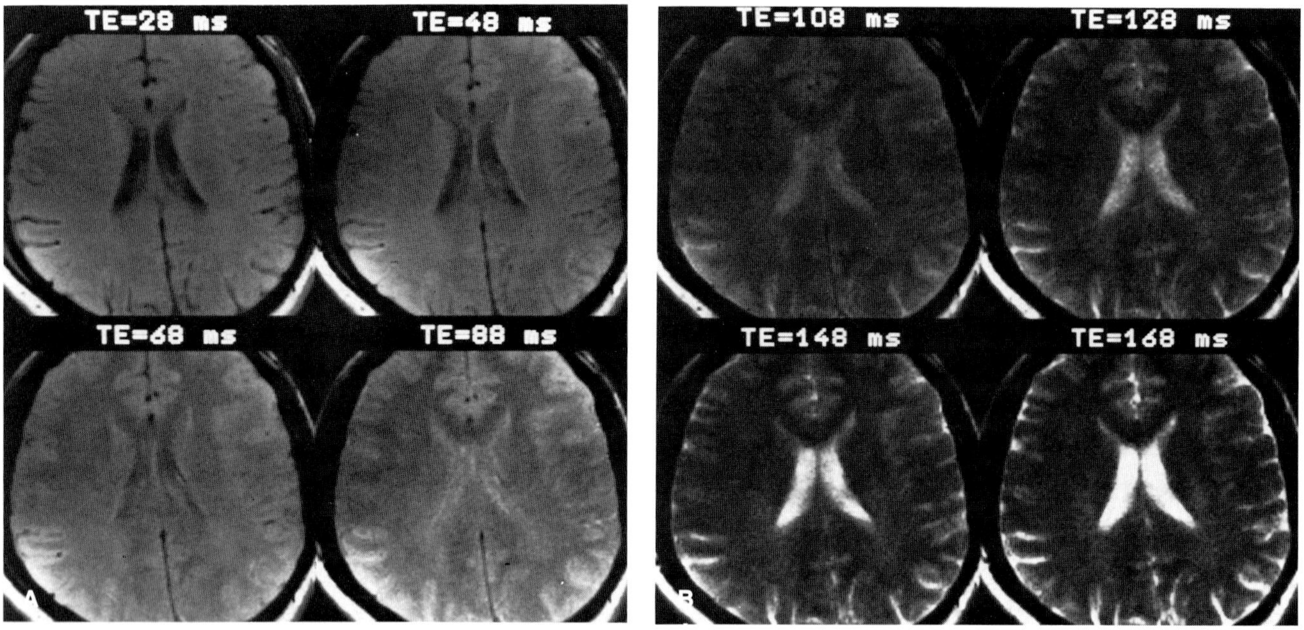

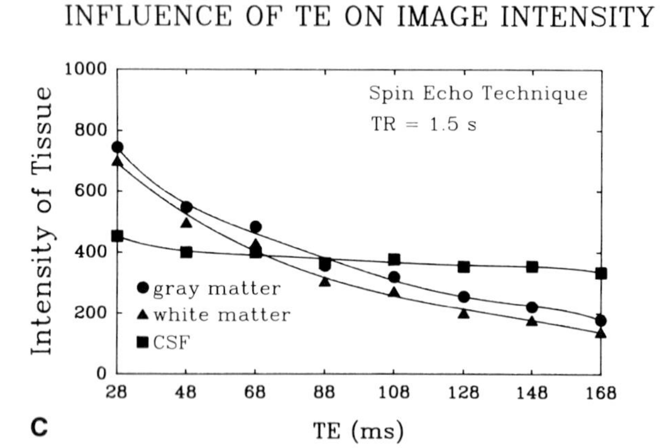

FIGURE 13–4. Influence of TE on the intensity of various cranial tissues for a relatively short TR of 1.5 seconds. All other conditions were similar to those in Figure 13–3.

There was less separation between the curves in Figure 13–4 than in Figure 13–3. In other words, there was generally poor contrast between gray matter and white matter, which is undesirable. Furthermore, the special values of TE at which two tissues become isointense changed. In particular, CSF remained less intense than gray matter for values of TE below about 90 ms when TR was 1.5 seconds. For comparison, CSF and gray matter became isointense at a TE close to 45 ms when TR was 3.0 seconds. Similarly, when TR was only 1.5 seconds, CSF and white matter became isointense at a TE of 70 ms, instead of about 20 ms, which was the case for the 3.0-second TR.

Direct comparison of the TR = 1.5 and TR = 3.0 images was unfair, because it took twice as long to produce the latter images. The extra time could have been used for averaging twice as much data with TR set at 1.5 seconds. Averaging twice as much data lowers the noise in images by $2^{1/2}$ (the square root of 2), which is approximately 1.4. Had twice as much data been averaged, the separation of intensity between the three tissues in Figure 13–4C would have increased by a factor of 1.4, if the noise was scaled to the same level. Still, the intensity difference between gray matter and white matter in Figure 13–4C would have been less than that in Figure 13–3C. Half of the lost intensity of CSF would have been recovered by averaging. Therefore, for the particular imaging technique considered, a 3.0-second TR produced greater contrast between cranial tissues than a TR of 1.5 seconds with twice as much data averaged.

The values of TR and TE that achieve the greatest contrast between two tissues depend on the proton density, T1, and T2 of the tissues. Figures 13–5 to 13–7 demonstrate the contrast change in axial abdominal images acquired at a field strength of 1.0 T. It is particularly informative to follow changes in the relative intensity of liver and spleen. The intensity of all abdominal tissues increased when TR was prolonged (Fig. 13–5). The spleen was more intense than

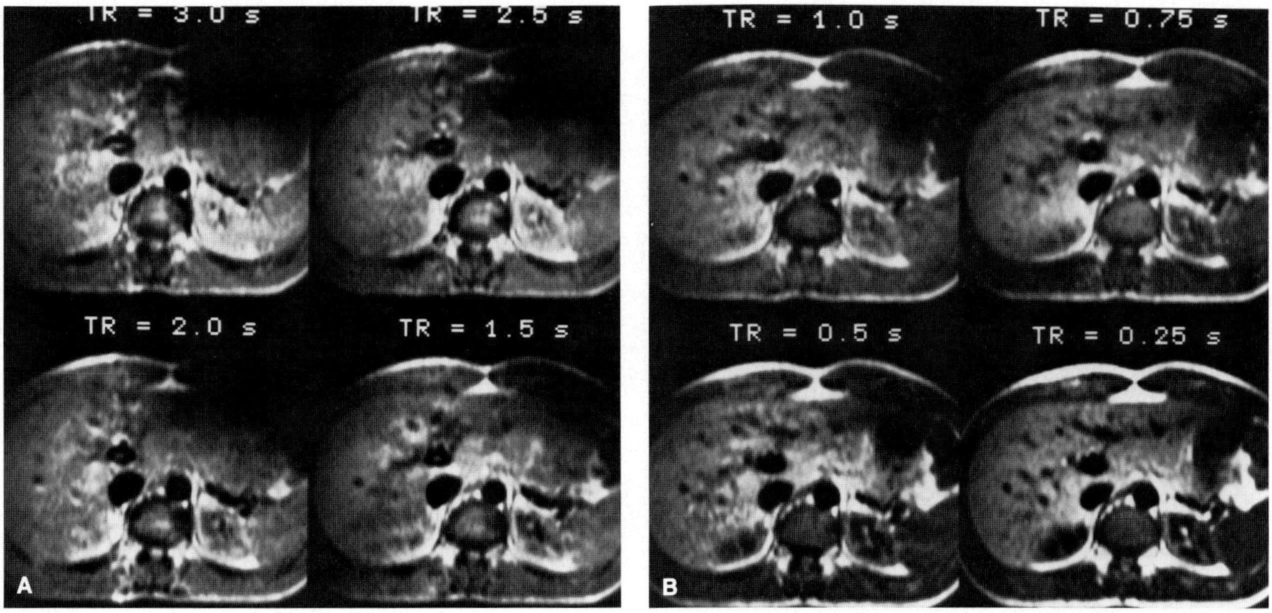

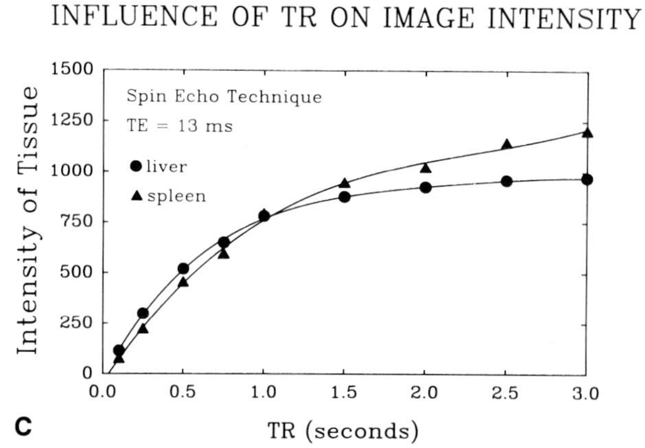

FIGURE 13–5. Influence of TR on the intensity of abdominal tissues. As in Figure 13–2, TR is indicated directly on each image **(A,B).** These axial images were acquired from a normal volunteer at 1.0 tesla. TE was 13 ms, and only one slice was imaged, which was 10 mm thick. The field of view was 500 mm, and the use of only 128 phase-encoding steps produced 2-mm × 4-mm rectangular pixels. There was no averaging of data. To facilitate visual comparison of the contrast between liver and spleen, the images were scaled to give liver a similar intensity. Intensity values of representative liver and spleen pixels measured **(A,B)** are plotted **(C).** The measurements were acquired before scaling the images relative to liver.

the liver in long TR images, but the reverse was true for values of TR below about 1.0 second. In fact, when TR was 2.0 seconds, spleen remained more intense than liver for all values of TE. Figure 13–6C shows that the intensity of spleen decreased the most slowly of the three tissues considered. Hence, spleen had the longest T2. Similarly, the T2 of liver was greater than that of muscle. These results agree with the nominal values presented in Figure 13–1B.

When TR was 2.0 seconds, the greatest separation between the intensity of spleen and liver occurred for a value of TE near 50 ms. The intensity of both tissues diminished in later echoes, as did the difference in intensity. Actually, the most notable feature in the later echoes is the enhancement of fluids, because fluids have long T2 values. Upon closer inspection of Figure 13–6, it appears that fluids were systematically more intense in every second echo. This is an example of a phenomenon known as even echo rephasing.[33,34]

The contrast between liver and spleen in Figure 13–5 vanished when TR was close to 1.0 second and TE was short. Therefore, the lack of contrast between liver and spleen in the TR/TE = 1000/28 ms image of Figure 13–7 is not surprising. Contrast between the two tissues returned in later echoes, however. Nevertheless, at this relatively short 1.0-second TR, the intensity difference between liver and spleen remained significantly less than for a TR of 2.0 seconds. Even considering the factor of 1.4 improvement that could be realized through averaging twice as much data, the difference between the intensity of liver and spleen remained less for the 1.0-second TR than for the longer TR.

Judging from the head and abdominal images, the intensity of tissues in spin echo MR images depends greatly on TR and TE. These two variables afford control over the relative contributions of proton density, T1, and T2. In general, proton density dominates when TR is long and TE is short. Longer values of TE

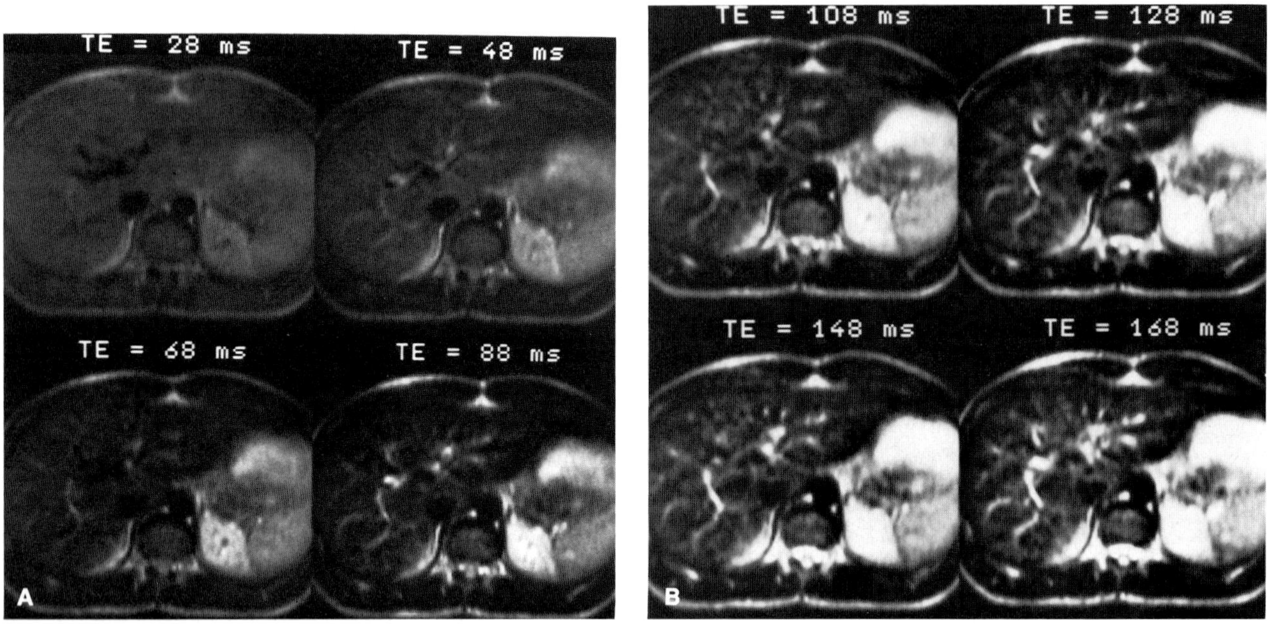

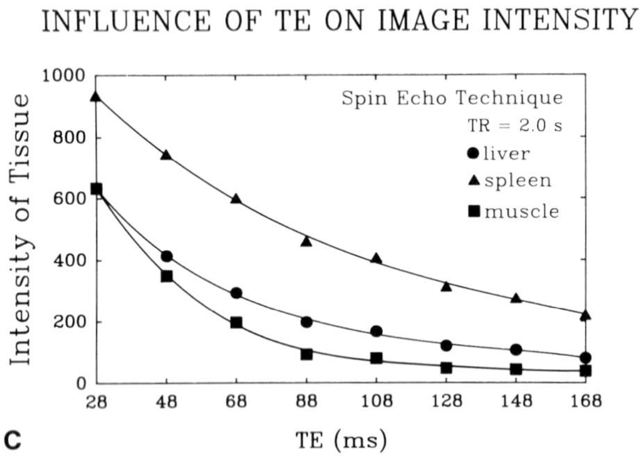

FIGURE 13–6. Influence of TE on the intensity of abdominal tissues for a TR of 2.0 seconds. The TE is indicated directly on each image **(A,B).** These axial images were acquired from a normal volunteer at 1.0 tesla. The imaging technique collected eight echoes from one slice, which was 10 mm thick. The field of view was 500 mm, and there were only 128 phase-encoding steps, creating pixels that were 2 mm × 4 mm. Two acquisitions of data were averaged to reduce motion artifacts. The intensity of liver, spleen, and muscle at different values for TE is plotted **(C).** Measurements were taken from the images **(A,B)** before they were scaled to give liver a common intensity.

introduce more T2 dependence, although the intensity of most tissues, and more importantly, their difference, decreases when TE becomes too long. The dependence of image intensity on T1 is maximized by short TR and short TE. A more subtle observation is that certain combinations of TR and TE cause two different tissues to become isointense. These conditions can be exploited to help resolve the identity of ambiguous anatomic structures.

Gradient-Echo Techniques

Gradient-echo techniques can be regarded as "stripped-down" versions of spin echo techniques. Most notably, gradient-echo techniques lack a 180° RF pulse that induces the formation of a spin echo. Instead, the refocusing of NMR signals into echoes is brought about entirely by the reversal of a magnetic field gradient (hence the name gradient echo). Short values of TR are generally used with gradient-echo techniques, and when TR is short, stronger NMR signals are produced when the RF tip angle is less than 90°.[37]

By convention in MRI, a magnetic field gradient called the read-out or frequency-encoding gradient is activated while each NMR signal is being measured. This gradient encodes spatial information into NMR signals by making components at each location along the gradient precess at different rates. In so doing, however, the gradient accelerates the decay of the transverse magnetization. The various components add destructively, thereby making the resultant magnetization shrink or become dephased. Of course, it would be best to measure the transverse magnetization when it is fully rephased and the strongest. For this reason, the gradient is first applied briefly with negative polarity before any measurements. Initially this gradient causes dephasing, but rephasing begins to occur when the gradient is applied with positive polarity during the measurement of an NMR signal. The transverse magnetization grows, attains a peak as

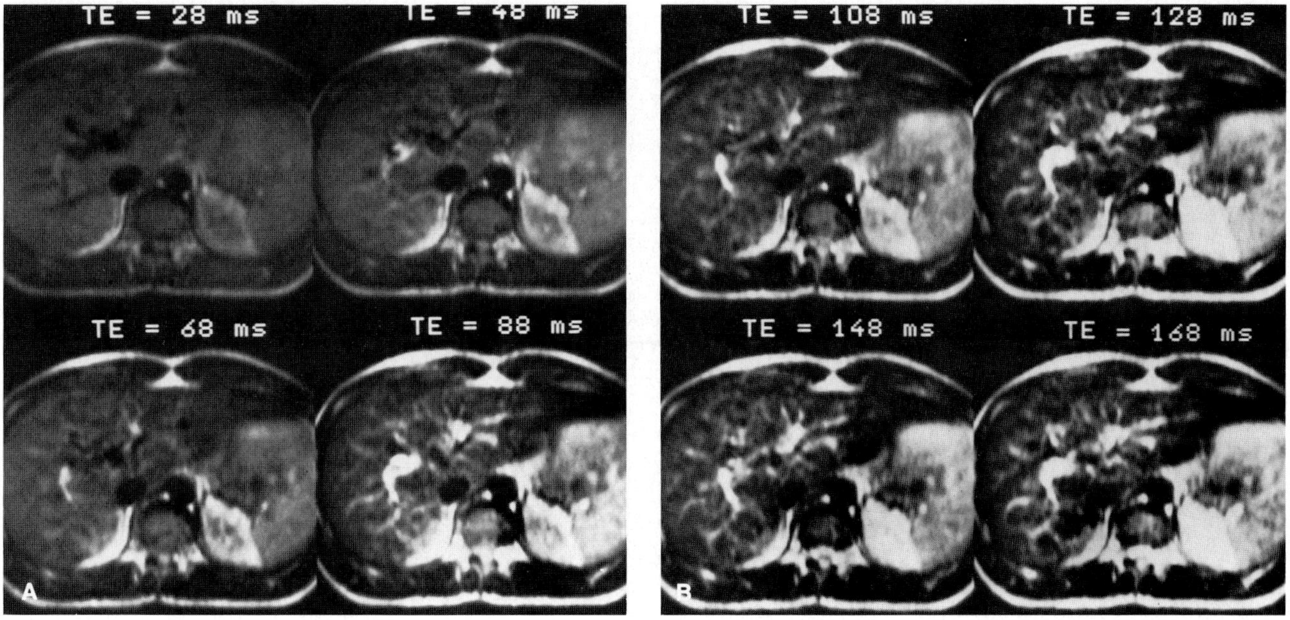

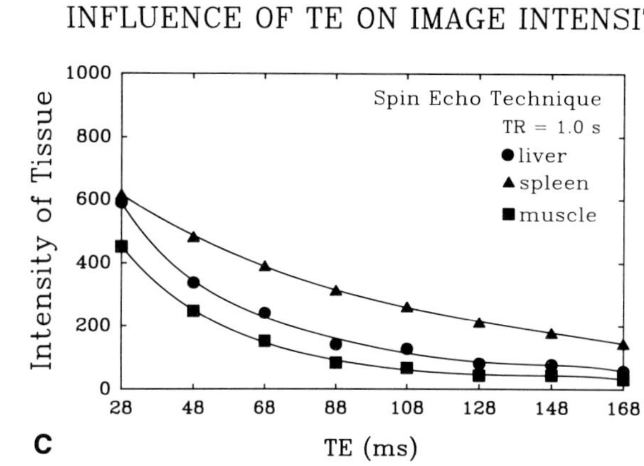

FIGURE 13–7. Influence of TE on the intensity of abdominal tissues for a relatively short TR of 1.0 seconds. All other conditions were similar to Figure 13–6.

an echo, and then decays again. It is customary to balance the size of the negative and positive gradient pulses so that the echo forms midway through the measurement process.

Gradient-echo techniques generally feature RF pulses with tip angles smaller than 90°. A 90° RF pulse converts all of the longitudinal magnetization into transverse magnetization. If TR is so short that negligible T1 relaxation can occur between RF pulses, there would be little longitudinal magnetization to convert to transverse magnetization by the next 90° RF pulse. However, by tipping only a fraction of the longitudinal magnetization, a reduced tip angle RF pulse leaves some available for the next RF pulse. Reduced tip angle RF pulses also deposit less heat into patients.[38]

Image intensity and contrast are highly sensitive to the RF tip angle.[39] In Figure 13–8, the image intensity increased for larger tip angles until it attained a maximum, after which it decreased again. At small tip angles, spleen was more intense than liver, but the contrast reversed to become more T1-weighted for larger tip angles. More importantly, the tip angle affected the difference between the intensity of liver and spleen. Under these conditions, notably TR/TE = 38/10 ms, tip angles near 50° maximized the difference in intensity between liver and spleen. Notice that the intensity difference remained large at higher tip angles, even though the intensity of both tissues decreased. If TR had been shorter, there would have been less time for T1 relaxation, and consequently, even smaller tip angles would have yielded the greatest intensity difference and contrast between liver and spleen. Similarly, structure with longer T1 (eg, metastases) would have gained intensity as the tip angle was reduced below 50°, resulting in less contrast compared to normal liver.

The images in Figure 13–8 arose from a gradient-echo technique called FLASH, which attempts to achieve predominantly T1-weighted contrast. In most

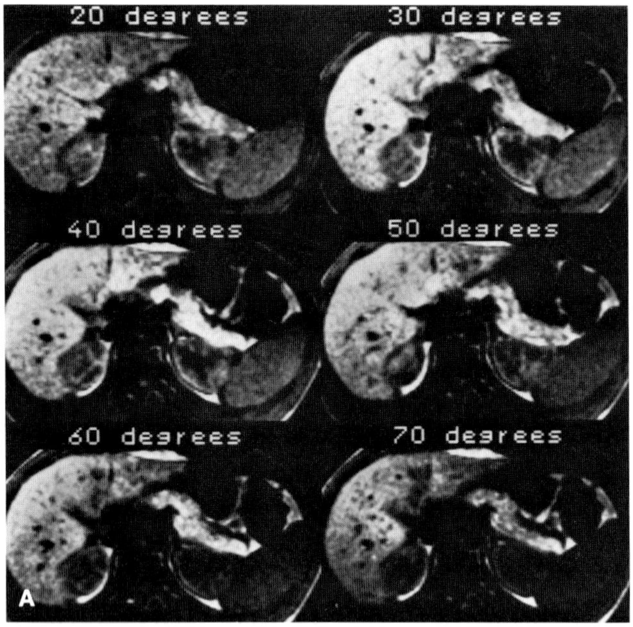

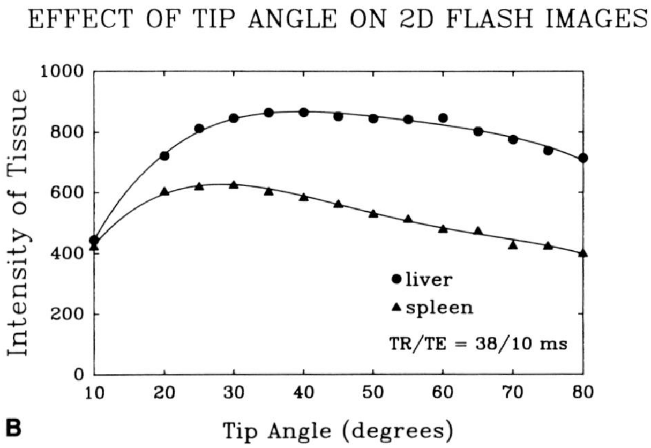

FIGURE 13–8. Effect of RF tip angle on the appearance of abdominal FLASH images. The tip angle is specified at the top of each image. Each axial image of a normal volunteer was acquired at 1.0 tesla during a 10-second breath-holding period. The imaging technique was characterized by a 38-ms TR and 10-ms TE. The slice was 10 mm thick, and there were 256 phase-encoding steps, with no data averaging. Artifacts from the pulsating flow of blood were minimized by a technique called presaturation, which uses additional RF pulses to reduce the intensity of blood flowing into the slice from either side. The images were displayed after they were scaled to give liver the same intensity. The graph **(B)** compares the image intensity of liver and spleen for various RF tip angles. The measurements were taken from the images **(A)** before they were scaled relative to liver.

implementations of FLASH, TR is much too short for the transverse magnetization to decay sufficiently before the next RF pulse. The residual transverse magnetization affects the contrast between tissues and generates an artifact that appears as a bright band through the center of an MR image.[40–42] To suppress this band artifact and achieve heavily T1-weighted contrast, it is necessary to eliminate the effect of residual magnetization. The most popular strategy involves activating strong magnetic field gradients, called spoiler gradients, for about 10 ms after the measurement of each NMR signal. Spoiler gradients, or equivalent schemes that use RF pulses, do not actually destroy residual magnetization, but they prevent it from contributing to subsequent measurements.[40–42]

The FLASH technique is only one of many gradient-echo techniques. Others, such as GRASS, FISP, or CE-FAST, attempt to maintain the transverse magnetization in a steady state.[43–45] Such steady state techniques tend to enhance the intensity of fluids, which contribute the most residual magnetization, due to their long T2. Residual transverse magnetization becomes partially converted into longitudinal magnetization by the next RF pulse. This increases the longitudinal magnetization available for the next RF pulse, which translates into enhanced image intensity.

Gradient-echo techniques provide two additional variables to manipulate, RF tip angle and residual transverse magnetization. Contrast can depend much less on TR and, hence, imaging time. For example, the influence of T1 can be reduced by using a small tip angle, instead of resorting to a long TR.

The short imaging times that are possible with gradient-echo techniques allow several unique applications. High-resolution images can be produced in less than 10 seconds, instead of several minutes. Most 10-second images are noisier than 5-minute images, but when a complete image can be acquired during a period of breath holding, the absence of the ghost artifacts and blurring caused by respiratory motion is an extremely desirable feature. Evidence suggests that fast gradient-echo abdominal images may be superior to the more time-consuming spin echo images. At the very least, images such as those in Figure 13–8 appear to be competitive in quality, especially when there is significant patient motion.

Gradient-echo techniques, because of their short TR, also allow imaging of entire 3D volumes in a few minutes instead of hours. The most compelling reason for choosing a 3D technique is the opportunity for both extremely thin slices and extensive coverage.[46-49] A common example is 128 slices, each of which is 1 mm thick. The slices in a 3D technique are created by phase encoding, analogous to one of the dimensions in the plane of each slice. Whereas the more familiar 2D images may be constructed from 128 phase-encoding steps, a 128-slice 3D image requires 128×128 steps, which takes 128 times longer. However, in return for the extra time, 3D techniques provide numerous thin slices. Thin slices afford high-resolution coverage of anatomic structures, such as the brain or knee. When the slices are as thin as the dimensions of the pixels in each slice, the visualization of anatomy can be improved by reformatting the images so that they can be displayed in another orientation (e.g., convert axial images into coronal images). Reformatting avoids the time-consuming acquisition of another set of differently oriented MR images.

A notable disadvantage of gradient echoes is that they reverse only the dephasing caused by a magnetic field gradient. Many other factors, such as magnetic field inhomogeneities, cause transverse magnetization to dephase. Consider the border between an air sinus and soft tissue. Because of differences in susceptibility, the magnetic field in the two regions is very different. Therefore, a magnetic field gradient exists between the two regions, which dephases the transverse magnetization analogously to the external gradients employed intentionally.[50]

As a result of the uncorrected dephasing of transverse magnetization, images experience a loss of intensity near the borders of structures that have different susceptibility.[51] In Figures 13-9 and 13-10, the supposedly circular interface between air and the copper sulfate solution became severely distorted in the gradient-echo images. More specifically, the diameter of the circle increased as a result of the dephasing. The distortion was clearly worse at longer values of TE. Fortunately, gradient-echo techniques can achieve shorter TE values than spin echo. Analysis of the 3D images in Figure 13-10 reveals less distortion for thinner slices. The number of partitions (slices) had no observable influence. Therefore, the ability to create thin slices with 3D techniques improves spatial resolution, and diminishes susceptibility effects.

Gradient echoes are certainly not unique. In fact, spin echo techniques feature gradient echoes in addition to echoes elicited by the 180° refocusing RF pulses. However, 180° RF pulses are avoided in gradient-echo techniques, because they invert the longitudinal magnetization, which may leave too little longitudinal magnetization after a short TR to tip over into transverse magnetization. The absence of a 180° RF pulse allows a shorter TE to be achieved, which compensates at least partially for the incomplete refocussing of gradient echoes.

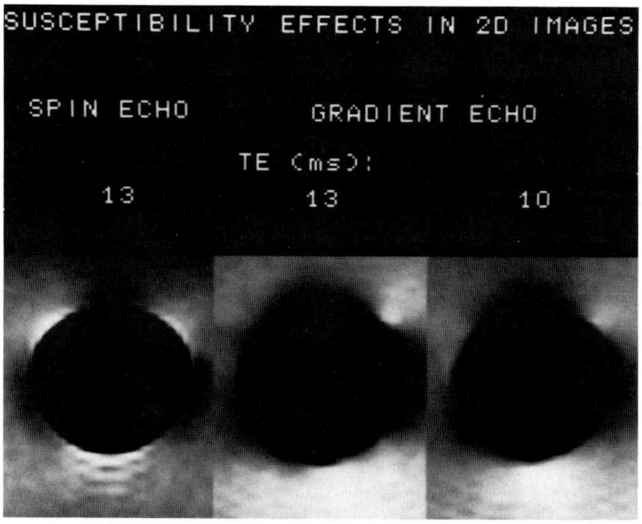

FIGURE 13-9. Image degradation near the borders of materials with greatly different magnetic susceptibility. Shown here are three images of a bottle containing a copper sulfate solution with an air-filled syringe imbedded inside. The dark area in each image is a cross-section through the 20-mm diameter syringe. Ideally, the dark area would be circular. Except where noted, imaging conditions were similar for the three images.

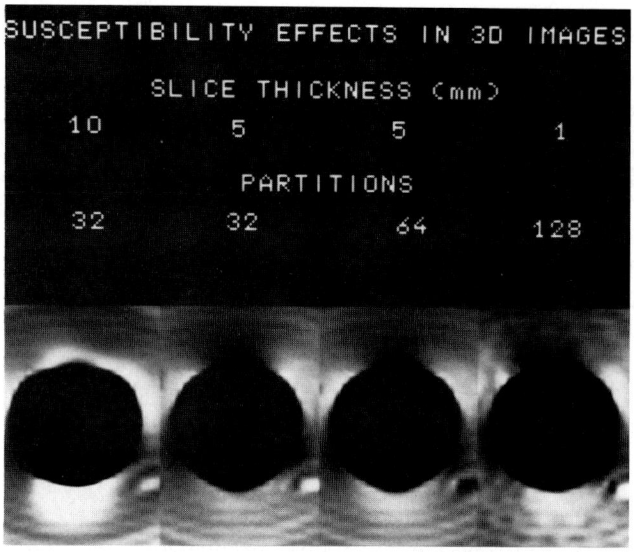

FIGURE 13-10. The distortion caused by magnetic susceptibility differences in various 3D MR images. The images show a cross-section through a 20-mm diameter syringe as a dark area. Except for the slice thickness and the number of partitions or slices produced in the 3D technique, imaging conditions were similar for the four images.

OVERCOMING NOISE

Certain imaging parameters, such as the field of view (FOV) and slice thickness, affect noise. When these parameters change, the consequences are essentially the same for all tissues. The level of noise is affected, but the intensity difference between various tissues remains unaltered.

Signal-to-Noise Ratio

When the level of noise is subject to change, it becomes necessary to analyze the CNR, rather than simply the difference in image intensities. If the changes affect all tissues similarly, it is easier to compare the signal-to-noise ratio (SNR). The SNR from a particular tissue is defined as the mean image intensity in a certain region of interest divided by the standard deviation of image intensity in a background region that contains no tissue. This definition of the SNR describes the graininess between pixels, and not surprisingly, it pertains to the visualization of small high-contrast lesions.[29]

Given that a high SNR or low level of noise is desirable, there are many parameters to consider.[52–56] At the top of the list is the equipment, because its state of function affects the quality of images. Furthermore, most MRI units include receiver coils specialized for various anatomic sites. In our experience, when a smaller coil was substituted for examining the head, the SNR was 40% greater than with the standard head coil. This is just one example of the possible improvements associated with the choice of a coil. For the remainder of this chapter, however, it will be assumed that the best hardware has been chosen, and all that remains to be decided on are details of a particular imaging technique.

In principle, a mathematical equation for the SNR could be formulated that specified every relevant parameter explicitly. The equation might reveal how the SNR depends on magnetic field strength, receiver coil, and other properties of MRI units and patients. Although such information could be interesting, much of it would have no impact on the routine clinical operation of an MRI unit. For example, if the SNR for a particular MRI protocol was too low, it would generally not be feasible to increase the magnetic field strength without moving to another MRI unit.

It would be useful to have a simplified equation for the SNR, which showed only those parameters that could be modified readily. The FOV, slice thickness, amount of data averaging, number of measurements of each signal, and number of phase-encoding steps influence the SNR. Because these parameters can be altered over a wide range, it is critical to appreciate their influence on the SNR. An equation for the SNR should help users of MRI respond to demands for higher SNR, higher resolution, or shorter imaging times.

The SNR is proportional to the volume of a voxel. The larger the voxel, the stronger the associated NMR signal and the greater the SNR. Voxels are large when the image covers a large FOV or when the FOV is divided into relatively few voxels. The volume of a voxel equals the product of the slice thickness and the area of a pixel. The dimensions of each pixel equal the FOV divided by the number of rows and columns of data, or equivalently, the number of samples of each NMR signal and the number of phase-encoding steps.

The SNR also depends on the number of repeated measurements. For example, averaging twice as many measurements of data generally increases the SNR by the square root of 2, denoted as $2^{1/2}$. The reason that the SNR does not become twice as large is because repetitive measurements contribute to signal and to noise. If the noise is uncorrelated, averaging would diminish its level by $2^{1/2}$, which would therefore raise the SNR by $2^{1/2}$. If measurements of noise were identical in both sets of measurements, averaging would not improve the SNR. Fortunately, most of the noise in MRI is random, except for contributions from patient motion or imperfections of the MRI system. Random noise is uncorrelated and distributed uniformly across an image.[57]

Another condition that affects the SNR is the length of time allocated to the measurement of each NMR signal. This characteristic is related to bandwidth, which is discussed later. If it takes 10 ms to collect 256 measurements of an NMR signal, there would be 39 μs between consecutive measurements. The time for each measurement is much less than 39 μs, so the NMR signal is actually observed for only a small fraction of the total measurement time. Therefore, brief glitches and other high-frequency noise during the space between measurements are missed. The noise that contaminates NMR signals occurs at all frequencies, with equal distribution. In other words, NMR signals are as likely to have slowly changing noise as high-frequency glitches. However, if more time elapses between consecutive samples of an NMR signal, it is more likely that high-frequency noise will be missed, and less noise will be measured overall. If less noise is measured, the entire image will be less noisy, because random noise is distributed uniformly across MR images. Therefore, the time taken to measure each NMR signal influences the SNR.

The dependence of the SNR on the parameters discussed above can be stated as follows:

$$SNR = k\,\frac{(FOV)^2\, W_{slice}\,(N_{av}\, T_s)^{1/2}}{N_{read}\,(N_{phase})^{1/2}}$$

where FOV = field of view,

W_{slice} = slice thickness,
N_{av} = number of data measurements averaged,
T_s = time to measure each NMR signal,
N_{read} = number of measurements of each NMR signal,
N_{phase} = number of phase-encoding steps

The "1/2" superscript denotes the square root, and k is a constant of proportionality that incorporates all of the other factors that contribute to the SNR, such as the type of imaging technique, tissue, and MRI unit. The term NEX is equivalent to N_{av}. As expected, the equation reveals that the SNR depends on the volume of each voxel and the number of repeated measurements. The equation is valid for most MRI techniques.

Manipulation of the SNR

Consider a reduction of the FOV. Frequently, a smaller FOV is desired for the superior resolution that it affords. The resolution in both directions of a 2D MR image equals the FOV divided by either N_{read} or N_{phase}.[58,59] It should not be surprising to find a lower SNR in images with a smaller FOV. The SNR equation indicates that the SNR drops as the square of the FOV, because the FOV influences two dimensions of a voxel. If the FOV became twice as small, as in Figure 13-11, the SNR would decrease fourfold.

Less drastic changes are the norm. If the resolution from a particular set of imaging conditions was slightly less than desired, and the SNR was not already a limiting factor, then a slight reduction in the FOV might be worthwhile. At the expense of a 40% reduction in the SNR, a 20% smaller FOV in Figure 13-12 provided 20% better resolution in both directions. The loss of SNR did not appear to hinder the visibility of the large mass, and in fact, its margins appear better defined in the higher-resolution image.

Certain choices of imaging technique, particularly thin slices or small FOVs, sometimes provide an insufficient SNR, and averaging is one of the most familiar ways to boost it. The equation shows that the SNR increases as the square root of the number of measurements that are averaged. Averaging reduces the level of uncorrelated noise, which fortunately describes most of the noise in MRI, and it reduces the ghost artifacts caused by motion. Of course, it takes longer to average more data. In Figure 13-13, averaging two sets of data took twice as long as no averaging at all, but it recovered the SNR that was lost in reducing the FOV by 20%.

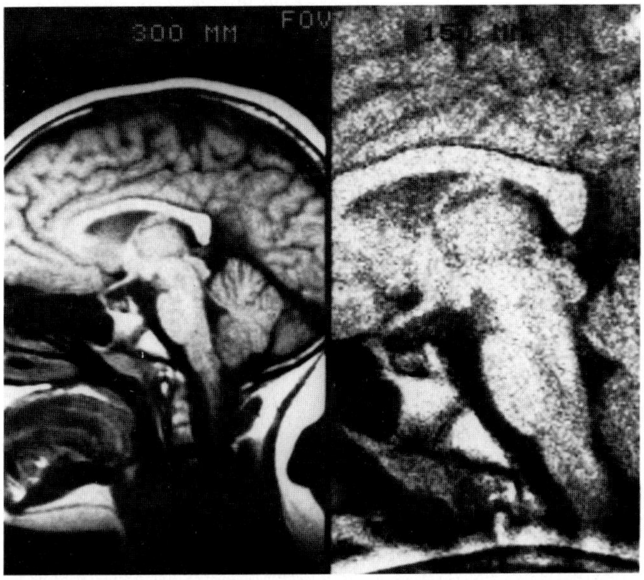

FIGURE 13-11. Two MR images illustrating that a reduction of the field of view improves spatial resolution at the expense of increased noise. Both images were acquired under similar conditions, except that the field of view for the right-hand image was only one-half of that on the left.

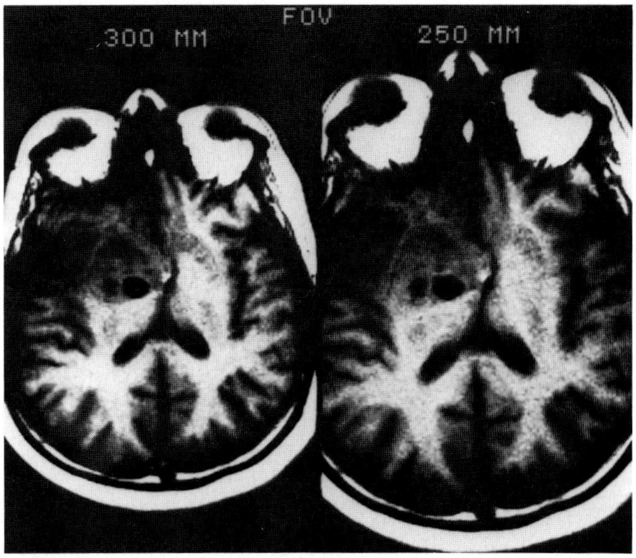

FIGURE 13-12. Two MR images similar except for the field of view, which was 1.2 times smaller for the right-hand image.

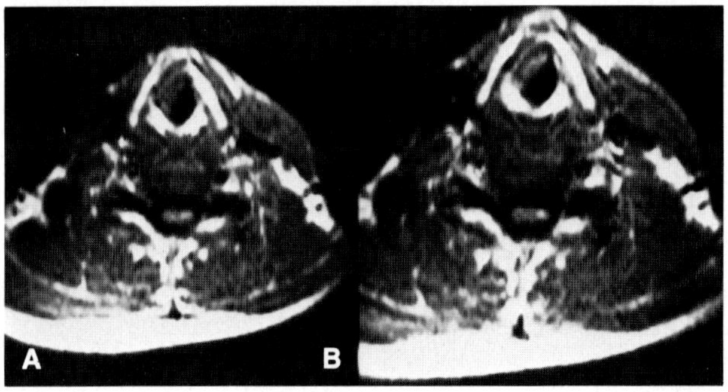

FIGURE 13-13. The use of averaging to raise the signal-to-noise ratio. A tumor of the right vocal cord is apparent in these axial MR images. Three hundred millimeter FOV, 1 average **(A);** 250 mm FOV, 2 averages **(B).**

Another way to boost the SNR is to accept lower spatial resolution, either through a larger FOV or fewer phase-encoding steps. Consider, for example, the use of 128 phase-encoding steps instead of 256. The SNR equation indicates that the SNR would increase by a factor equal to the square root of 2. Each voxel would become twice as large, because one of its dimensions would double in size. Also, only half as many uncorrelated measurements would be combined in producing an MR image, so the average noise in each voxel would be $2^{1/2}$ times greater. These two competing effects combine to provide a factor of $2^{1/2}$ improvement for the SNR in response to reducing by half the number of phase-encoding steps. Such an effect can be seen in Figure 13–14. The SNR in the right-hand image was actually twice as large as on the left. The other factor of $2^{1/2}$ arose from the 20% reduction of the FOV. Notice that the use of fewer phase-encoding steps caused rings in the right-hand image to become more conspicuous. These rings, caused by data truncation, could have been reduced, but the image would have become blurred.[60]

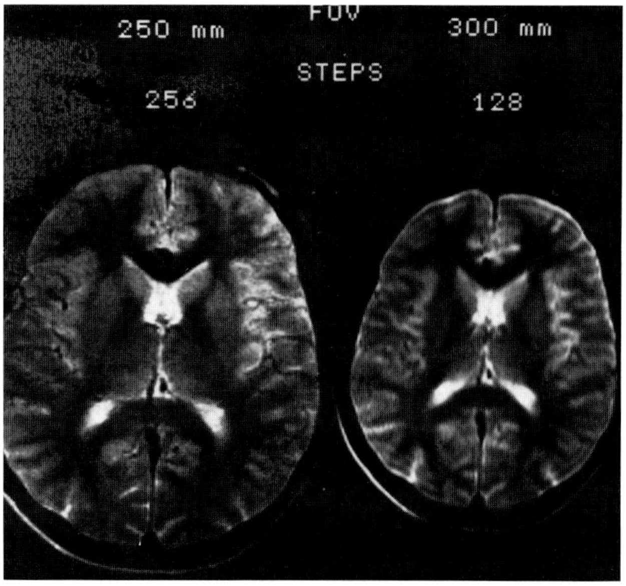

FIGURE 13–14. Two MR images of the same patient presenting two extremes of the tradeoff between high spatial resolution and a high signal-to-noise ratio. Except for the specified FOV and the number of phase-encoding steps, imaging conditions were similar.

Bandwidth

Images have less noise if more time elapses between consecutive samples of data. These techniques are said to have a lower bandwidth.[61] Bandwidth is defined as the reciprocal of the time between consecutive samples of data. The level of noise in an MR image is proportional to the square root of the bandwidth. If it takes a time T_s to acquire N_{read} samples of an MR signal, the bandwidth is given by N_{read}/T_s. For example, a technique in which 256 samples of data are acquired in 7.68 ms has a bandwidth of 33.3 kHz. The total noise is distributed uniformly into N_{read} voxels across the FOV. With all other variables fixed, a 33.3-kHz bandwidth technique would generate images in which noise was a factor of $(33.3/14.2)^{1/2}$, or 1.5, greater than that in images from a 14.2-kHz bandwidth technique. Measurements of the background noise in Figure 13–15 agree with this prediction.

An operational feature of low bandwidth techniques is their use of weaker frequency-encoding gradients during the measurement of NMR signals. The frequency-encoding gradient makes transverse magnetization components at the edges of the FOV precess either faster or slower than those in the middle. The difference between the highest and lowest precessional frequency is equal to the imaging bandwidth. The frequency-encoding gradient is reduced for a lower bandwidth technique, because it need not establish as large a range of precessional frequencies. In fact, a low bandwidth image would be "zoomed" if the gradient was not decreased.

When NMR signals are measured in the presence of weaker gradients, the associated images can be degraded more by magnetic field inhomogeneities, which can be created by imperfectly constructed magnets or differences in the susceptibility of adjoining tissues. Furthermore, the image of adipose tissue can become shifted noticeably relative to watery tissues, because the hydrogen protons attached to water molecules have a slightly greater Larmor frequency than their counterparts in adipose tissue. The frequency difference is about 150 Hz in a field strength of 1.0 T, which corresponds to 1.2 pixels in the 33-kHz bandwidth image of Figure 13–16A, and 2.7 pixels in the 14.2-kHz technique. Therefore, structures composed of fat are shifted spatially 2.3 times farther in the lower bandwidth image.

Slice Interference

It takes many slices to cover an extensive anatomic region for an MRI examination. Very few MRI techniques produce single slices. In the interest of efficiency, as many slices as possible are acquired during the free time after the end of measurement and before the production of another NMR signal. Because of the risk of missing small lesions between slices, the slices should be contiguous. However, the slices that are created in MRI are generally poor approximations to abrupt steps, and there can be appreciable overlap between adjacent slices.

If it were possible to view the side of a slice instead of its face, a slice profile would be displayed. Ideally, slice profiles would resemble abrupt steps. In reality, slice profiles in MRI feature a transition zone, in which the intensity climbs from a small value to its maxi-

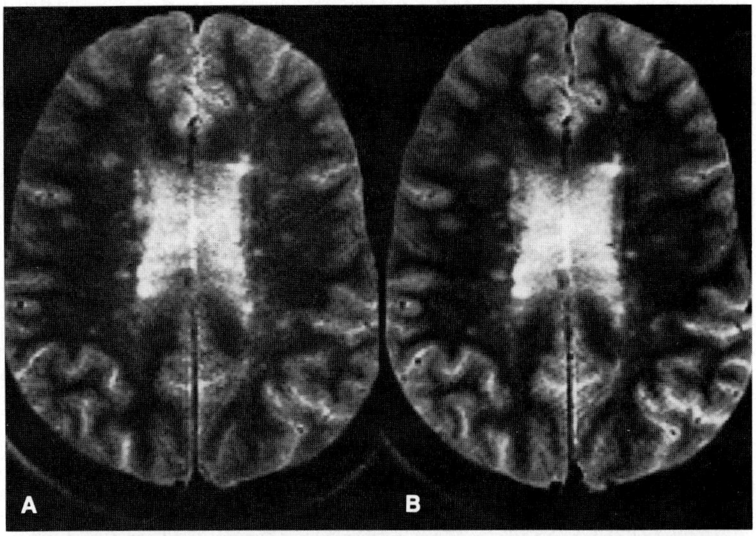

FIGURE 13–15. The effect of imaging bandwidth on the signal-to-noise ratio. These two images of a patient with MS were acquired under the same conditions (TR/TE = 3000/60). The slice was 10 mm thick, and the field of view was 250 mm. There were 256 phase-encoding steps and no averaging of data. The bandwidths were 33.3 kHz **(A)** and 14.2 kHz **(B).** Equivalently, 256 measurements of each NMR signal were collected in 7.68 ms **(A)** and in 17.92 ms **(B).** The standard deviation of random noise in the background was 9.0 **(A)** and 5.8 **(B).** (Runge VM, Wood ML, Kaufman DM, Traill MR, Nelson KL. The straight and narrow path to good head and spine MRI. Radiographics 1988;8:507)

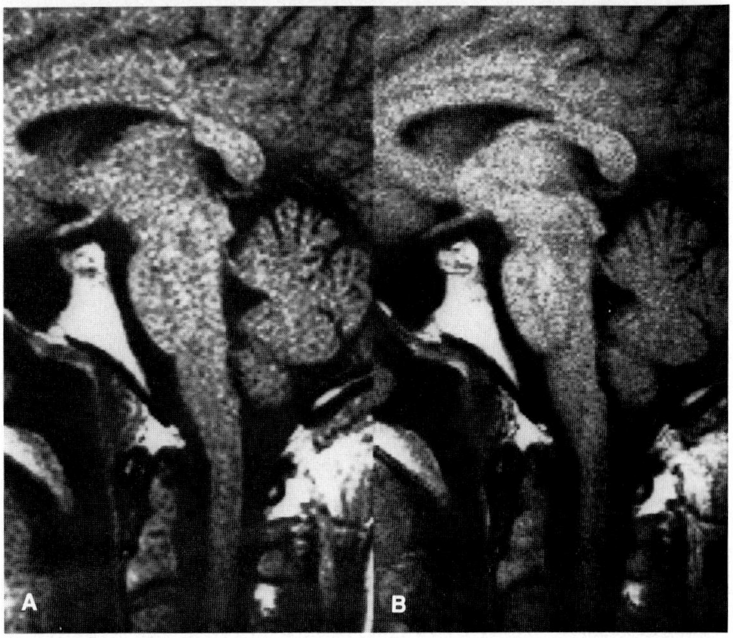

FIGURE 13–16. Illustration of the noise reduction realized through the use of a lower bandwidth imaging technique. Normal anatomy is depicted in these relatively T1-weighted MR images, for which TR was 600 ms. The imaging bandwidths were 33 kHz **(A)** and 20 kHz **(B).** It took 7.68 ms **(A)** or 12.8 ms **(B)** to measure each NMR signal. The TE was 17 ms for **(A),** but the longer measurement time for **(B)** stretched the minimum TE to 19 ms. Each slice was 5 mm thick, and the field of view was 214 mm. There were 256 phase-encoding steps, and no data was averaged. (Runge VM, Wood ML, Kaufman DM, Traill MR, Nelson KL. The straight and narrow path to good head and spine MRI. Radiographics 1988;8:507)

mum, producing a "tail" that can extend far beyond the intended boundaries of the slice. Because of these imperfect characteristics, it is customary to specify slice thickness as the full-width-at-half-maximum (FWHM) and sometimes even full-width-at-tenth-maximum (FWTM). The shape of a slice profile depends on several parameters, especially the shape of the RF pulse.[61–66] If the transition zone of one slice encroaches on another, RF pulses that were supposed to be confined to that first slice also affect neighboring slices.

The overlap of adjacent slices degrades the quality of MR images, because RF pulses interrupt T1 relaxation. The RF pulses actually tip over some of the longitudinal magnetization in adjacent slices, which hinders T1 relaxation in those slices. The outcome of such interruptions depend on TR. For example, if TR is short, as in a T1-weighted image, slice interference has the effect of reducing the SNR without altering contrast significantly. For example, the SNR was 15% less in Figure 13–17A than in Figure 13–17B, for which there was a greater gap between slices. Almost the same SNR reduction occurs for all tissues, because the RF pulses interrupt the relatively early phase of T1 relaxation, long before the longitudinal magnetization of any tissue can approach its equilibrium value.[61,64]

Slice interference at long TRs reduces the contrast between tissues (Fig.13–18).[61,62,64] The signal difference or contrast between gray matter and white matter was only half as large in Figure 13–18A as in Figure 13–18B, for which the slices were spaced farther

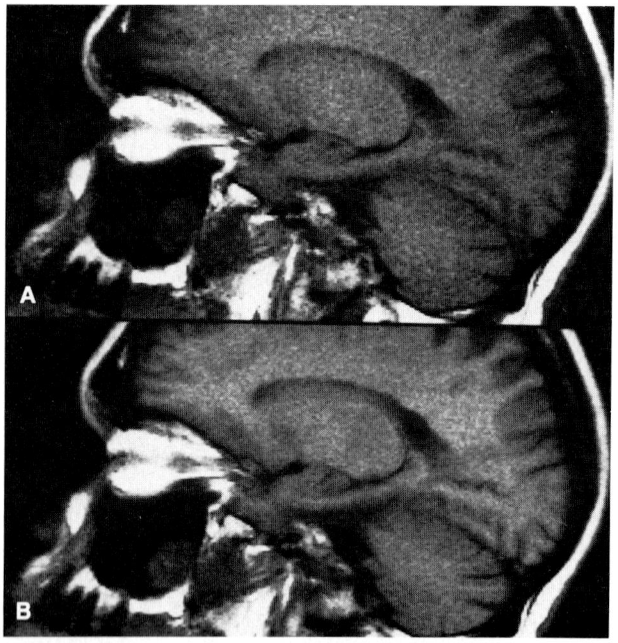

FIGURE 13–17. Demonstration of interference between adjacent slices in a predominantly T1-weighted MR image. Both sagittal images were acquired at 1.0 tesla (TR/TE = 650/28). The difference between the images was the distance between adjacent slices, which was negligible in **(A)** and one-half as wide as the slices in **(B).** Each slice was 5 mm thick, and the field of view was 214 mm. There were 256 phase-encoding steps and no data averaging.

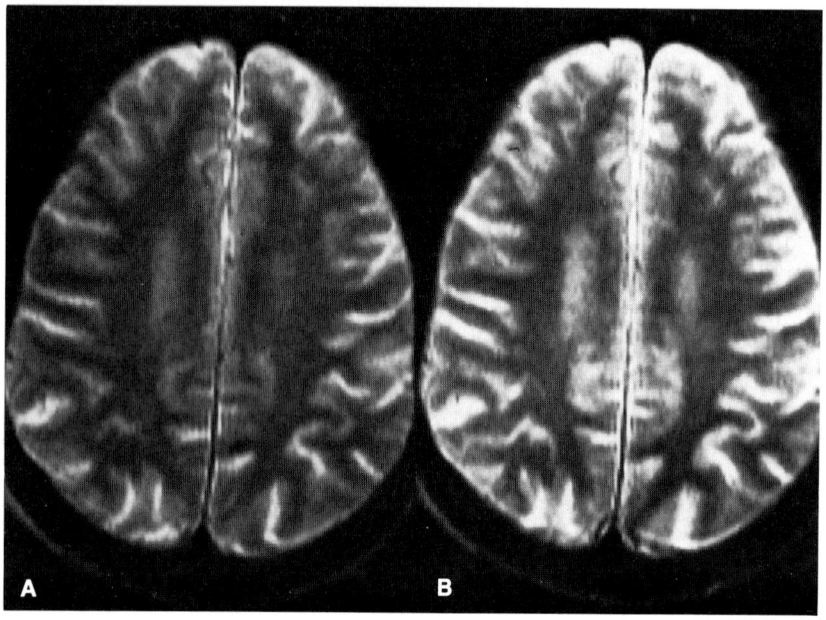

FIGURE 13–18. Slice interference in long TR images (TR/TE = 3000/70). There was essentially no space between adjacent slices in **(A)** and a separation of one slice width between slices in **(B).** Each slice was 10 mm thick, and the field of view was 250 mm. There were 128 phase-encoding steps and no averaging of data. The intensity difference between gray matter and white matter was 50 units **(A)** and 100 units **(B).** (Runge VM, Wood ML, Kaufman DM, Traill MR, Nelson KL. The straight and narrow path to good head and spine MRI. Radiographics 1988;8:507)

apart. A long TR provides more time for the longitudinal magnetization to recover from the interfering effects of RF pulses in adjacent slices. The longer time available can make a difference for tissues with different T1. A tissue with a shorter T1 can overcome the interference created by the RF pulses better than a longer T1 tissue. Therefore, when a new NMR signal is created for a particular slice, the longitudinal magnetization from tissues with shorter T1 have recovered more fully from previous RF pulses, and they contribute NMR signals as if no slice interference had occurred. The NMR signals from longer T1 tissues are still reduced. Because slice interference at long TRs preferentially reduces the intensity of tissues with longer T1s, contrast between tissues becomes more T1-weighted, which is not the objective of using a long TR.

An obvious way to reduce slice interference is to widen the gap between adjacent slices. The extreme case separates slices by one entire slice width and performs two separate scans, with the second scan designed to fill in the gaps. The drawback is that it takes twice as long to acquire all of the slices. Fortunately, there are other solutions.

The severity of slice interference depends on the slice profile. The more abrupt the slice profile, the less interference. Early in the development of MRI, slices were often defined using Gaussian-shaped RF pulses. Current MRI units can employ sinc-shaped RF pulses, which produce significantly sharper slice profiles. A sinc function of the variable t is defined mathematically as $\text{sinc}(t) = \sin(t)/(t)$. A sinc function possesses sidelobes, which become weaker for larger values of its argument. A long sinc pulse with many sidelobes produces a sharper slice. With long RF pulses, however, weaker magnetic field gradients are used and the shortest values of TE cannot be achieved. The motivation for using a sinc-shaped RF pulse is that the Fourier transform of a sinc function is a rectangular pulse, and as a very crude approximation, the Fourier transform of an RF pulse resembles a slice profile.

Slice profiles that arise from sinc-shaped RF pulses are not entirely satisfactory. Alternatives exist for the shape of RF pulses, many of which produce significantly sharper slice profiles than sinc pulses of similar length.[65,66] Consider the two images in Figure 13–19, which compare the performance of a sinc-shaped RF pulse to one that was crafted to create a sharper slice profile. Less slice interference is expected for the crafted RF pulse, which is manifested as greater contrast in a long TR image. In fact, the specially crafted RF pulse was responsible for about four times more contrast between gray matter and white matter in Figure 13–19A than in Figure 13–19B.

Two-dimensional multislice techniques are used most often. The overlapping of slices cannot be eliminated entirely, but it can be reduced through the use of specially designed RF pulses. Most imaging protocols need to use a gap that is large enough to avoid the degradation caused by slice overlap, yet small enough that structures between slices are not missed. These conflicting objectives make the optimization of MRI techniques an intriguing task.

OVERCOMING MOTION

Another source of noise, which often swamps the random component, are the so-called ghosts that are multiple images of moving structures. Anatomic structures that move periodically blur MR images and create multiple ghosts in the phase-encoding direction.[67–72] Ghosts are undesirable because they can mask lesions and mimic abnormalities. Moreover, ghosts extract intensity from moving structures, making them less intense than if they had been stationary, which alters the contrast between tissues.

Motion in any direction can cause ghosts, and any part of the body can move during an MRI examination. The abdominal motion that is part of respiration is the most detrimental factor in MRI of the body. Images of the head can be degraded by the flow of CSF and blood and any gross movement of the head. There are numerous methods to reduce the ghosts and blurring caused by motion.

Two well-known methods for reducing respiratory motion artifacts are gating and reordering. They require patient monitoring, which often is less reliable than desired and sometimes a burden to implement. Respiratory gating rejects data if the displacement of the abdomen becomes excessive, and although it reduces ghosts and blurring, it unfortunately prolongs the time for imaging.[73,74] The reordering methods, which have been named ROPE, COPE, and EXORCIST (trademark of General Electric Company, Milwaukee, WI), need not extend the imaging time.[70,75,76]

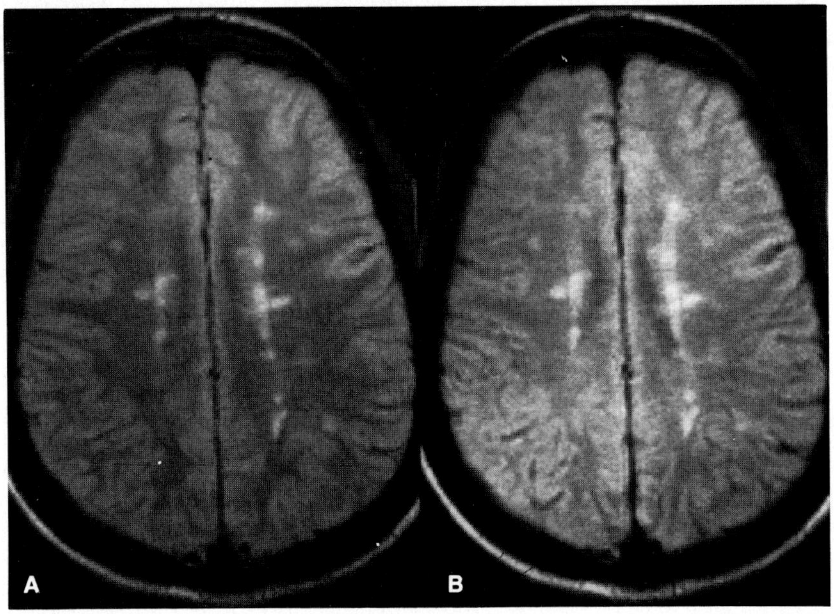

FIGURE 13–19. Characteristics of the RF pulses can affect interference between adjacent slices. These MR images were acquired from a patient with MS at 1.0 tesla (TR/TE = 3000/28). Specially optimized RF pulses were employed for **(A)**. Both the 90° and 180° RF pulses for **(B)** had the relatively conventional sinc shape. Each slice was 10 mm thick, and the field of view was 250 mm. There were 256 phase-encoding steps and no averaging of data. The intensity difference between gray matter and white matter was 200 units **(A)** and 50 units **(B)**. (Runge VM, Wood ML, Kaufman DM, Silver MS. MR imaging section profile optimization: improved contrast and detection of lesions. Radiology 1988;167:831)

These methods reorder the phase-encoding steps to make it appear as if a patient had simply inhaled once during imaging, which eliminates ghosts, but does not reduce blurring.

Other popular methods for reducing motion artifacts do not require monitoring. They reduce the displacement of anatomic structures or their intensity, or they attempt to correct for errors caused by the phase-encoding process. In the first category, the use of an inflexible band to restrain the expansion of the abdomen or prevent another relevant structure from moving can decrease blurring and reduce ghosts. Of course, the simplest method for overcoming abdominal motion is breath-holding, although it precludes imaging techniques that take much longer than 10 seconds.[77] Nevertheless, high-quality 10-second images of the abdomen are possible (Fig. 13–8).

Several methods that do not require patient monitoring diminish the intensity of moving structures, thereby reducing the associated ghosts. These include the use of surface coils or RF pulses that saturate moving tissue before imaging to weaken the corresponding MR signals. The latter method, called presaturation, has proven especially useful.[78,79] Short-tau-inversion-recovery (STIR) can make fat have little or no image intensity, which is desirable because often the most conspicuous ghosts arise from fat on the abdominal wall.[10] Averaging and gradient moment reduction (or, equivalently, gradient moment nulling) are methods that address errors in phase encoding.[75,80–82] Averaging of measured data reduces the intensity of ghosts, but not the blurring. Averaging also spreads ghosts farther apart, and it can even make the ghosts fold back on top of each other. Gradient moment reduction (GMR), which is similar to motion artifact suppression technique (MAST), reduces the effects of motion along magnetic field gradients by attempting to make MR signals produced by moving tissue similar to those from stationary tissue.[83] GMR does not prolong the time for imaging or patient preparation, but it sacrifices some flexibility in the choice of TE.

Theoretically, many methods are capable of superb performance in reducing the intensity of ghosts and reassigning it to the proper place. In practice, however, every method has a deficiency, such as requiring monitoring, prolonging the time for imaging, or imposing various constraints on the imaging technique. For convenient clinical use, a method should demand as little technical intervention as possible. Ideal methods would be transparent to the users. Even though no method is completely satisfactory, several methods can be combined for more complete suppression of motion artifacts. The methods known as gradient moment reduction and presaturation are generally easy to implement and can be combined effectively with other methods.

Gradient Moment Reduction

There are two consequences of motion that contribute to artifacts in MR images. The first is a misregistration of position from one phase-encoding step to another. Obviously, anatomic structures can change position during the several minutes that it usually takes to execute 256 phase-encoding steps. Measurements for an MR image occur during a relatively brief segment of each phase-encoding step, which lasts for a time TR. These measurements are completed after a time slightly longer than TE, typically between 10 and 100 ms, which is just a small fraction of TR. It generally makes no difference how fast a structure moves from the time after an NMR signal has been measured to when a new RF pulse is applied. All that matters is the total displacement of the structure. However, this is not the case for motion during the TE interval.

Motion from start of a phase-encoding step until after measurement of an NMR signal contributes significantly to artifacts, because it alters the characteristics of NMR signals, whether they are spin echoes or gradient echoes. The magnetic field gradients in MRI techniques cause the transverse magnetization to dephase, which means that the magnetization components lose synchrony. Dephasing is controlled through careful adjustments of the various gradient pulses. For example, a second gradient of opposite polarity can reverse the dephasing caused by one gradient. However, adjustments that would be correct for stationary structures might be inappropriate if there is movement during an MRI examination. The problem is that the dephasing caused by a gradient depends on the position of a structure, and if this position keeps changing, it is more difficult to reverse it. Figures 13–20A and 13–21A demonstrate images from a technique that fails to take into account motion during the TE interval.

The magnetization from a moving structure might still be dephased when it was supposed to be completely rephased. The extra dephasing depends on its velocity. Because the velocity of most anatomic structures varies over time, the dephasing attributed to motion is different in the echoes of each phase-encoding step, which contributes to ghosts in the phase-encoding direction. GMR, MAST, or gradient moment nulling add gradient pulses to undo the dephasing caused by motion.

The additional gradient pulses attempt to rephase the MR signal produced by moving tissue similarly to stationary tissue. The concept is similar to "even-echo rephasing," which describes a recovery of image in-

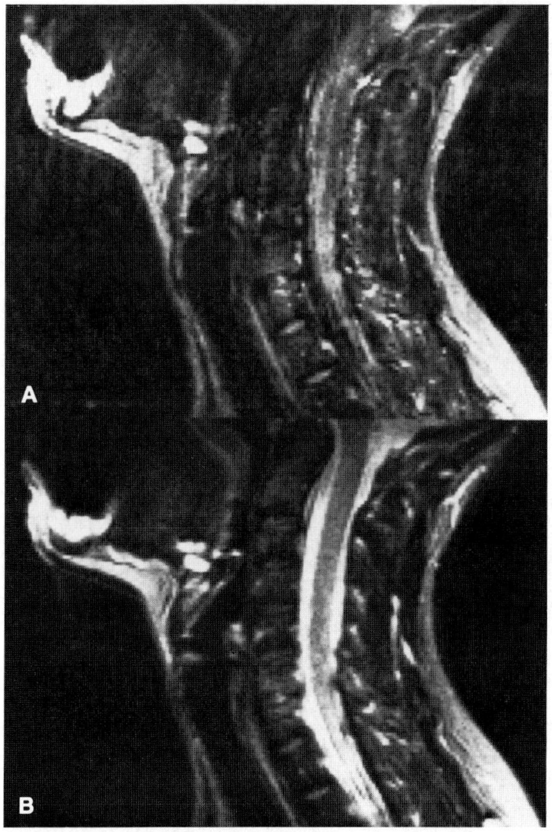

FIGURE 13–20. Ghost artifacts, primarily from CSF pulsation, at 1.0 tesla (TR/TE = 3000/100). The imaging techniques were similar, except that **(B)** employed a configuration of gradients that compensated for the dephasing of structures that moved at constant velocity in the slice selection and frequency-encoding directions during TE. Other imaging parameters included a slice thickness of 5 mm and 300-mm field of view. There were 256 phase-encoding steps and no averaging of data. (Runge VM, Wood ML, Kaufman DM, Traill MR, Nelson KL. The straight and narrow path to good head and spine MRI. Radiographics 1988;8:507)

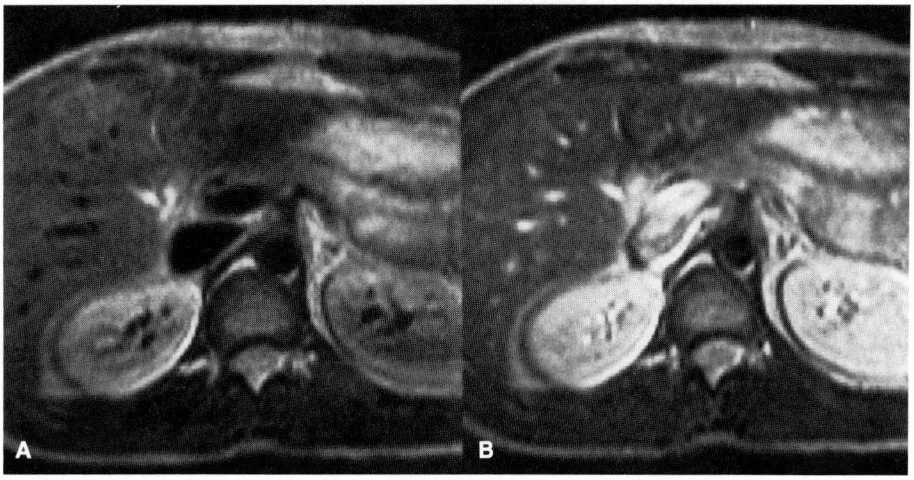

FIGURE 13–21. Demonstration of gradient moment reduction (GMR) similar to Figure 13–20. The imaging parameters for these axial abdominal MR images included TR/TE = 3000/45 ms, 8-mm slice thickness, 417-mm field of view, 128 phase-encoding steps, and averaging of two sets of data. The imaging technique for **(B)** featured a constant velocity GMR correction in the slice selection and frequency-encoding directions.

tensity for moving fluids in even-numbered echoes.[33,34] One or more additional gradient pulses can be included to compensate for the dephasing of moving tissue. The associated benefits often justify the complexity of the imaging technique, as Figures 13–20B and 13–21B demonstrate. The technique for these two images compensated for motion of constant velocity along the frequency-encoding and slice-selection directions. Measurements of ghost intensity in the background of Figures 13–20B and 13–21B were about four times smaller than in Figures 13–20A and 13–21A. Furthermore, the intensity that was extracted from the ghosts was restored to the associated anatomic structures.

GMR applies separately for motion along each of the three axes. The phase-encoding direction is the least critical, because the phase-encoding gradient is usually activated only briefly in each phase-encoding step. Any type of motion in the body can be broken down into components, the first two of which are constant velocity and acceleration. One additional gradient pulse can achieve complete rephasing for constant-velocity motion, but many more are needed for complex motion. In practice, the decision about the number of additional gradient pulses depends primarily on the shortest TE that is required. GMR can be employed in almost any imaging technique, and it can reduce artifacts from several moving structures simultaneously.

The inclusion of extra gradient pulses prolongs the minimal achievable TE, especially if a correction for complicated motion is desired. This is unfortunate for T1-weighted images, which use the shortest TE possible, but not necessarily restrictive for T2-weighted images. GMR requires no additional time for patient preparation.

Analogous to even-echo rephasing, GMR causes an enhancement of moving fluids, but not just for even echoes or constant-velocity motion. In principle, bright blood vessels that are imaged in cross-section could be confused for metastases in T2-weighted images. However, it should be possible to distinguish between blood and metastases by following the course of blood vessels through adjacent slices, as is the practice in x-ray CT, and also by comparing their appearance in images from different techniques. Therefore, bright blood need not be detrimental to image interpretation.

Presaturation

Ghosts are proportional in intensity to the associated moving anatomic structure.[72] Therefore, one way to reduce the intensity of ghosts is to make sure that moving structures are weak in intensity. This is the concept behind presaturation. The most common application of presaturation is to diminish the artifacts caused by the pulsatile flow of blood into a slice (Fig.13-22). Another established use for presaturation is to reduce the intensity of structures within a slice.

The objective is to reduce the longitudinal magnetization of certain structures, which diminishes the associated NMR signals. Presaturation employs RF pulses and magnetic field gradients as in selective excitation. The technique is widely applicable amid two drawbacks: greater power deposition and less "deadtime" after the measurement of data, both of which could limit the number of slices.

The use of presaturation to reduce ghosts from the flow of blood through the abdominal aorta and vena cava is illustrated in Figure 13-22. These ghosts are especially intense in single-slice gradient-echo images. The longitudinal magnetization of blood outside of the slice can be much greater than that of blood and other tissues inside the slice, because it has not been tipped over repeatedly by RF pulses. For the right-hand image in Figure 13-22, tissues within two wide slabs on either side of the imaged slice were subjected to RF pulses before generating NMR signals in each phase-encoding step. The intent was to reduce the longitudinal magnetization of blood that flows into the imaged slice. Blood in the aorta and vena cava became about 15 times less intense.

Presaturation is also used routinely to reduce the intensity of structures that are already in the imaged slice and which are undesirable for some reason. For example, the tissues anterior to the spine can be reduced in intensity, so that ghosts from their motion do not interfere with examination of the spinal cord in an axial or sagittal MR image. Another application minimizes the intensity of structures that extend beyond the edge of the desired FOV and which are folded back into an MR image (aliasing). Thus, presaturation can be useful when reducing the FOV.

Presaturation and GMR are two effective and convenient techniques for overcoming motion. Neither is completely sufficient, but it is difficult to imagine a single technique that could suppress motion artifacts perfectly. It is becoming clear that combinations of techniques are worthwhile, and strategic decisions for suppressing motion artifacts need to be reevaluated frequently, based on growing experience and new technology.

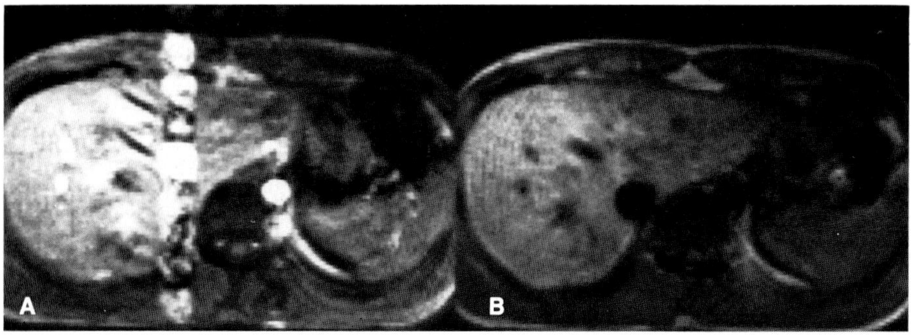

FIGURE 13-22. Ghost artifacts from blood flow through the aorta and vena cava in a single-slice gradient echo image **(A)** and their suppression by presaturation **(B).** Two 100° RF pulses were used for presaturation on both sides of the slice **(B).** Imaging conditions, which were common to both images, included TR/TE = 40/10 ms, 10-mm slice thickness, 500-mm field of view, 256 phase-encoding steps, and no averaging of data.

ACKNOWLEDGMENT

The author thanks Jim Rawson for assisting with the production of Figures 13-3 and 13-4.

REFERENCES

1. Wehrli FW, MacFall JR, Newton TH. Parameters determining the appearance of NMR images. In: Newton NH, Potts DG, eds. Modern neuroradiology, vol. 2. San Anselmo, CA: Clavadel Press, 1983.
2. Purcell EM, Torrey HC, Pound RV. Resonance absorption by nuclear magnetic moments in a solid. Phys Rev 1946;69:37.
3. Bloch F, Hansen WW, Packard ME. Nuclear induction. Phys Rev 1946;69:127.
4. Pykett IL, Newhouse JH, Buonanno FS, et al. Principles of nuclear magnetic resonance imaging. Radiology 1982;143:157.
5. Harms SE, Morgan TJ, Yamanashi WS, Harle TS, Dodd GD. Principles of nuclear magnetic resonance imaging. RadioGraphics 1984;4:26.
6. Pavlicek W, Modic M, Weinstein M. Pulse sequence and significance. RadioGraphics 1984;4:49.
7. Balter S. An introduction to the physics of magnetic resonance imaging. RadioGraphics 1987;7:371.
8. Kumar A, Welti D, Ernst RR. NMR Fourier zeugmatography. J Magn Reson 1975;18:69.
9. Edelstein WA, Hutchison JMS, Johnson G, Redpath T. Spin warp NMR imaging and applications to human whole-body imaging. Phys Med Biol 1980;25:751.
10. Bydder GM, Young IR. MR imaging: clinical use of the inversion recovery sequence. J Comput Assist Tomogr 1985;9:675.
11. Frahm J, Merboldt KD, Hanicke W, Hasse A. Stimulated echo imaging. J Magn Reson 1985;64:81.
12. Sattin W, Mareci TH, Scott KN. Exploiting the stimulated echo in nuclear magnetic resonance imaging: II. Applications. J Magn Reson 1985;65:298.
13. Mansfield P. Multi-planar image formation using NMR spin echoes. J Physiol 1977;C10:L55.
14. Pykett IL, Rzedzian RR. Instant images of the body by magnetic resonance. Magn Reson Med 1987;5:563.
15. Hawkes RC, Patz S. Rapid Fourier imaging using steady-state free precession. Magn Reson Med 1987;4:9.
16. Hahn EL. Spin echoes. Phys Rev 1950;80:580.
17. Le Bihan D, Breton E, Lallemand D, Grenier P, Cabanis E, Laval-Jeantet M. MR imaging of intravoxel incoherent motions: application to diffusion and perfusion in neurologic disorders. Radiology 1986;161:401.
18. Nyman R, Ericsson A, Hemmingsson A, Jung B, Sperber G, Thuomas KA. T1, T2, and relative proton density at 0.35 T for spleen, liver, adipose tissue, and vertebral body: normal values. Magn Reson Med 1986;3:901.
19. Henkelman RM, Hardy P, Poon PY, Bronskill MJ. Optimal pulse sequence for imaging hepatic metastases. Radiology 1986;161:727.
20. Wehrli FW, MacFall JR, Shutts D, Breger R, Herfkens RJ. Mechanisms of contrast in NMR imaging. J Comput Assist Tomogr 1984;8:369.
21. Fullerton GD. Physiologic basis of magnetic relaxation. In: Stark DD, Bradley WG, JR, eds. Magnetic Resonance Imaging. St. Louis: C.V. Mosby Co., 1988:36.
22. Bottomley PA, Foster TH, Argersinger RE, Pfeifer LM. A review of normal tissue hydrogen NMR relaxation times and relaxation mechanisms from 1-100 MHz: dependence on tissue type, NMR frequency, temperature, species, excision, and age. Med Phys 1984;11:425.
23. Breger RK, Wehrli FW, Charles HC, MacFall JR, Haughton VM. Reproducibility of relaxation and spin-density parameters in phantoms and the human brain measured by MR imaging at 1.5T. Magn Reson Med 1986;3:649.
24. Droege RT, Wiener SN, Rzeszotarski MS, Holland GN, Young IR. Nuclear magnetic resonance: a gray scale model for head images. Radiology 1983;148:763.
25. Young IR. Considerations affecting signal and contrast in NMR imaging. Brit Med Bull 1984;40:139.
26. Hendrick RE, Nelson TR, Hendee WR. Optimizing tissue contrast in magnetic resonance imaging. Magn Reson Imaging 1984;2:193.
27. Nelson TR, Hendrick RE, Hendee WR. Selection of pulse sequences producing maximum tissue contrast in magnetic resonance imaging. Magn Reson Imaging 1984;2:285.
28. Hardy PA, Bronskill MJ, Henkelman RM. Signal strength on a 0.15-T magnetic resonance imager. Med Phys 1985;12:581.
29. Bradley WG, Tsuruda JS. MR sequence parameter optimization: an algorithmic approach. AJR 1987;149:815.
30. McVeigh ER, Bronskill MJ, Henkelman RM. Optimization of MR protocols: a statistical decision analysis approach. Magn Reson Med 1988;6:314.
31. Dreher W, Boenert P. Pulse sequence and parameter choice in NMR imaging as a problem of constrained multidimensional optimization. Magn Reson Med 1988;8:16.
32. Hendrick E. Image contrast and noise. In: Stark DD, Bradley WG, JR, eds. Magnetic Resonance Imaging. St. Louis: C.V. Mosby Co., 1988:66.
33. Waluch V, Bradley WG. NMR even echo rephasing in slow laminar flow. JCAT 1984;8:594.
34. Axel L. Blood flow effects in magnetic resonance imaging. AJR 1984;13:1157.
35. van der Meulen P, Cuppen JJM, Groen JP. Very fast MR imaging by field echoes and small angle excitation. Magn Reson Imaging 1985;3:297.
36. Haase A, Frahm J, Matthaei D, Hanicke W, Merboldt KD. FLASH imaging. Rapid NMR imaging using low flip-angle pulses. J Magn Reson 1986;67:258.
37. Ernst RR, Anderson WA. Application of Fourier transform spectroscopy to magnetic resonance. Rev Sci Instrum 1966;37:93.
38. Mills TC, Ortendahl DA, Hylton NM, Crooks LE, Carlson JW, Kaufman L. Partial flip angle MR imaging. Radiology 1987;162:531.
39. Buxton RB, Edelman RR, Rosen BR, Wismer GL, Brady TJ. Contrast in rapid MR imaging: T1- and T2-weighted imaging. J Comput Assist Tomogr 1987;11:7.
40. Frahm J, Hanicke W, Merboldt KD. Transverse coherence in rapid FLASH NMR imaging. J Magn Reson 1987;72:307.
41. Wood ML, Silver M, Runge VM. Optimization of spoiler gradients in FLASH MRI. Mag Res Imaging 1987;5:455.
42. Crawley AP, Wood ML, Henkelman RM. Elimination of transverse coherences in FLASH MRI. Magn Reson Med 1988;8:248.
43. Wehrli FW, Perkins TG, Shimakawa A, Roberts F. Chemical shift-induced amplitude modulations in images obtained with gradient refocusing. Magn Reson Imaging 1987;5:157.
44. Oppelt A, Graumann R, Barfuss H, Fischer H, Hartl W, Schajor W. FISP—a new fast MRI sequence. Electromedica 1986;54:15.
45. Gyngell ML. The application of steady-state free precession in rapid 2DFT NMR imaging: FAST and CE-FAST sequences. Magn Reson Imaging 1988;6:415.
46. Sutherland RJ, Hutchison JM. Three-dimensional NMR imaging using selective excitation. J Phys E Sci Instrum 1978;11:79.
47. Johnson G, Hutchinson JM, Redpath TW, Eastwood LM. Improvements in performance time for simultaneous three-dimensional NMR imaging. J Magn Reson 1983;54:374.
48. Carlson J, Crooks L, Ortendahl D, Kramer D, Kaufman L. Signal-to-noise ratio and section thickness in two-dimensional versus three-dimensional Fourier transform MR imaging. Radiology 1988;166:266.
49. Frahm J, Haase A, Matthaei D. Rapid three-dimensional MR imaging using the FLASH technique. J Comput Assist Tomogr 1986;10:363.
50. Luedeke KM, Roeschmann P, Tischler R. Susceptibility artefacts in NMR imaging. Magn Reson Imaging 1985;3:329.
51. Czervionke LF, Daniels DL, Wehrli FW, et al. Magnetic suscep-

tibility artifacts in gradient-recalled echo MR imaging. AJR 1988;9:1149.

52. Edelstein WA, Bottomley PA, Hart HR, Smith LS. Signal, noise, and contrast in nuclear magnetic resonance (NMR) imaging. J Comput Assist Tomogr 1983;7:391.
53. Crooks LE, Arakawa M, Hoenninger J, McCarten B, Watts J, Kaufman L. Magnetic Resonance Imaging: Effects of magnetic field strength. Radiology 1984;151:127.
54. Hendrick RE, Newman FD, Hendee WR. MR imaging technology: maximizing the signal-to-noise ratio from a single tissue. Radiology 1985;156:749.
55. Hoult DI, Lauterbur PC. Sensitivity of the zeugmatographic experiment involving human samples. J Magn Reson 1979;34:425.
56. Edelstein WA, Bottomley PA, Pfeifer LM. A signal-to-noise calibration procedure for NMR imaging systems. Med Phys 1984;11:180.
57. McVeigh ER, Henkelman RM, Bronskill MJ. Noise and filtration in magnetic resonance imaging. Med Phys 1985;12:586.
58. Crooks LE, Kaufman L, Hoenninger J, Arakawa M, Watts J, Cannon CR. Spatial resolution in NMR imaging. IEEE Trans Med Imaging 1984;3:51.
59. Crooks LE, Hoenninger J, Arakawa M, et al. High-resolution magnetic resonance imaging-technical concepts and their implementation. Radiology 1984;150:163.
60. Wood ML, Henkelman RM. Truncation artifacts in magnetic resonance imaging. Magn Reson Med 1985;2:517.
61. Runge VM, Wood ML, Kaufman DM, Traill MR, Nelson KL. The straight and narrow path to good head and spine MRI. RadioGraphics 1988;8:507.
62. Kneeland JB, Shimakawa A, Wehrli FW. Effect of intersection spacing on MR image contrast and study time. Radiology 1986;158:819.
63. Kneeland JB, Knowles RJ, Cahill PT. Multi-section multi-echo pulse magnetic resonance techniques: optimization in a clinical setting. Radiology 1985;155:159.
64. Kucharczyk W, Crawley AP, Kelly WM, Henkelman RM. The effect of interslice gaps on signal-to-noise and contrast in multislice MRI (abstract). Presented at the 25th Annual Meeting of the American Society of Neuroradiology, May 1987.
65. Loaiza F, Lim KT, Warren WS, Silver MS, Egloff H, Laub G, Kiefer B. Crafted pulses and pulse sequences for MR imaging. Health Care Instrum 1986;1:188.
66. Runge VM, Wood ML, Kaufman DM, Silver MS. MR imaging section profile optimization: improved contrast and detection of lesions. Radiology 1988;167:831.
67. Schultz CL, Alfidi RJ, Nelson AD, Kopiwoda SY, Clampitt ME. Effect of motion on two-dimensional Fourier transformation magnetic resonance images. Radiology 1984;152:117.
68. Wood ML, Henkelman RM. MR image artifacts from periodic motion. Med Phys 1985;12:143.
69. Axel L, Summers RM, Kressel HY, Charles C. Respiratory effects in two-dimensional Fourier transform MR imaging. Radiology 1986;161:795.
70. Haacke EM, Patrick JL. Reducing motion artifacts in two-dimensional Fourier transform imaging. Mag Reson Imaging 1986;4:359.
71. Wood ML, Runge VM, Henkelman RM. Overcoming abdominal motion. AJR 1988;150:513.
72. Wood ML, Henkelman RM. The magnetic field dependence of the breathing artifact. Mag Reson Imaging 1986;4:387.
73. Ehman RL, McNamara MT, Pallack M, Hricak H, Higgins CB. Magnetic resonance imaging with gating: techniques and advantages. AJR 1985;143:1175.
74. Runge VM, Clanton JA, Partain CL, Everette J Jr. Respiratory gating in magnetic resonance imaging at 0.5 tesla. Radiology 1984;151:521.
75. Wood ML, Henkelman RM. Suppression of respiratory motion artifacts in magnetic resonance imaging. Med Phys 1986;13:794.
76. Bailes DR, Gilderdale DJ, Bydder GM, Collins AG, Fermin DN. Respiratory ordering of phase encoding (ROPE): a method for reducing respiratory motion artifacts in MR imaging. J Comput Assist Tomogr 1985;9:835.
77. Edelman RR, Hahn PF, Buxton R, et al. Rapid MR imaging with suspended respiration: clinical application in the liver. Radiology 1986;161:125.
78. Felmlee JP, Ehman RL. Spatial presaturation: a method for suppressing flow artifacts and improving depiction of vascular anatomy in MR imaging. Radiology 1987;164:559.
79. Edelman RR, Atkinson DJ, Silver MS, Loaiza FL, Warren WS. FRODO pulse sequences: a new means of eliminating motion, flow, and wraparound artifacts. Radiology 1988;166:231.
80. Stark DD, Hendrick RE, Hahn PF, Ferrucci JT. Motion artifact reduction by fast spin echo imaging. Radiology 1987;164:183.
81. Stark DD, Wittenburg J, Edelman RR, et al. Detection of hepatic metastases; analysis of pulse sequence performance in MR imaging. Radiology 1986;159:365.
82. Haacke EM, Lenz GW. Improving image quality in the presence of motion by using rephasing gradients. AJR 1987;148:1251.
83. Pattany PM, Phillips J, Chiu LC, et al. Motion artifact suppression technique (MAST) for MR imaging. J Comput Assist Tomogr 1987;11:369.

14

Day-to-Day Operations

Daphna Y. Gelblum
Martha I. Pacetti
Val M. Runge

Magnetic resonance imaging (MRI) is an innovative modality with a growing number of applications. Most radiologists encounter MR images in their daily practices. Unit operation requires a basic knowledge of the physics of MRI to understand the constraints imposed by magnetic fields and gradients. Most importantly, the radiologist must learn to interpret a new set of information. The image no longer represents variations in x-ray attenuation. Instead, the MR image represents variations in the proton environment based on the proton relaxation times of normal and pathologic tissue. The routine patient examination has been divided into eight steps in the following sections, highlighting new techniques and constraints encountered in MRI.

PATIENT EDUCATION

Proper patient education ensures better image quality. Patients are often unfamiliar with MRI, and they first learn about the modality from their referring physician, who usually describes it as an experience similar to CT. This information does little to prepare the patient for the spatial confinement, knocking sounds, or length of the examination.

A brief explanation of the examination can be given when the MR receptionist calls to schedule the appointment. The patient should be told about the absence of ionizing radiation, the "long tube," the potential for claustrophobia, the need to lie still for about an hour, and the contraindications of ferromagnetic objects. If time allows, an information booklet should be mailed to the patient.

Brochures discussing the principles involved in MRI, specifically magnetism and radiowaves and the necessity for patient screening, should be available in the waiting area. An illustration of the magnet room should also be included. After the paper work is completed, the technologist or physician's assistant can bring the patient and any accompanying family into a private area to answer questions or anxieties they may have and to discuss what to expect during the examination.

The tapping noises made during routine machine operation and the importance of holding still during these times should be explained. These tapping sounds are generated by the gradient coil wires being strained during the gradient magnetic field generation. The noise amplitude depends on the technique chosen and on the machine used. The sounds are loudest when the gradients are the strongest: with thin slices, small fields of view (FOV), or with multiple echoes. Ear plugs can be provided for increased patient comfort.

The patient is often reassured by hearing that there is no exposure to ionizing radiation. Instead, radio waves, much like those emitted in an FM broadcast, are used to generate the images. The static field aligns mobile protons in the body along one axis. Radio frequencies (RF) tuned to the resonance frequency of protons are then turned on for short bursts to excite the hydrogen nuclei. The time required for the nuclei to return to their preferred orientation (aligned with the static field) is distinctive for each tissue and is reflected in the image signal intensities.[1,2]

The importance of explaining the procedure in detail to the patient cannot be overemphasized. Creating a confident and cooperative patient assures better image quality and a completed examination.

EQUIPMENT PRECAUTIONS AND PATIENT SCREENING

MRI has introduced many new safety issues to radiology. These topics may be divided into two groups: equipment precautions and patient screening.

The static and time-varying gradient magnetic fields associated with the MR scanner require that precautions be taken in the immediate examination area. The scanner continuously generates a static magnetic field, which decreases in strength at a rate directly proportional to distance from the unit. Fringe fields differ in magnitude at equal distances, depending on magnet strength. The scan room walls generally demarcate the 10-gauss line. (This restriction varies from state to state.) In general it is not safe to bring ferromagnetic articles beyond this point.[3] Some cryogen tanks, oxygen tanks, metal encased monitors, and most wheel chairs and stretchers may be forcefully drawn into the bore of the magnet. Magnetic tapes will be erased if brought into a strong field.

Some patient-monitoring equipment is made of nonmagnetic materials and has a digital display, but it is still not compatible with the MR environment. The magnet and monitoring equipment each generate RF and thus may interfere with each other. The monitor may display a false reading or show nothing at all. The resulting scan may be noisy or have signal voids in the areas closest to the monitor and its leads. Some companies manufacture life support and resuscitative equipment that is shielded, permitting operation in a magnetic environment.[4,5] Similarly there are some MR systems that have lower field strengths or design configurations that allow monitors close to the magnet.[6] Specially constructed patient transport equipment has also been built for use in MRI.[7]

The most critical piece of medical equipment prohibited from the MR room is the code cart, which is often stocked with metallic and electronic devices.[7] Should a patient require emergency care, they must be removed from the scanner and brought out of the MR scan room into an adjacent room to be assisted by the code team. To provide optimal patient care in an emergency, all MR staff should be trained in CPR. A protocol should be instituted for the procedure taken in case of cardiac or respiratory arrest. This training is particularly important because there is often a delay in response time by the code team due to the remote location of some private imaging centers and of some MR departments within hospitals.

Proper screening is essential before allowing anyone to enter the MRI room.[8] Medical staff attending to patients in the scanner room must remove their beepers, stethoscopes, hemostats, keys, and radiation and hospital identification badges before entering; these are all potential projectiles. Credit cards and analog watches will be damaged by the magnetic field; digital watch operation is not affected. Patients must change out of any clothing containing metal (e.g., zipper, snaps, studs, underwire bras, or bra hooks) near the area being scanned. Dentures, bobby pins, earrings, and necklaces must also be removed. Ferromagnetic materials within the patient or any personnel entering the scanning environment can also be hazardous.

A brief explanation of the interaction of the magnetic field and gradients with metallic objects within the human body will help in understanding the mechanism for possible adverse effects. Potential harm may arise from one of three factors: local heating around the object, torquing of the object, or electrical interference between the RF pulses and the device's operation. How strongly the magnetic field affects the implant depends on the object's size, its location relative to the center of the bore, and its magnetic susceptibility, the ability of a material to concentrate magnetic field lines.[9] The magnetic gradients influence the electrical current distribution through the body. Gradient strength depends on the imaging technique and particular scan conditions chosen.

The Food and Drug Administration, before approving the routine clinical use of MRI, set maximal strengths allowed for the static field, the time-varying magnetic gradients, and the RF fields (see the display on this page). The static B_0 field is set by the manufacturer when the MR unit is installed. Today some manufacturers are installing magnets that have a variable range of operating fields (1.5–2.0 T). The maximum strength of the magnetic gradients depends on the pulse sequence and is typically on the order of 5 to 10

Maximum Permissible Field Strengths[72]

Static field (B_0)	2.0 T
Time-varying field	3 T/s (limited to levels insufficient to produce peripheral nerve stimulation or other adverse effects)*
Radio-frequency fields	SAR of 3.0 W/kg averaged over the whole body or 8.0 W/kg averaged over a spatially localized region or Fields insufficient to produce a core temperature increase in excess of 1°C and localized heating to greater than 38°C in head, 39°C in trunk, and 40°C in extremities*

* These limitations are set on the machine by the manufacturer

mT/m. The maximum rate of change in the new FLASH and FISP sequences, however, may reach 50 T/sec.[9] Even higher rates may be encountered with echo planar sequences. The most sensitive biologic reaction to time-varying magnetic fields are magnetophosphenes, characterized by the visualization of short bright bursts of light. There are no reports of patients experiencing these electric-current-evoked responses during an MR exam at field strengths of 2.0 T and below.[11] However, with the introduction of short TR sequences and echo planar imaging, the topic should be studied more closely.[6,9,10]

During the imaging sequence, RF pulses pass into body parts lying in the field of the transmitter coil. This causes tissue heating, which is measured as the specific absorption ratio (SAR; units are W/kg) and reflects the rate at which thermal energy is deposited into the body. The amount of heat deposited depends on the number of slices, flip angle magnitude, number of averages, TR, and shape and characteristics of the tissue being exposed.[6] The human thermoregulatory system dispels most of the heat through evaporative heat loss. This process is abetted by a cool scan room, relatively few layers of clothing on the patient, and a continuous air flow through the magnet tube. The SAR limitations are similar in infants and adults because the increased RF power required to create a 90° and 180° pulse in adults is offset by the greater body weight.

The greatest concern with RF absorption is the deposition of thermal energy in small anatomic regions, such as the lens of the eye or the testicles, which do not conduct heat, yet collect it efficiently. Both of these structures have their own compensatory mechanisms. The lens is continuously bathed in liquid, permitting evaporation to dissipate heat. The immediate surroundings of the testes provide shielding and the folds of skin allow for good surface-to-air heat transfer.

Magnetic fields can affect implanted devices (see the display on this page). The most familiar contraindicated internal electromechanical device is the heart pacemaker. The time-varying magnetic gradients used in MRI may affect the mechanical and electrical operations of this device.[12] The time-varying gradients applied during MR imaging may fool the pacemaker into pacing without an arrhythmia or cause a continuously pacing device to switch from synchronous to asynchronous mode. When screening patients for pacemakers, be aware that not all patients, the elderly in particular, are aware or remember that they have one. A thorough physical examination of debilitated patients covering both sides of the chest cavity and the abdominal cavity can avert a mistake.

Absolute Contraindications to MRI[10]

- Pacemakers
- Ferromagnetic aneurysm clips
- Metallic fragments in the eye
- Cochlear implants
- Starr-Edwards pre-6000 model prosthetic heart valve
- Internal drug infusion pumps
- Neurostimulators
- Bone-growth stimulators

Two other frequently encountered ferromagnetic surgical devices are brain aneurysm clips and middle ear prostheses (stapedectomies).[13–17] Although most surgical clips are made of nonmagnetic materials, when joined with other alloys and shaped for surgical use, they may adopt magnetic properties. Aneurysm clips are potentially more dangerous than surgical clips elsewhere in the body because they are not anchored by fibrosis in the brain. Furthermore, ferromagnetic aneurysm clips (i.e., Drake DR14,16, 301 SS; Heifetz 17-7PH, Elgiloy; Mayfield 301 SS, 304 SS) have been employed surgically in the past. A catastrophic event could occur because of the forces exerted on such a clip by the static magnetic field. Recently implanted surgical clips elsewhere in the body also may be hazardous. In general, a few weeks should pass between the surgical placement of nonmagnetic clips and the MR scan.[4]

Stapes prostheses are made with a small coil of wire running through them, which in the newest models is tantalum, a nonferromagnetic material. All of the Richard's stainless steel prostheses used through 1985 have been tested for torquing and found to be safe for MR scanning.[16–17] These implants are made of Teflon, gelfoam, and platinum. Cochlear implants, however, have been found to be unsafe in an electromagnetic field because of their electrical neurostimulation mechanism.[17]

Prosthetic cardiac valves have also been evaluated for heat deposition, torque, and the potential to induce stray electric currents.[18,19] With one exception, all have been found safe.[20] The one contraindication is the Starr-Edwards model pre-6000 prosthetic heart valve. Several other cardiac valves displayed minor deflection as well, but the torque was minimal when compared with the natural forces created by cardiac muscle contractions.[19] There are no accounts of heating, nor sporadic current generation, nor of any implant-created artifacts preventing visualization of surrounding tissue.[19]

Orthopedic implants are typically constructed from stainless steel or alloys and are generally safe for MR examination, as are the new graphite halos. External braces and Stryker frames, however, are often magnetic and must be removed to permit imaging. Other implants have been tested. All IUDs and all but one penile implant, the Omniphase by Dacomed, have been found to be acceptable.[20,21] In general it is a good rule to delay an examination if a prosthetic material is unknown until further information is collected. Strong hand-held magnets can be used to test exposed metallic parts (e.g., braces and orthopedic plates). Even if a brace is composed of nonmagnetic materials, removal is recommended to prevent the possibility of eddy current generation or local heating.

Another major concern is the existence of foreign metallic fragments within the globe due to occupational or recreational exposure. It is good practice to order orbital x-rays for former machine, auto, or metal workers to confirm the absence of metallic shavings in their orbits. Plain films are the most cost-effective and efficient means to screen for metallic orbital foreign bodies. Computed tomography (CT) scans are preferable but may not be time- or cost-effective. At least one case has been reported of blindness following MR imaging in a patient with an unsuspected intraocular metallic fragment.[22]

One other possible contraindication, which may be encountered more frequently in inner city hospitals or by those who treat prison inmates, is bullet fragments. An unpublished study performed at The New England Medical Center showed that only minimal torque is exerted on bullets at 1.0 T. A conservative approach is to allow a patient to be scanned if the bullet is lodged in abdominal fat or muscle, away from the spinal cord, and away from any major vessels or organs. These patients must be carefully screened and if any doubt exists, x-ray films should be taken to confirm bullet location.

In many imaging centers, pregnancy is considered a contraindication to an MR exam. There are no known harmful effects to the developing fetus or the mother, but the possibility of adverse effects remains. Research conducted to determine the utility of MR imaging of the fetus and mother shows that fetal motion during the first and second trimesters degrades pelvic image quality.[23,24] Scanning during the third trimester, however, has clearly shown maternal anatomy and the fetal brain and liver. It should be noted that most of these tests were performed on women whose pregnancies were being terminated because of sonographic findings. The status of scanning pregnant women will continue to evolve in the next few years, and MRI may find utility in those patients in whom obesity and oligohydramnios limit the effectiveness of ultrasound.[25]

One final source of complications encountered in MR imaging is unrelated to the magnetic field but concerns the use of contrast media. The only agent currently approved for clinical use is Gd DTPA, which is administered intravenously. Gadopentetate dimeglumine is cleared by glomerular filtration and thus should not be given to patients with renal failure. A transient rise in serum iron and bilirubin has been seen in a small percentage of patients.[26] It has been suggested that because of possible hemolysis, patients with hemolytic anemias should not receive the drug, pending further study. Concern about the possibility for gadolinium ion exchange with either zinc or copper suggests that it would be prudent not to give the drug to people with Wilson's disease.[27] Pediatric safety and efficacy is being reviewed.[28] There is only limited data collected on pregnant and nursing mothers. The finding that a small amount of the Gd DTPA is excreted in human milk suggests that nursing mothers should not receive the contrast agent.[29]

PATIENT PREPARATION

If contrast media are indicated, then the risk, benefits, and method of administration are explained to the patient. No major complications have been reported to date with Gd DTPA,[26] unlike those with iodinated contrast media as used in CT. In a recent report of 7000 patients who received Gd DTPA, only 1% experienced any side-effects, all of which were mild.[26] It should be explained to the patient that they may feel a slight warm sensation at the injection site during Gd DTPA administration.

Starting the intravenous line before the examination saves time and decreases the chance of a patient moving or changing his position between the preinjection and postinjection sequences. Usually a #20 or #22 angio catheter is inserted in a superficial vein, and intravenous tubing with 100 ml bag of normal saline is connected. The injection site should be checked for infiltration before contrast administration. Tissue sloughing is theoretically possible with Gd DTPA extravasation.

Gd DTPA is currently dispensed in 20-ml vials and given in a dose of 0.2 ml/kg (0.1 mmol/kg). Injection is performed at the tubing port closest to the vein. The rate of injection should not exceed 10 ml/min, followed by a saline flush, to insure complete delivery of the agent.[29] The patient is observed during and immediately after the contrast injection for possible reaction. After completion of the examination, the catheter is removed. The patient is asked if he has experienced any problems during the scan, either before or after injection. An instruction sheet is given, which includes the following information:

1. Resume regular diet.
2. Routine medication may be taken (ordered by physician).
3. Drink plenty of liquids (Gd DTPA is primarily excreted in the urine).

4. There will be no change in color or smell of urine.
5. May resume normal activities.
6. In 24 hours, 91% of Gd DTPA will be excreted from the body.[29]
7. The phone number of the department is given, in case there are any questions.

SEDATION AND MONITORING

Anxiety

Although MRI poses no known biologic risk, many patients experience apprehension and anxiety before and during the procedure.[30] The patient should be informed that they will be continuously monitored while in the magnet. A two-way communication line allows them to speak with the technologist during the examination.

Patients often experience claustrophobia inside the scanner. The sensation may trigger memory of a past negative experience. For example, one patient remembered being locked in a closet as a child. Some patients have known claustrophobia. Relaxation techniques, informing the patient about what to expect during the scan (e.g., tapping noise, the long scan duration, what is happening between the tapping periods) and showing that the magnet is open at both ends help.[31] If desired, the patient may be accompanied into the scan room by a family member, who must then also be screened. Music can be provided by a headset while inside the scanner.

Adult Sedation

Sedation may be used as a last resort. Often the patient is rescheduled and medication may be ordered by the referring physician or by the radiologist. No patient should be allowed to leave alone after sedation, and they must be informed not to drive or operate machinery for several hours and not to consume alcohol. If the patient requires sedation. Xanax (alprazolam, Upjohn Co.) has been found to be useful in a dose of 0.25 to 0.5 mg, given orally. It acts partly as a placebo, because often the drug has not had time to take effect by the start of the examination. Xanax is a benzodiazepine and caution must be used. Patients with acute angle closure (narrow) glaucoma should not be given a benzodiazepine; valium is also a benzodiazepine.[32]

Pediatric Sedation

Because the MR examination is very sensitive to motion and requires the patient to maintain a specific position for a lengthy time, a cooperative patient is necessary. This is not realistic in the pediatric population, specifically those between the ages of 3 months and 5 years. Some children younger than 3 months fall asleep without sedation if they are fed before the examination and wrapped snugly in a blanket. However, infants with neurologic problems that cause increased agitation (e.g., cocaine-addicted infants) and infants with gastric reflux should not be fed before the examination. The age parameter for sedation of pediatric patients is not fixed, and clinical judgment should be used.

PREPARATION OF CHILDREN

Preparation for the MR examination is for the child and the parent. Good communication between the staff and parent leads to a calm and trusting parent, which is reflected in the child (hopefully cooperative!).

A week before the examination, a letter should be sent to the family explaining briefly the scan, the preparation (i.e., NPO after midnight or 4–6 hours before scan), the sedation process, and the postscan procedure. This mailing can also include a coloring book or story book explaining the examination from a child's perspective. The day before, the parent should receive a call from either the physician or the nurse. At this time the information in the letter is reinforced, and additional information is obtained (i.e., weight, allergies, sedation history, medical history, surgical history, and current medications). The parent is told to dress the child in clothing that has no metal components. The parent should be encouraged to bring the child's favorite toy or blanket.

The child should arrive 1 hour before the examination. Explanations of the sedation procedure and the test are reiterated to both parent and child (depending on the child's age). The words used to describe the sedation process to the child should be carefully chosen. Children's cognition is literal and concrete.[33] An example is a 6-year-old girl who was scheduled for an MR examination and was told she should drink a "special drink" and she would "go to sleep." The child became very upset, fearing she would die. This fear in children may come from several life events, such as a death of a grandparent or family animal, or a message conveyed from television. The child should be reassured that he or she will wake up after the test.

Vital signs are obtained, and the lungs are auscultated. A general assessment of the child's physical state is obtained. A flow sheet specific for pediatric radiology sedation is necessary. The flow sheet contains the name and phone number of the responsible adult, a brief medical history (i.e., allergies, medications, and weight), vital signs, length of examination, medication given (i.e., time, route, and site), postexamination vital signs, color, responsiveness, time of discharge, condition on discharge, plus an area for follow up and problems. A verbal or written consent from the responsible adult should be obtained before sedation and documented on the flow sheet. This flow sheet is kept as a permanent part of the child's medical records.

A holding room that houses a crib and a rocking chair is desirable. A warm feeling may be created by having stuffed animals and children's posters and books. If a room is not available, a quiet area should be established in the department away from the reception area, but close to trained personnel in case of an emergency.

SEDATION OF CHILDREN

The perfect sedation medication probably does not exist. In our experience, the combination of chloral hydrate and Vistaril (hydroxyzine pamoate, Pfizer Pharmaceuticals) is 90% effective. Chloral hydrate is administered in a dosage of 50 to 100 mg/kg, not to exceed 2 gm, along with 1 tsp or 25 mg of Vistaril, both given orally.[34] The dosage of Vistaril is reduced to 1 mg/kg for children 1 year or younger. It is best to give the Vistaril first due to its pleasant lemon taste. The child is then more receptive to the unpleasant taste of the chloral hydrate that follows. Another helpful hint is to immediately cover the bottle of chloral hydrate, because it is volatile.[32]

A study in 582 pediatric cranial CT examinations found chloral hydrate (80 mg/kg) to be an effective sedative, with a failure rate of 15%. An important consideration is its safety and ease of administration.[35] Sander and Low studied 119 patients undergoing a CT scan who were sedated with 75 mg/kg of chloral hydrate. Of these 119 patients, only 1 patient required resedation.[36] In both studies, the drug appeared to be safe and produced no major complications.

One problem with chloral hydrate is the varying time to achieve sedation in children. In our experience, the range is 15 minutes to 1 hour (a reason for having the patient come 1 hour before examination). Because the time to sedate children cannot be controlled, it is wise to schedule sedations no more frequently than every other patient. The sedations should be done in the morning, allowing for several hours of parental observation after imaging. Therefore, late afternoon or early evening sedations are not appropriate. In our clinical series, chloral hydrate has not been found to be effective in the sedation of autistic and hyperactive children. If the child is not sedated with an adequate dosage of chloral hydrate, the exam is canceled and rescheduled for a stronger sedation medication.

The next drug of choice is MCP (meperidine, chlorpromazine, and promethazine). Each 2 ml vial contains 25.0 mg of meperidine, 6.25 mg of chlorpromazine, and 6.25 mg of promethazine.[37] MCP is premixed in the pharmacy and should be kept in a dark storage area, because chlorpromazine is light-sensitive. MCP should not be used if the solution is colored. MCP is administered in a dosage of 0.1 ml/kg intramuscularly. The primary age group for use is 2 to 5 years, although it can be used in children younger than 2 years.[32] The viscosity of the agent makes the injection painful. It should not be given to patients weighing more than 20 kg because two injections would be required. An intravenous heplock should be started as precaution for respiratory problems.

Along with its analgesic effect, meperidine (Demerol, Winthrop Pharmaceuticals) produces a euphoric sedative state. This sedative effect may be greater in meperidine than morphine when given in equianalgesic doses; however, the respiratory depression is the same.[32]

Chlorpromazine (Thorazine, Smith Kline and French) is a phenothiazine derivative. Its principle action in MCP is as a sedative and antiemetic.[38]

Promethazine (Phenergan, Wyeth) is also a phenothiazine derivative with sedating, antihistamine, and antiemetic action. Promethazine sustains the sedative action of meperidine up to 6 to 8 hours.[38]

Weir and colleagues evaluated 113 patients receiving MCP for various radiologic procedures. MCP was found to be effective in 86% of the patients, based on the authors' criteria.[39] In a clinical study of 95 patients, respiratory depression ensued in 4 patients.[40] The long half-life of MCP can lead to prolonged sedation and its accompanying potential for respiratory depression.[38,40]

Chloral hydrate with Vistaril and MCP are the two primary drug combinations we use for sedation. However, other institutions find Nembutal (pentobarbital sodium, Abbott Laboratories) effective. The drug is given intravenously. Nembutal is administered in a dosage of 2 to 6 mg/kg. An additional dose can be given. It is very quick-acting and lasts approximately 55 minutes.[32,41] Nembutal is used in the age group of 1 to 10 years. Slow administration is recommended to decrease the incidence of respiratory depression.[32]

In our experience, Midazolam is usually ineffective due to its short half-life.[37,42] Children have the tendency to wake up before the scan is over, becoming frightened and unable to complete the scan.

MONITORING

Two basic questions must be answered when monitoring children: Are they breathing and is there adequate oxygenation? To assure this, continuous noninvasive monitoring is necessary. An obvious monitoring device is the trained eye (nurse or physician) who is present in the scanner room during the examination. However, due to the length of the magnet bore, patient observation is hampered. Also visual changes of the sedated child (i.e., cyanosis of lips and nail beds, changes in respiration rate) become evident only after moderate hypoxia has set in.[43,44]

A useful instrument in monitoring the patient's breathing is an apnea monitor. The Biochem 515 CO_2 monitor works on the principle of measuring exhaled CO_2 in each breath.[45]

To determine if there is adequate exchange of O_2 and CO_2, a pulse oximeter can be used. This is a noninvasive device that measures oxygenated hemoglobin and reduced hemoglobin by means of light absorption by the vascular bed.[44]

Evaluation of the respiratory system is important in children because they have lower oxygen reserve than adults (i.e., infant's functional residual capacity is 80 and an adult's is 3000). For this reason, hypoxia occurs earlier in children.[46] The pulse oximeter can inform the observer of mild hypoxia before severe hypoxia occurs. It should be remembered that the oximeter is measuring O_2 saturation (SaO_2), not arterial oxygen (PaO_2). For example, an SaO_2 of 90% is approximately equal to PaO_2 of 60 mmHg.[47] The pulse oximeter also provides pulse rate.

There are pulse oximeters available that can be used in the magnetic field, but all have some limitations. Most appear to function 80 to 90% of the time, with problems in operation caused by the magnetic field and by RF interference. One such oximeter is the Nonin 8604 pulse oximeter (Nonin Medical, Inc.)

Although the traditional observation techniques are useful, the apnea monitor and the pulse oximeter add to the safety of monitoring the sedated pediatric patient. The pulse oximeter or apnea monitor should be used with sedated or debilitated adult patients.

An emergency crash cart with resuscitation equipment should be kept in the department. A good reference for stocking the cart is the *Standards and Guidelines for Cardiopulmonary Resuscitation and Emergency Care* by the American Heart Association.[48]

Post-Scan Recovery

A useful reference for protocol after the procedure is the *Guidelines for the Elective Use of Conscious Sedation, Deep Sedation, and General Anesthesia in Pediatric Patients,* formulated by the American Academy of Pediatrics and the American Academy of Pediatric Dentistry.[49]

The patient can be discharged after several criteria are met: the airway and cardiovascular status are stable; the patient is aware of the surroundings; the patient can verbalize; and the patient sits up independently, requiring only minimal assistance during ambulation. The child's age and developmental level should be taken into account when evaluating the readiness for discharge.[49] Depending on the medication and dose, vital signs should be taken every 15 minutes for the first hour and then every 30 minutes. Most of our patients stay for 30 minutes to 2 hours after the scan.

The following information should be charted on the same radiology flow sheet that the preassessment and sedation data were recorded on: the time of discharge, the name of the responsible adult to whom the child is being discharged, and confirmation that the post-scan instruction sheet has been explained and given to the responsible adult. The post-scan instruction sheet contains the following:

1. Do not take any medications, except those ordered by your physician.
2. Plan for child to have quiet activities for the remainder of the day.
3. Start with liquids or light foods and progress to the child's normal eating pattern.
4. Your child has received the following medications today in the MRI department: ______.
5. If you have any problems or questions, please call the MRI department at ______________.

The parents should be advised about the expected behavior of their child at home and how long the medication should last. Instruct the parent to place the child on his or her stomach or side when sleeping to prevent possible aspiration of vomitus if the child becomes ill.[50] The day after the scan, a follow-up phone call is recommended to assure that there were no problems at home and to assess the child's reaction to the medication.

SCAN PROTOCOLS

With the patient comfortably positioned on the table, scanning can begin. Prospectively assigned protocols aid the technologist in planning ahead during the scan process. Most examinations begin with a localizer to check positioning and help with proper slice selection. The localizer can be a quick, short TR spin echo or gradient-echo T1-weighted scan with one acquisition and a 256 × 192 (readout × phase encoding) matrix. This is performed in a plane perpendicular to that used for the remainder of the exam. Unlike CT, which allows rapid addition of a few slices, MRI currently cannot add additional cuts to an examination. Thus, the completeness of an MR scan is judged by whether the region of interest has been fully covered. Some scanners provide a grid to assist in centering, and others actually draw the slices over the image for easy visualization and recentering if necessary. For subsequent series, the sequence parameters can be entered into the computer while the current data acquisition is still under way. This is a time-saving step, benefiting both the patient and the department. Current-generation scanners also permit simultaneous image reconstruction and acquisition.

In many cases, the examination includes three sequences in the same plane following the localizer; T2-weighted and T1-weighted sequences, followed by a second T1-weighted series after contrast injection if necessary. The longer sequences (multi-echo series) are often prescribed first because the patient is usually able to lie still much longer early in the study, and if the exam is terminated prematurely, the T2-weighted scans, often the most important for disease detection, will have been completed. Scans are typically set up with an interslice gap to minimize cross-talk, which degrades the signal-to-noise ratio (SNR) of the T1-weighted series and the contrast of the T2-weighted series. Copies of some specific protocols used at our institution on both a 1.0 and a 1.5T scanner are included in Appendix I as an introduction to sequence selection.

Head scans are performed in a volume coil (preferably of quadrature design) using a high-resolution 256 × 256 matrix. The general protocol begins with a 2-minute sagittal scout for slice orientation and lesion localization. The next series is a T2-weighted axial examination, lasting almost 11 minutes. Gradient moment nulling (GMN) and low bandwidth techniques are employed in this series. GMN compensates for artifacts generated by eye movement, venous blood flow, and cerebrospinal fluid (CSF) pulsation. High-frequency noise is reduced with low bandwidth techniques, improving the overall SNR.[27] (See Chapter 13 for a more complete discussion of these techniques.) The T2 weighting (TR/TE = 3000/90) of this sequence gives excellent contrast between normal and pathologic tissue in most instances. The second series is a high-resolution T1-weighted sequence. After contrast injection, this same sequence is repeated.[51,52] The protocol for internal auditory canal imaging follows the same general outline, with an emphasis on thin sections through the region of interest for improved lesion detection and depiction. To maintain adequate SNR, the number of acquisitions is doubled on T1-weighted scans. The advent of quadrature coils permits 2- to 3-mm sections to be obtained with high SNR using only two data acquisitions.

MRI of the thoracic and lumbar spine requires the patient to lie supine with a planar coil located under the area in question. Contoured coils are available for cervical spine imaging. Scout images can be run in the sagittal and axial planes to aid in patient positioning. The basic diagnostic sequences include thin-section T1-weighted scans in both the sagittal and axial planes. For proper evaluation of potential intrinsic spinal cord abnormalities, a T2-weighted sequence should also be employed. Contrast media are useful in differentiating postoperative scar from recurrent disc and for the detection and delineation of neoplastic disease.[53] The postcontrast T1-weighted series is run in the plane most suitable for viewing the abnormality with the same parameters used in the precontrast sequence. Chapters 5 through 7 offer a more detailed discussion of spine imaging.

Detection of hip, or femoral head, disease has been greatly improved with MRI due to the excellent visualization of bone marrow. The patient is positioned supine in the body coil and a relatively quick T1-weighted sequence is obtained in the axial plane for orientation. This is followed by a thin-section, heavily T1-weighted coronal pulse sequence (TR/TE = 500/15) with four acquisitions to obtain a high SNR. This scan is used primarily for detection of bone marrow disease and depiction of anatomic detail. The final series is a coronal T2-weighted spin echo sequence (TR/TE = 3000/45,90) with one acquisition. The T2-weighted scan is used for delineation of fluid collections and soft tissue masses, as well as providing a second look at bone marrow.

The fifth and last protocol covers the knee. The patient is supine with the abnormal knee in a small-diameter volume coil. To avoid wrap-around artifacts, the unaffected knee should be wrapped in shielding material, for example aluminum foil (covered with a cloth layer for insulation), when using a receive-only coil. Use of the smallest available volume coil increases the SNR and thus the spatial resolution which can be achieved, allowing improved detection of small meniscal tears. Due to the high SNR obtained with the volume coil, a maximum of two acquisitions is required in any of these sequences. The knee is initially scanned with 10° to 20° external rotation, employing a T1-weighted series followed by a T2-weighted sagittal series. Low bandwidth and motion-compensation techniques are applied in conjunction with the T2-weighted sequence to further increase the SNR and to minimize the artifacts created by the popliteal vein and artery. Slice thickness is held constant at 4 mm for the entire set of sequences. The final series is a coronal T1-weighted scan with the knee in neutral position.

SPECIAL TECHNIQUES

To minimize the problems due to respiratory motion, peristalsis, blood flow, and CSF pulsation, an understanding of the tradeoffs in changing scan parameters is required. These potential problems have also spurred the development of fast imaging techniques. Motion suppression was initially addressed by using physical restraints, such as a band to limit abdominal excursion, and by gating data acquisition to the cardiac or respiratory cycles.

Other approaches model the motion and pulse the gradients to minimize such motion artifacts. GMN, as commonly employed in the clinical setting, applies a first-order correction for the velocity effects of moving tissue, typically along the slice select and read axes. The correction may be applied along any combination of the three gradient directions. Higher-order corrections (second order for acceleration correction and third order for "jerk" correction) may also be performed. This technique, however, requires additional gradient pulses, increasing the minimum possible TE. This tends to detract from the T1 contrast of an image in short TR scans. An additional obstacle is the resulting increased signal from flowing blood, making vessels isointense to hyperintense with the surrounding soft tissue in many instances.[54-58] GMN is a fixed feature on most machines and is most often used in conjunction with T2-weighted sequences, permitting the desired TE values to be used.

Low bandwidth is another technique used to improve image quality. Low bandwidth uses an extended sampling period, eliminating much of the high-frequency noise. The decrease in noise yields an increase in the SNR.[59] Unfortunately, the weaker gradients used with low bandwidth techniques amplify chemical shift artifacts. This increase does not diminish the diagnostic quality of head and spine scans.[28,53] The technique is also applicable to T2-weighted imaging in the abdomen and musculoskeletal system (see Chapters 12 and 13).

The balance of image resolution and SNR is an important tradeoff to comprehend. Different manufacturers have different terminology for expressing the size of the area being scanned. The FOV is a direct measure of the size of the imaging volume. Other companies refer to fractions of a standard window as a zoom factor. For example, one manufacturer uses as the reference standard a width of 500 mm for the body coil and 300 mm for all other coils. A zoom factor greater than 1 means that the actual FOV, equal to the base value divided by the zoom factor, has been reduced. The SNR is proportional to the square of the FOV and therefore a reduced FOV, or a greater zoom, reduces the SNR. With small FOVs there is a level beyond which, despite the theoretically improved resolution, lesion detection becomes difficult and the SNR is no longer acceptable. When an enlarged view of an area is desired (e.g., the pituitary), it is advisable to zoom only to acceptable SNR limits and then photographically magnify the image for easier interpretation.

Equipment currently being installed has advanced capabilities that affect pulse sequence parameter selection. The ability to acquire thinner sections (2 mm) may become routine with new quadrature head coil designs for imaging of the pituitary and internal auditory canal (IAC). The increased SNR available with such coils allows routine half-Fourier imaging. This technique produces an image from slightly more than half as much data as usual, producing a substantial savings in imaging time.

Advances in instrumentation allow the use of matrix sizes other than the conventional 256×256, 256×128, or 128×128 matrices, as well as asymmetrical matrices. Pulse sequences permitting acquisition of thick and thin slices in the same scan have been developed and may improve imaging of the head.[60] Thin sections can be acquired through the posterior fossa, especially the IAC, with thick sections covering the remainder of the head to assess for other abnormalities. New gradient-coil control mechanisms allow shorter echo times, making breath-hold imaging a routine abdominal technique.[61] This may also permit shorter TR times while preserving the maximal allowable number of slices. Short TR times lead to 3D fast imaging techniques with improved T1 contrast and scan times under 10 minutes.[60] This approach, which allows acquisition of contiguous 1-mm sections through the entire intracranial contents, may be particularly useful in the study of congenital abnormalities and space-occupying lesions.

Progress is also being made in imaging and quantitating flow in vessels. This is being studied from various approaches, such as time-of-flight methods and MR angiography with motion-artifact suppression.[63-65] The ability to noninvasively measure flow rates could help greatly in the detection and treatment of stenotic vessel disease.

INSTRUMENTATION

Good image quality depends as much on the choice of pulse sequence as on instrumentation. Clinical superconducting imagers today have field strengths ranging from 0.3 to 2.0 T. Once field strength is chosen, the appropriate imaging coil must be selected. The objective in both of these decisions regarding instrumentation is to optimize the SNR of the scan.

Several distinctions exist between low-field (0.04–0.5 T) and high-field strength (1.0–2.0 T) imagers. Many investigators have reported a decrease in motion artifacts with low-field imaging systems, most evident in the thorax and abdominal areas. Artifactual ghosts resulting from motion are less apparent because of the generally weak signal strength of these systems. T1 relaxation times change with field strength. T2 relaxation times are similar for the range of field strengths encountered in MRI. Signal strength is higher with the high-field systems, yielding images with increased SNR. A stronger signal necessitates fewer acquisitions, so scan times are shortened. Use of contrast enhancement will probably not affect selection of field strength. Although minor differences can be seen, paramagnetic agents such as Gd DTPA are effective across the entire range of field strengths from 0.04 to 2.0 T.[66,67]

Image quality also depends on proper coil selection. Many surface and volume coils are receive-only coils, employing the body coil as the transmitter. The advantage of using a separate receiver coil is the increased SNR achieved in a focused region permitting the use of a smaller FOV. Surface-coil sensitivity is not uniform with distance from the surface. As a general rule, sensitivity is satisfactory to a distance of one radius (the shorter radius for an elliptical or rectangular coil) from the coil.[68] This is advantageous in spinal cord imaging because the anterior abdominal fat pad is usually farther than one radius from the receiver coil. At this distance, the intensity of the fat signal is much weaker and the associated respiratory motion artifacts are even weaker, reducing image degradation.

In an attempt to improve the SNR of surface-coil images, coil shapes are designed to resemble anatomic parts closely. For this reason, different coils are used routinely for the head, extremities, temporomandibular joint, and spine. Three basic coil shapes are planar coils for the lumbar spine, contoured coils for the cervical spine, and cylindrical (either Helmholtz or saddle type), as in the head and extremity coils. Other configurations under development include transrectal and transvaginal probes and "potato chip" coils for gonadal work.

Attention should be given to the orientation of the receive-only coil relative to the transmitter coil. To induce a current in the coil, it must be perpendicular to the magnetic field established by the transmitter coil. The two coils must also be decoupled. In newer generation machines, active decoupling, made possible by added electronics altering the sensitivity of the receiver coils, permits a greater range of safe coil orientations. The receiver is designed to be sensitive to weak signals generated by tissues and will overload if it receives the frequencies being emitted by the transmitter. Unless decoupled, the receiver coil may serve as an antenna to the RF emitted by the transmitter coil and redirect these energies. These stray energies can cause apparent signal voids in the image.[51] Coils that both transmit and receive have a fast relay electronic switch, which switches one coil off while the other functions. The disadvantage in these coils is the nonuniformity of transmission across the FOV.

A recent advance in coil design, now standard in new-generation scanners, is the quadrature coil.[69] Such a configuration can lead to a gain in SNR of up to 40%. Unfortunately, these coils cannot be retrofitted to linearly polarized systems without substantial modification. Coils can also be designed for pediatric anatomy.[70,71]

Further instrumentation optimization will improve image acquisition and processing speeds. With breath-hold and FLASH scanning, the time required to reconstruct the data factors heavily into the overall examination time. Most MR systems do not permit new acquisitions before the previous data has been reconstructed.[27] As faster computers and secondary processors for increased raw data handling are added to MR systems, data acquisition and image reconstruction will be able to run concurrently.

IMAGE STORAGE AND PRESENTATION

Once acquired, images are commonly photographed on hard copy and archived to a storage device. The most common format for photography is 15 on 1 on a 14 × 17-inch sheet of film. Each image should be magnified to fill the entire frame. The slices can be anatomically arranged, and each series can be photographed separately. For a double-echo T2-weighted sequence, the images from each echo are photographed on separate sheets. This means that with a TR/TE = 3000/45,90 sequence, all of the TE 45 slices are arranged anatomically on one sheet and all of the 90-ms slices are anatomically arranged on a second sheet. During interpretation, the two sheets can be hung next to each other. When exams focus on small parts of the anatomy, as in the IAC, the images need to be further magnified before filming. These enlarged views can be photographed on a separate sheet of film.

Laser cameras have helped speed up photography and developing. Most laser cameras have a batch film process, featuring combined exposed and unexposed film magazines, eliminating individual sheet and cassette handling. At some sites the unit is connected directly to the processor, facilitating the development process as well.

In addition to hard-copy filming, images are typically archived on a computer storage device. The most familiar options are floppy disk, magnetic tape, or optical disk. Floppy disks will not hold a complete case and are only useful for minimal data transfer from one computer to another. Magnetic tapes have a capacity of approximately 180 images, the equivalent of four standard cases. The 12-inch optical disk is two-sided, with a combined memory of 2 gigabytes or 15,000 images. This memory capacity will increase with further developments in optical data handling. Disks are also limited in that they may only be written to once; if a file is erased, it cannot be replaced. Erasable disks are now entering the market. The optical system is economical, space-saving, and extremely fast for both archival storage and retrieval, and thus it is the most sensible option available today.

Additional data processing may be accomplished with a 3D workstation. A series of images can be reformatted from a 3D FLASH data set in any user-defined plane (Fig. 14-1), including curved planes to follow the spinal cord in a patient with scoliosis. These high-resolution slices are subject to minimal volume averaging effects. It is possible to perform gray-scale surface modeling to depict the tissue of interest in 3D in any orientation in space and at any depth (Figs. 14-2 and 14-3). Current developments allow vessel and tissue segmentation, producing venous angiograms or separated soft tissue structures. These workstations can also be used for cardiac cine display and for the display of MR angiograms.

Following in the path of 3D workstations is console examination reading. As picture archival stations (PACS) make their way into radiology departments, digital modalities such as MRI may become filmless. Auxiliary consoles could be located in reading rooms, scattered through the department and throughout the hospital, on patient floors and in operating rooms, permitting the physician to type in the hospital identification number and view images. When combined with a conventional word processing screen, the examination report would be available simultaneously.

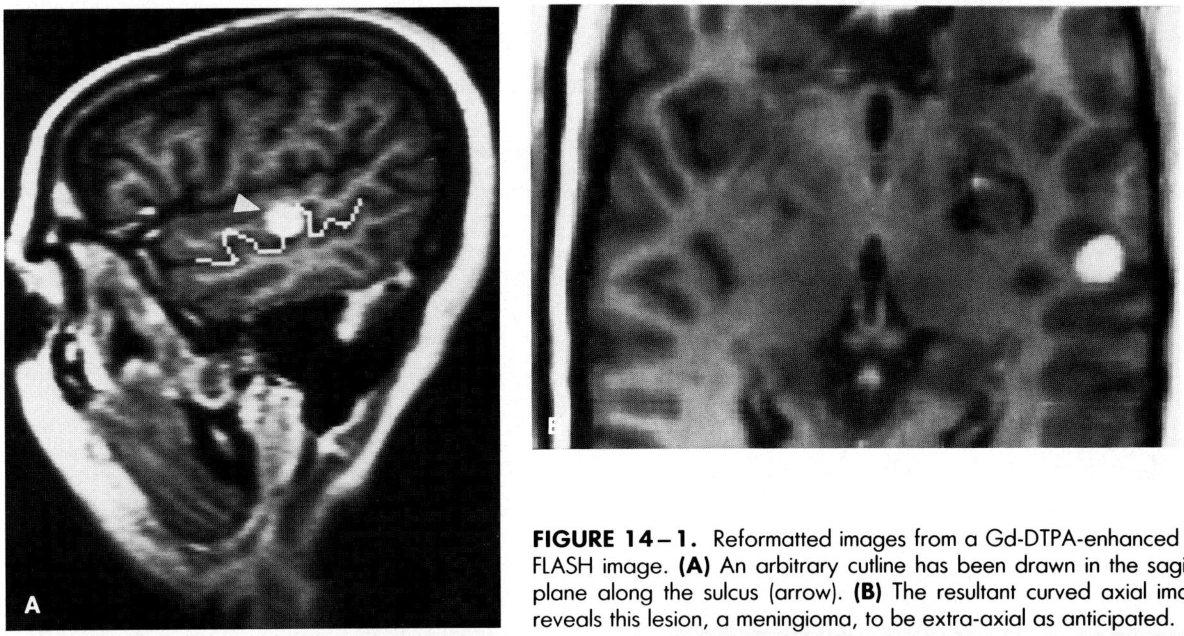

FIGURE 14-1. Reformatted images from a Gd-DTPA-enhanced 3D FLASH image. **(A)** An arbitrary cutline has been drawn in the sagittal plane along the sulcus (arrow). **(B)** The resultant curved axial image reveals this lesion, a meningioma, to be extra-axial as anticipated.

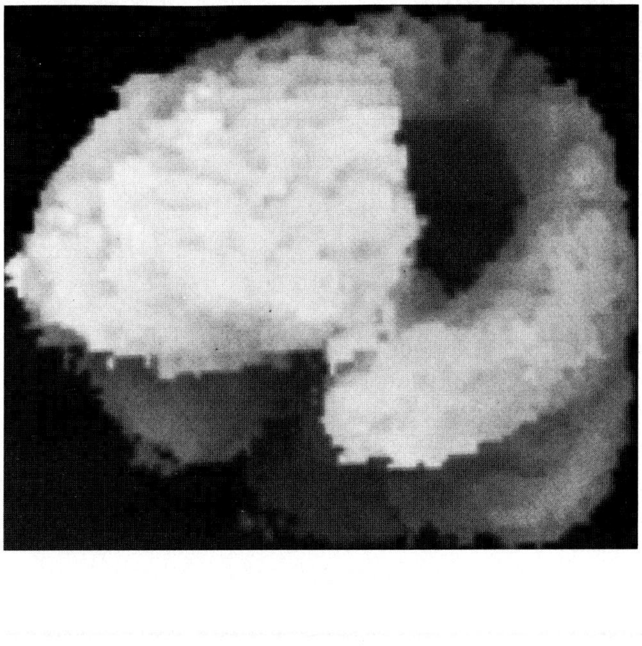

FIGURE 14-2. Tissue segmentation applied to a 3D FLASH study in a patient with schizencephaly. The data were collected in the sagittal plane, segmented to isolate the brain, and reformatted in rotations about the y-axis (45° rotation displayed).

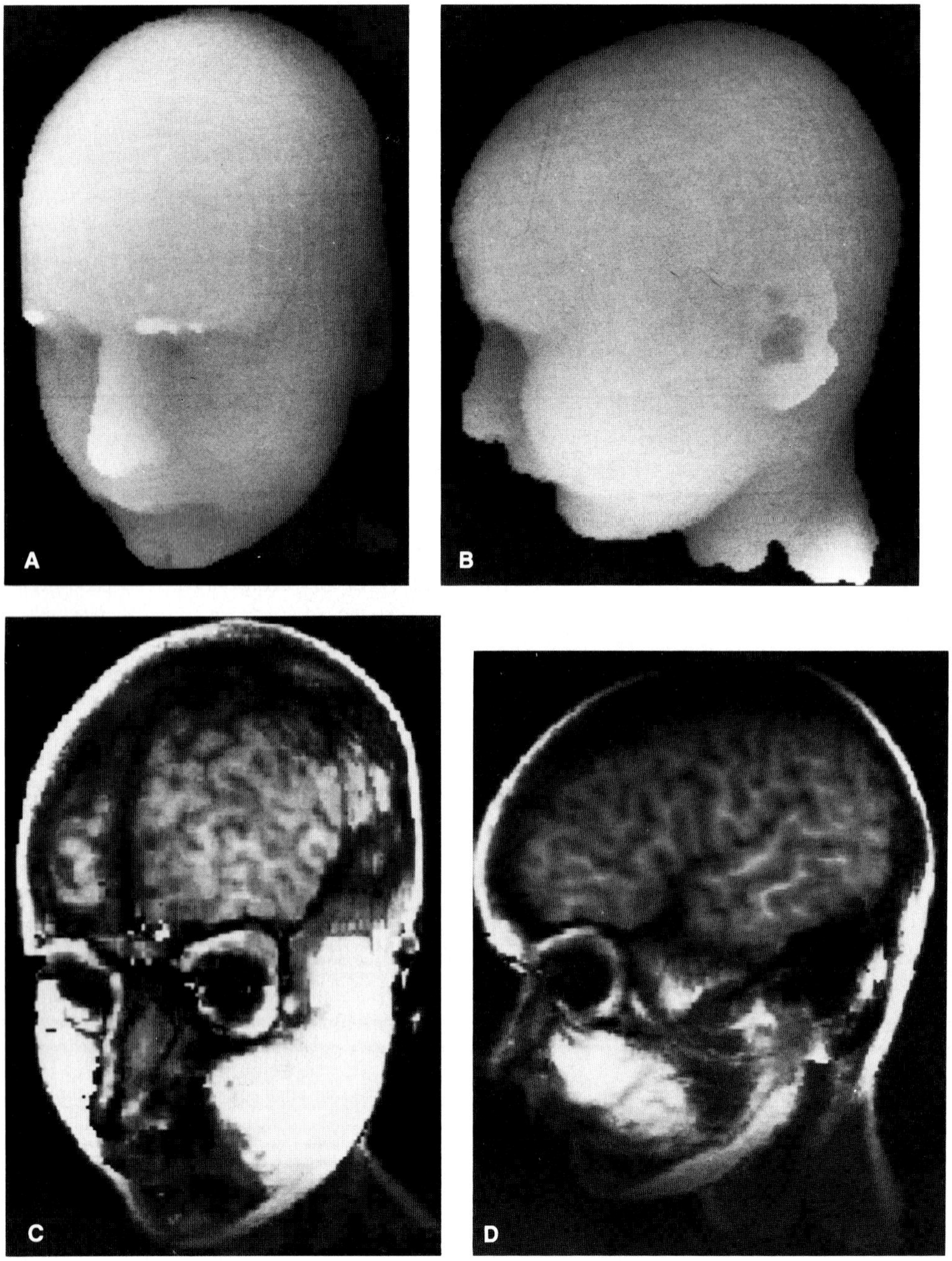

FIGURE 14–3. (A,B) Gray scale surface modeling performed with a 3D FLASH study of a pediatric patient. The data was collected in the sagittal plane and rotated after reconstruction to allow visualization from two perspectives. **(C,D)** Depiction of structures 12 mm below the skin surface as viewed from a point source, again using the surface modeling algorithm. (Runge VM. Flash: Clinical three-dimensional magnetic resonance imaging. Radiographics 1988;8:957)

Films will then be necessary only for mailing to other institutions.

CONCLUSION

As the field of MRI continues to expand, it is becoming increasingly important that radiologists be versed in the science behind it. Although hailed as a safe noninvasive modality, untoward events can occur if proper precautions are not followed. Simple preventative steps include the use of a strong hand-held magnet to test questionable metallic materials before bringing them within the 5-gauss line. Walk unsure patients slowly into the room, watching for any strange sensation in the region of their implant. When reviewing the literature for the safety of an implant in a magnetic field, check the field strength at which the device was tested. Much of the early testing was performed at 0.6T, whereas today many MR imagers operate at 1.0 and 1.5T.

An easy and effective risk-management program includes three steps:

1. Physical security around the high field area (e.g., a padlock)
2. Educating the people responsible for the area, including maintenance personnel

3. Screening everyone who enters the area: patients, family members, attending physicians and other visitors.

Optimal image quality is obtained with a cooperative patient when appropriate coil selection and positioning and pulse sequence choices are made.

REFERENCES

1. Fullerton GD. Basic concepts for nuclear magnetic resonance imaging. Magn Reson Imaging 1982;1:39.
2. Dixon RL, Ekstrand KE. The physics of proton NMR. Med Physics 1982;9:807.
3. Foster MA, Hutchinson JMS. Practical NMR imaging. Oxford: IRL Press, 1987.
4. Barnett GH, Ropper AH, Johnson KA. Physiological support and monitoring of critically ill patients during magnetic resonance imaging. J Neurosurg 1988;68:246.
5. Karlik SJ, Heatherley T, Pavan F, et al. Patient anesthesia and monitoring at a 1.5 T MRI installation. Magn Reson Med 1988;7:210.
6. Kanal E, Burk DL, Brunberg JA, et al. Pediatric musculoskeletal magnetic resonance imaging. Radiol Clin North Am 1988;26:211.
7. Weinreb JC, Maravilla KR, Peshock R, Payne J. Magnetic resonance imaging: improving patient tolerance and safety. AJR 1984;143:1285.
8. Merritt CRB. Magnetic resonance imaging—a clinical perspective: image quality, safety and risk management. Radiographics 1987;7:1001.
9. Stark DD, Bradley WG. Magnetic resonance imaging. St. Louis: CV Mosby, 1988.
10. Shellock FG, Crues JV. Safety considerations in magnetic resonance imaging. MRI Decisions 1988;2:25.
11. Kanal E, Shellock F, Sonenblick D. MRI clinical site survey: phase I results and preliminary data. Program and abstracts of the Seventh Annual Meeting of the Society of Magnetic Resonance Imaging, 1989, Los Angeles, CA.
12. Erlebacher JA, Cahill PT, Pamizzo F, et al. Effect of magnetic resonance imaging on DDD pacemakers. Am J Cardiol 1988;57:437.
13. Shellock FG, Crues JV. High-field-strength MR imaging and metallic biomedical implants. AJR 1988;151:389.
14. Davis PL, Crooks L, Arakawa M, et al. Potential hazards in NMR imaging: heating effects of changing magnetic fields and RF fields on small metallic implants. AJR 1981;137:857.
15. Leon JA, Gabriele OF. Middle ear prosthesis: significance in magnetic resonance imaging. Magn Reson Imaging 1987;5:405.
16. Applebaum EL, Valvassori GE. Effects of magnetic resonance imaging fields on stapedectomy prostheses. Arch Otolaryngol 1985;111:820.
17. Mattucci KF, Setzen M, Hyman R, Chaturvedi G. The effects of nuclear magnetic resonance imaging on metallic middle ear prostheses. Otolaryngol Head Neck Surg 1986;94:441.
18. Randall PA, Kohman LJ, Scalzetti EM, et al. Magnetic resonance imaging of prosthetic cardiac valves in vitro and in vivo. Am J Cardiol 1988;62:973.
19. Soulen RL, Budinger TF, Higgins CB. Magnetic resonance imaging of prosthetic heart valves. Radiology 1985;154:705.
20. Shellock FG. MR imaging of metallic implants and materials: a compilation of the literature. AJR 1988;151:811.
21. Mark AS, Hricak H. Intrauterine contraceptive devices: MR imaging. Radiology 1987;162:311.
22. Kelly WM, Paglen PG, Pearson JA, et al. Ferromagnetic unilateral blindness after MR study. AJNR 1986;7:243.
23. Powell MC, Worthington BS, Buckley JM, et al. Magnetic resonance imaging (MRI) in obstetrics. I. Maternal anatomy. Br J Obstet Gynaecol 1988;95:31.
24. Powell MC, Worthington BS, Buckley JM, et al. Magnetic resonance imaging (MRI) in obstetrics. II. Fetal anatomy. Br J Obstet Gynaecol 1988;95:38.
25. Hill MC, Lande IM, Larsen JW. Prenatal diagnosis of fetal anomalies using ultrasound and MRI. Radiol Clin North Am 1988;26:287.
26. Niendorf HP. Tolerance and safety of Gd-DTPA in 7000 patients: a review. Diagn Imag Int 1988;4:16.
27. Runge VR, Gelblum DY, Pacetti MI, et al. Optimizing MRI protocols: brain. MRI Decisions 1989;3:2.
28. Powers TA, Partain CL, Kessler RM, et al. Central nervous system lesions in pediatric patients: Gd-DTPA-enhanced MR imaging. Radiology 1988;169:723.
29. Magnevist—the first paramagnetic enhancement agent for MRI. Brochure: 890-07/July 1988. Wayne, NJ: Berlex Laboratories.
30. Brennan SC, Redd WH, Jacobsen PB, et al. Anxiety and panic during magnetic resonance scans. Lancet 1988;2:512.
31. Quirk ME, Letendre AJ, Ciottone RA, et al. Anxiety in patients undergoing MR imaging. Radiology 1989;170:463.
32. McEvoy GK. AHFS American Hospital Formulary Service: drug information 87. Bethesda: American Society of Hospital Pharmacists, 1987.
33. Ryan JF. A practice of anesthesia for infants and children. Orlando, FL: Grune & Stratton, 1986.
34. Whitehead BG, Durr DP, Adair SM, Proskin HM. Monitoring of sedated pediatric dental patients. ASDC J Dent Child 1988;55:329.
35. Thompson JR, Schneider S, Ashwal S, et al. The choice of sedation for computed tomography in children: a prospective evaluation. Radiology 1982;143:475.
36. Sander JE, Low W. Computed tomographic premedication in children [Letter]. JAMA 1983;249:2639.
37. Nahata MC. Sedation in pediatric patients undergoing diagnostic procedures. Drug Intell Clin Pharm 1988;22:711.
38. Benusis KP, Kapaun D, Furnam LJ. Respiratory depression in a child following meperidine, promethazine, and chlorpromazine premedication: report of a case. ASDC J Dent Child 1979;46:50.
39. Weir MR, Segapeli JH, Tremper LJ. Sedation for pediatric procedures. Milit Med 1986;151:181.
40. Nahata MC, Clotz MA, Krogg EA. Adverse effects of meperidine, promethazine, and chlorpromazine for sedation in pediatric patients. Clin Pediatr 1985;24:558.
41. Strain JD, Harvey LA, Foley LC, et al. Intravenously administered pentobarbital sodium for sedation in pediatric CT. Pediatr Radiol 1986;161:105.
42. Lucida R, Seleny FL, Goodarzi M, et al. Dose-finding study of intramuscular midazolam in children. Anesthesiol Rev 1985;12:40.
43. Anderson JA, Vann WF. Respiratory monitoring during pediatric sedation: pulse oximetry and capnography. Pediatr Dent 1988;10:94.
44. Mueller WA, Drummond JN, Pribisco TA, et al. Pulse oximetry monitoring of sedated pediatric dental patients. Anesth Prog 1985;32:237.
45. Shellock FG. Monitoring during MRI: an evaluation of the effect of high-field MRI on various patient monitors. Medical Electronics 1986;17:93.
46. Gregory GA. Pediatric anesthesia. Vol 1. New York: Churchill Livingstone, 1983.
47. Shapiro BA. Oxygenation: measurement and clinical assessment. Refresher course in anesthesiology. Philadelphia: JB Lippincott, 1979:195.
48. American Heart Association. Standards and guidelines for cardiopulmonary resuscitation and emergency care. JAMA 1986;255:2905.
49. American Academy of Pediatrics. Guidelines for the elective use of conscious sedation, deep sedation, and general anesthesia in pediatric patients. Pediatrics 1985;76:317.
50. ElBadrawy HE, Riekman GA. A survey of parental attitudes toward sedation of their child. Pediatr Dent 1986;8:206.
51. Runge VM, ed. Enhanced magnetic resonance imaging. St. Louis: CV Mosby, 1989.
52. Carollo BR, Wolf CR, Pacetti MI, et al. Prospective evaluation of Gd-DTPA in 105 consecutive cranial cases. Radiology 1988;169:339.

53. Runge VM, Wood ML, Kaufman DM, et al. The straight and narrow path to good head and spine MRI. Radiographics 1988;8:507.
54. Colletti PM, Raval JK, Benson RC, et al. The motion artifact suppression technique (MAST) in magnetic resonance imaging: clinical results. Magn Reson Imaging 1988;6:293.
55. Mitchell DG, Vinitski S, Burk DL, et al. Motion artifact reduction in MR imaging of the abdomen: gradient moment nulling versus respiratory-sorted phase encoding. Radiology 1988;169:155.
56. Ester AD. Motion artifact suppression technique (MAST) for cranial MR imaging: superiority over cardiac gating for reducing phase shift artifacts. AJNR 1988;9:671.
57. Quencer RM, Hinks RS, Pattany PH. Improved MR imaging of the brain by using compensating gradients to suppress motion-induced artifacts. AJR 1988;151:163.
58. Edelman RR, Atkinson DJ, Silver MS, et al. FRODO pulse sequences: a new means of eliminating motion, flow and wrap-around artifacts. Radiology 1988;166:321.
59. Wolf C, Carollo B, Runge V. MRI of the brain: new techniques for improving image quality. Siemens pamphlet (in press).
60. Runge VM, Wood ML, Carollo BR, et al. Combined acquisition of thin and thick sections within one imaging sequence. [Abstract] Magn Reson Imaging 1989;7:132.
61. Wolf CR, Wood ML, Runge et al. Artifact free MRI: two new breath-hold techniques. Proceedings of the Society of Magnetic Resonance Imaging annual meeting, 1989, Los Angeles, CA.
62. Runge VM, Wood ML, Kaufman DM, et al. FLASH: clinical three-dimensional magnetic resonance imaging. Radiographics 1988;8:947.
63. James TL, Margulis AR. Biomedical magnetic resonance. San Francisco: Radiology Research and Education Foundation, 1984.
64. Dumoulin CL, Hart HR. Magnetic resonance angiography. Radiology 1986;161:717.
65. Chenevert TL, Fechner KP, Gelblum DY. Utility of motion corrective gradients for MR angiography and motion artifact suppression. Proceedings of the Sixth Annual Meeting of the Society of Magnetic Resonance in Medicine, 1987, New York, NY.
66. Pearce RB. MRI at ultra-low fields—can less really be better? Diagn Imag 1988;10:112.
67. Runge VM, Clanton JA, Herzer WA, et al. The field strength dependence of contrast enhancement with gadolinium DTPA in MRI. Proceedings of the Third Annual Meeting of the Society of Magnetic Resonance in Medicine, 1987, New York, NY.
68. Lufkin R, Votruba J, Reicher M, et al. Solenoid surface coils in magnetic resonance imaging. AJR 1986;146:409.
69. Hyde JS, Jesmanowicz A, Grist TM, et al. Quadrature detection surface coil. Magn Reson Med 1987;4:179.
70. Requardt H, Offermann J, Kess H, et al. Surface coil with variable geometry: a new tool for MRI imaging of the spine. Radiology 1987;165:574.
71. Doornbos J, Grimbergen HAA, Booijen PE, et al. Application of anatomically shaped surface coils in MRI at 0.5 T. Magn Reson Med 1986;3:270.
72. Food and Drug Administration. Magnetic resonance diagnostic device: panel recommendation and report on petitions for MR reclassification. Rockville, MD, Center for Devices and Radiological Health, 1988.

APPENDIX

Table 14–1. **Head Screening Examination**

SCAN #	AX	TR	TE	MATRIX	ACQ.	SL*	TIME
Scout	sag	500	15	192	1	5–7/30%	1.6
1†	ax	2500	45,90	256	1	7–8/30%	10.7
2‡	ax	600	22	256	1	7–8/30%	2.6
3§	ax	600	22	256	1	7–8/30%	2.6

Acquisition time is given in minutes; FOV = 25 cm for all series.
* Slice thickness/interslice gap.
† This should be a low bandwidth, motion-compensated technique.
‡ This should be a motion-compensated technique.
§ With 0.1 mmol/kg I.V. Gd DTPA.

Table 14–2. **Internal Auditory Canal**

SCAN #	AX	TR	TE	MATRIX	ACQ.	SL*	TIME
Scout	sag	500	15	192	1	5/30%	1.6
1	ax	3000	45,90	256	1	3/30%	12.8
2	ax	500	22	256	4	3/30%	8.5
3†	ax	500	22	256	4	3/30%	8.5

Acquisition time is given in minutes; FOV = 25 cm for all series.
* Slice thickness/interslice gap.
† With 0.1 mmol/kg I.V. Gd DTPA.

Table 14–3. **Lumbar Spine (r/o HNP)**

SCAN #	AX	TR	TE	MATRIX	ACQ.	SL*	TIME
Scout	sag	125	10	128	1	5	0.2
1†	sag	450	20	256	4	4/30%	7.7
2‡	ax	550	10	256	3	3/30%	7.0
3	sag	3000	45,90	256	1	4/30%	12.8

Acquisition time is given in minutes; FOV = 25 cm for all series.
* Slice thickness/interslice gap.
† This should be a low bandwidth technique.
‡ Twenty-one slices should cover L3-4 to L5-S1 disc spaces.

Table 14–4. **Hips**

SCAN #	AX	TR	TE	MATRIX	ACQ.	SL*	TIME
Scout	ax	500	10	256	3	4/30%	6.4
1	cor	500	15	256	4	4–5/30%	8.5
2	cor	3000	45,90	256	1	4–5/30%	12.8

Acquisition time is given in minutes; FOV = 40 cm for all series.
* Slice thickness/interslice gap.

Table 14–5. **Knee**

SCAN #	AX	TR	TE	MATRIX	ACQ.	SL*	TIME
1†	sag	750	15	256	2	4/30%	6.4
2‡	sag	3000	45,90	256	1	4/30%	12.8
3†	cor	750	15	256	2	4/30%	6.4

Acquisition time is given in minutes; FOV = 15 cm for all series.
* Slice thickness/interslice gap.
† Meniscal windows also should be shot on film from the T1-weighted scans.
‡ This should be a low bandwidth, motion-compensated technique.

15

Contrast Media

Val M. Runge

This chapter focuses on the clinical use of gadolinium (Gd) DTPA for contrast enhancement in magnetic resonance imaging (MRI) of the head and spine. The structure of Gd DTPA (Fig. 15-1) is that of a paramagnetic metal ion (Gd^{3+}) bound firmly by a chelate (DTPA). The use of this type of agent for contrast enhancement was first suggested in 1982.[1-3] Clinical trials began in the United States during 1984, leading to FDA approval in 1988.[4-12]

The safety of this agent depends on the strength of the ionic bonds between Gd and DTPA. After intravenous injection, the compound is excreted intact by glomerular filtration. Gd^{3+} affects proton relaxation and reduces T1 and T2 relaxation times. This increases signal intensity on T1-weighted images.

To correctly interpret scans acquired after Gd DTPA administration, one should be familiar with normal patterns of enhancement. The choroid plexus and pituitary infundibulum are strongly enhanced after Gd DTPA, but the falx and meninges are not (Fig. 15-2). Enhancement of venous, but not arterial, structures is also typically observed after contrast administration. This phenomenon results from a combination of flow effects and the reduction in T1 by intravascular Gd DTPA.

To simplify the examination, we usually place an intravenous line before the patient enters the scan room. After acquiring precontrast images, Gd DTPA is injected over a 2- to 3-minute period by means of a peripheral port without moving the patient table. Lack of nausea with Gd DTPA permits this approach.

A prospective interpretation of 50 phase II and III examinations in 1986 revealed that intravenous Gd DTPA improved lesion visualization and characterization (Fig. 15-3).[10] Our experience, which included more than 700 patients by March 1989, can be used to confirm and expand these conclusions. For clarity, in most cases we present three spin echo images: the precontrast T2-weighted and T1-weighted images and the postcontrast T1-weighted images.

HEAD ABNORMALITIES

Extra-axial Neoplasia

Small meningiomas and acoustic neuromas can be isointense with surrounding normal structures, regardless of the choice of pulse technique.[13] There may also be little distortion of adjacent normal anatomy. Thus, these lesions can be difficult to diagnose on unenhanced MRI.

Gd DTPA improves the sensitivity of MRI in the diagnosis of intracanalicular acoustic neuromas. In a prospective study of 225 consecutive cranial cases at our institution, three intracanalicular acoustic neuromas were not visualized on unenhanced scans (Fig. 15-4). In each case, the T1-weighted Gd-DTPA-enhanced image was diagnostic. Gd DTPA can also be useful in large acoustic neuromas for defining the extent of intracanalicular disease and recognizing necrosis.[14,15]

All of 21 acoustic neuromas in a recent study dem-

Major portions of this chapter are reprinted with permission from Runge VM, Carollo BR, Wolf CR, et al. Gd DTPA: a review of clinical implications in the CNS. Radiographics 1989;9:929.

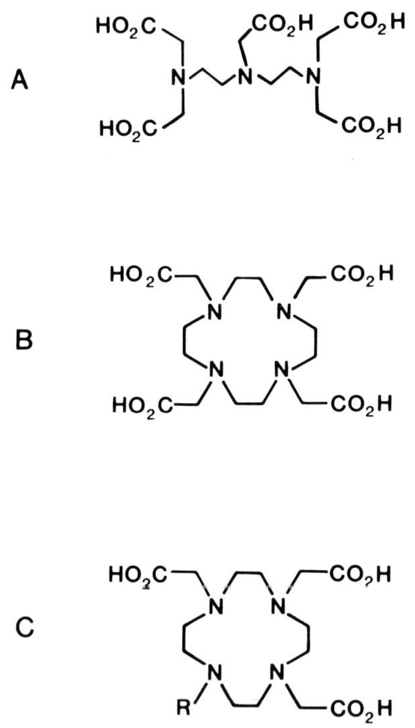

FIGURE 15–1. Ligand structures for *(A)* DTPA, *(B)* DOTA, and *(C)* DO3A-R. In the fully dissociated state, these three ligands carry charges of *(A)* -5, *(B)* -4, and *(C)* -3. Due to the 3+ charge of the gadolinium ion, the chelates of this metal with DTPA and DOTA must be prepared as salts, typically sodium or meglumine. Gd DO3A-R is a nonionic compound. Thus, the osmolality of these three MRI contrast agents, for a given gadolinium concentration, ranks as follows: Gd DTPA > Gd DOTA > Gd DO3A-R.

onstrated contrast enhancement with Gd DTPA on MRI.[15] Improved depiction of intracanalicular disease, compared with unenhanced MRI and enhanced computed tomography (CT), was shown, confirming our findings. The authors also concluded that, although necrotic or cystic changes within these lesions can be demonstrated on T2-weighted images, enhanced MRI may prove superior.

Small meningiomas can be missed on unenhanced exams due to the similarity of their T1 and T2 values with normal brain and to the frequent absence of substantial mass effect or accompanying cerebral edema (Figs. 15–5 and 15–6). With large lesions, Gd DTPA can be essential for identifying the extent of the lesion (Fig. 15–7). These lesions often grow along the skull base or cerebral convexity, two areas that have been poorly visualized in the past with x-ray CT due to beam-hardening artifacts. Although growth of meningiomas in this fashion can be visualized on unenhanced MRI, there is no question that contrast enhancement improves depiction of the full extent of the lesion.

Extra-axial lesions display contrast enhancement with Gd DTPA on the basis of vascularity. We strongly recommend use of this agent in any patient with suspicion of an extra-axial lesion, particularly in evaluating the internal auditory canal and meningeal disease. Intracanalicular acoustic neuromas, small meningiomas, and meningeal disease of any type can easily be overlooked on unenhanced MRI (Fig. 15–8).

Intra-axial Neoplasia

Contrast enhancement with Gd DTPA improves visualization of metastatic lesions in the brain.[17] With intra-axial neoplasia, enhancement occurs due to disruption of the blood-brain barrier.[18,19]

Small metastatic lesions, particularly those adjacent to cerebrospinal fluid (CSF), may be missed on unenhanced MRI. This is illustrated in a 61-year-old man with metastatic melanoma. Two lesions that enhanced after Gd DTPA (Fig. 15–9) were not observed prospectively on the unenhanced T1-weighted and T2-weighted images. Gd DTPA improved sensitivity and specificity in this case. The multiplicity of enhancing lesions favors the diagnosis of metastatic disease. Plans for treatment of this patient were changed, because he had been scheduled for resection of a large, presumed solitary, lesion in the right parietal lobe (not shown).

Gd DTPA is commonly employed for improved depiction of primary intracranial neoplastic disease (Figs. 15–10 and 15–11). Although contrast enhancement does aid in selecting a site for stereotaxic biopsy, it may not identify the true extent of the lesion. With

(text continues on page 524)

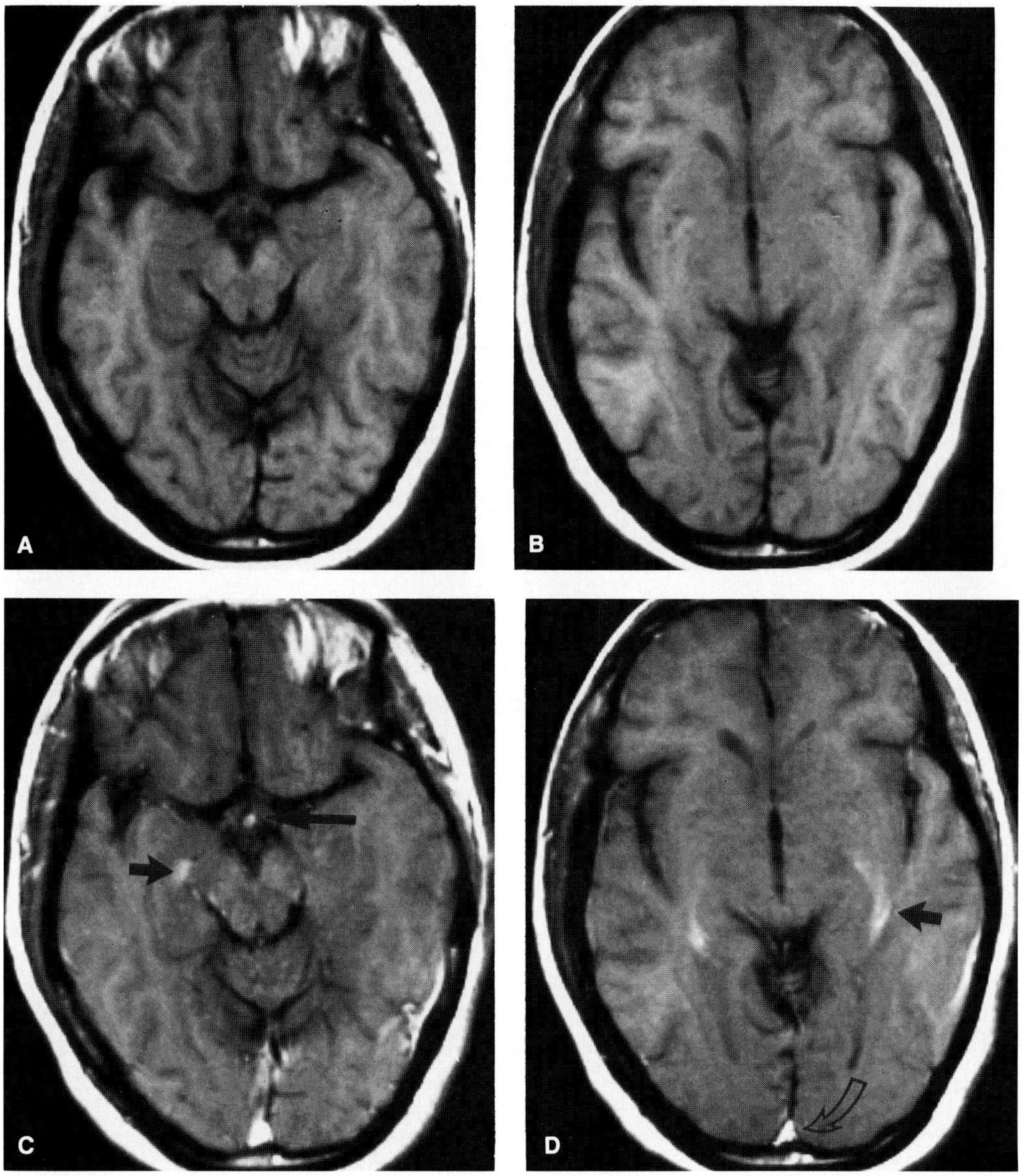

FIGURE 15–2. Normal brain: Comparison of **(A,B)** unenhanced and **(C,D)** enhanced T1-weighted brain images (TR/TE = 650/20). In this and all subsequent cases, the contrast agent used is meglumine Gd DTPA (Berlex Laboratories, New Jersey) in a dosage of 0.1 mmol/kg intravenously. Acquisition of the postcontrast scan begins approximately 1 minute after completion of the injection. Notice the normal enhancement of choroid (arrowhead), infundibulum (closed arrow), and venous structures like the superior sagittal sinus (open arrow). The falx and arterial vessels do not brightly enhance in the normal patient with spin echo technique; notice the lack of enhancement of the middle cerebral artery.

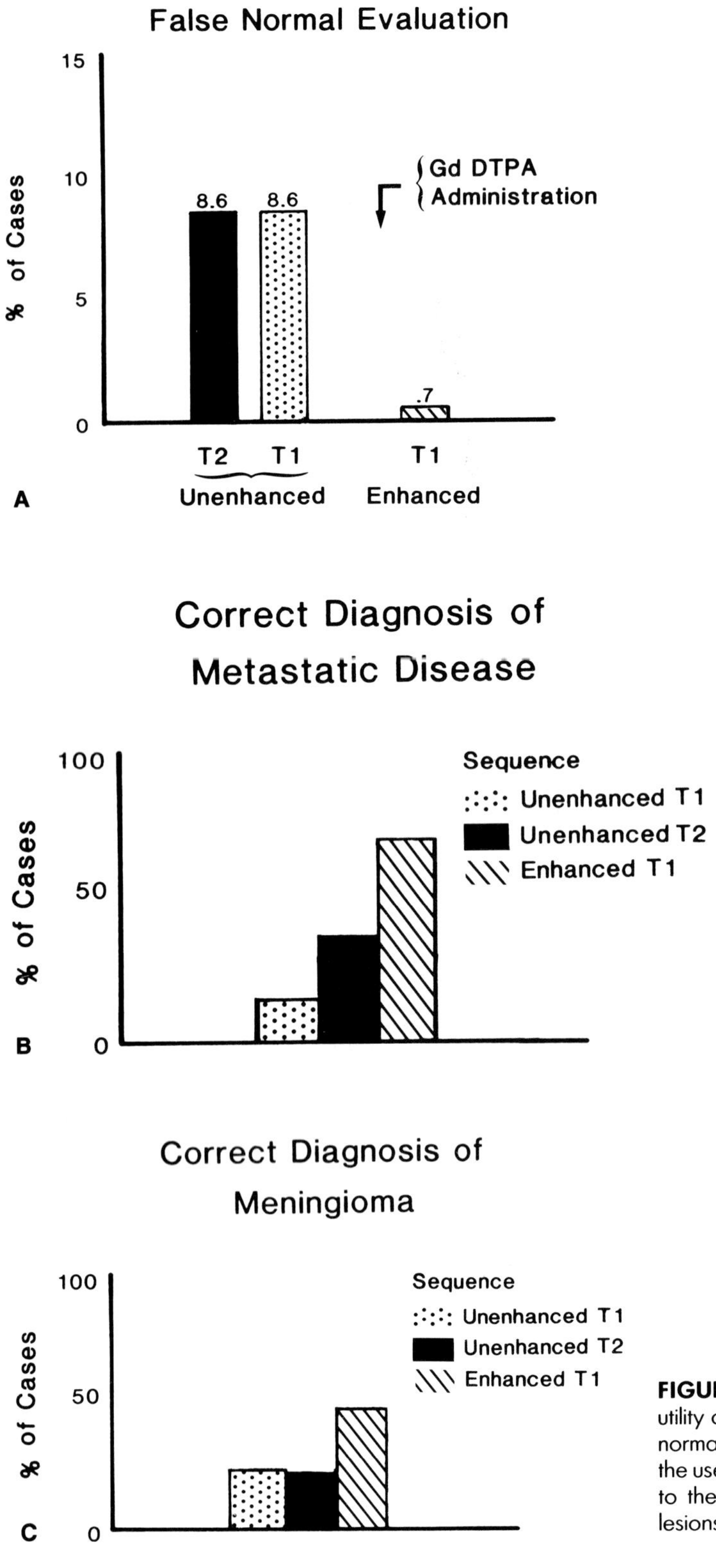

FIGURE 15–3. Results from a blind randomized study examining the utility of Gd DTPA administration in head scans. **(A)** The number of false normal results was reduced from approximately 9% to less than 1% by the use of Gd DTPA. **(B,C)** Diagnostic specificity was also improved, due to the pattern of enhancement and to the visualization of additional lesions in the case of metastatic disease.

FIGURE 15–5. Temporal fossa meningioma. **(A)** T2-weighted and **(B,C)** T1-weighted pre- and post-Gd DTPA images. Small meningiomas can be difficult to identify on unenhanced scans because these lesions are often isointense with normal brain tissue. The absence of secondary signs, such as mass effect or associated cerebral edema, make lesion recognition even more difficult. Diagnosis depends upon enhancement after intravenous Gd DTPA administration (arrow), which occurs because of abnormal vascularity. (Runge VM, ed. Enhanced magnetic resonance imaging. St. Louis: CV Mosby, 1989) ▶

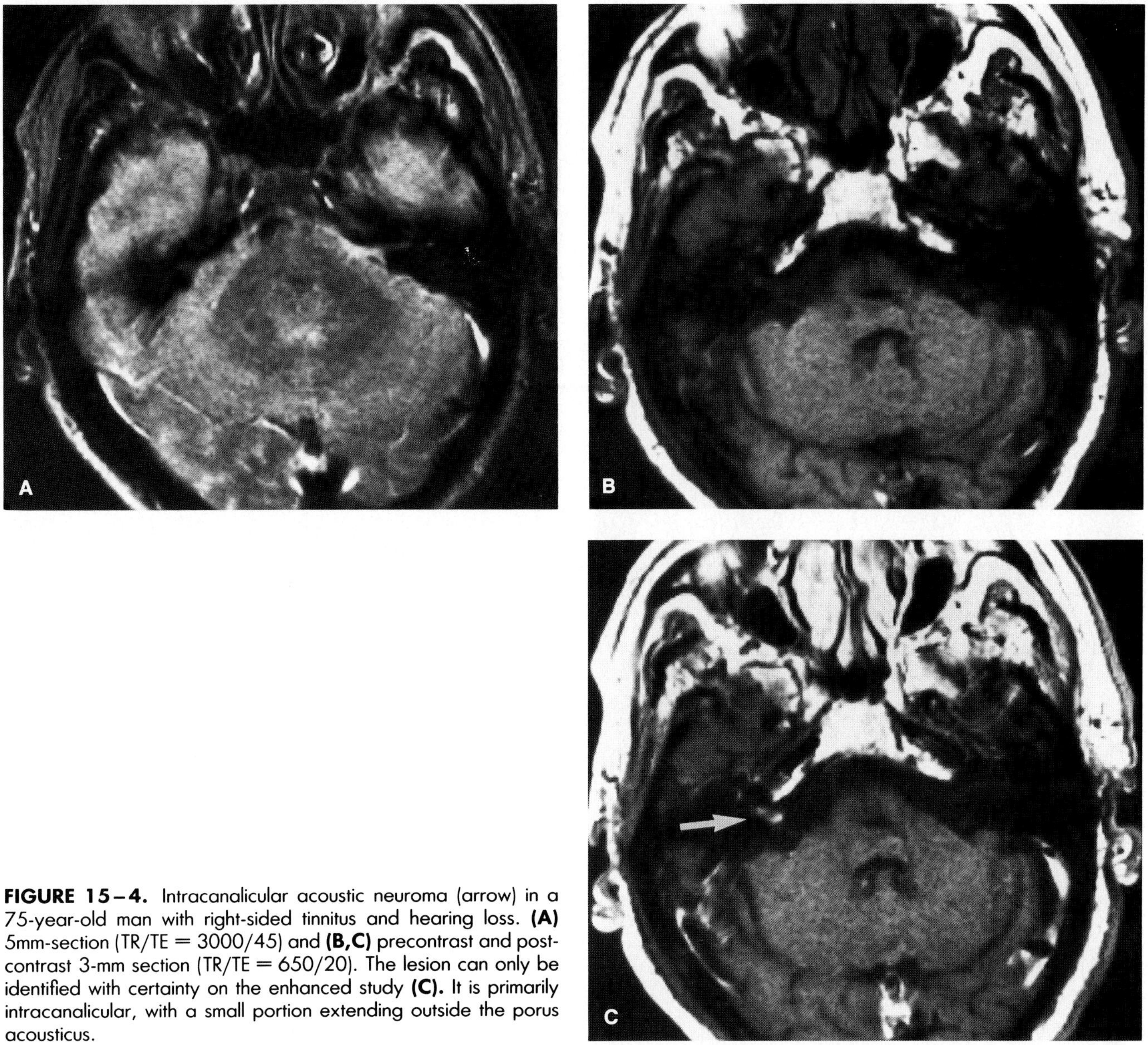

FIGURE 15–4. Intracanalicular acoustic neuroma (arrow) in a 75-year-old man with right-sided tinnitus and hearing loss. **(A)** 5mm-section (TR/TE = 3000/45) and **(B,C)** precontrast and post-contrast 3-mm section (TR/TE = 650/20). The lesion can only be identified with certainty on the enhanced study **(C).** It is primarily intracanalicular, with a small portion extending outside the porus acousticus.

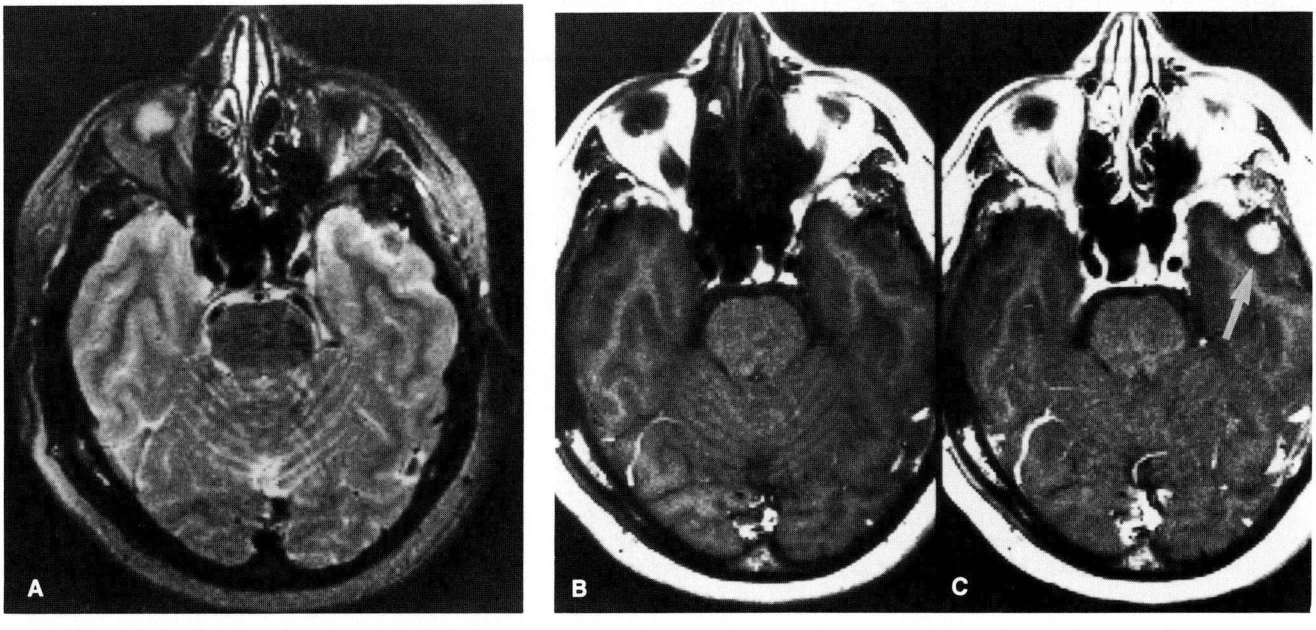

Figure 15–5.

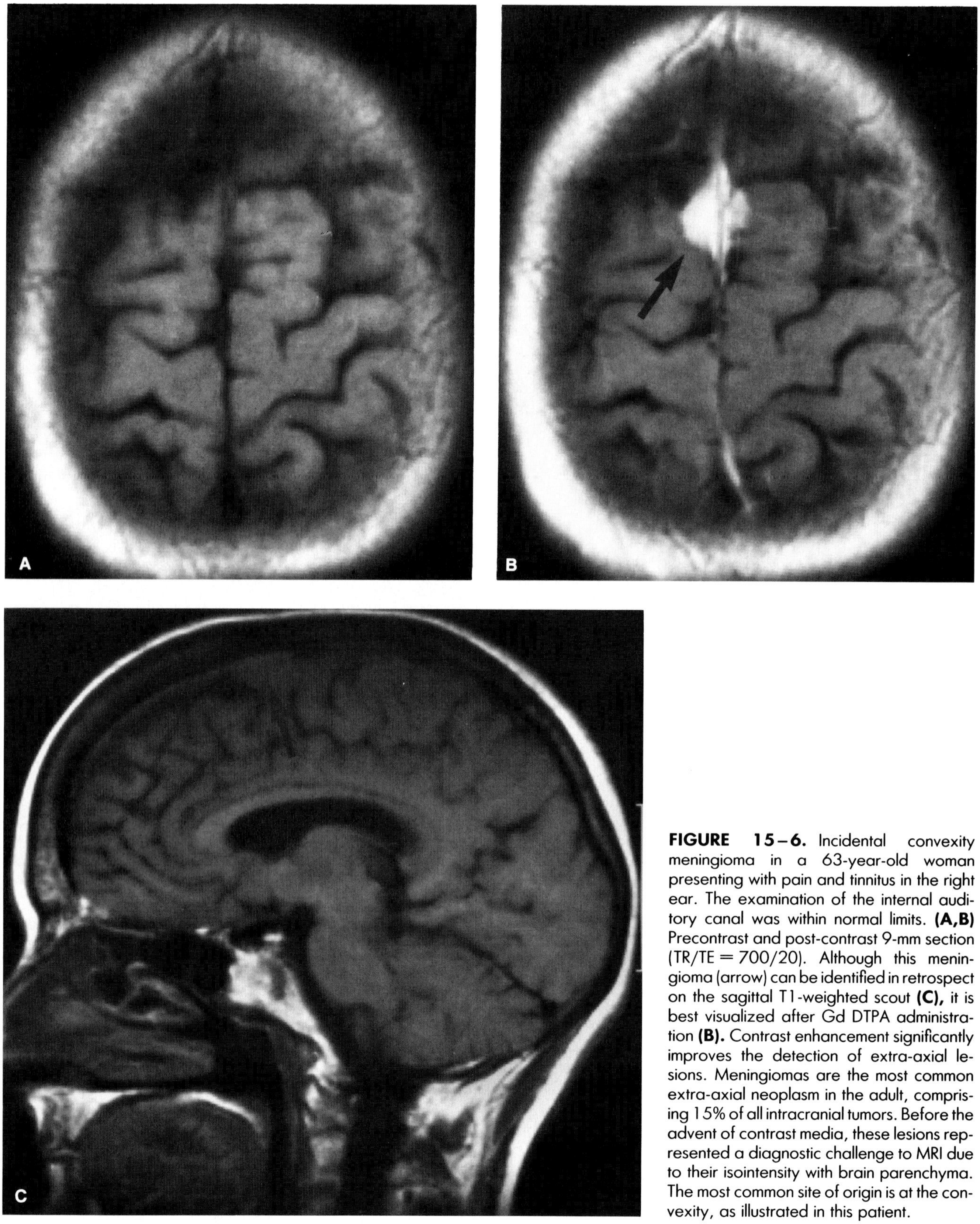

FIGURE 15–6. Incidental convexity meningioma in a 63-year-old woman presenting with pain and tinnitus in the right ear. The examination of the internal auditory canal was within normal limits. **(A,B)** Precontrast and post-contrast 9-mm section (TR/TE = 700/20). Although this meningioma (arrow) can be identified in retrospect on the sagittal T1-weighted scout **(C),** it is best visualized after Gd DTPA administration **(B).** Contrast enhancement significantly improves the detection of extra-axial lesions. Meningiomas are the most common extra-axial neoplasm in the adult, comprising 15% of all intracranial tumors. Before the advent of contrast media, these lesions represented a diagnostic challenge to MRI due to their isointensity with brain parenchyma. The most common site of origin is at the convexity, as illustrated in this patient.

FIGURE 15–7. Parasellar meningioma in a 66-year-old woman presenting for follow-up examination. **(A,B)** 3-mm section (TR/TE = 3000/90); **(C,D)** precontrast 3-mm section (TR/TE = 650/20); **(E,F)** postcontrast 3-mm section (TR/TE = 650/20). Although the bulk of the lesion can be identified on the unenhanced T1-weighted and T2-weighted images by virtue of its size and distortion of normal anatomy, contrast enhancement aids lesion recognition and characterization. Notice the encasement of the supraclinoid carotid artery (closed arrow). The principle value of contrast enhancement in this setting may be demonstrating lesion extent. **(F)** Extension of this meningioma posteriorly along the right tentorium can only be identified with certainty on the postcontrast image (open arrow). ▶

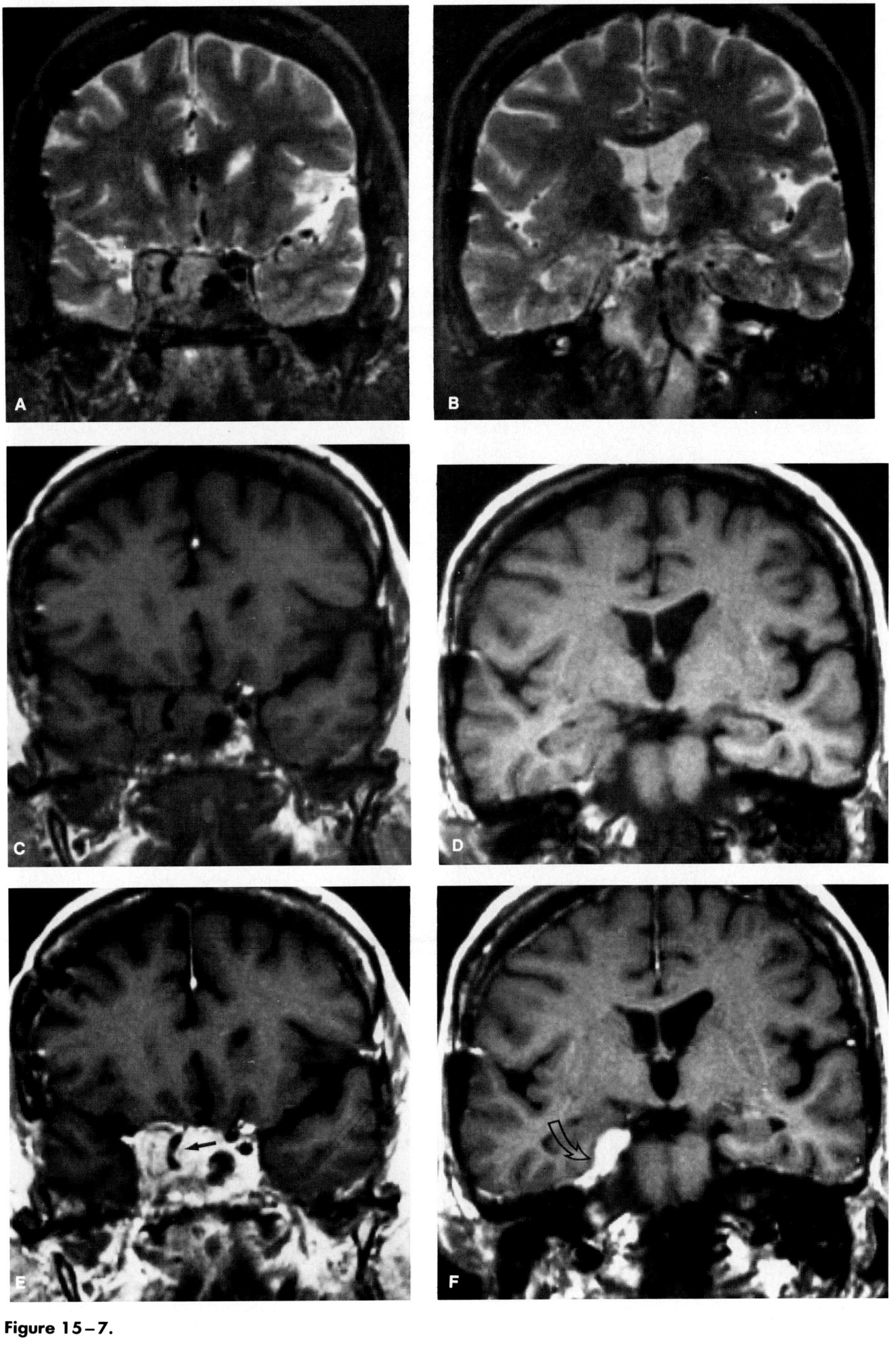

Figure 15–7.

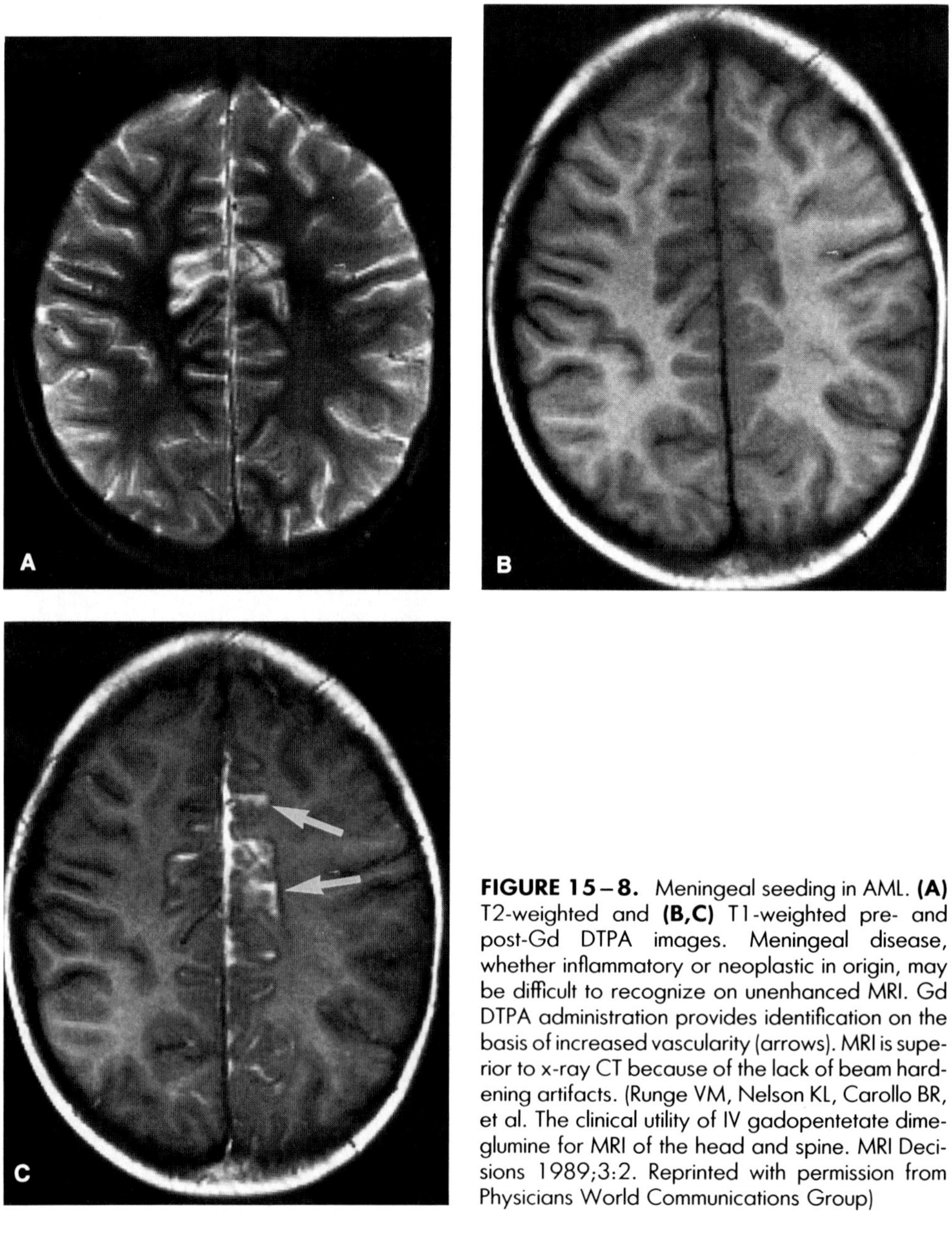

FIGURE 15–8. Meningeal seeding in AML. **(A)** T2-weighted and **(B,C)** T1-weighted pre- and post-Gd DTPA images. Meningeal disease, whether inflammatory or neoplastic in origin, may be difficult to recognize on unenhanced MRI. Gd DTPA administration provides identification on the basis of increased vascularity (arrows). MRI is superior to x-ray CT because of the lack of beam hardening artifacts. (Runge VM, Nelson KL, Carollo BR, et al. The clinical utility of IV gadopentetate dimeglumine for MRI of the head and spine. MRI Decisions 1989;3:2. Reprinted with permission from Physicians World Communications Group)

gliomas, it has been shown pathologically that neoplastic cells may extend far beyond the site of blood-brain-barrier disruption.

A logical extension of contrast use in MRI is for space-occupying intracranial lesions if neoplasia is a consideration (Fig. 15–12). The patterns of contrast enhancement established for x-ray CT generally hold true for MRI. Gd DTPA improves diagnostic specificity and aids in selection of biopsy sites. In the postoperative patient, unenhanced MRI is frequently difficult to interpret. Although enhancement with Gd DTPA merely identifies disruption of the blood-brain barrier, this information can be quite valuable in defining recurrent tumor, particularly if immediate postsurgical baseline studies are available (Fig. 15–13). A recent investigation of pediatric patients after brain tumor resection demonstrated the value of intravenous Gd DTPA (Fig. 15–14). In 6 of 15 patients, the contrast-enhanced scan depicted tumor not suspected on unenhanced MRI.[20]

One pitfall in the diagnosis of recurrent tumor should be mentioned. Brain irradiation can lead to necrosis and wallerian degeneration, which can demonstrate enhancement with Gd DTPA.[21] In surround-

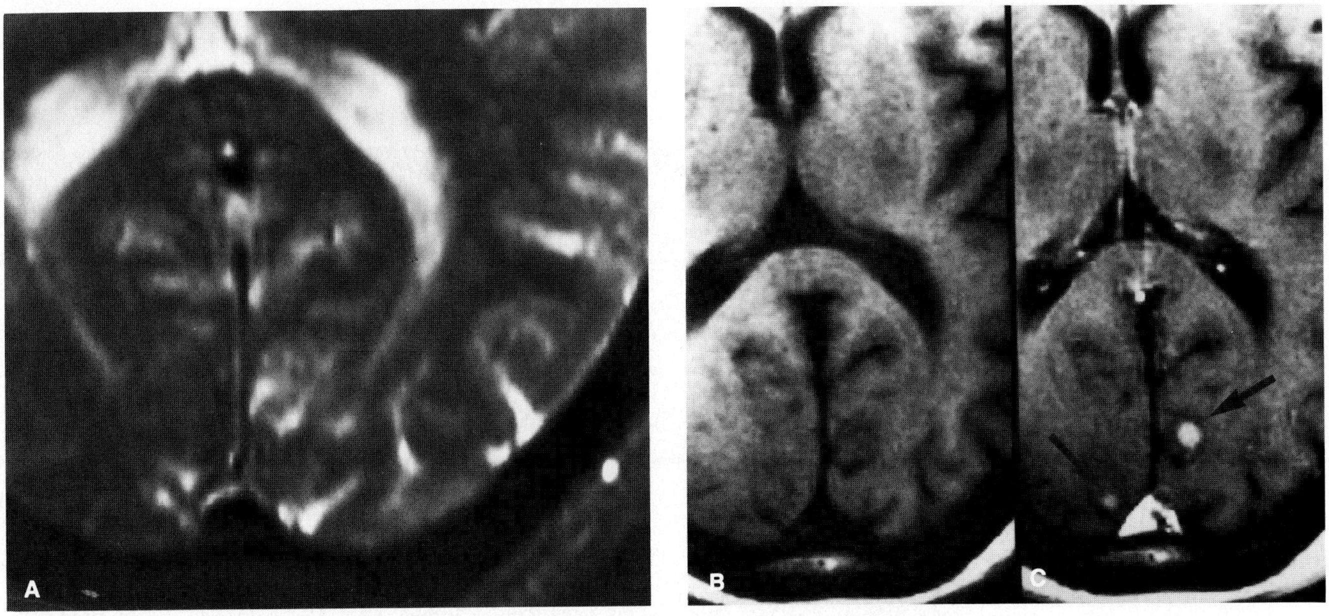

FIGURE 15–9. Metastatic melanoma in a 61-year-old man. **(A)** T2-weighted and **(B,C)** precontrast and postcontrast T1-weighted spin echo scans. Only the postcontrast image reveals the two metastases (arrows). The small size of these lesions, their peripheral location, and the lack of significant associated cerebral edema prevent their recognition on unenhanced scans. (Runge VM, ed. Enhanced magnetic resonance imaging. St. Louis: CV Mosby, 1989)

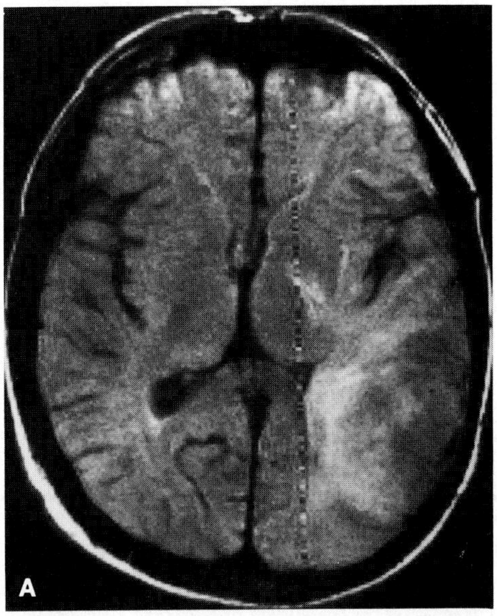

FIGURE 15–10. Glioblastoma multiforme. **(A)** Proton density and **(B–D)** T1-weighted precontrast, immediately postcontrast, and 4 hours post-Gd DTPA images. Enhancement identifies the bulk of the lesion (arrow), aiding plans for either stereotaxic biopsy or surgical debulking. Notice the diffusion of the contrast agent in the delayed scan **(D).** (Runge VM, Nelson KL, Carollo BR, et al. The clinical utility of IV gadopentetate dimeglumine for MRI of the head and spine. MRI Decisions 1989;3:2. Reprinted with permission from Physicians World Communications Group)

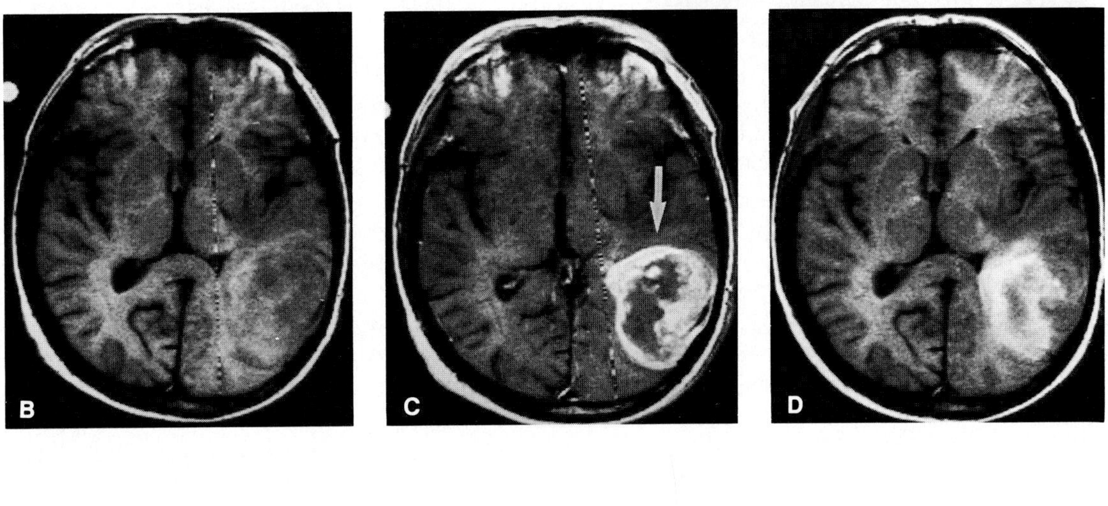

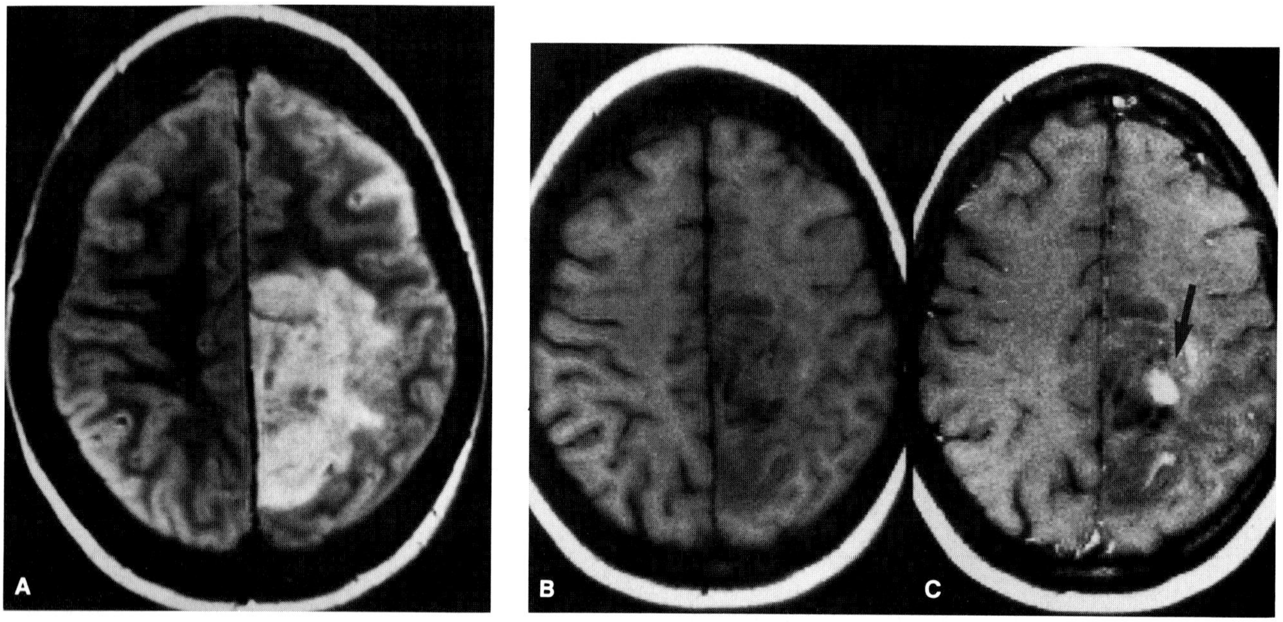

FIGURE 15–11. High-grade astrocytoma. **(A)** T2-weighted and **(B,C)** T1-weighted precontrast and post-Gd DTPA scans. Significant enhancement within the lesion (arrow) was only observed on MRI. CT scan is not shown, but previous studies have demonstrated superior contrast enhancement on MRI. Gd DTPA acts as an indirect contrast agent, and enhancement of the lesion depends on the concentration of the agent and the inherent relaxation times in the tissue of interest. (Runge VM, Nelson KL, Carollo BR, et al. The clinical utility of IV gadopentetate dimeglumine for MRI of the head and spine. MRI Decisions 1989;3:2)

ing tissue that does not enhance, there can be increased signal intensity on T2-weighted images. This corresponds to regions of demyelination without necrosis.

In the study of pituitary neoplasms, Gd DTPA may improve lesion detection and characterization (Fig. 15–15). In a study of eight patients with Cushing's disease and surgically proven pituitary microadenomas, visualization of the lesion was possible only on the contrast-enhanced scan in two cases.[22] However, there is need for caution. One lesion in this small study could not be diagnosed on MRI even after Gd DTPA administration. European study supports the use of Gd DTPA for evaluating pituitary microadenomas.[23] In examining the pituitary, special attention must be paid to imaging technique. High-resolution thin sections with an adequate signal-to-noise ratio (SNR) are mandatory, requiring the use of high magnetic fields.

In comparing CT and MRI, it has been demonstrated that contrast enhancement is superior on MRI in most intracranial mass lesions.[9] Although enhancement on CT depends solely on the concentration of agent achieved, enhancement on MRI depends also on intrinsic relaxation properties and tissue structure of the lesion.[12] These factors and the absence of beam-hardening artifacts account for the marked superiority of MRI in detecting lesion enhancement.

Infection

Gd DTPA enhancement improves the sensitivity of MRI to intracranial infection. Investigation in 1984 with a canine brain abscess model established that contrast-enhanced MRI was superior to unenhanced MRI and enhanced CT for detecting parenchymal infection.[24] Initial clinical experience indicates that contrast enhancement also improves the identification of epidural inflammatory disease.

For parenchymal disease, contrast enhancement demarcates the extent of blood-brain-barrier disruption. The abscess focus itself can thus be differentiated from surrounding edema (Fig. 15–16). Contrast enhancement can reveal extensive meningeal disease involving the basilar cisterns. Improved staging (i.e., early vs. late cerebritis or capsule formation) and evaluation of lesion activity are also provided by Gd DTPA injection.[24]

Meningeal enhancement on MRI is nonspecific and can be seen with both inflammatory and neoplastic disease.[25,26] In identifying these pathologic conditions,

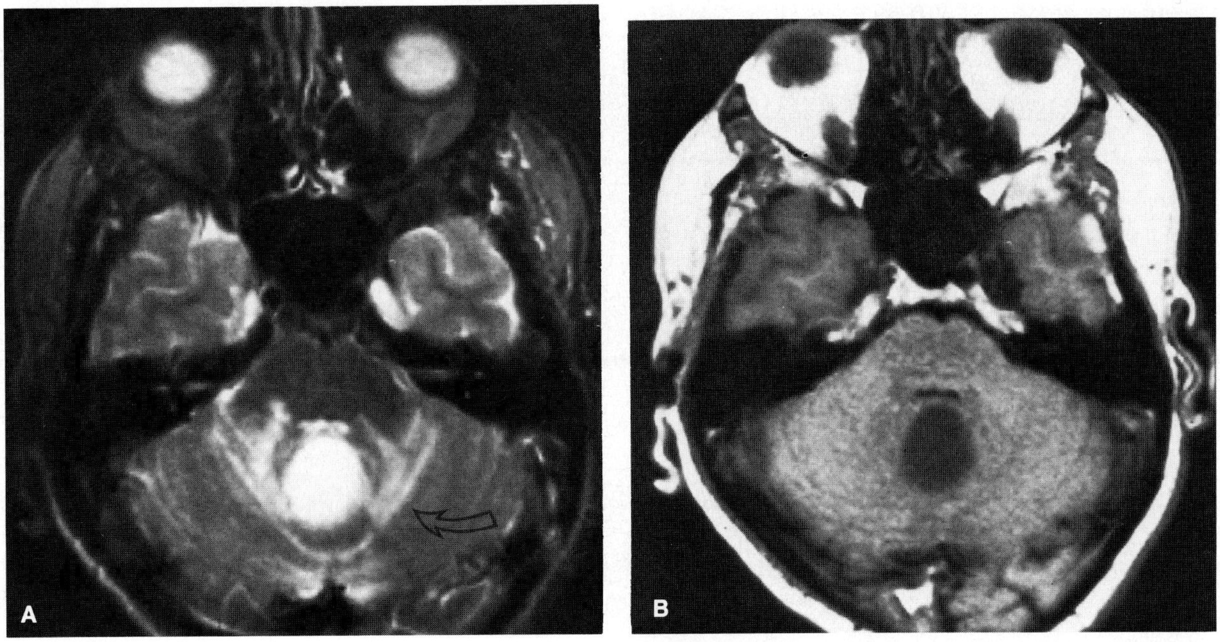

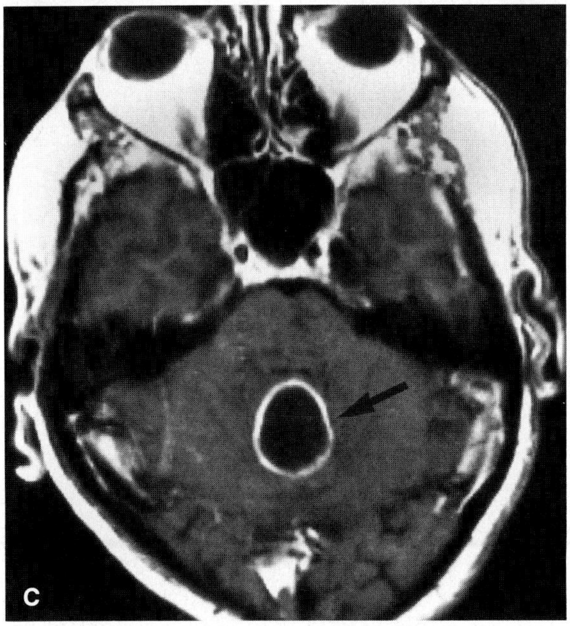

FIGURE 15–12. Metastatic, mucin-producing adenocarcinoma in the superior vermis of an unknown primary in a 54-year-old man presenting with nausea and imbalance. **(A)** 5-mm section (TR/TE = 3000/90) and **(B,C)** precontrast and postcontrast 5-mm section (TR/TE = 650/20). Ring enhancement (closed arrow) of this cystic metastasis is seen on the postcontrast image. Surrounding edema (open arrow) can be recognized by comparing the appearance of the lesion on the T2-weighted scan with that on the postcontrast T1-weighted scan.

which are often located in the posterior fossa or adjacent to the skull, enhanced MRI has proven superior to x-ray CT partially because of the lack of beam-hardening artifacts. Gd DTPA has provided an elegant means to detect meningeal disease that could not be visualized on unenhanced MRI.

In a canine model of bacterial meningitis, Gd-DTPA-enhanced MRI proved superior to x-ray CT for detecting disease.[26] Contrast enhancement on MRI enabled identification of ventriculitis, cerebritis, and meningitis. Enhanced CT was less effective in visualizing these abnormalities. In clinical studies, contrast-enhanced MRI has also proven superior to x-ray CT for detecting meningeal disease.[27] The relative lack of contrast enhancement of the falx and meninges in normal patients is responsible for the improved detection of meningeal abnormalities on contrast-enhanced MRI (Fig. 15–17).

Infarction

We feel that the value of Gd DTPA in evaluating ischemic disease has been largely unrecognized due to the emphasis in U.S. clinical trials on neoplastic dis-

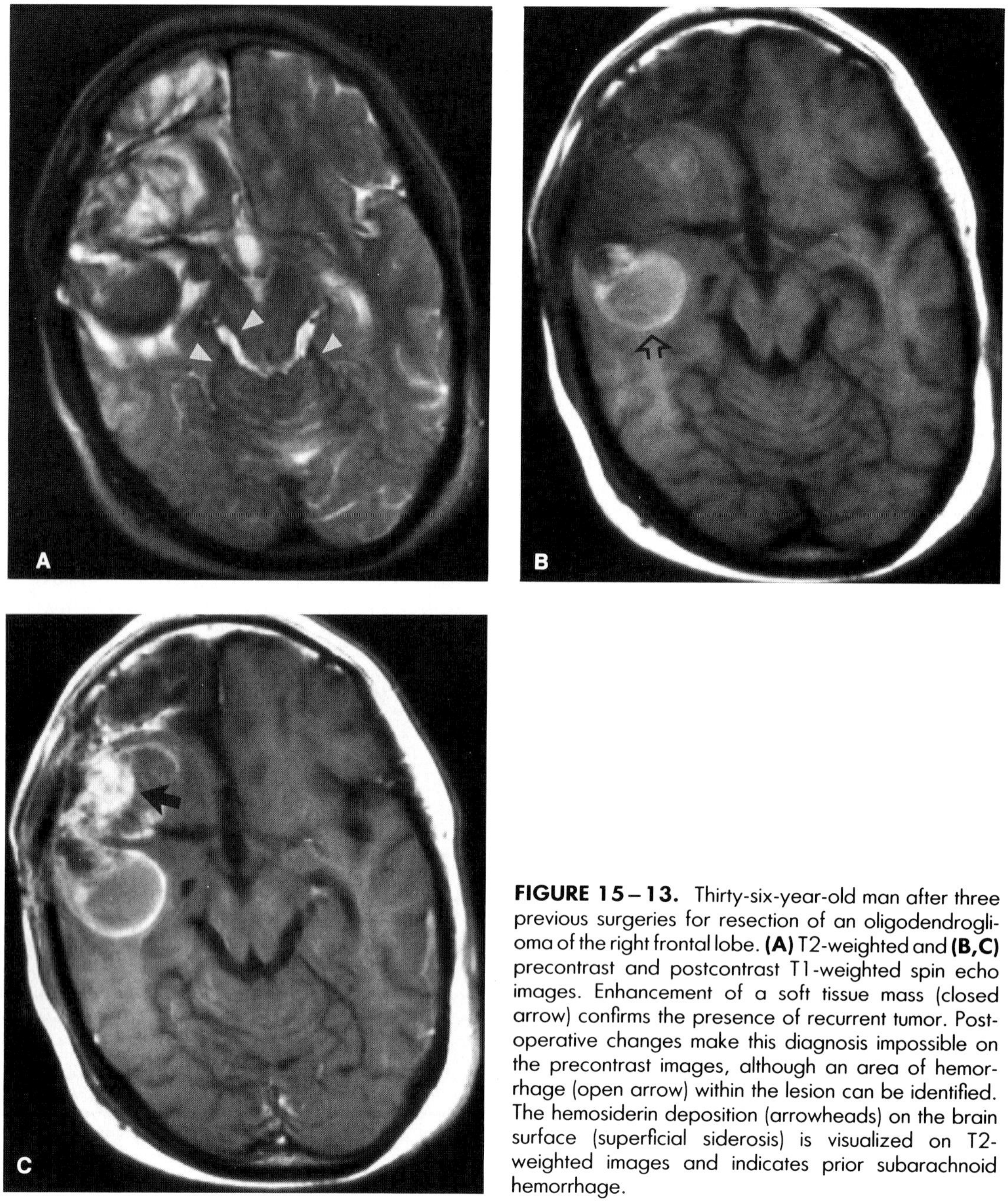

FIGURE 15–13. Thirty-six-year-old man after three previous surgeries for resection of an oligodendroglioma of the right frontal lobe. **(A)** T2-weighted and **(B,C)** precontrast and postcontrast T1-weighted spin echo images. Enhancement of a soft tissue mass (closed arrow) confirms the presence of recurrent tumor. Postoperative changes make this diagnosis impossible on the precontrast images, although an area of hemorrhage (open arrow) within the lesion can be identified. The hemosiderin deposition (arrowheads) on the brain surface (superficial siderosis) is visualized on T2-weighted images and indicates prior subarachnoid hemorrhage.

ease.[28,29] Within the first 2 months after an ischemic event, Gd DTPA administration can markedly improve detection of brain infarction (Figs. 15–18 and 15–19). The pattern of enhancement, often gyriform for cerebral infarction, also substantially aids lesion categorization.

In Japanese studies, Gd-DPTA-enhanced MRI was more sensitive to cerebral infarction than enhanced CT.[30] This was particularly true for cortical and subcortical lesions. Contrast enhancement increased gradually with time after injection.

In hypertensive or elderly patients, unenhanced images often reveal nonspecific ischemic changes in the deep white matter. Focal enhancement with Gd DTPA administration can be used to identify recent infarctions in these cases (Fig. 15–20). In ischemic disease of the brain, contrast enhancement on MRI

(text continues on page 536)

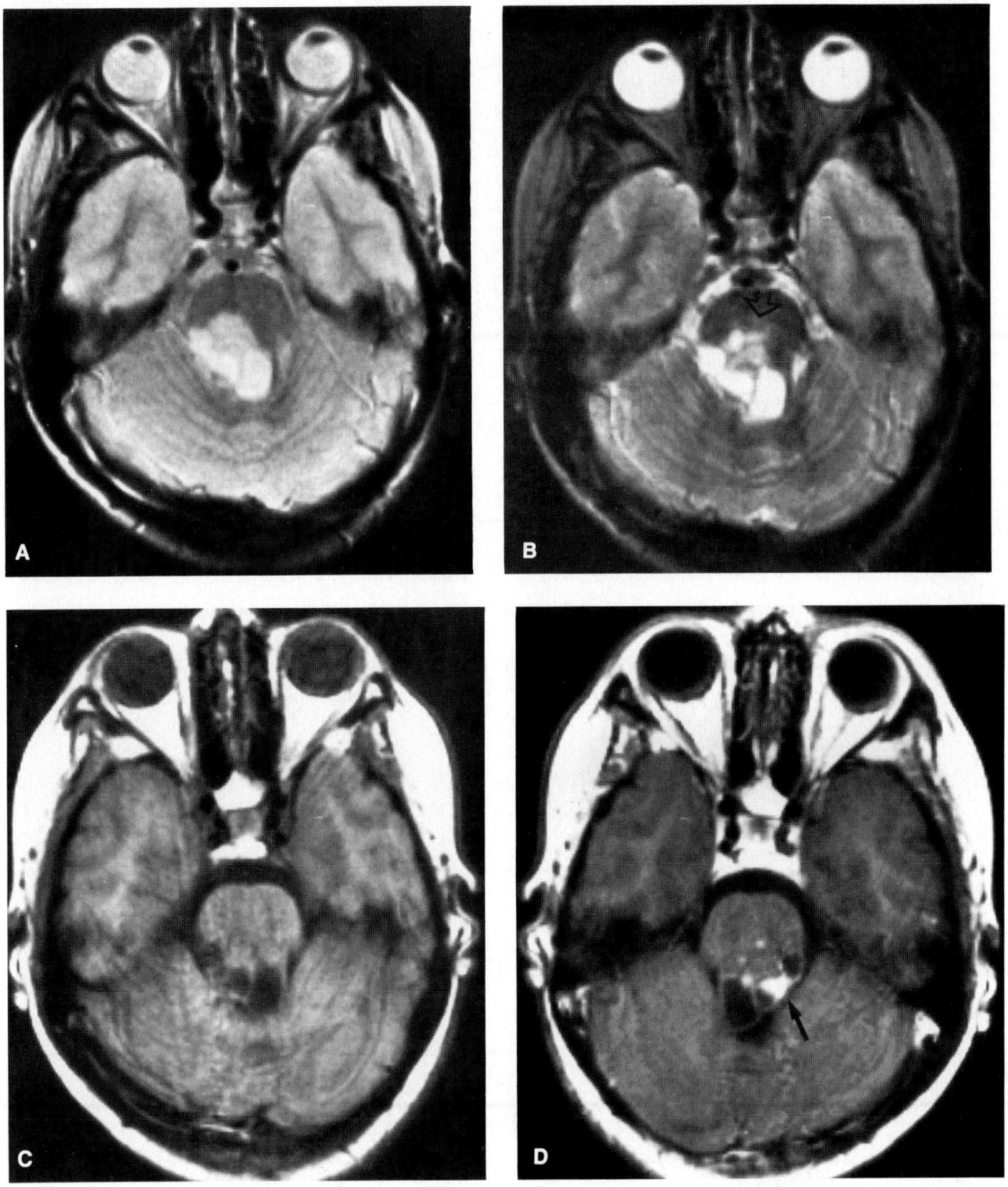

FIGURE 15–14. Postoperative brainstem astrocytoma with recurrence in a 16-year-old girl. **(A,B)** 5-mm section (TR/TE = 3000/45,90) and **(C,D)** precontrast and postcontrast 5-mm section (TR/TE = 650/20). The abnormal high signal intensity (open arrow) observed on the T2-weighted scans is nonspecific and may represent either recurrent tumor or postoperative change. Contrast enhancement reveals recurrent tumor (closed arrow) by delineation of abnormalities in the blood-brain barrier. This case illustrates the vital role that intravenous Gd DTPA plays in detection of recurrent primary neoplastic disease of the brain.

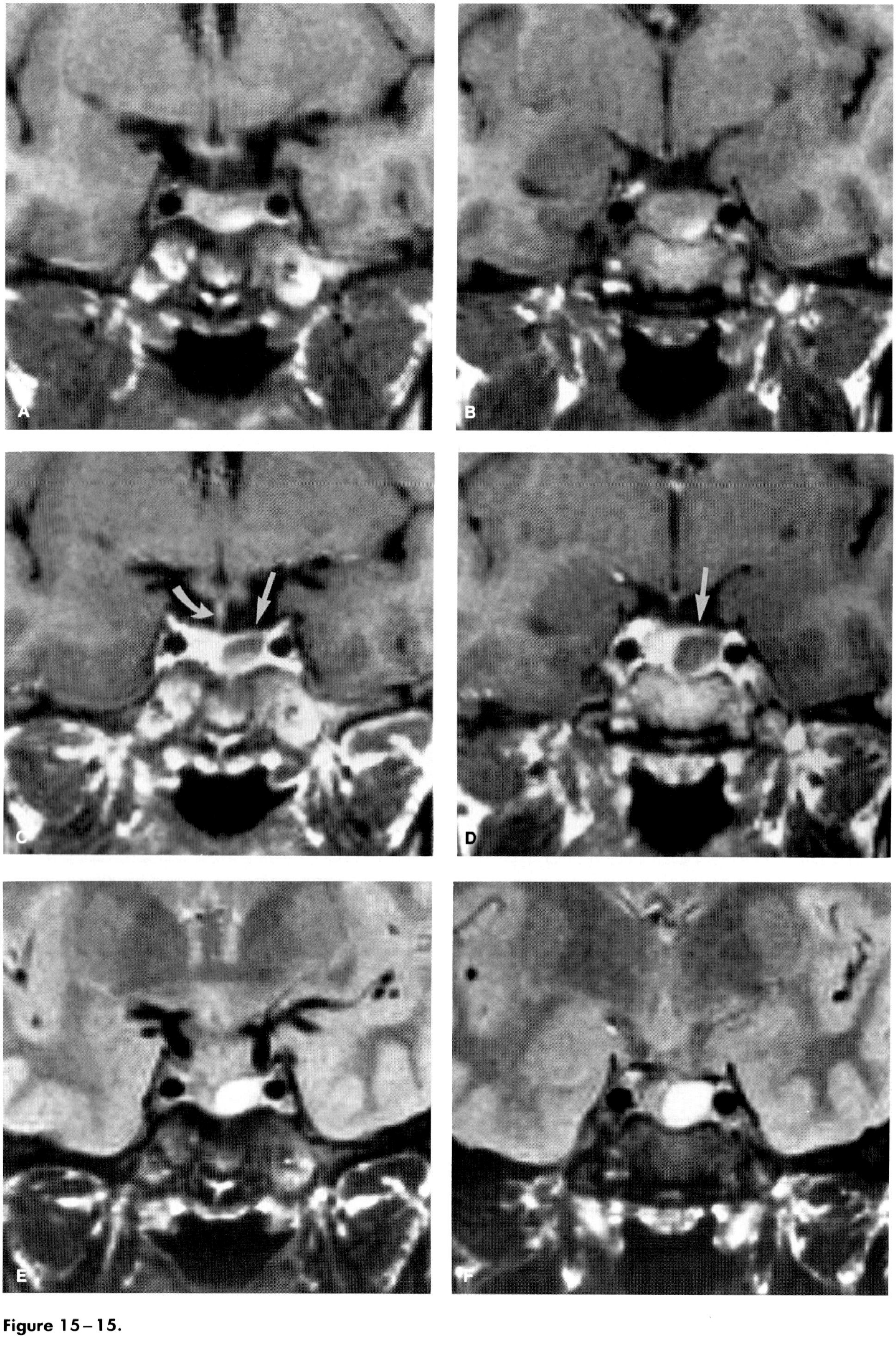

Figure 15–15.

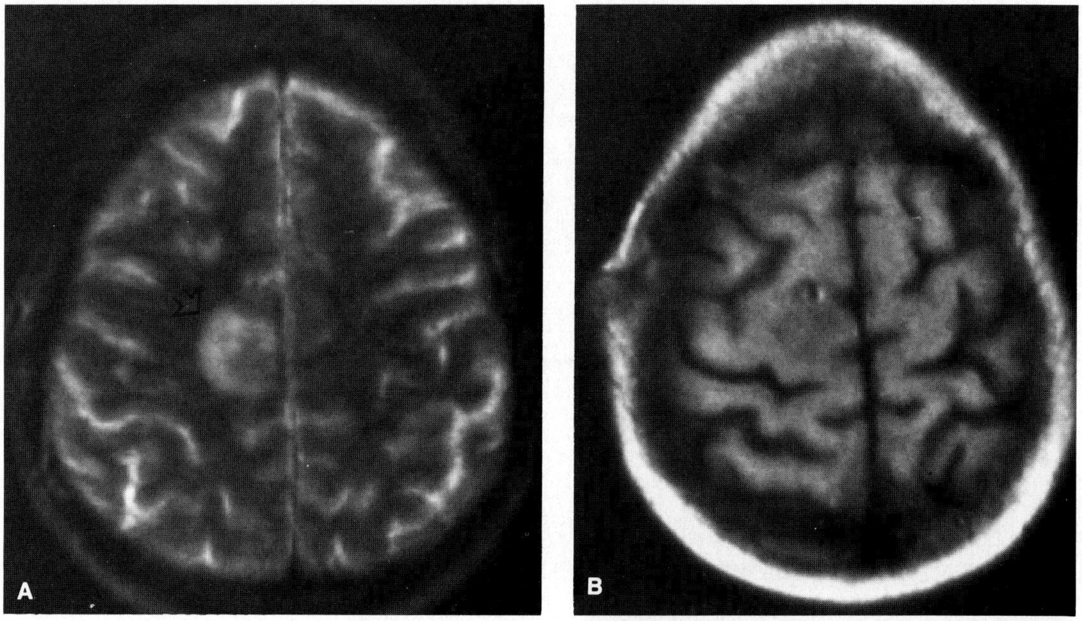

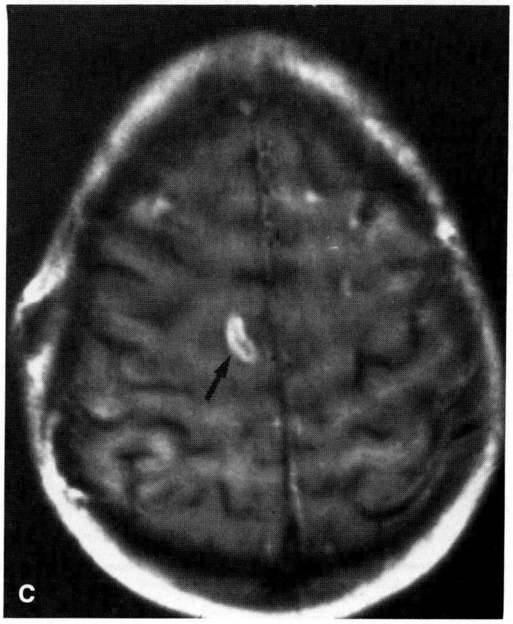

FIGURE 15–16. Tuberculoma within the supraventricular white matter in a 27-year-old woman with tuberculous meningitis and parenchymal infection. **(A)** 8-mm section (TR/TE = 3000/90) and **(B,C)** precontrast and postcontrast 8-mm section (TR/TE = 650/20). Contrast enhancement permits differentiation of the abscess capsule (closed arrow) on the T1-weighted image from surrounding cerebral edema (open arrow) on the T2-weighted image. Animal investigations have revealed that contrast-enhanced MRI is superior to both unenhanced MRI and enhanced CT for detecting parenchymal and meningeal inflammatory disease.

◀ **FIGURE 15–15.** Pituitary microadenoma in a 22-year-old woman, who first presented with elevated prolactin and amenorrhea. The patient received Bromocryptine therapy for 3 months before MRI. **(A,B)** Precontrast and **(C,D)** postcontrast coronal T1-weighted images (TR/TE = 650/20); **(E,F)** precontrast T2-weighted scans (TR/TE = 3000/45). This large microadenoma is not well demonstrated on the precontrast T1-weighted images. Like the majority of adenomas, it does not substantially enhance after administration of Gd DTPA if compared with the normal pituitary and cavernous sinus. This improves visualization of the lesion (arrow) on the postcontrast image. Notice the normal enhancement of the pituitary infundibulum (curved arrow). The use of Gd DTPA in imaging the pituitary improves lesion detection and delineates cavernous sinus invasion. Although some pituitary lesions are well depicted on T2-weighted scans, many centers have discontinued use of this technique because of the inability to routinely obtain high-quality thin sections.

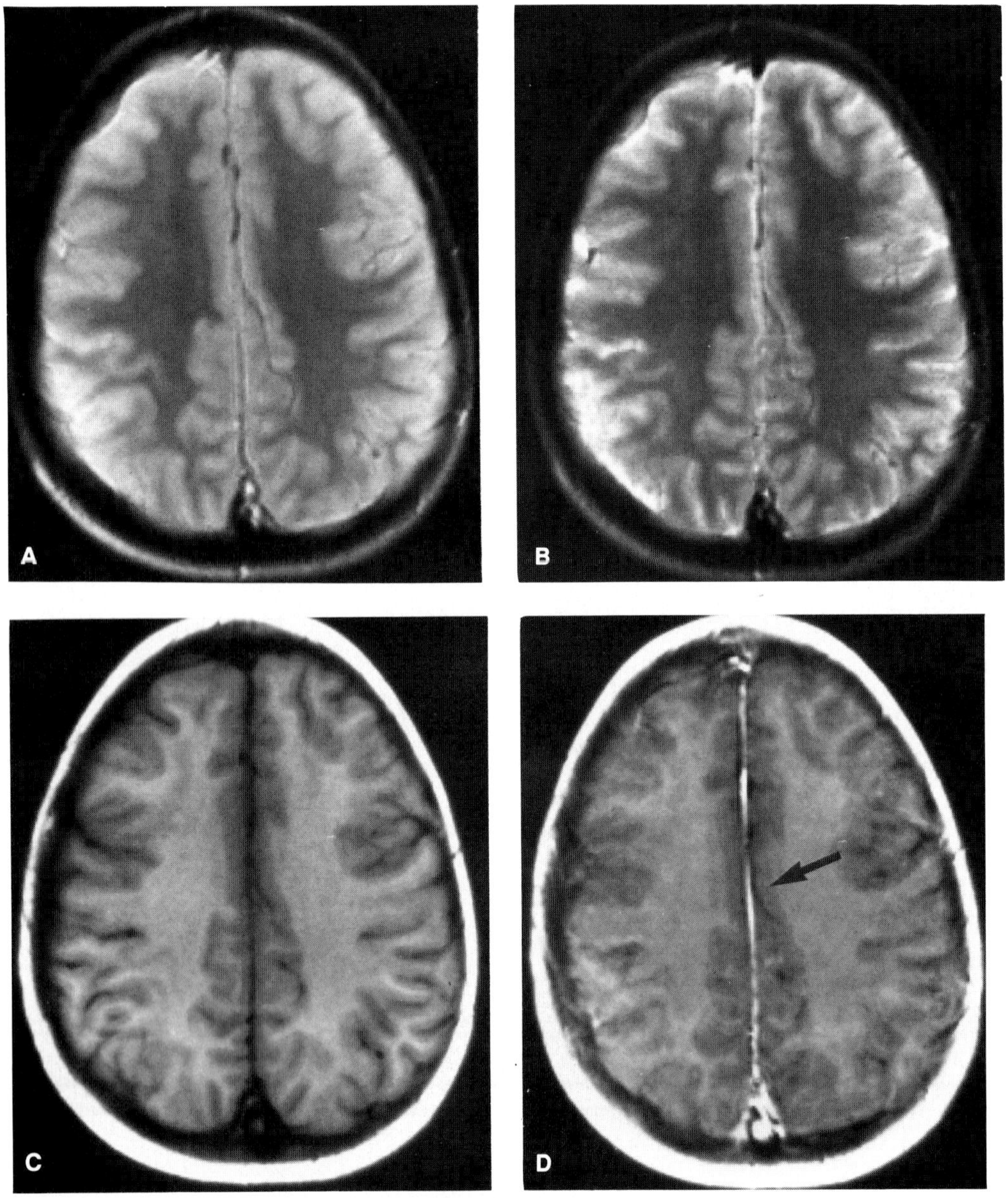

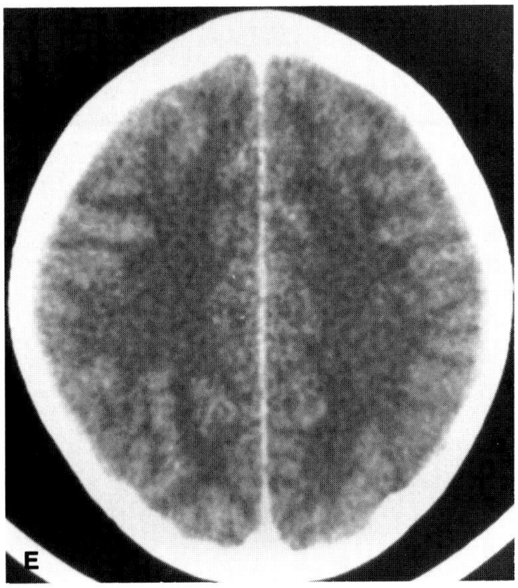

FIGURE 15–17. Chicken pox encephalitis in a 12-year-old boy. **(A,B)** 8-mm section (TR/TE = 3000/45,90); **(C,D)** precontrast and postcontrast 8-mm section (TR/TE = 650/20); **(E)** enhanced CT scan. Prominent enhancement of the falx (arrow) is seen on the postcontrast MRI scan enabling the diagnosis of meningeal inflammation. No abnormality can be detected on the T2-weighted image. This diagnosis also cannot be made on CT, because enhancement of the falx is normal with this modality. A subtle increase in signal intensity of the dura and falx can be detected in normal patients after Gd DTPA administration. Prominent enhancement of the meninges as illustrated in this case is abnormal. Unfortunately, this is a nonspecific finding, which can be seen in metastatic disease, in infection, following surgery, and secondary to trauma.

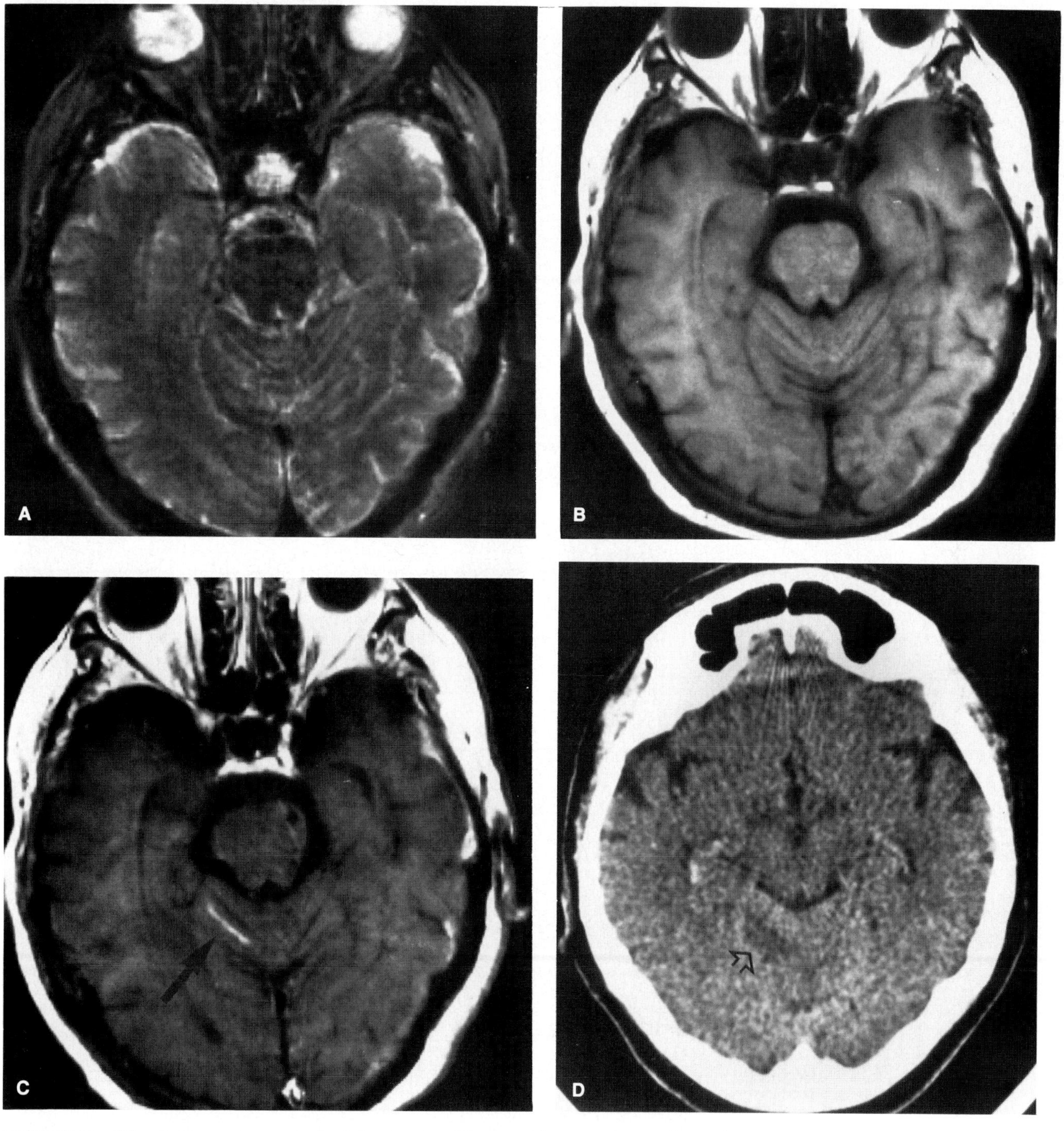

FIGURE 15–18. Right superior cerebellar infarction in a 73-year-old woman due to atherosclerotic disease of the posterior circulation. **(A)** 8-mm section (TR/TE = 3000/90); **(B,C)** precontrast and postcontrast 8-mm section (TR/TE = 650/20); **(D)** unenhanced CT scan. The CT and MRI scans were performed 4 and 11 days, respectively, after clinical presentation. CT demonstrates the lesion as an area of low attentuation (open arrow). By the time of the MRI scans, there was significant resolution of cerebellar edema, making diagnosis of this infarct possible only on the postcontrast image. The lesion can be identified as an area of linear contrast enhancement (closed arrow). Subacute infarction may be difficult to recognize on unenhanced MRI due to significant resolution of edema. Gd DTPA in this instance permits recognition of the lesion due to enhancement in the region of blood-brain barrier disruption. The pattern and distribution of enhancement (i.e., gyriform, vascular territory) can also enable a more specific diagnosis of infarction.

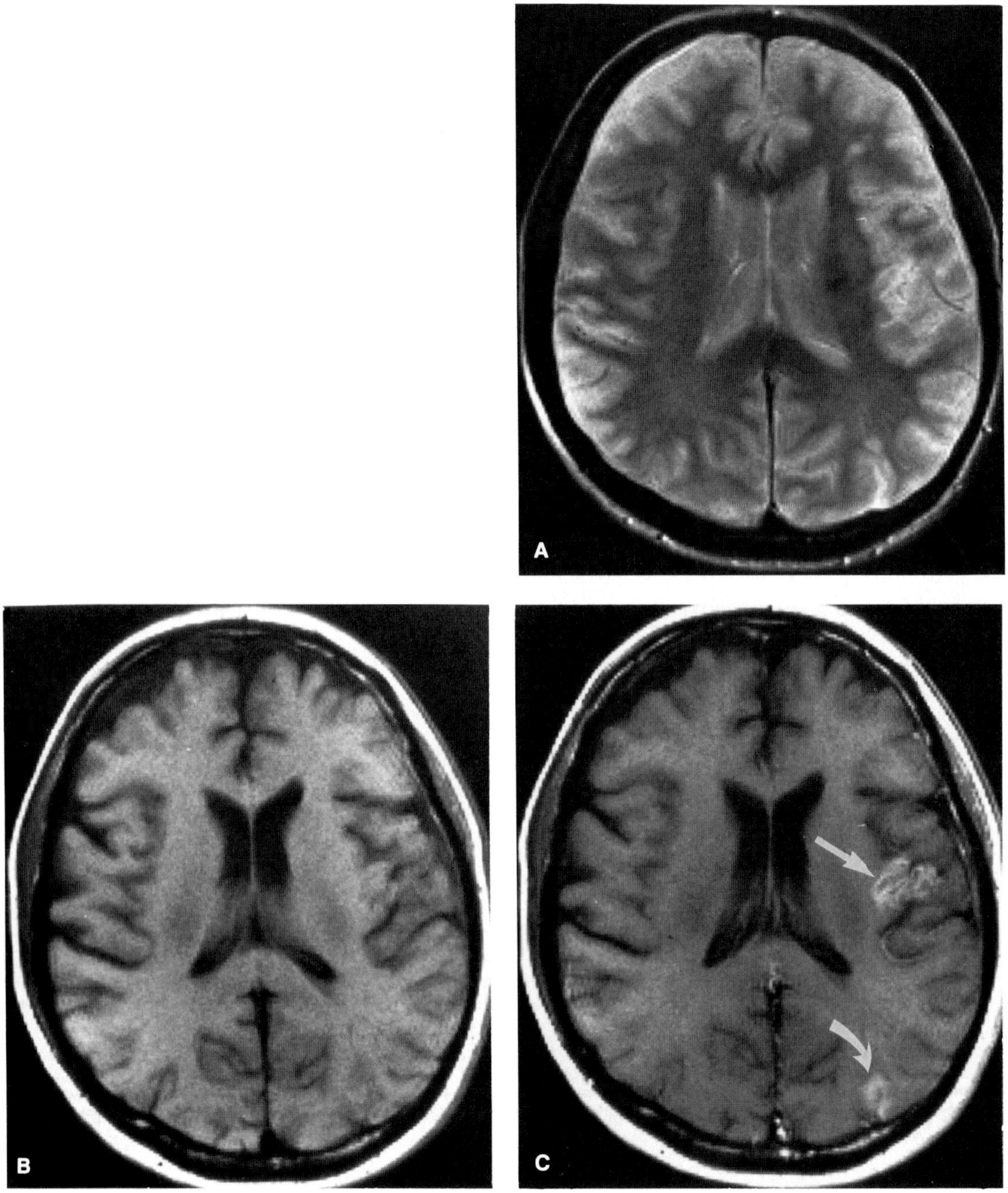

FIGURE 15–19. Infarction in the distribution of the middle cerebral artery, approximately 1 month after presentation. **(A)** T2-weighted and **(B,C)** T1-weighted pre- and post-Gd DTPA scans. Gyriform enhancement, due to blood-brain-barrier disruption, enables the diagnosis of infarction (closed arrow) to be made. With the unenhanced scans alone, only nonspecific white matter abnormalities can be recognized. Notice the watershed infarct (curved arrow). In a blinded, prospective reader evaluation, these lesions were only recognized on the postcontrast image. (Runge VM, Nelson KL, Carollo BR, et al. The clinical utility of IV gadopentetate dimeglumine for MRI of the head and spine. MRI Decisions 1989;3:2. Reprinted with permission from Physicians World Communications Group)

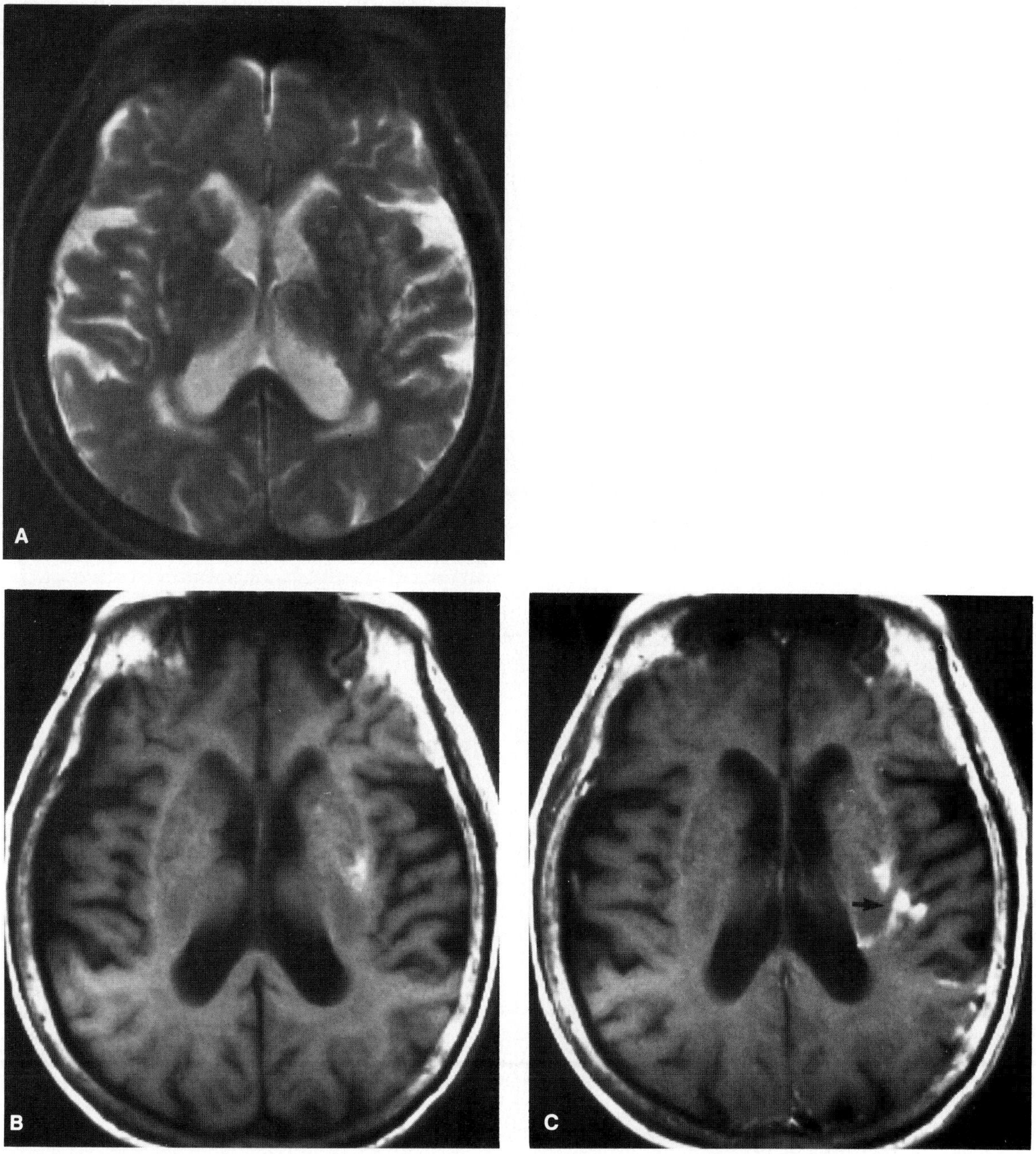

FIGURE 15–20. Hemorrhagic basal ganglia and deep white matter infarction in a 78-year-old woman with development of right hemiparesis and aphasia after a fall with loss of consciousness. The patient also had a 20-year history of hypertension. **(A)** 8-mm section (TR/TE = 3000/90) and **(B,C)** precontrast and postcontrast 8-mm section (TR/TE = 650/20). With significant deep white matter ischemia, recognition of recent brain infarction can be difficult. Enhancement with Gd DTPA (arrow) enables the diagnosis of subacute cerebral infarction due to identification of blood-brain-barrier abnormalities.

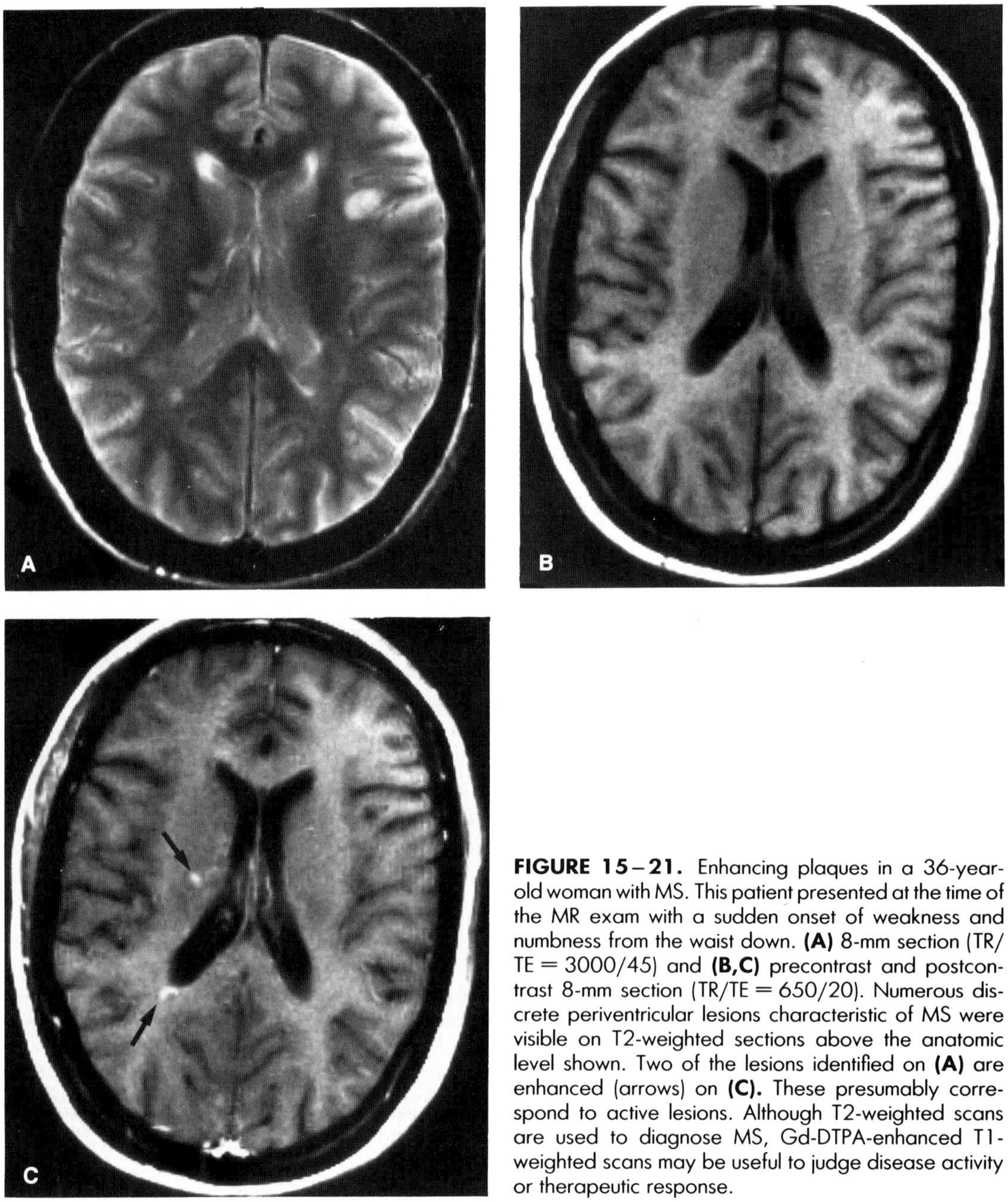

FIGURE 15–21. Enhancing plaques in a 36-year-old woman with MS. This patient presented at the time of the MR exam with a sudden onset of weakness and numbness from the waist down. **(A)** 8-mm section (TR/TE = 3000/45) and **(B,C)** precontrast and postcontrast 8-mm section (TR/TE = 650/20). Numerous discrete periventricular lesions characteristic of MS were visible on T2-weighted sections above the anatomic level shown. Two of the lesions identified on **(A)** are enhanced (arrows) on **(C)**. These presumably correspond to active lesions. Although T2-weighted scans are used to diagnose MS, Gd-DTPA-enhanced T1-weighted scans may be useful to judge disease activity or therapeutic response.

improves sensitivity, specificity, and dating of the lesion.

Multiple Sclerosis

In multiple sclerosis (MS), Gd DTPA can provide information concerning the status of the blood-brain barrier, which presumably reflects activity of the disease.[32-35] Although enhancement can be seen in MS, its value depends on the utility of these scans for assessment of disease progression with new therapeutic regimens (Fig. 15–21).

Vascular Abnormalities

Vascular lesions may become more evident after Gd DTPA administration due to enhancement of slow venous flow or to increased prominence of pulsation

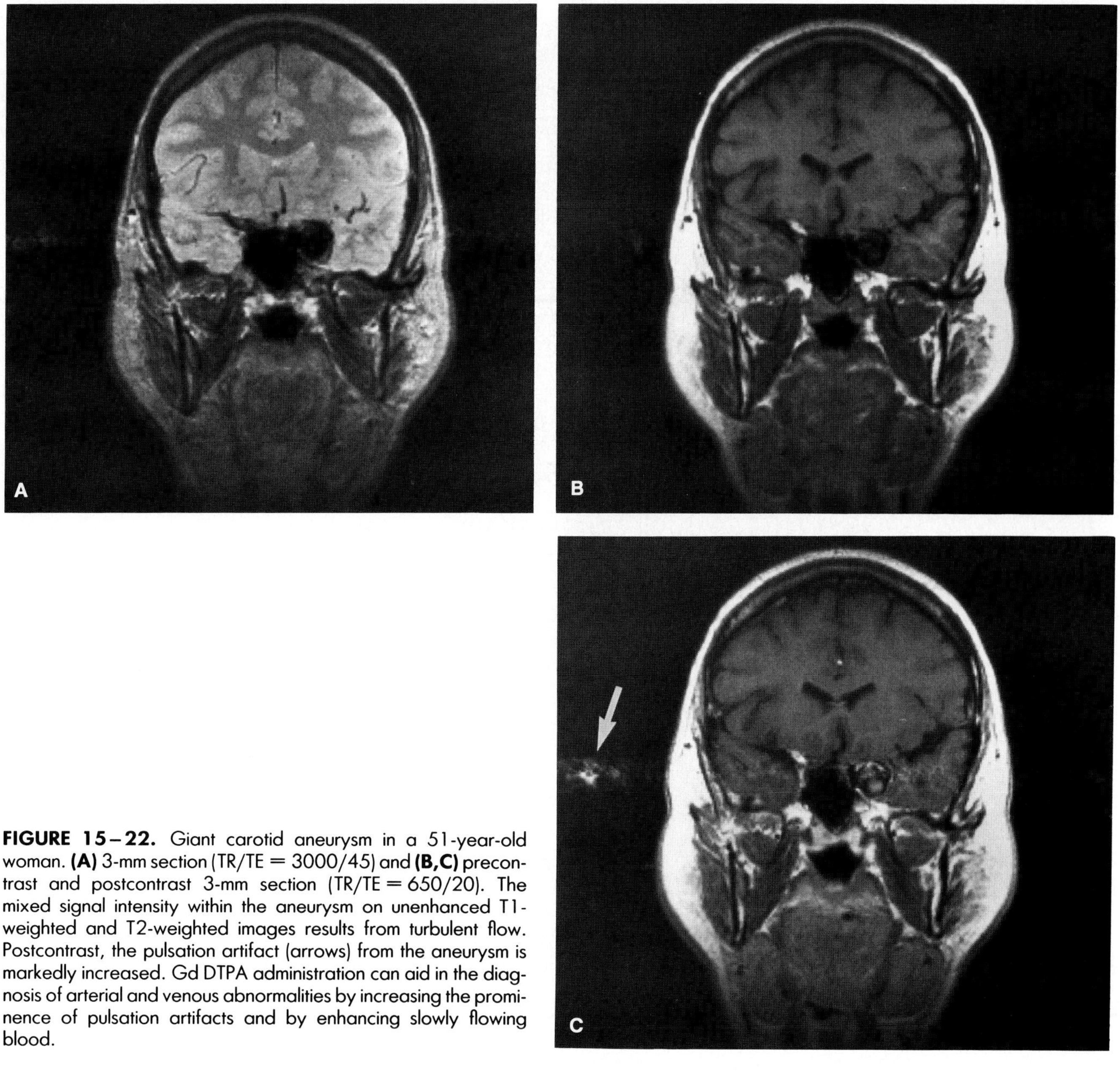

FIGURE 15–22. Giant carotid aneurysm in a 51-year-old woman. **(A)** 3-mm section (TR/TE = 3000/45) and **(B,C)** precontrast and postcontrast 3-mm section (TR/TE = 650/20). The mixed signal intensity within the aneurysm on unenhanced T1-weighted and T2-weighted images results from turbulent flow. Postcontrast, the pulsation artifact (arrows) from the aneurysm is markedly increased. Gd DTPA administration can aid in the diagnosis of arterial and venous abnormalities by increasing the prominence of pulsation artifacts and by enhancing slowly flowing blood.

artifacts (Figs. 15–22 and 15–23). Motion-correction techniques, such as gradient moment nulling (MAST), have been implemented to improve image quality. However, these techniques tend to make vascular abnormalities less evident, a trend that can be reversed with contrast use.

Venous angiomas in particular can become much more apparent after Gd DTPA administration. In a blinded prospective trial at our institution, one such lesion was more accurately characterized on the enhanced scan.

SPINE ABNORMALITIES

Disc Disease

Clinical trials in the United States have revealed the utility of Gd DTPA in the postoperative back for the differentiation of scar from recurrent disc.[36] In this evaluation, the acquisition of postcontrast images within 10 minutes after injection is essential. Scar enhances during this time, due to vascularity, but disc material should not (Fig. 15–24). The magnitude of

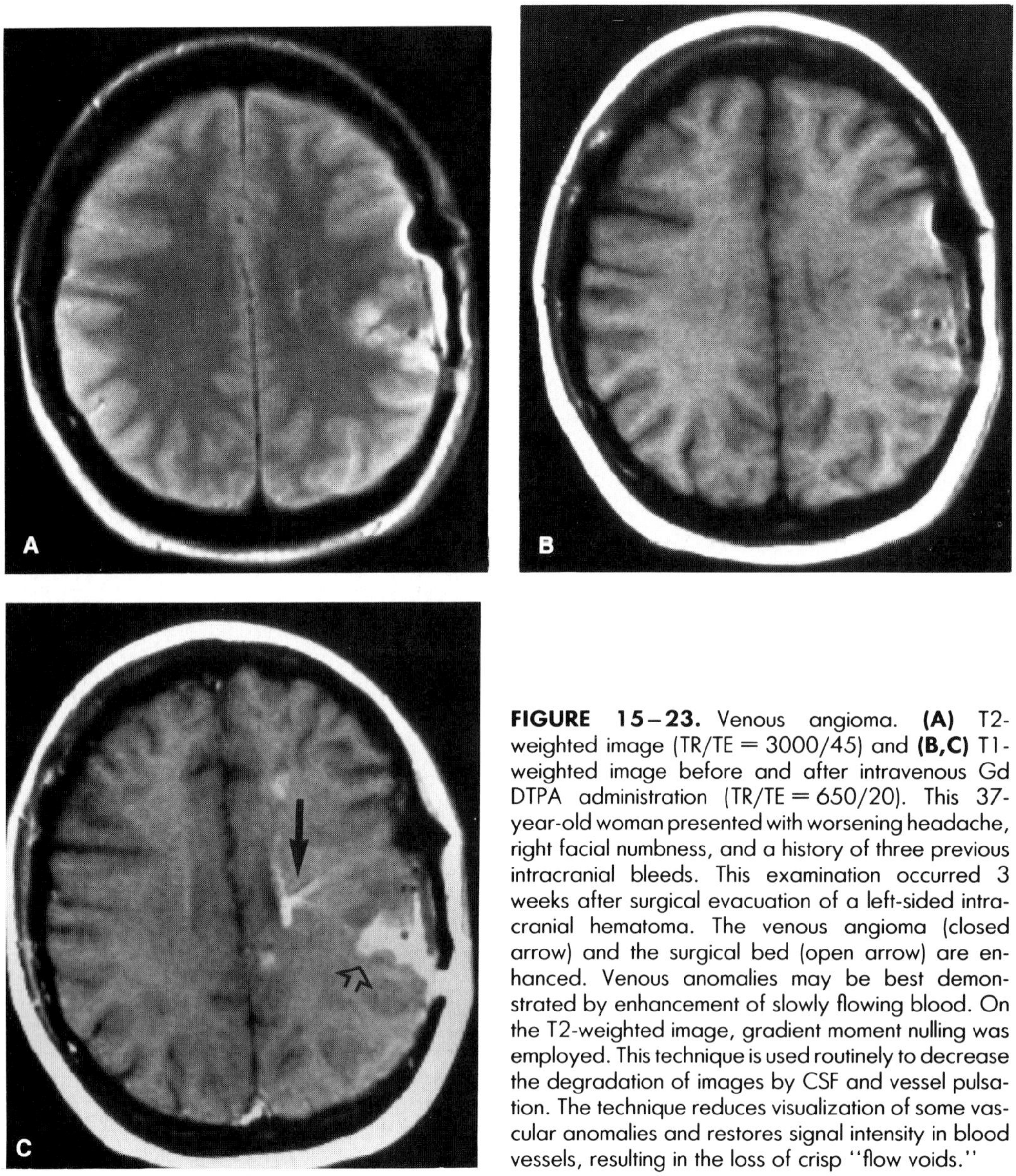

FIGURE 15–23. Venous angioma. **(A)** T2-weighted image (TR/TE = 3000/45) and **(B,C)** T1-weighted image before and after intravenous Gd DTPA administration (TR/TE = 650/20). This 37-year-old woman presented with worsening headache, right facial numbness, and a history of three previous intracranial bleeds. This examination occurred 3 weeks after surgical evacuation of a left-sided intracranial hematoma. The venous angioma (closed arrow) and the surgical bed (open arrow) are enhanced. Venous anomalies may be best demonstrated by enhancement of slowly flowing blood. On the T2-weighted image, gradient moment nulling was employed. This technique is used routinely to decrease the degradation of images by CSF and vessel pulsation. The technique reduces visualization of some vascular anomalies and restores signal intensity in blood vessels, resulting in the loss of crisp "flow voids."

enhancement seen with scar is much lower than that commonly encountered in cerebral neoplasia, emphasizing the need in spine examinations for close attention to imaging technique. Higher doses of new contrast agents may alleviate this problem.

Early reports have suggested the utility of enhancement in the diagnosis of "virgin" discs (i.e., before surgery) in the cervical spine.[12] In this instance, enhancement of the displaced epidural venous plexus outlines herniated disc material. The lack of enhancement of disc material can also be important for improved characterization of lesions (Fig. 15–25).

To properly interpret spine images after-Gd DTPA administration, the patterns of enhancement commonly seen in the normal patient should be appreciated. Both the dorsal root ganglion and Type I endplate disease (a degenerative condition) typically enhance.[12]

Intradural Neoplasia

Preliminary reports demonstrate great utility for Gd DTPA in intramedullary and intradural extramedullary disease.[37–41] Its application in extradural disease

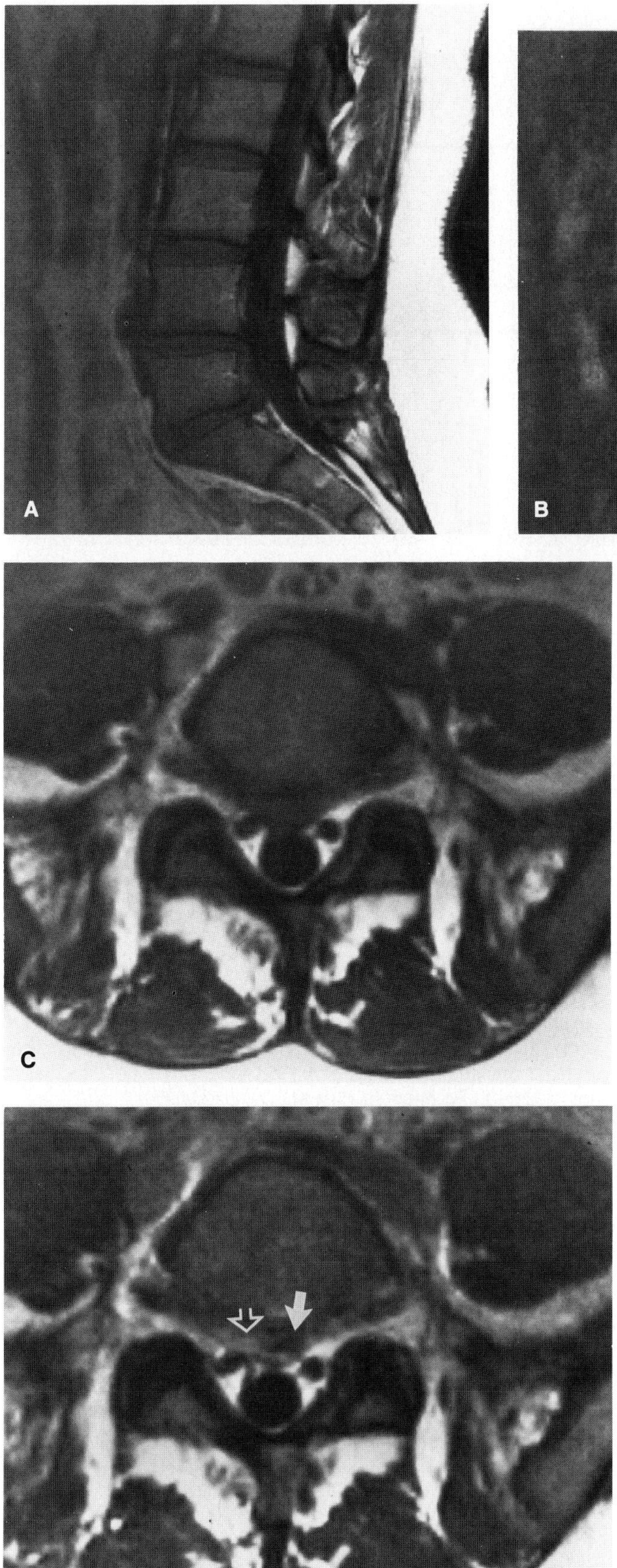

FIGURE 15–24. Recurrent disc herniation with adjacent enhancing scar in a 27-year-old woman after percutaneous discectomy. The patient presented with increased back pain and new right-sided radicular pain. **(A)** Sagittal 4-mm section (TR/TE = 450/20); **(B)** sagittal 5-mm section (TR/TE = 3000/90); **(C,D)** axial 4-mm section before and immediately after Gd DTPA administration (TR/TE = 450/20). A recurrent central disc herniation can be identified at L5-S1 and can be distinguished from postoperative fibrosis, due to its lack of contrast enhancement (closed arrow). There is marked surrounding epidural fibrosis and scar encasing the right L5 nerve root within the lateral recess. These areas (open arrow) enhance on the post-Gd DTPA scan.

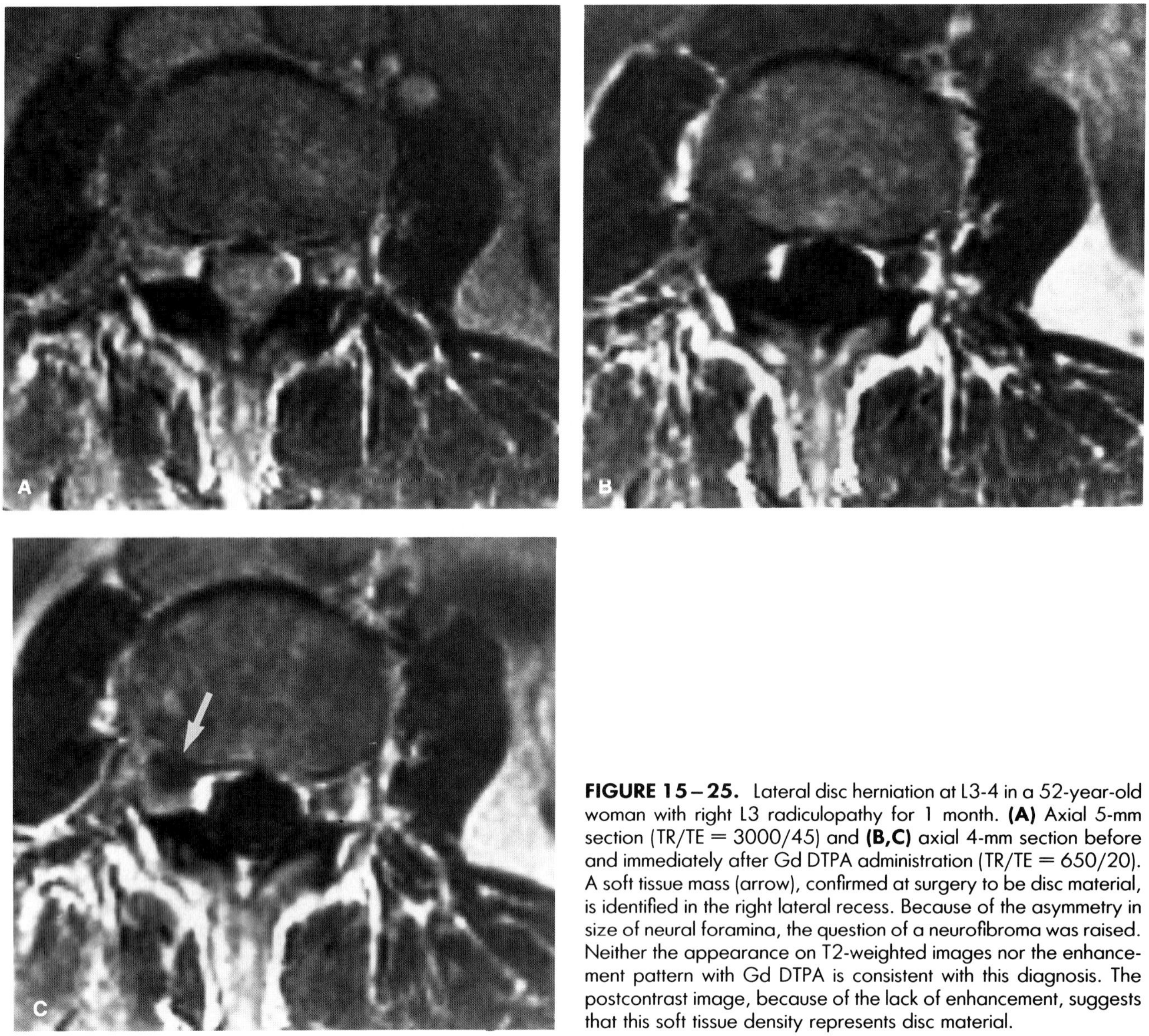

FIGURE 15–25. Lateral disc herniation at L3-4 in a 52-year-old woman with right L3 radiculopathy for 1 month. **(A)** Axial 5-mm section (TR/TE = 3000/45) and **(B,C)** axial 4-mm section before and immediately after Gd DTPA administration (TR/TE = 650/20). A soft tissue mass (arrow), confirmed at surgery to be disc material, is identified in the right lateral recess. Because of the asymmetry in size of neural foramina, the question of a neurofibroma was raised. Neither the appearance on T2-weighted images nor the enhancement pattern with Gd DTPA is consistent with this diagnosis. The postcontrast image, because of the lack of enhancement, suggests that this soft tissue density represents disc material.

appears to be somewhat more restricted. Gd DTPA use in intramedullary neoplastic disease has been advocated for the differentiation of simple and complex (neoplastic) syrinxes and for directing surgical biopsy (Fig. 15–26). Caution is advised because, by analogy with brain MRI, some neoplastic cord lesions may not enhance after contrast administration. In extramedullary disease, Gd DTPA provides exquisite recognition of drop metastases, an area in which unenhanced MRI has been disappointing (Fig. 15–27).[42,43] Nonneoplastic lesions of the cord may also display contrast enhancement with Gd DTPA (Fig. 15–28).

Extradural Neoplasia

In metastatic disease limited to bone, Gd DTPA may be of limited benefit.[44] Diagnosis in this situation can be made primarily on the basis of unenhanced T1-weighted images. The low signal intensity of metastatic lesions allows their visualization, distinguishing them from high-signal-intensity normal marrow on unenhanced scans. Contrast enhancement within metastatic lesions can confirm their presence. However on post-Gd-DTPA images alone, lesions can be difficult to appreciate because enhancement may make these areas isointense with normal marrow fat.

Conversely, Gd DTPA administration can be of great value for defining the soft tissue extent of extradural disease. The soft tissue extent of bony metastatic disease, especially compression of neural elements, is well depicted by enhanced T1-weighted images (Figs. 15–29 and 15–30).

Neurofibromas can be recognized by their very high signal intensity on T2-weighted images. These

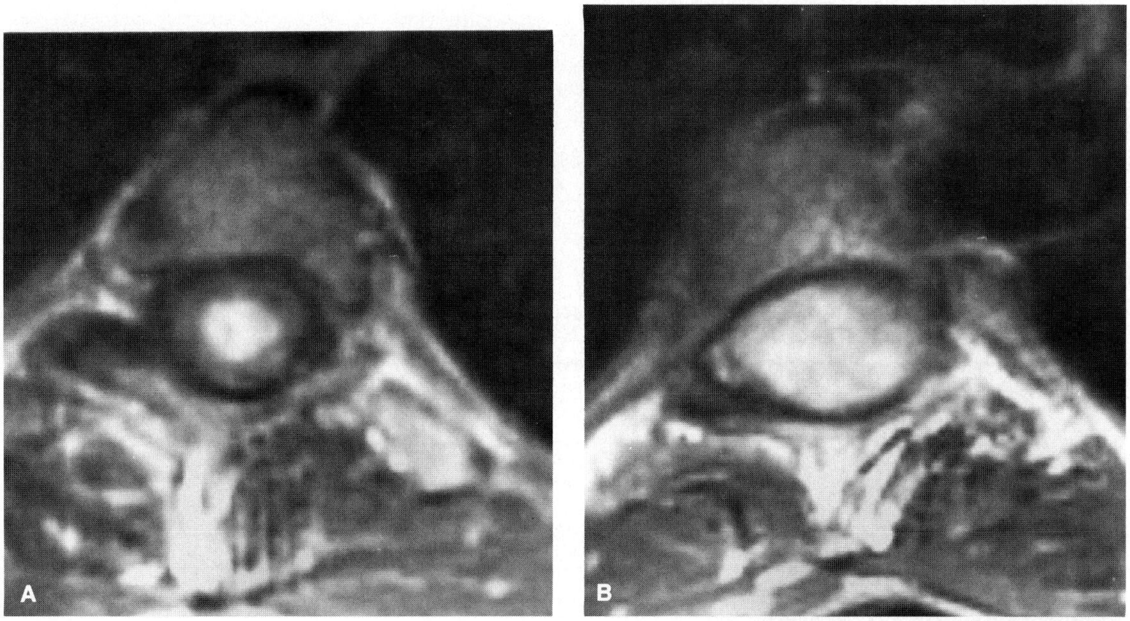

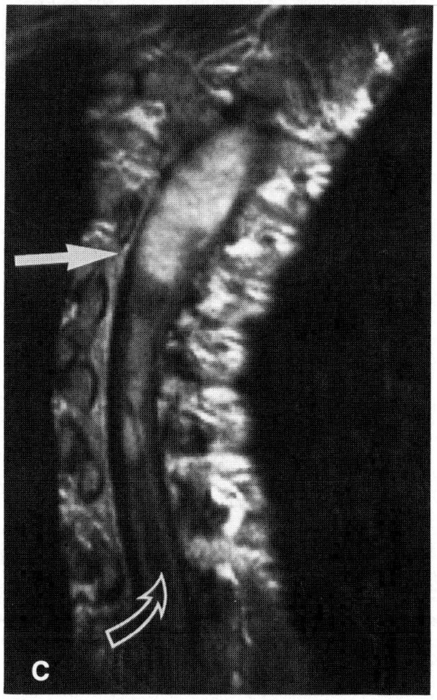

FIGURE 15–26. Surgically proven astrocytoma of the thoracic cord in a 27-year-old man. Postcontrast 5-mm **(A,B)** axial sections at T4 and T6 and **(C)** coronal section (TR/TE = 650/20). An enhancing mass (closed arrow) is seen extending from T3 through T7, easily differentiated from the accompanying syrinx (open arrow) due to contrast administration. At T4, the lesion seems to involve only the central portion of the cord, but at T6, there is homogeneous enhancement and marked cord expansion.

lesions also demonstrate homogeneous contrast enhancement. Enhanced T1-weighted images can offer advantages over T2-weighted images in resolution and SNR. This difference could be exploited to shorten the scan time for a single diagnostic sequence or to achieve thinner, higher-resolution sections. Taking this argument to its logical conclusion, small meningiomas and neuromas (intradural or extradural) should be best visualized on enhanced T1-weighted scans.

NON-CNS APPLICATIONS

Application of contrast media in other areas of the body remains primarily investigational. To some extent, this reflects the development of MRI itself. Clinical utility has been demonstrated in the neck, oropharynx, and nasopharynx.[45] By rim enhancement, Gd DTPA permits identification of necrotic lymph nodes. Early experience indicates that the extent of

(text continues on page 545)

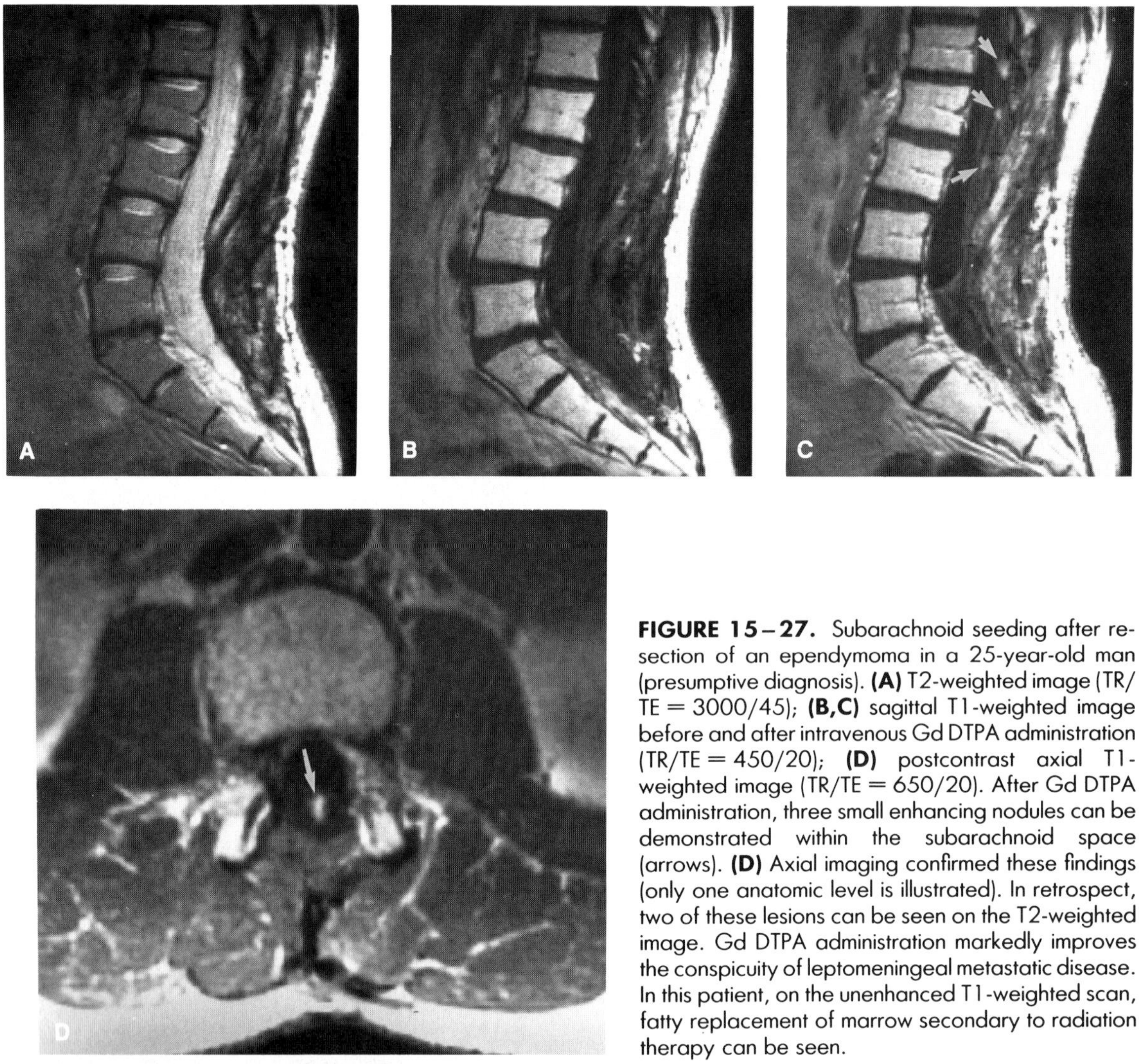

FIGURE 15–27. Subarachnoid seeding after resection of an ependymoma in a 25-year-old man (presumptive diagnosis). **(A)** T2-weighted image (TR/TE = 3000/45); **(B,C)** sagittal T1-weighted image before and after intravenous Gd DTPA administration (TR/TE = 450/20); **(D)** postcontrast axial T1-weighted image (TR/TE = 650/20). After Gd DTPA administration, three small enhancing nodules can be demonstrated within the subarachnoid space (arrows). **(D)** Axial imaging confirmed these findings (only one anatomic level is illustrated). In retrospect, two of these lesions can be seen on the T2-weighted image. Gd DTPA administration markedly improves the conspicuity of leptomeningeal metastatic disease. In this patient, on the unenhanced T1-weighted scan, fatty replacement of marrow secondary to radiation therapy can be seen.

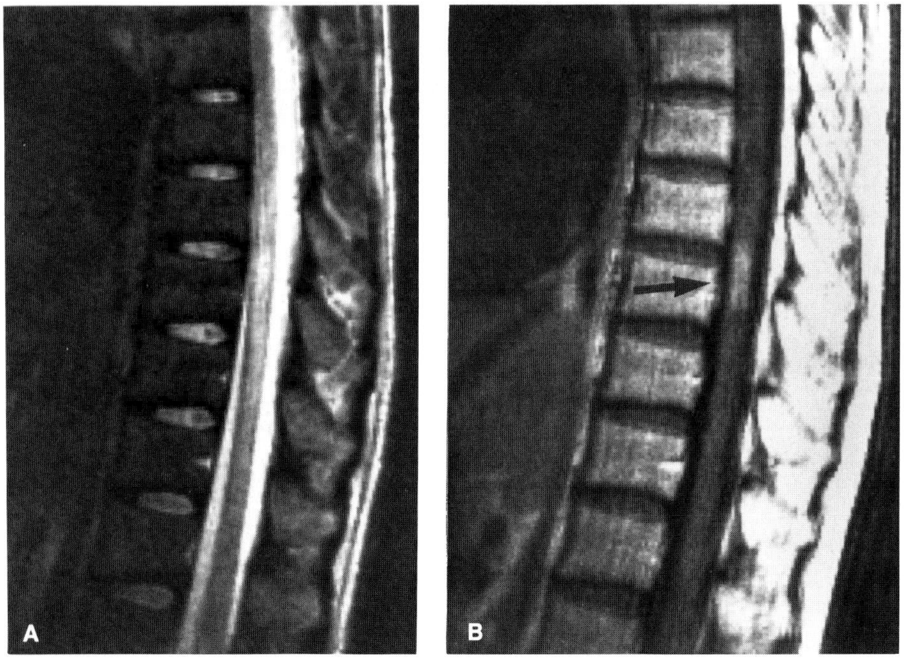

FIGURE 15–28. Enhancing T9 cord lesion (arrow) in a 39-year-old woman with midback pain, right leg weakness, and left leg numbness, presumed to represent MS. Cranial MRI scan was within normal limits. **(A)** 4-mm section (TR/TE = 3000/90) and **(B)** postcontrast 4-mm section (TR/TE = 450/20). The precontrast T1-weighted scan was normal. This lesion, which does not cause cord deformity, can be equally well identified on the T2-weighted or postcontrast T1-weighted scan. Enhancement of the lesion correlates with clinical activity.

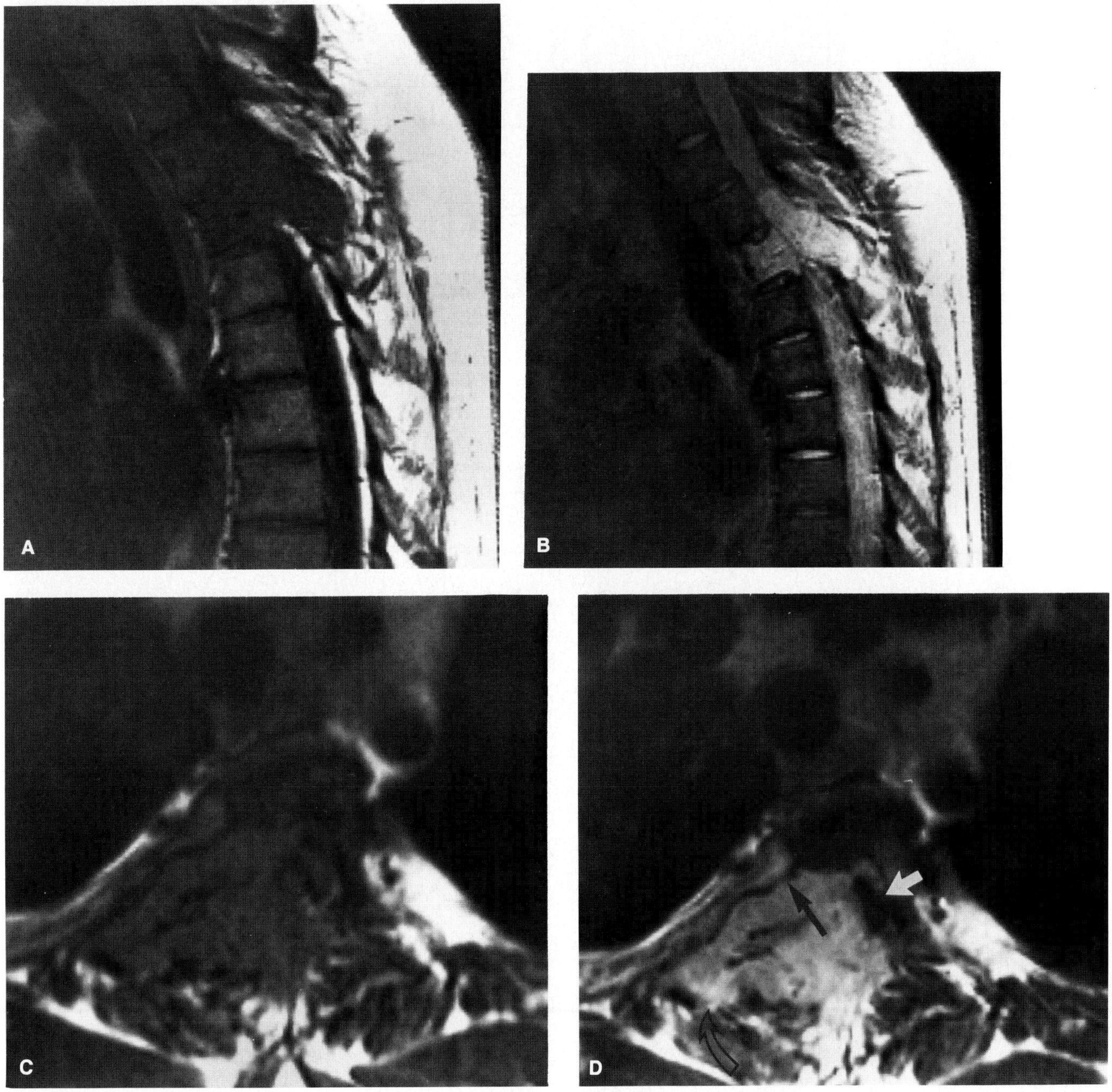

FIGURE 15–29. Malignant melanoma with metastases to T3 and T4 in a 28-year-old man presenting clinically with cord compression. **(A)** Sagittal 4-mm section (TR/TE = 650/20); **(B)** sagittal 5-mm section (TR/TE = 3000/45); **(C,D)** axial 4-mm section before and after contrast (TR/TE = 650/20). The location of the displaced thoracic cord (white arrow), extent of soft tissue metastatic disease (open arrow), and rib involvement (black arrow) are best appreciated on the postcontrast image. Although an axial T2-weighted scan might have provided similar information, the enhanced T1-weighted scan offers superior resolution and is less likely to be degraded by motion artifacts.

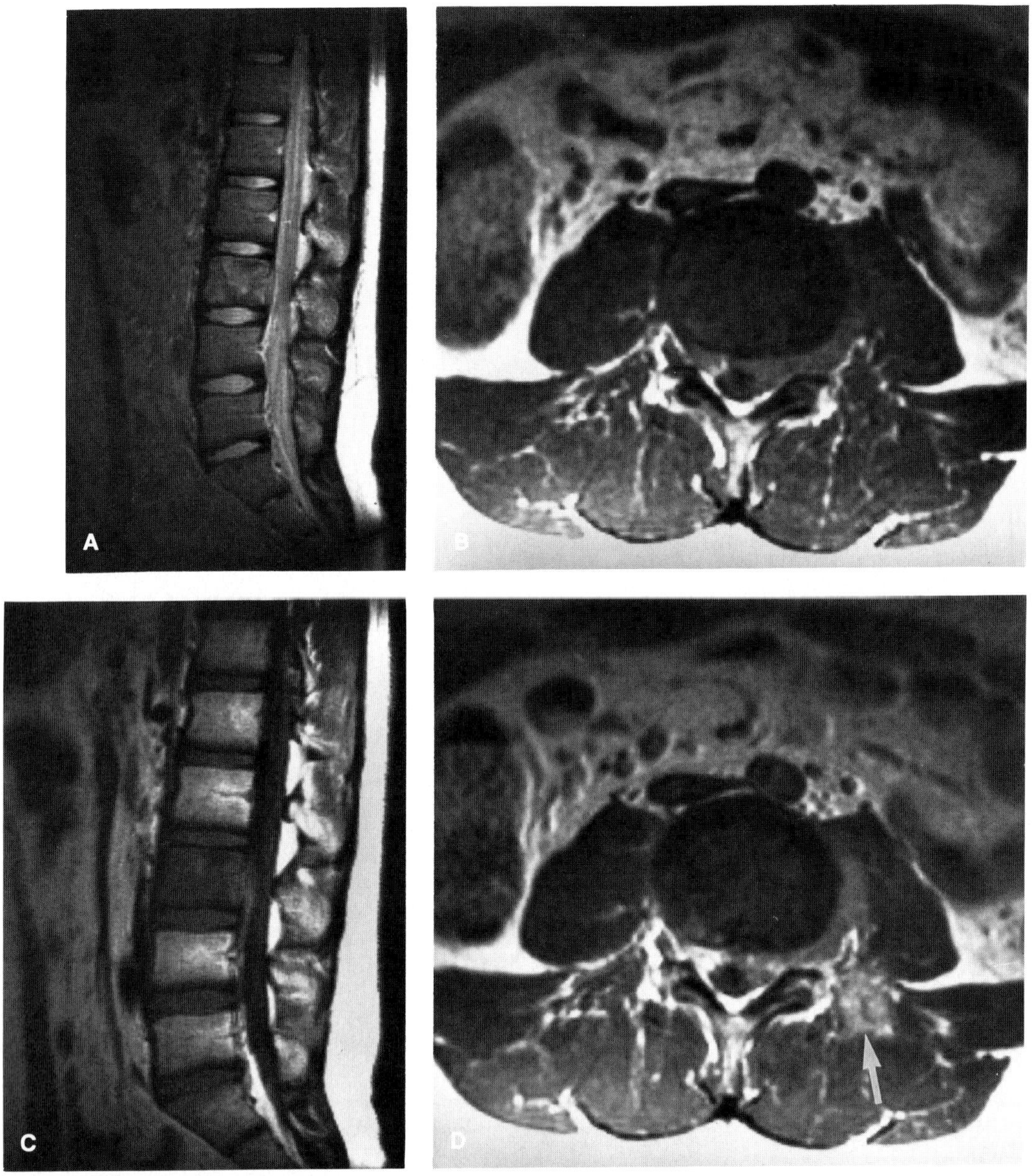

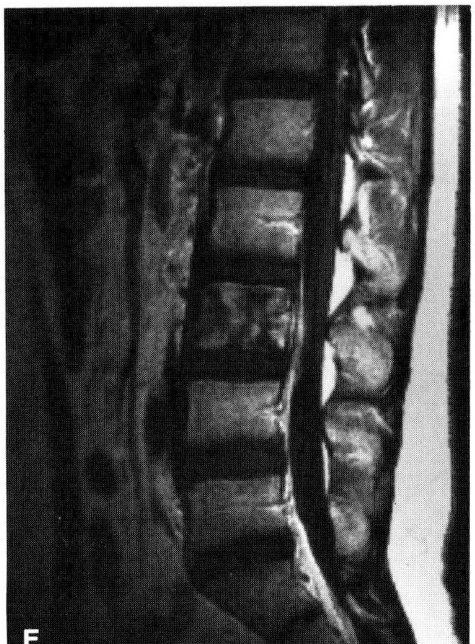

FIGURE 15–30. Metastatic Ewing's sarcoma, with soft tissue extension. **(A)** Sagittal T2-weighted scan; axial and sagittal T1-weighted scans **(B,C)** before and **(D,E)** after Gd DTPA. Contrast enhancement is advantageous for the recognition and delineation of extradural metastatic disease. As in Figure 15-29, soft tissue extension of neoplasia (beyond bony confines) is best demonstrated on enhanced scans (arrow). Replacement of normal bone marrow by neoplastic disease on unenhanced scans is often best identified on unenhanced T1-weighted scans. However, soft tissue involvement may be isointense with muscle on both T1-weighted and T2-weighted scans and therefore difficult to recognize. Enhancement of metastatic disease limited to bone need not lead to lower lesion contrast. Gd DTPA can improve detection of diploic space metastases. Enhancement may also aid differentiation of metastatic disease from osteoporosis as the cause of vertebral body collapse. (Runge VM, Nelson KL, Carollo BR, et al. The clinical utility of IV gadopentetate dimeglumine for MRI of the head and spine. MRI Decisions 1989;3:2. Reprinted with permission from Physicians World Communications Group)

disease spread in squamous cell carcinoma can be better delineated on postcontrast T1-weighted scans. Furthermore, contrast enhancement may play a role in distinguishing tumor recurrence from postoperative or postradiation fibrosis.

Acute myocardial infarctions enhance more than normal myocardium after Gd DTPA administration.[46,47] The greater the degree of cellular damage, the greater the observed enhancement. Enhancement does not aid in the demonstration of chronic myocardial infarction.

Initial studies of the breast have demonstrated that Gd DTPA improves visualization of tumors, due to their enhancement, within mammographically dense breast tissue.[48,49] Contrast enhancement also improves the distinction between nonproliferative dysplasia or scarring and carcinoma.[50]

In liver, information regarding lesion perfusion can be supplied by intravenous Gd DTPA administration.[51] Enhancement increases contrast between lesion and liver with fast imaging techniques.[52] Breath-hold techniques will probably play a major role in abdominal imaging. The use of paramagnetic metal ion chelates, like Gd DTPA will be critical, particularly if larger amounts of new contrast agents can be administered safely. Although T2-weighted MRI is still the preferred technique for diagnosing hemangiomas, administration of Gd DTPA is indicated in complex cases. In dynamic studies after contrast administration, hemangiomas are characterized by enhancement that progresses from the periphery toward the central portion of the lesion. On delayed postcontrast T1-weighted images, these lesions classically display homogeneous high signal intensity.

In the kidney, small neoplastic lesions may be difficult to detect due to their isointensity with normal parenchyma and the absence of contour deformity. Gd DTPA has improved detection of small renal tumors by providing enhancement of normal renal parenchyma.[53] Dynamic studies can demonstrate the hypervascularity of renal lesions, which is analogous to that seen in renal angiography and dynamic CT. Postcontrast images also clearly reveal internal lesion characteristics. Central nonenhancement suggests tumor necrosis or degeneration. Enhancing mural nodules in otherwise cystic masses support the diagnosis of neoplastic disease.

In pelvic tumors, the use of Gd DTPA does not significantly improve diagnosis or staging. In prostatic and endometrial carcinoma, tumor delineation is better after contrast administration than on unenhanced T2-weighted scans.[54] An advantage of the postcontrast T1-weighted exam is the higher SNR than on T2-weighted exams.

In musculoskeletal tumors, enhancement may prove useful in selecting the site for biopsy.[55] Little or no enhancement has been observed within areas of necrosis or edema. Contrast enhancement may also represent the best method for defining recurrent tumor. In infection, Gd DTPA administration can better delineate the extent of involvement.[56]

Opacification of the gastrointestinal system is important for the identification of intra-abdominal mass lesions and delineation of the pancreas.[57,58] Clinical trials have been performed with both positive and negative contrast agents.[59] It is important that agents (e.g., Gd DTPA and particulate iron oxides) are properly formulated for oral administration. Bowel peristalsis and resulting motion artifacts may limit the use of positive contrast agents like Gd DTPA.

PROSPECTIVE TRIALS

Six hundred adult patients have been enrolled in a prospective study at Tufts University examining the utility of Gd DTPA for the diagnosis of intracranial disease. This study is particularly impressive because FDA approval was based on fewer than 420 cases.

The MR scans in 108 of these patients with intracranial disease were interpreted in a blinded fashion. In 68%, the enhanced scan provided additional diagnostic information. In 33%, enhancement improved visualization of the lesion. Gd DTPA aided interpretation through enhancement (36%) and lack of enhancement (27%).

Gd DTPA significantly changed the physician's interpretation in 25% of cases (Fig. 15-31). Prominent in the group of lesions that were unrecognized on unenhanced images were neuromas, infarctions, and vascular abnormalities.

PRACTICAL CLINICAL USE

Gd DTPA use can be essential for lesion recognition.[12,60] Our recommendation for use in head examinations includes acoustic neuromas, metastatic disease, and infarction, particularly in deep white matter ischemia. In certain cases, meningiomas may only be diagnosed after contrast, and primary neoplastic disease often is more clearly depicted. The pattern of enhancement can improve specificity. There is also significant value in a negative enhanced scan, in ruling out metastatic disease. In spine examinations, contrast enhancement should be employed for detecting neoplastic disease (except lesions restricted to bone) and in differentiating scar from recurrent disc herniation in the postoperative patient.

In a study of 209 patients, Gd DTPA administration improved lesion visualization and definition of extent in intracranial and spinal neoplastic disease.[8] In inflammatory disease, contrast administration aided in differentiating active and chronic lesions.

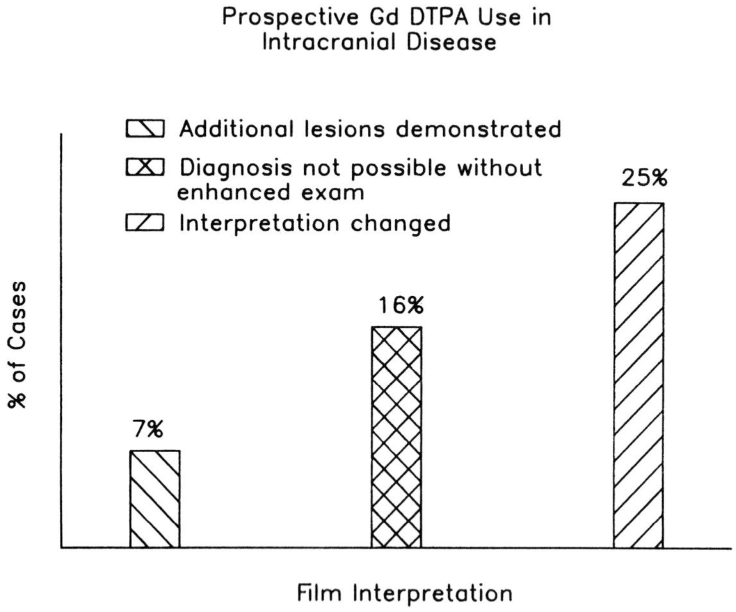

FIGURE 15–31. Preliminary results from a prospective trial of Gd DTPA use in adult head examinations.

At a dose of 0.1 mmol/kg of intravenous Gd DTPA, a slight transient increase in both serum iron and bilirubin can be observed.[61] From a blind, randomized, cross-over study in 12 volunteers using 0.25 mmol/kg Gd DTPA, this change was maximal between 6 and 12 hours, with recovery to baseline by 24 hours. No related clinical side-effects have been reported or observed. In personal experience with over 700 cases, no significant adverse reactions have been encountered. Hives have been observed (< 1% of all patients) immediately after intravenous Gd DTPA injection. Nausea, a common problem with iodinated agents, is virtually nonexistent when Gd DTPA is given as a slow infusion.

IMAGING TECHNIQUE

Rapid advances in imaging techniques influence the use of contrast media. Short TR, short TE spin echo sequences with mild T1-weighting have been used primarily for detecting contrast agents like Gd DTPA. Imaging technique must be optimized for contrast detection.[62]

It is important to be familiar with the normal pattern of enhancement in the brain, which may be sequence dependent. On spin echo images, the mucosal surfaces, veins, and the infundibulum show striking enhancement. Yet the dura does not prominently enhance, a major difference from x-ray CT. Newer techniques, such as 3D FLASH, may replace conventional spin echo techniques in certain instances due to superior sensitivity to T1 contrast and thus to Gd DTPA. Enhanced 3D FLASH may be particularly useful in imaging intracranial mass lesions, because it is possible to obtain by postprocessing high-resolution images in any plane, permitting tissue segmentation and lesion viewing in three dimensions. The 2D spin echo sequences may ultimately be replaced by 2D gradient-echo sequences (e.g., FLASH) for screening the brain as refinements in instrumentation continue to improve SNR. Fat-suppression sequences may also be employed following contrast enhancement, particularly for demonstrating epidural disease and meningeal disease and for detecting lesions within the orbit.

NEW AGENTS

New agents modeled on Gd DTPA are already nearing clinical use. These include two nonionic compounds, one derived from Gd DTPA and another based on Gd DO3A.[12] Certain agents, Gd HP-DO3A in particular, may allow significantly higher doses, opening new applications in the heart and upper abdomen.

Compounds based upon the 12-membered tetraaza macrocycle, such as Gd HP-DO3A and DOTA, may be favored due to their kinetic stability (Fig. 15–1). When the reactivity of Gd DOTA and Gd HP-DO3A was evaluated with respect to endogenously available ions, both proved to be kinetically inert.[63,64] Gd DTPA reacted with both Cu^{2+} and Zn^{2+}, a finding consistent with the known stability constants for these complexes. Animal studies have demonstrated that meglumine Gd DOTA behaves in an identical fashion with dimeglumine Gd DTPA in short-term biodistribution and excretion.[65] Both agents have an extravascular distribution. Relaxivity at high field strengths (1.0–1.5 T) is comparable for Gd DOTA, Gd HP-DO3A, and Gd DTPA.[66] Gd DOTA has already undergone clinical trials in Europe. Initial trials with Gd HP-DO3A have recently been completed in the United States.

CONCLUSION

Since approval for clinical use in 1988, Gd DTPA has found widespread application as a contrast agent in MRI. This paramagnetic metal ion chelate has been employed primarily for enhancement of head and spine lesions. Indications for use of contrast agents such as Gd DTPA have been summarized from results in more than 1500 patients and a review of the literature. Enhancement improves both lesion detection and categorization. In head exams, the use of Gd DTPA is recommended for studies of the IAC, metastatic disease, infarction, infection, meningeal disease, and primary neoplastic disease. In spine exams, contrast enhancement is employed both for detection of neoplastic disease and infection and for the differentiation of scar from disc herniation.

REFERENCES

1. Runge VM, Stewart RG, Clanton JA, et al. Paramagnetic NMR contrast agents: potential oral and intravenous agents. Work-in-progress paper presented at the Radiological Society of North America Meeting, November 1982, Chicago, IL.
2. Runge VM, Clanton JA, Lukehart CM, et al. Paramagnetic agents for contrast-enhanced NMR imaging: a review. AJR 1983;141:1209.
3. Weinmann HJ, Brasch RC, Press WR, Wesbey GE. Characteristics of Gadolinium-DTPA complex: a potential NMR contrast agent. AJR 1984;142:619.
4. Felix R, Schorner W, Laniado M, et al. Brain tumors: MR imaging with gadolinium-DTPA. Radiology 1985;156:681.
5. Carr DH, Brown J, Bydder GM, et al. Gadolinium DTPA as a contrast agent in MRI: initial clinical experience in 20 patients. AJR 1984;143:215.
6. Brant-Zawadzki M, Berry I, Osaki L, et al. Gadolinium DTPA in clinical MR of the brain. I. Intraaxial lesions. AJNR 1986;7:781.
7. Berry I, Brant-Zawadzki M, Osaki L, et al. Gd DTPA in clinical MR of the brain. II. Extraaxial lesions and normal structures. AJNR 1986;7:789.
8. Bauer WM, Fenzl G, Vogl T, et al. Indications for the use of Gd-DTPA in MRI of the central nervous system: experiences in patients with cerebral and spinal diseases. Invest Radiol 1988;23:S286.
9. Runge VM. Gd-DPTA: an i.v. contrast agent for clinical MRI. Int J Radiat Appl Instrum [B] 1988;15:37.
10. Runge VM, Schaible TF, Goldstein HA, et al. Gd DTPA—clinical efficacy. Radiographics 1988;8:147.
11. Runge VM, Wood ML, Kaufman DM, Price AC. Gd DTPA—future applications with advanced imaging techniques. Radiographics 1988;8:161.
12. Runge VM, ed. Enhanced magnetic resonance imaging. St. Louis: CV Mosby, 1989.
13. Haughton VM, Rimm AA, Czervionke LF, et al. Sensitivity of Gd-DTPA-enhanced MR imaging of benign extraaxial tumors. Radiology 1988;166:829.
14. Nelson KL, Runge VM. Radiologic evaluation of acoustic neuromas. Magn Reson Imag Decisions 1987;1:31.
15. Stack JP, Ramsden RT, Antoun NM, et al. Magnetic resonance imaging of acoustic neuromas: the role of gadolinium DTPA. Br J Radiol 1988;61:800.
16. Bydder GM, Kingsley DPE, Brown J, et al. MR imaging of meningioma including studies with and without gadolinium DTPA. JCAT 1985;9:690.
17. Healy ME, Hesselink JR, Press GA, Middleton MS. Increased detection of intracranial metastases with intravenous Gd DTPA. Radiology 1987;165:619.
18. Claussen C, Laniado M, Schorner W, et al. Gadolinium DTPA in MR imaging of glioblastomas and intracranial metastases. AJNR 1985;6:669.
19. Hesselink JR, Press GA. MR contrast enhancement of intracranial lesions with Gd-DTPA. Radiol Clin North Am 1988;26:873.
20. Bird CR, Drayer BP, Medina M, et al. Gd DTPA-enhanced MR imaging in pediatric patients after brain tumor resection. Radiology 1988;169:123.
21. Grossman RI, Hecht-Leavitt CM, Evans SM, et al. Experimental radiation injury: combined MR imaging and spectroscopy. Radiology 1988;169:305.
22. Doppman JL, Frank JA, Dwyer AJ, et al. Gadolinium DTPA enhanced MR imaging of ACTH-secreting microadenomas of the pituitary gland. J Comput Assist Tomogr 1988;12:728.
23. Wichmann W, Schubiger O, Valavanis A, Kasdaglis K. MR diagnosis of microadenomas of the pituitary gland. ROFO 1988;149:239.
24. Runge VM, Clanton JA, Price AC, et al. Evaluation of contrast-enhanced MR imaging in a brain abscess model. AJR 1985;6:139.
25. Frank JA, Girton M, Dwyer AJ, et al. Meningeal carcinomatosis in the VX2 rabbit tumor model: detection with Gd-DTPA-enhanced MR imaging. Radiology 1988;167:825.
26. Mathews VP, Kuharik MA, Edwards MK, et al. Gd-DTPA-enhanced MR imaging of experimental bacterial meningitis: evaluation and comparison with CT. Am J Neuroradiol 1988;9:1045.
27. Schorner W, Henkes H, Sander B, Felix R. MR demonstration of the meninges: normal and pathological findings. ROFO 1988;149:361.
28. Pykett IL, Buonanno RS, Brady TJ, Kistler JP. True three-dimensional nuclear magnetic resonance neuro-imaging in ischemic stroke: correlation of NMR, x-ray CT, and pathology. Stroke 1983;14:173.
29. Virapongse C, Mancuso AA, Quisling RG. Human brain infarcts: imaging by MR enhanced Gd DTPA. Radiology 1986;161:785.
30. Imakita S, Nishimura T, Yamada N, et al. Magnetic resonance imaging of cerebral infarction: time course of Gd-DTPA enhancement and CT comparison. Neuroradiology 1988;30:372.
31. Miyashita K, Naritomi H, Sawada T, et al. Identification of recent lacunar lesions in cases of multiple small infarctions by magnetic resonance imaging. Stroke 1988;19:834.
32. Miller DH, Rudge P, Johnson G, et al. Serial gadolinium enhanced magnetic resonance imaging in multiple sclerosis. Brain 1988;111:927.
33. Grossman RI, Gonzalez-Scarano F, Atlas SW et al. Multiple sclerosis: gadolinium enhancement in MR imaging. Radiology 1986;161:721.
34. Lukes SA, Crooks LE, Aminoff MJ, et al. Nuclear magnetic resonance imaging in multiple sclerosis. Ann Neurol 1983;13:592.
35. Runge VM, Price AC, Kirshner HS, et al. Magnetic resonance imaging of multiple sclerosis: a study of pulse technique efficacy. AJR 1984;143:1015.
36. Hueftle MG, Modic MT, Ross JS, et al. Lumbar spine: postoperative MR imaging with Gd-DTPA. Radiology 1988;167:817.
37. Sze G. Gadolinium DTPA in spinal disease. Radiol Clin North Am 1988;26:1009.
38. Bydder GM, Brown J, Niendorf HP, Young IR. Enhancement of cervical intraspinal tumors in MR imaging with intravenous gadolinium DTPA. J Comput Assist Tomogr 1985;9:847.
39. Sze G, Krol G, Zimmerman RD, Deck MDF. Intramedullary disease of the spine: diagnosis using gadolinium-DTPA-enhanced MR imaging. Am J Neuroradiol 1988;9:847.
40. Stimac GK, Porter BA, Olson DO, et al. Gadolinium-DTPA-enhanced MR imaging of spinal neoplasms: preliminary investi-

gation and comparison with unenhanced spin-echo and STIR sequences. Am J Neuroradiol 1988;9:839.
41. Valk J. Gd-DTPA in MR of spinal lesions. Am J Roentgenol 1988;150:1163.
42. Berns DH, Blaser S, Ross JS, et al. MR imaging with Gd-DTPA in leptomeningeal spread of lymphoma. J Comput Assist Tomogr 1988;12:499.
43. Sze G, Abramson A, Krol G, et al. Gadolinium-DTPA in the evaluation of intradural extramedullary spinal disease. Am J Neuroradiol 1988;9:153.
44. Sze G, Krol G, Zimmerman RD, Deck MDF. Malignant extradural spinal tumors: MR imaging with Gd-DTPA. Radiology 1988;167:217.
45. Schiller VL, Teresi L, Lufkin RB, Hanafee WN. Neck, oropharynx, and nasopharynx. In: Runge VM, ed. Enhanced magnetic resonance imaging. St. Louis: CV Mosby, 1989:211.
46. McNamara MT, Tscholakoff D, Revel D, et al. Differentiation of reversible and irreversible myocardial injury by MR imaging with and without gadolinium-DTPA. Radiology 1986;158:765.
47. Tscholakoff D, Higgins CB, Sechtem U, et al. Occlusive and reperfused myocardial infarcts: effect of Gd-DTPA on ECG-gated MR imaging. Radiology 1986;160:515.
48. Heywang SH, Fenzl G, Beck R, et al. Anwendung von Gd-DTPA bei der kernspintomographischen: untersuchung der Mamma. Fortschr Roentgenstr 1986;145:338.
49. Heywang SH, Hahn D, Schmidt H, et al. MR imaging of the breast using Gd-DTPA. J Comput Assist Tomogr 1986;10:199.
50. Revel D, Brasch RC, Paajanen H, et al. Gd-DTPA contrast enhancement and tissue differentiation in MR imaging of experimental breast carcinoma. Radiology 1986;158:319.
51. Hamm B, Wolf KJ, and Felix R. Conventional and rapid MR imaging of the liver with gadolinium-DTPA. Radiology 1987;1643:313.
52. Mano I, Yoshida H, Nakabayashi K, et al. Fast spin echo imaging with suspended respiration: gadolinium enhanced MR imaging of liver tumors. J Comput Assist Tomogr 1987;11:73.
53. Yashiro N, Iio M. Kidney and adrenal gland. In: Runge VM, ed. Enhanced magnetic resonance imaging. St. Louis: CV Mosby, 1989:268.
54. Schmidt H, Mayr B. Pelvis. In: VM Runge, ed. Enhanced magnetic resonance imaging. St. Louis: CV Mosby, 1989:276.
55. Traill MR, Sartoris DJ. Musculoskeletal system. In: Runge VM, ed. Enhanced magnetic resonance imaging. St. Louis: CV Mosby, 1989:290.
56. Reiser M, Erhardt W, Bauer R, et al. Gd DTPA enhanced magnetic resonance imaging in the diagnosis of inflammatory and neoplastic musculoskeletal lesions. In: Runge VM, Clausen C, Felix R, James AE Jr. Contrast agents in magnetic resonance imaging. Princeton: Excerpta Medica, 1986.
57. Runge VM, Foster MA, Clanton JA, et al. Particulate oral NMR contrast agents. Int J Nucl Med Biol 1985;12:37.
58. Laniado M, Felix R: Gastrointestinal system. In: Runge VM, ed. Enhanced magnetic resonance imaging. St. Louis: CV Mosby, 1989;301.
59. Laniado M, Kornmesser W, Hamm B, et al. MR imaging of the gastrointestinal tract: value of Gd-DTPA. AJR 1988;150:817.
60. Runge VM, Claussen C, Felix R, James AE Jr, eds. Contrast agents in magnetic resonance imaging: proceedings of an international workshop. Princeton: Excerpta Medica, 1986.
61. Niendorf HP, Seifert W. Serum iron and serum bilirubin after administration of Gd-DTPA-dimeglumine: a pharmacologic study in healthy volunteers. Invest Radiol 1988;23:S275.
62. Price AC, Runge VM. Optimization of pulse sequences in Gd DTPA tumor enhanced MRI. In Runge VM, Claussen C, Felix R, James AE Jr, eds. Contrast agents in magnetic resonance imaging. Princeton: Excerpta Medica, 1986:99.
63. Tweedle MF, Eaton SM, Eckelman WC, et al. Comparative chemical structure and pharmacokinetics of MRI contrast agents. Invest Radiol 1988;23:S236.
64. Meyer D, Schaefer M, Bonnemain B. Gd-DOTA, a potential MRI contrast agent: current status of physicochemical knowledge. Invest Radiol 1988;23:S232.
65. Allard M, Doucet D, Kien P, et al. Experimental study of DOTA-gadolinium: pharmacokinetics and pharmacologic properties. Invest Radiol 1988;23:S271.
66. Runge VM, Jacobson S, Wood ML, et al. MR imaging of rat brain glioma: Gd-DTPA versus Gd-DOTA. Radiology 1988;166:835.

16

Classic Diagnoses

Val M. Runge

This chapter gives an overview of clinical magnetic resonance imaging (MRI) and its utility in daily practice. The strengths and weaknesses of MR diagnosis are reviewed for each anatomic region. Practical tips about imaging technique and film interpretation are also provided, emphasizing disease entities for which a definitive diagnosis can be provided by MRI.

To obtain high-quality MR images routinely, attention must be paid to imaging technique.[1] An uncooperative patient, image artifacts, a poorly tailored study, and inappropriate hardware may lead to poor results. Caution is advised in translating the rules of conventional radiology to the sphere of MRI. Differential diagnosis with x-ray techniques is often based on recognition of dystrophic calcification. Computed tomography (CT) is exquisitely sensitive to calcium, as in craniopharyngiomas and oligodendrogliomas, but soft tissue calcification is poorly visualized on MRI. In the future, the recognition and characterization of hemosiderin deposition in pathologic processes on MR images may play as important a role as calcification on CT scans. Magnetic susceptibility and flow add additional information on MRI to that provided by proton density and T1 and T2 relaxation times, although signal intensity information can be nonspecific. For example, neoplasia may not be high signal intensity on T2-weighted exams.

MRI shares some common problems with more conventional x-ray-based modalities like CT. The sensitivity to pathologic processes constitutes its strength, but the lack of specificity remains a major weakness. Radiation necrosis can be difficult to differentiate from recurrent or residual tumor. Gd-DTPA-enhanced MRI is extremely sensitive to leptomeningeal disease, yet nonspecific. Enhancement of the dura and meninges can be seen with neoplastic disease, infection, and after trauma or surgery. The differentiation of osteophytic disease from disc herniation in the spine remains a significant problem, particularly in the cervical region.

The strengths of MRI include its sensitivity to disease, selective specificity, the ability to perform multiplanar imaging, the lack of ionizing radiation, the superior visualization of lesions adjacent to bone (e.g., in the posterior fossa), and the direct visualization of blood flow. MRI clearly represents a significant advance over CT for evaluating disease processes in the brain, spine, and extremities. The advent of imaging techniques that permit scans during breath holding should lead to routine use of MRI in the chest, abdomen, and pelvis. As with any diagnostic modality, the length of the examination and cost must also be considered.

DEMYELINATION AND INFECTION

MRI is the imaging modality of choice for detecting disease involvement in multiple sclerosis (MS) (Fig. 16–1). Foci of demyelination of various ages are well depicted on T2-weighted scans.[2] There is marked female predominance in MS. The disease also has a distinct geographic distribution, with increasing incidence at higher latitudes. Treatment remains essentially symptomatic. Although therapeutic trials continue, there is little evidence that administration of steroids or ACTH change the course of disease progression.

MRI is markedly superior to high-dose, delayed CT scanning for lesion detection in MS. Although the sudden onset of unilateral optic neuritis is a common clinical presentation of MS in young women, abnormalities of the affected optic nerve are rarely identified. Radiologic diagnosis depends on identification of

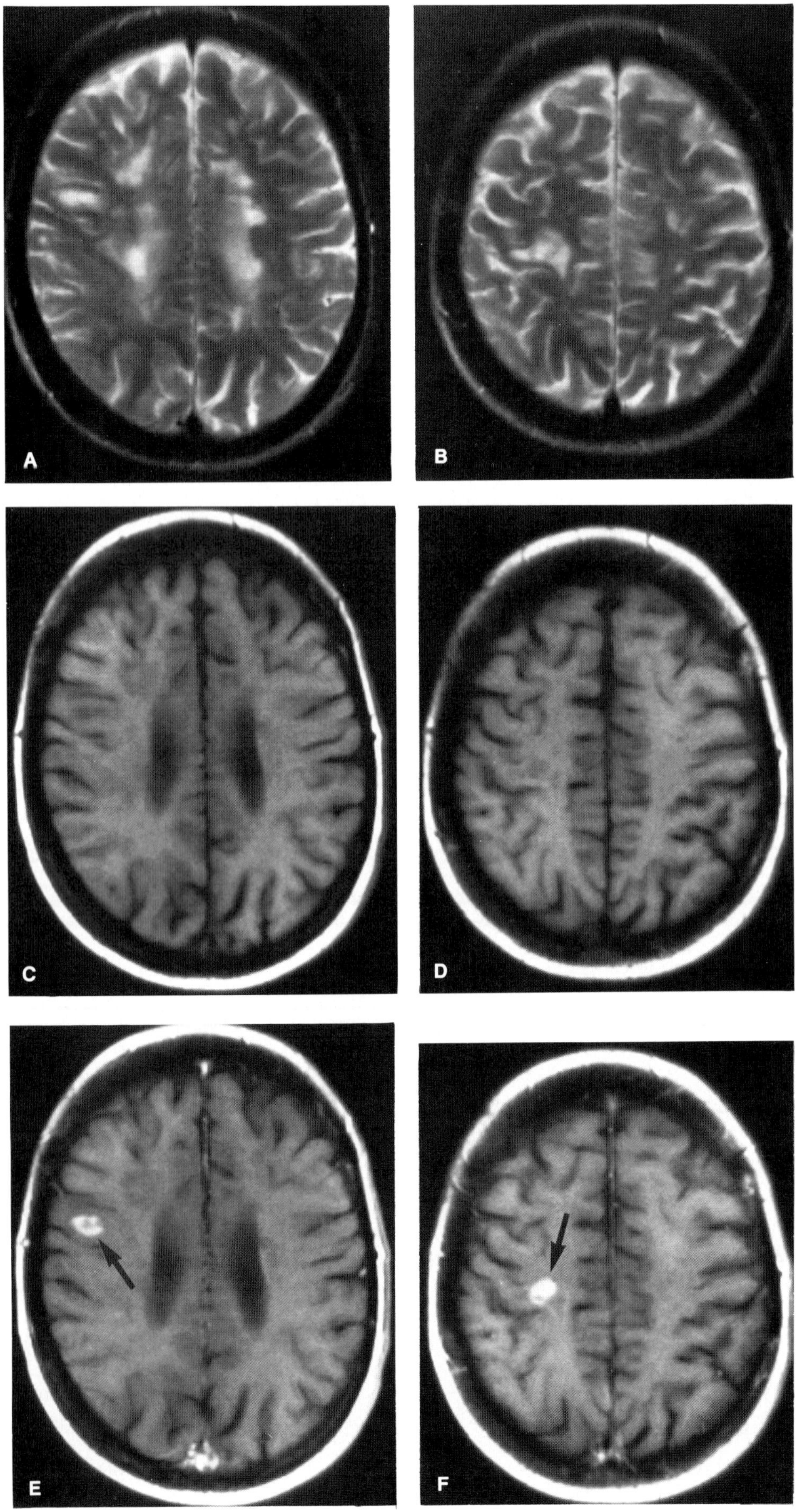

FIGURE 16–1. MS in a 38-year-old woman presenting with left arm weakness and a slight left facial droop. Images at two anatomic levels are presented. **(A,B)** T2-weighted images (TR/TE = 3000/90); T1-weighted images **(C,D)** before and **(E,F)** after intravenous Gd DTPA administration (TR/TE = 650/20). In advanced disease, periventricular plaques may become confluent. Clinically symptomatic lesions (arrows) are characterized by contrast enhancement.

disease plaques, with a characteristic appearance and distribution (i.e., punctate, periventricular, asymmetric) within the brain. Detection of lesions within the optic nerve and spinal cord requires careful attention to imaging technique.[3] Optic nerve lesions are best demonstrated with Short TI Inversion Recovery (STIR), a technique in which the prolongation of both T1 and T2 contribute to the high signal intensity of visualized lesions. With this imaging method, the signal intensity of fat is also decreased, improving visualization of the optic nerve within the orbital contents. For detecting spinal cord lesions, T2-weighted spin echo techniques with gradient moment nulling (GMN) are favored. At high field strengths (1 – 1.5 T), the addition of pulse or EKG gating may be required.

Clinical severity and course of the disease cannot necessarily be predicted from the appearance, number, or size of lesions. MS plaques do have elevated proton density, T1, and T2 values. The increased water content of plaques contributes to their excellent visualization on proton density weighted studies, which otherwise are relatively insensitive to tissue abnormalities on the basis of signal intensity differences. Disease activity can be assessed to some extent by contrast enhancement of plaques after intravenous Gd DTPA administration.[4,5] Cranial MRI may rarely be normal in MS. Many other pathologic processes, especially ischemic disease of white matter in elderly patients (Fig. 16–2), may mimic the appearance of MS on MRI.[6–8] For these reasons, MS continues to be a clinical diagnosis.

In the next decade, AIDS could become a major

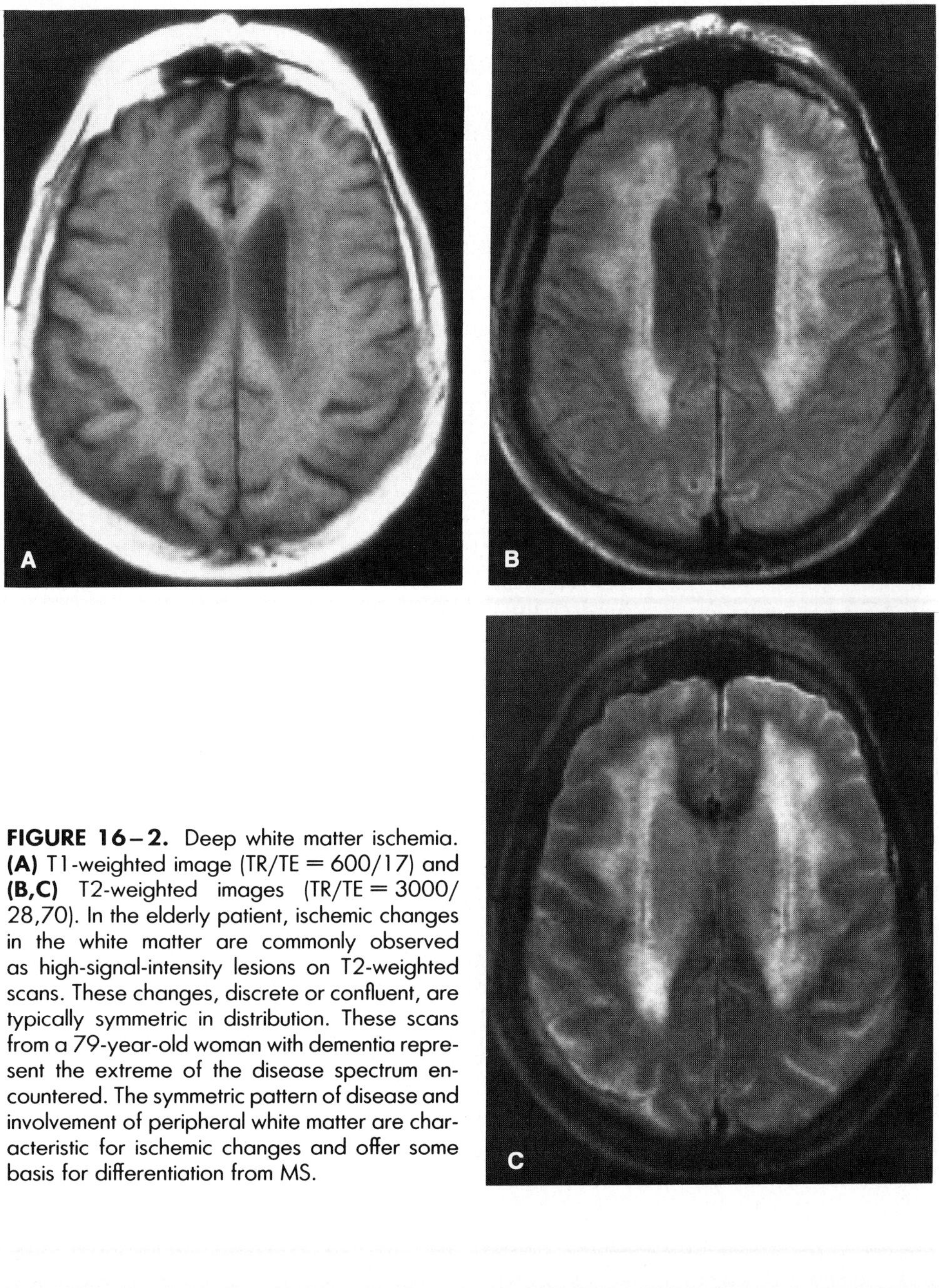

FIGURE 16–2. Deep white matter ischemia. **(A)** T1-weighted image (TR/TE = 600/17) and **(B,C)** T2-weighted images (TR/TE = 3000/28,70). In the elderly patient, ischemic changes in the white matter are commonly observed as high-signal-intensity lesions on T2-weighted scans. These changes, discrete or confluent, are typically symmetric in distribution. These scans from a 79-year-old woman with dementia represent the extreme of the disease spectrum encountered. The symmetric pattern of disease and involvement of peripheral white matter are characteristic for ischemic changes and offer some basis for differentiation from MS.

cause of death in the United States, with an incidence approaching that of cerebrovascular disease. Without substantial new developments in treatment, AIDS-related central nervous system (CNS) lymphoma is likely to become the third most common primary tumor of the brain, superseded only by glioma and meningioma. In this scenario, HIV encephalopathy would have a yearly incidence greater than that of MS by the early 1990s.

MRI is used in AIDS for differential diagnosis and to guide neurosurgical biopsy.[9] Toxoplasmosis is the most common intracranial mass lesion, with cryptococcus being the most common cause of meningeal disease. Caution should be exercised in attributing a specific pattern of disease involvement to a single cause, because several pathologic processes commonly involve the brain of the AIDS patient at any one time. Multiple, small, discrete disease foci are typically observed with toxoplasmosis infection, whereas a single, large lesion (> 3 cm) favors lymphoma. Diffuse atrophy is an ominous sign.

In part because of the lack of bone artifact, the outstanding anatomic detail presented by MRI is often best appreciated in the midbrain and brainstem. Ferritin-containing structures, such as the substantia nigra and red nuclei, can be distinguished by their low signal intensity on T2-weighted scans. Cranial nerves II, III, IV, and V can be routinely visualized on high-resolution scans with high signal-to-noise ratios (SNR). Cranial nerves VII and VIII can be directly visualized and distinguished within the internal auditory canal. In the young adult, the most common abnormality of the brainstem is MS. Vertebrobasilar infarction is more commonly encountered in older adults. Both are well depicted by T2-weighted spin echo images with GMN.

CEREBROVASCULAR DISEASE

Intracerebral hematomas follow a characteristic progression in signal intensity with time on MRI.[10,11] Acute hematomas (< 1 week old) appear hypointense on T2-weighted images at high field strength due to intracellular deoxyhemoglobin. These appear isointense or slightly hypointense relative to gray matter on T1-weighted scans. Surrounding cerebral edema appears hyperintense on T2-weighted images. At this stage, the plasma fraction of the initial hemorrhage has been resorbed, producing a hematocrit of 90% or greater within the hematoma, and the hemoglobin, having been deprived of oxygen, is in the deoxyhemoglobin state. In rare instances, the hematoma may be imaged before resorption of plasma. In this case, it will be hypointense on T1-weighted images and hyperintense on both proton density and T2-weighted images.

In avascular hypoxic regions, the appearance of acute hemorrhage can be different. The concentration of deoxyhemoglobin will be higher, causing greater hypointensity on T2-weighted scans. This appearance is likely with tumoral hemorrhage.

Although the time frame of the changes described is approximate, the sequence of changes on both MRI and pathologic examination are characteristic. The subacute stage (Fig. 16–3) occurs between 1 week and 1 month. Deoxyhemoglobin is converted to methemoglobin, initially at the periphery of the hematoma. A peripheral ring of variable hyperintensity can be demonstrated on T1-weighted images, with hypointensity on T2-weighted images. Over the next several weeks, the hyperintensity seen on T1-weighted scans extends to fill the entire hematoma, due to progressive conversion of deoxyhemoglobin to methemoglobin. There is subsequent red cell lysis and resorption, producing dilute, free methemoglobin that is hyperintense on all pulse sequences.

A chronic hematoma (after 1 month) appears hyperintense on all pulse sequences due to dilute, free methemoglobin. This pattern may persist for months and perhaps years. Digestion of hemoglobin by macrophages at the periphery of the hematoma deposits hemosiderin. If the blood-brain barrier is intact, these hemosiderin-laden macrophages are not removed from the brain, persisting indefinitely at the periphery of the hematoma.

As early as 1 week after hemorrhage, a ring of marked hypointensity on high-field T2-weighted images can be seen adjacent to the hematoma, corresponding to hemosiderin-laden reactive macro-

FIGURE 16–3. AVM with associated parenchymal hemorrhage in a 41-year-old woman. **(A,B)** ▶ T1-weighted and T2-weighted scans; **(C,D)** precontrast and postcontrast x-ray CT scans; **(E,F)** cerebral angiography of arterial and late venous phases. The angiogram **(E)** reveals a right temporal AVM (large arrow), with arterial supply from the middle cerebral artery and venous drainage via the superficial middle cerebral veins. The calcification (arrowhead) visible on x-ray CT cannot be identified on the MR scan, although the associated hemorrhage (open arrow) and major anomalous vessels (closed arrow) are well delineated. The signal intensity characteristics, high on T1-weighted scans and isointense on T2-weighted scans, are consistent with a subacute hemorrhage containing intracellular methemoglobin. Associated cerebral edema can also be identified on the T2-weighted scan (curved arrow).

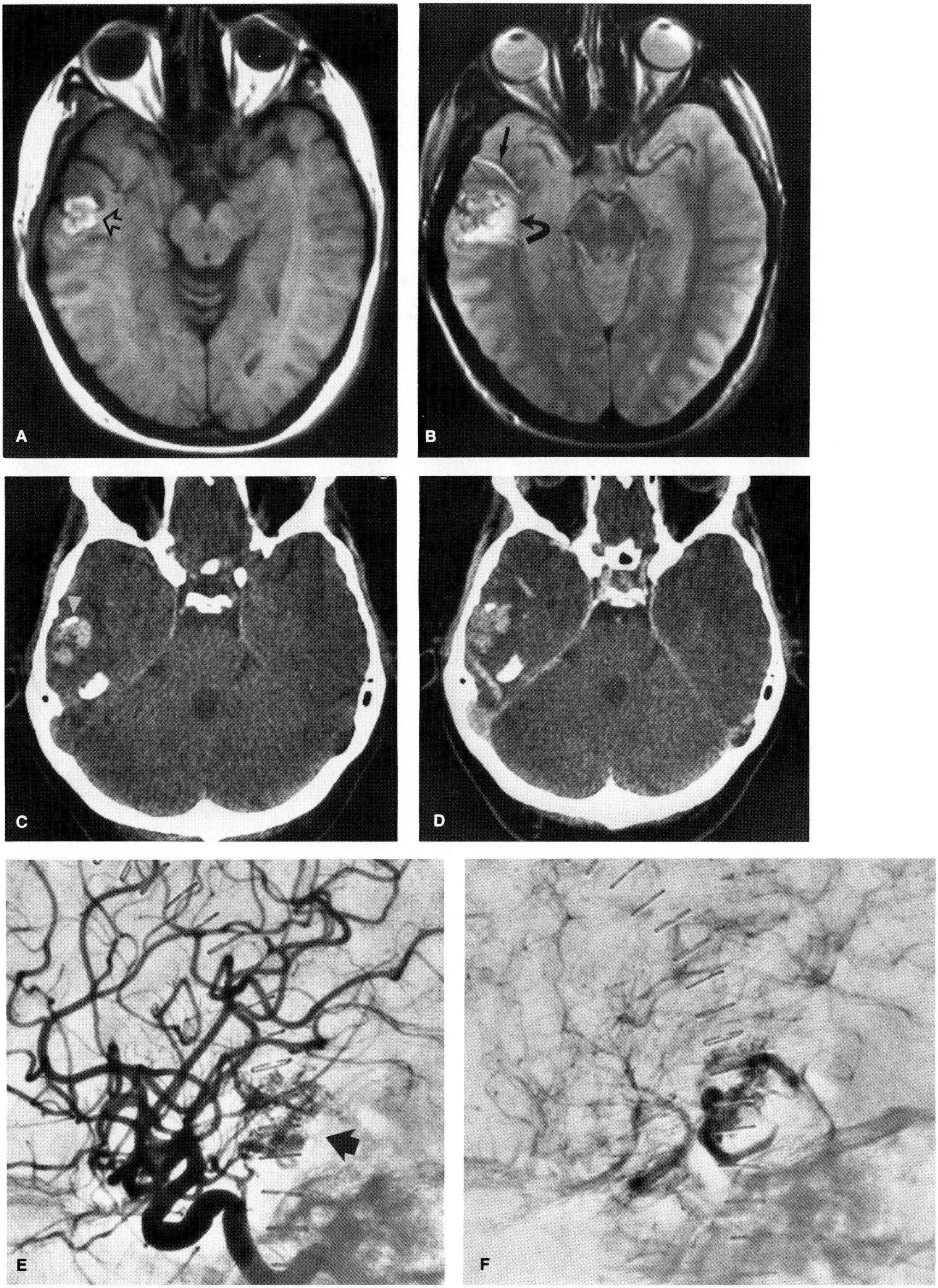

FIGURE 16–3.

phages. This rim may be isointense or mildly hypointense on T1-weighted images. If complete resorption of fluid from a chronic hematoma occurs, a hemosiderin-lined cleft is the only residual sign of previous hemorrhage. Edema surrounding an acute bleed resolves within a matter of weeks.

Hemorrhagic cortical infarctions are more common in watershed areas and may occur at the margin of a bland cortical infarct. There is a predilection for deeper cortical layers and gyral infolding. These also follow the temporal pattern of signal intensity change demonstrated by intracerebral hematomas. Edema and sulcal effacement accompanies the signal intensity characteristics of deoxyhemoglobin in acute hemorrhage. Acute hemorrhagic cortical infarction may appear less hypointense on T2-weighted scans at high field strengths than anticipated. Higher local oxygen tension, compared with intracerebral hematomas, is putatively responsible for this appearance. In the subacute stage, the high signal intensity on T1-weighted images of methemoglobin can be striking. Both the signal intensity characteristics and gyriform pattern improve differential diagnosis. In chronic infarction, hemosiderin deposition can be seen with the more common finding of localized atrophy.

Subdural hematomas undergo the same sequence of events in acute and subacute stages (Fig. 16–4). Hemosiderin deposition is not usually seen in chronic subdural hematomas, except after multiple bleeding episodes.

Acute subarachnoid hemorrhage is typically not visualized on MRI unless the collection of blood is quite large. Meningeal hypointensity can be observed at high field strength on T2-weighted images as a sequela of prior subarachnoid hemorrhage in a small number of cases. Hemosiderin deposition (e.g., superficial siderosis) is more common in chronic, recurrent subarachnoid hemorrhages. Recurrent or large intraventricular bleeds may also deposit hemosiderin along the ependyma.

MRI is the modality of choice for detecting occult cerebrovascular malformations (OCVM), due to the associated dense hemosiderin deposition.[12] These lesions are commonly cavernous angiomas and occur frequently in a supratentorial location. By definition, OCVM cannot be demonstrated by cerebral angiography. Circular deposits of hemosiderin are seen on MRI, a finding consistent with recurrent bleeding episodes. In contrast, old hematomas are visualized only as hemosiderin-lined clefts after resorption of fluid. A smooth, continuous rim of hypointensity, a central nonresorbable nidus, the lack of mass effect and edema, and the presence of similar noncontiguous lesions are consistent with a diagnosis of an OCVM.

Care must be exercised in distinguishing normal vessel flow from thrombosis. Imaging in multiple planes can be useful. For example, a blood vessel filled with methemoglobin is hyperintense, regardless of imaging plane. This appearance is unlikely to be mimicked by flow phenomena. Phase images are another simple and widely available alternative for demonstrating flow (Fig. 16–5). On T2-weighted images, vascular malformations are best depicted if motion-compensation techniques like GMN are not employed (Fig. 16–6). Gradient-echo techniques can be used to depict flow as high signal intensity, although results are highly technique-dependent and may only detect a limited range of velocities. MRI can be used to differentiate the thrombosed from patent portions of an intracranial aneurysm. In giant aneurysms, a multi-

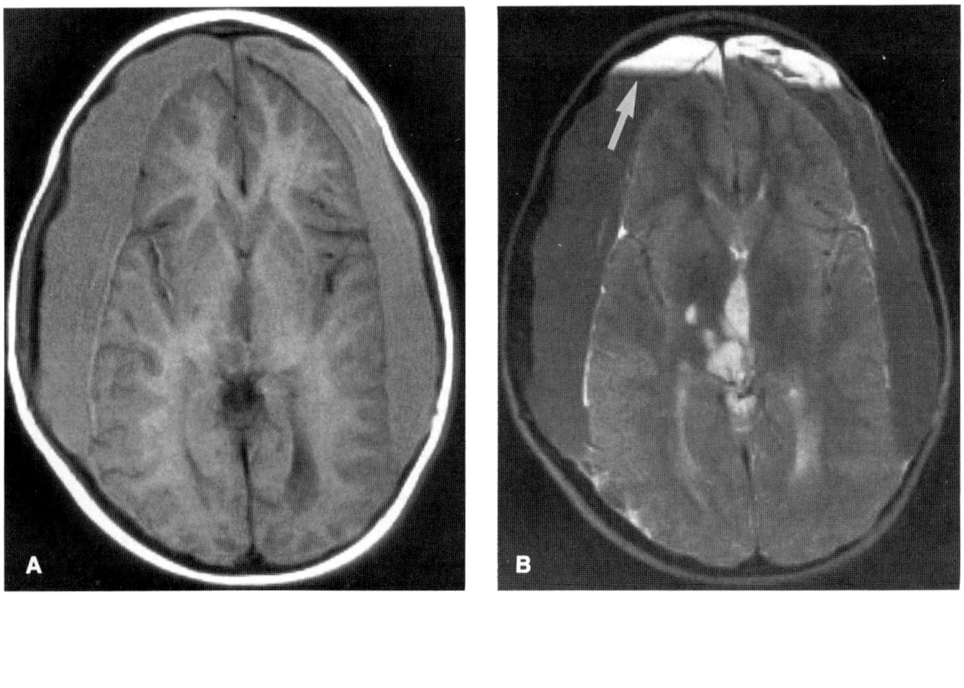

FIGURE 16–4. Bilateral subdural hematomas in a pediatric patient with a midbrain tumor. **(A)** T1-weighted image (TR/TE = 650/19) and **(B)** T2-weighted image (TR/TE = 3000/90). MRI is superior to x-ray CT for depicting subdural and epidural hematomas, due to the lack of partial volume effects from the bony calvarium. Fluid layers (arrow) represent different forms of hemoglobin. Hemosiderin, typically absent in extra-axial fluid collections, is removed by macrophages. The effects of hemoglobin dilution can markedly affect the signal intensity of blood-containing solutions, as in this patient.

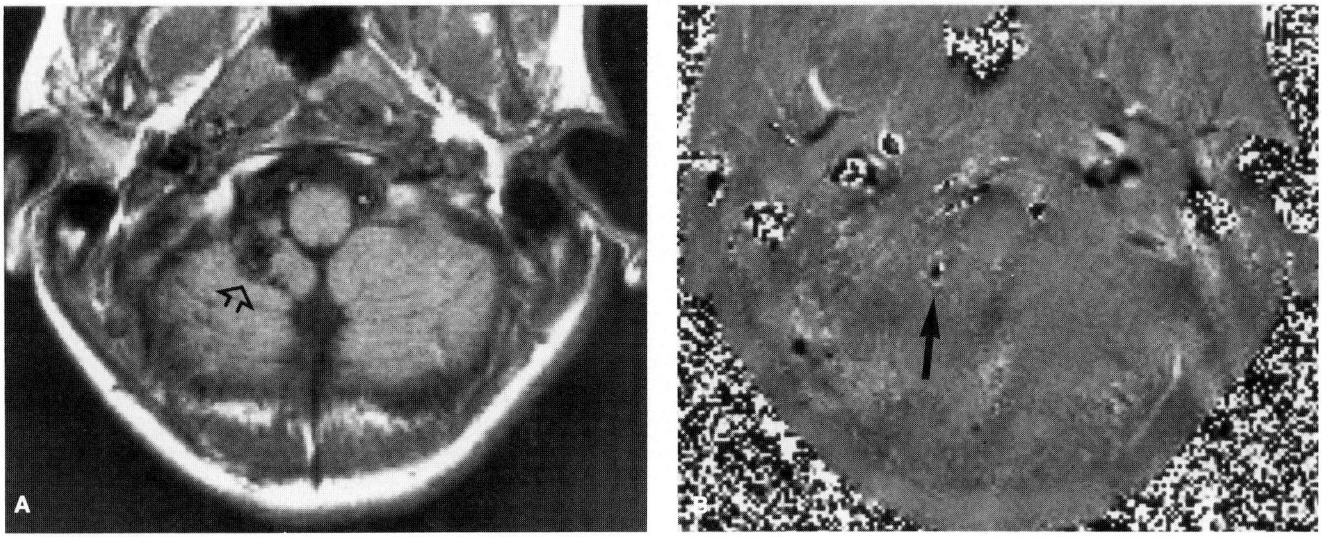

FIGURE 16–5. Right cerebellar AVM (presumptive diagnosis) in an 18-year-old boy. **(A)** Axial T1-weighted spin echo image (TR/TE = 650/20) and **(B)** corresponding phase image. Nonspecific low signal intensity is identified in a portion of the right cerebellum (open arrow) on the spin echo scan, with flow demonstrated within the lesion (closed arrow) on the phase image.

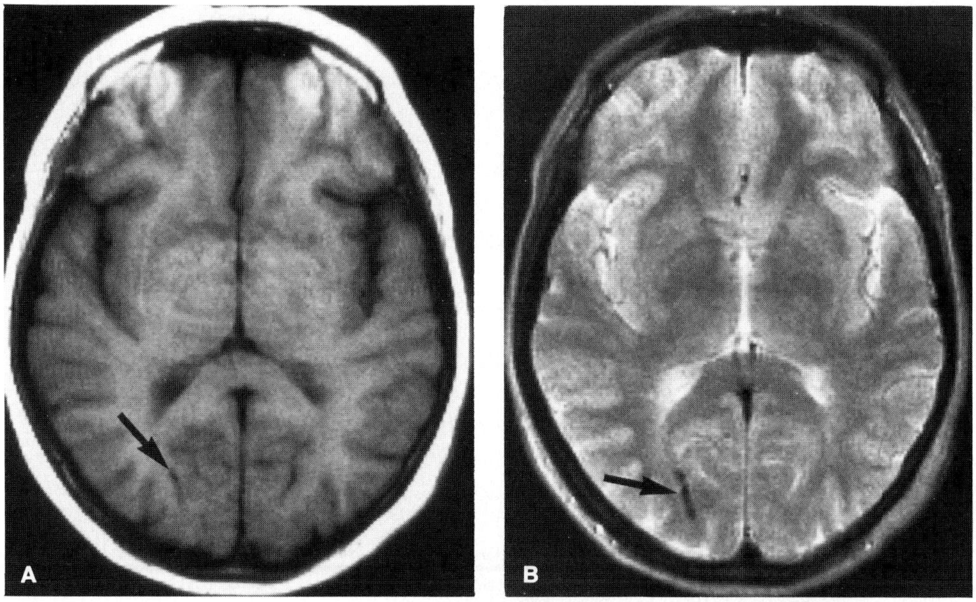

FIGURE 16–6. Venous angioma. **(A)** T1-weighted spin echo image (TR/TE = 600/17); **(B)** T2-weighted spin echo image (TR/TE = 3000/70); **(C)** gradient echo FLASH image (TR/TE = 40/9). A venous angioma can be identified in the right occipital lobe due to the presence of a flow void (closed arrow) on spin echo scans. The use of T2-weighted scans without gradient moment nulling improves visualization of vascular lesions. Flow-related enhancement (open arrow) is seen on gradient echo scans. Use of the gradient echo technique is limited primarily by magnetic susceptibility effects. For example, the difference in susceptibility between air and brain tissue leads to an artifactual low signal intensity in the frontal region above the ethmoid sinuses (curved arrow) on this gradient echo scan.

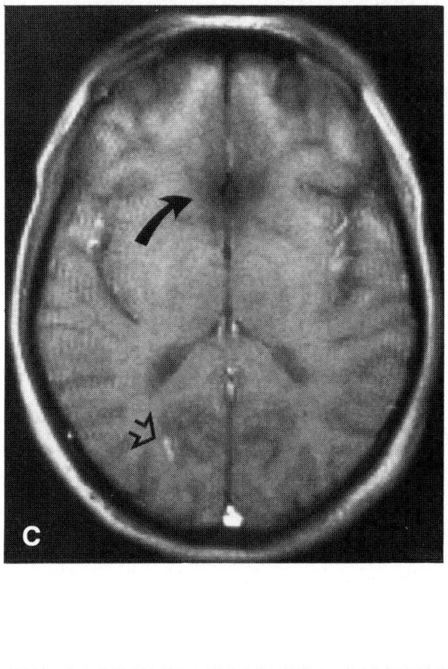

laminated appearance can be seen, with peripheral layers representing various stages of methemoglobin formation and hemosiderin deposition. In the future, MR angiography may play a significant role in the study of vascular disease.[13]

Sinus hemorrhage can be observed in head trauma, barotrauma, and after surgery. As with most extracerebral hemorrhages, hemosiderin deposition is typically absent in chronic lesions. Otherwise the progression of signal intensity changes follows that of intracerebral hemorrhage. Dilute, free methemoglobin may also be layered above more dependent, intact red blood cells.

Calcium and melanin can produce low signal intensity on T2-weighted images. However, these substances should be differentiated on MRI from hemosiderin. MRI is much less sensitive than CT to calcium deposition. Hemosiderin is much more hypointense than calcium on long TE T2-weighted images at high field strengths. Comparison of different pulse sequences reveals that hemosiderin deposits appear more extensive on T2-weighted than on T1-weighted images. Gradient-echo imaging may improve detection of hemosiderin, due to the inherent sensitivity of this technique to magnetic susceptibility effects. In deeply pigmented melanomas, the paramagnetic effect of melanin may mimic the signal intensity changes encountered with methemoglobin. However, melanotic melanomas typically are neither as hyperintense on T1-weighted images nor as hypointense on T2-weighted images as intracellular methemoglobin.

Cerebral ischemia and infarction represent the most common disease process to affect the brain. MRI provides exquisite sensitivity due to its ability to detect small changes in the water content of tissues.[14] The anatomic detail provided by MRI in both the brainstem and posterior fossa has required a greater understanding of vascular distributions for proper image interpretation (see Chapter 2). The depiction of disease in this region was poor before the advent of MRI, with x-ray CT being restricted by beam-hardening artifacts. Intravenous paramagnetic contrast agents like Gd DTPA provide a sensitive marker of blood-brain-barrier disruption in ischemic disease. Early clinical experience indicates that contrast agent administration may improve diagnostic sensitivity and specificity in the subacute phase of cerebral infarction (see Chapter 15).

BRAIN NEOPLASTIC DISEASE

MRI is more sensitive to many pathologic processes than x-ray CT, especially to intracranial neoplasia.[15-17] Low-grade astrocytomas can be difficult to detect on CT, due to small differences in x-ray attenuation. These lesions are easily demonstrated on T2-weighted spin echo images. MRI is particularly superior to CT in areas where bony artifacts create problems, including the vertex, middle fossa, posterior fossa, and craniovertebral junction. Not only is the contrast sensitivity of MRI greater than that of x-ray CT, but the multiplanar imaging capability improves anatomic localization. Acquisition of images in multiple planes is particularly important for aiding the neurosurgeon in operative planning.

In a few cases, CT remains the imaging modality of choice. Ferromagnetic aneurysm clips are an absolute contraindication to MRI. Because of its rapid scan time and greater accessibility, CT is the correct choice for uncooperative patients. CT can improve diagnostic specificity due to detection of calcification. The spatial resolution of early MRI scanners was markedly inferior to that of CT, but recent developments have made the resolution of MRI comparable to CT.

Gd DTPA is the first intravenous contrast agent approved by the FDA for clinical use in MRI.[18,19] Although the mechanisms of action are markedly different from those of iodinated agents, the trends and patterns of enhancement tend to parallel those of CT. In extra-axial lesions, specifically acoustic neuromas (Figs. 16–7 and 16–8) and meningiomas (Figs. 16–9 and 16–10), Gd DTPA administration is important for lesion recognition and definition of the extent of disease.[20] With intra-axial neoplasms, Gd DTPA administration can also improve lesion detection. Contrast enhancement is essential to rule out metastatic disease, given the existence of small lesions that otherwise cannot be detected due to the absence of mass effect and significant surrounding cerebral edema.[21] The observed side-effects are significantly less than those encountered with iodinated agents, although experience is limited. In a series of 700 patients at Tufts University, hives were observed in only a single patient (unpublished data). If given as a slow infusion, nausea is virtually nonexistent.

Before Gd DTPA, CT with intravenous contrast enhancement was superior to unenhanced MRI for detecting meningeal disease, but enhanced MRI is now recognized as more sensitive than CT.[22]

Before high-field imagers, CT was used exclusively for the radiologic evaluation of pituitary microadenomas. Technologic improvements have subsequently made similar slice thicknesses possible for MRI and CT. The ability to do multiplanar imaging, the contrast sensitivity of MRI, and the lack of artifacts due to dental fillings or bone interfaces have led to the acceptance of MRI over x-ray CT for evaluating the pituitary. The normal pituitary enhances after Gd DTPA administration, improving lesion contrast with most microadenomas (which usually do not enhance) on high-resolution T1-weighted images. Coronal and

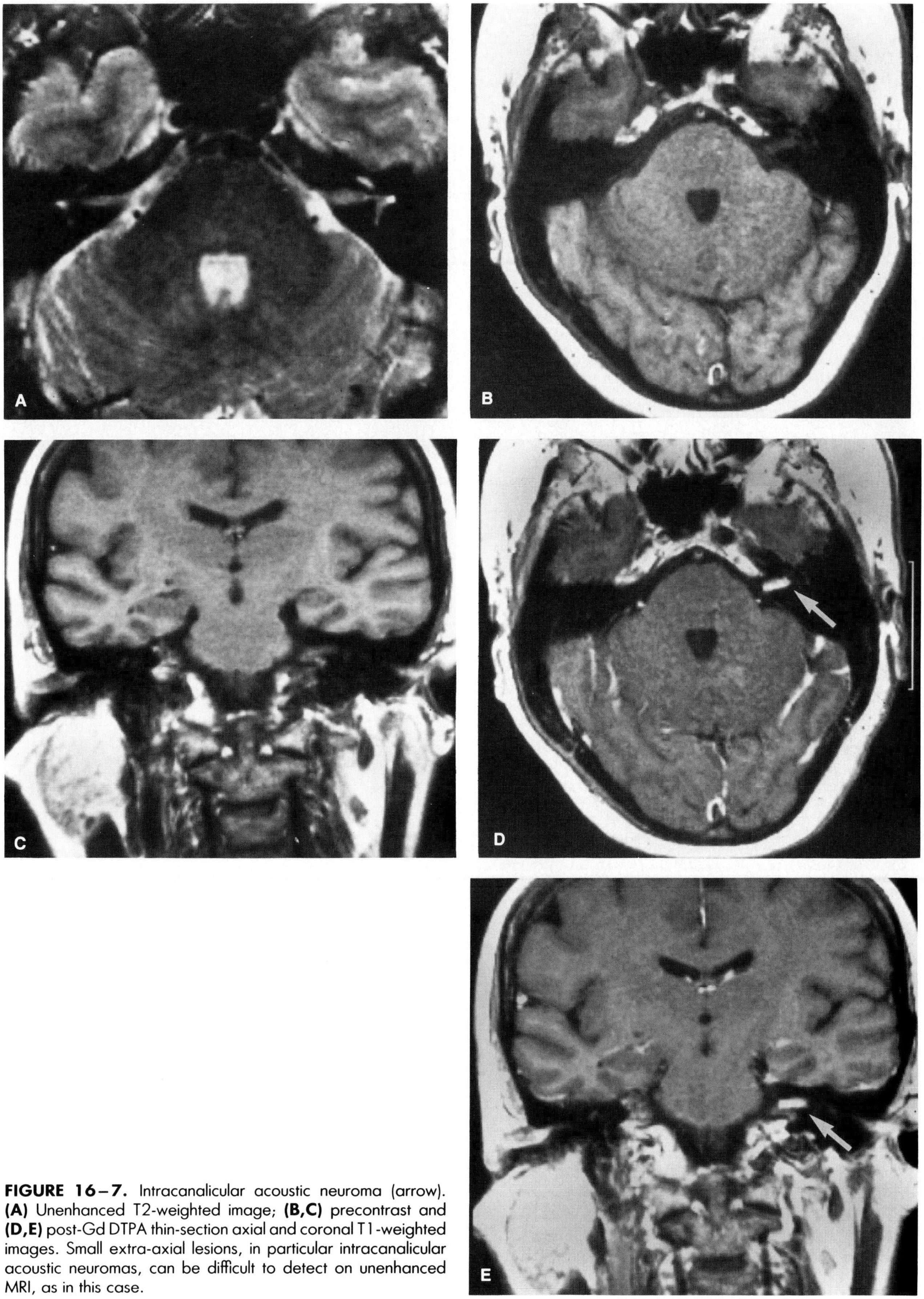

FIGURE 16–7. Intracanalicular acoustic neuroma (arrow). **(A)** Unenhanced T2-weighted image; **(B,C)** precontrast and **(D,E)** post-Gd DTPA thin-section axial and coronal T1-weighted images. Small extra-axial lesions, in particular intracanalicular acoustic neuromas, can be difficult to detect on unenhanced MRI, as in this case.

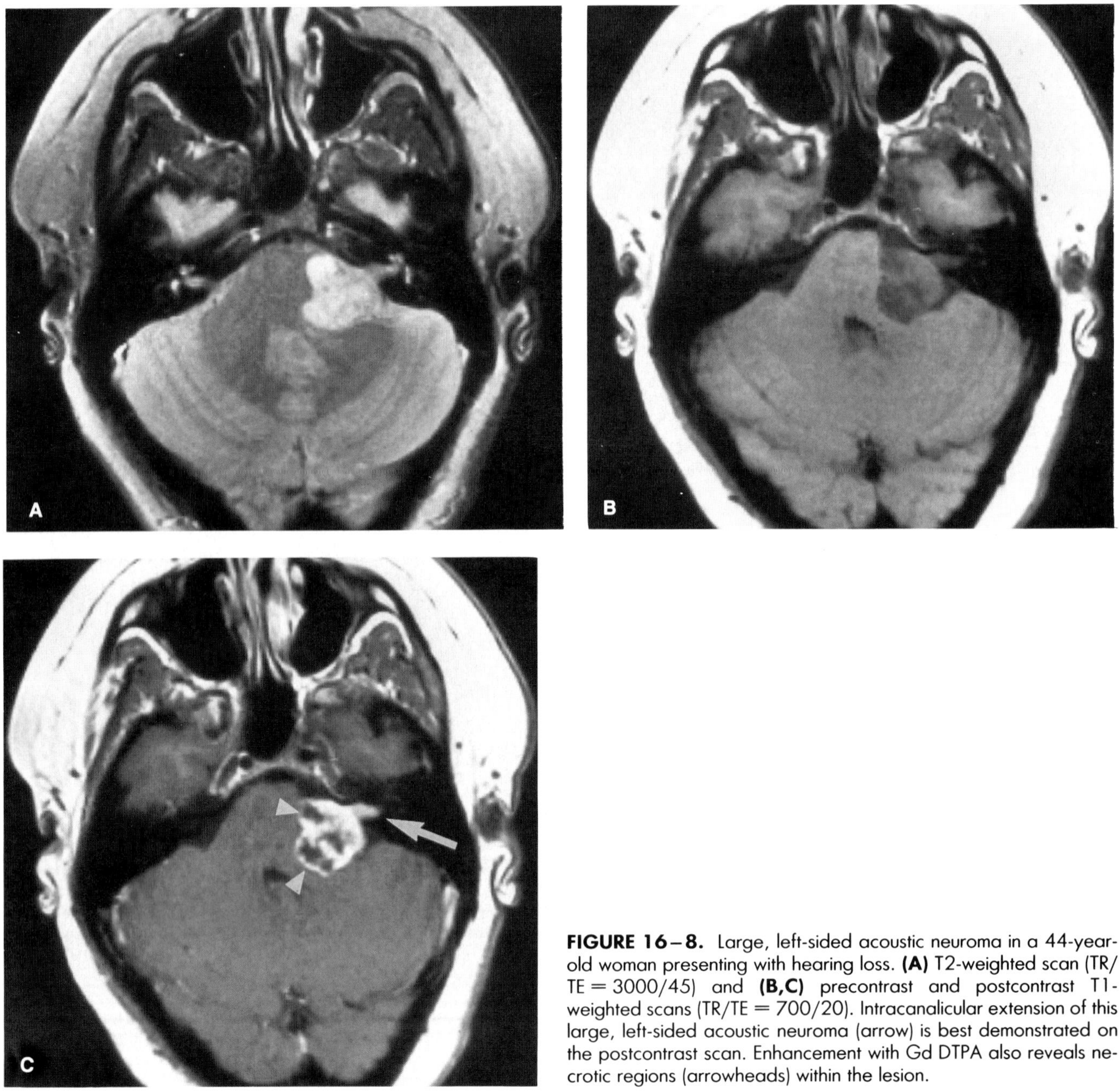

FIGURE 16–8. Large, left-sided acoustic neuroma in a 44-year-old woman presenting with hearing loss. **(A)** T2-weighted scan (TR/TE = 3000/45) and **(B,C)** precontrast and postcontrast T1-weighted scans (TR/TE = 700/20). Intracanalicular extension of this large, left-sided acoustic neuroma (arrow) is best demonstrated on the postcontrast scan. Enhancement with Gd DTPA also reveals necrotic regions (arrowheads) within the lesion.

sagittal images depict the relationship of sellar lesions to the optic chiasm. Large suprasellar aneurysms can also be diagnosed due to the presence of flow voids and pulsation artifacts, without angiography.

Contrast-enhanced MRI (precontrast T2-weighted, precontrast and postcontrast T1-weighted images) is the single best first examination for patients suspected of intracranial malignancy (Fig. 16–11). MRI offers increased contrast sensitivity, the absence of bone artifacts, and high-resolution multiplanar imaging. In the postoperative patient, contrast administration improves detection of recurrent or residual tumor (Fig. 16–12). Unfortunately, MR shares with CT the difficulty in differentiating neoplasia and postoperative change. Immediate postoperative scans combined with interval follow-up exams may assist in this evaluation. Caution is advised in the use of contrast media with suspected metastatic disease to the calvarium (Fig. 16–13). It is possible for the contrast between diploic space metastases and surrounding normal

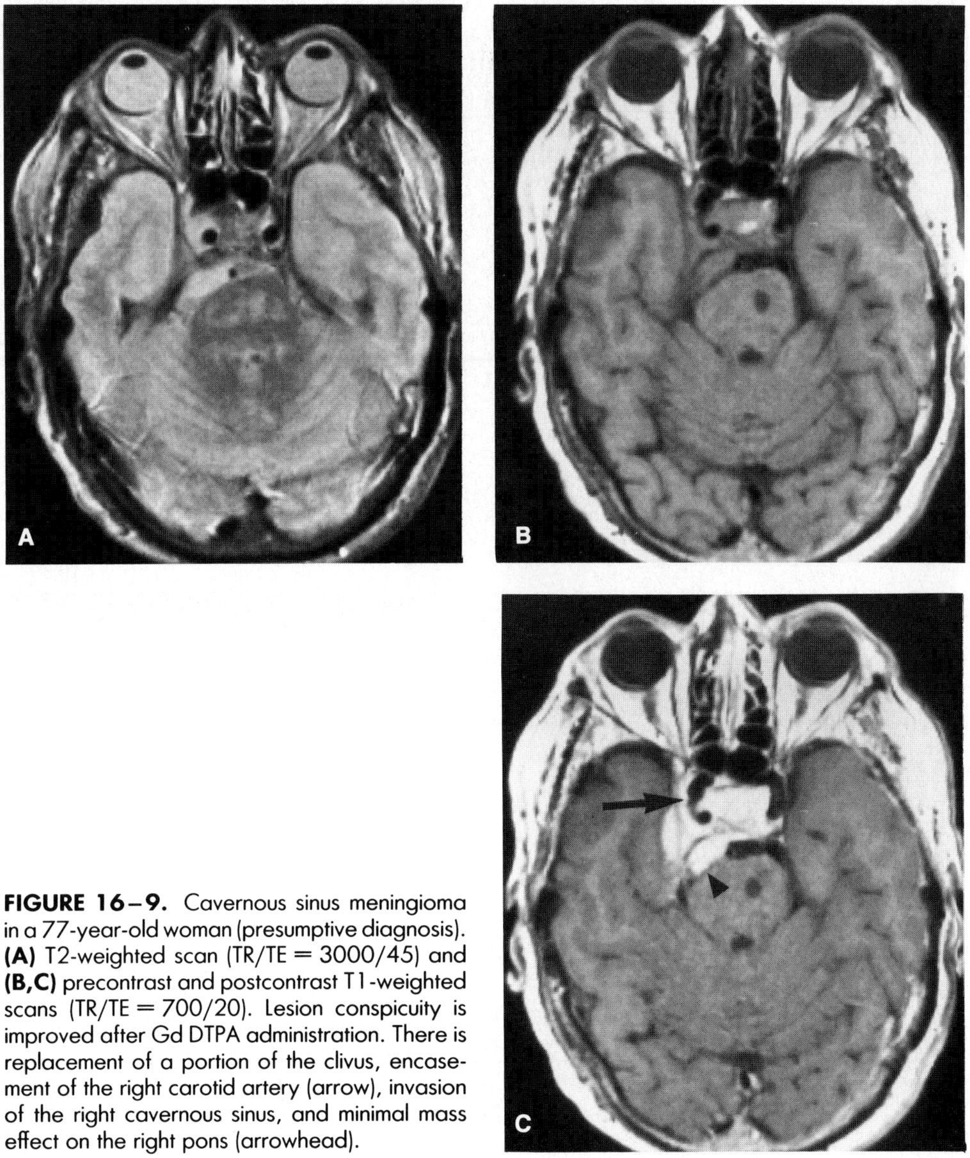

FIGURE 16–9. Cavernous sinus meningioma in a 77-year-old woman (presumptive diagnosis). **(A)** T2-weighted scan (TR/TE = 3000/45) and **(B,C)** precontrast and postcontrast T1-weighted scans (TR/TE = 700/20). Lesion conspicuity is improved after Gd DTPA administration. There is replacement of a portion of the clivus, encasement of the right carotid artery (arrow), invasion of the right cavernous sinus, and minimal mass effect on the right pons (arrowhead).

marrow to decrease on enhanced T1-weighted images. The data base for differential diagnosis with MRI is not as great as with x-ray CT, but over the next few years, much more will be learned about the characteristic changes exhibited on MRI by various pathologic processes, improving differential diagnosis.

CONGENITAL ABNORMALITIES OF THE CNS

MRI has emerged as the modality of choice for the examination and diagnosis of congenital abnormalities of the brain (Fig. 16–14) and spine.[23,24] The acquisition of high-resolution T1-weighted images in multiple planes is recommended. In the Chiari malformation, Dandy-Walker malformation, and Dandy-Walker variants, T1-weighted imaging alone may be sufficient for delineation of structural abnormalities. In the infant population, an appreciation of the changes in relaxation rates that occur with normal brain maturation (Fig. 16–15) is required for proper interpretation of scans.[25]

In the spine, MRI has provided new insight in the study of syringohydromyelia and spinal dysraphism (Fig. 16–16). Imaging of the congenital spine in two perpendicular planes is advocated. In particular, diastematomyelia may be difficult to visualize on sagittal images alone (Fig. 16–17). The diagnosis of retether-

(text continues on page 564)

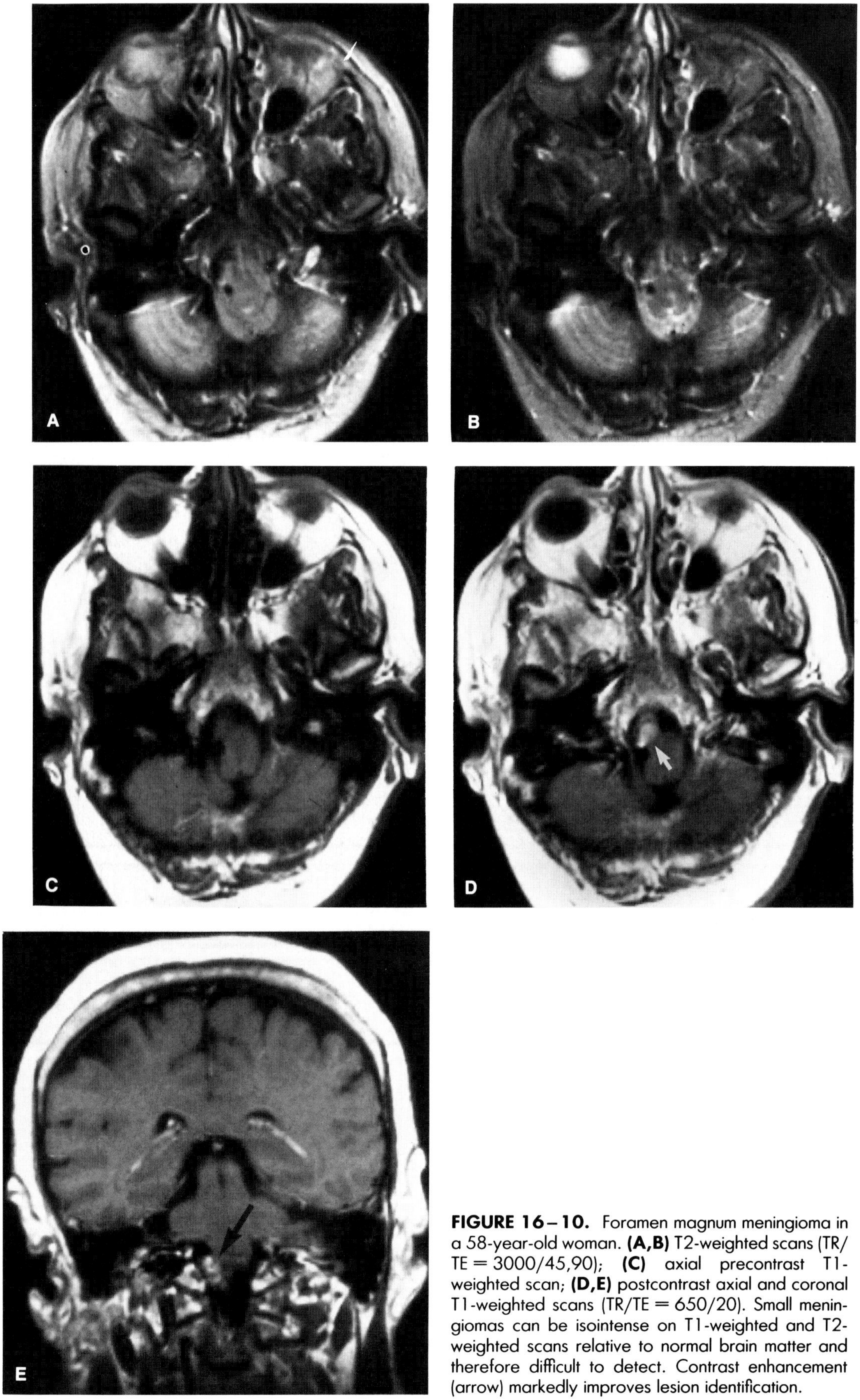

FIGURE 16–10. Foramen magnum meningioma in a 58-year-old woman. **(A,B)** T2-weighted scans (TR/TE = 3000/45,90); **(C)** axial precontrast T1-weighted scan; **(D,E)** postcontrast axial and coronal T1-weighted scans (TR/TE = 650/20). Small meningiomas can be isointense on T1-weighted and T2-weighted scans relative to normal brain matter and therefore difficult to detect. Contrast enhancement (arrow) markedly improves lesion identification.

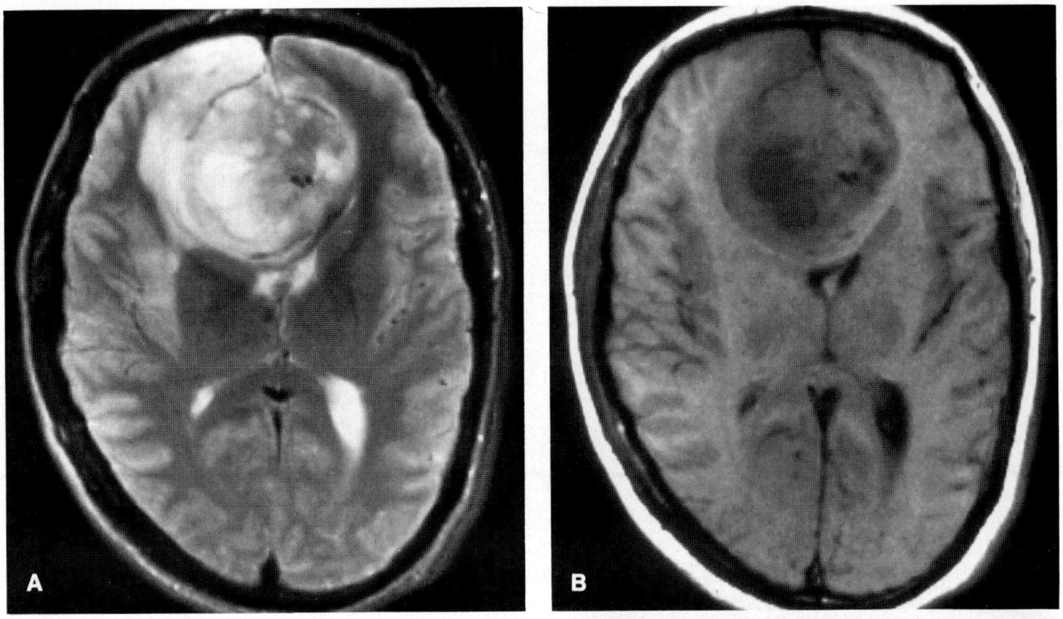

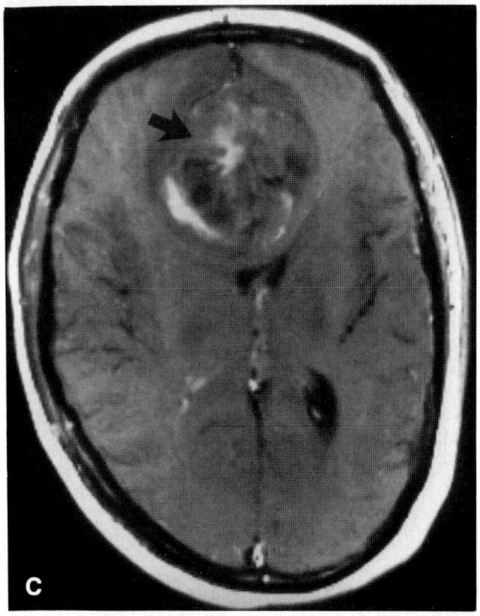

FIGURE 16–11. Frontal glioma (Grade 2/3) in a 31-year-old man with a history of headaches of progressive severity. **(A)** T2-weighted image (TR/TE = 3000/90) and **(B,C)** T1-weighted images before and after intravenous administration of 0.1 mmol/kg Gd DTPA (TR/TE = 650/20). A large mass can be identified in the anterior cranial fossa. In contrast to CT, the differentiation between extra-axial and intra-axial lesions can be made directly. This mass is within the frontal lobe and spans the falx anteriorly. Gyri are not displaced away from the lesion, a feature that would be identified if this lesion were a meningioma. The inhomogeneity of contrast enhancement (arrow) also identifies this lesion as a glioma. Even with calcification, significant and uniform contrast enhancement should be anticipated in meningiomas on MRI. With intra-axial lesions, contrast enhancement only identifies disruption of the blood-brain-barrier. This does serve as a marker for biopsy, but the true extent of the lesion, in the case of a glioma, is not indicated by contrast enhancement.

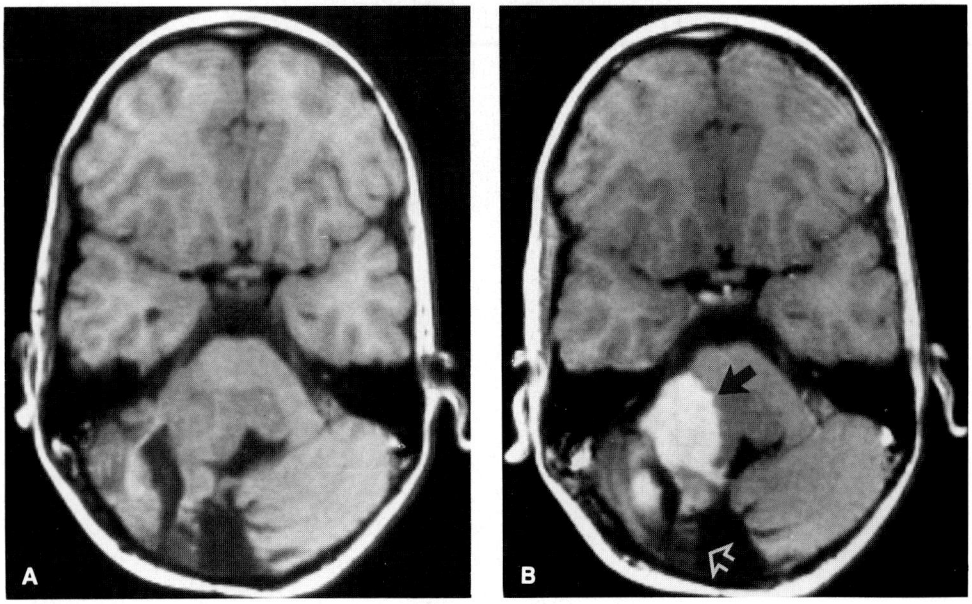

FIGURE 16–12. Recurrent cerebellar astrocytoma in a 6-year-old girl. **(A,B)** T1-weighted scan (TR/TE = 650/20) before and after intravenous Gd DTPA administration. Enhancement (closed arrow) identifies recurrent tumor. Postoperative changes are also seen in the right posterior cerebellum (open arrow). Contrast administration is essential for detecting recurrence after treatment of intracranial neoplastic disease. Changes on T2-weighted scans, although sensitive to disease pathology, are nonspecific and may indicate findings secondary to radiation, surgery, or recurrent tumor.

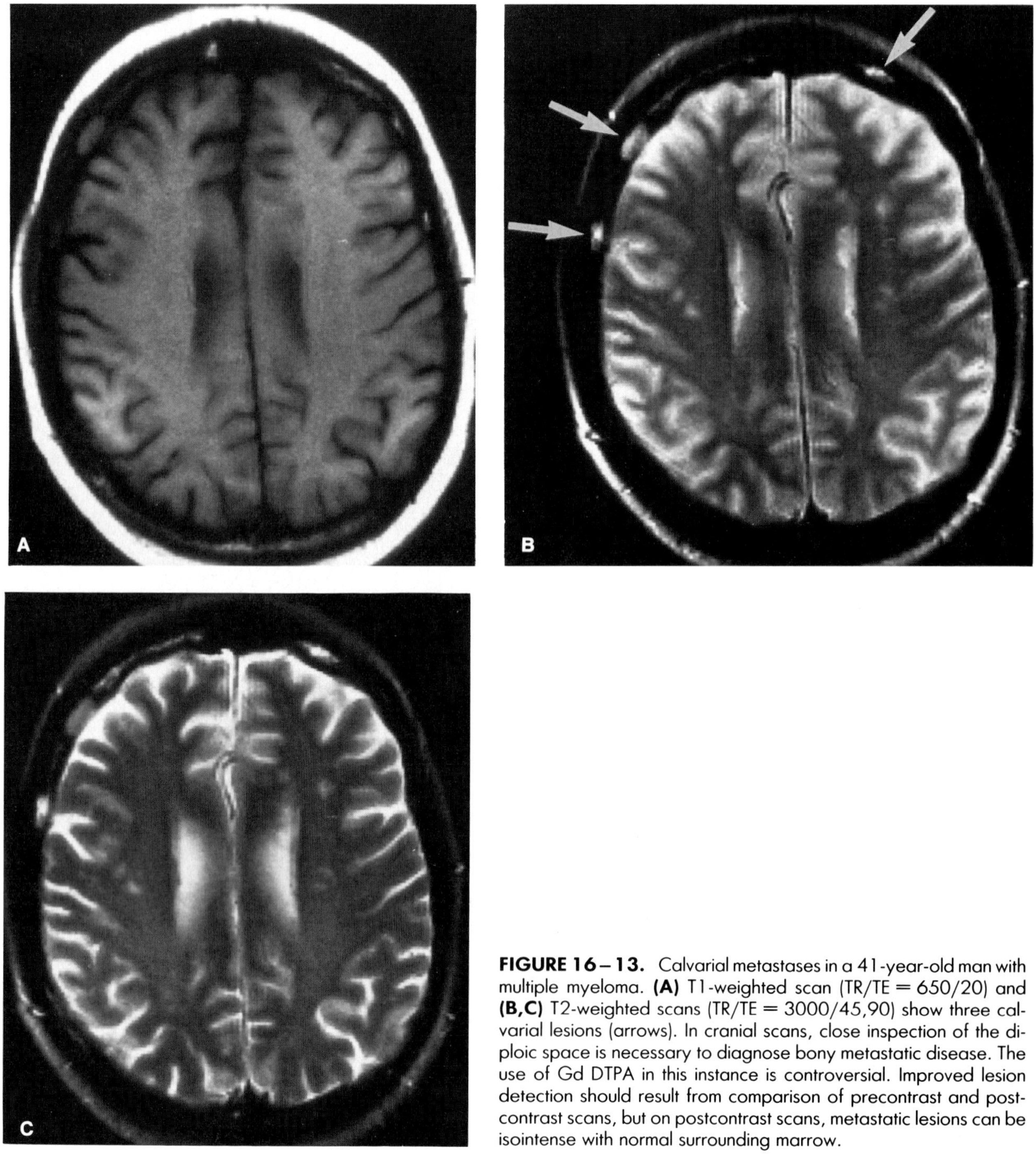

FIGURE 16–13. Calvarial metastases in a 41-year-old man with multiple myeloma. **(A)** T1-weighted scan (TR/TE = 650/20) and **(B,C)** T2-weighted scans (TR/TE = 3000/45,90) show three calvarial lesions (arrows). In cranial scans, close inspection of the diploic space is necessary to diagnose bony metastatic disease. The use of Gd DTPA in this instance is controversial. Improved lesion detection should result from comparison of precontrast and postcontrast scans, but on postcontrast scans, metastatic lesions can be isointense with normal surrounding marrow.

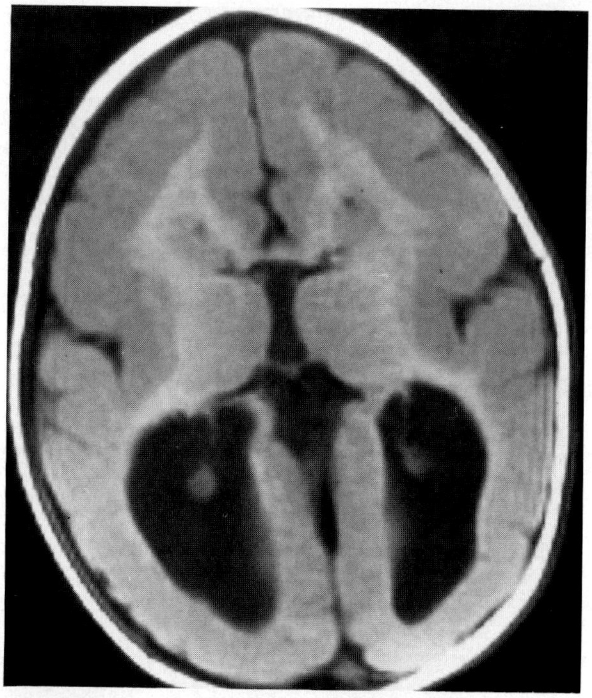

FIGURE 16–14. Pachygyria in a 7-year-old boy. Axial T1-weighted scan (TR/TE = 650/20). This patient presented with developmental delay and microcephaly. The gray matter is thickened, with limited gyral formation. There is enlargement primarily of the posterior portion of the lateral ventricles (culpocephaly). MRI is the diagnostic modality of choice for the examination of congenital brain malformations.

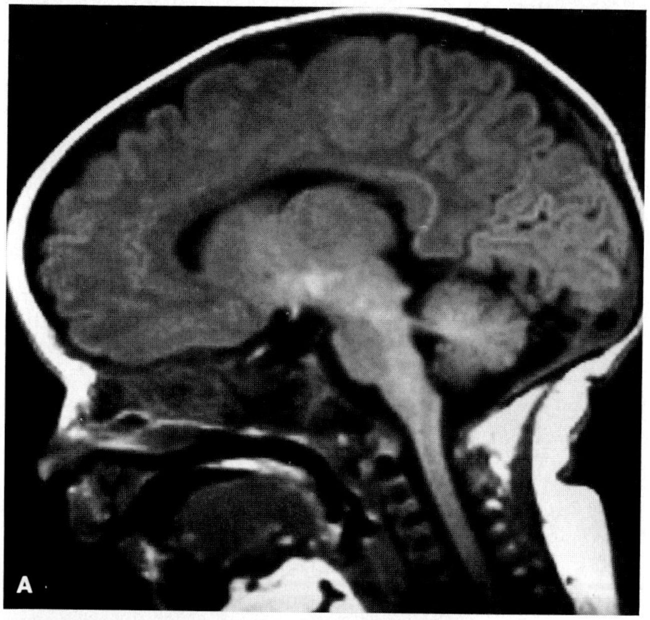

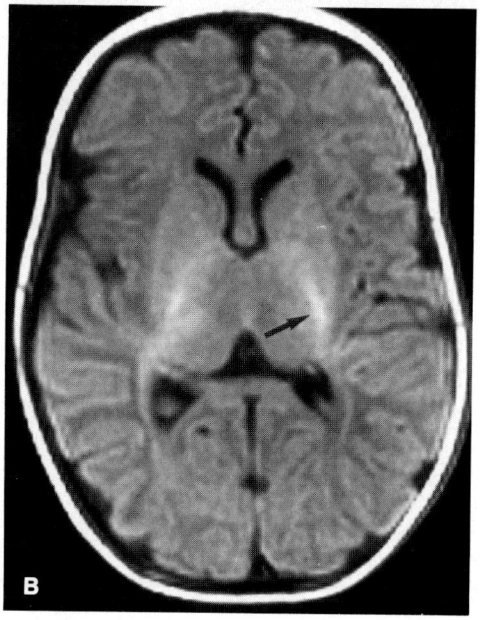

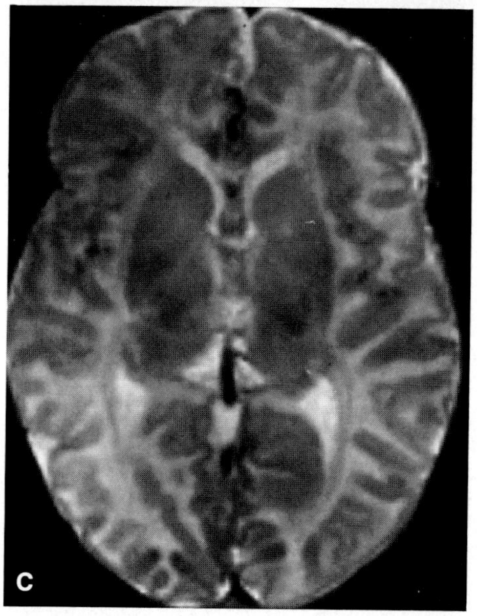

FIGURE 16–15. Normal 21-day-old girl, illustrating the pattern of early myelination on MRI. **(A,B)** Sagittal and axial T1-weighted scans (TR/TE = 650/20) and **(C)** T2-weighted scan (TR/TE = 3000/140). In the newborn, myelination can be demonstrated in the brainstem and internal capsule (arrow) on T1-weighted images. Otherwise, the white matter has lower signal intensity than gray matter, a reversal of the pattern seen in adults. On T2-weighted scans, long TEs are required for good differentiation of gray and white matter in the infant. The adult signal intensity ratio of gray and white matter is also reversed in newborns on T2-weighted exams. These findings are a consequence of the prolonged T1 and T2 relaxation times in the infant brain.

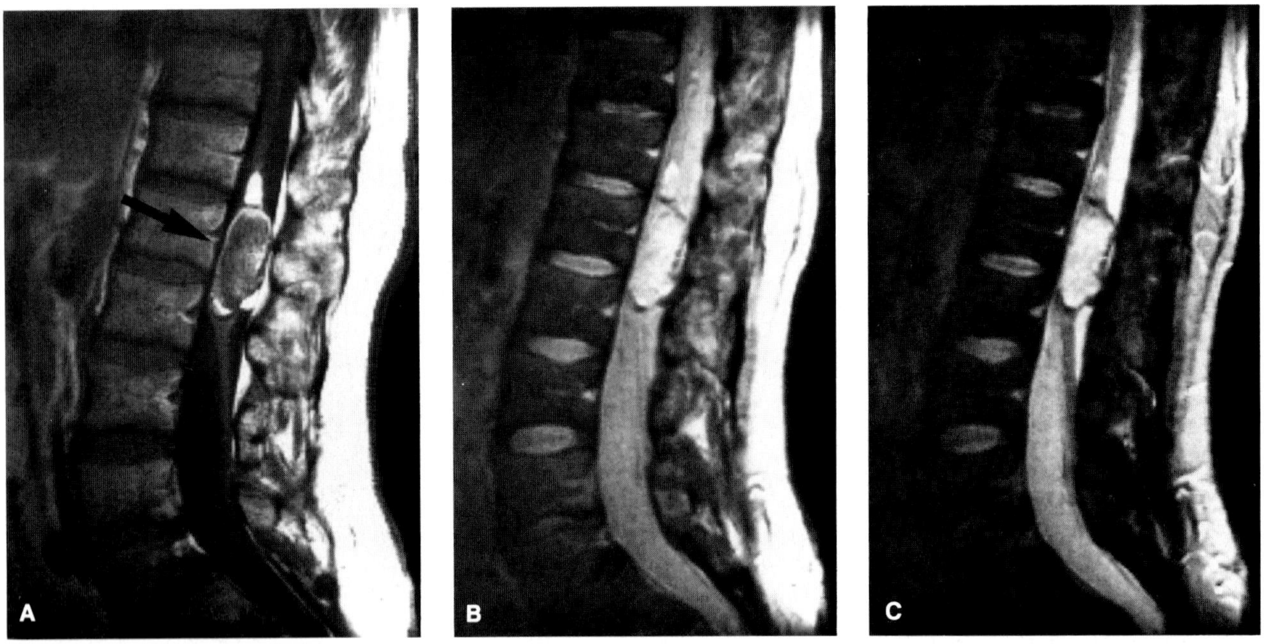

FIGURE 16–16. Tethered cord with associated epidermoid in a 43-year-old man presenting with long tract and conus signs (no previous medical history). On physical examination, a dermal sinus and hairy patch were seen in the sacral area, and plain films revealed spina bifida. **(A)** T1-weighted scan (TR/TE = 650/20) and **(B,C)** mildly and moderately T2-weighted scans (TR/TE = 3000/45,90). A mass containing fatty elements is seen at the L1-2 level (arrow). The cord extends at least to the L5 level. In general, axial T1-weighted images best demonstrate the dorsal termination of the cord, as well as associated lipomas.

ing in patients after meningomyelocele repair remains difficult, with clinical findings crucial to appropriate image interpretation (Fig. 16–18).

SPINE ABNORMALITIES

Cervical Spine

In degenerative disease of the cervical spine, the two primary considerations are disc herniation and spinal stenosis.[26] Bony hypertrophic changes may manifest clinically as narrowing of the central spinal canal with resultant myelopathy or stenosis of the foramina, which presents as a radiculopathy. Hypertrophy of the facet joints and the ligamentum flavum, bony spurs, and a congenitally small canal may contribute to spinal stenosis.

Cervical disc herniation most frequently presents acutely and is often not related to a significant traumatic episode. The most common location of a herniated disc is paracentral, typically presenting as a single-level radiculopathy. Central disc herniation with cord compression may present with myelopathy or radiculopathy (Fig. 16–19). CT is superior for evaluating hypertrophic spurring, particularly encroachment on the lateral neural canal. The disadvantages of MRI include the time required for the examination, poor visualization of bony abnormalities, and inconsistency in diagnostic quality from scan to scan due primarily to motion. Overall, myelographic CT remains superior to MRI for evaluating cervical degenerative disease, although recent improvements in surface-coil technology and imaging techniques have narrowed the gap between CT and MRI.

Conversely, MRI is markedly superior to x-ray CT for examining spinal cord lesions. T1-weighted imaging is recommended in two orthogonal planes, combined with high-quality T2-weighted spin echo imaging. For T2-weighted imaging, suppression of motion artifacts induced by cerebrospinal fluid (CSF) pulsation and blood flow is crucial. At 1 T, GMN is adequate in most cases for motion suppresion, but the addition of pulse or EKG gating may be required at higher fields.[27] Gradient-echo imaging is reserved primarily for extradural lesions.[28,29] The T2 weighting achieved with gradient echoes may be insufficient for detecting intramedullary lesions.

MRI should be the first examination ordered for patients with myelopathy (Fig. 16–20). Congenital abnormalities are effectively imaged by T1-weighted techniques. However, neoplasia, demyelination, and inflammatory processes require both T1-weighted and T2-weighted imaging. Signal intensity abnormali-

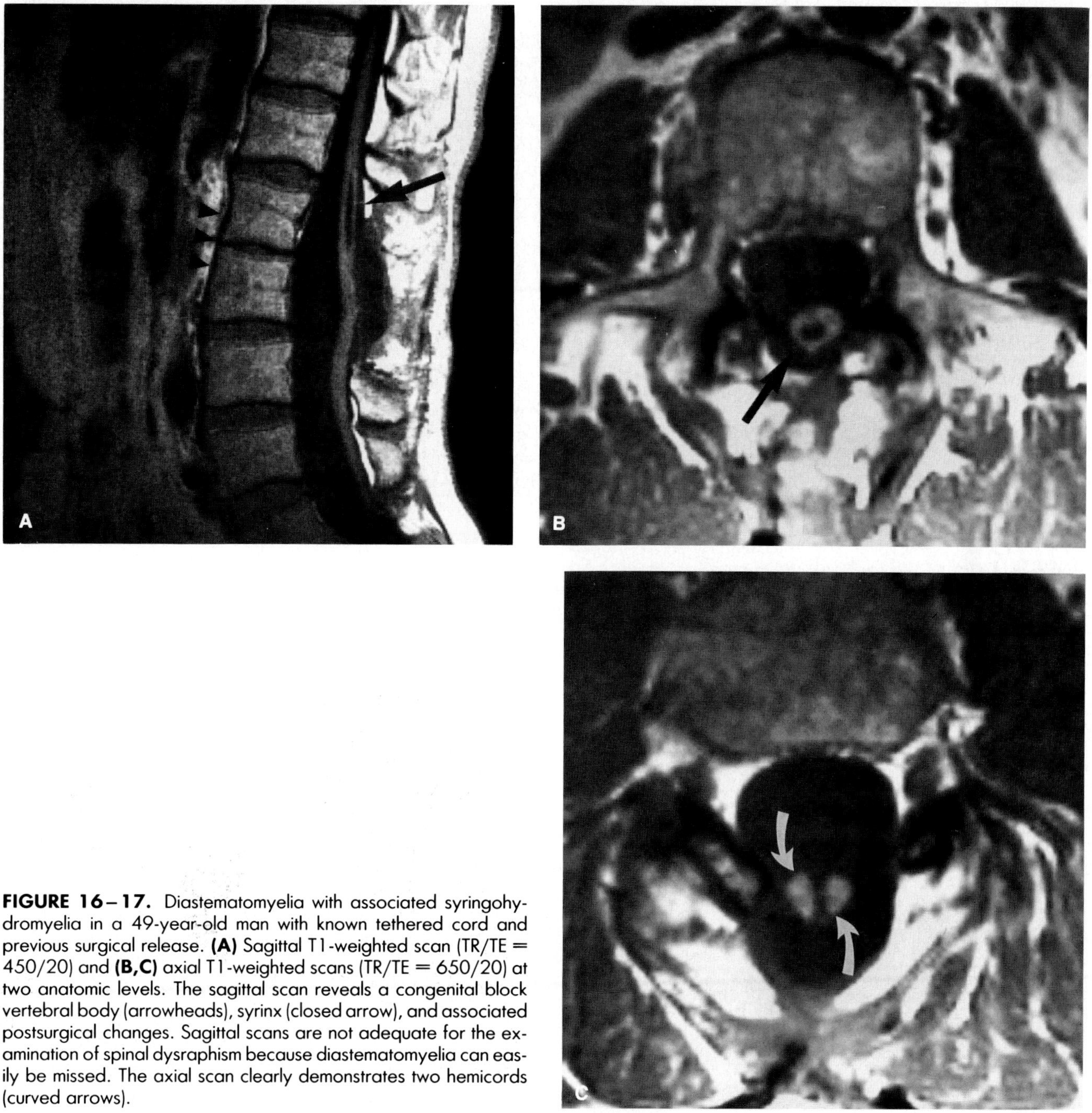

FIGURE 16–17. Diastematomyelia with associated syringohydromyelia in a 49-year-old man with known tethered cord and previous surgical release. **(A)** Sagittal T1-weighted scan (TR/TE = 450/20) and **(B,C)** axial T1-weighted scans (TR/TE = 650/20) at two anatomic levels. The sagittal scan reveals a congenital block vertebral body (arrowheads), syrinx (closed arrow), and associated postsurgical changes. Sagittal scans are not adequate for the examination of spinal dysraphism because diastematomyelia can easily be missed. The axial scan clearly demonstrates two hemicords (curved arrows).

ties within the cord may be the result of edema, gliosis, or neoplasia. Gd DTPA administration is particularly valuable for identifying neoplasia within a complex syrinx.

Suppression or minimization of motion-induced artifacts is critical for successful imaging of the spinal cord. CSF pulsation, blood flow, swallowing, cardiac motion, and respiration can contribute to image degradation. GMN is a technique that is transparent to the user and compensates for motion occurring during the time interval TE. This technique has been successfully employed with both T1-weighted and T2-weighted images, primarily for the reduction of artifacts associated with CSF pulsation and respiration. At high field strengths, it may be necessary to use pulse gating in addition to GMN to achieve satisfactory T2-weighted spin echo images. Saturation pulses can be employed to eliminate artifacts from swallowing in cervical spine examinations and from cardiac and respiratory motion in thoracic spine examinations.[30]

Syrinx cavities may be congenital, traumatic, neo-

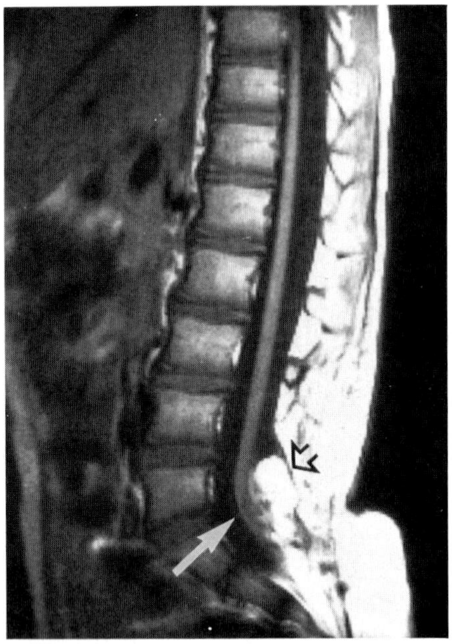

FIGURE 16–18. Retethered cord in a 7-year-old girl with new onset of night incontinence. Sagittal T1-weighted image (TR/TE = 450/20). No distinct conus can be identified. The cord terminates at the L5-S1 level (closed arrow) and has an associated intradural lipoma (open arrow). MRI provides a noninvasive means for evaluating lipomyeloschisis. MRI findings must be correlated with clinical symptoms, because retethering can be difficult to differentiate by imaging alone from a tethered cord after surgical release.

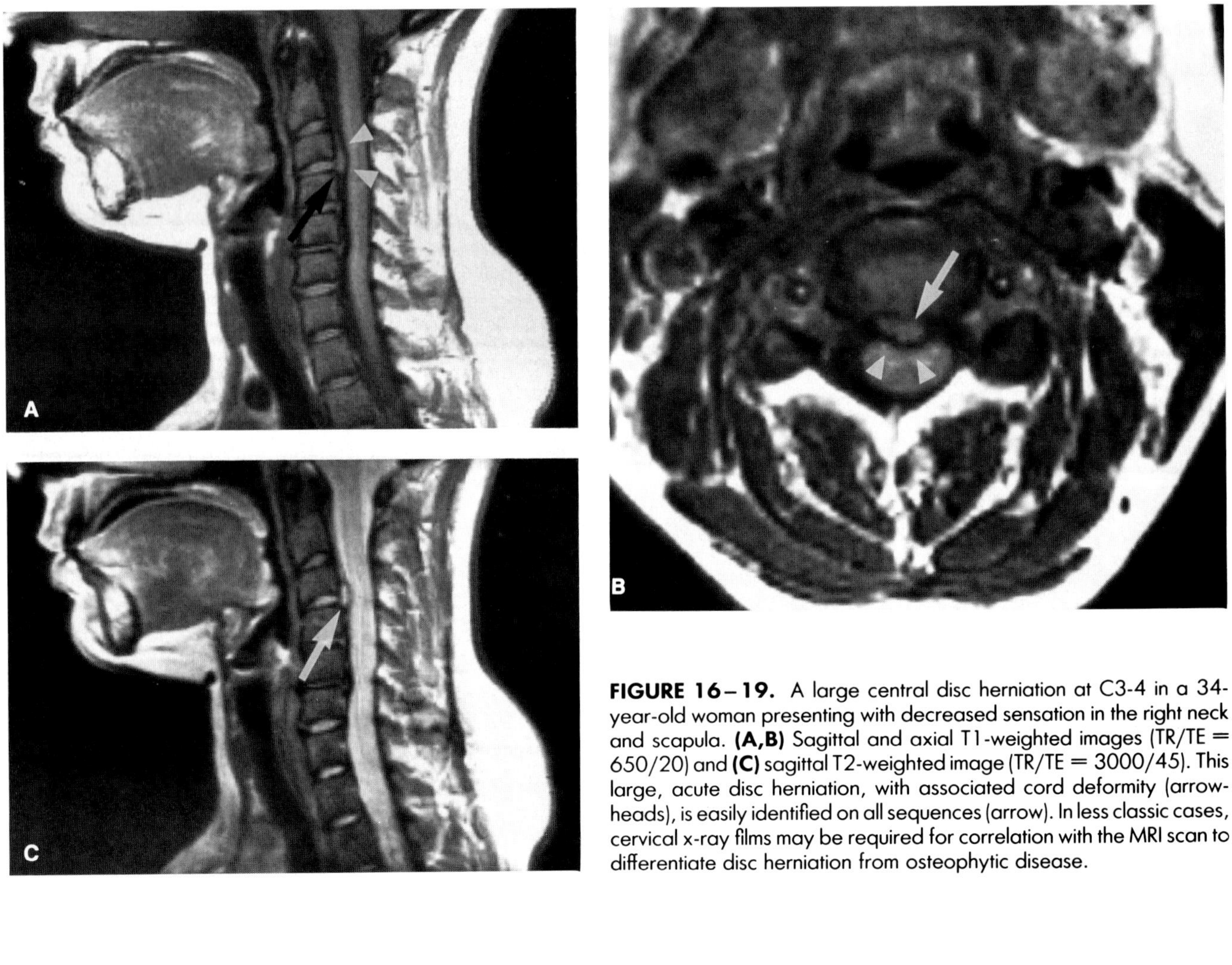

FIGURE 16–19. A large central disc herniation at C3-4 in a 34-year-old woman presenting with decreased sensation in the right neck and scapula. **(A,B)** Sagittal and axial T1-weighted images (TR/TE = 650/20) and **(C)** sagittal T2-weighted image (TR/TE = 3000/45). This large, acute disc herniation, with associated cord deformity (arrowheads), is easily identified on all sequences (arrow). In less classic cases, cervical x-ray films may be required for correlation with the MRI scan to differentiate disc herniation from osteophytic disease.

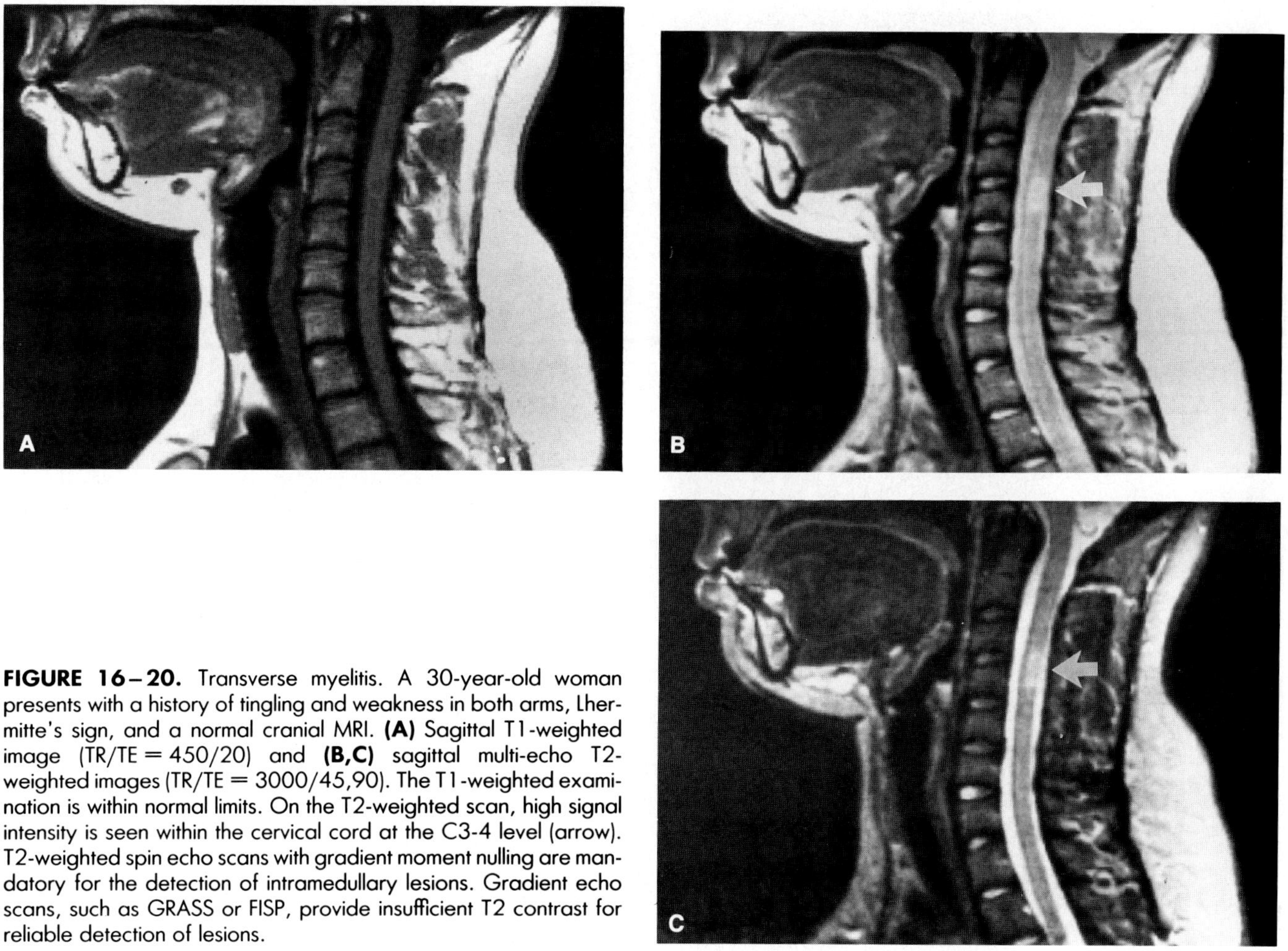

FIGURE 16–20. Transverse myelitis. A 30-year-old woman presents with a history of tingling and weakness in both arms, Lhermitte's sign, and a normal cranial MRI. **(A)** Sagittal T1-weighted image (TR/TE = 450/20) and **(B,C)** sagittal multi-echo T2-weighted images (TR/TE = 3000/45,90). The T1-weighted examination is within normal limits. On the T2-weighted scan, high signal intensity is seen within the cervical cord at the C3-4 level (arrow). T2-weighted spin echo scans with gradient moment nulling are mandatory for the detection of intramedullary lesions. Gradient echo scans, such as GRASS or FISP, provide insufficient T2 contrast for reliable detection of lesions.

plastic, inflammatory, or postoperative in origin. MRI can document flow or pulsation within in a syrinx. In syringohydromyelia, associated hind-brain anomalies must be ruled out.

Thoracic Spine

MRI has demonstrated that thoracic disc herniations are much more common than previously thought.[31] Myelography is an insensitive technique for detecting subtle thoracic disc herniations. In the thoracic spine, MRI can also detect and delineate other extradural lesions. These are frequently metastatic tumors, commonly from breast or prostate. The need for radiation therapy can be judged on the basis of MRI alone. Common intradural extramedullary lesions involving the thoracic spine include schwannomas, meningiomas, and neurenteric cysts. Intramedullary lesions include astrocytomas, ependymomas, dermoid cysts, and hemangioblastomas. After trauma, MRI can be critical in demonstrating extradural hematomas and traumatic disc herniation. In infection, MRI can demonstrate epidural spread and the loss of vertebral body end-plates and collapse of vertebral bodies. Differentiation of metastatic disease from osteoporosis in vertebral body collapse can be difficult. If marrow signal intensity is preserved on T1-weighted images, metastatic disease is unlikely. In the acute case, contrast enhancement with Gd DTPA suggests neoplastic disease.

Spinal Cord Trauma

MRI can be used for examining acutely injured patients who are medically stable.[32] Intramedullary lesions, including hemorrhagic contusion and cord edema, are well delineated by MRI, and extradural lesions can also be visualized (e.g., compression of the cord by disc material, bone fragments, or hematoma). MRI has replaced both myelography and CT for evaluating previously injured cords. Myelomalacia is commonly demonstrated adjacent to the area of spine injury. MRI may play a particularly important role in paraplegic or quadriplegic patients with recent clini-

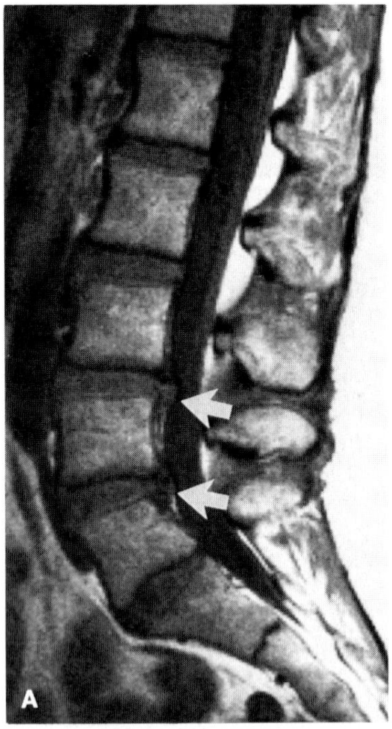

FIGURE 16–21. Lumbar disc herniation in a 33-year-old woman presenting with radiculopathy. **(A)** Sagittal T1-weighted scan (TR/TE = 450/20); **(B)** axial T1-weighted scan at the L3-4 interspace; **(C)** sagittal T2-weighted scan (TR/TE = 3000/45). The T2-weighted scan reveals dehydration of both the L3-4 and L4-5 discs (open arrows). Predominantly central disc herniations can be identified at both levels (closed arrows). The posterior longitudinal ligament appears intact (arrowheads).

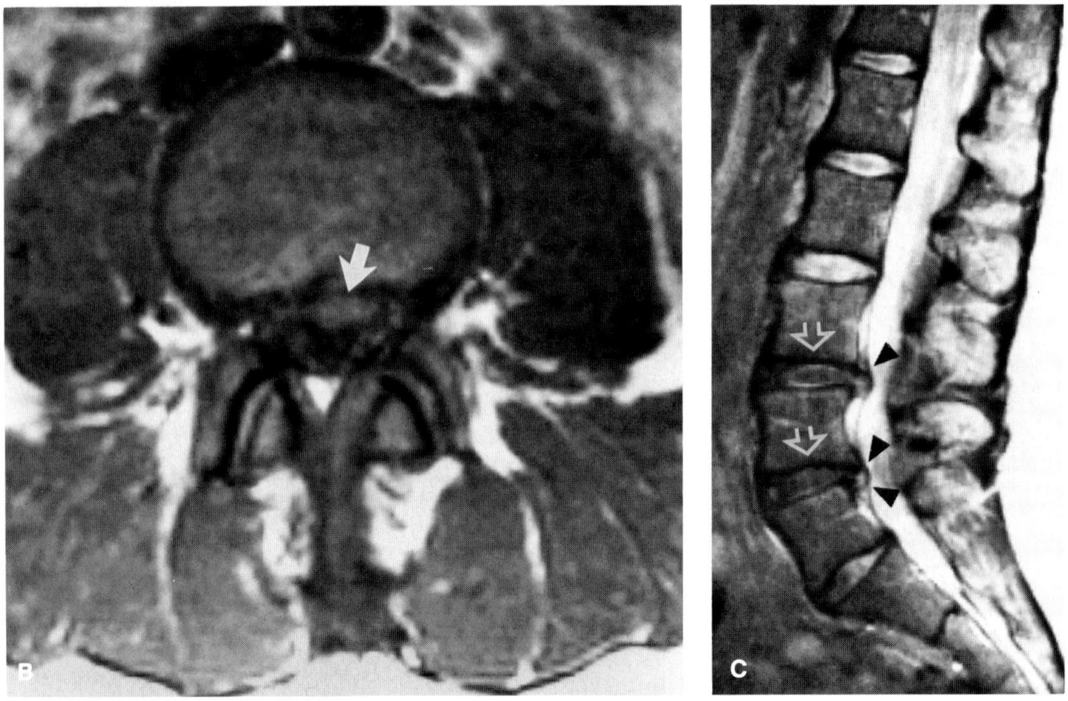

cal deterioration. Previously undiagnosed cord compression or expansion of cysts within the cord may be demonstrated.

Lumbar Spine

Extruded disc material may be contained (i.e., subligamentous herniation) or may rupture through the posterior longitudinal ligament (i.e., free fragment). In the latter case, the disc fragment can migrate superiorly or inferiorly in the spinal canal. Rupture of a free fragment through the dura into the thecal sac is rare. In the lumbar spine, 60% of disc herniations are posterolateral (paracentral), 30% are directly posterior (central), and approximately 10% are lateral (foraminal).

A paracentral disc herniation at the L5-S1 level that compresses the thecal sac usually presents clinically with an ipsilateral S1 radiculopathy. This is due to compression of the nerve root at the point where it exits from the thecal sac. A foraminal disc herniation at L5-S1 will most likely present as an ipsilateral L5 radiculopathy due to compression of the more peripheral portion of the L5 nerve root as it exits beneath the pedicle. Disc herniations can occur without radicular findings, and disc herniations can decrease in size with time without surgical treatment.

About 90% of disc herniations occur at L4-5 and L5-S1, with approximately 10% at L3-4. For this reason, it is important to routinely examine the lower three lumbar disc spaces in all patients evaluated for disc herniation (Fig. 16–21). High-resolution x-ray CT is considered to be more accurate than myelography alone for the diagnosis of lumbar disc herniation. The choice between MRI and CT for examining lumbar disc disease should be based on availability, quality of equipment, and relative cost. When state-of-the-art equipment is used, the best first examination is either MRI or CT. Continued improvement in MRI software and instrumentation may eclipse CT in the diagnosis of lumbar disc disease.

In the lumbar region, our standard practice is to perform thin-section sagittal T1-weighted and T2-weighted images with axial T1-weighted images covering the lower three disc spaces or as directed by findings on the sagittal scan or clinical presentation. On sagittal T1-weighted images, acute disc herniation often resembles "squeezed toothpaste," with disc material contacting the thecal sac and extending superiorly and inferiorly. This appearance is commonly observed in the cervical region. Changes in the vertebral body marrow commonly accompany degenerative disc disease.[33] Pantopaque resembles fat in its appearance and should be recognized as such, preventing possible confusion with a lipoma (Fig. 16–22). The 3D fast imaging performed with techniques like FLASH may soon be applied for thin-section (1 mm) imaging, providing high-resolution reformatted images in any desired plane.

In the postoperative spine, Gd DTPA use can be essential for differentiating scar from recurrent disc herniation.[34] On immediate postcontrast images, scar shows heterogeneous enhancement, but disc material fails to demonstrate significant enhancement.

In addition to epidural fibrosis and recurrent or residual disc material, spondylolisthesis, stenosis, and arachnoiditis are possible causes for recurrent pain after surgery. In severe arachnoiditis, thickened, clumped, irregular nerve roots can be readily demonstrated by MRI. More subtle changes, including mild irregularities, are better visualized by myelography, with or without CT.

NECK, OROPHARYNX, AND NASOPHARYNX

Screening for head and neck abnormalities on MRI is performed in the axial plane. This is supplemented by imaging in the coronal plane for determining cephalocaudal extent and mediastinal involvement. The sagittal plane is useful for midline lesions involving the tongue base, epiglottis, and hypopharynx. The initial axial examination should include T1-weighted and T2-weighted images. The value of intravenous contrast administration is becoming increasingly recognized, with particular importance for the demonstration of lesion margins and tumor recurrence.

Endoscopy remains the technique of choice for evaluating superficial nasopharyngeal and laryngeal

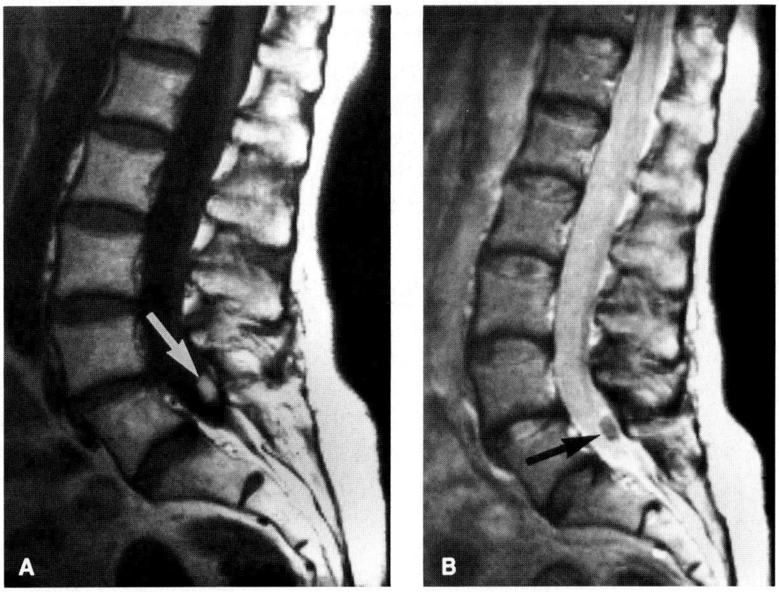

FIGURE 16–22. Pantopaque. **(A)** Sagittal T1-weighted scan (TR/TE = 450/20) and **(B)** T2-weighted scan (TR/TE = 3000/45). This patient had pantopaque myelography and laminectomy at L5-S1 in 1978. Pantopaque (arrow), because of its oily consistency, largely parallels the signal intensity characteristics of fat on T1-weighted and T2-weighted spin echo imaging.

lesions. For abnormalities of the salivary glands and infratemporal fossa, MRI is the best initial imaging modality.[35,36]

CHEST

In the chest, ECG gating is essential to obtain diagnostic images with current MR instrumentation. Although extracardiac applications remain limited, MRI has been used for evaluating aortic aneurysms and dissection. The size of the pulmonary arteries can be easily determined by MRI, a useful adjunct in the examination of congenital heart malformations. Thrombi or tumor invasion within the superior and inferior vena cava and jugular veins can be easily demonstrated on T1-weighted images.

Evaluation of ischemic heart disease by MRI remains investigational.[37,38] Abnormal wall thickness and discrete signal intensity changes of the myocardium can be seen. MRI can assess cardiac function, with calculation of end-diastolic and end-systolic volumes, as well as ejection fraction. Studies with animal models of acute myocardial infarction have revealed significant increases in myocardial signal intensity and T2 relaxation time within hours after coronary occlusion. This must be distinguished from other causes of increased signal intensity, such as respiratory or cardiac motion artifacts, stagnant blood adjacent to the endocardium, and partial voluming with epicardial fat. MRI may prove useful for quantitating myocardial infarct size, but the sensitivity and specificity in acute infarction is yet to be determined. In chronic ischemic disease, wall thinning can be demonstrated, which correlates with the site of infarction as determined by ECG. Cine MR may be performed with either spin echo or gradient-echo techniques. This technique is being investigated for the detection of regional wall motion abnormalities.[39]

MRI complements echocardiography in evaluating congenital heart abnormalities. Although echocardiography remains the technique of choice, MRI can demonstrate the size of hypoplastic central pulmonary arteries. MRI is also used for clarification of great vessel and intracardiac anatomy in complex congenital anomalies.

In valvular heart disease, low flip angle gradient-echo images can demonstrate stenotic and regurgitant lesions.[40] This approach also can assess ventricular septal defects and shunt size.[41]

MRI more effectively demonstrates intracardiac and paracardiac masses than 2D echocardiography. The large field of view, imaging of adjacent noncardiac structures, and the definition of myocardial walls are advantages of MRI. Assessment of cardiac tumors is a major area of cardiac MRI application.

The normal pericardium ($\leq$ 2 mm thick) appears on MRI as a low-signal-intensity structure due to its fibrous composition. MRI is accurate for the diagnosis of constrictive pericarditis, with thickening and abnormal signal intensity demonstrated. Often the cause of constriction, such as a loculated pericardial effusion or hematoma, can be better demonstrated by MRI. MRI is also superior to echocardiography for distinguishing the various types of pericardial effusions.

ABDOMEN

Compensation for motion is particularly important for imaging of the upper abdomen.[42] Successful approaches include the use of physical restraints and GMN. T1-weighted breath-hold scans have been developed, with lesion contrast-to-noise ratio (CNR) comparable to conventional spin echo techniques (Fig. 16-23). MRI has been used primarily as an adjunct to other imaging modalities for studying the abdomen, but with the advent of high CNR and high-resolution breath-hold scans, MRI may supplant x-ray CT due to its superior tissue contrast.[43-45]

In renal disease, one drawback to MRI has been the difficulty in detecting small tumors (< 3 cm). Breath-hold scans and the use of contrast media may markedly improve renal imaging in the future. MRI offers the advantages of multiple imaging planes and the ability to directly determine renal vein or caval involvement.

MRI has not proven specific for the differentiation of benign and malignant adrenal masses.[46] Although a lesion isointense with liver is less likely to be malignant, there is significant overlap in signal intensities between benign lesions and malignant disease on T2-weighted scans. Pheochromocytomas typically demonstrate very high signal intensity on T2-weighted images.

PELVIS

MRI is ideal for the evaluation of pelvic abnormalities.[47,48] Images are typically not degraded by respiratory artifact (Fig. 16-24). The internal architecture of organs can be visualized due to the superb soft tissue contrast provided by MRI, with the organs themselves highlighted by surrounding fat. The patient is instructed to take only clear liquids or to fast for at least 4 hours before pelvic MRI. Intravenous or intramuscular glucogon can be given immediately before imaging to decrease bowel motion. For suspected rectosigmoid disease, air can be instilled. The vagina can be seen without the use of a tampon, which is necessary for

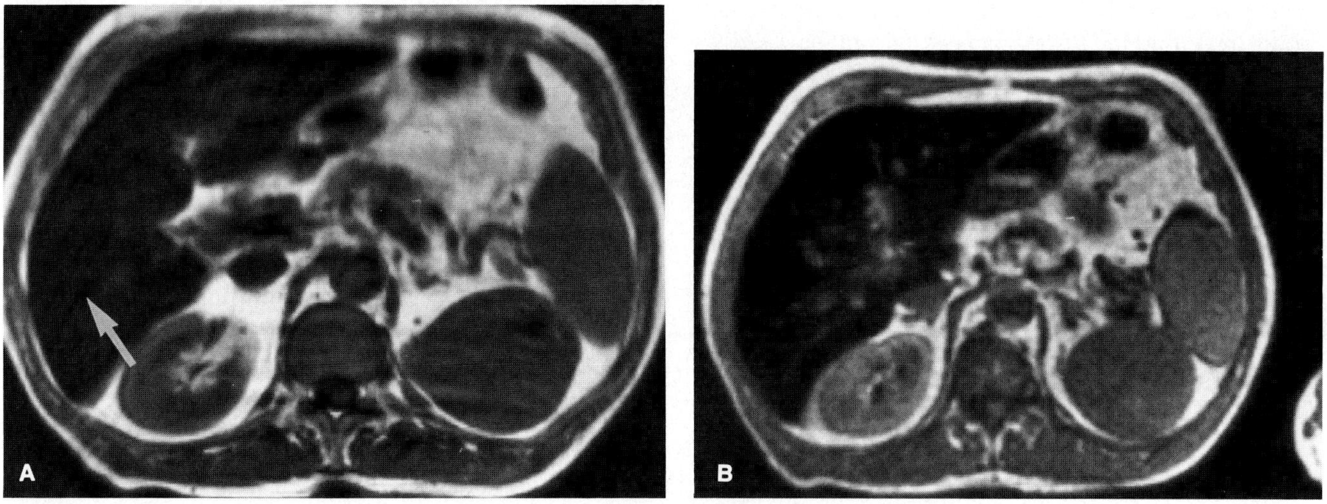

FIGURE 16–23. Hemosiderosis in a 60-year-old man with left renal cell carcinoma. **(A)** T1-weighted spin echo scan (TR/TE = 600/17, four data acquisitions; scan time of 10.2 minutes) and **(B)** T1-weighted breath-hold FLASH scan (TR/TE = 40/10, a 50° tip angle; scan time of 10 seconds). Iron deposition in the liver is clearly depicted on both the spin echo and FLASH images as abnormal low signal intensity, but the gradient echo technique (FLASH) is more sensitive to iron deposition. The left kidney is markedly abnormal in both images. Renal cell carcinoma, as in this case, is often isointense with respect to normal renal tissue and therefore difficult to identify on the basis of signal abnormality alone. The spin echo scan **(A)** does suffer from respiratory artifact (arrow). Routine abdominal imaging in the future is likely to be performed with breath-hold techniques such as that illustrated.

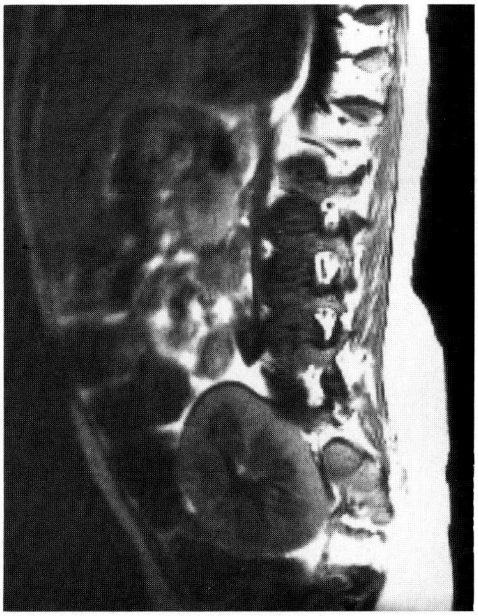

FIGURE 16–24. Single pelvic kidney in a 5-year-old girl. MRI (TR/TE = 650/20) is excellent for delineation of pelvic anatomy because significant pulsation and respiratory artifacts are absent. Surface coils, as used in this exam, may further improve image quality.

CT. For examination of the prostate, seminal vesicles, uterus, cervix, and bladder, thin-section images (3–5 mm) may be required. Surface-coil imaging may aid in evaluating pelvic abnormalities.

Knowledge of the internal architecture of the prostate is important. Prostatic carcinoma primarily originates within the peripheral zone. Benign prostatic hypertrophy (BPH) originates primarily in the transitional zone. Differentiation between these two zones can be obtained on T2-weighted images. Although MRI is very sensitive for detecting abnormalities, it cannot differentiate between prostatic carcinoma and BPH. The appearance of BPH is variable on MRI, reflecting its heterogeneous composition. The nodular form of hyperplasia may be demonstrated as higher or lower signal intensity than the surrounding gland on T2-weighted images. Enlargement and low signal intensity of the seminal vesicles on T2-weighted images occurs with neoplastic involvement. T1-weighted imaging can detect invasion of the periprostatic fat.

T1-weighted scans are used to determine gross involvement of the perivesical fat by bladder malignancies. Because of the ability to obtain coronal and sagittal planes, MRI is slightly better than CT for staging bladder tumors. Like CT, MRI is unable to determine nodal involvement if nodes are of normal size.

Sonography remains the initial screening technique for uterine and ovarian abnormalities. The junctional zone demonstrated on T2-weighted images of the uterus is believed to represent vascular structures within the inner third of myometrium. The appearance of leiomyomas depends on their composition. Diffuse adenomyosis is seen as a low-signal-intensity band on T2-weighted images surrounding the normal high-signal-intensity endometrium. Focal adenomyosis can simulate leiomyomas. Endometriosis typically is seen as high signal intensity on both T1-weighted and T2-weighted images, suggesting blood.

On T2-weighted images, the cervix is seen as two separate zones. The central zone is high signal intensity, representing the cervical epithelium and mucous. The fibrous cervical stroma is seen as low signal intensity surrounding the central canal. Small nabothian cysts are commonly demonstrated.

On T2-weighted images, the vaginal epithelium and mucosa are seen as high signal intensity. The surrounding vaginal wall is of lower signal intensity. Ovaries may be difficult to distinguish from bowel loops on T1-weighted sequences but appear as high signal intensity on T2-weighted images. The inability to detect microscopic tumor extension into the pericervical fat or microscopic involvement of normal-sized lymph nodes remains a downfall of MR evaluation of cervical carcinoma.

MUSCULOSKELETAL SYSTEM

MRI has replaced arthrography for the detection of meniscal tears.[49] Demonstration of high signal intensity within the meniscus connecting to the articular surface is necessary for the diagnosis of a tear (Fig. 16–25). Joint effusions can be easily recognized on T2-weighted spin echo or gradient-echo images. Hyaline cartilage, which lines the articular surface, is of higher signal intensity than the fibrocartilage of the meniscus and can be exquisitely depicted on gradient-echo imaging. The posterior and anterior cruciate ligaments are best evaluated in sagittal images with 10° to 20° external rotation and direct coronal images.[50] The coronal plane best demonstrates the collateral ligaments of the knee. Thin-section 3D gradient-echo imaging may soon play a significant role in evaluating meniscal and ligament abnormalities.[51] Pathologic marrow is commonly detected in knee examinations performed to establish a cause for joint pain (Figs. 16–26 and 16–27).

MRI remains the diagnostic modality of choice for detecting avascular necrosis of the femoral head.[52,53] Common causes include trauma, steroids, and alcohol. Idiopathic cases are also common. Core decompression is generally recommended for stage I and II disease. Later stages are treated with arthroplasty. Early detection and diagnosis by MRI may significantly affect the long-term prognosis in this patient population.

Complete tears of the rotator cuff are well depicted

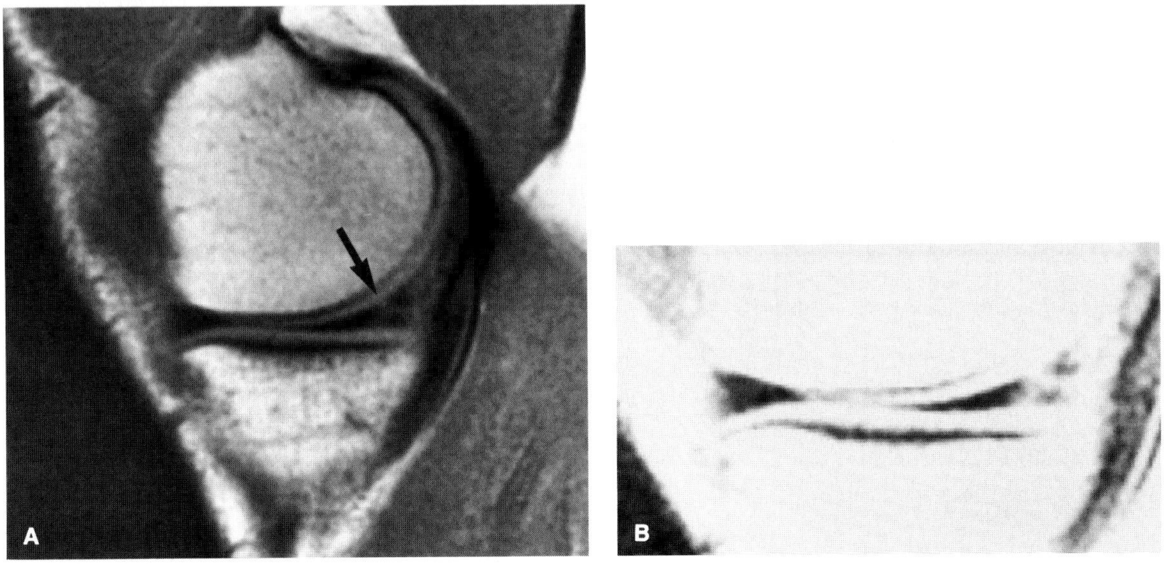

FIGURE 16–25. Full thickness tear of the posterior medial meniscus in a 45-year-old soccer player. T1-weighted image (TR/TE = 800/17) displayed with **(A)** standard and **(B)** meniscal windows. A meniscal tear can be diagnosed when a linear area of increased signal intensity extends to at least one articular surface (arrow). Lesion conspicuity may be increased by filming with high contrast, a narrow window, and large magnification **(B)**.

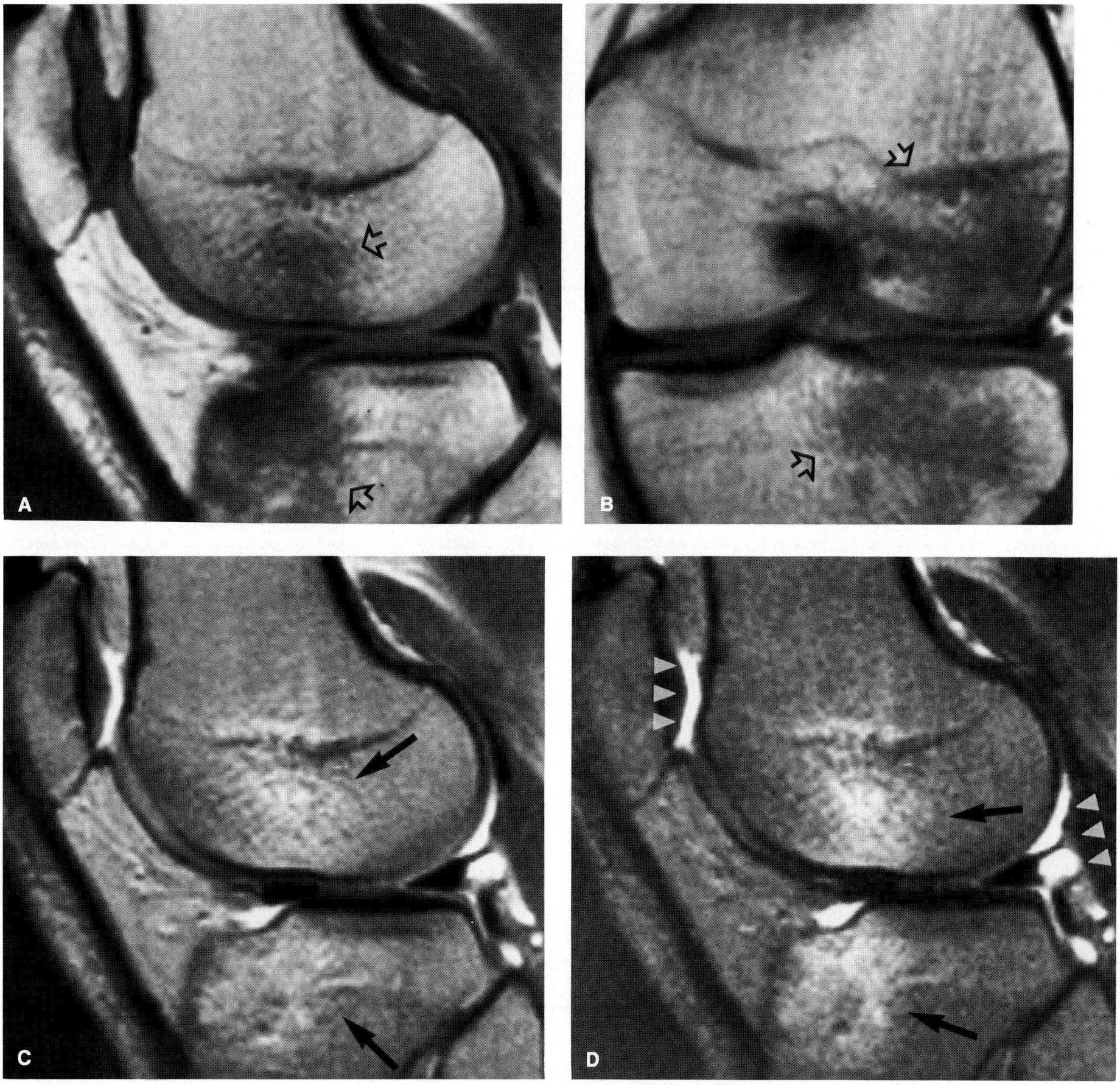

FIGURE 16–26. Femoral and tibial contusions in a 19-year-old woman. **(A,B)** Sagittal and coronal T1-weighted images (TR/TE = 800/17) and **(C,D)** sagittal T2-weighted images (TR/TE = 3000/ 45,90). The location of the low signal intensity (open arrows) within the marrow seen on the T1-weighted scans corresponds to the high-signal-intensity abnormality (closed arrows) seen on the T2-weighted scans. In cases of trauma, this finding can represent either osteonecrosis or microfractures with associated edema. Correlative radiographs are usually within normal limits. A small effusion can also be seen on the T2-weighted scan (arrowheads).

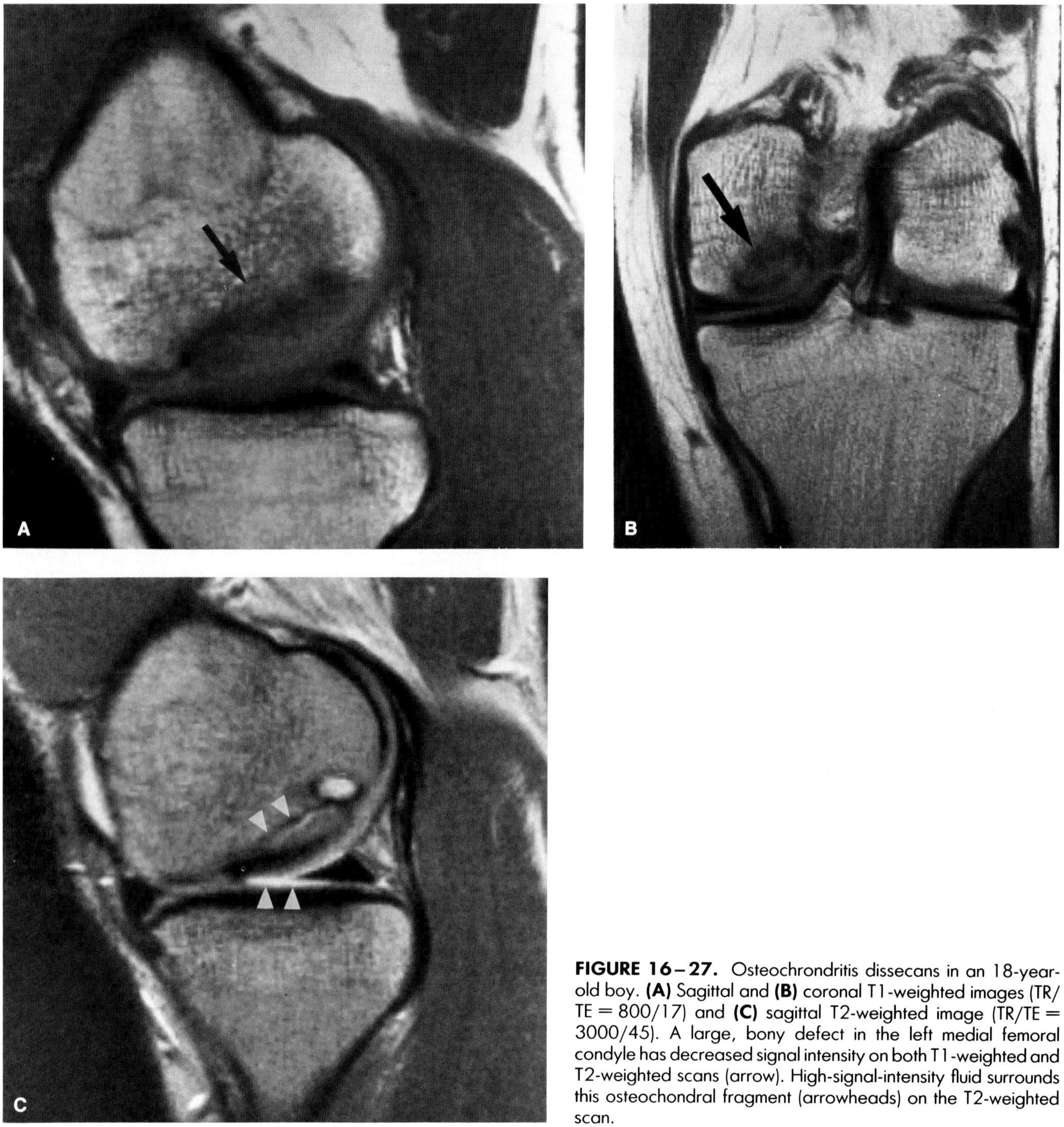

FIGURE 16–27. Osteochrondritis dissecans in an 18-year-old boy. **(A)** Sagittal and **(B)** coronal T1-weighted images (TR/TE = 800/17) and **(C)** sagittal T2-weighted image (TR/TE = 3000/45). A large, bony defect in the left medial femoral condyle has decreased signal intensity on both T1-weighted and T2-weighted scans (arrow). High-signal-intensity fluid surrounds this osteochondral fragment (arrowheads) on the T2-weighted scan.

on MRI.[54] Investigation continues in the application of MRI for evaluating incomplete tears and other shoulder disorders, such as inflammatory changes (i.e., tendonitis) and impingement syndrome.

MRI has become the major screening technique for TMJ pain.[55,56] The most common abnormality is an anterior dislocation of the meniscus, which can be either reducible or fixed.

In evaluating musculoskeletal disorders, MRI provides better soft tissue contrast than x-ray CT.[57] Because of this increased contrast, lesion identification and definition of disease extent are improved. There is superior visualization of disease processes involving the marrow space. MRI also allows acquisition of images in any plane, including sagittal and coronal, while maintaining high in-plane resolution.

Contrast media is not needed in MRI for vessel depiction. Vitamin E capsules serve as convenient

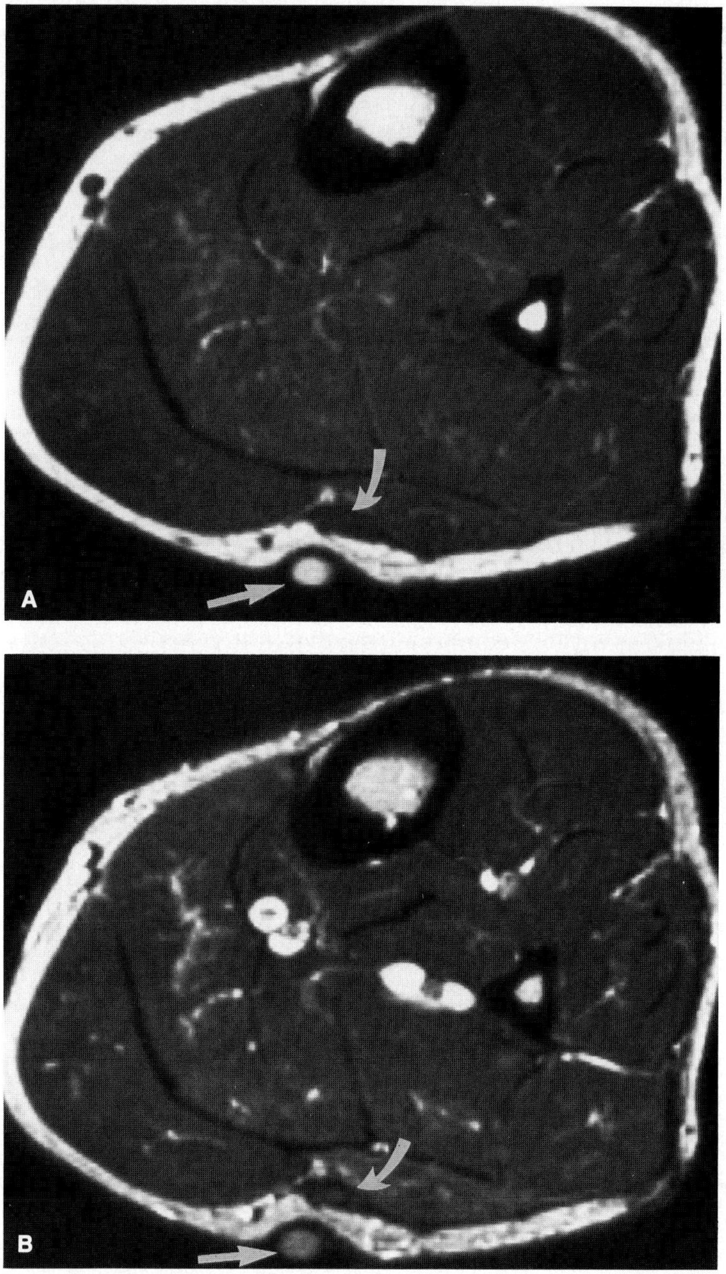

FIGURE 16–28. Use of vitamin E markers. **(A)** T1-weighted image (TR/TE = 600/17) and **(B)** T2-weighted image (TR/TE = 3000/45). A vitamin E capsule (arrow) has been used to mark the site of a recurrent fibrous tumor in this exam of the calf. Vitamin E capsules serve as a convenient marker on both T1-weighted and T2-weighted images because of their fat content. Fibrous lesions (curved arrow) have low signal intensity on both T1-weighted and T2-weighted imaging techniques.

markers for localizing soft tissue masses in the musculoskeletal system (Fig. 16–28), with similar applications in other anatomic regions. Although some distortion of the image occurs in scanning patients with metal prostheses, this is typically less than with CT. CT offers the advantages of a more detailed evaluation of cortical bone, a quicker examination, requiring less cooperation by the patient, and compatibility with ventilatory and monitoring equipment.

Although MRI does offer improved soft tissue contrast, distinction between benign and malignant disease cannot be made.[58,59] Benign lesions tend to be more homogeneous and sharply defined. Exceptions include infection and slowly growing malignant tumors. For definition of tumor extent and for detection of soft tissue lesions on the basis of contrast, MRI is preferred. If detection of soft tissue calcification, gas, or small bony changes are required, or if the patient is uncooperative, CT can provide a superior examination.

TECHNICAL CONSIDERATIONS

Imaging Technique

Advances in instrumentation and imaging techniques have decreased degradation of images from bowel peristalsis, vascular pulsation, respiration, and patient motion.[60] GMN has markedly improved the image quality of T2-weighted head and spine scans. As with all techniques, there can be pitfalls in its application (Fig. 16–29). Newer MR systems offer significantly greater flexibility in imaging parameters than in the past. For example, the number of phase-encoding steps can be chosen freely between 128 and 512, instead of being restricted to the choice of 128, 192, or 256. Half-Fourier imaging is also now a routine option. The slice thickness need not be the same for each acquired section, permitting simultaneous thin-section imaging of the posterior fossa with thicker sections of the cerebral hemispheres (Fig. 16–30). In analogy with CT, this approach may become the standard for screening of intracranial abnormalities. Quadrature coils are now available for both head and body imaging. Improvements in gradient design have allowed TEs as short as 3 ms for gradient-echo techniques and 10 ms for spin echo techniques. These developments can be used to improve SNR and CNR on routine scans, offering the potential for decreasing scan time without compromising diagnostic quality.

The primary magnetic field can be distorted by iron oxide in mascara, metal sutures, shunts, prostheses, and foreign bodies. Image artifacts result, which are typically greater on gradient-echo than spin echo technique.

High-resolution, T1-weighted, contiguous thin sections can be obtained with 3D FLASH. This pulse sequence is superior to T1-weighted spin echo technique for detecting contrast media, abnormal iron deposition, and pneumocephalus. The potential for high-resolution reformatted images in any desired plane, as well as tissue segmentation and three-dimensional display, may prompt adoption of this technique for the preoperative study of intracranial neoplastic disease (Fig. 16–31). This approach can also be adopted in the spine and extremities. Similar pulse techniques can be used to produce 3D angiographic-type studies. The 3D gradient-echo scans have placed new requirements on instrumentation, spurring advances in image reconstruction time and adoption of independent 3D workstations.

System Selection and Operation

It is difficult to objectively evaluate the strengths and weaknesses of an MRI system due to the aggressive marketing atmosphere. Rapid advances continue to be made in both hardware and software, dictating selection of a company with the resources needed to adequately fund research and development. Superconducting magnet systems continue to dominate the MRI market and produce consistently superior image quality.

Selection of an architect and construction company familiar with MRI can lead to a significant savings in time and money. The cost and coverage provided by the service contract should also be carefully considered before purchase.

Most existing MRI units are best able to image am-

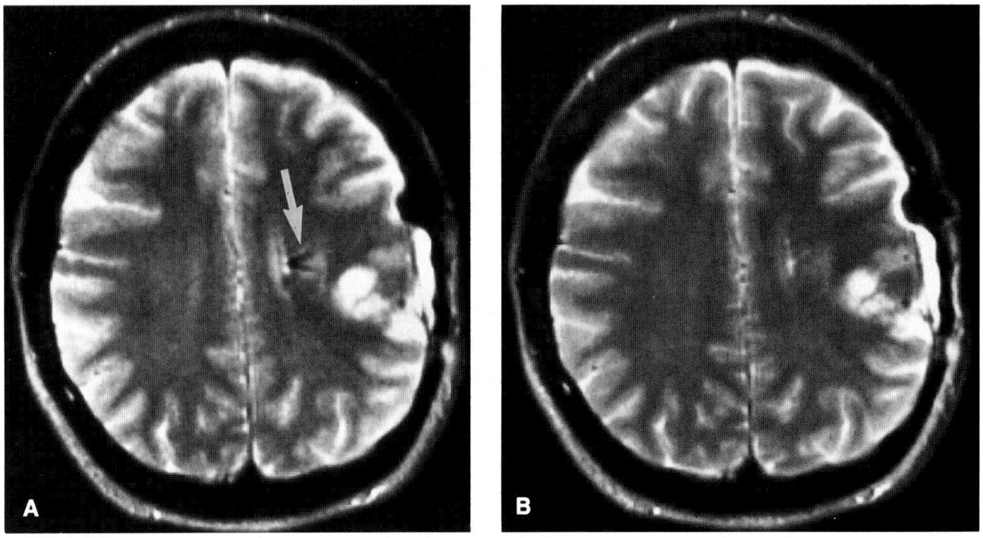

FIGURE 16–29. Venous angioma. T2-weighted images (TR/TE = 3000/90) with **(A)** no motion compensation or with **(B)** two-axis, first-order gradient moment nulling. The use of gradient moment nulling may reduce the visualization of arterial and venous abnormalities. On the uncompensated image, the venous angioma is well depicted as a flow void (arrow). The application of gradient moment nulling or ECG gating restores signal intensity to vessels and thus lowers the contrast with surrounding tissue, making detection of AVMs difficult **(B)**. Gradient moment nulling is essential for routine high-quality images of the posterior fossa and cervical spine. In the search for abnormal vessels, gradient moment nulling should not be employed.

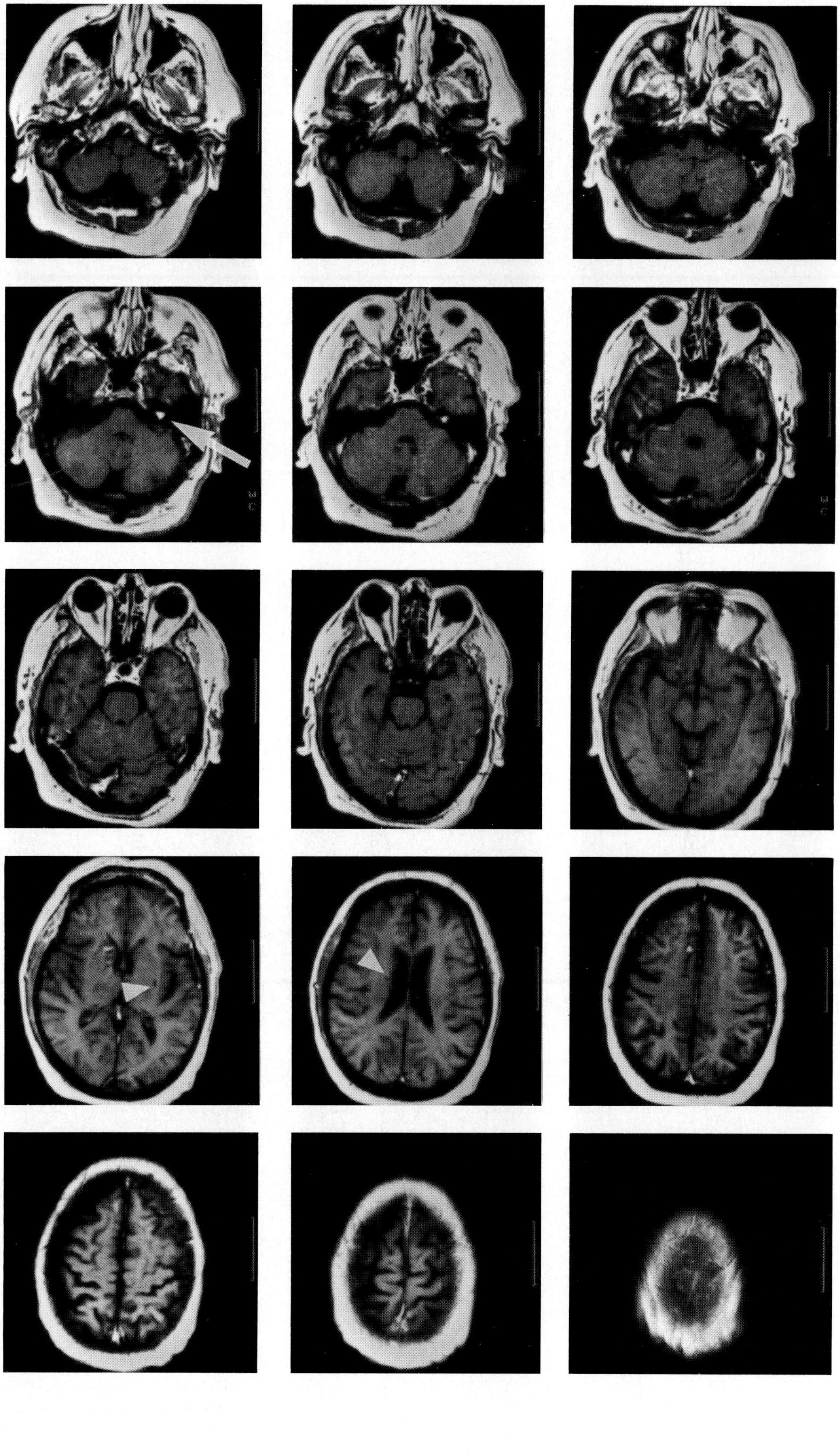

FIGURE 16–30. Simultaneous acquisition of thin and thick axial T1-weighted sections in a 70-year-old man 18 months after resection of a left-sided acoustic neuroma. There is marked enhancement in this postcontrast image of intracanalicular soft tissue (closed arrow), consistent with recurrent tumor. There is sufficient flexibility with MRI technique to permit acquisition of sections with different thicknesses during the same scan. Thin (2–3 mm) sections through the posterior fossa are acquired simultaneously with thick (7–9 mm) sections through the cerebral hemispheres. This approach allows thin-section, high-resolution imaging of the posterior fossa to be combined with a screening exam of the entire brain. Fifteen of the 16 cuts obtained with the combined thin and thick section technique after contrast enhancement are displayed. The first 8 slices illustrated are 3 mm thick; the subsequent 7 slices are 9 mm thick. In this patient, the additional thick sections reveal two lacunar infarcts (arrowheads).

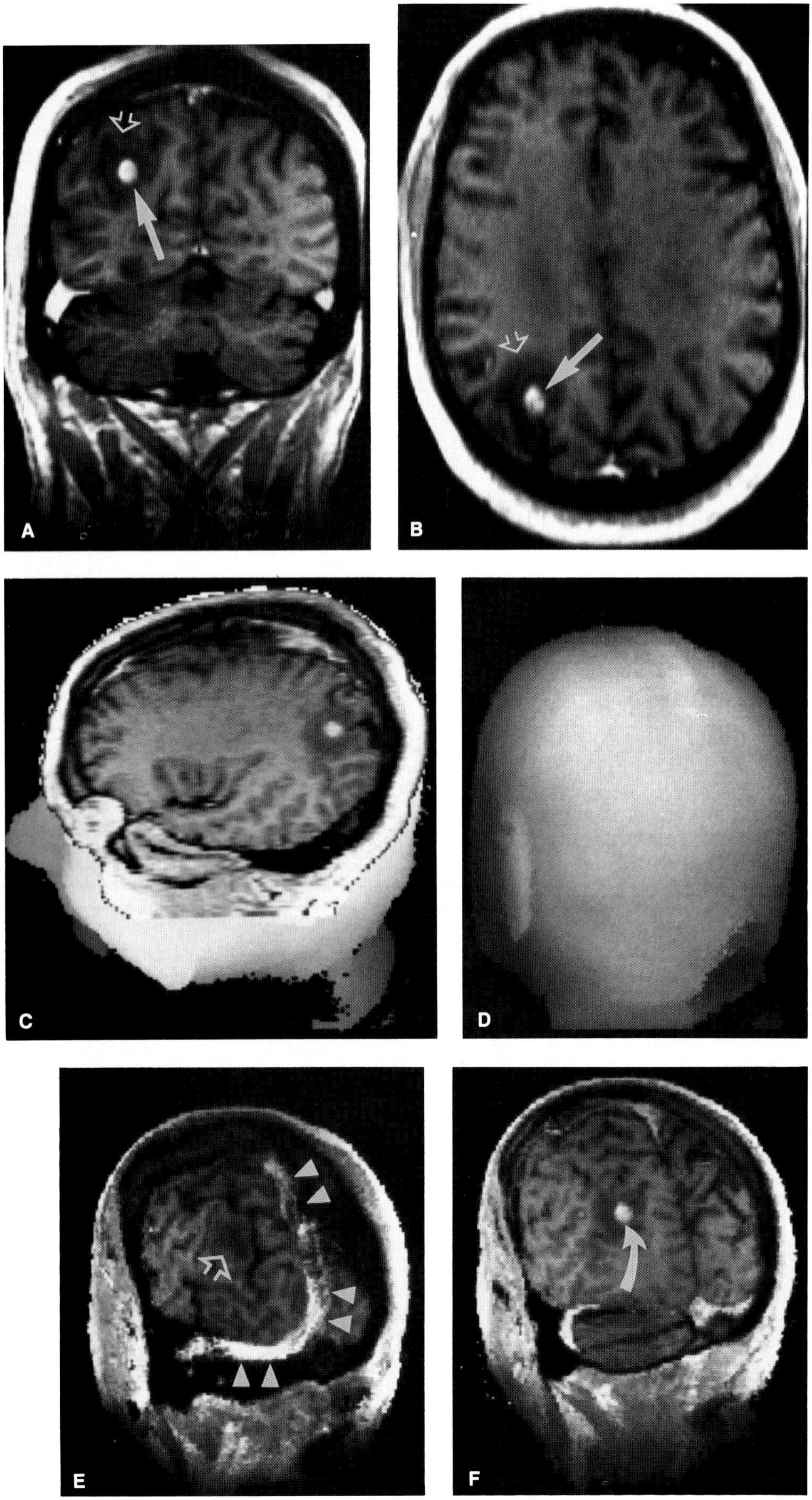

FIGURE 16–31. Metastatic melanoma in a 60-year-old man. The images **(A–F)** are reformatted from a single 11-minute 3D FLASH acquisition. This scan was acquired after intravenous Gd DTPA administration. **(A)** Coronal, **(B)** axial, **(C)** combined tilted axial and surface reformat, **(D–F)** 3D display at different tissue depths as viewed from a point source posterior and to the right of the patient. The metastatic lesion (closed arrow) is well demonstrated due to enhancement. The 3D FLASH image provides superior T1 contrast, compared with a conventional 2D spin echo scan, providing excellent visualization of edema surrounding the lesion (open arrow). From a single 3D FLASH acquisition, high-resolution cuts can be reconstructed in any desired plane, together with surface and 3D projections. By displaying the surface and the layers beneath **(D–F),** lesions can be more precisely localized for biopsy or resection. In this case, display of surface anatomy **(E)** demonstrates the superior sagittal and transverse sinuses (arrowheads). Edema (open arrow) surrounding the metastasis can be seen near the brain surface, with the metastatic focus itself identified **(F)** on a deeper cut (curved arrow).

bulatory individuals. MRI is also well suited for outpatient studies. Due to the many options available for imaging, significant physician input is required for proper development and evaluation of protocols. Attention must also be paid to patient safety, to avoid possible untoward events.[61]

Contrast Media

Gd DTPA is the only FDA-approved intravenous contrast agent for MRI. The chelation of the gadolinium ion by DTPA provides for rapid renal excretion, crucial to the clinical safety of this agent. Indications are broad in both the head and spine for contrast agent use.[19] Improved identification and definition of lesion extent is generally provided by intravenous Gd DTPA administration for neoplasia and infection. Within the next several years, second-generation nonionic paramagnetic metal ion chelates will become available for clinical use, making higher doses and broader clinical applications possible.

CONCLUSION

Clinical application of MRI continues to expand, accompanied by rapid changes in software and instrumentation. The sensitivity of MRI to pathologic tissue is superior to other imaging modalities, including CT, ultrasound, and nuclear medicine. With the introduction of Gd DTPA, MRI is becoming a modality that is routinely used before and after contrast administration. Improvements in diagnostic specificity await sufficient clinical experience and recognition of characteristic patterns of disease involvement. MRI has developed as the imaging modality of choice for a broad range of disease in less than a decade, compared with conventional x-ray techniques, which evolved over a century.

REFERENCES

1. Runge VM, Wood ML, Kaufman DM, et al. Straight and narrow path to good head and spine MRI. Radiographics 1988;8:507.
2. Ormerod IE, Miller DH, McDonald WI. The role of NMR imaging in the assessment of multiple sclerosis and isolated neurologic lesions. A quantitative study. Brain 1987;110:1579.
3. Miller DH, Newton MR, van der Poel JC, et al. Magnetic resonance imaging of the optic nerve in optic neuritis. Neurology 1988;38:175.
4. Grossman RI, Braffman BH, Brorson JR, et al. Multiple sclerosis: serial study of gadolinium-enhanced MR imaging. Radiology 1988;169:117.
5. Miller DH, Rudge P, Johnson G, et al. Serial gadolinium enhanced magnetic resonance imaging in multiple sclerosis. Brain 1988;111:927.
6. Braffman BH, Zimmerman RA, Trojanowski JQ, et al. Brain MR: pathologic correlation with gross and histopathology. 1. Lacunar infection and Virchow-Robin spaces. AJR 1988;151:551.
7. Braffman BH, Zimmerman RA, Trojanowski JQ, et al. Brain MR: pathologic correlation with gross and histopathology. 2. Hyperintense white-matter foci in the elderly. AJR 1988;151:559.
8. Marshall VG, Bradley WB, Marshall CE, et al. Deep white matter infarction: correlation of MR imaging and histopathologic findings. Radiology 1988;167:517.
9. Ramsey RG, Geremia GK. CNS complications of AIDS: CT and MR findings. AJR 1988;151:449.
10. Gomori JM, Grossman RI. Mechanisms responsible for the MR appearance and evolution of intracranial hemorrhage. Radiographics 1988;8:427.
11. Grossman RI. Hemorrhage. In: MR imaging, a categorical course in diagnostic radiology. Radiological Society of North America, 1988:189.
12. Atlas SW. Intracranial vascular malformations and aneurysms, current imaging applications; imaging in neuroradiology, part I. Radiol Clin North Am 1988;26:821.
13. Masaryk TJ, Ross JS, Modic MT, et al. Carotid bifurcation: MR imaging. Radiology 1988;166:461.
14. Drayer BP. Brain infarction. In: MR imaging, a categorical course in diagnostic radiology. Radiological Society of North America, 1988:39.
15. Zimmerman RA. Infratentorial neoplasms. In: Categorical course in diagnostic radiology. Radiological Society of North America, 1987:125.
16. Ramsey RG. Supratentorial neoplasms. In: Categorical course in diagnostic radiology. Radiological Society of North America, 1987:133.
17. Brant-Zawadzki N. MR imaging of the brain. Radiology 1988;166:1.
18. Runge VM, Clanton JA, Price AC, et al. Evaluation of contrast-enhanced MR imaging in a brain-abscess model. AJNR 1985;6:139.
19. Runge VM, ed. Enhanced magnetic resonance imaging. St. Louis: CV Mosby, 1989.
20. Breger RK, Papke RA, Pojunas KW, et al. Benign extraaxial tumors: contrast enhancement with Gd-DTPA. Radiology 1987;163:427.
21. Healy ME, Hesselink JR, Press GA, Middleton MS. Increased detection of intracranial metastases with intravenous Gd-DTPA. Radiology 1987;165:619.
22. Mathews VP, Kuharik MA, Edwards MK, et al. Gd-DTPA-enhanced MR imaging of experimental bacterial meningitis: evaluation and comparison with CT. AJNR 1988;9:1045.
23. Barkovich AJ, Chuang SH, Norman D. MR of neuronal migration anomalies. AJNR 1987;8:1009.
24. Braffman BH, Bilaniuk LT, Zimmerman RA. The CNS manifestations of the phakomatoses on MR. In: Lee SH, Zimmerman RA, eds. Radiologic Clinics of North America: Imaging in neuroradiology, part I. Philadelphia: WB Saunders, 1988:733.
25. Barkovich AJ, Kjos BO, Jackson DE, et al. Normal maturation of the neonatal and infant brain: MR imaging at 1.5 T. Radiology 1988;166:173.
26. Haughton VM. MR imaging of the spine. Radiology 1988;166:297.
27. Haacke EM, Lenz GW. Improving MR image quality in the presence of motion by using rephasing gradients. AJR 1987;148:1251.
28. Enzmann DR, Rubin JB. Cervical spine: MR imaging with a partial flip angle gradient refocused pulse sequence. I. General considerations and disc disease. Radiology 1988;166:467.
29. Enzmann DR, Rubin JB. Cervical spine: MR imaging with a partial flip angle gradient refocused pulse sequence. II. Spinal cord disease. Radiology 1988;166:473.
30. Edelman RR, Atkinson DJ, Silver MS, et al. FRODO pulse sequences: a new means of eliminating motion, flow, and wraparound artifacts. Radiology 1988;166:231.
31. Ross JS, Perez-Reyes N, Masaryk TJ, et al. Thoracic disk herniation: MR imaging. Radiology 1987;165:511.
32. Quencer RM, Beasley RE, Cammisa FJ, et al. MR in nonpenetrating spine injuries: use in clinical management. AJNR 1988;9:1001.

33. Modic MT, Steinberg PM, Ross JS, et al. Degenerative disk disease: assessment of changes in vertebral body marrow with MR imaging. Radiology 1988;166:193.
34. Hueftle MG, Modic MT, Ross JS, et al. Lumbar spine: postoperative MR imaging with Gd-DTPA. Radiology 1988;167:817.
35. Teresi LM, Lufkin RB, Vinuela F, et al. MR imaging of the nasopharynx and floor of the middle cranial fossa. Part I. Normal anatomy. Radiology 1987;164:811.
36. Teresi LM, Lufkin RB, Vinuela F, et al. MR imaging of the nasopharynx and floor of the middle cranial fossa. Part II. Malignant tumors. Radiology 1987;164:817.
37. Reed JD, Soulen RL. Cardiovascular MRI: current role in patient management. Radiol Clin North Am 1988;26:589.
38. Higgins CB. MR of the heart: anatomy, physiology, and metabolism. AJR 1988;151:239.
39. Pflugfelder PW, Sechtem UP, White RD, et al. Quantification of regional myocardial function by rapid cine MR imaging. AJR 1988;150:523.
40. Utz JA, Herfkens RJ, Heinsimer JA, et al. Valvular regurgitation: dynamic MR imaging. Radiology 1988;168:91.
41. Sechtem U, Pflugfelder P, Cassidy MC, et al. Ventricular septal defect: visualization of shunt flow and determination of shunt size by cine MR imaging. AJR 1987;149:689.
42. Wood ML, Runge VM. Combination of suppression technique helps reduce MRI motion artifacts. Diagn Imag 1988;6:139.
43. Ferruci JT, Freeny PC, Stark DD, et al. Advances in hepatobiliary radiology. Radiology 1988;168:319.
44. Rummeny E, Weissleder R, Start DD, et al. Primary liver tumors: diagnosis by MR imaging. AJR 1989;152:63.
45. Hamm B, Wolf KJ, Felix R. Conventional and rapid MR imaging of the liver with Gd-DTPA. Radiology 1987;164:313.
46. Chang A, Glazer HS, Lee JKT, et al. Adrenal gland: MR imaging. Radiology 1987;163:123.
47. Heiken JP, Lee JKT. MR imaging of the pelvis. Radiology 1988;166:11.
48. Hricak H. MRI of the female pelvis: review. AJR 1986;146:1115.
49. Mink JH, Levy T, Crues JV III. Tears of the anterior cruciate ligament and menisci of the knee: MR imaging evaluation. Radiology 1988;167:769.
50. Lee JK, Yao L, Phelps CT, et al. Anterior cruciate ligament tears: MR imaging compared with arthroscopy and clinical tests. Radiology 1988;166:861.
51. Tyrrell RL, Gluckert K, Pathria M, et al. Fast three-dimensional MR imaging of the knee: comparison with arthroscopy. Radiology 1988;166:865.
52. Beltran J, Herman LJ, Burk JM, et al. Femoral head avascular necrosis: MR imaging with clinical-pathologic and radionuclide correlation. Radiology 1988;166:215.
53. Coleman BG, Kressel HY, Dalinka MK, et al. Radiographically negative avascular necrosis: detection with MR imaging. Radiology 1988;168:525.
54. Zlatkin MB, Dalinka MK, Kressel HY. Magnetic resonance imaging of the shoulder. Magn Reson Q 1989;5:3.
55. Mafee MF, Heffez L, Campos M, et al. Temporomandibular joint: role of direct sagittal CT air-contrast arthrogram and MRI. Otolaryngol Clin North Am 1988;21:575.
56. Schellhas KP, Wilkes CH, Omile MR, et al. The diagnosis of temporomandibular joint disease: two-compartment arthrography and MR. AJR 1988;151:341.
57. Ehman RL, Berquist TH, McLeod RA. MR imaging of the musculoskeletal system: a 5-year appraisal. Radiology 1988;166:313.
58. Haggar AM, Froelich JW. MR imaging strategies in primary and metastatic malignancy. Radiol Clin North Am 1988;26:689.
59. Cohen EK, Kressel HY, Frank TS, et al. Hyaline cartilage-origin bone and soft-tissue neoplasms: MR appearance and histologic correlation. Radiology 1988;167:477.
60. Wood ML, Runge VM, Henkelman RM. Overcoming abdominal motion. AJR 1988;150:513.
61. Shellock FG, Crues JV. High field strength MR imaging and metallic biomedical implants: An ex vivo evaluation of deflection forces. AJR 1988;151:389.

Index

Page numbers in italics *indicate figures, those followed by* t *indicate tabular material.*

B

C

D

H

I

J

K

L

M

N

Q

R

S

W

X

Z

ISBN 0-397-50989-8

90000

9 780397 509898